Dennis J. McKenna, PhD
Kenneth Jones
Kerry Hughes, MSc
with Sheila Humphrey, IBCLC

Botanica

The Desk Reference for Major Herbal Supplements

Second Edition

*Pre-publication
REVIEWS,
COMMENTARIES,
EVALUATIONS . . .*

"This book is a marvelous compilation of information about dietary supplements derived from plants that is fully referenced and written in a lively, yet straightforward manner. It is an invaluable resource for historical and traditional use along with the research supporting the medicinal applications of dietary supplements.

Health care practitioners, especially pharmacists interested in the chemistry of dietary supplements, will find this text contains accurate and complete descriptions of constituents and their chemical classes. This information along with standards for the amount of constituents commonly associated with efficacy, dosing considerations, side effects, contraindications, drug interactions, toxicology, and special precautions make this text an excellent single resource for health care practitioners who need to respond to their patients' questions about dietary supplements.

Botanical Medicines is one of the only dietary supplement texts available to practitioners that covers the pharmacognosy, therapeutics, and toxicology of plant-derived medicines. The book is not only comprehensive, but also clearly written with extensive referencing, making it one of the most valuable texts to have on hand in a clinician's office or medical library."

June Riedlinger, PharmD
Assistant Professor
of Clinical Pharmacy;
Director, Center for Integrative
Therapies in Pharmaceutical Care,
Massachusetts College of Pharmacy
and Health Sciences

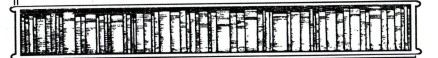

More pre-publication
REVIEWS, COMMENTARIES, EVALUATIONS . . .

"**A** detailed guide to the most common herbal supplements. An excellent resource for serious students, informed consumers, and health care professionals."

Andrew Weil, MD
Author, *Spontaneous Healing,*
Eight Weeks to Optimum Health,
and *Eating Well for Optimum Health*

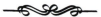

"**F**inally, a comprehensive reference book on botanical medicine that is well-referenced, science-based, authoritative, and comprehensive, summarizing the current state of the science for the most common botanicals in clinical use. This book covers herbal medicines from astragalus to vitex, providing the clinician, scientist, and pharmacist with concise information on the history and traditional uses, the botanical description, chemistry, and therapeutic applications including preclinical and clinical studies. Invaluable too is the information on drug interactions and toxicology and precautions in clinical use. This is, by far, the best available reference book on botanical medicine. No physician's or allied health care provider's desk should be without it. Please send me my copy as soon as possible."

Leanna J. Standish, ND, PhD
Senior Research Scientist,
Bastyr University Research Institute,
Kenmore, WA

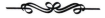

"**I**t has been my pleasure to review *Botanical Medicines.* This book examines common medicinal supplements of herbal origin, from astragalus to vitex.

Each is treated in monographic form, in a highly organized and systematic fashion that allows ready discovery of facts of interest, whether they pertain to the biochemistry, traditional uses, or clinical studies for a variety of indications. The information is accurate and up-to-date, including extensive bibliographies for each agent.

This book will be recognized as a standard work in the field, and a valuable addition to the libraries of interested physicians, naturopaths, scientists, herbal healers, and students of those disciplines. It will serve as a valuable text and reference source for multidisciplinary study."

Ethan Russo, MD
Neurologist/Medicinal Plant
Researcher; Author, *Handbook*
of Psychotropic Herbs

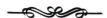

"**T**his is the most thoroughly referenced, most authoritative scientific reference on the top dietary supplements in the United States. All health professionals will benefit from its careful delineation of the common safety issues in clinical care, including dietary supplement–drug interactions and supplement use in pregnancy and lactation."

Gregory A. Plotnikoff, MD, MTS
Medical Director,
Center for Spirituality and Healing;
Associate Professor of Clinical
Medicine and Pediatrics,
University of Minnesota
Academic Health Center

Botanical Medicines
The Desk Reference for Major Herbal Supplements
Second Edition

Botanical Medicines
The Desk Reference
for Major Herbal Supplements
Second Edition

Dennis J. McKenna, PhD
Kenneth Jones
Kerry Hughes, MSc
with Sheila Humphrey, IBCLC

The Haworth Herbal Press®
An Imprint of The Haworth Press, Inc.
New York • London • Oxford

Published by

The Haworth Herbal Press®, an imprint of The Haworth Press, Inc., 10 Alice Street, Binghamton, NY 13904-1580.

The information contained in this publication is intended to supplement the knowledge of health care professionals regarding the use of herbal medicine. The information is educational only and is not intended to replace sound clinical judgment or individualized patient care. The authors disclaim all warranties, whether expressed or implied, including any warranty as to the quality, accuracy, safety, or suitability of this information for any particular purpose. The information in this book is also not a substitute for diagnosis or treatment by a professional health care provider. While information is given regarding herbal medicine usages and outcomes, the book is intended for educational purposes only. The authors, editor, and publisher do not accept liability in the event of negative consequences incurred as a result of information presented in this book.

Second edition of *Natural Dietary Supplements: A Desktop Reference* (Institute for Natural Products Research, 1998).

The herbal illustrations appearing on the cover and in the book are by Tristan Berlund and are used with her permission.

Cover design by Marylouise E. Doyle.

Library of Congress Cataloging-in-Publication Data

McKenna, Dennis, J.
    Botanical medicines : the desk reference for major herbal supplements / Dennis J. McKenna, Kenneth Jones, Kerry Hughes.— 2nd ed.
        p. cm.
    Includes bibliographical references and index.
    ISBN 0-7890-1265-0 (alk. paper) — ISBN 0-7890-1266-9 (alk. paper)
    1. Dietary supplements—Handbooks, manuals, etc. 2. Herbs—Handbooks, manuals, etc. I. Jones, Kenneth. II. Hughes, Kerry. III. Title.

RM258.5 .M38 2002
615'.32—dc21

                                                                            2001039101

CONTENTS

ABOUT THE AUTHORS

Dennis McKenna, PhD, has worked in the interdisciplinary fields of pharmacognosy, ethnopharmacology, and ethnobotany for over twenty years. Dr. McKenna received post-doctoral research fellowships in the Laboratory of Clinical Pharmacology, National Institute of Mental Health (NIMH), and in the Department of Neurology, Stanford University School of Medicine. In 1990, he joined Shaman Pharmaceuticals as Director of Ethnopharmacology and later worked as Senior Research Pharmacognosist for the Aveda Corporation. He is currently a Senior Lecturer at the Center for Spirituality and Healing in the Academic Health Center at the University of Minnesota. Dr. McKenna serves on the Advisory Board of the American Botanical Council and on the Editorial Board of *Phytomedicine, The International Journal of Phytotherapy and Phytopharmacology.*

Kenneth Jones is a medical writer specializing in food and medicinal plants. His work has appeared in both lay and professional publications, including *The Journal of Alternative and Complementary Medicine, Alternative and Complementary Therapies,* and others. He is the author of various books on specific medicinal plants: *Cordyceps: Tonic Food of Ancient China; Reishi: Ancient Herb for Modern Times; Cat's Claw: Healing Vine of Peru; Shiitake: The Healing Mushroom;* and *Pau d'arco.* As President of Armana Research, Inc., he has provided product development consulting services as well as written and research materials to botanical supplement companies in North America and abroad since 1986. He also serves as Educational Director and Assistant Editor for the Institute of Natural Products Research, a nonprofit organization in the United States.

Kerry Hughes, MSc, is an ethnobotanist specializing in product development, plant commercialization, and medical writing for the natural products industry. She founded EthnoPharm Consulting as a platform to bring new plants and plant uses to market, and to help widen our medicinal knowledge of plants in health care. Kerry has worked with natural product companies throughout the United States and in South America, Europe, and Asia on the development of plant products for the functional food, dietary supplement, specialty food, and cosmetic markets. She writes and speaks frequently on the subject of botanicals, their use in medicine and science, and the development of botanical products from indigenous cultures. Kerry currently serves as the Director of EthnoPharm Consulting, and is a Contributing and Field

Editor for *Prepared Foods* and *Nutrasolutions* magazines. She continues to serve as Assistant Editor to the Institute for Natural Products Research (INPR), and is the Product Development Advisor for Rockland Food Ingredients (RFI). She serves on the Journal Advisory Board for *Current Topics in Nutraceutical Research,* and is a Scientific Advisor for Supplement Watch.com.

Sheila Humphrey received a BSc from the University of British Columbia, Canada, in 1996, majoring in Botany. After graduate work in plant ecology, she switched to professional nursing, receiving her RN in 1984. She has been a certified La Leche League Leader since 1990, counseling breastfeeding mothers seeking information and support. In 1996, she qualified as an International Board Certified Lactation Consultant (IBCLC). She has continued her work with La Leche League as an information resource for complex breastfeeding situations, particularly questions involving medications including herbs. Over the last five years, she has made an intensive evaluation of both the lactation and botanical literature, focusing on safety and efficacy issues of herb use during pregnancy and lactation. She has presented continuing education lectures on herbs and breastfeeding for health care professionals including a co-presentation with Dennis McKenna at the La Leche League International Conference in 2001. She has lectured at the University of Minnesota on the ethnopharmacology of herbs traditionally used for reproductive health. She continues to act as an information resource on herbs for La Leche League International, as well as lactation professionals in the United States and abroad. She is currently writing a book for mothers on the use of herbs and other dietary supplements during lactation.

Foreword

Despite the wide use of coffee, cocaine, heroin, and tobacco for their physiologic effects, the medicinal properties of plant-derived substances have until recently been overlooked by American health professionals. Of the best-selling 150 prescription drugs, 86 contain at least one major active compound from natural sources. In addition to aspirin, digoxin, and antibiotics, plant-derived medications include numerous anticholinergic agents, anticoagulants, antihypertensives, and antineoplastic agents. Surprisingly, of the top 150 pharmaceuticals, only 35 plant species are represented.[1]

The most recent national survey documented that 44.6 million Americans use herbal remedies on a regular basis and that more than 90 million Americans had used an herbal remedy in the past 12 months. Thirty-six percent of those who use herbal medicines do so instead of prescription medicines and 31 percent do so with prescriptions. The leading reason for substitution is preference for a natural or organic product. Leading sources for information are, in order of preference, friends, magazines, product labels, and advertising. Ironically, health professionals are the least frequently consulted for information.[2]

At this time, there is a profound knowledge gap with significant public health implications. The lay public appears to distrust the knowledge base of health professionals regarding natural, plant-derived medicines. And, the health professionals who do seek to counsel on herbal medicines from an evidence-based perspective may not be aware that such evidence exists. This gap represents a serious challenge.

Thankfully, the authors/editors of this new volume, *Botanical Medicines: The Desk Reference for Major Herbal Supplements,* have now bridged the evidence gap using the dialect of the scientific community. They have provided us with the scientific rationale for 34 of the most popular and widely consumed herbal medicines. The evidence is comprehensively presented here; preclinical and clinical studies, as well as safety precautions, descriptions of active constituents, and dosage information for each of the botanicals profiled are all included within this volume. The focus and rationale of

---

[1]Grifo, F. (1997). *Biodiversity and human health.* Washington, DC: Island Press.

[2]Johnson, B.A. (2000). Prevention magazine assesses use of dietary supplements. *HerbalGram* 48: 65.

this volume is to provide comprehensive coverage of a limited set of botanical supplements, namely, those that the patients of health care providers are most likely to be using, and regarding which they are most likely to seek advice. The book's exhaustive references, inclusion of current literature, comprehensive coverage, and standardized organization make it a powerful reference tool, further enhancing its utility for practitioners, researchers, and the interested public.

With the publication of this book, there is no longer any excuse for ignorance of the scientific basis for the use of herbal medicines. The evidence is there, and it is clearly and thoroughly presented in this volume.

Gregory A. Plotnikoff, MD, MTS
Associate Professor
Clinical Medicine and Pediatrics;
Medical Director
Center for Spirituality and Healing
University of Minnesota

Preface

The volume you hold in your hands (or perhaps, in view of its size, have placed on your desk), *Botanical Medicines: The Desk Reference for Major Herbal Supplements*, is the outcome of a project that began nearly five years ago, in 1997. At that time, my co-editors, Kenneth Jones and Kerry Hughes, had been working as independent consultants to the supplement and pharmaceutical industries. We were presented with an attractive offer: to develop a series of detailed, up-to-date scientific monographs on thirty-four of the most popular herbal dietary supplements used in the United States. The monographs were to cover the botany, chemistry, preclinical studies, clinical studies, and safety profiles of these most widely used herbal supplements, comprehensively and in exhaustive detail. The offer came from Pharmanex, Inc., at that time a relatively new player in the field of botanical and other dietary supplements. To carry out this project, they proposed to give our small team, which was organizing a new educational organization, called INPR, an unrestricted educational grant.

Pharmanex was committed to what was then a rather new concept in the field of dietary supplements, to only sell supplements of the highest quality, backed by sound scientific evidence of safety, efficacy, and clinical validity as reflected in peer-reviewed scientific publications. Pharmanex's retail sales strategy was that its supplements would only be sold in pharmacies, and they would look to pharmacists to provide consumers with informed advice and recommendations regarding appropriate use. What quickly became apparent, however, was that a significant "information gap" regarding dietary supplements existed even among this educated group of professionals. It became apparent that there was a need to compile this information in a form that was readable, comprehensive, and current, a need resulting in the creation of such a comprehensive reference resource. With this resource, pharmacists could educate themselves, and in turn provide informed advice to their customers regarding the appropriate uses of these supplements.

We all agreed that a reference of this kind would raise the quality and tone of available information to a higher and more honest level, and thus would benefit the entire supplement industry along with more informed consumers. Science and evidence would replace marketing hype. Where safety issues were found, we would identify them and provide an honest assessment of the risks. Where efficacy was open to question or where equivocal or contradictory results were apparent, we would provide summaries of those studies to invite informed and educated professionals to form their own judgments. That is largely the tack we adopted when we undertook this project and the one we adhered to in creating this new, revised, expanded, and updated edition.

Our initial effort appeared in 1998 under the title *Natural Dietary Supplements: A Desktop Reference.* It was published under the imprimatur of the Institute for Natural Products Research. INPR is an organization that my colleagues and I established primarily to foster education, research, and development in the field of botanical medicines. The mission of INPR is to create educational tools and resources to provide the most complete, accurate, and impartial information possible on botanical medicines, and to conduct pioneering research and development for the natural products industry. While creating the original *Desktop Reference,* we also created the *Natural Dietary Supplements Pocket Reference,* which continues to be popular with professionals and consumers alike. These works represent our first steps toward fulfilling the mission of INPR.

Since the publication of the first edition of the *Desktop Reference* in 1998, the pace of scientific investigations has accelerated. Hundreds of new studies on the topics we covered appeared in rapid succession in the literature. Our commitment to producing a high-quality, accurate, and up-to-date text was challenged when we faced the fact that the first edition now required major updating and revision. The volume before you is the result of at least three complete revisions, as we struggled to keep up with and integrate the flood of new information on our chosen topics. Given the pace of discovery in these times, it is the nature of scientific publications that any book that purports to summarize the state of current science will be out of date by the time it finds its way to the shelves of your local bookstore. Ours will not escape that fate either. At a certain point, one must commit the manuscript to the hands of a sympathetic and at times long-suffering publisher, who must, sooner or later, freeze the information for all time into a galley proof, and then into a completed volume between two covers. However, given those constraints, we have spared no effort to include the most important, current publications we could find. We hope to continue covering the new research on herbal medicines through INPR, and perhaps in the future offer versions of this book in electronic formats.

As the text went through successive iterations and revisions, we made some major changes in the organizational structure of the chapters. Specifically, we developed a set of standardized major headings and subheadings that are utilized consistently in all chapters. Thus, the information in each chapter is distributed under nine major headings: 1. Botanical Data; 2. History and Traditional Uses; 3. Chemistry; 4. Therapeutic Applications; 5. Preclinical Studies; 6. Clinical Studies; 7. Dosage; 8: Safety Profile; 9. References. The subheadings under each major heading are similarly consistently organized. Thus, for example, each section on Botanical Data includes subheadings on Classification and Nomenclature, and another subheading under which a detailed Botanical Description is provided. The subheadings under the Chemistry section are organized according to the chemical class of the constituents under discussion, e.g., Carbohydrates, Lipid Compounds, Phenolics, Nitrogenous Compounds, etc. Each of these, in turn, includes subheadings as appropriate for the metabolites found in the particular botanical discussed. The subheadings under the Preclinical and Clinical studies sections are constructed in parallel and emphasize systems, functionalities, and disorders. Under Preclinical Studies, for example, the reader will find the following main subheadings: Cardiovascular and Circulatory Functions; Digestive, Hepatic, and Gastrointestinal Functions; Endocrine and Hormonal Functions; Genito-urinary and Renal Functions; Immune Functions, Inflammation and Disease; Integumentary, Muscular, and Skeletal Functions; Nutritional and Metabolic Functions; Neurological, Psychological, and Behavioral Functions; Reproductive Functions; Respiratory and Pulmonary Functions; and Miscellaneous Pharmacological Activities. The Clinical Studies sections are similarly organized, and each of these major headings has subheadings, as appropriate for the particular disorder or functionality under discussion, and for the particular botanical. There is admittedly some overlap in these heading categories and in some cases it was a judgment call as to where to place information. For example, does one discuss diabetes and insulin modulation under Endocrine and Hormonal Functions or under Metabolic and Nutritional Functions? Although discussion under either heading would be appropriate, once we made such a judgment we applied it consistently.

There is a massive amount of information in these chapters, and our hope is that the consistent application of headings will enhance their clarity and make comparisons between them that much easier. Unfortunately, pharmacology and physiology involve multifaceted, multirelational systems, with the result that some readers may find fault with our arrangement of the headings. Our intention was to make the consistent headings useful. For instance, when it comes to comparing similar pharmacological and systemic effects of different botanicals, our heading structure allows one to quickly compare the effects of ginkgo, garlic, green tea, and grape seed extract on cardiovascular and circulatory functions.

Another small but important change has been made in this edition. Of thirty-four chapters in the first edition, only one was not a botanical supplement, and that was Co-Q10. In order to make the current edition live up to its new name, we eliminated the chapter on Co-Q10 and substituted an entirely new chapter on Ephedra. In view of the current controversy surrounding the safety of this herb, we felt it was important to include it in this new edition.

Any project of this magnitude and duration is not accomplished in a vacuum. It was accomplished with the help, support, and encouragement of a large number of people whose names do not appear on the title page. Barb Apps, Ray Cooper, and Joe Chang were our initial project managers at Pharmanex when this work was initiated, and we thank them for their steady support and good advice from the beginning and throughout the publication of the first edition. As we became immersed in this project, we came to understand the merits of their original vision and grew to share in their passion for it. We thank them for giving us the opportunity to undertake this project, and for giving us the chance to make something more of it than at first they may have imagined it could be. I want to thank my colleague and good friend Janice Thompson, who was Director of Natural Products Research at Pharmanex at the time, for bringing this project to us. During the initial writing of the monographic reviews, and the subsequent extensive revisions and re-revisions, we occasionally employed the services of other colleagues and consultants in the supplement industry. While most of the content in the chapters was written by Kenneth Jones, Kerry Hughes, or myself, some significant contributions to the content were made by others, including Sheila Humphrey, Dennis Awang, Kathleen Harrison, Uzondu Jibuike, Connie Grauds, and Maggie George. We also gratefully acknowledge and thank our many friends and colleagues in the supplement industry and academia who provided mentorship, encouragement, and very often, just the right piece of information, reference, or commentary when it was most needed: Mark Blumenthal, Rob McCaleb, Jim Duke, Norman Farnsworth, Roy Upton, Mike McGuffin, Marilyn Barrett, Trish Flaster, Andy Weil, Ethan Russo, Greg Plotnikoff, and others. Wonderful people all. We are proud to share their passion for botanical medicine, and honored that they consider us friends and colleagues. We give special thanks to Tristan Berlund, a talented and gifted botanical illustrator, for providing the beautiful and technically accurate illustrations of the plants in each chapter. Her compensation was woefully inadequate, and it was ultimately her love of the subject that produced such stunning illustrations. Also, we owe much thanks to Maxim Hurwicz, our always good-humored web designer who created our site at <www.naturalproducts.org> and continues to keep the site running smoothly.

We also thank Jim Simon, of the Department of Horticulture at Purdue University, for seeing the merit of our work and representing it to The Haworth Herbal Press. It was Jim who brought it to the attention of the late, great Dr. Varro (Tip) Tyler, Emeritus Professor of Pharmacognosy at Purdue University, and the Editor in Chief at The Haworth Herbal Press at the time. Dr. Tyler advocated for its publication by Haworth, and thanks to him, they appreciated its merits. We are grateful for his confidence in our work. Many people at Haworth have provided so much help in guiding this publication through its long and sometimes frustrating evolution into an authoritative reference. None have been more steadfast in this respect than Peg Marr, Haworth's Senior Production Editor. Her patience, good humor, and unwavering support during a revision and correction process that must have at times seemed both doomed to fail and destined to continue forever, has been an inspiration and a much-deserved goad to all of us when we needed it most, which was often.

I want to give special thanks to my wife, Sheila Humphrey, who has been an incredibly patient and understanding spouse at times when obsession with this work has caused marriage and family priorities to be pushed, too often, to the back burner. I also want to give special acknowledgment to her as a respected colleague for the contributions she made to this work. As a botanist, herbalist, RN, and International Board Certified Lactation Consultant, her vast knowledge of this field puts my own to shame, though she has not the degrees to show for it. The sections on the safety of these supplements in pregnancy and lactation, and large parts of the monographs on Vitex and Black Cohosh, are hers, and it has been invaluable to have the benefit of her expertise. Her insistence on evidence, and not just because "Commission E says so," has forced us to cleave to a higher standard. As a result, I'm happy to say that the information presented herein on the use of these supplements during pregnancy or lactation is some of the most accurate and evidence-based to be found anywhere.

Finally, I want to thank my colleagues and co-editors, Kerry Hughes and Kenneth Jones. We've worked together closely over the last five years, and we have proven that our various backgrounds fit together synergistically to make a great team. Kerry has been fun to work with, and her extensive revision of the section on DSHEA has made it much more accurate and current. To Ken, especially, I give my heartfelt thanks for his devotion, long hours, and unstinting dedication. It is largely thanks to his persistence and nearly obsessional attention to detail that this work is as timely, thoroughly referenced, and accurate as it is. Ken, it's been great working with you, and I'm sure you are as relieved as I am that you will not have to send any more of those midnight faxes haranguing me for this or that citation or page reference; I know we're both going to sleep better.

Thanks go out also to anyone else, whom I may have overlooked by name, but who helped make this book possible in one way or another. It has been a great, long adventure, and could not have reached fruition without the support and input of many caring people. Thanks to everyone for being part of the team.

Dennis J. McKenna, PhD
Editor in Chief
Marine on St. Croix, Minnesota

A Note on the Interpretation of Information on Pregnancy, Lactation, and Pediatrics in This Desk Reference

Sheila Humphrey, RN, BSc (botany), IBCLC

The chapters in this book include sections discussing safety issues during pregnancy and lactation. Much of the herbal literature has dealt with these core issues in human reproduction in one of two ways: some herbal literature, including that written in antiquity, is bereft of any discussion of safety issues, while more modern works suggest that pregnant or breastfeeding mothers should not use any herbs at all, "just to be safe."

This desk reference employs standard sources of pharmacological information regarding chemical use during pregnancy and lactation and applies this considerable body of knowledge to herbal and plant chemical information. The following interpretive notes attempt to introduce the reader to this medical literature; the reader is further referred to more detailed works. To evaluate the safety of pediatric herb use, that is, the direct feeding of herbal preparations to children, is beyond the scale of this work. The slim but fascinating book by the pediatrician Dr. Heinz Schilcher is a fair introduction to how and when herbs are currently prescribed for children's health concerns, at least in Germany.[1] I further refer readers to reflect on the Lactation sections that follow whenever they are considering giving an herbal remedy directly to a young exclusively breastfed infant. Direct feeding of anything other than mother's milk is an introduction of risk that cannot be embarked upon without full consideration of alternative actions.

Since the chapters were completed, several very pertinent research reports have crossed my desk with information that would have changed some information in the pregnancy and lactation sections, but recalling what Dennis McKenna wrote in the preface, one must simply stop somewhere in order to ever publish a book. It is sincerely hoped that these interpretive notes will enable a better immediate grasp of the information presented for pregnancy and lactation.

---

[1]Schilcher, H. (1997). *Phytotherapy in paediatrics: Handbook for physicians and pharmacists*. Stuttgart: Medpharm Scientific Publishers.

PREGNANCY

Using herbs during pregnancy requires extra caution because a developing fetus is at the most vulnerable state to chemical influence. Following the thalidomide tragedies of the early 1960s, a great sea change occurred in the prescribing of pharmaceuticals to the pregnant woman. The new paradigm was no medication—OTC or prescription—for pregnant women, with few exceptions. Ironically, medication use during labor itself has simultaneously soared since then. Animal studies searching for teratogenic and mutagenic effects were started, and as information accumulated, classification schemes were developed to rate a drug's dangers in pregnancy and to the fetus.[2] Yet, today it is understood that many serious medical problems in the mother must be treated to ensure a healthy pregnancy and fetal health. Because the ethics of scientific experimentation with pregnant (and lactating) women are challenging if not impossible, and with many drugs having few animal studies to refer to, information has accumulated anecdotally: the medically necessary study of one (plus fetus). In general, what has been learned is what has been known since antiquity: the impact of a medicine depends to a great extent on the trimester of the pregnancy. Some medicines may show no interaction in the first trimester yet speed labor in the third, while others cause a toxic effect in the first trimester but at the same dose have little or no impact on the fetus when used in labor. Herbs are often attended with no or very sketchy animal studies on pregnancy, not unlike the case with many drugs.[2] Many herbs have been used since before antiquity for pregnancy and labor conditions; traditional use records provide a valuable piece of information but do not allow total assurance. Blanket contraindications for both pregnancy and lactation are often made in the herbal literature, often without providing a rationale. The blood:placenta barrier is unique, allowing a different set of chemicals to pass when compared to the blood:breast barrier; thus what may be unsafe in pregnancy may be safe in lactation. Further, other safety considerations of pregnancy are not those of lactation. As long as the pregnancy is maintained, the fetus depends on the mother to metabolize and eliminate chemicals. Herbs that have oxytocic effects, i.e., inducing birth in the pregnant uterus, may be risky for a mid-term pregnancy yet may provide a very useful mechanism of action to assist birth. As well, the same herbs may aid milk removal during lactation. Herbs used in labor are metabolized by the mother up to the point of delivery; after the cord is cut, the baby must now take over this elimination. An infant's liver will take two weeks to become fully able to metabolize certain chemicals. For all these

---

[2]See Briggs, G.G, Freeman, R.K., and Jaffe, S.J. (1998). *Drugs in pregnancy and lactation: A reference guide to fetal and neonatal risk,* Fifth edition. New York: Lippincott Williams and Wilkins.

reasons, medicines given late in labor are expected to have the greatest impact on the newborn infant. It is well known that some pharmaceuticals used during labor can affect a baby after birth; some are controversially considered to interfere with a baby's ability to breastfeed in the critical post-partum days. The relative risk of herb versus pharmaceutical use during pregnancy and labor may be difficult, as relatively little definitive information is available; yet the need to treat can be imperative.

The chapters in this book provide what is known or recognized to be pertinent about a herb regarding pregnancy; the information is summarized in the Pregnancy section.

LACTATION

Sufficient knowledge has accumulated with pharmaceuticals and lactation so that in most cases a reasoned prediction of the risk can be made. Modern analyses include the risks and benefits of maternal medicinal use for both mother and baby. It is not whether a chemical enters milk, because most things a mother can take up into her bloodstream, whether food, herb or pharmaceutical in origin, will enter milk to some degree. The question is how much enters milk and what are the consequences for this particular mother-baby pair? Clinical application of such knowledge requires an individualized assessment, because every mother and baby pair or dyad is unique. The first question is always: how much is the baby nursing (dose) and how old is the baby (impact)? Risk factors with a neonate and a toddler are not the same. The blood:breast barrier acts much like the blood:brain barrier. The amount of constituents that can enter the milk compartment is a function of many factors, starting with oral bioavailability and maternal serum level. The current depth of knowledge gathered over the whole spectrum of medications and milk entry has verified the general validity of this rule of thumb: only a tiny fraction of any oral maternal dose of a chemical will enter into breast milk, which for most is about 1 percent. This amount usually represents a physiologically inactive dose. Milk and infant serum levels often cannot be detected; many chemicals may have poor bioavailability or are immediately handled by the liver. However, local GI effects in the infant are known. The American Association of Pediatrics (AAP) 2002 statement on medications during lactation does not contraindicate the vast majority of drugs as the known benefits of breastfeeding to mother and child usually far outweigh the theoretical or known clinical risks.[3] It is generally agreed that the *Physician's Desk Reference* is considered more a tool to ward off litigation than a counseling resource.[4] Herbal pharmacokinetics, particularly bioavailability and serum level quantification of specific substances, would be definitive in predicting risk, though such data are usually not available. However, overall, there are very few reports of herbal adverse effects exerted through breast milk alone. Not that all herbal substances can be consumed without consequence. Experience with both pharmaceuticals and herbs shows that if an adverse reaction will occur in the baby, it will be similar to reactions known in adults, information that every mother needs before use. Another area to consider is the potential for a medicine or herb to alter milk synthesis and production or to alter the natural amenorrhea state of lactation. These factors are only now gaining the attention of lactation researchers; these effects can be a desired outcome of lactation management or an unpleasant way to learn about how a substance may interact with lactation. In many cases the alternative to an herb is a pharmaceutical. Herb authority James A. Duke's perennial challenge is also yours: is the herb safe or unsafe as compared to what? I refer the reader to the AAP statement,[3] as well as to Hale[4] for a more detailed but quick overview of lactation pharmacology. Hale's book has approached each herb using principles of lactation pharmacology, considering clues from traditional knowledge as well as the knowledge gained through working with many mothers. A summary of the lactation-related information in each chapter of the *Desk Reference* is provided in the Lactation section of the Safety Profile. It may be considered as a starting information resource when working with a mother-baby or dyad.

---

[3]American Academy of Pediatrics Committee on Drugs (2001). The transfer of drugs and other chemicals into human milk. *Pediatrics* 108: 776-789. The full article is available on the Web: <www.aap.org/policy>.

[4]Hale, T. (2002). *Medications and mother's milk,* Tenth edition. Amarillo, TX: Pharmasoft Medical Publications.

DIETARY SUPPLEMENTS

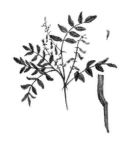

Astragalus

BOTANICAL DATA

Classification and Nomenclature

Scientific name: *Astragalus membranaceus* (Fisch.) Bunge and *Astragalus membranaceus* var. *mongholicus* (Bunge) Hsiao. (syn. *A. mongholicus* Bunge) (Zhu, 1998)

Family name: Fabaceae (formerly Leguminosae)

Common names: astragalus, milk vetch (United States), huang-ch'i (China), ogi (Japan), hwanggi (Korea) (Bensky et al., 1986)

Description

The genus *Astragalus* is a member of the Fabaceae or legume family. This xerophytic perennial is native to northern China and Mongolia. It inhabits mostly pine forests and sandy soils and is widely distributed in China, Siberia, and northern Korea, where it is cultivated for medicinal use (Morazzoni and Bombardelli, 1994). Morphological, chemical, and genetic means of distinguishing species of *Astragalus* used in Chinese commerce are available (Foster and Yue, 1992; Li et al., 1994; Lin et al., 2000; Ma et al., 1999; Wadlington et al., 1999; Cheng et al., 2000).

Astragalus *(Astragalus membranaceus)* grows to a height of 25-40 cm. The fernlike fronds are approximately 20-35 cm long with sulcated, angled stems covered with appressed white hairs. The leaves are 3-6 cm long, with obsolete petioles. The flowers are light yellow and resemble peas. The leaflets, numbering 12-24, are oblong-obovate, oval, or oblong-oval, and glabrous on the leaf surface and vested beneath. The peduncles are firm, axillary, and 4-7 cm long. *Astragalus membranaceus* has a long, branched tap root and two-valved seed pods (16-19 mm long and 11-15 mm wide) with short, dark hairs. The seeds are kidney-shaped, dark brown, and resemble miniature soybeans (Foster and Yue, 1992; Pedersen, 1994; Morazzoni and Bombardelli, 1994). *Astragalus membranaceus* (Fisch.) Bunge var. *mongholicus* (Bunge) Hsiao is found in the mountains and sunny grasslands of northeast China and may be distinguished from *A. membranaceus* by triangular-ovate stipules, dark yellow flowers, 25-37 leaflets, and hairless seed pods (Foster and Yue, 1992).

HISTORY AND TRADITIONAL USES

The first mention of *Astragalus* spp. is in the *Divine Husbandman's Classic of the Materia Medica,* an ancient Chinese medical text (Bensky et al., 1986). In traditional Chinese medicine (TCM), the dried root of *A. membranaceus* is used primarily as a tonic, especially for the spleen and lungs (Bensky et al., 1986; Hsu et al., 1986). It is said to benefit the deficiency of *qi* (vital energy) of the spleen that symptomatically presents with fatigue, diarrhea, and lack of appetite. *Astragalus membranaceus* is also important traditionally for the treatment of infections of the mucous membranes, especially the urinary and respiratory tracts. In China, it is used as a prophylactic against colds (Zhu, 1998). Astragalus is also believed to function as a cardiotonic and to increase contraction in normal hearts. In hearts affected by fatigue or poison, the improvement is reportedly more dramatic (Hsu et al., 1986).

CHEMISTRY

Carbohydrates

Polysaccharides

Astragalus membranaceus contains polysaccharides that are thought to play an important role in the immunomodulatory actions of the plant. Polysaccharide A was identified as an $\propto$-(1,4) and $\propto$-(1,6) glucan (5:2); polysaccharides B and C were identified as $\propto$-(1,4) glucans; and polysaccharide D as a heteropolysaccharide with a glucose, arabinose, and rhamnose in a 9:3:2 ratio (Morazzoni and Bombardelli, 1994).

Lipid Compounds

Saponifiable Lipids

Astragalosides I to VII (saponins) were isolated by an extraction of roots in methanol, followed by fractionation on silica gel. The structure of astragaloside VII was determined to be 3-*O*-β-D-xylopyranosyl-6-*O*-β-glucopyranosyl-25-*O*-β-glucopyranosylcycloastragenol, a rare example of a triterpene tridesmoside saponin. These saponins differ primarily in the location of sugar units (Morazzoni and Bombardelli, 1994; Lacaille-Dubois and Wagner, 1996).

Phenolic Compounds

Flavonoids

The isoflavones formononetin, calycosin, *L*-3-hydroxy-9,10-dimethoxypterocarpan-3-*O*-β-D-glucoside and 3,7-dihydroxy-3',4'-dimethoxyisoflavone 7-*O*-glucoside, among others, were isolated from the nonroot parts of the plant (Morazzoni and Bombardelli, 1994). The flower tops contain quercetin, isorhamnetin, and kaempferol (Cheshuina, 1990). In addition, a methanol extract of the roots contained the flavone kumatakenin (4',5-dihydroxy-3, 7-dimethoxy-flavone), along with additional flavonoids, aglycones, and glucosides (Morazzoni and Bombardelli, 1994), and 13 isoflavones including calycosin, calycosin-7-*O*-β-glucopyranoside, formononetin, odoratin-7-*O*-β-F-glucopyranoside, and 8,3'-dihydroxy-7,4'-dimethoxyisoflavone (Song et al., 1997a,b). Other flavonoids have been identified in the roots, including ononin and (3*R*)-7,2'-dihydroxy-3',4'-dimethoxyisoflavan-7-*O*-β-D-glucoside, in addition to flavonoid glycoside malonates: calycosin-7-*O*-β-D-glucoside-6"-)-malonate, astraisoflavanglucoside-6"-*O*-malonate, astrapterocarpanglucoside-6"-*O*-malonate, and formononetin-7-*O*-β-D-glucoside-6"-*O*-malonate (Lin et al., 2000).

Terpenoid Compounds

Triterpenes

As part of a series of studies undertaken to determine the bioactive constituents of astragalus, triterpene-oligoglycoside constituents of *A. membranaceus* were isolated by means of enzymatic and chemical degradation. These included the 9, 19-cyclolanostane-type triterpene, cycloastragenol, which was the common genuine aglycone of the astragalosides, and the lanost-9(11)-ene-type counterpart, astragenol, which was an artifact aglycone secondarily formed from cycloastragenol and soyasapogenol B, a genuine aglycone (Kitagawa et al., 1983a,b; Kitagawa, Wang, Saito, et al., 1983; Kitagawa, Wang, Yoshikawa, 1983).

Other Constituents

In the roots of Astragalus, zinc, copper, iron, magnesium, manganese, calcium, sodium, potassium, cobalt, rubidium, molybdenum, chromium, vanadium, tin, and silver have been found, as well as traces of europium, tantalum, hafnium, and thorium. Organic compounds identified in the roots include choline, betaine, gluconic acid, and β-sitosterol, as well as aromatic compounds, linoleic acid, essential oil, α-aminobutyric acid, bitter compounds (Bensky et al., 1986; Leung and Foster, 1996; Pedersen, 1994; Hsu et al., 1986; Yen, 1992), and asaparagine (0.2%) (Hikino et al., 1976).

THERAPEUTIC APPLICATIONS

The current primary applications of Astragalus are in immune system potentiation and cardiovascular disease. However, the main application of the plant in Chinese medicine is for influenza and the common cold. The herb has also been used in the treatment of chronic glomerulonephritis. An ointment containing 10% astragalus is used to treat wounds and in Chinese folk medicine the decoction and ointment have been applied on chronic ulcerated wounds (Huang, 1999).

PRECLINICAL STUDIES

Cardiovascular and Circulatory Functions

Cardiotonics; Cardioprotection

Zhang et al. (1997) reported evidence to suggest that the saponin astragaloside IV (1 μg/mL) could significantly increase the fibrinolytic potential of cultured human endothelial cells in vitro by downregulating PAI-1 (plasminogen activator inhibitor type 1) expression and upregulating tPA (tissue-type plasminogen activator) expression. tPA is believed to be the substance mainly responsible for breaking up blood clots in the vascular system and is regulated by PAI-1. Elevated levels of PAI-1 activity are associated with myocardial infarction (heart attack), coronary heart disease, and thrombotic disorders.

Hong et al. (1994) showed that a relatively strong concentration of the root extract (2 mg/mL) in vitro could inhibit adenosine 5'-diphosphate/ $FeSO_4$-induced lipid peroxidation in rat heart mitochondria. Of 13 other Chinese medicinal plants tested, only *Polygonum multiflorum* showed comparable activity at the same dose. The other 12, at up to three times the concentration, were considerably weaker.

Astragalus membranaceus root extract (1 g/day, i.p. × 35), following a model of congestive heart failure induced in rats, was reported to demonstrate diuretic, cardiotonic, and natriuretic activities. The extract was also found to ameliorate blunted kidney response to atrial natriuretic peptide (ANP), and partly ameliorate abnormal AVP (arginine vasopressin) system mRNA expression. Plasma ANP levels were lower in rats treated with extract and the amelioration of abnormal mRNA expression of both the AVP system and AQP2 (aquaporin-2) were found consistent with alleviations of reduced urinary sodium secretion, free water clearance, urinary volume, glomerular filtration rate, and renal plasma flow (Ma et al., 1998).

Hypertension

Astragalus membranaceus exhibits hypotensive activity. A few authors credit this to the direct vasodilatory action which seems to be induced by the root extract (Bensky et al., 1986). This vasodilation has been partially attributed to the presence of GABA (γ-aminobutyric acid) (Morazzoni and Bombardelli, 1994; Chang and But, 1987). GABA has also shown diuretic and anticonvulsant activity (Hikino et al., 1976).

Dogs administered an extract of astragalus (0.5 g/kg i.p.) showed no immediate effects on heart rate. However, 3-4 h postinjection, inverted and biphasic T waves and slightly prolonged sinus tachycardia (ST) intervals were recorded (Chang and But, 1987).

Zhang, Wang, et al. (1984) reported inhibitory activity against the increase in capillary permeability induced by 5-hydroxytryptamine plus histamine after administration of a saponin (saponin 1) derived from astragalus in rats. Administered orally (50 mg/kg) in the form of a liposome, the rate of inhibition (38.02%) from the saponin was comparable to that of cortisone administered by injection (25mg/kg i.p., 34.64% inhibition). At 5 mg/kg i.v., the saponin showed hypotensive activity when administered to anesthetized cats. A lower dose (0.25 mg/kg) was ineffective (Zhang, Wang, et al., 1984). However, earlier activity-guided fractionation studies on the hypotensive activity of the root (1 mL/kg, i.v.) in anesthetized rats showed a strong correlation with GABA (0.024% from dried root) (Hikino et al., 1976).

Digestive, Hepatic, and Gastrointestinal Functions

Hepatic Functions

Zhang et al. (1992) isolated a saponin (unidentified) from the root that protected liver cells from damage induced by acetaminophen, carbon tetrachloride, or D-galactosamine in mice. The authors reported that the saponin (6 mg/kg, p.o. b.i.d. × 5 days) could also significantly decrease elevations of SGPT (serum glutamic-pyruvic transaminase or alanine transaminase), increase the liver concentration of glutathione, and cause a decrease in liver concentrations of MDA (malondialdehyde) of mice. In primary rat hepatocytes, the saponin lowered the average level of GPT (glutamic-pyruvic transaminase or guanosine triphosphate) compared to the control. The authors concluded that the liver-protectant activity of the saponin was probably related to antioxidant activity, especially since the liver protein content of the saponin-treated mice showed a tendency to be higher compared to untreated control mice. In addition, there was a significant increase in the level of liver microsomal cytochrome P-450 in every mouse treated with the saponin (12 or 50 mg/kg p.o. b.i.d. × 4 days) compared to control mice, indicating both an immunoregulating and a liver metabolism enhancing activity. Zhang et al. (1990) showed that an ethanolic extract of the root (3 g/kg, p.o.) could significantly ameliorate stilbenemidine-induced liver injury in rats. Stilbenemidine is an anticancer agent. The authors speculated that the constituent betaine may have been responsible for the liver-protectant activity found. In addition, Zhang, Shen et al. (1984) reported a significant increase in liver DNA content in partially hepatectomized rats after administration of a saponin derived from astragalus (saponin 1, 10 mg/kg i.p.). The increase in plasma accumulation of cAMP was maximal 0.5~4.0 h after treatment.

Immune Functions; Inflammation and Disease

Cancer

Antiproliferative activity. Lau et al. (1994) showed that a water extract of *A. membranaceus,* when combined with a water extract of the Chinese herb *Ligustrum lucidum* (500 µg each, i.p.), could significantly inhibit the growth of renal cell carcinoma in mice. The authors reported that whereas 85.7% of the control mice died, 100% of the herbal extract-treated mice survived longer than 150 days with a cure rate of 100%. The herbal extract combination restored depressed oxidative burst activity of splenic macrophages from tumor-bearing mice and improved the generation of lymphokine-activated killer (LAK) cells of splenocytes in response to IL-2 in vitro.

Chemotherapy adjunct treatments. Wang et al. (1992) reported recombinant interleukin-2 (rIL-2) potentiated 10-fold from coincubation with a fraction of astragalus extract designated F3. They noted that by reducing the dosage required in treating cancer patients, the severe side effects of rIL-2 therapy (e.g., acute renal failure, capillary leakage syndrome, myocardial infarction, and fluid retention) might also be reduced.

Immune Functions

Immunopotentiation. Chu et al. (1988) obtained 3 polysaccharide fractions (50% carbohydrates, <1% protein) from the air-dried roots of astragalus which augmented the local xenogeneic graft-versus-host reaction (local XGVHR) of circulating monocytes in vitro derived from healthy normal donors. The local XGVHR also served as a model assay for testing the T cell function of circulating monocytes derived from 13 cancer patients. Two of the fractions induced highly significant increases in the local XGVHR compared to untreated monocytes from normal subjects, and the immunopotentiating activity was able to fully correct in vitro the deficient T cell function found in cancer patients.

Kajimura et al. (1997) found no significant enhancement of immuno-globulin G (IgG) production in young mice administered a crude poly-saccharide fraction of the root (p.o.), whereas in old mice they found IgG significantly increased. Productivity levels of IgG in the elderly mice were restored to levels found in young mice. The authors isolated two active poly-saccharides (F8 and F9) with molecular masses estimated at 120,000 and 220,000. Tomoda et al. (1992) reported that a polysaccharide (molecular mass of 60,000) isolated from a water extract of the root caused a highly sig-nificant immunopotentiating activity (phagocytosis) in the carbon clearance test.

A water extract of the root was shown by Yoshida et al. (1997) to mark-edly stimulate the proliferation of murine spleen cells of mice in vitro. The root extract also caused a significant stimulation in the production of tumor necrosis factor-α and IL-6 production by peritoneal exudate macrophages and significantly enhanced the activity of cytotoxic T cells in vitro.

A crude extract of astragalus (0.2 mL i.p.) enhanced the antibody re-sponse to a T-dependent antigen in healthy mice, immunodepressed mice (by irradiation or cyclophosphamide), and in aged mice. In the immuno-depressed and normal mice, the enhanced response was associated with an increase in T-helper cell activity (Zhao et al., 1990). Astragalus restored in vitro lymphocyte blastogenic responses (Sun, Hersh, Lee, et al., 1983) and graft-versus-host reaction (Sun, Hersh, Talpaz, et al., 1983) in mononuclear cells taken from cancer patients. In one study, the response of T cells from cancer patients treated with the root extract surpassed that of healthy indi-viduals. The most bioactive constituent in this study was identified as frac-tion F3, a polysaccharide fraction (Morazzoni and Bombardelli, 1994).

Jiao et al. (2001) demonstrated that the flavonoid fraction from the leaf and stem of *A. membranaceous* increased cell-mediated immunological re-sponses in mice. Treatment with the flavonoid fraction (0.2 mL i.p. daily for five days of a solution containing the fraction at a concentration 2.5 mg/mL) ameliorated hydrocortisone-induced immunosuppression of T cell and T cell subset counts. In vitro studies found a weak stimulatory effect on the proliferation of lymphocytes stimulated by concanavalin A (ConA) in spleen cells from the flavonoid fraction at low doses (3.9 to 62.5 µg/mL) and significant stimulatory activity at high doses (125 to 250 µg/mL). Lympho-kine-activated killer (LAK) cell activity in mice was not stimulated by the flavonoid fraction unless it was combined with recombinant interleukin-2 (rIL-2). In previous studies of the flavonoid fraction of the leaf and stem, in-dications of macrophage stimulation and an antibody-increasing effect were found.

Immunosuppression. Khoo and Ang (1995) found that a water extract of *A. membranaceus* root (240 mg p.o./rat per day × 12) could not prevent cyclophosphamide-induced myelosuppression in rats at a dosage approximately equivalent to a daily dose traditionally recommended for adults (30 g/day).

Infectious Diseases

Viral infections. Kajimura et al. (1996) administered a methanolic extract of the root to mice (0.1 mL/mouse, p.o.) infected with Japanese encephalitis virus and found survival rates of 30-40%, versus 20% in the untreated controls. Comparing *A. membranaceus* root extracts prepared from plant material collected in different regions of Japan revealed a significant difference in results. Based on the comparatively higher rate of active oxygen found in the peritoneal exudate cells of mice in the treated group, the authors suggest that the protective role of the root extract administered orally against Japanese encephalitis virus is due to the activity of macrophages.

A decoction of the root given to mice by gavage (daily for one to two weeks) increased phagocytic activity of the reticuloendothelial system. It was also shown that oral doses or nose drops of the root decoction protected mice against parainfluenza virus type I (Morazzoni and Bombardelli, 1994). Although the herb itself does not appear to be a direct interferon inducer, it may indirectly promote the production of interferon, perhaps due to immunomodulating polysaccharides or large lipids (Zhao et al., 1990).

Yang, Jin, Guo, Wu, et al. (1990) reported smaller and less severe lesions in the myocardium of mice with Coxsackie B-3-induced myocarditis that were treated with an alcoholic extract of the root (1 g/day, i.p.) shortly after infection compared to untreated controls. Both the relative area covered by lesions and the virus titer were less than those of the controls.

Animal studies have shown that in very high doses (25 g/kg p.o. per day × 4) astragalus can increase the interferon titer in response to infection on day two of the treatment period by Sendai virus (BB-1 strain, intranasal) or Newcastle disease virus (f and II strains) compared to placebo-treated control mice (Hou et al., 1981).

Inflammatory Response

Zhang, Wang, et al. (1984) tested a saponin derived from *A. membranaceous* against carrageenin-induced edema in rats (50 mg/kg p.o.). The saponin produced a rate of inhibition (63.1%) comparable to that of hydrocortisone (25 mg/kg i.p., 56.4% inhibition).

Metabolic and Nutritional Functions

Antioxidant Activity

Astragalus membranaceus has been shown to promote cell proliferation and survival (Morazzoni and Bombardelli, 1994; Chang and But, 1987). The addition of 0.5% astragalus extract to monolayer cultures of embryonic renal cells from hamsters and mice increased cell survival, induced cell proliferation, and doubled the life span of the cells (Chang and But, 1987). These effects are conceivably due to antioxidant activity. Both an extract of the root and a triterpene (cycloastragenol-xylosyl-glucoside) derived from it inhibited lipid peroxide production in vitro and inhibited the increase in lipid peroxidation induced by the anticancer agent adriamycin in mice (Rios and Waterman, 1997). In vitro antioxidant activity was also shown from a decoction of the root against copper-induced lecithin peroxidation (IC_{50} 117 µg/mL) and against copper-induced oxidative modification of albumin (IC_{50} 12.5 µg/mL) (Toda and Shirataki, 1999).

Reproductive Functions

Infertility (Male)

In screening crude water extracts of 18 major Chinese medicinal plants for sperm motility-enhancing activity in vitro, Hong et al. (1992) reported that only *A. membranaceus* showed significant activity (133%), both in washed and unwashed sperm of healthy donors (10 mg/mL, maximally). Lack of sperm motility is a major factor in male infertility.

CLINICAL STUDIES

Cardiovascular and Circulatory Disorders

Thrombosis, Hemostasis, and Embolism

Liao et al. (1988) conducted a study to evaluate the efficacy of *A. membranaceus* in the treatment of coronary heart disease (CHD). In combination with *Codonopsis pilosula* (0.5 gm of each per mL, called CP-A), *A. membranaceus* was administered intravenously to 37 patients with CHD and 14 cases of acute myocardial infarction (AMI). Patients were divided into three groups: condonopsis pilosula-Astragalus (CP-A) i.v., a dextrose group (20 mL 10% dextrose i.v.), and a Cedilanid-D (0.6 mg i.v.) group. The drugs were administered at a single dose. Before treatment and 1h following, the systolic time intervals (STI) were measured. STI parameters were evaluated as the mean values of five cardiac cycles. The results indicated that following administration of CP-A or Cedilanid-D, there was a significant increase in left ventricular performance and a decrease in PEP and PEP/LVET ratio. This suggests that CP-A exerts a positive inotropic action in patients with CHD, which may be responsible for improving dyspnea and fatigue.

In a large placebo-controlled clinical study in Beijing, 30 g of *A. membranaceus* was administered with a mixture of other herbs (15 g *C. pilosula,* 15 g *Polygonatum sibiricum,* 30 g *Salvia miltiorrhiza,* 15 g *Paeonia obovata,* and 15 g *Curcuma aromatica*) to patients who had suffered AMI. In the 208 cases treated over 29 months, 181 of the patients improved, and 27 died. The mortality rate in the treated group was 13.0% compared to 19.0% for those in the placebo group. Before complementary, traditional, and western medical treatments were combined in Chinese medical practice, the rate of mortality from AMI in China ranged as high as 33-56.5%. Once traditional techniques were combined, the mortality rate fell rapidly to 14.6% (Guo et al., 1983).

Genitourinary and Renal Disorders

Renal Disorders

Studies on humans indicate that *A. membranaceus* has a moderate diuretic action (Chang and But, 1987; Bensky et al., 1986). The clinical dose of 0.2 g/kg increased urine output by 64% and sodium excretion by 14.5% (Chang and But, 1987).

Immune Disorders; Inflammation and Disease

Immune Modulation

Cellular immune response. A controlled clinical treatment study of chronic cervicitis by Qian et al. (1990) reported that *A. membranaceus* has a "synergistic" effect with recombinant interferon (rINF-α1). In a double-blind study of 235 cases of typical chronic cervicitis, a combination treatment was applied which consisted of 30 μg INF-α1, plus *A. membranaceus,* 3 mL locally using a double-layered gauze soaked in a solution of the drugs. The researchers found that at a six-month follow-up examination the combined treatment had produced complete cures in 16% and markedly improved 51% of cases. INF-α1 alone (30 μg locally) produced cures in 6% and markedly improved 33%. The difference was statistically significant ($p < 0.05$). Further evidence of a "synergistic" effect was found when *A. membranaceus* extract was used alone (100% w/v, 3 mL locally). At the six-month follow-up, there were no cures and a rate of marked improvement of only 15%. At double the dosage (60 μg locally), INF-α1 alone produced the best results with a cure rate of 19% and marked improvement in 53% at the six-month follow-up. This was an overall success rate not much different ($p > 0.05$) from the combination treatment using half the dosage of INF-$\alpha 1$. In addition, the researchers detected a dramatic drop in the herpes simplex virus isolation rate in the combination treatment group (30.4% prior to therapy and 3.8% after), which was greater than that of the low dose INF-$\alpha 1$ group (33.3% prior and 10% after therapy) (Qian et al., 1990).

In a study to evaluate the effect of *A. membranaceus* root extract, patients suffering from Coxsackie B viral myocarditis with depressed natural killer cell (NK) activity were treated with *Astragalus* versus conventional Chinese therapy. Ten patients (seven male, three female, ages 15-48 years old) were injected with an extract of the herb (8 g/day i.m. for three to four months). Another six patients (three male, three female, ages 27-40) were treated with the conventional therapies of glucose, insulin, potassium chloride (polarized therapy), or vitamin C, coenzyme A, DNA, and Sheng Mai Chong Ji (not explained) for three to four months. NK cell activity was measured at the beginning and at the end of the therapy. In the *A. membranaceus* group, NK activity increased significantly, while the same activity remained unchanged in those on conventional therapy. The authors concluded that the results suggest *A. membranaceus* could partially regulate the loss of cellular immunity in patients with viral myocarditis (Yang, Jin, Guo, Wang, et al., 1990).

In a pilot study on astragalus (8 g p.o./day × 60) in 28 adults with 14 serving as the placebo control group, Hou et al., 1981 found the interferon-inducing ability of blood leucocytes significantly higher in the astragalus group and baseline measurements taken before the treatment period. The effect persisted for 2 months after the treatment period ended compared to the placebo controls. Similar results were found against the common cold in field studies in China from 1974-1978 in 1,137 volunteers. Subjects received interferon alone (intranasal spray, 0.5 mL every other day), or combined with astragalus (intranasal spray, 0.5 mL interferon mixed with 50 percent astragalus aqueous extract, or interferon spray plus 8 g astragalus p.o., every other day), using an inactive influenza vaccine as the treatment for the controls. Courses of treatment lasted two to four months and the combination of interferon and astragalus was superior to interferon or the inactive vaccine. In one cohort (141 placebo, 40 interferon plus astragalus), the course of illness lasted 4.6 days in the placebo group versus 2.6 days in the interferon plus astragalus group (Hou et al., 1981).

DOSAGE

In China, the officially recognized daily dose of astragalus is from 9 to 30 g (Tu et al., 1992).

SAFETY PROFILE

Contraindications

Astragalus membranaceus is classified as an herb that when used appropriately is safe (McGuffin et al., 1997). The only contraindications mentioned are those found in the TCM literature (Bensky et al., 1986), which suggest that it may not be appropriate during acute sickness with fever and thirst.

No detrimental effects were found in mice within 48 h of oral administration of 75 g/kg or 100 g/kg. The LD_{50} in mice was found to be 39.82 g/kg i.p. Prostration, paralysis, dyspnea, and cyanosis were observed before death, as was some contraction of extremities. At 0.5 g/kg i.per/day in mice, the root elicited no significant toxic reactions in terms of activity, defecation, micturation, and food intake (Chang and But, 1987).

Drug Interactions

In a double-blind study of 235 cases of typical chronic cervicitis, Qian et al. (1990) reported that *A. membranaceus* has a "synergistic" effect with recombinant interferon ($rINF-\alpha 1$) when applied as combination treatment ($INF-\alpha 1$, 30 µg plus *A. membranaceus* 3 mL locally; double-layered gauze soaked in a solution of the drugs).

Pregnancy and Lactation

No special precautions are mentioned in the literature for either pregnancy or lactation. Reports in the ethnobotanical literature show three other species of *Astragalus* being used as galactogogues in dairy animals or humans (Bingel and Farnsworth, 1994).

Side Effects

None known.

Special Precautions

None known.

Toxicology

In Vitro Toxicity

Mutagenicity. Yamamoto et al. (1982) reported that a methanol/water extract of the root showed no mutagenic effects. However, Yin et al. (1991) reported that a water extract of the root of *Astragalus mongholicus* Bge. exhibited mutagenic activity in the Ames test using *Salmonella typhimurium* TA98 with S9 mix, but not in TA 100 and not in either without S9 mix. The effect appeared to be dose-dependent from 5-40 mg/plate. Tadaki et al. (1995) rexamined the effect of astragalus in the Ames test with S9 mix and found the mutagenic effect was modest, with a concentration of 1.25 mg/mL causing only a 16% increase in aberrant cell incidence.

Toxicity in animal models. The LD_{50} of *A. membranaceus* in mice was found to be 39.82 g/kg i.p. (Chang and But, 1987). Prostration, paralysis, dyspnea, and cyanosis were observed before death, as was some contraction of extremities (Bensky et al., 1986). At 0.5 g/kg i.per/day (for 30 days in mice), the root elicited no significant toxic reactions in terms of activity, defecation, micturation, and food intake (Chang and But, 1987).

In a bone marrow-chromosomal and a bone marrow-micronucleus assay in TAI (inbred strain) mice of either sex, evidence of mutagenicity was found from an intraperitoneal dose of the extract (1 g/kg) that the authors calculated to be equivalent to "the dosage used in medication" and from higher amounts (Yin et al., 1991). These effects also appeared to increase with increasing dosages; however, it remains to be seen whether any mutagenic effects are found when the herb is administered by the traditional, oral route.

REFERENCES

Bensky, D., Gamble, A., and Kaptchuk, T. (1986). *Chinese Herbal Medicine Materia Medica,* Seattle, WA: Eastland Press.

Bingel, A.S. and N.R. Farnsworth (1994). Higher plants as potential sources of galactogogues. In: Wagner, H., Hikino, H. and Farnsworth, N.R. (Eds.). *Economic and Medicinal Plant Research,* Volume 6. NY: Academic Press, pp. 1-54.

Chang, H.M. and But, P.P.H. (Eds.) (1987). *Pharmacology and Applications of Chinese Materia Medica,* Volume 2. Hong Kong: World Scientific.

Cheng, K.T., Su, B., Chen, C.T., and Lin, C.C. (2000). RAPD analysis of *Astragalus* medicines marketed in Taiwan. *American Journal of Chinese Medicine* 28: 273-278.

Cheshuina, A.I. (1990). Flavonol aglycons of *Astragalus membranaceus. Chemistry of Natural Compounds* 26: 712.

Chu, D.T., Wong, W.L., and Mavligit, G.M. (1988). Immunotherapy with Chinese medicinal herbs. I. Immune restoration of local xenogeneic graft-versus-host reaction in cancer patients by fractionated *Astragalus membranaceous* in vitro. *Journal of Clinical and Laboratory Immunology* 25: 119-123.

Foster, S. and Yue, C. (1992). *Herbal Emissaries: Bringing Chinese Herbs to the West.* Rochester, VT: Healing Arts Press, pp. 27-33.

Guo S.K., Chen, K.J., Yu, F.R., Li, X.G., and Tu, X.H. (1983). Treatment of acute myocardial infarction with AMI-mixture combined with western medicine. *Planta Medica* 48: 63-64.

Hikino, H., Funayama, S., and Endo, K. (1976). Hypotensive principle of *Astragalus* and *Hedysarum* roots. *Planta Medica* 30: 297-302.

Hong, C.Y., Ku, J., and Wu, P. (1992). *Astragalus membranaceus* stimulates human sperm motility in vitro. *American Journal of Chinese Medicine* 20: 289-294.

Hong, C.Y., Lo, Y.C., Tan, F.C., Wei, Y.H., and Chen, C.F. (1994). *Astragalus membranaceus* and *Polygonum multiflorum* protect rat heart mitochondria against lipid peroxidation. *American Journal of Chinese Medicine* 22: 63-70.

Hou, Y., Ma, G., Wu, S., Li, Y., and Li, H. (1981). Effect of radix Astragali seu hedysari on the interferon system. *Chinese Medical Journal* 94: 35-40.

Hsu, H.Y., Chen, Y.P., Shen, S.J., Hsu, C.S., Chen, C.C., and Chang, H.C. (Eds.) (1986). *Oriental Materia Medica: A Concise Guide.* Long Beach, CA: Oriental Healing Arts Institute.

Huang, K.C. (1999). *The Pharmacology of Chinese Herbs,* Second Edition. Boca Raton, FL: CRC Press, p. 387.

Jiao, Y., Wen, J., Yu, X.H., and Zhang, D.S. (2001). Influence of flavonoid of *Astragalus membranaceous'* stem and leaf on the function of cell mediated immunity in mice. *Chinese Journal of Integrated Traditional and Western Medicine* 7: 117-120.

Kajimura, K., Takagi, Y., Miyano, K., Sawabe, Y., Mimura, M., Sakagami, Y., Yokoyama, H., and Yoneda, K. (1997). Polysaccharide of *Astragali radix* enhances IgM antibody production in aged mice. *Biological and Pharmaceutical Bulletin* 20: 1178-1182.

Kajimura, K., Takagi, Y., Ueba, N., Yamasaki, K., Sakagami, Y., Yokotama, H., and Yoneda, K. (1996). Protective effect of *Astragali radix* by oral administration against Japanese encephalitis virus infection in mice. *Biological and Pharmaceutical Bulletin* 19: 1166-1169.

Khoo, K.S. and Ang, P.T. (1995). Extract of *Astragalus membranaceus* and *Ligustrum lucidum* does not prevent cyclophosphamide-induced myelosuppression. *Singapore Medical Journal* 36: 387-390.

Kitagawa, I., Wang, H.K., Saito, M., Takagi, A., and Yoshikawa, M. (1983a). Saponin and sapogenol, XXXIV. Chemical constituents of *Astragali radix,* the root of *Astragalus membranaceus* Bunge (1). Cycloastragenol, the 9,19-cyclolanostane-type aglycone of the astragalosides and the artifact aglycone astragenol. *Chemical and Pharmaceutical Bulletin* 31: 689-697.

Kitagawa, I., Wang, H.K., Saito, M., Takagi, A., and Yoshikawa, M. (1983b). Saponin and sapogenol, XXXV. Chemical constituents of *Astragali radix,* the root of *Astragalus membranaceus* Bunge (2). Astragalosides I, II, and IV, acetylastragaloside I and isoastragalosides I and II. *Chemical and Pharmaceutical Bulletin* 31: 698-708.

Kitagawa, I., Wang, H.K., Saito, M., and Yoshikawa, M. (1983). Saponin and sapogenol. XXXVI. Chemical constituents of *Astragali radix*, the root of *Astragalus membranaceus* Bunge. (3). Astragalosides III, V, and VI. *Chemical and Pharmaceutical Bulletin* 31: 709-715.

Kitagawa, I., Wang, H.K., and Yoshikawa, M. (1983). Saponin and sapogenol, XXXVII. Chemical constituents of *Astragali radix,* the root of *Astragalus membranaceus* Bunge (2). Astragalosides I, II, and IV, acetylastragaloside I and isoastragalosides I and II. *Chemical and Pharmaceutical Bulletin* 31: 716-722.

Lacaille-Dubois, M.A. and Wagner, H. (1996). A review of the biological and pharmacological activities of saponins. *Phytomedicine* 2: 363-386.

Lau, B.H.S., Ruckle, H.C., Botolazzo, T., Botolazzo, T., and Lui, P.D. (1994). Chinese medicinal herbs inhibit growth of murine renal cell carcinoma. *Cancer Biotherapy* 9: 153-161.

Leung, A.Y. and Foster, S. (1996). *Encyclopedia of Common Natural Ingredients Used in Foods, Drugs, and Cosmetics*. New York: John Wiley and Sons, Inc.

Li, M., Qin, X.Q., Chen, S.B., and Feng, Y.X. (1994). Morphological and microscopical identification of genus *Astragalus* on mainly used commercial huang qi. *Acta Pharmaceutica Sinica* 29: 862-871.

Liao, J.Z., Chai, Z.N., Li, W.S., Liu, X.F., Wang, S., Qin, L., and Guo, W.Q. (1988). Pharmacologic effects of *Codonopsis pilosula-Astragalus* injection in the treatment of CHD patients. *Journal of Traditional Chinese Medicine* 8: 1-8.

Lin, L.Z., He, X.G., Lindenmaier, M., Nolan, G., Yamg, J., Cleary, M., Qiu, S.X., and Cordell, G.A. (2000). Liquid chromatography-electrospray ionization mass spectrometry study of the flavonoids of the roots of *Astragalus mongholicus* and *A. membranaceus*. *Journal of Chromatography* A 876:87-95.

Ma, J., Peng, A., and Lin, S. (1998). Mechanisms of the therapeutic effect of *Astragalus membranaceus* on sodium and water retention in experimental heart failure. *Chinese Medical Journal* 111: 17-23.

Ma, X.Q., Duan, J.A., Zhu, D.Y., Dong, T.T.X., and Tsim, K.W.K. (1999). Species identification of Radix Astragali (Huang qi) by DNA sequence of its 5S-rRNA spacer domain. *Phytochemistry* 54: 363-368.

McGuffin, M., Hobbs, C., Upton, R., and Goldberg, A. (Eds.) (1997). *American Herbal Products Association's Botanical Safety Handbook*. Boca Raton, FL: CRC Press, p. 17.

Morazzoni, P.E. and Bombardelli, E. (1994). *Indena Scientific Documentation*. Milan, Italy: Indena.

Qian, Z.W., Mao, S.J., Cai, X.C., Zhang, X.L., Gao, F.X., Lu, M.F., and Shao, X.S. (1990). Viral etiology of chronic cervicitis and its therapeutic response to a recombinant interferon. *Chinese Medical Journal* 103: 647-651.

Rios, J.L. and Waterman, P.G. (1997). A review of the pharmacology and toxicology of *Astragalus*. *Phytotherapy Research* 11: 411-418.

Song, C.Q., Zheng, Z.R., Liu, D., and Hu, Z.B. (1997a). [Antimicrobial isoflavans from *Astragalus membranaceus* (Fisch.) Bung.]. *Acta Botanica Sinica* 39: 486-488.

Song, C.Q., Zheng, Z.R., Liu, D., and Hu, Z.B.(1997b). [Isoflavones from *Astragalus membranaceus*]. *Acta Botanica Sinica* 39: 764-768.

Sun, Y., Hersh, E.M., Lee, S.L., McLaughlin, M., Loo, T.L., and Mavligit, G.M. (1983). Preliminary observations on the effects of the Chinese medicinal herbs *Astragalus membranaceus* and *Ligustrum lucidum* on lymphocyte blastogenic responses. *Journal of Biological Response Modifiers* 2: 227-237.

Sun, Y., Hersh, E.M., Talpaz, E.M., Lee, S.L., Wong, W., Loo, T.L., and Mavligit, G.M. (1983). Immune restoration and/or augmentation of local graft versus host reaction by traditional Chinese medicinal herbs. *Cancer* 52: 70-73.

Tadaki, S., Yamada, S., Miyazawa, N., Nozaka, T., and Tanaka, A. (1995). [Clastogenicity of Eucommiae and Astragali Radix]. *Japanese Journal of Toxicology and Environmental Health* 41: 463-469.

Toda, S. and Shirataki, Y. (1999). Inhibitory effects of Astragali Radix, a crude drug in Oriental medicines, on lipid peroxidation and protein oxidative modification by copper. *Journal of Ethnopharmacology* 68: 331-333.

Tomoda, M., Shimizu, N., Ohara, N., Gonda, R., Ishii, S., and Otsuki, H. (1992). A reticuloendothelial system-activating glycan from the roots of *Astragalus membranaceus*. *Phytochemistry* 31: 63-66.

Tu, G., Fang, Q., Guo, J., Yuan, S., Chen, C., Chen, J., Chen, Z., Cheng, S., Jin, R., Li, M., et al. (Eds.), (1992). *Pharmacopoeia of the People's Republic of China*. Guangzhou, China: Guangdong Science and Technology Press, pp. 153-154.

Wadlington, C., Graff, A., Williamson, E., Sudberg, S., Sudberg, E., Upton, R., Roberts, J., Reich, E., Wang, X.P., Wagner, H., et al. (1999). Astragalus root. *Astragalus membranaceus* & *Astragalus membranaceus* var. *mongholicus*. In Upton, R. (Ed.), *Analytical, Quality Control, and Therapeutic Monograph*, Santa Cruz, CA: American Herbal Pharmacopoeia.

Wang, Y., Qian, X.J., Hadley, H.R., and Lau, B.H.S. (1992). Phytochemicals potentiate interleukin-2 generated lymphokine-activated killer cell cytotoxicity against murine renal cell carcinoma. *Molecular Biotherapy* 4: 143-146.

Yamamoto, H., Mizutani, T., and Nomura, H. (1982). Studies on the mutagenicity of crude drug extracts. I. *Yakugaku Zasshi* 102: 596-601.

Yang, Y.Z., Jin, P.Y., Guo, Q., Wang, Q.D., Li, Z.S., Ye, Y.C., Shan, Y.F., Zhao, H.Y., Zhu, J.R., Pu, S.Y. (1990). Effect of *Astragalus membranaceus* on natural killer cell activity and induction of α- and γ-interferon in patients with Coxsackie B viral myocarditis. *Chinese Medical Journal* 103: 304-307.

Yang, Y.Z., Jin, P.Y., Guo, Q., Wu, W.Z., Pu, S.Y. Chen, H.Z., Yang, J.H., Wang, K.Q., Shi, J.Y., Gong, Z.X., et al. (1990). Treatment of experimental Coxsackie B-3 viral myocarditis with *Astragalus membranaceus* in mice. *Chinese Medical Journal* 103: 14-18.

Yen, K.Y. (1992). *The Illustrated Chinese Materia Medica Crude and Prepared.* Taipei, Taiwan: SMC Publishing Inc., p. 29.

Yin, X.J., Liu, D.X., Wang, H., and Zhou, Y. (1991). A study on the mutagenicity of 102 raw pharmaceuticals used in Chinese traditional medicine. *Mutation Research* 260: 73-82.

Yoshida, Y., Wang, M.Q., Liu, J.N., Shan, B.E., and Yamashita, U. (1997). Immunomodulating activity of Chinese medicinal herbs and *Oldenlandia diffusa* in particular. *International Journal of Immunopharmacology* 19: 359-370.

Zhang, W.J., Wojta, J., and Binder, B.R. (1997). Regulation of the fibrinolytic potential of cultured human umbilical vein endothelial cells: Astragaloside IV downregulates plasminogen activator inhibitor-1 and upregulates tissue-type plasminogen activator expression. *Journal of Vascular Research* 34: 273-280.

Zhang, Y.D., Shen, J.P., Song, J., Wang, Y.L., Shao, Y.N., Li, C.F., Zhou, S.H., Li, Y.F., and Li, D.X. (1984). [Effects of Astragalus saponin 1 on cAMP and cGMP level in plasma and DNA synthesis in regenerating liver]. *Acta Pharmaceutica Sinica* 19: 619-621.

Zhang, Y.D., Shen, J.P., Zhu, S.H., Huang, D.K., Ding, Y., and Zhang, X.L. (1992). [Effects of *Astragalus* (ASI, SK) on experimental liver injury]. *Yao Hsueh Hsueh Pao* [*Acta Pharmaceutica Sinica*] 27: 401-406.

Zhang, Y.D., Wang, Y.L., Shen, J.P., and Li, D.X. (1984). [Effects on blood pressure and inflammation of Astragalus saponin 1, a principle isolated from *Astragalus membranaceous* Bge]. *Acta Pharmaceutrica Sinica* 19: 333-337.

Zhang, Z.L., Wen, Q.Z., and Liu, C.X. (1990). Hepatoprotective effects of *Astragalus* root. *Journal of Ethnopharmacology* 30: 145-149.

Zhao, K.S., Mancini, C., and Doria, G. (1990). Enhancement of the immune response in mice by *Astragalus membranaceus* extracts. *Immunopharmacology* 20: 225-234.

Zhu, Y.P. (1998). *Chinese Materia Medica. Chemistry, Pharmacology and Applications.* Amsterdam, The Netherlands: Harwood Academic, pp. 560-564.

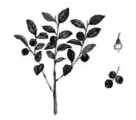

Bilberry

BOTANICAL DATA

Classification and Nomenclature

Scientific name: *Vaccinium myrtillus* L.

Family name: Ericaceae

Common names: Bilberry, whortleberry, black whortles, shinberry, trackleberry, hurts, bleaberry, airelle (French), hurtleberry (English), heidelbeeren (German)

Description

Vaccinium myrtillus L. is a small perennial shrub closely related to the blueberry. Included in the same family (Ericaceae) are many other berry-producing plants, such as cranberries and huckleberries, which obtain their color from anthocyanidins (flavonoid pigments). Generally, members of the Ericaceae family are native to the forests of Europe and also tend to grow well in the temperate areas of the United States (Cunio, 1993).

With wiry, angular branches and globulous, waxlike flowers, the stems of bilberry are 15-60 cm high, erect and freely branched, glabrous and green in color. The leaves are alternate, 1-2.5 cm long, oval to elliptic, shortly petiolate and slightly dentate. In the autumn, the leaves change color from rosy to yellowish-green and then to red. The flowers are borne solitary in the leaf axils, and are shortly stalked and pendulous. The greenish-pink tipped corolla is 3-6 mm, with a globose tube and short lobes. The fruit is a bluish-black globular berry with a flat top, approximately the same size as a currant

19

(6-10 mm). The bilberry shrub rarely reaches over 30 cm in height. The flowering season is May to June, and the ripe fruits are collected between July and September (Cunio, 1993; Morazzoni and Bombardelli, 1996).

HISTORY AND TRADITIONAL USES

The common name bilberry is derived from *bollebar,* a Danish word which means dark berry. Both as a food and a therapeutic remedy, bilberry has a long history of use. Therapeutically, bilberry was mentioned as far back as Dioscorides, and several North American Native tribes are known to have used seven different species of indigenous *Vaccinium* (Cunio, 1993). Traditionally, bilberry has been used for digestive disorders (diarrhea, dyspepsia, dysentery, gastrointestinal infections, and inflammations), poor night vision, scurvy, urinary infections, and stones, bruising, capillary fragility, varicose veins, poor circulation, Raynaud's disease, circulatory complications of diabetes, rheumatoid arthritis, gout, periodontal disease, and hemorrhoids (Morazzoni and Bombardelli, 1996; Cunio, 1993). The cosmetic use of bilberry is mostly attributable to its astringent activity. Bilberry is reported to protect against the harmful effects of sunburn and sudden changes in temperature. Other topical uses of bilberry preparations include the healing of bruises and wounds, and lessening the visual marks of cellulitis (Cunio, 1993).

Interest in the use of bilberry for ophthalmologic disorders appears to have begun during World War II when British Royal Air Force pilots noted improved night vision after eating the berries (Werbach and Murray, 1994).

CHEMISTRY

The main active constituents in bilberry are the carotenoids zeaxanthin and lutein, and flavonoids in the form of anthocyanidins.

Lipid Compounds

Oils

The volatile oils present in bilberry include methyl and ethyl 2-hydroxy-3-methylbutanoate, methyl and ethyl 3-hydroxy-3-methylbutanoate, 2-phenylethyl formate, farnesol, farnesyl acetate, vanillin, myristicin, 4-vinylphenol, 2-methoxy-5-vinylphenol, citronellol, hydroxycitronellol, methyl salicylate, and some lactones (Cunio, 1993).

Nitrogenous Compounds

Alkaloids

Bilberry contains the quinolizidine alkaloid myrtine (Cunio, 1993).

Phenolic Compounds

Polyphenolics

Over 15 different anthocyanosides are found in *Vaccinium myrtillus*. Anthocyanosides are anthocyanidins bound to one of three glycosides composed of an aglycone (Cunio, 1993; Baj et al., 1983). Madhavi et al. (1998) reported a proanthocyanidin content of over 1,800 mg/g (dry weight) in an extract of the fruits, which was largely composed of polymeric proanthocyanidins (1613 mg/g by dry weight). The anthocyanin content of the dried fruits (27.3 mg/g) was reported to mainly consist of cyanidin-3-galactoside, cyanidin-3-arabinoside, and cyanidin-3-glucoside.

Terpenoid Compounds

Tetraterpenes

The main carotenoids in the hexane extract of the fruits are zeaxanthin and lutein (Madhavi et al., 1998).

Other Constituents

On a dry weight basis per 100 g, bilberry is relatively high in aluminum (31.8 mg), magnesium (390 mg), potassium (1,673 mg), selenium (0.28 mg), thiamin (0.78 mg), vitamin A (7,800 IU), and vitamin C (165 mg); it is also very high in iron (15.1 mg), manganese (9.10 mg), phosphorus (1,070 mg), tin (5.0 mg), and zinc (0.87 mg). In addition, bilberry contains 15% sugars (glucose, fructose, galactose, and arabinose) (Pedersen, 1994). The leaves contain the flavonoids hyperin and isoquercitrin (Smolarz et al., 2000) and a relatively high amount of chromium (9 ppm) (Wichtl, 1994).

THERAPEUTIC APPLICATIONS

Pharmacological and clinical studies show that bilberry holds promise for the treatment of diverse conditions, mostly due to its beneficial effect on the microcirculatory system.

PRECLINICAL STUDIES

Bilberry is reported to be vasoprotective, antiedemic, antioxidant, anti-inflammatory, antiulcer and astringent (Cristoni and Magistretti, 1987; Magistretti et al., 1988). The anthocyanosides in bilberry, like some other flavonoids, have been shown to increase the contractile energy of the myocardium, stimulate urinary output, induce relaxation of the visceral and vascular smooth musculature, reduce capillary permeability (Bettini et al., 1993), and inhibit the aggregation of platelets (Bottecchia et al., 1987). These anthocyanosides have demonstrated collagen-stabilizing/strengthening activity, which is thought to be due to several interactive mechanisms (Cunio, 1993; Lietti et al., 1976). Anthocyanidins also have antiedemic and arterial vasomotive effects (Cunio, 1993; Lietti et al., 1976; Colantuoni et al., 1991). The efficacy of bilberry has been shown through clinical studies on peripheral vascular disorders, venous disorders, and microcirculatory conditions (Morazzoni et al., 1991).

Cardiovascular and Circulatory Functions

Atherosclerosis

Kadar et al. (1979) studied the effect of anthocyanosides from bilberry on the development of vascular lesions in the brains and aortas of male rabbits which were fed a 1% cholesterol-supplemented diet. Compared to the untreated rabbits on the same high-cholesterol diet, the group that received bilberry anthocyanosides (100 mg/kg i.p. daily for six weeks) showed considerably less extracellular matrix development, considerably thinner intima, a complete absence of calcium deposits, and cells involved in intimal proliferation appeared morphologically much closer to normal in orientation, size, shape, and lipid content in the thoracic aorta. Serum cholesterol levels were unaffected; however, cholesterol contents of thoracic aorta in the untreated high-cholesterol diet group were twice that of the anthocyanoside-treated group on the same diet. In their other findings, vessel wall DNA contents were significantly increased in the untreated group and normal in the anthocyanoside-treated group. Lipid contents of brain microvessels were normal in the treated group versus increased in the untreated group and DNA contents of brain microvessels showed a strong increase in the untreated group versus a strong decrease in the treated group. Brain microvessels of the treated group showed significant decreases in protein and total collagen content, as did aortic wall hexose content, and comparatively more moderate decreases in the treated group (each not significantly different from that of the normal control group).

Cardiotonic; Cardioprotection

Anthocyanosides in bilberry may promote prostacyclin A and endothelium A-derived relaxing factor-release from the coronary artery vessel wall. In support of this hypothesis, the anthocyanosides from bilberry have been shown to increase the methacholine-induced relaxation of isolated coronary arteries (Bettini et al., 1993).

Cerebrovascular Dysfunctions

Increased permeability of the blood-brain barrier (BBB) can result in toxicity when either degradation products from the body or certain drugs pass through. Robert et al. (1977) showed that when male rats were administered anthocyanosides from bilberry (50 mg/kg i.per/day × 5), the collagenase injection-induced increase in BBB permeability was reduced by about 25%, an effect apparently resulting from a protective effect against enzymatic attack on collagen. Similar experiments using dimethyl sulfoxide (DMSO) combined with collagenase and pronase found that the anthocyanoside treatment abolished the effect of DMSO almost completely. It was also shown that recovery of the BBB in the anthocyanoside-treated rats occurred in one-third the time (after 24 h versus 72 h) of the untreated collagenase-injected rats. The increase in hydroxyproline levels following collagenase injection was also inhibited by the anthocyanoside treatment by 28% compared to controls.

Cholesterol and Lipid Metabolism

Clinical and pharmacological studies have suggested the use of bilberry leaf in the treatment of type I diabetes, especially in the vascular complications associated with diabetes. After administration to rats with streptozocin-diabetes placed on a cholesterol-enriched diet, high dosages (1.2 g/kg and 3 g per kg p.o. daily × 4) of a hydroalcoholic extract of the leaves (Indena, Milan, Italy) caused triglyceride levels to decrease by 39%. When compared to a well-established lipid-lowering drug (ciprofibrate), both the extract and the drug were able to lower triglyceride levels in a dose-dependent fashion over the same period of treatment. Bilberry leaf extract was unable to affect the rise in plasma triglycerides induced by fructose, and did not affect free fatty acid levels. When tested on rats treated with triton WR-1339, the results of bilberry leaf extract administration suggested that its cholesterol-lowering action may reflect improved triglyceride-rich lipoprotein catabolism. The authors concluded that bilberry leaf extract may be useful for the treatment of dyslipidosis associated with impaired triglyceride-rich lipoprotein clearance (Cignarella et al., 1996). In spite of these results, chronic administration of bilberry leaf in animals (1.5 g/kg per day) caused toxic symptoms and eventually death (Blumenthal et al., 1998).

Digestive, Hepatic, and Gastrointestinal Functions

Gastric Functions

In rats dosed orally with Myrtocyan VMA, and in later studies with another standardized product (IdB 1027), a significant preventive and curative effect was seen against gastric ulcers in several animal models. Bilberry's anthocyanidins did not affect gastric secretion, but increased gastric mucus (Mertz-Nielsen et al., 1990; Cristoni and Magistretti, 1987; Magistretti et al., 1988).

Endocrine and Hormonal Functions

Carbohydrate Metabolism; Antidiabetic Activity

In an attempt to assess the putative antidiabetic action of bilberry, a hydroalcoholic extract of the leaves was tested on streptozocin-diabetic rats for four days (1.2 g/kg and 3 g per kg p.o.). Plasma glucose levels showed a consistent drop of approximately 26% (Cignarella et al., 1996).

Immune Functions; Inflammation and Disease

Cancer

Chemopreventive activity. In vitro screening of bilberry extract revealed potential anticarcinogenic activity by components of the hexane/chloroform and proanthocyanidin fractions (Bomser et al., 1996). Studies by Madhavi et al. (1998) on the main fractions of bilberry fruits in a hexane extract showed the constituents that were active against the growth of human breast cancer cell lines (BT-20 and MCF-7) were the carotenoids zeaxanthin and lutein, and to a lesser degree, the plant sterol β-sitosterol. Fractions of the fruit extract and the crude extract itself were devoid of quinone reductase (QR)-inducing activity, an enzyme that assists in detoxifying potential carcinogens in the body. However, the hexane-extractable fraction was active and produced a substantial twofold increase in QR activity. The highest concentration tested caused a 3.5-fold increase in QR activity, which was comparable to that reported for extracts of bok choy or broccoli; however, at that concentration the hexane extract showed some cytotoxicity. The main constituents of the hexane extract were shown to be the carotenoids zeaxanthin and lutein, which demonstrated significant QR-inducing activity. β-sitosterol, also found in the hexane extract, was only slightly active. The content of the active QR-inducing fraction of the hexane extract amounted to 4 mg/g dry weight (Madhavi et al., 1998).

Infectious Diseases

Microbial infections. Ofek et al. (1991) reported that of seven commonly ingested fruit juices (blueberry, cranberry, grapefruit, guava, mango, orange, and pineapple), only juices prepared from *Vaccinium* species (blueberry and cranberry) inhibited *Escherichia coli* adhesions which are hairlike pili protruding from the surface of the bacteria which allow the bacteria to adhere to urinary tract walls and other internal organs.

Inflammatory Response

Anthocyanosides have shown in vitro platelet antiaggregatory activity greater than that of acetylsalicylic acid (Zaragoza et al., 1985). An anthocyanoside-rich extract of bilberry (Inverni della Beffa S.p.A., Milan, Italy, (MyrtocyanVMA, 25% anthocyanosides) inhibited platelet aggregation induced by ADP (adenosine 5'-diphosphate), collagen, PAF (platelet activating factor), or arachidonic acid (Bottecchia et al., 1987).

In an ex vivo study, 30 clinically healthy volunteers of either sex averaging 45 years of age were divided into three groups and treated for 30 and 60 days with either a bilberry extract alone (Myrtocyan, 160 mg p.o. 3 ×/day) alone, the extract plus 1,000 mg ascorbic acid p.o. 3 ×/day, or ascorbic acid alone. For eight weeks before the start of treatment, patients had abstained from ingesting corticoids, NSAIDs, and acetylsalicylic acid, although there were no restrictions on diet. Blood samples collected after each treatment period and 120 days after the treatments were discontinued were tested for antiaggregatory changes against adenosine 5'-diphosphate (ADP) and collagen-induced aggregation. In the group that received the bilberry extract alone, ADP-induced platelet aggregation was inhibited after 30 and 60 days of treatment and more so in those taking the additional ascorbic acid, whereas ascorbic acid alone was less inhibitory than either of the other treatments. In all the groups, platelet aggregation had returned to baseline 120 days after discontinuation of the treatments. The results from the collagen-induced aggregation tests were virtually the same. The researchers hypothesized that like other flavonoids, the antiaggregatory action of the anthocyanosides from bilberry depends on an increase in cyclic adenosine monophosphate (AMP) and/or a decrease in platelet thromboxane A_2 (Pulliero et al., 1989).

Integumentary, Muscular, and Skeletal Functions

Connective Tissue Functions

The capillaries of rats administered an extract of bilberry containing 25% anthocyanosides (5 mg intradermally) were studied using a foreign body granuloma test (cotton pellet method). The results showed that the anthocyanosides provided a protective effect on the capillary walls by stabilizing membrane phospholipids and by increasing connective tissue biosynthesis (Mian et al., 1977).

Studies on the effects of *V. myrtillus* anthocyanosides (VMA) on smooth muscle have found the relaxant effect of VMAs not to be associated with β-adrenergic mediation, but rather with metabolic functions involving the release of vasodilating prostaglandins (Bettini et al., 1984).

An anthocyanoside-rich extract of *V. myrtillus* berries (Myrtocyan) consisting of a 36% anthocyanoside complex was studied on microvascular permeability in a hamster cheek pouch model of ischemia reperfusion injury. After four weeks of administration (100 mg/kg, p.o.), researchers found a significant reduction in microvascular impairment, preservation of arteriolar tone, a decreased number of leukocytes adhering to venular walls, preservation of capillary perfusion, and a significant increase in microvascular permeability. The researchers noted a statistically significant difference in improvements in hamsters treated with the extract for four weeks versus the lesser degree of improvements found after four weeks ($p < 0.05$). Anthocyanosides of the berries may modulate arteriole microvascular tone and serve an important role in therapy designed to improve capillary perfusion. Inhibition of vasoconstriction caused by oxygen-derived free radicals was significantly lessened by oral administration of the berry anthocyanosides, indicating that the extract may serve to help preserve free radical scavenger mechanisms (Bertuglia et al., 1995).

Working from the premise that increased vascular permeability is a feature of hypertension, Detre et al. (1986) administered bilberry anthocyanosides (MercK-Sharp and Dohme-Chibret, Paris, dry, flavonoid-rich extract of *V. myrtillus*) to male rats at a dosage of 500 mg/kg by stomach tube for 12 days prior to inducing experimental hypertension by ligation. Results were compared using two groups of controls: normotensive rats and hypertensive rats (experimental renovascular hypertension). As indicated by tryptan blue staining, there was greater clearance of the dye in tissues of rats pretreated with the extract compared to untreated controls. Compared to untreated normotensive rats, the same rate of clearance was achieved in the bilberry anthocyanoside-pretreated rats. Similarly, the blood-brain barrier permeability of the pretreated ligation-induced hypertensive rats was decreased compared to the untreated hypertensive control group. After one week, the permeability index of the pretreated group was close to that of normotensive rats. In the hypertensive control rats (renovascular hypertensives) treated with the bilberry extract, blood-brain barrier permeability reached the same level as that of nonoperated, normotensive controls seven days after the operation. Edema resulting from increased water content in the brains of the hypertensive control (ligation-induced) rats was also inhibited by the bilberry extract pretreatment. Aortic wall permeability showed a strong eightfold increase in the untreated hypertensive control group by day 7. In a separate experiment, the normotensive rats pretreated with the extract showed a 40 percent inhibition of the permeability index compared to untreated normotensive rats. In another study, the skin capillary permeability index reached six times the normal level and fell to twice normal at day 14 in untreated (ligation-induced) hypertensive rats, whereas the increase was inhibited by 20% in the hypertensive rats pretreated with the extract. The greatest benefit from the bilberry extract was seen in cerebral vessels of the ligation-induced hypertensive rats. The pretreatment caused a complete normalization of the otherwise increased permeability index.

Elastase is an enzyme involved in vascular disorders. It contributes to the deterioration of elastic fibers and conjunctive tissue as is seen in atherosclerosis. In a study by Jonadet et al. (1983), the in vitro noncompetitive inhibition of elastase required less grape seed anthocyanidin than anthocyanidin derived from either bilberry or pine bark (50% inhibiting doses, 13 mg/mL, 0.20 mg per mL, and 0.31 mg/mL, respectively). The same order of potency was demonstrated in capilllary permeability-reducing (angioprotective) activity in rats with dosages of 50 mg/kg to 200 mg per kg i.p. (Jonadet et al., 1983).

Metabolic and Nutritional Disorders

Antioxidant Activity

In mice, the antioxidant activity of an anthocyanoside-rich extract of bilberry fruits (Sima Tau, Alcalá de Henares, Madrid, Spain) as a pretreatment before the induction of liver lipid peroxidation was significant at doses of 250 and 500 mg/kg p.o., but not at 100 mg/kg. Vitamin E was significantly effective at a dose of 25 mg/kg p.o., reducing the malondialdehyde content of the liver as much as 500 mg/kg of the bilberry extract (Martín-Aragón et al., 1999).

Pharmacokinetics

Morazzoni et al. (1991) reported that after i.v. administration of *V. myrtillus* anthocyanosides in the male rat, a rapid body distribution was followed by disappearance in the blood through a three-compartment pharmacokinetic model. The urine and bile were mostly responsible for their elimination, with an approximate 5% absorption. After one oral dose, the plasma concentrations of the anthocyanosides reached a peak level after 15 min., and then declined over a period of about 2 h. No hepatic first pass metabolism was observed, and the plasma peak levels (2-3 µg/mL) after oral treatment were in the range of biological activity reported for anthocyanosides (Morazzoni et al., 1991). Intravenous and intraperitoneal route administration of bilberry anthocyanins in the rat were investigated by Lietti and Forni

(1976) who found a greater affinity for these compounds in the skin and kidney compared to the plasma.

Neurological, Psychological, and Behavioral Functions

Neurodegenerative Disorders

Retinopathies. The increased sensitivity of the retina to light with bilberry administration was first suggested in 1964 by French scientists (Morazzoni and Bombardelli, 1996). The anthocyanosides in bilberries are known to have capillary-strengthening and capillary-permeability properties, and their activity in the retina is believed to be due to three main activities: (1) increasing the sensitivity of the retina to light; (2) increasing the rate of blood flow in the microcirculatory system; and (3) interference with prostaglandin synthesis (Vannini et al., 1986). In comparative studies using retinograms, Wegmann et al. (1969) determined that various different enzyme systems in the outer and inner segments and pigment layer were affected by anthocyanosides in vitro and in vivo in rabbit retinae exposed to light and dark.

CLINICAL STUDIES

Digestive, Hepatic, and Gastrointestinal Disorders

Gastric Disorders

Dyspepsia. In an observatory study, Tolan et al. (1969) administered concentrated bilberry powder (2.5:1 to 5:1) to infants with acute dyspepsia. The results were reported as so favorable and the preparation so well-tolerated that the researchers suggested large-scale use of commercially prepared bilberry powder for acute infantile dyspepsia. The beneficial effects were attributed to pectin, vitamin A, invertose, and acidic substances. However, since this time, no placebo-controlled studies of bilberry in the treatment of dyspepsia have been conducted.

Neurological, Psychological, and Behavioral Functions

Retinopathies. In a randomized, double-blind, placebo-controlled trial, Bravetti et al. (1987) administered vitamin E (dl-tocopherol, 100 mg) plus bilberry extract (180 mg, 25% anthocyanosides) combined in tablets taken twice daily for four months to 50 outpatients of both sexes (ages 48-81) diagnosed with mild senile cortical cataract. The combination of vitamin E and bilberry anthocyanosides stopped lens opacity in 97% of the eyes examined without causing adverse effects or drug reactions.

Perossini et al. (1987) reported benefits from bilberry extract (Tegens, 160 mg twice daily) in the treatment of vascular retinopathy in 40 outpatients diagnosed with diabetes and/or hypertension. The one-month, double-blind, placebo-controlled crossover study found that patients improved by 77% to 90%. No adverse reactions or side effects from bilberry were evident. The researchers concluded that the bilberry extract appeared to be a safe and effective therapy for hypertensive or diabetic retinopathy.

Sala et al. (1979) conducted a placebo-controlled study of a bilberry anthocyanoside preparation (300 mg/day) in the treatment of 46 subjects in normal health and found significant results in adaptive ability to light and dark, macular recuperation time, and chromatic discrimination compared to placebo. In another placebo-controlled trial, Jayle and Aubert (1964) administered an anthocyanoside-rich extract of bilberry (C 116) to 37 normal subjects (8 men and 29 women, average age 32), half of whom received an identical-appearing placebo. After testing the subjects for darkness adaptation, when compared to the placebo group, significant improvement in the bilberry group was seen in the following tests: visual field with high mesopic lighting; macular sensitivity to low mesopic lighting; and "adapto-cinematographic thresholds" (a psychosensory test). These effects were noticeable even during the first 4 h after administration. The benefits lasted 24 h. No signs of adverse effects were noted.

Recent, randomized, double-blind, placebo-controlled trials on the benefits of bilberry preparations on night vision have all reported a lack of any significant benefits. Dosages ranged from single oral doses of 12, 24, and 36 mg/day in an acute dosage study (Levy and Glovinsky, 1998) to 24 or 48 mg of anthocyanosides/day for four days, also with a concentrated European bilberry extract with 2 mg β-carotene/12 mg anthocyanosides (Strix tablets, Halsoprodukter, Forserum, Sweden) (Zadok et al., 1999), to 420 mg/day for 21 days using a bilberry extract standardized to contain 25% anthocyanosides (Muth et al., 2000). All these trials were conduced in healthy males with good vision who ranged in age from 21 to 47 years.

A number of clinical studies during the 1960s sought to confirm the reported beneficial effects of bilberry on vision following studies on British Royal Air Force pilots of World War II who noted improved night vision (Jünemann, 1967; Belleoud et al., 1966; Gloria and Perla, 1966; Jayle and Aubert, 1964). One of these was Belleoud et al. (1966), who conducted an open study on the effect of long-term administration of Difrarel 100 (100 mg anthocyanosides) on the night vision of 14 air traffic controllers from a French military base. All of the subjects were tested before administration of Difrarel 100 and were given four tablets/day for eight consecutive days. They were each tested the day after the last dose, again at 15 days, and one month after the last dose. The vision test consisted of dazzling the subjects with a white lamp to impair visual purple and then administering a reading test which was conducted in darkness with a screen distance of 75 cm. The use of Difrarel 100 lowered the night vision threshold in all subjects, and was found particularly effective in those diagnosed with poor night vision at the start of the treatment. Overall, improvement in night vision leveled off in all the subjects, so that those with poor night vision attained the levels of those with good sight. Among the results were (1) a decreased effect of dazzle; (2) decreased visual fatigue; and (3) in some subjects, a quicker adaptation of scotopic vision. Belleoud et al. (1966) concluded that the anthocyanoside-rich extract of bilberry was a fast and effective means to promote night vision for specialized personnel in the Air Force, although the data had not been replicated in a controlled study.

DOSAGE

The German Commission E gives the dosage for the dried, ripe fruit in the treatment of nonspecific, acute diarrhea as 20-60 g/day. For external applications in the treatment of mild inflammations of the mucous membranes of the mouth and throat, a 10% decoction or equivalent preparations have been used (Blumenthal et al., 1998). See Clinical Studies for dosages of bilberry extracts.

SAFETY PROFILE

Contraindications

The German Commission E states that there are no known contraindications for the dried, ripe fruit (Blumenthal et al., 1998).

High doses of bilberry are cautioned against in patients taking warfarin or antiplatelet drugs (Bone and Morgan, 1997). In an ex vivo study, volunteers taking an extract of bilberry standardized to contain a mixture of anthocyanosides (Myrtocyan) at a dosage of 480 mg/day for 30 and 60 days showed inhibited blood platelet aggregation which returned to baseline 120 days after discontinuation of the extract (Pulliero et al., 1989).

Drug Interactions

The platelet antiaggregatory activity of bilberry extract is potentiated by high doses of ascorbic acid (1,000 mg 3 ×/day) (Pulliero et al., 1989). See also Contraindications.

Pregnancy and Lactation

Bilberry has been used by pregnant women with no ill effects noted to either the mother or infant (Cunio, 1993). It is thought to be safe for use during pregnancy, and is prescribed for gestational hemorrhoids. The researchers concluded that the treatment was effective and safe for hemorrhoids and venous insufficiency in pregnancy in two or three divided doses of 160 to 240 to 340 mg according to the intensity of the clinical condition (Teglio et al., 1987).

Use of bilberry fruit in appropriate doses during lactation is not known to cause adverse effects in mother or infant. No contraindication for lactation is noted in the German Commission E monograph for doses of the fruit up to 60 grams/day (Blumenthal et al., 1998). Bilberry fruit is commonly consumed as a food in Europe.

Side Effects

The German Commission E states that side effects from the dried, ripe fruits of bilberry are unknown (Blumenthal et al., 1998). In the case of bilberry leaf, the *American Herbal Products Association's Botanical Safety Handbook* (McGuffin et al., 1997) gives it a class 4 rating, meaning that it is an herb for which insufficient data are available for safety classification.

Special Precautions

Generally, precautions with bilberry use are few, and mostly related to very high doses or poor quality supplements. The German Commission E monograph on bilberry leaf (rather than the fruit) states that chronic intoxication may accrue from prolonged use or higher dosage (Blumenthal et al., 1998).

The ascorbic acid content of bilberry varies depending on the source. *Vaccinium* grown in the forests of Poland was found to contain very high amounts of aluminum due to aluminum smelter contamination. Also, residues of the herbicides 2,4,D, and 2,4,5,T, as well as 4-chlor-2-methyl-phenoxyacetic acid have been detected in some products. *V. myrtillus* is known for its ability to adapt to polluted environments (Cunio, 1993).

Toxicology

Mutagenicity

No mutagenic or teratogenic effects were found (Cunio, 1993).

Toxicity in Animal Models

A standardized bilberry extract (36% anthocyanins) showed low acute toxicity with an oral LD_{50} equivalent to 720 mg/kg anthocyanins in rats and mice. The i.p. and i.v. LD_{50} in rats was found to be 2.35-4.11 g/kg and 0.24-0.85 g/kg, respectively. Long-term studies found no toxic effects with oral administration of the equivalent of up to 180 mg/kg anthocyanins per day for six months. No mutagenic or teratogenic effects were found (Bone and Morgan, 1997; Cunio, 1993).

REFERENCES

Baj, A., Bombardelli, E., Gabetta, B., and Martinelli, E.M. (1983). Qualitative and quantitative evaluation of *Vaccinium myrtillus* anthocyanins by high-resolution gas chromatography and high-performance liquid chromatography. *Journal of Chromatography* 279: 365-372.

Belleoud, L., Leluan, D., and Boyer, Y. (1966). [Study on the effects of anthocyanin glucosides on the nocturnal vision of air traffic controllers]. *Revue de Medecine Aeronautique et Spatiale* 3: 45.

Bertuglia, S., Malandrino, S., and Colantuoni, A. (1995). Effect of *Vaccinium myrtillus* anthocyanosides on ischemia reperfusion injury in hamster cheek pouch microcirculation. *Pharmacological Research* 31: 183-187.

Bettini, V., Aragno, R., Bettini, M.B., Braggion, G., Calore, L., Morimando, I., Penada, G., and Sabbion, P. (1993). Facilitating influence of *Vaccinium myrtillus* anthocyanosides on the acetylcholine-induced relaxation of isolated coronary arteries: Role of the endothelium-derived relaxing factor. *Fitoterapia* 64: 45-57.

Bettini, V., Mayellaro, F., and Zanella, P. (1984). Effects of *Vaccinium myrtillus* anthocyanosides on vascular smooth muscle. *Fitoterapia* 55: 265-272.

Blumenthal, M., Busse, W.R., Goldberg, A., Gruenwald, J., Hall, T., Riggins, C.W., and Rister, R.S. (Eds.) (1998). *The Complete German Commission E Monographs*. Austin, TX: American Botanical Council, pp. 88 and 311.

Bomser, J., Madhavi, D.L., Singletary, K., and Smith, M.A.L. (1996). In vitro anticancer activity of fruit extracts from *Vaccinium* species. *Planta Medica* 62: 212-216.

Bone, K. and Morgan, M. (1997). Bilberry—The vision herb. *Medi-Herb Professional Review* 59 (August): 1-4.

Bottecchia, D., Bettini, V., Martino, R., and Camerra, G. (1987). Preliminary report on the inhibitory effect of *Vaccinium myrtillus* anthocyanosides on platelet aggregation and clot reaction. *Fitoterapia* 58: 3-8.

Bravetti, G.O., Fraboni, E., and Maccolini, E. (1987). Valutazione clinica dell'associazione vitamina E-antocianosidi del mirtillo nel trattamento medico preventivo della cataratta senile [Preventive medical treatment of senile cataract with vitamin E and *Vaccinium myrtillus* anthocyanosides: Clinical evaluation]. *Annali di Ottalmologia e Clinica Oculistica* 115: 109-116.

Cignarella, A., Nastasi, M., Cavalli, E., and Puglisi, L. (1996). Novel lipid-lowering properties of *Vaccinium myrtillus* L. leaves, a traditional antidiabetic treatment, in several models of rat dyslipidaemia: A comparison with ciprofibrate. *Thrombosis Research* 84: 311-322.

Colantuoni, A., Bertuglia, S., Magistretti, M.J., and Donato, L. (1991). Effects of *Vaccinium myrtillus* on arterial vaso-motion. *Arzneimittel-Forschung/Drug Research* 41: 905-909.

Cristoni, A. and Magistretti, M.J. (1987). Anti-ulcer and healing activity of *Vaccinium myrtillus* anthocyanosides. *Il Farmaco* 42: 29-43.

Cunio, L. (1993). *Vaccinium myrtillus. Australian Journal of Medical Herbalism* 5: 81-85.

Detre, Z., Jellinek, H., Miskulin, M., and Robert, M. (1986). Studies on vascular permeability in hypertension: Action of anthocyanosides. *Clinical Physiology and Biochemistry* 4: 143-149.

Gloria, E. and Perla, A. (1966). Effetto degli antocianosidi sulla soglia visiva assoluta [Effect of anthocyanosides on the absolute visual threshold]. *Annali di Ottalmologia e Clinica Oculistica* 92: 595-607.

Jayle, G.E. and Aubert, L. (1964). Action des glucosides d'anthocyanes sur la vision scotopique et mésopique du sujet normal [Action of anthocyanin glucosides on scotopic and mesopic vision in normal subjects]. *Thérapie* 19: 171-185.

Jonadet, M., Meunier, M.T., and Bastide, P. (1983). Anthocyanosides extraits de *Vitis vinifera,* de *Vaccinium myrtillus* et de *Pinus maritimus.* I. Activités inhibitrices vis-à-vis de l'élastase in vitro. II. Activités angioprotectrices comparées in vivo [Anthocyanosides extracted from *Vitis vinifera, Vaccinium myrtillus* and *Pinus maritimus.* I. Elastase-inhibiting activities in vitro. II. Compared angioprotective activities in vivo]. *Journal de Pharmacie Belgique* 38: 41-46.

Jünemann, G. (1967). Über die wirkung der anthozyanoside auf die hemeralopie nach chininintoxikation [About the effect of the anthocyanosides on hermeralopia after quinine intoxication]. *Klinische Monatsblatter für Augenheilkunde* 151: 891-896.

Kadar, A., Robert, L., Miskulin, M., Tixier, J.M., Brechemier, D., and Robert, A.M. (1979). Influence of anthocyanosides treatment on the cholesterol-induced atherosclerosis in the rabbit. *Paroi Artérielle/Arterial Wall* 5: 187-206.

Levy, Y. and Glovinsky, Y. (1998). The effect of anthocyanosides on night vision. *Eye* 12: 967-969.

Lietti, A., Cristoni, A., and Picci, M. (1976). Studies on *Vaccinium myrtillus* anthocyanosides. *Arzneimittel-Forschung/Drug Research* 26: 829-832.

Lietti, A. and Forni, G. (1976). Studies on *Vaccinium myrtillus* anthocyanosides. II. Aspects of anthocyanins pharmacokinetics in the rat. *Arzneimittel-Forschung/Drug Research* 26: 832-835.

Madhavi, D.L., Bomser, J., Smith, M.A.L., and Singletary, K. (1998). Isolation of bioactive constituents from *Vaccinium myrtillus* (bilberry) fruits and cell cultures. *Plant Science* 131: 95-103.

Magistretti, M.J., Conti, M., and Cristoni, A. (1988). Anti-ulcer activity of an anthocyanidin from *Vaccinium myrtillus*. *Arzneimittel-Forschung/Drug Research* 38: 686-690.

Martín-Aragón, S., Basabe, B., Benedi, J.M., and Villar, A.M. (1999). In vitro and in vivo antioxidant properties of *Vaccinium myrtillus*. *Pharmaceutical Biology* 37: 109-113.

McGuffin, M., Hobbs, C., Upton, R., and Goldberg, A. (1997). *American Herbal Products Association's Botanical Safety Handbook.* Boca Raton, FL: CRC Press, p. 119.

Mertz-Nielsen, A., Munck, L.K., Bukave, K., and Rask-Madsen, J. (1990). A natural flavonoid, IdB 1027, increases gastric luminal release of prostaglandin E_2 in healthy subjects. *Italian Journal of Gastroenterology* 22: 288-290.

Mian, E., Curri, S.B., Lietti, A., and Bombardelli, E. (1977). Antocianosidi e parete dei microvasi nuovi aspetti sul modo d'azione dell'effetto protettivo nelle sindromi da abnorme fragilità capillare [Anthocyanosides and microvessels wall: New findings on the mechanism of action of their protective effect in syndromes due to abnormal capillary fragility]. *Minerva Medica* 68: 3565-3581.

Morazzoni, P. and Bombardelli, E. (1996). *Vaccinium myrtillus* L. *Fitoterapia* 69: 3-29.

Morazzoni, P., Livio, S., Scilingo, A., and Malandrino, S. (1991). *Vaccinium myrtillus* anthocyanosides pharmacokinetics in rats. *Arzneimittel-Forschung/Drug Research* 41: 128-131.

Murray, M. (1997). Bilberry *(Vaccinium myrtillus). American Journal of Natural Medicine* 4: 18-22.

Muth, E.R., Laurent, J.M., and Jasper, P. (2000). The effect of bilberry nutritional supplementation on night visual acuity and contrast sensitivity. *Alternative Medicine Review* 5: 164-173.

Ofek, I., Goldhar, J., Zafriri, D., Lis, H., Adar, R., and Sharon, N. (1991). Anti-*Escherichia coli* adhesin activity of cranberry and blueberry juices. *New England Journal of Medicine* 324 (May 30): 1599 (letter).

Pedersen, M. (1994). *Nutritional Herbology: A Reference Guide to Herbs.* Warsaw, IN: Wendell W. Whitman Company.

Perossini, M., Guidi, G., Chiellini, S., and Siravo, D. (1987). Studio clinico sull'impiego degli antocianosidi del mirtillo (Tegens) nel trattamento delle microangiopatie retiniche di tipo diabetico ed ipertensivo [Diabetic and hypertensive retinopathy therapy with *Vaccinium myrtillus* anthocyanosides (Tegens): Double-blind, placebo-controlled clinical trial]. *Annali di Ottalmologia e Clinica Oculistica* 113: 1173-1190.

Pulliero, G., Montin, S., Bettini, V., Martino, R., Mogno, C., and Lo Castro, G. (1989). *Ex vivo* study of the inhibitory effects of *Vaccinium myrtillus* anthocyanosides on human platelet aggregation. *Fitoterapia* 60: 69-74.

Robert, A.M., Godeau, G., Moati, F., and Miskulin, M. (1977). Action of antho-cyanosides of *Vaccinium myrtillus* on the permeability of the blood-brain barrier. *Journal of Medicine* 8: 321-332.

Sala, D., Rolando, M., Rossi, P.L., and Pissarello, L. (1979). Effetto degli antocianosdi sulle "performances" visive alle basse luminanze [Effect of anthocyanosides on visual performances at low lumination]. *Minerva Oftalmologica* 21: 283-285.

Smolarz, H.D., Matysik, G., and Wojciak-Kosior, M. (2000). High-performance thin-layer chromatographic and densitometric determination of flavonoids in *Vaccinium myrtillus* L. and *Vaccinium vitis-idaea* L. *Journal of Planar Chromatography: Modern TLC* 13: 101-105.

Teglio, L., Mazzanti, C., Tronconi, R., and Guerresi, E. (1987). Impiego degli antocianosidi del mirtillo (Tegens) nella terapia della insufficienza venosa e nella sindrome emorroidaria in gravidanza [*Vaccinium myrtillus* anthocyanosides (Tegens) in the treatment of venous insufficiency of the lower limbs and acute hemorrhoids in pregnancy]. *Quaderni di Clinica Ostetrica e Ginecologica* 42: 221-231.

Tolan, L., Barna, V., Szigeti, I., Tecsa, D., Gavris, C., Csernatony, O., and Buchwald, I. (1969). Utilizarea prafului de afine in dispepsiile sugarului [Use of bilberry powder in infantile dyspepsia]. *Pediatria* 18: 375-379.

Vannini, L., Samuelly, R., Coffano, M., and Tibaldi, L. (1986). Study of the pupillary reflex after anthocyanoside administration. *Bollettino di Oculistica* 65(Suppl. 6): 11-12.

Wegmann, R., Maeda, K., Tronche, P., and Bastide, P. (1969). Effets des antho-cyanosides sur les photoréceptoeurs. Aspects cytoenzymologiques [Effects of anthocyanosides on photoreceptors. Cytoenzymatic aspects]. *Annales d'Histochemie* 14: 237-256.

Werbach, M.R. and Murray, M.T. (1994). *Botanical Influences on Illness*. Tarzana, CA: Third Line Press, pp. 14-15.

Wichtl, M. (1994). *Herbal Drugs and Phytopharmaceuticals*. Boca Raton, FL: Medpharm Scientific/CRC Press.

Zadok, D., Levy, Y., and Glovinsky, Y. (1999). The effect of anthocyanosides in a multiple oral dose on night vision. *Eye* 13: 734-736.

Zaragoza, F., Iglesias, I., and Benedi, J. (1985). Estudio comparativo de los efectos antiagregantes de los antocianósidos y otros agentes [Comparsion of thrombocyte antiaggregant effects of anthocyanosides with those of other agents]. *Archives of Pharmacology and Toxicology* 11: 183-188.

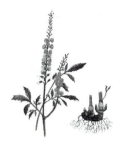

Black Cohosh

BOTANICAL DATA

Classification and Nomenclature

Scientific name: *Actaea racemosa* L.*; synonyms: *A. monogyna* Walt, *Cimicifuga racemosa* (L.) Nutt.; *C. sepentaria* Pursh, *Macrotys actaeoides* Rafin., *Botrophis serpentaria* Rafin., *B. actaeoides* Fisch. & C.A. Mey

Family name: Ranunculaceae

Common names: black cohosh, black snakeroot, squaw root, rattleroot, rattleweed, rattle top, bugbane, cimicifuga (United States and Canada), frauenwurzel, Amerikanisches wanzenkraut (Germany), actée à grappes (France)

Description

Following its first description by Leonard Plukenet in 1696, Carl Linnaeus first classified black cohosh as *Actaea racemosa*. It was later reclassified by Pursh as *Cimicifuga* after a temporary placement in the genus *Macrotys* (Foster, 1999). Recently, however, the genus *Cimicifuga* was changed back to *Actaea* following extensive DNA sequence mapping and morphological studies (Compton et al., 1998). Accordingly, in this book, we revert to *Actaea racemosa.*

The genus *Actaea* comprises 15 species of erect perennial plants of northern temperate distribution. *Actaea racemosa,* commonly called black cohosh, is native to eastern North America. Black cohosh, familiar to herb-

---

*Actaea racemosa (black cohosh) should not be confused with *Caulophyllum thalictroides* (L.) Michaux (Berberidaceae) (blue cohosh), an entirely different plant.

alists and gardeners, is a wildflower of moist or dry woods cultivated as an ornamental. It is typically found in shady, rich soil in woods from Maine to Ontario and Wisconsin and south to Georgia. The hardy perennial produces clumps of quadrangular stems up to 3 m tall. The cylindrical rhizomes (1-2.5 cm thick and 2-15 cm long) appear knotted and show deep radiating scars. Thin roots extend from their sides. Black cohosh has large, alternate, three-pinnately compound leaves with toothed edges, the middle lobe being the largest. The terminal leaflet is three-lobed. The flowers are petalless with greenish-white sepals borne in tall racemes well above the foliage. Blooming from June through September, the flowers are thought to be pollinated by flesh flies (Strauch, 1995; Leung and Foster, 1996; Snow, 1996).

The previous generic name, *Cimicifuga,* is from the Latin *cimex,* (a kind of insect), and *fuga,* (to put to flight.) The English equivalent is "bugbane" and refers to the belief that the plant's strong odor repels insects. In Europe and Siberia, pillows and mattresses were formerly stuffed with the dried tops of the Eurasian species *(Actaea foetida)* for this purpose. "Racemosa" refers to the arrangement of individual flowers on an elongated stalk. "Cohosh" comes from an Algonquian word meaning "rough" and refers to the plant's lumpy, blackish rhizomes. The common name, "rattleweed," refers to the sound made by the dry seeds when shaken in their pods atop the flower stalks (Strauch, 1995).

HISTORY AND TRADITIONAL USES

Native Americans used the rhizomes for general malaise, kidney ailments, malaria, rheumatism, sore throat, and, notably, to relieve menstrual cramps and to ease labor. *Actaea racemosa* was traditionally used by the Cherokee and Iroquois nations for general malaise, gynecopathy (diseases particular to women), kidney ailments, malaria, rheumatism, and sore throat. *Actaea racemosa* was used by American colonists for amenorrhea, bronchitis, chorea, dropsy, fever, hysteria, itch, lumbago, malaria, nervous disorders, snakebite, uterine disorders, and yellow fever (Duke, 1985). The Cherokee also used black cohosh to "stimulate menstruation" and used an infusion to treat colds, coughs, constipation, and fatigue. The plant was also used to "make babies sleep." An infusion of the root in alcohol for internal use against rheumatic pains was used by the Cherokee and the Iroquois prepared a decoction of the plant or root for use in steam baths and as a soak for treating rheumatism. Iroquois women used an infusion of the roots as a galactagogue, and both the Micmac and Penobscot tribes used the roots to treat kidney ailments (Moerman, 1998).

The rhizome of black cohosh is considered by herbalists to be alterative, antispasmodic, antidotal to snakebite, astringent, antitussive, expectorant, aphrodisiac, diaphoretic, stomachic, diuretic, emmenagogue, narcotic, nervine, sedative, and tonic (Duke, 1985). Black cohosh was an ingredient of Lydia Pinkham's Vegetable Compound, a patent remedy sold for "female complaints" which was very popular in the earlier part of the twentieth century (Riddle, 1997). Black cohosh was proposed as a specific antidote to rattlesnake bite and St. Vitus' dance (chorea) and has also been prescribed for various infantile disorders, including diarrhea, whooping cough, and paroxysmal (suddenly recurring or intensifying) cough. It has also been used as a homeopathic preparation for "stimulating the female system" (e.g., amenorrhea, dysmenorrhea, menorrhagia, difficulties of menopause), rheumatism and arthritic complaints, and in parturition (Duke, 1985). It should be noted that these uses are anecdotal in nature, and are based on the experiences of herbalists and not from clinical studies.

Black cohosh was an official herb in the *United States Pharmacopoeia* from 1820 to 1920 (Boyle, 1991). Proprietary herbal formulations containing black cohosh are currently listed in Europe, South Africa, and Australia for the treatment of premenstrual, menopausal, and postmenopausal symptoms, nervous irritability, fluid retention, cough, respiratory tract disorders, muscular pain, and pain and inflammation (Reynolds et al., 1996).

Current detailed descriptions of the use of black cohosh in obstetrics draw from the medical practices of the Eclectics. Black cohosh came into general use around 1850 in the United States, becoming one of the most popular remedies, and was given a prominent place in the American *Eclectic Dispensatory* published in 1854. It was used specifically for rheumatoid muscular pains, menstrual pain, neuralgic pain, headache, and inflammation. The resinous concentrate was highly regarded for the treatment of amenorrhea as well as other female "disorders," as an aid to appetite, and as a sedative. A tincture made from the fresh rhizomes was considered useful before, during, and after labor, and was commonly given in small doses (Ellingwood, 1983) during the last four weeks of pregnancy as a *partus* preparator. Black cohosh was believed to reduce irritability of the uterus or false labor. The Eclectics wrote of its specific use in multiparas with histories of difficult labors, and in cases in which the uterus was lax. A report written in 1885 on 160 childbirths stated that the tincture was mildly sedating, reduced discomforts in the first stage of labor, increased rhythmicity of contractions in the second stage, but specifically relaxed the cervical tissues, thus reducing lacerations (Brinker, 1996).

The rhizomes of several Eurasian species of *Actaea* [*A. heracleifolia* Kom., *A. dahurica* (Turcz.) Maxim., or *A. foetida* L.], all known as *shengma* in China, are officially used in traditional Chinese medicine as analgesic (for headache and sore throat), anti-inflammatory (for mouth ulcers), and pyretic (fever-inducing) agents (Tu et al., 1992). They are used officially in China to treat prolapsed uterus or rectum as a consequence of chronic diarrhea, measles in cases of insufficient eruptions, other febrile diseases accompanied with eruptions, gingivitis, aching gums (Tu et al., 1992; Zhu, 1998), and to "cure" drooping and ptosis (Tu et al., 1992), presumably referring to drooping of the upper eyelid. Other principle indications for *shengma* in TCM include vaginal discharge, uterine bleeding, chronic diarrhea, and maculopapular eruption (Yen, 1992). Curiously, the American species, *A. racemosa,* is an ingredient of *Qingwei San* (Stomach Heat Clearing Powder), a multicomponent herbal preparation used for gum swelling and erosion, and acute periodontal and pharyngeal diseases. *Shengma* species, *A. dahurica* rhizome tincture, and cimifugin are all reported to have sedative effects (Chang and But, 1986). The rhizomes of *shengma* species are reported to often cause vomiting, a side effect attributed to gastric irritation (Zhu, 1998).

CHEMISTRY

Phenolic Compounds

Flavonoids

Formononetin, an estrogenic isoflavone isolated from black cohosh by Jarry et al. (1985) has failed to show up in more recent analyses of commercial black cohosh extract products prepared from dried rhizome, although other flavonoids (undisclosed) were present (Struck et al., 1997). A survey of 13 rhizomes collected in various eastern states in the United States also failed to find formononetin (Kennelly et al., 2001). The isoflavone biochanin was identified in alcohol preparations of black cohosh (McCoy and Kelly, 1996); however, Hagels et al. (2000) reported the absence of flavonoids in extracts of the rhizome, although kaempferol glycosides were present in the leaves and flowers. They also identified large amounts of petasiphenol and cimiciphenol (3,4-dihydroxyphenyl-2-oxopropyl esters) in rhizomes harvested late in the summer, which were only found in minor amounts in the autumn (Hagels et al., 2000).

Organic Acids

Salicylic acid occurs in black cohosh (Jarry, et al., 1985). (Note: low concentrations of salicylates are widely distributed in many plants. The small amounts in black cohosh are unlikely to cause any allergic reaction in individuals sensitive to acetylsalicylic acid.) From the dried rhizome, Kruse et al. (1999) isolated hydroxycinnamic acid esters of fukiic and piscidic acids, along with fukinolic and cimicifugic acids A, B, E, and F, ferulic, isoferulic, and caffeic acids.

Terpenoid Compounds

Black cohosh principally contains the following xylosides: actein (aglycone: acetylacteol), cimicifugoside (cimigoside) (aglycone: cimigenol) (He et al., 2000; Zheng et al., 1999), cimicifugoside M (He et al., 2000), cimiracemoside A, and others (Bedir and Khan, 2000, 2001). The xylosides 27-deoxyactein and 27-deoxyacetylacteol (He et al., 2000; Zheng et al., 1999) were recently found to instead be 26-deoxyactein and 26-deoxyacetylacteol (Awang, 2001). The rhizome also contains the cycloartane triterpene glycoside actaeaepoxide 3-*O*-β-D-xylopyranoside and cimigenol 3-*O*-β-D-xylopyranoside which is also found in Asian species of *Cimicifuga* (Wende et al., 2001).

Bedir and Khan (2000) identified cimiracemoside A as a new cyclolanostanol xyloside (triterpene glycoside) from the powdered rhizome. From a standardized extract of black cohosh (Finzelberg GmbH and Co. Ltd., Andernach, Germany), Shao et al. (2000) identified cimiracemosides A to H (arabinosides and xylosides), and acetylshengmanol xyloside. However, their description of cimiracemoside A is different from that of Bedir and Khan (2000), which is identical to cimiracemoside F (Shao et al., 2000; Awang, 2001). In addition, the recently identified cimiracemoside B of Bedir and Kahn (2001) is not the same as that described as cimiracemoside B by Shao et al. (2000) and is different from any others described. The chemical makeup of black cohosh is not completely known; however, the triterpene glycosides are considered the main active constituents (Liske, 1998) (see Figure 1).

Other Constituents

Other constituents include tannin, resins, volatile oils, acetic, formic, palmitic, gallic, butyric, and oleic acids, starches and sucrose (Jarry, et al., 1985; Duke, 1985). Duke (1985, p. 121) recounted that the roots contain 15% to 20% of cimicifugin, "an amorphous resinous substance" (cimicifugin = macrotin), and a bitter principle, racemosin. He et al. (2000) identified cimicifugoside M as being unique to *A. racemosa* and suggested that it may serve as a marker to distinguish the species.

THERAPEUTIC APPLICATIONS

The primary therapeutic application of black cohosh is in the treatment of menopausal symptoms. It is also used for postoperative functional deficits following ovariectomy or hysterectomy, for the treatment of premenstrual syndrome, and for juvenile menstrual disorders. The herbal extract, as well as homeopathic preparations, are used as an emmenagogue (a substance that

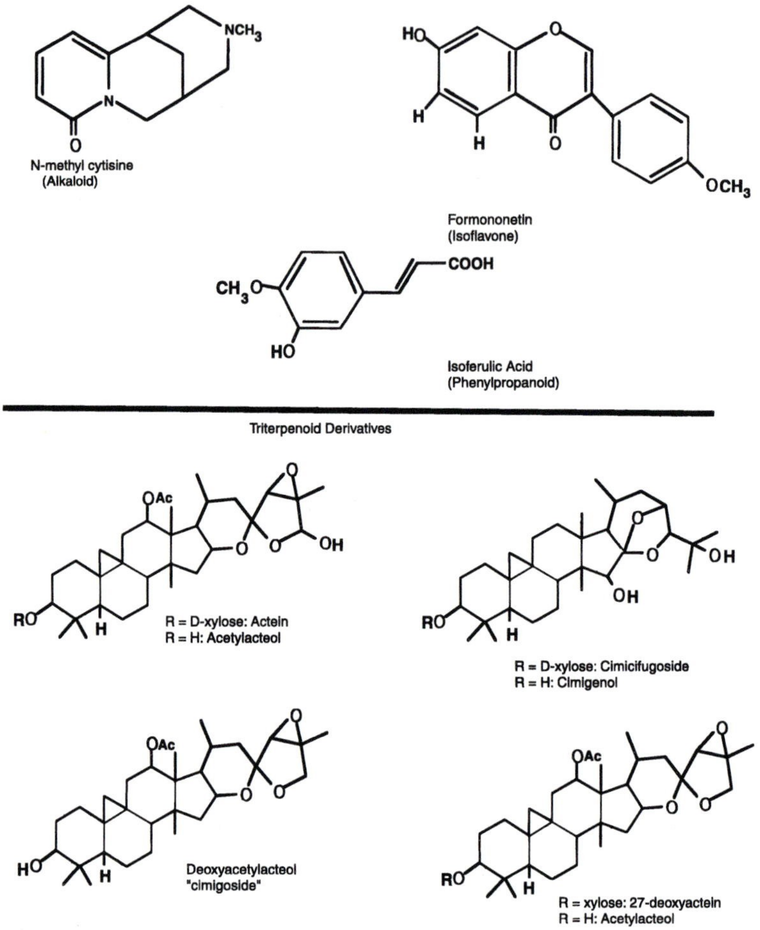

N-methyl cytisine
(Alkaloid)

Formononetin
(Isoflavone)

Isoferulic Acid
(Phenylpropanoid)

Triterpenoid Derivatives

R = D-xylose: Actein
R = H: Acetylacteol

R = D-xylose: Cimicifugoside
R = H: Cimigenol

Deoxyacetylacteol
"cimigoside"

R = xylose: 27-deoxyactein
R = H: Acetylacteol

FIGURE 1. Major Constituents of Black Cohosh

promotes menstrual flow) (NAPRALERT, 1997). The German Commission E cites evidence for the efficacy of black cohosh in its use for dysmenorrhea or painful menstruation (Blumenthal et al., 1998).

PRECLINICAL STUDIES

Cardiovascular and Circulatory Functions

Actein is hypotensive in cats and rabbits, but not consistently in dogs (Newall et al., 1996; Duke, 1985). Newall et al. (1996) cited a study showing that actein causes peripheral vasodilation and an increase in peripheral blood flow in patients diagnosed with peripheral arterial disease; their blood pressure (normal or hypertensive) was unchanged by this treatment.

Endocrine and Hormonal Functions

Hypothalamic and Pituitary Functions

Studies in rats (Eagon et al., 1997, 1998) as well as menopausal women (Jarry and Harnischfeger, 1985) have demonstrated reduced luteinizing hormone (LH) levels from black cohosh. An alcoholic extract of black cohosh administered to ovariectomized rats as part of their diet at one-third the human dose equivalent for three weeks was reported to increase the hypothalamic/pituitary response of the test animals. Eagon et al. (1998) quantified luteinizing hormone (LH) levels. Black cohosh extract produced a significant ($p < 0.05$) decrease in LH of 25%. However, a proprietary isopropanolic extract of the rhizome (Remifemin) did not produce a significant decrease in LH (Liske, 1998) (see Clinical Studies), at least with the new lower dose now recommended by the manufacturers of the extract (Schaper and Brümmer GmbH, 1997).

Düker et al. (1991) characterized pharmacological responses to various chromatographically separated fractions of black cohosh lipophilic extract in ovariectomized rats. These studies resulted in the isolation of three endocrinologically-active fractions: fraction I inhibited luteinizing hormone (LH) secretion but did not bind to estrogen receptors; fractions IV to VI were active in both assays, while fraction VIII displayed the most potency in estrogen receptor assays, without suppressing LH secretion after chronic treatment. This fraction did inhibit LH after a single acute injection; single injections of estradiol showed a similar activity profile. The lack of an effect on follicle-stimulating hormone (FSH) inhibition is due to FSH secretion being under the control of steroids plus inhibin, while LH secretion is mediated only by gonadal steroids. It was speculated that fraction VIII, which acutely but not chronically inhibited LH secretion, may contain estrogenically active compounds which are rapidly metabolized so that only a transient suppressive effect on LH secretion is produced. This may provide a rationale for the demonstrated clinical efficacy of black cohosh in the treatment of menopausal hot flashes; the pulsatile release of LH is inhibited, but overall LH levels are not suppressed. At present, this explanation is speculative. Fraction I, which was nonestrogenic but did suppress LH secretion, may have contained alpha-2 agonists similar to clonidine, which suppresses LH secretion without binding to the estrogen receptor (Düker et al., 1991; Jarry and Harnischfeger, 1985).

Reproductive Hormone Interactions

Conclusions regarding the hormonal effects of black cohosh must be tempered by recent research findings of the existence of two types of estrogen receptors, alpha and beta (ERα and ERβ) (Shughrue et al., 1998). Researchers note that this previously unrecognized complexity has, in all likelihood, been a significant source of the many conflicting reports of estrogenic and anti-estrogenic activities for a large number of plants and their constituents (Cassidy 1999; Davis et al., 1999). Conflicting results from black cohosh preparations may also be due to all the usual conditions that apply to plant extracts, including differences in solvents and lack of standardization of plant materials.

Zava et al. (1998) reported only little estrogenic and estrogen receptor-binding bioactivity from a 50% ethanol/water extract of black cohosh in vitro. Liu, Burdette et al. (2001) reported that a methanolic extract of black cohosh rhizome (wild-harvested) failed to exhibit any activity in a number of in vitro assays for estrogenic activity. These include: estrogen-competitive binding for human recombinant ERα and ERβ; alkaline phosphatase-inducing activity; progesterone receptor gene *(PR)*-up-regulating activity in estrogen-positive endometrial adenocarcinoma (Ishikawa) cells; and stimulation of *presenelin*-2 *(pS2)* gene expression in an estradiol-responsive breast cancer cell line (S30 cells), suggesting that the effects of the herb in menopausal women may have little or nothing to do with estrogenic effects.

Contrary to the findings of Liu, Burdette et al. (2001), Liu, Yang et al. (2001) reported that black cohosh caused a significant increase in estrogen receptor levels of human breast cancer (MCF-7) cells in vitro at a concentration of 4.75 µg/mL. The time at which cell growth doubled was comparable to that of cells treated with 17β-estradiol at 0.3 µM/L. Administered to immature female mice by feeding tube (75, 150, and 300 mg/kg for 14 days), black cohosh caused a dose-dependent increase in their uterine weights, and at 300 mg/kg, significantly prolonged the number of days of estrus.

An increase in uterine weight was also reported in ovariectomized rats fed an alcohol extract of black cohosh as part of a standard liquid diet (one-third the human dose equivalent for three weeks) (Eagon, 1999; Eagon et al., 1997). According to changes in serum ceruloplasmin, the hepatic estrogenic response was also increased by black cohosh (Eagon et al., 1997). However, a study by Einer-Jensen et al. (1996) indicated a lack of estrogenic effects in mice and rats.

Constituents of black cohosh rhizome can bind to estrogen receptors in rat uteri and pituitary glands, but some controversy exists as to what estrogenic effects result from the binding of these sites (Düker et al., 1991). The effects of a black cohosh extract (BNO 1055, 62.5 mg/day for 1 or 12 weeks) on the expression of genes in estrogen-dependent tissue in rats was compared to those of estradiol (3.5 µg/rat for 1 or 12 weeks). Some similar and different results were found. In contrast to estradiol, the black cohosh extract at either dosing schedule failed to effect uterine weight and exhibited no effect on various estrogen-regulated genes of the uterus. However, its effects on gene expression in the liver, aorta, and bone were in most instances like those of estradiol (Seidlova-Wuttke et al., 2000). Further studies, using ERα knockout (ERKO) mice, found that the extract contains yet-to-be-identified phytoestrogens that exhibit estrogenic effects on the aorta, bone, and hypothalamo-hypophysial system, but not on the uterus (Seidlova-Wuttke et al., 2001). Estrogenic effects of the extract were also found in the bone of orchidectomized male rats, as evidenced by significantly increased gene expressions of osteocalcin and tumor necrosis factor-α (TNFα) (Wuttke et al., 2001).

Knuvener et al. (2000) examined estrogenic effects of a 50% ethanolic extract of the rhizome using the Allen-Doisy test. In this test, changes in cornification in vaginal smears are used as an index of estrogenicity. Three groups of female castrated mice, uniformly sensitive to estrogen after priming for three weeks with mestranol (100 mg/kg per day p.o. × 3), were treated either with oral doses of the black cohosh extract (50-600 mg/day), water, or 17-β estradiol or mestranol (each 75 μg/kg per day p.o.). After cessation of treatment, the mice treated with 17-β estradiol developed a stage of estrus for 0.4-0.7 days, but only in half their group. For the mice treated with mestranol, the entire group developed a stage of estrus which lasted 3.5 days. For the black cohosh group however, estrogenic effects were absent. Checking the possibility of an antiestrogenic activity from the extract, researchers then treated a group of the mice with a combination of the black cohosh extract (50-250 mg/kg per day p.o.) and mestranol (75 μg/kg per day p.o.). Compared to the group treated with mestranol alone, the combination treatment produced a significant increase in the period of positive vaginal smears and the results were much the same when black cohosh extract was combined with 17-β estradiol. An increase in estrogenic activity was also indicated from the combination treatments in significantly increased urinary excretions of LH compared to mice treated with mestranol or 17-β estradiol alone.

IMMUNE FUNCTIONS; INFLAMMATION AND DISEASE

Cancer

Antiproliferative Activity

Kruse et al. (1999) have noted conflicting reports of an increased proliferation of estrogen-dependent MCF-7 cells in vitro by black cohosh. In this study, the caffeic acid ester constituent, fukinolic acid, isolated from an aqueous-ethanolic extract of the rhizome, caused a significant increase in the proliferations of MCF-7 cells in vitro. However, such activity was not shown by other researchers when an extract of black cohosh was administered to mice or rats. On the surface, this may infer that differences in the contents of fukinolic acid in black cohosh extracts may be responsible for conflicting results in assays of estrogenic activity. However, other constituents, or the lack of them, may also bear upon such results.

Dixon-Shanies and Shaikh (1999) examined the in vitro activity of an ethanolic extract of black cohosh on the growth of an estrogen- and progesterone-positive human breast cancer cell line, T-47D. At a concentration of 0.1%, growth of T-47D cells was significantly decreased by 22% and by 61% at a concentration of 1% (each $p < 0.001$).

Freudenstein et al. (2000) also reported that an isopropanolic extract of black cohosh (Remifemin) failed to stimulate proliferation of estrogen receptor-positive breast cancer cell lines. In a further investigation, they administered three oral doses of the extract to female rats with dimethylbenz [a] anthracene (DMBA)-induced mammary gland tumors after allowing the tumors to grow for 5-9 weeks (one comparable to a human therapeutic dose, one 10 times and one 100 times the human therapeutic dose). The results were as follows: the rats treated with black cohosh showed no significant differences in tumor size or number compared to the vehicle-treated control group; no regrowth of tumors from black cohosh was evident in ovariectomized mice treated with black cohosh; no estrogenic effects compared to controls were evident in uterine tissue; and in plasma hormone levels of LH, FSH, and prolactin, no estrogen agonist effects were found from treatment with black cohosh. However, compared to the vehicle-treated controls, those receiving black cohosh showed a trend towards a reduction in the size of estrogen-positive mammary tumors.

Nesselhut et al. (1993) reported that isopropanolic aqueous extracts of black cohosh inhibited in vitro proliferation of estrogen-dependent breast cancer cell lines in a dose-dependent manner, an activity interpreted as an estrogen-receptor blockade. Foster (1999) referred to a study by Freudenstein and Bodinet in which an extract of black cohosh rhizome was shown not to stimulate proliferation of estrogen receptor-positive MCF-7 breast cancer cells. The extract was also found to increase the growth-inhibitory effect of tamoxifen on the cells. The authors concluded that extracts of the herb can be safely taken by patients who are susceptible to breast cancer (see Contraindications).

Infectious Diseases

Microbial Infections. Black cohosh extracts are mostly without antibacterial, antifungal, or antiviral activity, although they have shown activity against *Staphylococcus aureus,* according to NAPRALERT (1997).

Inflammatory Response

Löser et al. (2000) noted that the Native Americans used black cohosh for rheumatoid arthritis, and traditional Chinese and Japanese medicine practitioners use *shengma* to treat inflammatory conditions. One of the typical aspects of an active state of inflammation is found in elevated plasma levels of a proteinase released by neutrophils known as elastase. Because cinnamic acid esters isolated from a Japanese species of *shengma* (*Actaea simplex* Wormsk., or *shoma*) were reported to inhibit the activity of enzymes (carboxypeptidase and α-amylase), Löser et al. (2000) tested the in vitro inhibitory effects of cinnamic acid esters from black cohosh rhizomes on neutrophil elastase. Using human leukocyte elastase, a particularly destructive enzyme, varying degrees of inhibitory activity were found from each of the cinnamic acid esters. The most potent by far was fukinolic acid (IC_{50} 0.1 µg/mL) with two free catechol moieties, followed by cimicifugic acid A (IC_{50} 2.2 µM/L), and cimicifugic acid B (11.4 mg/mL) with less than two free catechol moieties. Cimicifugic acids E and F, ferulic acid, and isoferulic acid were comparatively much weaker and are devoid of unsubstituted catechol units.

Sakai et al. (1999) reported that ferulic and isoferulic acid inhibit the in vitro production of a macrophage inflammatory protein (MIP-2) which is produced in response to infection with respiratory syncytial virus. Hirabayashi et al. (1995) showed that isoferulic acid inhibited both in vitro and in vivo production of MIP-2 induced by influenza virus. In an animal model of lethal influenza virus pneumonia, Sakai et al. (2001) compared the effect of isoferulic acid to dexamethasone, also an inhibitor of MIP-2, for possible changes in the rate of survival. Groups of female mice infected with influenza virus (a lung-adapted strain, H1N1 subtype) were administered isoferulic acid (0.25 mg to 1 mg p.o.) once a day for four days starting just prior to infection. Dexamethasone was administered i.p. in the same schedule at doses of 0.04 mg to 4.0 mg. Compared to controls, mice treated with isoferulic acid showed a significant increase in the rate of survival and less weight loss from the lowest dose ($p = 0.016$), but not from the highest dose. Dexamethasone failed to improve either survival rates or weight loss.

Integumentary, Muscular, and Skeletal Functions

Osteoporosis

Wuttke et al. (2000) reported evidence of organ-specific effects of a black cohosh extract (BNO 1055) in ovariectomized (ovx) rats. As with a control group treated with estradiol, the black cohosh extract inhibited and prevented the development of osteoporosis. Nisslein and Freudenstein (2000) found that treatment of ovx rats with a standardized isopropanolic extract of black cohosh rhizomes caused indicators of bone metabolism to drop to levels seen in untreated female rats and by as much as ovx rats treated with the selective estrogen receptor modulator (SERM) raloxifene, a drug prescribed for the treatment and prevention of postmenopausal osteoporosis. Similar effects have been reported from *shengma*. Two recent studies of *Actaea foetida* and *A. heracleifolia* demonstrated inhibition of parathyroid hormone-induced bone resorption in tissue culture and in ovariectomized rats (Li et al., 1995, 1996). Li et al. (1996/1997) reported a significant (approximately 10%) increase in spinal bone mineral density in ovariectomized rats fed a low-calcium diet following administration of ethyl acetate-soluble fractions of *A. heracleifolia* and *A. foetida* (100 mg/kg per day, p.o.). The fractions prevented osteoporosislike bone loss. Four triterpenoids derived from these species also showed calcium level-decreasing activity in low-calcium diet rats (25 mg/kg, p.o.), implicating them as the active constituents.

Neurological, Psychological, and Behavioral Functions

Receptor- and Neurotransmitter-Mediated Functions

Löhning and Winterhoff (2000) have conducted animal studies with black cohosh to elucidate effects on neurotransmitters. Their findings portend a new era of investigation into the still "controversially discussed" mechanism of action of black cohosh in the treatment of hot flashes and psychical symptoms of menopausal disorders (Löhning and Winterhoff, 2000, p. 13). They report that acute treatments with black cohosh in animals produced marked CNS effects in the form of prolongation of ketamine-induced sleeping times and decreases in body temperature; effects which were blocked when animals were pretreated with a dopamine antagonist (sulpiride). After a 21-day pretreatment with black cohosh, serotonin turnover in the striatum of the animals showed a significant decrease while dopamine levels showed a significant increase. Levels of HVA (homovanillic acid) and DOPAC (dihydroxyphenylacetate) were both reduced, indicating inhibition of MAO (monoamine oxidase). After long-term (eight days) treatment with black cohosh, female mice subjected to the tail suspension test showed a significant decrease in immobility time, thereby suggesting an antidepressant effect which may well be facilitated by an MAO-inhibitory activity.

Reproductive Functions

Pregnancy and Labor

Black cohosh has a documented uterine stimulant effect and can induce labor (NAPRALERT, 1997). Although it was extensively used by the Eclectic medical doctors of North America for specific conditions of pregnancy, labor, and postpartum, there are no recent studies clarifying the pharmacological effects of black cohosh during pregnancy and labor. Studies from the 1920s showed that black cohosh stimulated the nonpregnant uterus of the guinea pig and cat, but depressed the pregnant uterus. The resinous cimicifugin had no effect on isolated intestine or uterus of animals (Brinker, 1996).

CLINICAL STUDIES

Endocrine and Hormonal Disorders

Hypothalamic and Pituitary Functions

Jacobson et al. (2001) conducted a randomized, double-blind, placebo-controlled trial of black cohosh in the treatment of hot flashes in 85 women who had undergone primary treatment for breast cancer. The majority of women with a history of breast cancer report hot flashes, which are also the most common climacteric symptom in menopause and are closely related to pulsatile LH release. Eligible participants were those who had completed radiation and chemotherapy at least 8 weeks before entry into the trial. Ineligible patients were either pregnant, diagnosed with metastatic or recurrent breast cancer, suffering from a major psychiatric illness, or taking hormone replacement therapy for the treatment of hot flashes. At the time of enrollment, and again at the last visit, patients completed a menopausal symptom index questionnaire and a visual analogue scale rating of their well-being and health overall. They were also to complete a four-day hot flash diary before treatment and at days 30 and 60 of the treatment period. (At the end of the trial, diaries of 68 study participants were usable for evaluation.) Nonhormonal medications were allowed, but no new treatments for hot flashes were permitted. Patients were randomly assigned to treatment groups of either black cohosh (Jacobson et al., 2001) (Remifemin, two 20 mg tablets daily, one each with the morning and evening meal, for 60 days) (Jacobson, 2001) or placebo. Tamoxifen was not taken by 26 patients while 59 patients also took tamoxifen so that there were two arms made up of the following groups: placebo/tamoxifen, black cohosh/tamoxifen, black cohosh/no tamoxifen, and placebo/no tamoxifen. A subset of patients were tested for changes in levels of LH and FSH at the first and last visits. When the data obtained from the black cohosh group was compared to the placebo group, the results showed no significant differences in reports of decreased incidences and intensity of hot flashes, which, however, showed an overall decrease of about 27% compared to baseline. Improvements in symptoms of menopause and changes in levels of LH and FSH in the black cohosh group also showed no significant differences compared to placebo or tamoxifen, except in the symptom of sweating, which showed a significant decrease in the black cohosh group ($p = 0.04$). Nearly all the adverse events reported were from tamoxifen users, yet a clear association to the drug was not apparent.

Reproductive Disorders

Menopause

The majority of clinical studies on black cohosh in the treatment of menopausal symptoms have, to date, been open-label trials (e.g., Lehmann-Willenbrock and Riedel, 1988; Pethö, 1987; Warnecke, 1985; Vorberg, 1984; Daiber, 1983; Stolze, 1982) or controlled trials lacking a placebo control (Schaper and Brümmer GmbH, 1997). As such, they are of questionable value, especially in treating patients with psychogenic complaints (Freeman and Rickels, 1999). Given that the use of black cohosh in Europe for the treatment of menopausal complaints is about 50 years old, the lack of placebo-controlled clinical trials is remarkable. Since black cohosh recently became the largest-selling herbal supplement used for menopausal symptoms in the United States (Blumenthal et al., 2000), this situation may soon change.

Stoll (1987) conducted a randomized, double-blind, placebo-controlled study of a standardized extract of black cohosh (Remifemin) in 80 female volunteers (ages 46-54 years) suffering from symptoms of menopause. This extract is standardized to contain triterpene glycosides calculated as 27-deoxyactein (1 mg/tablet) (see Dosage). Five were excluded from the final statistical analysis due to failure to appear for the follow-up visits, improper use of the black cohosh extract, and treatment with a hormone injection. Exclusion criteria included osteoporosis; use of sex hormone in the four-week period preceding entry to the trial; contraindications for treatment with hormone therapy; use of antihypertensive agents; gonadal failure subsequent to irradiation, castration, or bilateral ovariectomy; and complaints that could be ascribed to "other causes of menopause." For 12 weeks, patients ($n = 75$) received tablets containing either Remifemin (two tablets twice daily, each containing 2 mg of black cohosh powder extract), conjugated estrogens (0.625 mg/day plus placebo three times daily for 21 days followed by placebo twice daily for seven days) or placebo (two tablets twice daily). All preparations were equal in taste and appearance. To gauge efficacy, the study employed the 14-item Hamilton Anxiety Scale to measure outcomes in psychic disturbances and the Kupperman Menopausal Index to assess primarily neurovegetative complaints. In addition, researchers checked for changes in proliferation of the vaginal epithelium to measure somatic changes. Before treatment, all the patients were assessed as suffering from moderate to severe menopausal symptoms; however, none were found with cohabitation problems, pruritus vulvae, or genital inflammation (Stoll, 1987).

After 12 weeks of treatment, patients in the Remifemin group showed a significant decrease in mean (median) Hamilton Anxiety Scale scores compared to those on estrogens or placebo ($p < 0.001$). The results showed that the improvement was already apparent after four weeks of treatment. A significant increase ($p < 0.01$) in the proliferation of the vaginal epithelium was found in the black cohosh group whereas no changes were found in either the estrogen or placebo group. The black cohosh group also showed significant improvements of somatic and psychological parameters (Kupperman Menopausal Index values) compared to estrogen or placebo ($p < 0.001$). Symptoms changed from moderate-severe to slight after four weeks and thereafter became nil in the black cohosh. In the placebo and estrogen groups, symptoms showed a trend toward improvement, but after 12 weeks were still in the moderate range. The average number of hot flashes dropped from 4.9/day to 0.7/day in the black cohosh group, from 5.2/day to 3.2/day in the estrogen group, and from 5.1/day to 3.1/day in the group treated with placebo.

Side effects reported by the patients were minor. In the placebo group, one patient complained of headaches. Among those treated with estrogen, there were complaints of heaviness in the legs ($n = 1$), mastodynia ($n = 1$), eventual tachycardia ($n = 1$), and weight problems ($n = 1$). Patients in the black cohosh group reported heaviness in the legs ($n = 1$), mastodynia ($n = 1$), feeling pepped up ($n = 1$), weight gain ($n = 3$), headaches, or an increase in symptoms present before entry to the trial ($n = 6$). In all, 16 patients dropped out of the trial before its completion due to several factors. In the black cohosh group these factors were: nonconformation to the trial criteria due to the development of thrombophlebitis ($n = 1$); in the placebo group: inefficacy ($n = 1$), headache and weight gain ($n = 2$); and in the estrogen group: inefficacy ($n = 12$). It was concluded that the extract of black cohosh is an effective alternative to hormone-based treatments for menopausal complaints and that without their side effects, is a more desirable treatment with characteristics of a first-choice therapy (Stoll, 1987).

Düker et al. (1991) compared the effect of a standardized Remifemin ethanolic extract to placebo in an open-controlled study on LH and FSH secretion in 110 menopausal women. None of the women had received previous hormonal therapy for the preceding six months or more. Patients received placebo or black cohosh tablets to be taken at a dosage of two tablets twice daily. After eight weeks, LH, but not FSH, levels (by radioimmunoassay) were significantly reduced in patients receiving Remifemin, but not in those given placebo; FSH levels were similar in both groups.

An open multicenter, multiclinic, retrospective study was published in Germany in 1982 (Stolze, 1982). In total, 131 general practitioners provided data on 629 female patients with menopausal complaints. Some of the patients ($n = 367$) had received no previous treatment, 204 had been previously treated with hormones, 35 had received psychopharmaceutical treatments, 11 had been treated with a combination of psychopharmaceuticals and hormone therapy, and no specific pretreatment data was available for 12 subjects. Clear improvements in neurovegetative complaints (hot flashes, profuse perspiration, headache, vertigo, heart palpitation, ringing in the ears) and psychological disturbances (nervousness, irritability, sleep disturbances, depressive moods) were experienced by approximately 80% of the patients after four weeks of therapy. After six to eight weeks, all symptoms abated in approximately 40% to 50% of the patients, and were markedly reduced or improved in an additional 30% to 40%. Overall improvement rates (abolished or ameliorated symptoms) ranged from 76% to 93% of patients. The dosage regime (40 drops of Remifemin standardized extract twice daily for six to eight weeks) lacked side effects, or had only minor side effects in 93% of the patients (Stolze, 1982).

A recent product surveillance study of 911 post-, pre-, and perimenopausal women with psychovegetative complaints reported putative synergistic effects for the combination of black cohosh and St. John's wort *(Hypericum perforatum)* standardized extracts in the management of psychological symptoms (Liske et al., 1997).

DOSAGE

Clinical studies of *C. racemosa* have almost all utilized Remifemin, a standardized extract containing triterpene glycosides calculated as 27-deoxyactein (1 mg/tablet). The usual dose had been two tablets twice/day (equivalent to 4 mg triterpene glycosides per day). Dosages twice and three times this amount have been used in some studies (Schaper and Brümmer GmbH, 1997; Liske and Wüstenberg, 1998). Recent information from the makers of Remifemin claims that half this dose (i.e., one tablet, twice daily or a total of 2 mg triterpene glycosides) is just as effective as two tablets twice daily for the relief of climacteric symptoms. For Remifemin liquid extract, 40 drops are equivalent to 40 mg of herbal drug, and contain a total of 2 mg triterpene glycosides, equal to two tablets (Schaper and Brümmer GmbH, 1997; Liske, 1998). Most studies of the liquid extract used 40 drops twice a day for a total daily dose equivalent to 80 mg of the herbal drug and containing 4 mg triterpene glycosides.

Liske and Wüstenberg (1998) reported that a randomized double-blind clinical study of a special isopropanolic extract of the rootstock of black cohosh in the treatment of climacteric complaints found similar efficacy and results from a dosage of 40 mg/day as from 127 mg/day for six months, adding that the Kupperman-Menopausal Index values already showed improvement after two weeks of treatment.

The *British Herbal Compendium* recommends a dose of 40-200 mg dried rhizome, or 0.4-2 mL of a 1:10 60% ethanol tincture (Bradley, 1992). However, Newall et al. (1996) recommend a dose range of 2-4 mL for this tincture, based on the *British Pharmacopoeial Compendium* (1934). Newall and colleagues further describe a dose range of a liquid extract (BPC 1898) of 1:1 in 90% alcohol as 0.3-2.0 mL. The dosage for the decoction of the rhizome is given as 0.3-2.0 g t.i.d.

SAFETY PROFILE

In human studies with the fluid extract, up to 890 mg/day was given with no evidence of toxic effects (Novitch and Schweiker, 1982).

Ames test (*Salmonella* microsomal assay) results showed no in vitro evidence of mutagenic potential of the isopropanolic extract of black cohosh (Liske, 1998). Dosages of 0.32 to 1,000 µg/plate were used with negative and positive controls (Schaper and Brümmer GmbH, 1997).

Contraindications

Certain estrogens, notably estradiol, are associated with an increased risk of breast, ovarian, or endometrial cancers. In contrast, the estrogen estriol is associated with some degree of protection against these cancers because it acts as a weak partial antagonist to estradiol. The action of Remifemin is interpreted as "estriol-like" by the manufacturers, and the German Commission E has not included any contraindications for use in patients with estrogen-dependent tumors. Although it has been recommended that such patients should consult their physicians prior to use (Schaper and Brümmer GmbH, 1997), Freudenstein et al. (2000) reported an antiproliferative effect of a black cohosh extract (isopropanolic/aqueous) on breast cancer cells (MCF-7, an estrogen receptor-positive cell line). In a study of 50-day-old female rats with estrogen-receptor-positive mammary gland tumors, oral administration of the extract (Remifemin) at one, ten, and 100 times the equivalent therapeutic dose used by humans also failed to show stimulatory activity. These results appear to contradict those of Liu, Yang et al. (2001), who reported that oral administration of black cohosh to immature female mice (300 mg/kg) produced various indications of an estrogenic effect, such as significantly prolonging the days of estrus and uterine weight. In human estrogen receptor-positive breast cancer cells (MCF-7), black cohosh (4.75 µg/mL) caused the rate of cell growth to increase by as much as 64.7% and produced a significant increase in estrogen receptor levels. Also, the time required for the cancer cells treated with black cohosh to double was comparable to that of cells treated with 17β-estradiol. Although details of this study were not available in English, differences in the results compared to those of Freudenstein et al. (2000) may be due to a host of factors including the chemical makeup of the two plants, laboratory procedures, the type and state of the animals, and/or dosage parameters.

In a review of black cohosh research, Liske (1998) states that the therapeutic efficacy of the commercial extract is not attributable to hormonal (estrogenic) effects. The latest Remifemin brochure (Schaper and Brümmer GmbH, 1997) makes no claims regarding any estrogenic effects, such as increased vaginal epithelium thickness or alteration in hormone levels, including prolactin, estrogen, progesterone, FSH and, notably, LH-inhibition. A previous clinical study had demonstrated a decline in LH attributed to Remifemin at the formerly recommended higher dose (two tablets twice daily) (Düker et al., 1991). In another trial of Remifemin (two tablets twice daily, each containing 2 mg of black cohosh powder extract), Stoll (1987) reported a significant increase ($p < 0.01$) in the proliferation of the vaginal epithelium, whereas no changes were found in either the estrogen or placebo group.

In a randomized double-blind clinical trial of patients (ages 43-60) treated for climacteric complaints ($n = 152$) with a special isopropanolic extract of black cohosh root (40 mg/day and 127 mg/day for 6 months) (apparently manufactured by the makers of Remifemin), indications of an estrogenlike effect were absent in all tests (changes in levels of estradiol, prolactin, FSH, and LH). The degree of cellular proliferation of the vagina was also not affected by the treatment (Liske and Wüstenberg, 1998). FSH and LH also showed no change in breast cancer patients taking tamoxifen and black cohosh or black cohosh alone compared to controls administered placebo (Jacobson et al., 2001).

Drug Interactions

Standardized extracts have been used in conjunction with physician-monitored estrogen replacement therapy with minimal side effects (Liske, 1998; Warnecke, 1985).

A multicenter postmarketing surveillance study of a standardized combination product (Schaper and Brümmer GmbH & Co.) containing an extract of black cohosh (1 mg triterpene glycoside/tablet) and St. John's wort (0.25 mg hypericin/tablet) reported very good tolerability in menopausal patients in 99% of cases, according to physician assessment of global tolerability in over 800 women ages 46-55 (Liske, 1997).

The report of MAO-inhibiting activity in rodents administered black cohosh (Löhning and Winterhoff, 2000), however portentous of caution in patients taking MAO inhibitors, serotonergic antidepressant agents, and other drugs, must be balanced with the fact that no specific drug interactions have been identified with black cohosh (Blumenthal et al., 1998) and that confirmation of significant MAO-inhibiting activity has yet to be reported in humans.

A case of nocturnal seizures was reported in a 45-year-old woman, who, for about four months had combined black cohosh, *Vitex agnus-castus,* and evening primrose oil to regulate her menstrual cycle (Shuster, 1996). Her sister had been taking the same regimen for one to two years and had recommended that she try it. Within a period of three months while taking the herbal products, the woman recalled having some fatigue and facial flushing and had experienced three nocturnal seizures, as witnessed by her sister and boyfriend. Their description of the events matched that of the general tonic-clonic type of seizure. The seizures stopped upon her discontinuation of the products for three days and she was prescribed carbamazepine as a prophylactic measure. Upon a further review, nothing remarkable was evident in her medical history. She added that one or two days preceding each of the seizures, she had drunk one or two beers; however, alcohol was something she claimed only to partake of on special occasions and weekends. The investigating pharmacist stated that ingesting alcohol so far in advance seemed an unlikely cause of the seizures. The pharmacist found nothing in the literature indicating seizures or central nervous system effects from the herbs, and the manufacturer of two of the products (Nature's Herbs, American Fork, Utah) had no such information either (Shuster, 1996). In the end, the cause of the reported seizures was unresolved.

Pregnancy and Lactation

Black cohosh alone does not at this time have an established safe dosage for any indication of use during pregnancy or labor. The *American Herbal Products Association's Botanical Safety Handbook* (1997) lists black cohosh as a class 2b herbal medicine, meaning that it is an herb that should not be taken during pregnancy unless otherwise directed by an expert qualified in its use (McGuffin et al., 1997). An assessment of risks and benefits of use during pregnancy or labor should be undertaken with the assistance of an informed health care provider. Brinker (1998, p. 137) contraindicates use during the first trimester of pregnancy, "due to its emmenagogue effects (empirical)." Moerman (1998, p. 162) notes that the Cherokees used black cohosh "to stimulate menstruation."

The *American Materia Medica* of 1919 noted that large doses of black cohosh given prenatally could induce labor prematurely. As an aid to labor (*partus* accelerator), 130-325 mg of "a fluid extract" was employed. Postpartum hemorrhage was thought to be prevented by the herb, and it was suggested that a special single dose of 30 minums (1.8 mL) be administered upon the delivery of the baby's head (Ellingwood, 1983).

Black cohosh is sometimes used by herbalists in combination with blue cohosh *(Caulophyllum thalictroides)* to induce and aid labor. An anecdotal report of a child born with no spontaneous breathing who subsequently suffered brain hypoxia in which unknown/unreported oral doses of a combination of black cohosh and blue cohosh was taken by the mother to induce labor has been documented. The authors of this report queried the possible role of the herb in contributing to the infant's initial low APGAR scores, but also raised the question of postbirth resuscitation mismanagement (Gunn and Wright, 1996). Unfortunately, no indication of dose was given, so conclusions about the toxicity of either herb in labor cannot be definitive. The pharmacological contribution of black cohosh when used in conjunction with blue cohosh is unknown. However, blue cohosh *(Caullophyllum)* was implicated in a case of an infant who suffered the chance of permanent injury, possibly related to the third trimester overdosage by the mother from taking blue cohosh at two times the recommended dose for three weeks (Jones and Lawson, 1998).

Little information exists regarding the use of *Actaea (=Cimicifuga)* species during lactation. Ethnobotanical records of use indicate that an infusion of the rhizome was used postpartum by Iroquois women to promote milk flow (Moerman, 1986). No current descriptions of use as a lactagogue exist and no record of adverse effects on lactation, or breastfeeding are available (NAPRALERT, 1997). No evidence from animal or human studies exist regarding the entry of constituents of *Actaea* into breast milk. No reports of negative effects on the neonate were found associated with the use of black cohosh during labor or in the immediate postpartum period to prevent or lessen uterine hemorrhage.

A monograph on black cohosh published in 1989 by the German Commission E provided no contraindications for use during lactation (Blumenthal et al., 1998). Brinker (1998, p. 37) cites "empirical evidence" of black cohosh having "potential toxicity in large doses" without providing further details. The *American Herbal Products Association's Botanical Safety Handbook* (1997) classified *Cimicifuga foetida (shengma)* as 2d (i.e., other specific use restrictions as noted, providing a list of adverse effects of overdose), without restriction of use during lactation. *Cimicifuga racemosa* is classified as 2c, (i.e., not to be used while breastfeeding unless otherwise directed by an expert qualified in its use). The *Handbook* cites gastrointestinal (GI) discomfort, the negative effects of overdose, and "estrogenic effect" as the rationales for this classification. GI discomfort and any other known side effects of an herb should be watched for in the breastfeeding infant; risk of side effects would be greatest in the neonate. The documented estrogen-blocking receptor activity of black cohosh (Liske, 1998) has as yet unclear implications for lactation, although other herbs with similar phyto-estrogenic effects are reputed to promote milk flow. Several studies provide evidence that prolactin levels are not affected with use of black cohosh; however, these studies were conducted with nonlactating subjects (Schaper and Brümmer GmbH, 1997).

Side Effects

In 1892 Jean Brunton claimed that doses of up to 890 mg/day of black cohosh fluid extract appeared to be safe (Brunton, 1892). Currently, occasional gastric discomfort is the only noted side effect (Blumenthal et al., 1998).

Special Precautions

The German Commission E recommends that the duration of use of black cohosh should not exceed six months (based on a lack of toxicology studies available at the time of their review in 1989) (Blumenthal et al., 1998).

Willard (1991) describes effects from large doses, including a mild, emetic property which can cause nausea as well as giddiness and headache. McGuffin et al. (1997) list the following side effects from large doses: vertigo, vomiting, nausea, headache, and impaired circulation and eyesight.

Overdoses may produce gastrointestinal irritation, prostration, headache, (Reynolds et al., 1996), nausea, vomiting, and dizziness, and may reduce pulse rate and induce perspiration. Overdosing during pregnancy can cause premature birth (Duke, 1985). Although not listed as toxic, black cohosh is classified by the FDA as an herb of undefined safety. Brinker (1998) cites empirical evidence contraindicating large doses in nursing mothers and pregnancy.

Toxicology

Mutagenicity

Ames test (*Salmonella* microsomal assay) results showed no in vitro evidence of mutagenic potential of the isopropanolic extract of black cohosh (Liske, 1998). Dosages of 0.32 to 1,000 µg/plate were used with negative and positive controls (Schaper and Brümmer GmbH, 1997).

Toxicity in Animal Models

Toxicity assessments for the minimum lethal dose of the chloroform extract range from as low as >3.0 mg/kg s.c. for 30 days in the rabbit, to as high as >1 g/kg p.o. for 30 days in the rat (NAPRALERT, 1997). In one study, the minimum acute, lethal dose of a tincture of black cohosh in mice was >500 mg/kg i.p. In the rat, the minimum acute, lethal dose was >1 g/kg p.o. and for the rabbit, >70 mg/kg p.o. In a 30-day test for subchronic toxicity, the minimum lethal dose in mice was >10 mg/kg i.p. and in rabbits, >6 mg/kg p.o. (Schindler, 1952). In Wistar rats given up to 5,000 mg Remifemin granulate/kg for 26 weeks, no conspicuous chemical or organ toxicities were observed (Korn, 1991). In human studies with the fluid extract, up to 890 mg/day was given with no evidence of toxic effects (Novitch and Schweiker, 1982).

REFERENCES

Awang, D.V.C. (2001). MediPlant Consulting, Inc., White Rock, B.C., Canada, personal communication with Kenneth Jones, June 2001.

Bedir, E. and Khan, I.A. (2000). Cimiracemoside A: A new cyclolanostanol xyloside from the rhizome of *Cimicifuga racemosa*. *Chemical and Pharmaceutical Bulletin* 48: 425-427.

Bedir, E. and Khan, L.A. (2001). A new cyclolanostanol arabinoside from the rhizome of *Cimicifuga racemosa*. *Pharmazie* 56:268-269.

Blumenthal, M., Busse, W.R., Goldberg, A., Gruenwald, J., Hall, T., Riggins, C.W., and Rister, R.S. (Eds.) (1998). *The Complete German Commission E Monographs*. Austin, TX: American Botanical Council, p. 90.

Blumenthal, M., Goldberg, A., and Brinckmann, J. (Eds.) (2000). *Herbal Medicine. Expanded Commission E Monographs*. Newton, MA: Integrated Medicine Communications, p. 22.

Boyle, W. (1991). *Official Herbs. Botanical Substances in the United States Pharmacopoeia 1820-1990*. East Palestine, OH: Buckeye Naturopathic Press, pp. 22-23.

Bradley, P.R. (Ed.) (1992). *British Herbal Compendium,* Volume 1. Bournemouth, Dorset, England: British Herbal Medicine Association, pp. 34-36.

Brinker, F. (1996). Macrotys. *The Eclectic Medical Journals* 2 (February-March): 2-4.

Brinker, F. (1998). *Herb Contraindications and Drug Interactions,* Second Edition. Sandy, OR: Eclectic Medical Publications, p. 137.

Brunton, J. (1892). The use of *Actaea racemosa* in dysmenorrhea and ovarian irritation. *Practitioner* 48: 265-268.

Cassidy, A. (1999). Potential tissue selectivity of dietary phytoestrogens and estrogens. *Current Opinion in Lipidology* 10: 47-52.

Chang, H.M. and But, P.P.H. (1986). *Pharmacology and Applications of Chinese Materia Medica,* Volume 1. Singapore: World Scientific.

Compton, J.A., Culham, A., and Jury, S.L. (1998). Reclassification of *Actaea* to include *Cimicifuga* and *Souliea* (Ranunculaceae): Phylogeny inferred from morphology, nrDNA ITS, and cpDNA *trn*L-F sequence variation. *Taxo* 47: 593-634.

Daiber, W. (1983). Klimakterische heschwerden: Ohne hormone [Climacteric related symptoms: Success without hormones]. *Ärztliche Praxis* 35: 1946-1947.

Davis, S.R., Dalais, F.S., Simpson, E.R., and Murkies, A.L. (1999). Phytoestrogens in health and disease. *Recent Progress in Hormone Research* 54: 185-211.

Dixon-Shanies, D. and Shaikh, N. (1999). Growth inhibition of human breast cancer cells by herbs and phytoestrogens. *Oncology Reports* 6: 1383-1387.

Duke, J.A. (1985). *Handbook of Medicinal Herbs.* Boca Raton, FL: CRC Press, pp. 120-121.

Düker, E.M., Kopanski, L., Jarry, H., and Wuttke, W. (1991). Effects of extracts from *Cimicifuga racemosa* on gonadotropin release in menopausal women and ovariectomized rats. *Planta Medica* 57: 420-424.

Eagon, C.L., Teepe, M.S., and Eagon, P.K. (1997). Medicinal botanicals: Estrogenicity in rat uterus and liver. *Proceedings of the American Association for Cancer Research* 38: 293 (abstract 1967).

Eagon, P.K. (1999). University of Pittsburgh School of Medicine, personal communication with Kenneth Jones, August 23, 1999.

Eagon, P.K., Swafford, D.S., Elm, M.S., Ayer, H.A., Rich, C., Tress, N.B., and Eagon, C.L. (1998). Estrogenicity of medicinal botanicals. *Proceedings of the American Association for Cancer Research* 39 (March): abstract 2624.

Einer-Jensen, N., Zhao, J., Anderson, K.P., and Kristoffersen, K. (1996). *Cimicifuga* and Melbrosia lack oestrogenic effects in mice and rats. *Maturitas* 25: 149-153.

Ellingwood, F. (1983). *American Materia Medica, Therapeutics and Pharmacognosy,* Eleventh Edition. Sandy, OR: Eclectic Medical Publications.

Foster, S. (1999). Black cohosh: *Cimifuga racemosa,* a literature review. *HerbalGram* (45): 35-50.

Freeman, E.W. and Rickels, K. (1999). Characteristics of placebo responses in medical treatment of premenstrual syndrome. *American Journal of Psychiatry* 156: 1403-1408.

Freudenstein, J., Dasenbrock, T., and Nisslein, T. (2000). Lack of promotion of estrogen dependent mammary gland tumors in vivo by an isopropanolic black cohosh extract. *Phytomedicine* 7(Suppl. 2): 13-14 (abstract SL-14).

Gunn, T.R. and Wright, I.M. (1996). The use of black and blue cohosh in labour. *New Zealand Medical Journal* 109: 410-411.

Hagels, H., Baumert-Krauss, J., and Freudenstein, J. (2000). Composition of phenolic constituents in *Cimicifuga racemosa.* In International Congress and 48th Annual Meeting of the Society for Medicinal Plant Research, 8th International Congress on Ethnopharmacology of the International Society for Ethnopharmacology, Zurich, Switzerland, Abstracts (abstract P1B/03).

He, K., Zheng, B., Kim, C.H., Rogers, L., and Zheng, Q. (2000). Direct analysis and identification of triterpene glycosides by LC/MS in black cohosh, *Cimifuga racemosa,* and in several commercially available black cohosh products. *Planta Medica* 66: 635-640.

Hirabayashi, T., Ochiai, H., Sakai, S., Nakajima, K., and Terasawa, K. (1995). Inhibitory effect of ferulic and isoferulic acid on murine interleukin-8 production in response to influenza virus infections *in vitro* and *in vivo. Planta Medica* 61: 221-226.

Jacobson, J.S. (2001). Division of Epidemiology, Mailman School of Public Health, Columbia University, New York, NY, letter to Kenneth Jones, June 20.

Jacobson, J.S., Troxel, A.B., Evans, J., Klaus, L., Vahdat, L., Kinne, D., Lo, K.M., Moore, A., Rosenman, P.J., Kaufman, E.L., et al. (2001). Randomized trial of black cohosh for the treatment of hot flashes among women with a history of breast cancer. *Journal of Clinical Oncology* 19: 2739-2745.

Jarry, H. and Harnischfeger, G. (1985). [Studies on the endocrine effects of the contents of *Cimicifuga racemosa*: 1. Influence on the serum concentration of pituitary hormones in ovariectomized rats]. *Planta Medica* 51: 46-49.

Jarry, H., Harnischfeger, G., and Düker, E. (1985). [Studies on the endocrine effects of the contents of *Cimicifuga racemosa*: 2. In vitro binding of compounds to estrogen receptors]. *Planta Medica* 51: 316-319.

Jones, T.K. and Lawson, B.M. (1998). Profound neonatal congestive heart failure caused by maternal consumption of blue cohosh herbal medication. *Journal of Pediatrics* 132: 550-552.

Kennelly, E.J., Baggett, S., Nuntanakorn, P., Osoki, A.L., Mori, S.A., Duke, J., and Kronenberg, C.M. (2001). Analysis of thirteen populations of black cohosh for formononetin. *Alternative Therapies in Health and Medicine* 7: S18 (abstract).

Knuvener, E., Korte, B., and Winterhoff, H. (2000). Cimicifuga and physiological estrogens. *Phytomedicine* 7(Suppl. 2): 12 (abstract SL-11).

Korn, W.D. (1991). Six-month oral toxicity study with Remifemin granulate in rats followed by an eight-week recovery period. Hannover, Germany: International Bioresearch.

Kruse, S.O., Löehning, A., Pauli, G.F., Winterhoff, H., and Nahrstedt, A. (1999). Fukiic and piscidic acid esters from the rhizome of *Cimicifuga racemosa* and the *in vitro* estrogenic activity of fukinolic acid. *Planta Medica* 65: 763-764.

Lehmann-Willenbrock, E. and Riedel, H.H. (1988). Clinical and endocrinologic examinations of climacteric symptoms following hysterectomy with remaining ovaries. *Zentralblatt für Gynäkologie* 110: 611-618.

Leung, A.Y. and Foster, S. (1996). *Encyclopedia of Common Natural Ingredients Used in Food, Drugs, and Cosmetics,* Second Edition. New York: John Wiley and Sons, Inc., pp. 88-89.

Li, J.X., Kadota, S., Li, H.Y., Miyahara, T., and Namba, T. (1996). [The effect of traditional medicines on bone resorption induced by parathyroid hormone (PTH) in tissue culture: A detailed study on *Cimicifuga rhizoma*]. *Wakan Iyakugaku Zasshi [Journal of Traditional Medicine]* 13: 50-58.

Li, J.X., Kadota, S., Li, H.Y., Miyahara, T., Wu, Y.W., Seto, H., and Namba, T. (1996/1997). Effects of *Cimicifugae* rhizoma on serum calcium and phosphate levels in low calcium dietary rats and on bone mineral density in ovariectomized rats. *Phytomedicine* 3: 379-385.

Li, J.X., Li, H.Y., Miyahara, T., Kadota, S., Wu, Y.W., Seto, H., Kakishita, M., and Namba, T. (1995). [Anti-osteoporotic activity of traditional medicines: active constituents of *Cimicifuga* rhizoma]. *Wakan Iyakugaku Zasshi* [*Journal of Traditional Medicine*] 12: 316-317.

Liske, E. (1998). Therapeutic efficacy and safety of *Cimicifuga racemosa* for gynecological disorders. *Advances in Therapy* 15: 45-53.

Liske, E., Gerhard, I., and Wüstenberg, P. (1997). Klimacterium: Phytokombination lindert psychovegetative leiden [Menopause: Herbal combination product for psychovegetative complaints]. *Therapiewosche Gynäkologie* 10: 172-175.

Liske, E. and Wüstenberg, P. (1998). Therapy of climacteric complaints with *Cimicifuga racemosa*: Herbal medicine with clinically proven evidence. *Menopause* 5: 250 (abstract).

Liu, J., Burdette, J.E., Xu, H., Gu, C., van Breemen, R.B., Bhat, K.P., Booth, N., Constantinou, A.I., Pezzuto, J.M., Fong, H.H., et al. (2001). Evaluation of estrogenic activity of plant extracts for the potential treatment of menopausal symptoms. *Journal of Agricultural and Food Chemistry* 49: 2472-2479.

Liu, Z., Yang, Z., Zhu, M., and Huo, J. (2001). [Estrogenicity of black cohosh *(Cimicifuga racemosa)* and its effect on estrogen receptor level in human breast cancer MCF-7 cells]. *Wei Sheng Yan Jiu* 30(2): 77-80 (in Chinese).

Löhning, A. and Winterhoff, H. (2000). Neurotransmitter concentrations after three weeks treatment with *Cimicifuga racemosa*. *Phytomedicine* 7(Suppl. 2): 13 (abstract SL-13).

Löser, B., Kruse, S.O., Melzig, M.F., and Nahrdstedt, A. (2000). Inhibition of neutrophil elastase activity by cinnamic acid derivatives from *Cimicifuga racemosa*. *Planta Medica* 66: 751-753.

McCoy, J. and Kelly, W. (1996). "Survey of *Cimicifuga racemosa* for phytoestrogenic flavonoids." Paper presented at the 212th American Chemical Society National Meeting, Orlando, FL, August 25-29 (abstract O82).

McGuffin, M., Hobbs, C., Upton, R., and Goldberg, A. (1997). *American Herbal Products Association's Botanical Safety Handbook*. Boca Raton, FL: CRC Press, pp. 29-30.

Moerman, D.E. (1986). *Medicinal Plants of Native America*, Volume 1. Ann Arbor, MI: University of Michigan Museum of Anthropology, pp. 162-163.

Moerman, D.E. (1998). *Native American Ethnobotany*. Portland, OR: Timber Press, Inc., pp.162-163.

NAPRALERT database (1997). The NAPRALERT database is owned by the Board of Trustees, University of Illinois at Chicago, and administered by the Department of Medicinal Chemistry and Pharmacognosy, Program for Collaborative Research in the Pharmaceutical Sciences, University of Illinois at Chicago. <http://www.cas.org/ONLINE/DBSS/napralertss.html>.

Nesselhut, T., Schellhase, T., Dietrich, C., and Kuhn, W. (1993). Untersuchungen zur proliferativen potenz von phytopharmaka mit ostrogenahnlicher wirkung bie mammakarzinom-zellen [Examination of the proliferative potential of phytopharmaceuticals with estrogen-mimicking activity on mammary carcinoma cells]. *Archives of Gynecology and Obstetrics* 254: 817-818.

Newall, C.A., Anderson, L.A., and Phillipson, J.D. (1996). *Herbal Medicines: A Guide for Health Care Professionals.* London: Pharmaceutical Press, pp. 80-81.

Nisslein, T. and Freudenstein, J. (2000). Effects of black cohosh on urinary bone markers and femoral density in OVX-rat model. *Osteoporosis International* 11(Suppl. 2): S191 (abstract 504).

Novitch, M. and Schweiker, R.S. (1982). Orally administered oral drug products for over-the-counter human use, establishment of a monograph. *Federal Register* 47: 55076-55101.

Reynolds, J.E.F., Parffitt, K., Parsons, A.V., and Sweetman, S.C. (Eds.) (1996). *Martindale. The Extra Pharmacopoeia,* Twenty-First Edition. England: Royal Pharmaceutical Society.

Riddle, J.M. (1997). *Eve's Herbs: A History of Contraception and Abortion in the West.* Cambridge, MA: Harvard University Press, p. 250.

Sakai, S., Kawamata, H., Kogure, T., Mantani, N., Teresawa, K., Umatake, M., and Ochiai, H. (1999). Inhibitory effect of ferulic acid and isoferulic acid on the production of macrophage inflammatory protein-2 in response to respiratory syncytial virus infection in RAW264.7 cells. *Mediators of Inflammation* 8: 173-175.

Sakai, S., Kawamata, H., Mantani, N., Kogure, T., Shimada, Y., Teresawa, K., Sakai, T., Imanishi, N., and Ochiai, H. (2000). Therapeutic effect of anti-macrophage inflammatory protein 2 antibody on influenza virus-induced pneumonia in mice. *Journal of Virology* 74: 2472-2476.

Sakai, S., Ochiai, H., Mantani, N., Kogure, T., Shibahara, N., and Teresawa, K. (2001). Administration of isoferulic acid improved the survival rate of lethal influenza virus pneumonia in mice. *Mediators of Inflammation* 10: 93-96.

Schaper and Brümmer GmbH (1997). *Remifemin: A Plant-Based Gynecological Agent.* Scientific Brochure.

Schindler, H. (1952). Die inhaltsstoffe von heilpflanzen und prüfungsmethoden für pflanzliche tinkturen [The contents of medicinal plants and a method for verifying plant tinctures]. *Arzneimittel-Forschung/Drug Research* 2: 547-549.

Seidlova-Wuttke, D., Jarry, H., Heiden, I., Hellmann, T., Christoffel, V., Spengler, M., and Wuttke, W. (2001). Evidence for selective estrogen receptor modulator (SERM) effects of the *Cimicifuga racemosa* (CR) extract BNO 1055. *Experimental and Clinical Endocrinology and Diabetes* 109(Suppl. 1): S17 (abstract v066).

Seidlova-Wuttke, D., Jarry, H., Heiden, I., and Wuttke, W. (2000). Effects of *Cimicifuga racemosa* on estrogen-dependent tissues. *Phytomedicine* 7(Suppl. 2): 11-12 (abstract SL-9b).

Shao, Y., Harris, A., Wang, M., Zhang, H., Cordell, G.A., Bowman, M., and Lemmp, E. (2000). Triterpene glycosides from *Cimicifuga racemosa. Journal of Natural Products* 63: 905-910.

Shughrue, P.J., Lane, M.V., Scrimo, P.J., and Merchenthaler, I. (1998). Comparative distribution of estrogen receptor-alpha (ER-α) and beta (ER-β) mRNA in the rat pituitary, gonad, and reproductive tract. *Steroids* 63: 498-504.

Shuster, J. (1996). ISMP adverse drug reactions. *Hospital Pharmacy* 31: 1553-1554.

Snow, J.M. (1996). *Cimicifuga racemosa* (L.) Nutt. (Ranunculaceae). *Protocol Journal of Botanical Medicine* (Spring): 17-19.

Stoll, W. (1987). [Phytopharmacon influences atrophic vaginal epithelium. Double-blind study - *Cimicifuga* versus estrogenic substances]. *Therapeuticon* 1: 23-31.

Stolze, H. (1982). Der andere weg, klimakterische beschwerden zu behandlung [The other way to treat symptoms of menopause]. *Gyne* 3: 14-16.

Strauch, B. (1995). An herb to know: Black cohosh. *The Herb Companion* (October/November): 24-25.

Struck, D.M., Tegtmeier, M., and Harnischfeger, G. (1997). Flavones in extracts of *Cimicifuga racemosa*. *Planta Medica* 63: 289.

Tu, G., Fang, Q., Guo, J., Yuan, S., Chen, C., Chen, J., Chen, Z., Cheng, S., Jin, R., Li, M., et al. (Eds.) (1992). *Pharmacopoeia of the People's Republic of China*. Guangzhou, China: Guangdong Science and Technology Press, pp. 198-199.

Vorberg, G. (1984). Therapie kilmaktarischer beschwerden. Erfolgreiche hormonfreie therapie mit Remifemin [Therapy of climacteric complaints. Successful hormone-free therapy with Remifemin]. *Zeitschrift für Allegemeinmedizin* 60: 626-629.

Warnecke, G. (1985). Beeinflussung klimakterischer beschwerden durch ein phyto-therapeutikum [Influencing menopausal symptoms with a phytotherapeutic agent]. *Medizinische Welt* 36: 871-874.

Wende, K., Mügge, C., Thurow, K., Schöpke, T., and Lindequist, U. (2001). Actaeaepoxide-3-O-β-D-xylopyranoside, a new cycloartane glycoside from the rhizomes of *Actaea racemosa (Cimicifuga racemosa)*. *Journal of Natural Products* 64: 986-989.

Willard, T. (1991). *The Wild Rose Scientific Herbal*. Calgary, Alberta, Canada: Wild Rose College of Natural Healing Ltd.

Wuttke, W., Jarry, H., Heiden, I., Westphalen, S., Seidlova-Wuttke, D., and Christoffel, V. (2000). Selective estrogen receptor modulator (SERM) activity of the *Cimicifuga racemosa* extract BNO 1055: Pharmacology and mechanisms of action. *Phytomedicine* 7(Suppl. 2): 12 (abstract SL-10).

Wuttke, W., Jarry, H., Hellmann, T., Heiden, I., Christoffel, V., Spengler, M., and Seidlova-Wuttke, D. (2001). Effects of estradiol (E2), testosterone (T) and of 2 plant extracts on expression of various estrogen-regulated genes in the heart and bone of orchidectomized (orchex) rats. *Experimental and Clinical Endocrinology and Diabetes* 109(Suppl. 1): S22 (abstract v088).

Yen, K.Y. (1992). *The Illustrated Chinese Materia Medica: Crude and Prepared*. Taipei, Taiwan: SMC Publishing Inc., p. 79.

Zava, D.T., Dollbaum, C.M., and Blen, M. (1998). Estrogen and progestin bio-activity of foods, herbs, and spices. *Proceedings of the Society for Experimental Biology and Medicine* 217: 369-378.

Zheng, Q.Y., He, K., Pilkington, L., Shao, Y., and Zheng, B. (1999). CimiPure *(Cimicifuga racemosa):* A standardized black cohosh extract with novel triterpene glycoside for menopausal women. In Shahidi, F. and Ho, C.T. (Eds.), *Phytochemicals and Phytopharmaceuticals* (pp. 360-370). Champaign, IL: AOCS Press.

Zhu, Y.P. (1998). *Chinese Materia Medica: Chemistry, Pharmacology and Applications*. Amsterdam, The Netherlands: Harwood Academic, pp. 102-105.

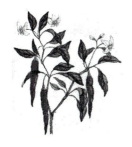

Capsicum

BOTANICAL DATA

Classification and Nomenclature

Scientific name: *Capsicum annuum* L., *Capsicum frutescens* L.

Family name: Solanaceae

Common names: capsicum, chile or chili pepper, hot pepper, cayenne, red pepper, tabasco paprika pepper, sweet pepper, bell pepper, green pepper (Rosengarten, 1969), Spanish pepper, gach-mirichi or lal-mirichi (Hindi) (Nadkarni, 1976), piment de cayenne (French), cayennepfeffer (German)

Description

Capsicum annuum is native to the tropical Americas and widely cultivated throughout the tropics and elsewhere (Rosengarten, 1969). There is confusion regarding the classification of *Capsicum* species. Currently, all varieties of mild and hot peppers (not to be confused with black and white pepper derived from *Piper nigrum* and related species) are considered as the fruits of a single species, *C. annuum* and its many varieties, or of two species, *C. annuum* and *C. frutescens*. Current practice is to classify the pungent varieties of pepper (chile peppers or cayenne peppers) as *C. frutescens,* and the milder-flavored sweet peppers (bell peppers, sweet peppers, green peppers) as varieties of *C. annuum* (Vaughan and Geissler, 1997); however, most botanists agree that they should properly be regarded as varieties of a single species (Rosengarten, 1969). Bell peppers are mild in flavor, whereas "paprikas" are slightly pungent or mild and "cayennes" or "chilies" are the hot cultivars (Vaughan and Geissler, 1997).

Capsicum annuum is an annual herb that grows to a height of 1-5 m with singly borne greenish or white flowers 10-15 mm wide. The leaves greatly

65

vary in length, from 1.5 to 12 cm, as do the fruits (0.8-30 cm), which are hollow berries containing many seeds. Their shape also varies, from nearly spherical to elongated, and may be found in colors of red, brownish-purple, or yellow, and green when unripe. *Capsicum frutescens* is widely cultivated for its extremely pungent fruits, which are small (2-3 cm long) and have a conical shape. Unlike *C. annuum,* its flowers are borne in groups (Vaughan and Geissler, 1997). Early authorities differentiated the species by the rather shrubby stem of *C. frutescens* which is absent in *C. annuum* (Dasgupta and Fowler, 1997).

HISTORY AND TRADITIONAL USES

Archaeologists estimate that in Mexico, *Capsicum* was used as a food as long as 9,000 years ago (Rumsfield and West, 1991) and that it was first cultivated sometime between 5,000 and 3,000 B.C.E. (Vaughan and Geissler, 1997). In Peru, where chilies were grown as early as around 2,000 B.C.E., the Incas are said to have prespiced their fish by throwing chilies into the lakes they fished (Dasgupta and Fowler, 1997). Columbus brought the plant to Europe whereafter it spread south to Africa and eventually reached Asia (Vaughan and Geissler, 1997), and was then exported from Pernambuco, Brazil to India at the end of the fifteenth century (Dasgupta and Fowler, 1997). Today, it is estimated that *Capsicum* is consumed by close to 25% of the population worldwide (Szallasi and Blumberg, 1999).

In folk medicine, *Capsicum* is regarded as an aphrodisiac, depurative, digestive, stomachic, carminative, antispasmodic, diaphoretic, antiseptic, counterirritant, rubefacient, astringent, and tonic. Internally, *Capsicum* has been used to treat asthma, pneumonia, diarrhea, cramps, colic, toothache, and flatulent dyspepsia without inflammation; insufficiency of peripheral circulation; as a gargle for sore throat, chronic pharyngitis and laryngitis; and externally as a lotion or ointment to treat neuralgia, including rheumatic and arthritic pain, and unbroken chilblains (cold injuries) (Duke, 1985; Leung and Foster, 1996; Newall et al., 1996).

The medicinal use of a number of *Capsicum* species, including *C. annuum* by the Mayans, is described in an article by Chichewicz and Thorpe (1996). The Mayans used the roots, leaves, as well as the fruits in applications for infections, fresh burns, respiratory complaints, earaches, and sores. The Aztecs combined chilies with honey to treat coughs. An infusion of salt and chilies was drunk for treating persistent cough (Dasgupta and Fowler, 1997).

Moerman (1998) records that nursing women of the Ramah-Navajo tribe applied the powdered fruits [*C. annuum* var. *frutescens* (L.) Kuntze] to their breasts as a weaning agent. The Cherokee used the same plant to remedy colds and colics, and as a powerful stimulant. They applied a poultice of the plant to treat gangrene and to the soles of the feet to treat low fevers. The Ramah-Navajo used the fruits (*C. annuum* L. var. *annuum*) as a condiment or spice in stews and soups, as did the Pima and Papago, and the Hopi, Keresan, Navajo, and Sia tribes (*C. annuum* L.).

Traditional Indian medicinal uses of *C. annuum* include: a plaster consisting of storax, garlic, pepper, and *Capsicum* for the treatment of lumbago; lozenges containing tragacanth, sugar, and *Capsicum* for hoarseness; a tincture for the treatment of flatulence or poor appetite; combined with *Cinchona* bark for the treatment of advanced rheumatism and gout; and snakebites (Nadkarni, 1976).

The root of *Capsicum* is used as an Indonesian folk remedy for gonorrhea. In central Africa *Capsicum* is used as a calming medicine, and in Hawaiian folk medicine it is used for backaches, rheumatism, and swollen feet. Regular ingestion of hot red pepper is recommended by some practitioners for anorexia, hemorrhoids, liver congestion, varicose veins, and vascular conditions (Duke, 1985).

The well-known characteristic of capsaicinoids to induce temporary pain has led to the use of crude extracts of hot peppers in sprays as a self-defense weapon. These sprays typically contain a 10% solution diluted in solvents (Reilly, Crouch, Yost, and Fatah, 2001).

CHEMISTRY

Phenolic Compounds

The most potent and predominant chemical entity in *Capsicum* is capsaicin (0.14%) (Cordell and Araujo, 1993). A series of homologous branched- and straight-chain alkyl vanillylamides, collectively known as capsaicinoids, is present in lesser concentrations than the parent compound, capsaicin. Of the capsaicinoid fraction, capsaicin (48.6%) is quantitatively followed by 6,7-dihydrocapsaicin (36%), nordihydrocapsaicin (7.4%), homodihydrocapsaicin (2%), and homocapsaicin (2%) (Duke, 1985) (see Figure 1). Capsaicinoids in *Capsicum* are collectively found in amounts of 0.1% to 2%, with quantities varying according to soil, climate, *Capsicum* variety, and harvest time. These conditions also affect the proportions of capsaicin analogues (Cordell and Araujo, 1993; Rumsfield and West, 1991; Govindarajan and Sathyanarayana, 1991; Govindarajan, 1985).

Capsaicin, a colorless crystalline substance, was first synthesized in 1930. Capsaicin has been studied since the mid-nineteenth century and its structure is elucidated as 8-methyl-6-nonenoyl vanillylamide (Cordell and Araujo, 1993). Most pharmacological studies performed with isolated constituents of chile pepper have focused on capsaicin, which is the major pungent constituent.

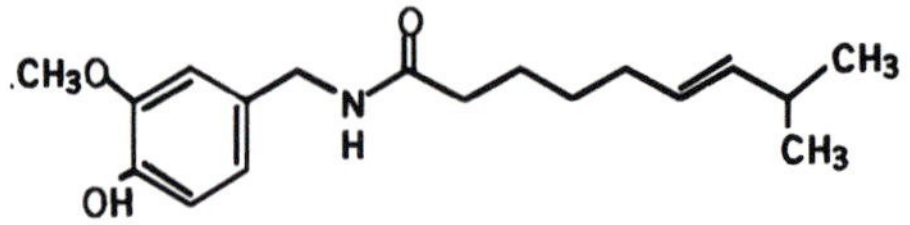

Capsaicin

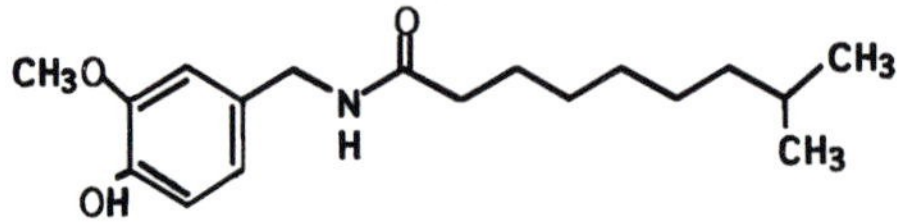

6,7-dihydrocapsaicin

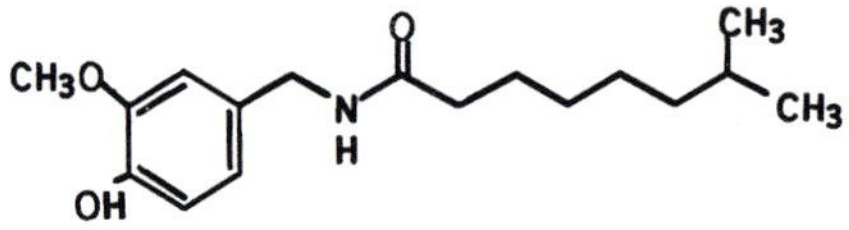

Nordihydrocapsaicin

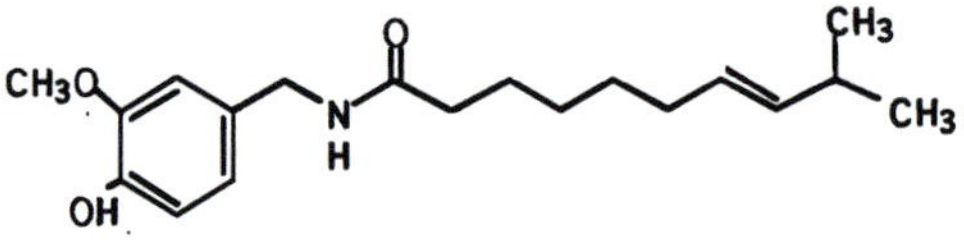

Homocapsaicin

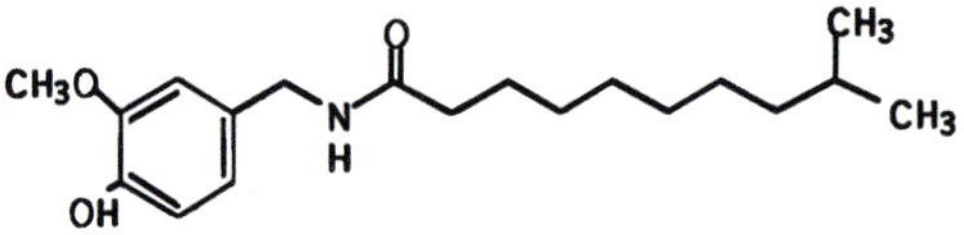

Homodihydrocapsaicin

FIGURE 1. Major Capsaicinoids in *Capsicum*

The crude extract of *Capsicum* fruits, known as *Capsicum* oleoresin, contains at least 100 different volatile chemical constituents, and therefore may function in differing ways from pure capsaicin. Thus, it is important to distinguish between studies using capsaicin and those employing *Capsicum* oleoresin (Cordell and Araujo, 1993).

Nonivamide (pelargonic acid vanillylamide) is a common synthetic adulterant of *Capsicum* products. Although structurally different from capsaicin, its presence in *Capsicum* or capsaicin samples can be detected spectrographically (Cordell and Araujo, 1993). Until recently, there was no evidence that this compound occurred naturally in *Capsicum* (Reilly, Crouch, and Yost, 2001).

Lipid Compounds

Oils

Volatile oils are present as a trace component, including over 125 individual constituents, 24 of which have been identified (Marsh, 1977).

Terpenoid Compounds

Steroids

Other parts of the plant contain steroidal alkaloid glycosides (solanine, solanidine, solasodine) (Newall et al., 1996). The seeds contain the steroidal glycosides capsicoside A through D, all of which are furostanol glycosides (Yahara et al., 1994).

Other Constituents

Capsicum annuum is rich in carotenoid pigments, including capsanthin, capsorubrin, carotene, lutein, zeaxanthin, and cucurbitaxanthin A (Leung and Foster, 1996; Hornero-Méndez and Mínguez-Mosquera, 1998).

Capsicum is also rich in fats (9-17%) and protein (12-15%) (Leung and Foster, 1996) and is an excellent source of vitamin C (~370 mg/100 g) and vitamin A (77,000 IU/100 g, equivalent to 7,700 RE/100 g) (Ensminger et al., 1993).

Scopoletin, a coumarin, also occurs in the plant (Newall et al., 1996).

THERAPEUTIC APPLICATIONS

Despite the widespread use of chili peppers in the diet, little is known about the pharmacological activities of capsaicin in humans. Much of the pharmacological information has been obtained from animals with intravenous or intraperitoneal injections, or direct application of capsaicin to exposed nerves. Intravenous administration of capsaicin has been observed to induce bradycardia, hypotension, and apnea in animals; effects from administration to humans has been unclear (Rumsfield and West, 1991). Numerous studies on the effect of capsaicin on pain exist (Szallasi and Blumberg, 1999) while the actions of *Capsicum* remain less well understood.

PRECLINICAL STUDIES

Cardiovascular and Circulatory Functions

Cholesterol and Lipid Metabolism

As demonstrated in a study by Kawada Hagihara, et al. (1986), capsaicin affects lipid metabolism. Male rats fed a diet containing 30% lard with capsaicin at 0.14% of the diet developed serum triglyceride levels that were significantly lower than those of animals receiving a high-fat diet without capsaicin. Levels of free fatty acids, cholesterol, and pre-β-lipoprotein were not affected. Activities of liver enzymes involved in lipid synthesis (acetyl-CoA carboxylase) and in carbohydrate metabolism (glucose-6-phosphate dehydrogenase) were inhibited in the rats fed the high-fat diet. The activity of glucose-6-phosphate dehydrogenase was restored to control levels in the capsaicin-fed rats. The weight of perirenal adipose tissue was reduced in a dose-dependent manner by capsaicin. These results suggest that capsaicin did not interfere with lipid biosynthesis but rather, that capsaicin might stimulate lipid metabolism, and possibly facilitate mobilization of lipid from adipose tissue.

Peripheral Vascular Functions

Yamato et al. (1996) showed that capsaicin produced a marked concentration-dependent decrease in the amplitude, the rate of rise, and the rate of relaxation of the contractile tension of rat ventricular papillary muscles; however, the half-life of the relaxation and the time to peak tension were only slightly affected. Calcium release and shortening of action potential duration in ventricular myocytes was profoundly reduced by capsaicin, perhaps resulting from the nonspecific membrane-stabilizing effects of capsaicin.

Kaygisiz et al. (1990) reported that capsaicin treatment caused a biphasic effect on contractile force, left ventricular systolic blood pressure, and heart rate of isolated perfused rat hearts. A transient initial increase in contractile force and left ventricular systolic pressure was observed, followed by a prolonged depression of both parameters. Heart rate was increased, but this effect was not followed by a subsequent reduction. The initial increases in contractile force and blood pressure could have been induced by the release of calcitonin gene related peptide (CGRP) from local sensory nerves. The negative inotropic effects following the initial increase may be due to a direct inhibitory effect of capsaicin on ventricular cells, or to nonspecific membrane-stabilizing effects. The increased heart rate was attributed to the release of CGRP (Kaygisiz et al., 1990).

Capsaicin elicits a vasoconstrictive response in the large cerebral arteries of the cat (Saito et al., 1988), and in the middle and basilar cerebral arteries, an effect was attributed to a direct contraction of smooth muscle, since the response was independent of the presence of endothelium and nerve components. However, Saito and colleagues found results suggesting that while capsaicin releases and depletes vasodilator peptides from perivascular nerves, the direct vasoconstrictor effects overwhelm the vasodilator effects of these peptides.

Digestive, Hepatic, and Gastrointestinal Functions

Gastric Functions

In tests using cultured human intestinal epithelial cells, Jensen-Jarolim et al. (1998) found sufficient in vitro evidence to suggest that *Capsicum* may increase the permeability of the gastrointestinal tract to allow transport of macromolecules and ions across the epithelium, an effect, they add, that might have importance to food intolerance and allergic reactions to food. The transepithelial electrical resistance (TER) of confluent human intestinal epithelial cells was significantly reduced ($p < 0.001$) by paprika powder *(C. annuum),* chili pepper ($p < 0.001$), or cayenne pepper *(C. frutescens; $p < 0.005$).* A sustained decrease in TER by paprika correlated with an increase in permeability for ≤ 40 kDa-sized macromolecules, which are sufficient for important plant-derived allergenic proteins to pass (i.e., MW 14 and 17 kDa). However, while chili pepper, cayenne pepper, and paprika may loosen cell contacts to increase permeability of the intestinal epithelium, other spices (bay leaf, black pepper, and nutmeg) were found to decrease permeability (Jensen-Jarolim et al., 1998). This is interesting because in diets in which these spices are used most commonly they are typically combined in dishes, a practice that could conceivably counteract an increase in gastrointestinal epithelial cell permeability.

Graham et al. (1988) concluded on the basis of direct visualization of the human stomach that ingestion of a spicy meal by normal individuals was not associated with acute damage to the stomach mucosa.

A number of studies have shown that capsaicin exerts gastroprotective effects in rodents (Holzer and Lippe, 1988; Holzer et al., 1989, 1990). Administered concomitantly with aspirin (25 mM), capsaicin dose-dependently (160 μm by intragastric perfusion) inhibited aspirin-induced injury to the gastric mucosa of rats, resulting in 62% less lesion formation and 92% less bleeding (Holzer et al., 1989). Intragastric administration of capsaicin (160 μm) to rats reduced the formation of mucosal lesions caused by 25% ethanol and enhanced blood flow of the gastric mucosa by 89% (Holzer et al., 1990).

The stimulatory effect of orally administered capsaicin on gastric acid secretion and mucosal blood flow was studied in rats using amounts roughly equivalent to a normal Thai diet. The protective effect of capsaicin against ethanol-induced gastric lesions was attenuated upon pretreatment with indomethacin and disappeared in capsaicin-sensitive nerve-degenerated rats, suggesting that enhanced prostaglandin formation inhibited lesion formation (Uchida et al., 1991); however, others reported no interference against the gastroprotective effect of capsaicin in rats from pretreatment with indomethicin (Holzer et al., 1990). Further study found decreased stomach motility and increased mucosal blood flow with intragastric capsaicin treatment, whereas capsaicin pretreatment desensitized the afferent neurons, thereby mitigating this protective effect (Uchida et al., 1991).

Either intragastric or subcutaneous administration of capsaicin (2 mg i.g. or s.c.) was found to exert gastroprotective effects against ethanol-induced damage in rats. When administered intragastric pretreatment doses of chili powder comparable to those consumed by humans (200 mg/day for four weeks or ≥ 200 mg i.g. acutely), rats also showed protection from ethanol-induced damage to the gastric mucosa, although not to the extent of protection provided by capsaicin at 5 mg i.g. The gastric mucosa and juice of capsaicin- and chili-treated rats showed higher contents of mucus compared to controls, which may be fundamental to the protective effect (Kang, Yeoh et al., 1995).

Anuras et al. (1977) demonstrated effects of capsaicin on electrical slow waves in the isolated cat colon that paralleled the reported effects of other laxative agents. It has long been observed that oral ingestion of *Capsicum* can result in a laxative effect in humans, especially if the individual is unaccustomed to the dose taken.

Endocrine and Hormonal Functions

Adrenal Functions

Kawada, Watanabe, et al. (1986) measured the effect of capsaicin (6 mg/kg i.p.) on the general energy metabolism of rats, including oxygen consumption, respiratory quotient, and substrate utilization. Capsaicin had a general stimulatory effect on metabolism, similar to that of epinephrine; oxygen consumption was elevated, respiratory quotient was initially elevated, then decreased; and serum glucose and insulin levels were elevated, concomitant with a rapid decrease in liver glycogen, and a gradual increase in serum triglycerides. The response was blocked by β-adrenergic blockers, but was not affected by α-adrenergic or ganglion blockers. These results suggest that capsaicin affects metabolism either as a direct β-adrenergic agonist, or indirectly by stimulating catecholamine release.

Carbohydrate Metabolism; Antidiabetic Activity

Monsereenusorn (1980) measured a hypoglycemic effect of crude *Capsicum* on blood glucose levels in the rat. Oral administration at 1,200 mg/kg resulted in an 18% reduction in fasting blood glucose levels, while i.p. administration resulted in a similar reduction (16.9%) at 700 mg/kg. In glucose tolerance tests, pretreatment with *Capsicum* (500 mg/kg p.o.) flattened the oral glucose tolerance curve compared to controls. A small but significant reduction in blood glucose levels was observed when the glucose load was administered intracardially, suggesting that capsaicin induced changes in systemic glucose metabolism. In earlier studies (Monsereenusorn, 1979; Monsereenusorn and Glinsukon, 1979), using everted sacs of rat and hamster jejunum, capsaicin caused a significant inhibition of glucose transport across the intestinal wall at pH 7.4, but only a slight inhibition at pH 5.0. Capsaicin at pH 7.4 increased the conversion of glucose to lactic acid, indicating a stimulatory effect on glucose metabolism; however, at the lower pH value of 5.0, glucose metabolism was suppressed with a concomitant increase in glucose transport across the intestinal wall. The authors speculated that at the lower pH oxidative glucose metabolism was disturbed, with the mucosal cells compensating by enhancing anaerobic glucose metabolism with a consequent increase in lactic acid formation (Monsereenusorn, 1979; Monsereenusorn and Glinsukon, 1979).

A partial mechanism for the inhibition of glucose transport across the intestinal wall was suggested in experiments by Monsereenusorn and Glinsukon (1979). In everted sac preparations, capsaicin (14 mg/100 mL) produced a 22.6% inhibition of the intestinal Na^+-K^+-ATPase sodium pump in hamsters, although not in the rat. In the small intestine of hamsters and rats, there are high levels of these pumps. In addition to their potential involvement in active transport of cations across cell membranes, these pumps have been implicated in the sodium-dependent active transport of amino acids and sugar (Monsereenusorn and Glinsukon, 1979).

Immune Functions; Inflammation and Disease

Cancer

Chemopreventive activity. An in vitro chemopreventive activity of capsaicin was shown by Morré et al. (1995). When capsaicin was added to cultured cells of Caov-3 human ovarian carcinoma, MCF-10A human mammary adenocarcinoma, HL-60 human promyelocytic leukemia, and HeLa cervical carcinoma cells, a preferential growth inhibition was evident as cells became smaller and underwent cell death. Condensed and appearing fragmented, the nuclear DNA of these cells suggested that capsaicin had induced apoptosis. Miller et al. (1993) reported that capsaicin (0.5 μm) inhibited the in vitro formation of liver enzyme metabolites of NKK or nitrosamine 4-(methylnitrosamino)-1-(3-pyridyl)-1-butanone, a carcinogen found in tobacco smoke. Since capsaicin inhibited the formation of all NKK metabolites, the authors suggest that it acts as an anticarcinogen and antimutagenic.

Zhang et al. (1997) administered single doses of capsaicin (2 mg/kg and 10 mg/kg p.o. in olive oil) to male Syrian golden hamsters in a study of its potential chemopreventive effects against liver and lung metabolism of NKK. The doses were calculated to approximate the estimated daily intake of capsaicinoids by people in Thailand and Korea (8 mg/kg) and Mexico (1.6 mg/kg). Liver microsomes obtained 6 and 24 h after the administration of capsaicin showed significantly enhanced in vitro inhibition of keto aldehyde formation at both harvest times. In the lung microsomes, in vitro metabolism of NKK also showed significant changes. Either dose of capsaicin inhibited N-oxidation of NKK and in microsome harvest at either time. Both doses also caused a significant inhibition of total α-carbon hydroxylation of NKK and a significant increase in unmetabolized NKK was observed, although only in microsomes harvested at 6 h posttreatment. Keto aldehyde and keto alcohol formation were also inhibited by capsaicin at both times, but from the higher dose only at 6 h posttreatment. These results suggest that capsaicin would produce a greater chemopreventive effect against NKK-induced lung cancer cells than NKK-induced liver cancer cells.

Jung et al. (2001) reported the chemopreventive activity of capsaicin (IC_{50} 90 μm) against the in vitro growth of SK-Hep-1 hepatocarcinoma cells. Dose-dependent inhibition of SK-Hep-1 cell growth was found to involve upregulation of Bax, a key apoptosis-linked gene. Noncancerous cells and human breast epithelial cells showed no growth inhibition from treatment with capsaicin (100 μm), suggesting that it may function as a tumor-specific growth inhibitor. Kim et al. (1997) reported that capsaicin induced cell death (apoptosis) and inhibited the growth of human stomach tumor cells (SNU-1) in vitro at concentrations of >1 mM, an effect that appears to have been at least partly facilitated by inducing overexpression of c-myc and/or p53 genes.

Capsaicin added to the diet of mice (0.01%) significantly inhibited the development of lung tumors induced by polycyclic aromatic hydrocarbons (benzo[a]pyrene and DMBA). Greatest inhibition was found against DMBA-induced tumor development in female mice (Jang et al., 1989). In a nitrosamine-induced multiorgan model of carcinogenesis in rats, capsaicin added to the diet (0.01%) significantly decreased the incidence of lung tumors and induction of GST-P+ hepatic foci, whereas the incidence of tumors in other organs was no different compared to controls, except that in the urinary bladders of capsaicin-treated rats there was a higher incidence of nodular or papillary hyperplasia (Jang et al., 1991). In theory, this may have resulted from an interaction of capsaicin with the high amount of nitrosamines in the drinking water of the rats (0.05%), in addition to the high amounts they received by injection (total dose, 180 mg/kg i.p.).

Infectious Diseases

Microbial infections. In Mayan herbal medicine, *Capsicum* species were used as antimicrobials. Including capsaicin and dihydrocapsaicin, Chichewicz and Thorpe (1996) used a filter-disk assay to assess the antimicrobial activity of several varieties of five species (*C. annuum, C. baccatum, C. chinense, C. frutescens,* and *C. pubescens*) against a range of pathogenic bacteria and one yeast, *Candida albicans.* The pure capsaicinoids showed no antimicrobial activity. In general, the extracts displayed varying degrees of inhibition against *Bacillus cereus, B. subtilis, Clostridium sporogenes, C. tetani,* and *Streptococcus pyogenes.* In some cases, heating the extracts to 100°C for 20 min resulted in a complete or partial loss of activity. Most significantly, uncooked extracts of all species and varieties produced complete or partial inhibition of the growth of *Clostridium sporogenes* and *C. tetani,* indicating that the use of *Capsicum* species in Mayan medicine may have been related to the prevention or treatment of *Clostridium*-related diseases. Growth of *Bacillus* species in general was stimulated by the extracts, except for the leaves of the jalapeño and red chile varieties of *C. annuum,* which partially inhibited the growth of *B. cereus* and *B. subtilis.*

Capsaicin has shown little growth-inhibitory activity in vitro against *Escherichia coli* (DH5α Difco ATCC 25922), *Pseudomonas solanacearum* (ssp. Kodiak), or *Saccharomyces cerevisiae* (wild strain 288C) even at high concentrations (200 or 300 μg/mL). Against *Bacillus subtilis* (ssp. Kodiak), capsaicin showed potent inhibitory activity at a concentration of 25 μg/mL (Mollina-Torres et al., 1999).

Capsaicin has shown significant dose-dependent inhibitory activity (10-50 μg/mL) on the growth of *Helicobacter pylori* strain LC-11 at a broth pH value of 7.4. At the highest concentration, capsaicin also inhibited in vitro growth of *H. pylori* at pH values of 6.4 (72%) and 5.4 (92%); however, ten times that concentration was necessary to inhibit the growth of clinical strains of *H. pylori* (LC 28 and LC 32), which were inhibited by 89.9% and 91.4%, respectively (Jones, Shabib et al., 1997).

Tsuchiya (2001) proposes that the antibacterial activity of capsaicin is mediated by its ability to fluidize the outer cellular membrane of bacteria, which was demonstrated in lipids using concentrations of capsaicin previously shown to inhibit the in vitro growth of bacteria (50-100 μM). The ability to fluidize membranes may also help to elucidate the mechanism whereby capsaicin inhibits platelet aggregation.

Inflammatory Response

The immunomodulatory effects of capsaicin are varied and may be related to interactions with the neuropeptides somatostatin and SP, a peptide made up of 11 amino acids which is found throughout the body in nerve cells and certain endocrine cells in the gut. Payan et al. (1984) hypothesized that exposure to noxious stimuli or injury of sufficient magnitude stimulates the release of SP and somatostatin from peripheral terminals of primary afferent neurons. SP triggers vasodilation, increases permeability of regional microcirculation, and activates mast cells which release histamine, leukotactic peptides, and leukotrienes. Histamine and leukotrienes LTC_4 and LTD_4 increase vascular permeability, and peptide leukotactic factors stimulate the influx of polymorphonuclear leukocytes (PMNs) and monocytes that have adhered to venular walls. SP also magnifies the functional responses elicited by the leukotriene LTB_4. In addition, increased vascular permeability promotes the local delivery of both the protein and cellular components of adaptive immunity, so that SP could augment the activity of T lymphocytes that accumulate at the site of reaction (Payan et al., 1984). However, opposite of what might have been expected, capsaicin pretreatment was shown to block the localized immune and inflammatory response. This effect was observed in studies described previously, in which capsaicin prevented the SP-mediated increase in vascular permeability and inflammation in lung tissue exposed to noxious stimuli (Biggs and Ladenius, 1990; Krishna and Ghosh, 1989; Lundberg and Saria, 1983). Other studies focusing on the role of SP and other neuropeptides in mediating the antigenic response have, in general, supported this hypothesis. For example, SP stimulates synthesis of lymphocytes and stimulates production of immunoglobulins (Stanisz et al., 1986; Helme et al., 1987). Pretreatment of neonatal rats with capsaicin reduced by more than 80% the number of lymphocytes secreting antigenic antibodies in response to a subcutaneous antigenic stimulus of sheep red blood cells. This was reversed by a subcutaneous infusion of SP at the injection site immediately following antigen stimulation (Helme et al., 1987).

The arachidonic acid cascade is an important component of inflammation and the associated localized immune response. The release of arachidonic acid (AA) from membrane phospholipids and subsequent leukotriene biosynthesis occurs during inflammation, and products formed by arachidonic acid oxidation act in concert with numerous other factors, including cytokines, PAF (platelet-activating factor), nitrogen oxide, and histamine, all of which are important mediators of the immune response. An in vitro study (Panossian et al., 1996) found that at low concentrations, capsaicin stimulated the production of interleukin-1∝, while at higher doses it inhibited this response. Capsaicin caused a dose-dependent release of arachidonic acid from PMNs (poly-morphonuclear leukocytes), and a similar concentration-dependent conversion of the arachidonic acid metabolites, prostaglandin E_2 (PGE_2) and LTB_4. When incubated with granulocytes, capsaicin caused an increased synthesis of 12-HETE, an eicosanoid metabolite of arachidonic acid, but at the same time was found to cause a dose-dependent decrease of all products of 5-lipoxygenase. These results suggested that the dose-dependent reversible effects of capsaicin on immune cells and interleukin-1$\propto$ are closely associated with arachidonic acid metabolism (Panossian et al., 1996).

Capsaicin (278 µM) inhibited collagen-induced platelet aggregation of rat platelets (Wang et al., 1984), and by action(s) separate from sensory afferent neurons, inhibited the aggregation of rabbit platelets by 50% at a concentration of 39-88 µM (Hogaboam and Wallace, 1991). As to what these actions are, Tsuchiya (2001) has produced evidence to suggest that capsaicin fluidizes lipid membranes (50-250 µM), and with a potency greater than benzyl alcohol or lidocaine and comparable to that of 4-ethylphenol or geraniol.

In a guinea pig model of arthritis, treating the animals with capsaicin at gradually larger doses every two to three days (0.5-10 mg/kg s.c.; total 27.5 mg/kg s.c.) for 14 days before inducing inflammation significantly ameliorated the progression of arthritis compared to vehicle-treated controls. The capsaicin group showed 20% less footpad swelling, fewer T cells (but not macrophages) in their inflamed joints, and an overall 28% reduction in scores of bone demineralization, soft tissue swelling, the formation of new bone (periostitis), erosions, and cartilage spacing in their inflamed limbs (Hood et al., 2001). However, comparatively greater reductions in joint diameters from capsaicin have been observed in rat models of arthritis (Hood et al., 2001 citing Cruwys et al., 1995 and Levine et al., 1987).

Metabolic and Nutritional Functions

Antioxidant Activity

In a quantitative HPLC method of determining antioxidant activity, capsaicin inhibited the formation of lipid hydroperoxides by about 30% at a concentration of 0.001 M and by 60% at double that concentration. At the same respective concentrations, BHT (butylated hydroxytoluene) inhibited lipid peroxide formation by 80% and 90% (Henderson et al., 1999).

Pharmacokinetics

Oral dosing of rats with capsaicin and dihydrocapsaicin results in an 85% absorption in the jejunum after 3 h (Rumsfield and West, 1991; Kawada et al., 1984).

The distribution and metabolism of capsaicin and/or dihydrocapsaicin has been studied in rats. Capsaicin is distributed to the brain, spinal cord, liver and blood within 20 min of i.v. administration. Oral doses of dihydrocapsaicin in the rat showed metabolic activity associated with its absorption into the portal vein. Capsaicin and dihydrocapsaicin are metabolized in the liver by the mixed-function oxidation system (cytochrome P-450-dependent system). It is assumed that capsaicin is excreted in urine. In rats, most of dihydrocapsaicin is known to be rapidly metabolized and excreted in the urine (Rumsfield and West, 1991).

Neurological, Psychological, and Behavioral Functions

Receptor- and Neurotransmitter-Mediated Functions

In a study by Lee (1954), ripe red chili paste was applied to the mouth or lips of 46 apparently experienced chili eaters and was used to measure gustatory sweating. Flushing and venous engorgement of the head and neck areas were noted, as well as lacrimation and nasal discharge. However, after repeated applications in close succession, sweating and reports of pain or pungency were reduced, notably after the fourth round. Application to the lips only elicited sweating, which led to the conclusion that pain sensors were involved more than taste sensors. When peppers were ingested after the mouth was numbed with a local anesthetic, no sweating was elicited; an application of atropine also abolished sweating, demonstrating that the nerve fibers affected were cholinergic. Lee (1954) concluded that the same nerve fibers that controlled emotional, thermal, or other forms of sweating also controlled gustatory sweating, and noted that gustatory sweating and factors promoting sweating acted in an additive way.

The ability of capsaicin-sensitive afferent fibers to innervate joints, muscles, and various areas of the genitourinary, respiratory, and cardiovascular systems, led to new understandings of the mechanisms of pain (Wood, 1993). Over the past 20 years, research has shown that primary afferent neurons of the pain pathway, known as nociceptors, are the selective target of capsaicin, the majority being C fibers (Caterina and Julius, 2001), a population of unmyelinated primary afferent sensory neurons. Capsaicin- or vanilloid-sensitive neurons are found in abundance in the cornea, mucous membrane of the oral cavity, and the skin (Fuller, 1990).

Many of capsaicin's cardiovascular effects and effects on respiratory reflex functions can be attributed to its excitation of a distinct population of these neurons in the vagus nerve (pneumogastric or tenth cranial nerve). Intact sensory supply is required for many of the actions of capsaicin. For example, deafferentiation of the skin areas and guinea pig ileum abolishes many capsaicin-induced responses, such as the inflammatory response and smooth muscle contraction (Nagy, 1982). Some of the unmyelinated sensory fibers sensitive to capsaicin contain the neuropeptide substance P (SP) and somatostatin. SP is a highly potent vasoactive substance which appears to be a neurotransmitter. It mediates sensory pain, temperature, and touch. Capsaicin can stimulate the release of these neuropeptides (Szolcsányi et al., 1998). Prolonged exposure to capsaicin results in a gradual desensitization to capsaicin's acute effects. This may be due to diverse mechanisms, including: increased production of nitric oxide in the spine; glutamate release from terminals of vanilloid-sensitive nerves facilitating release of SP; increased levels of cAMP allowing for the release of SP from vanilloid-sensitive nerves, and others (Meyer et al., 1994). The role of SP in topical applications of capsaicin-containing preparations is complicated by the fact that capsaicin has shown poor bioavailability in human skin, and biopsy samples of skin treated with topical capsaicin show insignificant immunoreactivity to SP (Munn et al., 1997). In addition, because the pronounced irritating effect of capsaicin has limited its use in the treatment of pain, research is being devoted to related compounds with less irritating effects, which still retain its beneficial actions (Kasting et al., 1997; Cruz, 1998).

CLINICAL STUDIES

Digestive, Hepatic, and Gastrointestinal Disorders

Gastric Disorders

Gastroprotection. The intraesophageal administration of a suspension of red pepper sauce (total capsaicinoid content, 0.35 mg/mL; capsaicin 0.168 mg/mL) compared to saline in seven healthy volunteers produced a significant delay in the gastric emptying rate without affecting the ororececal time, implying that intestinal transit was increased. It was reasoned that the changes on the upper gastrointestinal motility induced by red pepper sauce could improve clearance of the esophagus (Gonzalez et al., 1998).

Yeoh et al. (1995) examined the protective effect of chili pepper against aspirin-induced damage to the gastroduodenal mucosa reported in rats in 18 nonsmoking, healthy adult volunteers, none of whom had recently used NSAIDs. Subjects abstained from using chili for two weeks prior to the treatment period. In this study, 20 g of chili powder (capsaicin content, 0.478 mg/g) in 200 mL water was ingested and 30 min later, a single 600-mg dose of aspirin with the same amount of water was ingested. Two weeks later, the experiment was repeated with 200 mL water with no chili powder followed by aspirin with water and endoscopic examination 6 h later as before. The endoscopist was blinded as to which patients had taken chili powder. The results showed a significant difference in median lesion scores between the two treatments, with a score of 1.5 for the chili group and 4 in the control group. In another study, the gastroprotective effect of chili was associated with a lower incidence of peptic ulcer among the population of India and Malaysia compared to Chinese residents of Singapore who have traditionally consumed comparatively less chili (Yeoh et al., 1995 citing Kang et al., 1995).

A study of the effect of chili powder on the healing of duodenal ulcers was conducted in 50 inpatients. The patients were randomly assigned to one of two groups: a group that would consume regular hospital food without chili powder and six times daily take a liquid antacid (Aludrox MH, 15 mL at one and 6 h after each meal); and a group that would receive 1,000 mg chili powder in each of three daily hospital meals, in addition to receiving the antacid treatment. After four weeks, endoscopic examination showed that the addition of chili powder to the antacid regimen, which was administered in a dosage previously found to be optimal for healing duodenal ulcers, had no effect on healing the ulcers. No evidence of damage to the gastric mucosa such as erosions or hyperemia was found (Kumar et al., 1984).

Integumentary, Muscular, and Skeletal Disorders

Skin Disorders

Ellis et al. (1993) reported their results of a placebo-controlled, double-blind study in 197 patients with pruritic (itchy) psoriasis treated with a cream containing 0.025% capsaicin or vehicle (q. i. d. topical applications for six weeks). The capsaicin group showed significantly superior improvement in relief from pruritis ($p = 0.60$), improvement in physician's global evaluation ($p = 0.030$), and in combined severity of psoriasis scores (pruritis, scaling, erythema, and thickness scores combined) ($p = 0.036$) compared to placebo. The side effect most reported by both groups was a "transient burning sensation" at the sites of application. It was concluded that topical capsaicin is an effective treatment for pruritic psoriasis. Bernstein et al. (1986) reported similar benefits compared to vehicle-treated controls in a six-week, double-blind trial of capsaicin-containing cream in 44 patients with moderate to severe psoriasis.

Munn et al. (1997) conducted a double-blind study of topical capsaicin in the treatment of prurigo nodularis in which two concentrations were compared. A weaker concentration of 0.025% was just as effective as one containing 0.075% capsaicin. For 5/14 patients, skin lesions completely flattened and itching was resolved after just 14 days of treatment.

Metabolic and Nutritional Disorders

Metabolism and Nutrient Utilization

In an open-label, comparative study of 12 individuals accustomed to eating spicy foods (ages 19-22), the resting metabolic rate (RMR) after ingesting spicy (3 g mustard and chili sauce) or nonspicy meals was measured. A statistically significant increase of 25% in the postspicy meal RMR was measured, peaking at around 75-90 min postmeal. The peak increase in the nonspicy meal was smaller and came earlier at 60-75 min. After 180 min, the length of the study, the metabolic rate after the spicy meal was still relatively elevated (Henry and Emery, 1986).

The addition of hot red pepper to the breakfast meals of eight male middle and long distance runners (ages 21-23 years) was also reported to increase carbohydrate oxidation, whether the runners were exercising or resting. The ingestion of an acute dose of hot red pepper (10 g) also caused a significant increase in plasma norepinephrine and epinephrine 30 min after the meal, and in blood lactate concentrations at 60 and 150 min after the meal compared to controls; however, energy expenditure and oxygen consumption showed a nonsignificant increase at 30 min after the chili breakfast (Lim et al., 1997).

In a pilot study, a ~30% increase in energy expenditure and oxygen consumption in men right after consuming a meal containing hot red peppers was attributed to β-adrenergic stimulation since these effects were absent after β-adrenergic blockade (Yoshioka et al., 1995). In a small follow-up study in 13 healthy Japanese women (mean age 25.8; mean weight 54.2 kg; mean body fat 25.3%), researchers measured differences in lipid oxidation, carbohydrate oxidation, and energy expenditure before and during 210 min after subjects ate experimental breakfasts containing varying proportions of hot red pepper, fat, carbohydrates, and combinations thereof, or control meals. A significant increase in postprandial oxygen consumption was observed after meals containing hot red pepper. The postprandial resting quotient (RQ) of the women showed a significant decrease right after they consumed high-fat or high-carbohydrate meals containing the capsicum (Yoshioka et al., 1998), the opposite effect found in the pervious study in men (Yoshioka et al., 1995). This is possibly due to the greater numbers of type I fibers in the muscle tissue of women, which contain a greater density of β-adrenergic receptors, thereby allowing greater skeletal muscle β-adrenergic stimulation than in men. Diet-induced thermogenesis, which was significantly higher after subjects ate the high-carbohydrate meals compared to the high-fat meals, was significantly increased for up to 150 min after meals containing capsicum. The effect was more pronounced when the capsicum was added to the high-fat meals and enough to obviate the difference in diet-induced thermogenesis between the high-fat and high-carbohydrate meals.

Changes in lipid oxidation showed much the same pattern. Between 30 and 150 min after ingestion of high-fat meals containing capsicum, lipid oxidation showed a significant increase, between 50 and 210 min, more so than when added to the high-carbohydrate meal. Conversely, for 30-60 min after ingesting a high-carbohydrate meal containing hot red peppers, there was a significantly greater decrease in carbohydrate oxidation compared to its addition in high-fat meals. It was concluded that the addition of hot red peppers to the diet is beneficial to postprandial energy expenditure and that it favorably changes the comparatively weak thermogenic effects of high-fat meals (Yoshioka et al., 1998).

Neurological, Psychological, and Behavioral Disorders

Psychological and Behavioral Disorders

Headaches/Migraine. The desensitizing action of topical capsaicin on sensory neurons may be mediated through depletion of SP in nerve endings. The release of substance P (SP) from nerve terminals of trigeminal sensory neurons in an activated state has been theorized to cause cluster headache (Sicuteri et al., 1988).

Marks et al. (1993) conducted a randomized, double-blind, placebo-controlled trial of capsaicin in the treatment of cluster headache. They treated 17 patients diagnosed with either chronic or episodic types of cluster headache using a capsaicin cream (Zostrix, GenDerm, Lincolnshire, IL, 0.025% capsaicin plus 3% camphor) or placebo (Cetaphil cream containing 3% camphor) applied twice daily for seven days by cotton-tipped applicator, 1.27 cm up the nostril corresponding to the same side of the head that patients experienced headaches. Using a visual analogue scale (VAS), patients rated the severity of their headaches and compared them to headaches they had during the three days prior to the start of treatment, during the trial, and for seven days after the last treatment. Owing to incomplete records, three patients were excluded and one from the placebo group dropped out before the treatment period started. With only 13 patients remaining, the weight of the results were therefore compromised. The authors reported that the results were favorable, with less severe headaches experienced by the capsaicin group compared to the placebo group from days 8-15, but no difference on days 1-7. The capsaicin group also showed more patients who reported headache-free days compared to the placebo group, especially during days 8-15; however, because of the small number of patients left in each treatment group, the results failed to become statistically significant.

Receptor- and Neurotransmitter-Mediated Functions

Double-blind clinical studies of topical capsaicin creams have shown significant pain relief in patients suffering from intractable chronic postherpetic neuralgia (Lynn, 1990), osteoarthritis, and rheumatoid arthritis (Deal et al., 1991), and in diabetics with painful diabetic neuropathy (Capsaicin Study Group, 1991). There are at least 50 clinical trials of topical capsaicin in the treatment of neuropathic pain. However, as Szallasi and Blumberg (1999) have pointed out, when combined with the high rate of placebo response and the high number of dropouts in these trials, plus the near impossibility of blinding something as pungent as capsaicin, the value of capsaicin for treating neuropathic pain is difficult to evaluate. Therefore, only a small selection of these trials are discussed in this review.

Oral capsaicin's gustatory and olfactory effects on habitual and non-habitual users of chili pepper were studied by Lawless et al. (1985). They found that gustatory and olfactory sensations are partially masked by capsaicin in both nonhabituated and habitual users. They also found that flavor identification was not interfered with, although habitual users were best able to discern flavors. As expected, regular users reported less intensity of what the researchers described as oral irritation from capsaicin.

Frerick et al. (2000) conducted a double-blind, placebo-controlled, parallel group multicenter trial of a standardized extract of cayenne pepper in the form of a plaster in the treatment of chronic, nonspecific low back pain of at least a 12 weeks' duration. Using a pain index, the three-week trial quantified changes in pain of maximum and average intensity during the last 14 days in which patients had to experience a reduction of pain measuring at least 30 percent. The results showed that 60.8% of those in the active (cayenne) treatment group responded to the therapy compared to 42.9% in the placebo group, and that reports of improvement were twice as frequent in the cayenne plaster group versus the placebo group. Global evaluations of physicians and patients closely matched each other, with physicians rating the active cayenne treatment as good or excellent in 75.7% cases versus the same efficacy rating for the placebo in 47.4% of cases. The only side effects were local reactions related to initial hyperemic action of the cayenne. It was concluded that the cayenne plaster presented a genuine alternative to other treatments for low back pain of a nonspecific nature and that the absence of systemic side effects highlight its positive profit-risk profile.

McCarthy and McCarthy (1992) studied the potential benefit of topical capsaicin (0.075%) in the treatment of painful hand joints in rheumatoid arthritis. They conducted a randomized, placebo-controlled, double-blind trial in 21 patients suffering from pain in the hands whose conditions were diagnosed as either osteoarthritis ($n = 14$) or rheumatoid arthritis ($n = 7$). Capsaicin was applied 4 times/day and assessments were made of pain, morning stiffness, joint swelling, functional capacity, grip strength, and tenderness, before and once-weekly during the four-week treatment period. Although one patient failed to complete the trial, the results showed no significant benefit in patients with rheumatoid arthritis treated with capsaicin compared to placebo, whereas the osteoarthritis patients showed significant improvements in pain and tenderness (each $p < 0.02$), at only four weeks. Tenderness and pain was reduced by about 40% compared to the control group, but no improvement was found in joint swelling, period of morning stiffness, or function. The sole side effect was a local burning sensation in the capsaicin group. These results indicated that topical capsaicin is both safe and of potential use in the treatment of pain associated with osteoarthritis of the hands.

Studies on the treatment of postmastectomy pain syndrome (PMPS) have reported good results with topical capsaicin (Dini et al., 1993; Watson and Evans, 1992). Watson and Evans (1992) conducted a randomized, parallel, double-blind, vehicle-controlled trial of a 0.075% capsaicin cream (Zostrix-HP, applied q.i.d. for six weeks) in 25 patients with PMPS. The results showed that steady pain only developed a trend to improvement compared to vehicle (placebo), whereas visual analogue scale (VAS) ratings for jabbing pain showed a significant improvement compared to vehicle ($p < 0.05$), as did pain relief ($p < 0.04$). However, no significant improvements were found compared to placebo in skin pain. Still, the number of patients who improved by ≥50% according to global ratings were significantly greater with capsaicin (62%) compared to placebo (30%) ($p < 0.007$).

The Capsaicin Study Group (1991) performed a multicenter randomized, double-blind, vehicle-controlled study of topical capsaicin (0.075%) cream in the treatment of patients diagnosed with diabetic neuropathy. Patients ranging in age from 27 to 92 were enrolled who met the criteria of stable diabetes with moderate to severe pain or either a peripheral radiculopathy or neuropathy experienced daily and of sufficient intensity to have interfered with their sleep or daily activities, exclusive of psychological causes. The majority of patients in both the capsaicin ($n = 106/138$) and vehicle ($n = 120/139$) groups taking prescription drugs, including oral analgesics were permitted to continue their medication as long as the dosages were maintained. However, topical agents were discontinued for ≥7 days before the start of the eight-week treatment period. Among those who failed to complete the trial ($n = 58$), there were more in the capsaicin group ($n = 38$) than the vehicle group ($n = 20$), and most of them withdrew because of side effects ($n = 18$ versus $n = 5$ in the vehicle group). These side effects were mostly due to a burning sensation in the skin ($n = 14/18$) versus $n = 2$ in the vehicle group, and occurred during the first two weeks of the treatment period ($n = 11/14$). Therefore, efficacy was based on results obtained from 252 patients who applied the treatment for at least two weeks and were evaluated at least once. The study was completed by 219 patients. An "intent-to-treat" analysis showed a significant difference between the groups ($p = 0.06$). The results of the physician's global evaluation showed that a significantly greater number of patients in the capsaicin group improved during each of four evaluation periods compared to vehicle-treated patients ($p = 0.05$). Patient-rated scores (visual analogue scale for pain relief and visual analogue scale for pain intensity) showed similar improvements compared to the physician's global evaluation. At week 8, relief from pain in the patient score showed the greatest difference compared to vehicle ($p = 0.005$), while the decrease in pain intensity was also greater versus vehicle ($p = 0.014$). The most frequent side effect reported in both groups was "burning" (87 versus 23 in the vehicle-treated group). Other notable side effects reported in the capsaicin- versus the vehicle-treated group were, respectively: rash-erythema (10 versus 4), exposure-irritation to other areas of the body (9 versus 1), and coughing-sneezing (16 versus 2). Capsaicin-containing cream was concluded to be both safe and effective for the treatment of painful diabetic neuropathy.

Deal et al. (1991) studied the pain-relieving effect of a cream containing capsaicin (0.025%) in the treatment of knee pain in 101 patients diagnosed with either osteoarthritis ($n = 70$) or rheumatoid arthritis ($n = 31$). In a randomized, double-blind, placebo-controlled trial, patients applied the capsaicin or vehicle (placebo) cream to their knees q.i.d. daily for four weeks. Mean reductions of pain of 33% in the osteoarthritis patients and of 57% in the rheumatoid arthritis patients were significantly greater than their respective controls using the vehicle cream ($p = 0.033$ and $p = 0.003$, respectively). Physician's global evaluations showed 80% of the capsaicin group experienced less pain after the first two weeks of the treatment. The most common side effect was a transient burning sensation where the cream was applied and was reported by 23/52 of the capsaicin group. It was concluded that the treatment was both safe and effective against arthritic pain.

Following positive results in a pilot study of capsaicin (0.075%) in a topical cream in the treatment of postherpetic (Herpes zoster) neuralgia, Bernstein et al. (1989) conducted a randomized double-blind, vehicle-controlled study in 32 patients with the disorder, all diagnosed with severe intractable postherpetic neuralgia. All had suffered from this pain for a duration of at least 12 months and experienced partial or poor control of pain using neuroleptic agents, oral analgesics, and antidepressants. Topical preparations used by the patients were discontinued for ≥7 days prior to the start of the treatment period. Oral medications were allowed provided that the dosage remained as before throughout the trial. The patients were randomized to receive either a vehicle cream or a capsaicin-containing cream of identical appearance which they were to apply locally to painful areas, three to four times daily for six weeks. Results based on the 29 patients who com-

pleted the full trial showed that according to the physician's global evaluation, 62% of those in the capsaicin group experienced less pain after two
weeks, compared to 31% of those in the vehicle group. After four weeks,
31% of the vehicle group showed reduction in pain which they maintained
throughout the rest of the trial, versus 77% maintained by the capsaicin
group ($p < 0.05$ at all time points). Pain severity ratings using the visual analogue scale for pain showed 46% of the capsaicin-treated group experienced
less pain by week 6, versus 6% of the vehicle-treated group ($p < 0.01$). Mean
decreases in initial pain scores according to the visual analogue scale (VAS)
were 30% after six weeks in the capsaicin group and 1% in the vehicle group
($p < 0.05$). On the pain relief scale, 54% of those treated with capsaicin
reported a 40% or better reduction in pain after six weeks versus 6% of the
vehicle-treated group ($p < 0.02$). Side effects of erythema and/or stinging
and burning at application sites were reported by 5/16 in the capsaicin group
and by 2/16 in the vehicle group. These results show that capsaicin cream
represents a safer approach to treating postherpetic pain than other agents
and that it may be a more effective treatment.

Miscellaneous Pharmacological Activities

The use of capsaicin by intravesical instillations (1-2 mmol/L) to treat
urge incontinence, both in patients with hypersensitivity disorders and those
with spinal detrusor hyperreflexia, was reported to be effective in the majority of cases (Cruz, 1998). In one open-label study of 79 patients diagnosed
with intractable urinary incontinence, the majority of which multiple sclerosis patients with spinal cord disease, complete continence was found in 44%
of patients with phasic detrusor hyperreflexia, improvement was satisfactory in 36%, and the treatment failed for 20%. Benefits persisted for three to
five years after treatments (De Ridder et al., 1997). Others have reported
less successful results with this treatment (Chancellor, 1997). Because of its
unpleasant side effects (burning pain leading some patients to abandon the
therapy; severe episodic autonomic dysreflexia in patients with spinal cord
lesions; unknown long-term carcinogenicity), the use of capsaicin for urinary incontinence and neurogenic pain is likely to fall into disuse (Cruz,
1998). Another vanilloid agent (RTX or resiniferatoxin, derived from
Euphorbia resinifera) which has no carcinogenicity, similar activity, and far
greater potency with little or no irritation to the bladder, is being investigated as a possible alternative to capsaicin. (Appendino and Szallasi, 1997).

DOSAGE

Dosage of the whole fruits or red pepper powder for medicinal purposes
varies between 30-120 mg, t.i.d. (Newall et al., 1996), and 30 mg to 1.2 g,

with the usual dose at 60 mg (Willard, 1991). (Note: do not bite, chew, or open capsules.)

The German Commission E provides dosages only for external use of the dried fruits of *Capsicum* (rich in capsaicin) in the treatment of adults or school-age children who have painful spasms of the muscles in the spine, shoulders, and arms: liquid preparations: 0.005-0.01% capsaicinoids; semi-liquid preparations: 0.02-0.05% capsaicinoids; poultices: 10-40 g capsa-icinods/cm^2 (Blumenthal et al., 1998).

The *British Pharmaceutical Codex* (BPC) of 1968 lists the dose of *Capsicum* tincture as between 0.3-1.0 mL; the BPC for 1934 lists the dose of "Stronger Tincture" of *Capsicum* at between 0.06-2.0 mL (Newall et al., 1996).

According to a U.S. governmental nutrition survey, the average daily consumption of hot pepper in Thailand is 60-70 mg (U.S. Interdepartmental Committee on Nutrition for National Defense, 1962; quoted in Anuras et al., 1977). Otherwise, in tropical countries human consumption of caps-aicin is usually 0.5-1.0 mg/kg (Szallasi and Blumberg, 1999).

The oleoresin dosage is listed as 0.6-2.0 mg in the BPC of 1934. Other sources (cited in Newall et al., 1996) list a dose of 1.2-1.8 mg for the oleoresin internally, and state that topical preparations should contain a maximum strength of 2.5%.

The content of capsaicin in creams used in clinical trials has ranged from 0.025 to 0.075% with the cream being applied four to five times a day to the affected area for at least four weeks (Rumsfield and West, 1991; Lynn, 1990; Capsaicin Study Group, 1991; Robbers et al., 1996).

SAFETY PROFILE

Malignant or premalignant changes were absent in the bladders of 20 patients with intractable detrusor hyperreflexia (bladder hypersensitivity) who were treated with instillations of intravesical capsaicin (1-2 μm/L) for five years (Dasgupta et al., 1998).

A case control study in India that compared incidences of stomach cancer in users and nonusers of hot chili powder reported a significant trend of association with the risk of gastric cancer in users (Notani and Jayant, 1987). A study in Mexico reported similar results in chili pepper consumers who were at a 5.5-fold greater risk for developing gastric cancers than those who abstained from its use (López-Carillo et al., 1994). However, a larger study in Italy found the opposite result. Regular consumption of chili peppers showed a significant ($p < 0.001$) trend of protection against the formation of gastric carcinoma, as did grapes, fresh fruit, tomatoes, and cooked garlic (each $p < 0.001$) (Buiatti et al., 1989). Balachandran and Sivara-mkrishnan (1995) found that the method of cooking chili peppers has a significant bearing on its potential carcinogenicity. Azizan and Blevins (1995) found that chlorophyll suppressed the albeit weak mutagenicity of capsaicin (see Toxicity in Animal Models and Mutagenicity). Closer scrutiny of differences in methods of food preparation with chili peppers among populations may help to resolve these seemingly conflicting results.

Contraindications

Capsicum has been cited as contraindicated in topical applications on damaged skin and near the eyes, and for internal use by individuals who are sensitive to the herb and may in some cases develop gastrointestinal irritations. Further contraindications in the German Commission E are found in topical applications by individuals who are allergic (sensitive) to *Capsicum* (Blumenthal et al., 1998).

Relatively mild capsaicin topical treatment has been reported to worsen contact dermatitis and allergic contact dermatitis in some individuals (Lynn, 1990).

Drug Interactions

Capsicum may interfere with antidepressant therapy utilizing MAOI (monoamine oxidase inhibitors), or with antihypertensive therapy, and may stimulate the hepatic metabolism of drugs (Newall et al., 1996).

Pregnancy and Lactation

No documented cases of adverse effects from the use of capsaicin during pregnancy have been found. Brinker (1983) states that *Capsicum* oleoresin was found to be a uterine stimulant in animals.

No information has been found regarding the entry of capsaicin into breast milk, though anecdotal information suggests that it does. Based on informal observation, children nursed by habitual users of chili peppers will eat chili pepper-seasoned solids at an early age (less than 12 months). No reports of adverse effects from the consumption of *Capsicum* related to breast-feeding have been found in the literature or from anecdotal sources. Unpublished anecdotes from lactation consultants suggest occasional isolated episodes of diarrhea/irritated perineums in young infants, but only when the mother consumed a large amount of spicy food in an episodic manner.

Side Effects

Initial topical application of capsaicin creams results in burning sensations for most, but not all people, which lessens or disappears with repeated applications. Erythema often accompanies the burning, sometimes with rash. Coughing and sneezing from aerosolized particles from dried cream residues has also been noted in some studies. These effects fade with repeated daily use (see Clinical Studies for references). Accidental contamination of other body parts, particularly the eyes, mouth, or perineal regions, can occur without careful hand washing or the use of rubber gloves for cream application (Mitchell and Rook, 1979). In a controlled study, Jones, Tanberg, et al. (1997) found that cool tap water was more effective at providing immediate relief from the pain of chili burns of the hands than room temperature vegetable oil. Immersing the hands in the vegetable oil provided significantly better long-term pain relief, as long as the hands were immersed in the oil for at least 60 min. Further studies of using cold temperature oil may reveal the effect of temperature on pain relief from chili burn.

Capsaicin and capsaicinoids are strongly irritant to mucous membranes and can produce dermatitis. Inhalation can produce allergic alveolitis (Mitchell and Rook, 1979). Oral use of *Capsicum* and its extractives may cause gastrointestinal irritation, though it does not inhibit the healing of duodenal ulcers and does not need to be avoided by persons with such a condition (Leacock, 1985). Sugar is widely believed to quell the burning sensation in the mouth caused by foods containing hot chili pepper.

Special Precautions

Sneezing and coughing occurred in 11.6% of patients topically applying capsaicin-containing cream versus 1.4% of subjects medicating with a topical placebo (Capsaicin Study Group, 1991) and may also occur in health care workers. Regular washing of the area to which the cream is applied, or at least once daily, may help to avoid exposure to airborne particles of capsaicin. In a case report, a nurse with a history of asthma experienced such severe symptoms (rhinitis, coughing, shortness of breath, and congestion) during application of a 0.025% capsaicin cream to the feet of a patient that she had to resort to using an albuterol inhaler for relief (Marciniak et al., 1995).

Use of topical capsaicin by a parent or caretaker of an infant or young child requires special care in regard to hand washing to avoid any direct transfer to the child's mucous membranes.

No information on overdosage is available.

Toxicology

Mutagenicity

Capsaicin is reported to show mutagenic activities in strains of *Salmonella typhimurium* (Toth et al., 1984; Nagabhushan and Bhide, 1985), and in the mammalian system in V79 cells, capsaicin and dehydrocapsaicin were both mutagenic (Lawson and Gannett, 1989).

Azizan and Blevins (1995) reported that although capsaicin was weakly mutagenic in the Ames test, using *Salmonella typhimurium* strains TA97, TA98, and TA100, with or without S9 metabolic activation, when combined with an acetone extract of *C. annuum* fruit, it became nonmutagenic. They also found that chlorophyll could suppress capsaicin's mutagenicity.

Toxicity in Animal Models

The dermal LD_{50} of capsaicin in dimethylsulfoxide (DMSO) in male mice was >512 mg/kg and there were no deaths or signs of toxicity (Glinsukon et al., 1980). Other LD_{50} values reported for capsaicin in mice are: intravenous, 0.56 mg/kg; intraperitoneal, 7.56 mg/kg; subcutaneous, 9 mg/kg; oral, 190 mg/kg. The acute toxicity of capsaicin and related capsaicinoids may be reduced through their metabolism (Srinivasan et al., 1980). However, in an acute toxicity study in mice, capsaicin was fourfold more toxic in a *Capsicum* extract (*C. minimum*, capsaicin content 1.82 mg/g dry wt.) than pure capsaicin (each administered i.p. dissolved in DMSO). The i.p. LD_{50} of capsaicin in adult female mice (6.50 mg/kg) was lower than in adult male mice (7.65 mg/kg), and the *Capsicum* extract in female mice produced an LD_{50} of 1.51 mg/kg i.p. (Glinsukon et al., 1980).

In female rats, the i.p. LD_{50} of capsaicin dissolved in DMSO was 10.40 mg/kg. Male guinea pigs showed a much lower i.p. LD_{50} of 1.10 mg/kg, and in male hamsters the LD_{50} of capsaicin was much higher (>120 mg/kg i.p.), as it was in male or female rabbits (>50 mg/kg i.p.) (Glinsukon et al., 1980). Toxicity of capsaicin in dogs and cats from i.v. administration has been attributed to a combination of respiratory failure, hypotension, and bradycardia (Monsereenusorn et al., 1982). A dose of 10 mg/kg p.o. is ten times the human consumption of capsaicin usually found in tropical countries (Szallasi and Blumberg, 1999).

Toth and Gannett (1992) reported that randomly bred female Swiss albino mice were fed capsaicin for their entire life at 0.03125% of the diet starting from the age of six weeks. Results showed a statistically significant increase ($p < 0.05$) in benign polypoid adenomas of the cecum. Male mice also showed an increase in these adenomas compared to controls, but the incidence failed to reach statistical significance.

Park et al. (1998) found no tumor-promoting activity from capsaicin in a two-stage skin carcinogenesis model in mice. Instead, when administered at the same time as the tumor promoter TPA (12-*O*-tetradecanoylphorbol-13-acetate), *Capsicum* was found to inhibit mouse skin carcinogenesis. However, an extract of chili (capsaicin content of 2.5 mg/mL) applied to the tongue or administered in the drinking water of mice was reported to promote oral and stomach tumor development initiated by TPA plus DMN-OAc (methyl-acetoxy methyl nitrosamine). Mice administered the chili extract plus a carcinogenic pesticide commonly used in India (BHC or benzene hexachloride) showed a higher incidence of hepatocarcinoma and hepatomas than controls (29% versus 5% untreated and 8% BHC-treated). Among the population of India, the use of chili powder may promote the carcinogenic activity of nitrosamines which are provided by the chewing of betel quid, obtained from fruits of *Areca* species, and by the use of tobacco (Agrawal et al., 1986).

Chronic administration of a *Capsicum* extract (20 mL to cheek pouch until death) was reported to be toxic in hamsters, producing reduced life span, and eye abnormalities. The latter effect was attributed to the depletion of SP by capsaicin in primary afferent neurons, causing a loss of corneal pain sensation and consequent loss of protective corneal reflexes (Agrawal et al., 1985).

Chili prepared by sun-drying, salting, and deep-frying in groundnut oil contains a high amount of carcinogenic 3,4-benzo[*a*]pyrene. Long-term feeding studies in male mice with chili prepared in this way (100 mg/day) and added to a laboratory rodent diet found that none of the controls developed tumors; however, the chili group showed a 35% incidence of adenocarcinoma in the abdomen over two years. These results suggest that the 16% incidence of gastric cancer found among the male population of Madras reported by the Indian government in 1992 may be due to the consumption of salted, sun-dried, and oil-fried red chili (Balachandran and Sivaramkrishnan, 1995).

In a nitrosamine-induced multiorgan model of carcinogenesis in rats, capsaicin added to the diet (0.01%) significantly decreased the incidence of lung tumors and induction of GST-P+ hepatic foci, yet the urinary bladders of capsaicin-treated rats showed a higher incidence of nodular or papillary hyperplasia compared to controls (Jang et al., 1991). This may have been a result of an interaction of capsaicin with the high amount of nitrosamines in their drinking water (0.05%), plus what they received by injection (total nitrosamines, 180 mg/kg i.p.).

Rabbits fed high levels of red pepper (0.2% capsicum-containing peppers constituting 14% of the diet) for one year showed adverse nutritional effects starting at six months, which was attributed to the large proportion of *Capsicum* used in this study (Srinivasan et al., 1980). A long-term, comparative, controlled feeding study of rats given various levels of red *Capsicum* peppers (0.3% capsaicin), capsaicin, and a synthetic analogue of capsaicin (*N*-vanillyl nonanamide) was carried out with short- and long-term evaluations of effects. The animals fed red pepper in amounts varying from 0.05% to 5.0% of their diet did not show any adverse effects in food intake, growth, nitrogen balance, or blood constituents. Both the rats fed capsaicin (at 3 mg/100 g and 15 mg/100 g) and those fed the synthetic analogue of capsaicin (at 15 mg/100 g) showed slower food intake in the first month. An increase to control levels by eight weeks was found in the capsaicin group, and overall weight gain was depressed, especially at the higher dose level of 15 mg/100 g of feed (Srinivasan et al., 1980).

In India, where dietary intake of *Capsicum* is common, submucous fibrosis of the palate and fauces (opening of the mouth and oral pharynx) has been reported (Duke, 1985). A 10% *Capsicum,* protein-deficient diet fed to rats led to a 54% increase in the incidence in hepatomas, suggesting that capsaicin may contribute to the development of liver cancer (Buchanan, 1978). Rats fed a diet containing red chili (8 mg/day per 100 g body weight) alone or with a carcinogenic substance (DMH, 1,2-dimethyl hydrazine, 20 mg/kg, s.c.) showed tumor incidences of 83.3% and 93.3%, respectively (Nalini et al., 1998). Histopathological examination of the colons of the DMH plus red chili group showed a significant increase in β-glucuronidase activity. This was not found in the red chili alone group. β-glucuronidase is an enzyme that enhances the breakdown of glucuronides which conjugate toxins, drugs, and hormones in the liver, thereby rendering them soluble and detoxified. Although over 90% of these conjugated toxins are excreted via the colon, if the colonic microflora becomes stimulated by procarcinogens (e.g., DMH, red chili) the glucuronides could be broken down and, therefore, liberate toxins and drugs. Mucinase in the colon and fecal contents of the DMH plus red chili group was also significantly higher than in the controls, but not in the red chili alone group. Mucinase is found in the intestinal flora where it breaks down protective mucins (glycoproteins) which serve as lubricants and possibly as a barrier to the damaging effects of toxins, bacteria, and viruses.

A full review of capsaicin's carcinogenic and anticarcinogenic potential (Surh and Lee, 1996) provided theoretical evidence for both effects. Ernst and Barnes (1998) refer to the study by Surh and Lee with the comment that "Taken orally in regular high doses it may act as a *carcinogen* and could promote gastric cancer, but in low doses it seems to have anticarcinogenic activity" (p. 490).

REFERENCES

Agrawal, R.C., Sarode, A.V., Lalitha, V.S., and Bhide, S.V. (1985). Chili extract treatment and induction of eye lesions in hamsters. *Toxicology Letters* 28: 1-7.

Agrawal, R.C., Wiessler, M., Hecker, E., and Bhide, S.V. (1986). Tumor promoting effects of chilli extracts in BALB/c mice. *International Journal of Cancer* 38: 689-695.

Anuras, S., Christiansen, J., and Templeman, D. (1977). Effect of capsaicin on electrical slow waves in the isolated rat colon. *Gut* 18: 666-669.

Appendino, G. and Szallasi, A (1997). Euphorbium: Modern research on its active principle, resiniferatoxin, revives an ancient medicine. *Life Sciences* 60: 681-696.

Azizan, A. and Blevins, R.D. (1995). Mutagenicity and antimutagenicity testing of six chemicals associated with the pungent properties of specific spices as revealed by the Ames *Salmonella*/microsomal assay. *Archives of Environmental Contamination and Toxicology* 28: 248-258.

Balachandran, B. and Sivaramkrishnan, V.M. (1995). Induction of tumours by Indian dietary constituents. *Indian Journal of Cancer* 32: 104-109.

Bernstein, J.E., Korman, N.J., Bickers, D.R., Dahl, M.V., and Millikan, L.E. (1989). Treatment of chronic postherpetic neuralgia with topical capsaicin. *American Journal of Dermatology* 21: 265-270.

Bernstein, J.E., Parish, L.C., Rapaport, M., Rosenbaum, M.M., and Roenigk, H.H. Jr. (1986). Effects of topically applied capsaicin on moderate and severe psoriasis vulgaris. *Journal of the American Academy of Dermatology* 15: 504-507.

Biggs, D.F. and Ladenius, R.C. (1990). Capsaicin selectively reduced airway responses to histamine, substance P, and vagal stimulation. *European Journal of Pharmacology* 175: 29-33.

Blumenthal, M., Busse, W.R., Goldberg, A., Gruenwald, J., Hall, T., Riggins, C.W., and Rister, R.S. (Eds.) (1998). *The Complete German Commission E Monographs*. Austin, TX: American Botanical Council, p. 178.

Brinker, F.J. (1983). *The Toxicology of Botanical Medicines,* Second Edition. Sandy, OR: Eclectic Medical Publications.

Buchanan, R.L. (1978). Toxicity of spices containing methylenedioxybenzene derivatives: A review. *Journal of Food Safety* 1: 275-293.

Buiatti, E., Palli, D., Decarli, A., Amadori, D., Avellini, C., Bianchi, S., Biserni, R., Cipriani, F., Cocco, P., Giacosa, A., et al. (1989). A case control study of diet and cancer in Italy. *International Journal of Cancer* 44: 611-616.

Capsaicin Study Group (1991). Treatment of painful diabetic neuropathy with topical capsaicin. *Archives of Internal Medicine* 151: 2225-2229.

Caterina, M.J. and Julius, D. (2001). The vanilloid receptor: A molecular gateway to the pain pathway. *Annual Review of Neuroscience* 24: 487-517.

Chancellor, M.B. (1997). Should we be using chili pepper extracts to treat the overactive bladder? *Journal of Urology* 158: 2097 (editorial).

Chichewicz, R.H. and Thorpe, P.A. (1996). The antimicrobial properties of chile peppers (*Capsicum* species) and their uses in Mayan medicine. *Journal of Ethnopharmacology* 52: 61-70.

Cordell, G.A. and Araujo, O.E. (1993). Capsaicin: Identification, nomenclature, and pharmacotherapy. *Annals of Pharmacotherapy* 27: 330-336.

Cruwys, S.C., Garrett, N.E., and Kidd, B.L. (1995). Sensory denervation with capsaicin attenuates inflammation and nociception in arthritic rats. *Neuroscience Letters* 193: 205-207.

Cruz, F. (1998). Desensitization of bladder sensory fibers by intravesical capsaicin or capsaicin analogs. A new strategy for treatment of urge incontinence in patients with spinal detrusor hyperreflexia or bladder hypersensitivity disorders. *International Urogynecology Journal* 9: 214-229.

Dasgupta, P., Chandiramani, V., Parkinson, M.C., Beckett, A., and Fowler, C.J. (1998). Treating the human bladder with capsaicin: Is it safe? *European Urology* 33: 28-31.

Dasgupta, P. and Fowler, C.J. (1997). Chillies: From antiquity to urology. *British Journal of Urology* 80: 845-852.

De Ridder, D., Chandiramani, V., Dasgupta, P., Van Poppel, H., Baert, L., and Fowler, C.J. (1997). Intravesical capsaicin as a treatment for refractory detrusor hyperreflexia: A dual center study with long-term follow up. *Journal of Urology* 158: 2087-2092.

Deal, C.L., Schnitzer, T.J., Lipstein, E., Seibold, J.R., Stevens, R.M., Levy, M.D., Albert, D., and Renold, F. (1991). Treatment of arthritis with topical capsaicin: A double-blind trial. *Clinical Therapeutics* 13: 383-395.

Dini, D., Bertelli, G., Gozza, A., and Forno, G.G. (1993). Treatment of the post-mastectomy pain syndrome with topical capsaicin. *Pain* 54: 223-226.

Duke, J.A. (1985). *Handbook of Medicinal Herbs.* Boca Raton, FL: CRC Press.

Ellis, C.N., Berberian, B., Sulica, V.I., Dodd, W.A., Jarratt, M.T., Katz, H.I., Prawer, S., Krueger, G., Rex, I.H. Jr., and Wolf, J.E. (1993). A double-blind evaluation of topical capsaicin in pruritic psoriasis. *Journal of the American Academy of Dermatology* 29: 438-442.

Ensminger, E.H., Ensminger, M.E., Konlande, J.E., and Robson, J.R. (1993). *Foods and Nutrition Encyclopedia,* Second Edition. Boca Raton, FL: CRC Press.

Ernst, E. and Barnes, J. (1998). Treatments used in complementary medicine. *Side Effects of Drugs Annual* 21: 489-495.

Frerick, H., Schmidt, U., Keitel, W., Kuhlmann, M., Bredehprst, A., and Kuhn, U. (2000). Capsicum pain plaster in chronic low back pain—Results of a treatment of 3 weeks duration. *Phytomedicine* 7(Suppl. 2): 52 (abstract SL-107).

Fuller, R.W. (1990). The human pharmacology of capsaicin. *Archives Internationales de Pharmacodynamie* 303: 147-156.

Glinsukon, T., Stitmunnaithum, V., Toskulkao, C., Buranawuti, T., and Tangkrisanavinont, V. (1980). Acute toxicity of capsaicin in several animal species. *Toxicon* 18: 215-220.

Gonzalez, R., Dunkel, R., Koletzko, B., Schusdziarra, V., and Allescher, H.D. (1998). Effect of capsaicin-containing red pepper sauce suspension on upper gastrointestinal motility in healthy volunteers. *Digestive Diseases and Sciences* 43: 1165-1171.

Govindarajan, V.S. (1985). Capsicum production, technology, chemistry, and quality. Part I: History, botany, cultivation, and primary processing. *Critical Reviews in Food Science and Nutrition* 22: 109-176.

Govindarajan, V.S. and Sathyanarayana, M.N. (1991). Capsicum production, technology, chemistry, and quality. Part V: Impact on physiology, pharmacology, nutrition, and metabolism; structure, pungency, pain, and desensitization sequences. *Food Science and Nutrition* 29: 435-474.

Graham, D.Y., Smith, J.L., and Opekun, A.R. (1988). Spicy food and the stomach. Evaluation by videoendoscopy. *Journal of the American Medical Association* 260: 3473-3475.

Helme, R.D., Eglezo, A., Dandie, G.W., Andrews, P.V., and Boyd, R.L. (1987). The effect of substance P on the regional lymph node antibody response to antigen stimulation in capsaicin pretreated rats. *Journal of Immunology* 139: 3470-3473.

Henderson, D.E., Slickman, A.M., and Henderson, S.K. (1999). Quantitative HPLC determination of the antioxidant activity of capsaicin on the formation of lipid hydroperoxides of linoleic acid: A comparative study against BHT and melatonin. *Journal of Agricultural and Food Chemistry* 47: 2563-2570.

Henry, C.J.K. and Emery, B. (1986). Effect of spiced food on metabolic rate. *Human Nutrition: Clinical Nutrition* 40C: 165-168.

Hogaboam, C.M. and Wallace, J.L. (1991). Inhibition of platelet aggregation by capsaicin. An effect unrelated to actions on sensory afferent neurons. *European Journal of Pharmacology* 202: 129-131.

Holzer, P. and Lippe, I.T. (1988). Stimulation of afferent nerve endings by intragastric capsaicin protects against ethanol-induced damage of gastric mucosa. *Neuroscience* 27: 981-987.

Holzer, P., Pabst, M.A., and Lippe, I.T. (1989). Intragastric capsaicin protects against aspirin-induced lesion formation and bleeding in the rat gastric mucosa. *Gastroenterology* 96: 1425-1433.

Holzer, P., Pabst, M.A., Lippe, I.T., Peskar, B.M., Livingstone, E.H., and Guth, P.H. (1990). Afferent nerve-mediated protection against deep mucosal damage in the rat stomach. *Gastroenterology* 98: 838-848.

Hood, V.C., Cruwys, S.C., Urban, L., and Kidd, B.L. (2001). The neurogenic contribution to synovial leucocyte infiltration and other outcome measures in a guinea pig model of arthritis. *Neuroscience Letters* 299: 201-204.

Hornero-Méndez, D. and Mínguez-Mosquera, M.I. (1998). Isolation and identification of the carotenoid capsolutein from *Capsicum annuum* as curcurbitaxanthin A. *Journal of Agricultural and Food Chemistry* 46: 4087-4090.

Jang, J.J., Cho, K.J., Lee, J.H. and Bae, J.H. (1991). Different modifying responses of capsaicin in a wide-spectrum initiation model in F344 rats. *Journal of Korean Medical Science* 6: 31-36.

Jang, J.J., Kim, S.H., and Yun, T.K. (1989). Inhibitory effect of capsaicin on mouse lung tumor development, in vivo. *Journal of Korean Medical Science* 3: 49-53.

Jensen-Jaorlim, E., Gajdzik, L., Haberl, I., Kraft, D., Scheiner, O., and Graf, J. (1998). Hot spices influence permeability of human intestinal epithelial monolayers. *Journal of Nutrition* 128: 577-581.

Jones, L.A., Tanberg, D., and Troutman, W.G. (1997). Household treatment for "chile burns" of the hands. *Clinical Toxicology* 25: 483-491.

Jones, N.L., Shabib, S., and Sherman, P.M. (1997). Capsaicin as an inhibitor of the growth of the gastric pathogen *Helicobacter pylori*. *FEMS Microbiology Letters* 146: 223-227.

Jung, M.Y., Kang, H.J., and Moon, A. (2001). Capsaicin-induced apoptosis in SK-Hep-1 hepatocarcinoma cells involves Bcl-2 downregulation and caspase-3 activation. *Cancer Letters* 165: 139-145.

Kang, J.Y., Teng, C.H., Wee, A., and Chen, F.C. (1995). The effect of capsaicin and chili on ethanol-induced gastric mucosal injury in the rat. *Gut* 36: 664-669.

Kang, J.Y., Yeoh, K.G., Chia, H.P., Lee, H.P., Chia, Y.W., Guan, R., and Yap, I. (1995). Chili—Protective factor against peptic ulcer? *Digestive Diseases and Sciences* 40: 576-579.

Kasting, G.B., Francis, W.R., Bowman, L.A., and Kinnett, G.O. (1997). Percutaneous absorption of vanilloids: *In vivo* and *in vitro* studies. *Journal of Pharmaceutical Sciences* 86: 142-146.

Kawada, T., Hagihara, K.I., and Iwai, K. (1986). Effects of capsaicin on lipid metabolism in rats fed a high fat diet. *Journal of Nutrition* 116: 1272-1278.

Kawada, T., Suzuki, T., Takahashi, M., and Iwai, K. (1984). Gastrointestinal absorption and metabolism of capsaicin and dihydrocapsaicin in rats. *Toxicology and Applied Pharmacology* 72: 449-456.

Kawada, T., Watanabe, T., Takaishi, T., Tanaka, T., and Iwai, K. (1986). Capsaicin-induced β-adrenergic action on energy metabolism in rats: Influence of capsaicin on oxygen consumption, the respiratory quotient, and substrate utilization. *Proceedings of the Society for Experimental Biology and Medicine* 183: 250-256.

Kaygisiz, Z., Cingi, M.I., and Cingi, E. (1990). Effect of capsaicin on contractility, left ventricular systolic pressure and rate of isolated perfused rat heart. *Fitoterapia* 61: 266-269.

Kim, J.D., Kim, J.M., Puo, J.O., Kim, S.Y., Kim, B.S., Yu, R., and Han, I.S. (1997). Capsaicin can alter the expression of tumor forming related genes which might be followed by induction of apoptosis of a Korean stomach cell line, SNU-1. *Cancer Letters* 120: 235-241.

Krishna, A. and Ghosh, J.J. (1989). Capsaicin pretreatment protects free radical induced rat lung damage on exposure to gaseous chemical lung irritants. *Phytotherapy Research* 3: 159-161.

Kumar, N., Vij, J.C., Sarin, S.K., and Anand, B.S. (1984). Do chillies influence healing of duodenal ulcer? *British Medical Journal* 288(June 16): 1803-1804.

Lawless, H., Rozin, P., and Shenker, J. (1985). Effects of oral capsaicin on gustatory, olfactory and irritant sensations and flavor identification in humans who regularly or rarely consume chili peppers. *Chemical Senses* 10: 579-589.

Lawson, T. and Gannett, P. (1989). The mutagenicity of capsaicin and dihydrocapsaicin in V79 cells. *Cancer Letters* 48: 109-113.

Leacock, R.A. (1985). *Capsicum. Canadian Pharmaceutical Journal* 118: 517-519.

Lee, T.S. (1954). Physiological gustatory sweating in a warm climate. *Journal of Physiology* 124: 528-542.

Leung, A.Y. and Foster, S. (1996). *Encyclopedia of Common Natural Ingredients Used in Food, Drugs, and Cosmetics.* New York: John Wiley and Son, Inc.

Levine, J.D., Goetzl, E.J., and Basbaum, A.I. (1987). Contribution of the nervous system to the pathophysiology of rheumatoid arthritis and other polyarthritides. *Rheumatic Diseases Clinics of North America* 13: 369-383.

Lim, K., Yoshioka, M., Kikuzato, S., Kiyonaga, A., Tanaka, H., Shindo, M., and Suzuki, M. (1997). Dietary red pepper ingestion increases carbohydrate oxidation at rest and during exercise in runners. *Medicine and Science in Sports and Exercise* 29: 355-361.

López-Carillo, L., Avila, M.H., and Dubrow, R. (1994). Chili pepper consumption and gastric cancer in Mexico: A case control study. *American Journal of Epidemiology* 139: 263-271.

Lundberg, J.M. and Saria, A. (1983). Capsaicin-induced desensitization of airway mucosa to cigarette smoke, mechanical and chemical irritants. *Nature* 302: 251-253.

Lynn, B. (1990). Capsaicin: Actions on nociceptive C-fibres and therapeutic potential. *Pain* 41: 61-69.

Marciniak, B.H., Brown, B., Peterson, B., Boult, L., and Guay, D. (1995). Adverse consequences of capsaicin exposure in health care workers. *Journal of the American Geriatrics Society* 43: 1181-1182 (letter).

Marks, D.R., Rapoport, A., Padla, D., Weeks, R., Rosum, R., Sheftell, F., and Arrowsmith, F. (1993). A double-blind placebo-controlled trial of intranasal capsaicin for cluster headache. *Cephalalgia* 13: 114-116.

Marsh, A.C. (1977). Composition of Food, Spices, and Herbs: Raw, Processed, and Prepared. *USDA Agricultural Handbook* No. 8-2. Washington, DC: Agricultural Research Service, USDA.

McCarthy, G.M. and McCarty, D.J. (1992). Effect of topical capsaicin in the therapy of painful osteoarthritis of the hands. *Journal of Rheumatology* 19: 604-607.

Meyer, R.A., Campbell, J.N., and Raja, S.N. (1994). Peripheral neural mechanisms of nociception. In Wall, P.D. and Melzack, R. (Eds.), *Textbook of Pain* pp. 13-43. London: Churchill Livingstone.

Miller, C.H., Zhang, Z., Hamilton, S.M., and Teel, R.W. (1993). Effects of capsaicin on liver microsomal metabolism of the tobacco-specific nitrosamine NNK. *Cancer Letters* 75: 45-52.

Mitchell, J. and Rook, A. (1979). *Botanical Dermatology: Plants and Plant Products Injurious to the Skin*. Vancouver, BC: Greengrass.

Moerman, D.E. (1998). *Native American Ethnobotany*. Portland, OR: Timber Press, p. 136.

Mollina-Torres, J., Garcia-Chávez, A., and Ramirez-Chávez, E. (1999). Antimicrobial properties of alkamides present in flavouring plants traditionally used in Mesoamerica: Affinin and capsaicin. *Journal of Ethnopharmacology* 64: 241-248.

Monsereenusorn, Y. (1979). Effect of capsaicin on intestinal glucose metabolism in vitro. *Toxicology Letters* 3: 279-283.

Monsereenusorn, Y. (1980). Effect of *Capsicum annuum* on blood glucose level. *Quarterly Journal of Crude Drug Research* 18: 1-7.

Monsereenusorn, Y. and Glinsukon, T. (1979). The inhibitory effect of capsaicin on intestinal glucose absorption in vitro. II. Effect of capsaicin upon intestinal Na^+-K^+-ATPase activities. *Toxicology Letters* 4: 399-406.

Monsereenusorn, Y., Kongsamut, S., and Pezella, P.D. (1982). Capsaicin—A literature survey. *CRC Critical Reviews in Toxicology* 10: 321-339.

Morré, D.J., Cheuh, P.J., and Morré, D.M. (1995). Capsaicin inhibits preferentially the NADH oxidase and growth of transformed cells in culture. *Proceedings of the National Academy of Sciences, USA* 92: 1831-1835.

Munn, S.E., Burrows, N.P., Abadia-Molina, F., Springall, D.R., Polak, J.M., and Russell Jones, R. (1997). The effect of topical capsaicin on substance P immunoreactivity: A clinical trial and immunohistochemical analysis. *Acta Dermato-Venereologica* 77: 158-159 (letter).

Nadkarni, A.K. (1976). *Indian Materia Medica,* 1, Third Edition. Bombay, India: Popular Prakashan, pp. 268-269.

Nagabhushan, M. and Bhide, S.V. (1985). Mutagenicity of chili extract and capsaicin in short-term tests. *Environmental Mutagenesis* 7: 881-888.

Nagy, J.I. (1982). Capsaicin's action on the nervous system. *Trends in the Neurosciences* 5: 362-365.

Nalini, N., Sabitha, K., Viswanathan, P., and Menon, V.P. (1998). Influence of spices on the bacterial (enzyme) activity in experimental colon cancer. *Journal of Ethnopharmacology* 62: 15-24.

Newall, C.A., Anderson, L.A., and Phillipson, J.D. (1996). *Herbal Medicines: A Guide for Health Care Professionals.* London: The Pharmaceutical Press, pp. 60-61.

Notani, P.N. and Jayant, K. (1987). Role of diet in upper aerodigestive tract cancers. *Nutrition and Cancer* 10: 103-113.

Panossian, A., Gabrielian, E., and Wagner, H. (1996). Dose-dependent reversible effects of capsaicin on interleukin-1 $\propto$ production is associated with the metabolism of arachidonic acid (leukotriene B_4 and prostaglandin E_2) as well as nitric oxide production in human leucocytes. *Phytomedicine* 3: 169-174.

Park, K.K., Chun, K.S., Yook, J.I., and Surh, Y.J. (1998). Lack of tumor promoting activity of capsaicin, a principle pungent ingredient of red pepper, in mouse skin carcinogenesis. *Anticancer Research* 18: 4201-4206.

Payan, D.G., Levine, J.D., and Goetzl, E.J. (1984). Modulation of immunity and hypersensitivity by sensory neuropeptides. *Journal of Immunology* 132: 1601-1604 (opinion).

Reilly, C.A., Crouch, D.J., and Yost, G.S. (2001). Quantitative analysis of capsaicinoids in fresh peppers, oleoresin capsicum and pepper spray products. *Journal of Forensic Sciences* 46: 502-509.

Reilly, C.A., Crouch, D.J., Yost, G.S., and Fatah, A.A. (2001). Determination of capsaicin, dihydrocapsaicin, and nonivamide in self-defense weapons by liquid chromatography-mass spectrometry and liquid chromatography-tandem mass spectrometry. *Journal of Chromatography* A 912: 259-267.

Robbers, J.E., Speedie, M.K., and Tyler, V.E. (1996). *Pharmacognosy and Pharmacobiotechnology*. Baltimore, MD: Williams and Wilkins, pp. 134-135.

Rosengarten, F., Jr. (1969). *The Book of Spices*. Wynnewood, PA: Livingston.

Rumsfield, J.A. and West, D.P. (1991). Topical capsaicin in dermatological and peripheral pain disorders. *Annals of Pharmacotherapy* 25: 381-387.

Saito, A., Masaki, T., Lee, T.J.F., and Goto, K. (1988). Effects of capsaicin on large cerebral arteries of the cat. *Japanese Journal of Pharmacology* 46(Suppl.): 285P (abstract).

Sicuteri, F., Fanciullacci, M., Nicolodi, M., Geppetti, P., Fusco, B.M., Marabini, S., Alessandri, M., and Campagnolo, V. (1990). Substance P theory: A unique focus on the painful and painless phenomena of cluster headache. *Headache* 30: 69-79.

Sicuteri, F., Fusco, B.M., Marabini, S., and Fanciullacci, M. (1988). Capsaicin as a potential medication for cluster headache. *Medical Science Research* 16: 1079-1080.

Srinivasan, M.R., Sambaiah, K., Satyanarayana, M.N., and Rao, M.V.L. (1980). Influence of red pepper and capsaicin on growth, blood constituents and nitrogen balance in rats. *Nutrition Reports International* 21: 455-467.

Stanisz, A.M., Befus, D., and Bienenstock, J. (1986). Differential effects of vasoactive intestinal peptide, substance P, and somatostatin on immunoglobulin synthesis and proliferations by lymphocytes from Peyer's patches, mesenteric lymph nodes, and spleen. *Journal of Immunology* 136: 152-156.

Surh, Y.J. and Lee, S.S. (1996). Capsaicin in hot chili pepper: Carcinogen, cocarcinogen or anticarcinogen? *Food and Chemical Toxicology* 34: 313-316.

Szallasi, A. and Blumberg, P.M. (1999). Vanilloid (capsaicin) receptors and mechanisms. *Pharmacological Reviews* 51: 159-212.

Szolcsányi, J., Nemeth, J., Oroszi, G., Helyes, Z., and Pinter, E. (1998). Effect of capsaicin and resiniferatoxin on the release of sensory neuropeptides in the rat isolated trachea. *British Journal of Pharmacology* 124: 8P.

Toth, B. and Gannett, P. (1992). Carcinogenicity of lifelong administration of capsaicin of hot pepper in mice. *In Vivo* 6: 59-64.

Toth, B., Rogan, E., and Walker, B. (1984). Tumorigenicity and mutagenicity studies with capsaicin of hot peppers. *Anticancer Research* 4: 117-120.

Tsuchiya, H. (2001). Biphasic membrane effects of capsaicin, an active component in *Capsicum* species. *Journal of Ethnopharmacology* 75: 295-299. See also erratum in volume 76, p. 313.

Uchida, M., Yano, S., and Watanabe, K. (1991). The role of capsaicin-sensitive afferent nerves in protective effect of capsaicin against ethanol-induced gastric lesions in rats. *Japanese Journal of Pharmacology* 55: 279-282.

U.S. Interdepartmental Committee on Nutrition for National Defense (1962). *The Kingdom of Thailand: Nutrition Survey*. Washington, DC: Government Printing Office.

Vaughan, J.G. and Geissler, C. (1997). *The New Oxford Book of Food Plants*. New York: Oxford University Press, pp. 138-139.

Wang, J.P., Hsu, M.F., and Teng, C.M. (1984). Antiplatelet effect of capsaicin. *Thrombosis Research* 36: 497-507.

Watson, C.P.N. and Evans, R.J. (1992). The postmastectomy pain syndrome and topical capsaicin: A randomized trial. *Pain* 51: 375-379.

Willard, T. (1991). *The Wild Rose Scientific Herbal*. Calgary, Alberta: Wild Rose College of Natural Healing.

Wood, J.N. (Ed.) (1993). *Capsaicin in the Study of Pain*. San Diego, CA: Academic Press, Inc.

Yahara, S., Ura, T., Sakamoto, C., and Nohara, T. (1994). Steroidal glycosides from *Capsicum annuum*. *Phytochemistry* 37: 831-835.

Yamato, T., Aomine, M., Ideda, N., Noto, H., and Ohta, C. (1996). Inhibition of contractile tension by capsaicin in isolated rat papillary muscle. *General Pharmacology* 27: 129-132.

Yeoh, K.G., Kang, J.Y., Yap, I., Guan, R., Tan, C.C., Wee, A., and Teng, C.H. (1995). Chili protects against aspirin-induced gastroduodenal mucosal injury in humans. *Digestive Diseases and Sciences* 40: 580-583.

Yoshioka, M., Lim, K., Kikuzato, S., Kiyonaga, A., Tanaka, H., Shindo, M., and Suzuki, M. (1995). Effects of red-pepper diet on the energy expenditure in men. *Journal of Nutritional Science and Vitaminology* 41: 647-656.

Yoshioka, M., St. Pierre, S., Suzuki, M., and Tremblay, A. (1998). Effects of red pepper added to high-fat and high-carbohydrate meals on energy metabolism and substrate utilization in Japanese women. *British Journal of Nutrition* 80: 503-510.

Zhang, Z., Huynh, H., and Teel, R.W. (1997). Effects of orally administered capsaicin, the principal component of *Capsicum* fruits, on the in vitro metabolism of the tobacco-specific nitrosamine NNK in hamster lung and liver microsomes. *Anticancer Research* 17(2A): 1093-1098.

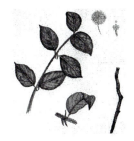

Cat's Claw

BOTANICAL DATA

Classification and Nomenclature

Scientific name: *Uncaria tomentosa* (Willd.) DC. *Uncaria tomentosa* (Willd.) DC. and *U. guianensis* (Aubl.) Gmel.

Family name: Rubiaceae

Common names: cat's claw, uña de gato, jipotatsa, garabato amarillo (Jones, 1995), rangayo, bejuco de agua, tua juncara (Standley, 1930), hawk's claw, uña de gavilán, paraguayo (Duke and Vasquez, 1994).

Description

Uncaria tomentosa is a massive climbing vine with curved, sharp, highly pungent, protruding spines on the branches. The main stem (stalk) can reach over 27 meters in length with a diameter of close to 15 cm for most of its length (Jones, 1995), although 20 cm and larger diameters are known (Keplinger et al., 1999). The roots are porous, bitter-tasting, and astringent. They usually measure several meters in length and as much as 7 cm in diameter (Laus and Keplinger, 1997). The leaves, measuring 10 cm in length (Reinhard, 1999), are opposite, ovate oblong, with eight to ten pairs of lateral veins; the underside of the leaves shows minute hairs, hence the term *tomentosa*. The seeds are winged, 2.5 - 3.5 mm in length and less than 1 mm in width. The flowers are fragrant, five-lobed, yellowish-white and tiny, occurring in globose heads (ball-shaped clusters) at the end of the vine (Woodson and Schery, 1980; Reinhard, 1999; Keplinger et al., 1999). *Uncaria tomentosa* is native to tropical South America and occurs in Colombia, Ecuador, Venezuela (Ridsdale, 1978), Costa Rica, Guatemala, Panama (Standley, 1930), and Peru (Teppner et al., 1984).

Two chemotypes were identified for Peruvian *U. tomentosa:* a tetracyclic oxindole alkaloid type and a pentacyclic oxindole alkaloid type (Laus et al., 1997). Researchers have noted that the pentacyclic oxindole alkaloid type is named *savéntaro* (powerful plant) by shamans of the Asháninka tribe of Peru (Keplinger et al., 1999). The pentacyclic chemotype (PC) contains isomeric pentacyclic oxindole alkaloids and the precursor indole alkaloids in the leaves, while the tetracyclic chemotype (TC) contains predominately tetracyclic oxindole alkaloids and their precursor indole alkaloids in small amounts (Keplinger et al., 1996; Laus et al., 1997). These differences were confirmed in analyses of progeny sprouted from the seeds of the two chemotypes (Laus et al., 1998).

The only other tropical American species, *Uncaria guianensis* (Aubl.) Gmel., also known as "uña de gato," can be readily distinguished from *U. tomentosa* by its alternating, recurving to spiralling spines, rather than the slightly curved, opposite spines of the former (Keplinger et al., 1999). The leaves are glabrous whereas those of *U. tomentosa* are hairy and generally less elongated. The inflorescence of *U. guianensis* is reddish-orange, spherical, three-lobed, and 2 to 4 cm in diameter, whereas those of *U. tomentosa* are yellowish-white, five-lobed, and 1.5 to 2.5 cm in diameter. The leaf veins number six to seven pairs whereas those of *U. tomentosa* have eight to ten pairs. In addition, the seeds (8 mm in length) are much larger than those of *U. tomentosa. Uncaria guianensis* is the smaller of the two species. At the adult stage, it attains a length of 4 to 10 m and a base of 4 to 15 cm in diameter, versus 10 to 30 m and 5 to 40 cm, respectively, in *U. tomentosa. Uncaria guianensis* appears to be found in wider distribution in Peru and at comparatively lower altitudes (Zavala Carrillo and Zevallos Pollito, 1996). Finally, *U. guianensis* is almost exclusively found in secondary forests whereas *U. tomentosa* is also found in closed, mature forests (de Jong et al., 1999). Besides Peru, this species is reported to occur in Paraguay, Bolivia, Venezuela, Guiana, and Trinidad (Ridsdale, 1978).

HISTORY AND TRADITIONAL USES

The use of *Uncaria tomentosa* and *U. guianensis* by indigenous healers of tropical South America has not been traced to any particular time in history, but extends for untold past generations as part of an oral tradition of healing. The inner bark of the main stem or stalk bark and that of the root and root bark share some common uses in Peru, the source country of practically all commercially available cat's claw (Jones, 1995). The use of *U. tomentosa* followed the early investigations of Peruvian and later Austrian researchers who brought the vine into pharmacies and clinics of their own countries. Later,

Germany, Italy, and several other European centers of phytopharmacy provided the root (Wagner, 1987a; Jones, 1995; Anonymous, 1997).

In the region of the eastern incline of the Peruvian Andes to the Amazon rainforest, indigenous healers prepare a decoction of the bark of *U. tomentosa* or *U. guianensis* for internal use to treat gastric ulcers. They regard the preparations as antitumor, anti-inflammatory, antirheumatic, and contraceptive (De Feo, 1992). In central Peru, indigenous people primarily use the bark of *U. tomentosa* to relieve inflammations, including those associated with rheumatism, arthritis, urinary tract inflammations, and gastric ulcers. Other central Peruvian indigenous uses of cat's claw bark include the relief of side effects from antibiotics and chemotherapy, and other treatments of cancer, weakness, bone pain, and deep wounds. It is also used to cleanse the kidneys, and for recovery from childbirth. External application of the bark decoction or tea is applied to wounds using the preparation as a wash twice daily (Jones, 1995).

The Asháninka Indians of central Peru are noted to use the root bark in the treatment of cancer (Montenegro de Matta et al., 1976). The highest order of Asháninka shaman priests use the root bark of *U. tomentosa*-PC, known to them as *savéntaro* or powerful plant, to remove the main cause of disease in the Asháninka medico-religious system of healing: a disturbance between the spirit and the body, or an "anxiety." Accordingly, *U. tomentosa*-PC is used by Asháninka shamans in the treatment of psychological disorders, and is regarded as being inhabited by "good spirits." It is placed among plants they use for religious purposes which include *Banisteriopsis caapi* (Spruce ex Griseb.) Morton (Malpighiaceae) and *Erythroxylum coca* Lamarck (Erythroxylaceae). The "good spirits" of the vine are said to remove the anxiety state interfering with spirit-body communication, thereby restoring health (Keplinger et al., 1999). Other uses of *U. tomentosa* by the Indians of Peru include the treatment of skin "impurities," "blood purification," "bone pains," fevers, asthma (sap with water), disease prevention, hemorrhages, menstrual irregularity, recovery from childbirth, contraception, "loose" stomach, fevers, and for a normalizing effect on the body. The main stem (stalk) holds potable water which is obtained by cutting it open (Jones, 1995).

Traditional uses of *U. guianensis* in Peru are similar to *U. tomentosa* (De Feo, 1992) and include treatment of arthritis, rheumatism, gastric ulcers, gastritis, female contraception, female genitourinary tract cancers, tumors, cirrhosis, and diabetes (Jovel et al., 1996; Duke and Vasquez, 1994; De Feo, 1992). In Brazil, the Yanomami drink an infusion of the stem to treat diarrhea and stomachache which is also treated by wrapping the crushed stem around the waist (Milliken and Albert, 1996). Indians of Colombia use the vine to treat gonorrhea and dysentery (Duke and Vasqez, 1994; Schultes and Raffauf, 1990). In Guiana the vine is used to treat dysentery (Uphof, 1968), and in Suriname the leaves are used as an extract to treat intestinal infections in children and dysentery. The Surinamese dry the leaves in a hot pan and then powder them before they are applied to wounds (Ostendorf, 1962). Compared to *U. tomentosa,* this species remains scarcely studied. The chemical composition of the plant shows some similarity to *U. tomentosa* (Lee et al., 1999; Yepez et al., 1991; Phillipson et al., 1978), yet, whereas *U. guianensis* is reported to contain nearly only tetracyclic oxindole alkaloids (Lavault et al., 1983), *U. tomentosa* contains largely pentacyclic oxindole alkaloids or both forms (see Chemistry).

Uncaria is a pantropical genus composed of approximately 60 species. Many are used medicinally. The young shoots and leaves of "Bengal gambir" (*U. gambir* Roxb.) are used to make a tannin-rich aqueous extract used in powder form in the treatment of gastrointestinal disorders, including diarrhea. Known as catechu or gambier, proprietary preparations are sold in Australia, England, Germany, France, and South Africa (Reynolds, 1996). In Equatorial Africa, the bark of *U. africana* G. Don var. *africana* (syn. *U. talbotii* Wernh.) is used to treat syphilis, stomach pains, and colds, and chewed to remedy coughs. The leaves are used to treat inflammatory conditions of the lungs, and in Ivory Coast the leaf juice is used to treat jaundice (Irvine, 1961; Oliver-Bever, 1986). In Papua New Guinea, the stem sap of *U. ferrea* (B1.) DC. is added to vegetable soup to relieve stomachache and fevers (Holdsworth and Mahana, 1983). In Malaysia the leaves are decocted to provide a cleansing liquid for the treatment of ulcers and wounds, and a tea made from the injured roots is used to treat intestinal inflammation (Perry and Metzger, 1980). In the Moluccas, the leaves of *U. longiflora* var *longiflora* are reported to be used to treat rheumatism and when rubbed into the skin are used to relieve pain (Phillipson et al., 1978). In Mizoram, India near the border of Myanmar, the native people decoct the root of *U. laevigata* Wall. for a gargle to treat tonsillitis and topically apply the root juice to treat herpes (Sharma et al., 2001). In the Pharmacopoeia of China, five species of *Uncaria* are listed interchangeably under the official medicine *gou teng: U. sinensis* (Oliv.) Havil., *U. hirsuta* Havil., *U. rynchophylla* (Miq.) Jacks., *U. sessilifructus* Roxb., and *U. macrophylla* Wall. A decoction of the dried stem with spine ("hook") is prescribed in the treatment of hypertension, headache, dizziness, and eclampsia (Tu et al., 1992). Otherwise, *gou teng* is used in the treatment of fevers, childhood epilepsy, and for adults as a sedative and antispasmodic (Huang, 1993; Zhu, 1998). *Uncaria rynchophylla* and *U. sinensis* are also used in traditional Japanese medicine *(Kampo)* for the treatment of hypertension and the associated symptoms of dizziness and headache (Yano et al., 1991).

CHEMISTRY

Carbohydrates

Glycosides

Various quinovic acid glycosides have been identified by Cerri et al. (1988) and Aquino et al. (1989, 1991, 1997) (see Figure 1) in the barks of *U. tomentosa* and *U. guianensis* (Yepez et al., 1991). Due to manufacturing procedures (e.g., aqueous-acid), quinovic acid derivatives are not extracted without undergoing chemical modification (Keplinger, 1999).

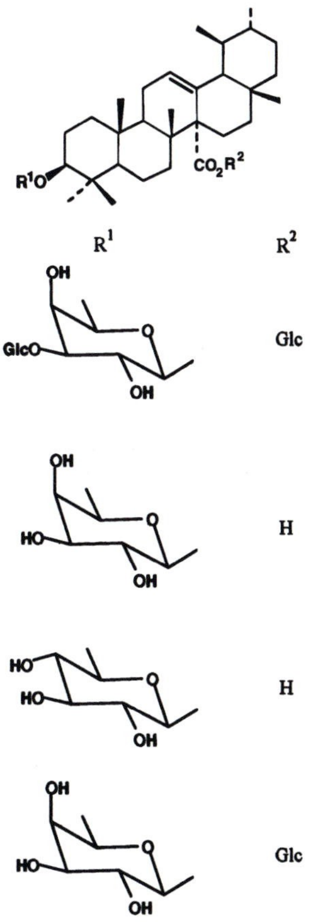

FIGURE 1. Major Active Constituents of *Uncaria tomentosa* (Cat's Claw): Quinovic Acid Derivatives

Nitrogenous Compounds

Alkaloids

The main active constituents of the root and stalk bark are thought to be oxindole alkaloids (Wagner, Kreutzkamp et al., 1985; Reinhard, 1999; Wurm et al., 1998). The major pentacyclic oxindole alkaloids (POAs) identified in the root and stalk bark of Peruvian *Uncaria tomentosa* are pteropodine (uncarine C), isopteropodine (uncarine E), speciophylline (uncarine D), uncarine F (methyl-2-oxo-formosanan-16-carboxylic acid-methyl ester), mitraphylline, and isomitraphylline. The tetracyclic oxindole alkaloids (TOAs) rynchophylline and isorynchophylline also occur in the root (see Figure 2). Like the POAs, their concentrations fluctuate widely (Stuppner et al., 1993; Laus and Keplinger, 1994; Laus et al., 1997) and appear to show seasonal variations. The TOAs occur in small amounts in *Uncaria tomentosa*-PC and in relatively large amounts in *Uncaria tomentosa*-TC. Variations in the concentration and occurrence of both indole alkaloid structures are further compounded by the fact that these alkaloids readily isomerize (Laus et al., 1996; Laus and Keplinger, 1994).

The main alkaloids in the stalk of *Uncaria tomentosa*-PC are POAs (0.5%) (Keplinger et al., 1996). The POA content of the roots (*Uncaria tomentosa*-PC) ranges from 0.5-3% (Laus and Keplinger, 1997). Minor oxindole and indole alkaloids occurring in the roots of either chemotype are as follows: hirsuteine, dihydrocorynantheine, hirsutine, akuammigine, isocorynoxeine, and corynoxeine (Laus et al., 1997).

The leaves, stalk, and root barks of *U. guianensis* contain predominantly tetracyclic oxindole alkaloids (TOAs), the major one being rynchophylline. POAs, speciopyhllline, and pteropodine were found in the root bark along with the TOA mitraphylline. Total alkaloid content of the leaves was 0.14% and that of the root bark, 0.04% (Lavault et al., 1983). TOAs found in the leaves and stalk of this species include: angustine, hirsutine, hirsuteine, dihydrocorynantheine, mitraphylline, rynchophylline, and isorynchophylline (Phillipson et al., 1978).

The indole alkaloid patterns of 50 representative cat's claw products sold commercially in the United States, Canada, Germany, the Netherlands, Austria, Spain, Peru, and New Zealand were analyzed for alkaloid contents. These products were mostly stalk bark preparations in the form of teas, extracts, crude material, tablets, drops, gel capsules, and hard gelatin capsules containing powder extracts. Tests revealed that of the total indole alkaloid content (0.02-4.39 mg/unit of capsules and tablets), TOAs occurred in amounts from 0-81% (Laus et al., 1998). These samples would therefore conform to the tetracyclic chemotype (TC) of *Uncaria tomentosa,* since samples of the PC have shown no TOAs, or only very little (Laus et al., 1997).

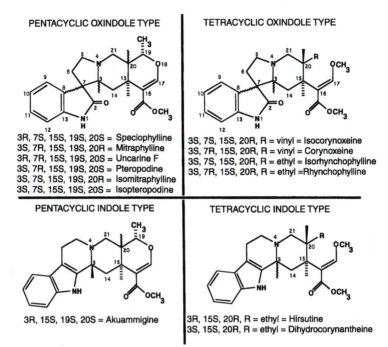

PENTACYCLIC OXINDOLE TYPE

3R, 7S, 15S, 19S, 20S = Speciophylline
3S, 7R, 15S, 19S, 20R = Mitraphylline
3R, 7R, 15S, 19S, 20S = Uncarine F
3S, 7R, 15S, 19S, 20S = Pteropodine
3S, 7S, 15S, 19S, 20R = Isomitraphylline
3S, 7S, 15S, 19S, 20S = Isopteropodine

TETRACYCLIC OXINDOLE TYPE

3S, 7S, 15S, 20R, R = vinyl = Isocorynoxeine
3S, 7R, 15S, 20R, R = vinyl = Corynoxeine
3S, 7S, 15S, 20R, R = ethyl = Isorhynchophylline
3S, 7R, 15S, 20R, R = ethyl =Rhynchophylline

PENTACYCLIC INDOLE TYPE

3R, 15S, 19S, 20S = Akuammigine

TETRACYCLIC INDOLE TYPE

3R, 15S, 20R, R = ethyl = Hirsutine
3S, 15S, 20R, R = ethyl = Dihydrocorynantheine

FIGURE 2. Major Active Constituents of *Uncaria tomentosa* (Cat's Claw): Alkaloids

Most cat's claw products contain varying mixtures of TOAs and POAs (Keplinger et al., 1999), and possibly mixtures of the two species of *Uncaria* indigenous to Peru: *U. tomentosa* and *U. guianensis*.

Several gluco indole alkaloids were recently found in the stem of Peruvian *U. tomentosa* (chemotype not determined): lyaloside, 5(*S*)-5-carboxystrictosidine, and 3-4-dehydro-5-carboxystrictosidine, a gluco monoterpenoid indole alkaloid with a 3,4-dihydro-β-carboline ring system (Kitajima, Hashimoto, Yokoya, Takayama, Aimi et al., 2000).

Phenolic Compounds

Tannins

The stalk bark of *U. tomentosa* contains a high amount (20%) of tannins (De Ugaz, 1995).

Polyphenolics

The root bark of *Uncaria tomentosa* contains proanthocyanidins 1b, 2b, 3b, 4b and 1a and (–)-epicatechin (Montenegro de Matta et al., 1976; Wirth and Wagner, 1997).

Terpenoid Compounds

Triterpenes

The root bark of *U. tomentosa* contains triterpenes (Aquino et al., 1990, 1991, 1997), including ursolic acid, oleanolic acid (Aquino et al., 1991), and hydroxylated ursenes (Aquino et al., 1990). Four hydroxyursolic acid-type triterpenes were identified in the stem bark (Kitajima, Hashimoto, Yokoya, Takayama, and Aimi, 2000).

Steroids

Stigmasterol and campesterol were identified in the bark of *U. tomentosa* (plant part not stated), and β-sitosterol was found to comprise 60% of the total sterolic fraction (Senatore et al., 1989).

Other Constituents

The inner bark of the stalk contains β-sitosteryl glucoside and 7-deoxyloganic acid, the C-8-(*S*)-isomer of 7-deoxyloganic acid, a newly reported natural product structurally similar to deoxyloganic acid isomers found in *Nepeta cataria* (Muhammad et al., 2001).

THERAPEUTIC APPLICATIONS

Applications of cat's claw in clinical settings have largely been made in immunological conditions, including inflammatory states (Jones, 1995).

PRECLINICAL STUDIES

Digestive, Hepatic, and Gastrointestinal Functions

Gastric Functions

The stalk bark of *Uncaria tomentosa* has shown beneficial effects against nonsteroidal anti-inflammatory drug (NSAID) enteropathy. In rats subjected to indomethacin-induced chronic intestinal inflammation (enteritis), administration of cat's claw bark to the drinking water at 5 mg/mL resulted in significantly lower levels of liver metallothionein as an index of inflammation (Sandoval et al., 1997). In a similar study, the intestinal morphology of indomethacin-treated rats was fully restored, and liver metallothionen expression and inflammatory indices were suppressed by cat's claw. In vitro experiments indicated that the anti-inflammatory action of cat's claw is primarily mediated through the inhibition of inflammatory gene expression involving a suppression of nuclear factor Kappa B (NF-κB) (Miller et al., 1999).

Endocrine and Hormonal Functions

Reproductive Hormone Interactions

Although the use of cat's claw in Peru as a contraceptive (De Feo, 1992; Jones, 1995) remains to be closely examined in pharmacological studies, recent research has shown definite reproductive hormone modulating activity. An aqueous extract of dried *U. tomentosa* bark from Peru (Alexander von Humbolt forest preserve) was tested against tamoxifen for the purpose of detecting possible estrogen receptor binding activity in vitro. Salazar and Jayme (1998) used tumor tissues from women diagnosed with infiltrating ductal carcinoma III (poorly differentiated), which were then incubated with radiolabelled estrogen in various concentrations. Sets of these cells were subsequently incubated with tamoxifen or 10 μg and 20 μg of the bark extract. In a specific binding assay, the addition of cat's claw significantly and dose-dependently inhibited [^{3}H]estradiol binding to the cell receptor of the estrogen-dependent tumor cytosol after 1 h incubation. In a competitive binding assay, cat's claw further reduced the [^{3}H]estradiol binding in a dose-dependent manner. In another test, using the cytosol pretreated with tamoxifen or cat's claw prior to adding [^{3}H]estradiol, the bark extract (20 μg) reduced [^{3}H]estradiol binding by 47.2%, while tamoxifen reduced binding by 69.3%. Additional tests using either concentration of the bark extract showed that the inhibition of [^{3}H]estradiol binding was definitely noncompetitive. These results suggest that cat's claw bark can interact with "distinct binding sites" on the estrogen receptor and that the receptor molecule then undergoes "different conformational modifications" (Salazar and Jayme, 1998, p. 124).

Rodriguez et al. (1998) reported that in human granulosa cells obtained from patients undergoing in vitro fertilization, cat's claw extracts (presumably stalk bark) at amounts equivalent to dietary doses, dose-dependently (100 pg/mL to 10 μg/mL) caused a statistically significant inhibition of progesterone production. Administered orally to sexually mature female rats for eight weeks, a low dose of cat's claw extract (2 mg/day), equivalent to the manufacturer's suggested daily dosage, produced no significant changes in profiles of electrolytes, kidney, liver, or glucose. For six weeks, no changes were noticed in circulating hormone levels compared to the untreated controls. By the eighth week however, serum progesterone (P_4) and estradiol (E_2) levels were reduced by 68% and 71%, respectively, in both the high-dose group (20 mg/day) and the low-dose group (2 mg/day). Rodriguez and colleagues concluded that these results indicate that cat's claw has the potential to selectively alter ovarian hormone production and therefore should be used with care.

Mice administered an aqueous extract of the root in their drinking water (6.25 mg/kg and 25 mg/kg p.o.) showed no signs of toxicity; however, the female mice, when caged with male mice, produced no offspring (Keplinger, 1982).

Immune Functions; Inflammation and Disease

Cancer

Cytotoxicity. Cat's claw is reported to inhibit tumor cell DNA polymerase, an enzyme that allows the proliferation of abnormal cells (Peluso et al., 1993). In other in vitro studies, a proprietary cat's claw extract (CampaMed, New York, NY, C-MED-100), consisting of a low molecular weight water-soluble fraction of *U. tomentosa* stalk bark, has been shown to both repair DNA in damaged, normal cells (Sheng, Bryngelsson et al., 2000) and to fragment DNA in tumor cells. The same water-soluble extract inhibited proliferation of human B lymphoma (Raji) and two types of human leukemic cells (HL60 and K562). The mechanism responsible appeared to be apoptosis (DNA fragmentation). Double and single strand breaks in the tumor cells were dose-dependently (50-400 μg/mL) increased after 24 h exposure to the extract. The authors point out that maximum apoptosis occurred at 48 or 72 h, a time course similar to that of betulinic acid derived from beech and birch trees (Sheng et al., 1998). This extract is standardized to contain 8% or more carboxyl alkyl esters and is prepared by hot water extraction and depletion of indole alkaloids (< 0.05%) and other high molecular weight (>10,000 MW) conjugated compounds such as tannins (Sheng, Bryngelsson, et al., 2000; Sheng, Pero, et al., 2000).

Pteropodine and isopteropodine showed only weak activity in yeast assays for DNA damage. An ethanolic extract of *U. guianensis* bark was even weaker (Lee et al., 1999).

The POA uncarine F showed pronounced antiproliferative activity in vitro in HL60 and U-937 leukemic cells in a dose-dependent fashion. At the IC_{50} for U-937 leukemic cells (29.0 μmol/L), there was no inhibition of normal human bone marrow progenitor cells. This lack of inhibition to normal cells made this compound a candidate for further consideration as a possible antileukemic drug. Isopteropodine was approximately 25% less potent, and the other POAs of cat's claw showed still less potency (Stuppner et al., 1993). However, research by others (Wurm et al., 1998) appears to refute this activity, for no antiproliferative effect on U937 cells with POAs in noncytotoxic concentrations were found.

Against the in vitro growth of three human cancer cell lines (nonsmall cell lung carcinoma, H460; prostate carcinoma, DU145; cervical carcinoma, ME180) and two mouse cancer cell lines (C3H stomach cancer, C678; reticular lymphosarcoma, LSR), pteropodine and isopteropodine showed moderate cytotoxic activity (38-51 μg/mL and 17-42 μg/mL) (Lee et al., 1999). When used against the in vitro growth of four human cancer cell lines (ductal carcinoma, BT549; epidermoid carcinoma, KB; ovarian carcinoma, SK-OV-3; and malignant melanoma, SK-MEL), isopteropodine showed no cytotoxicity activity; however, speciophylline was weakly active (30-35 μg/mL) and pteropodine was weakly active (IC_{50} 37 μg/mL) only against the ovarian carcinoma cell line. In a normal cell line (African green monkey kidney fibroblast cells, VERO; nontransformed), only speciophylline was active, however weakly (39 μg/mL), while the other two alkaloids were inactive (Muhammad et al., 2001).

Riva et al. (2001) examined the in vitro antiproliferative activity of cat's claw against the human breast cancer cell line MCF7. A freeze-dried water decoction and a methanolic extract of the powdered bark were tested along with a methanolic extract of the air-dried leaves, in addition to various fractions of both the leaves and bark. The methanolic extract of the bark was far more potent at inhibiting the proliferation of MCF7 cells (IC_{50} 38 μg/mL) than the water extract (270 μg/mL), with cell growth inhibited by 85% from 100 μg/mL of the methanolic extract. Fractions of the water extract proved less effective whereas two fractions of the methanolic extract showed good activity with IC_{50}s of 18 and 45 μg/mL. The methanolic extract of the leaves also inhibited cellular proliferation of the breast cancer cells (IC_{50} 38 μg/mL), and one fraction showed exceptional activity (IC_{50} 10 μg/mL) and inhibited cell growth by 90% at a concentration of 100 μg/mL. The leaf extract was clearly more potent than the bark extracts, but what constituted the active fractions had yet to be elucidated.

Immune Functions

Immunopotentiation. Sheng, Bryngelsson, et al. (2000) showed that female mice pretreated daily with an extract of *U. tomentosa* (C-MED-100 80 mg/kg by gavage for eight weeks) showed a greater increase in white blood cells after whole body irradiation than irradiated controls ($p < 0.01$), but not from a dose of 40 mg/kg. In separate experiments in nonirradiated female mice, the extract also caused a significant increase ($p < 0.05$) in white blood cells from a dose of 160 mg/kg (by gavage) for four weeks and from 40 mg/kg for eight weeks. Significant increases in lymphocyte proliferation were found in nonirradiated female mice administered daily doses of 40 mg/kg ($p < 0.05$) or 80 mg/kg ($p < 0.01$) for eight weeks, but not from doses of 20 mg/kg and lower.

Sheng, Pero, et al. (2000) examined the effects of C-MED-100 in a rat model of drug-induced leukopenia using the chemotherapy agent doxorubicin (DXR). The effects of the cat's claw extract were compared to a positive control, Neupogen, a granulocyte colony-stimulating agent used to counter-act and restore immune cells in chemotherapy patients, and to a group of fe-male rats treated only with DXR. A day after the last injection of DXR, the rats received consecutive daily treatment with either the cat's claw extract (80 mg/kg p.o. by gavage for 16 days) or Neupogen (5 and 10 µg/kg s.c. for 10 days). The recovery of white blood cells from treatment with the cat's claw extract was significant and dose-dependent, and while Neupogen also caused a rapid recovery of WBCs, the spectrum was more limited with no significant effect on recovery of mononuclear leukocyte fractions. Whereas the cat's claw extract allowed rapid recovery of all the WBC fractions in a proportional manner, with Neupogen only nonlymphocyte fractions showed significant recovery. No significant differences in organ or body weights were found in rats that received the cat's claw extract compared to controls other than those associated with DXR treatment.

Lemaire et al. (1999) worked with two commercial stalk bark extracts of *U. tomentosa* sold in Peru: a freeze-dried water extract (Pacifico), and an at-omized water extract (La Molina). Both extracts produced comparable re-sults in their ability to stimulate production of IL-1 and IL-6 of alveolar macrophages in vitro, which increased 10-fold and 7.5-fold, respectively; however, only from extremely high concentrations (>100 µg/mL) of little relevance to human use of cat's claw. HPLC analysis showed that both bark samples contained characteristic POAs of *U. tomentosa* but the study failed to include an analysis of the TOA contents. Total oxindole alkaloid contents of the extracts were reported as 5.57 mg/g (La Molina) and 6.98 mg/g (Pacifico).

A mixture of the immunologically-active POAs from *U. tomentosa*-PC induced the release of a lymphocyte-growth factor from endothelial cells that significantly stimulated the proliferation of normal resting hu-man T-lymphocytes and B-lymphocytes in vitro. However, the activity was antagonized by the presence of the TOAs rynchophylline and isoryncho-phylline (Keplinger et al., 1999). Incubating both alkaloid types together with endothelial cell lines resulted in supernatants (SNs) influencing the proliferation of normal human T lymphocytes at only $94 \pm 14\%$ of the con-trol. Similarly, when TOAs were admixed with POAs, the resulting SNs showed a dose-dependent reduction in lymphoblast antiproliferation activ-ity. Alone, TOAs showed no antiproliferating activity and even the opposite effect. Wurm et al. (1998) postulate that the antagonizing effects between the two types of oxindole alkaloids on the yet-to-be characterized immunoregulating factor(s) in cat's claw warrant greater control of mixed plant chemotypes in therapeutic preparations of the plant, for their use would be of doubtful benefit if the TOAs in cat's claw also show antagonistic activity in vivo.

When freshly isolated resting normal human B and T lymphocytes were incubated with diluted (1:4) SN-POAs, resting T lymphocyte proliferation increased 110% and 137% from a 1:8 dilution. Further dilutions resulted in smaller increases in proliferation. B cell proliferation increased 82% (1:4), 53% (1:8), and 43% (1:16 dilution). SN-TOAs showed proliferation activity not significantly different from the control (Wurm et al., 1998).

An immunoregulatory effect has been proposed for the action of the POAs which is not found from the TOAs of *U. tomentosa*-PC. The lymphocyte proliferation-regulating or "immunoregulatory" effect was found with noncytotoxic concentrations of POAs in POA-induced SNs, and cell viability was not adversely affected compared to controls (Wurm et al., 1998). SNs produced by incubating normal human endothelial cells (producers of T cell activators and B cell differentiating factors, interleukin-1α, IL-8, IL-6, and interleukin-1β) with POAs from *U. tomentosa*-PC (SN-POAs) showed significant antiproliferation activity on highly active human T lymphocytes and B blasts, compared to control cells (medium-treated SN and TOA-treated cells). Curiously, in the SNs treated with POAs and in the supernatant medium (medium-treated cells), Il-6 was detected (ELISA) in equal concentrations (Wurm et al., 1998).

Lymphoblasts are lymphocytes in a state ready to begin mitosis (cell division). The cells produced, known as effector cells, undergo maturation and show immune cell functions akin to their cellular lineage for a few days afterward. Therefore, the lymphocyte proliferation-regulating effect of POA SNs may have therapeutic bearing on immunological states in which immune cells are overly active, such as in autoimmune disorders. The yet-to-be elucidated factor(s) produced in the endothelial cells incubated with POAs appear(s) to be novel and to have a weight of 30 kDa (Wurm et al., 1998).

An aqueous extract in the form of a water-soluble hydrochloride of the mixed alkaloids of *Uncaria tomentosa* administered to rats (10 mg/kg, i.p.) caused a pronounced enhancement of granulocyte phagocytosis, as measured by the carbon clearance test. The same test substance in two different strengths (0.1 and 0.001 mg/kg i.p.) was much less active than the same substance at a higher dose (10 mg/kg i.p.). In vitro (chemoluminescence model), the POAs are immunologically active. But in vivo studies (carbon clearance test) have shown that they are not active without the presence of the catechin tannin fraction of the root bark, even though these catechins were shown to be immunologically inactive. Therefore, the catechin tannin content of the root bark in vivo contributes in some undetermined synergistic way to the immunological activity present (Wagner, Kreutzkamp, et al., 1985; Wirth and Wagner, 1997).

In the granulocytic test, the average increase in phagocytic activity shown by the stalk bark was found to be 10% to 20%, while that of the root bark (*U. tomentosa*-PC) was on average 30% to 40%. The difference in potency was attributed to the low alkaloid content of the stalk bark and to differences in patterns of the oxindole alkaloids present (Keplinger, 1994). Although a greater content of oxindole alkaloids occurs in the root compared to the stalk (Keplinger et al., 1996), the proposed chemotypes of *Uncaria tomentosa* could explain the differences in alkaloid patterns and immunological activity (Laus et al., 1997), which is pronounced from the POAs versus the TOAs (Wurm et al., 1998).

Wagner, Kreutzkamp, et al. (1985) tested the alkaloid-containing aqueous macerate and the individual OAs derived from the root of *Uncaria tomentosa* for phagocytosis-modulating activity in vitro, using two chemoluminescence models (granulocyte activation and phagocytosis), and the in vivo carbon clearance test of phagocytosis. The most active alkaloids (granulocyte-phagocytosis and a chemoluminescence model of granulocyte activity with opsonized zymosan), along with their respective activity as percent increases in phagocytic activity, were as follows: isopteropodine (55%), pteropodine (26%), isomitraphylline (27%), and isorynchophylline (27%); each producing a pronounced enhancing effect on phagocytosis. Mitraphylline and the TOA rynchophylline were inactive (Wagner, Kreutzkamp et al., 1985; Wagner, Proksch et al., 1985).

More extensive research with the root showed that the mixture of raw alkaloids (in water-soluble form) produce an average increase in phagocytic activity of 20%. Pteropodine (methyl-2-oxoformosanan-16-carboxylic acid-methyl ester) and isopteropodine (methyl-2-oxo-formosanan-18-carboxylic acid-methyl ester) in a concentration of 27 ng/mL stimulated phagocytic activity in vitro by 27% and 66%, respectively, and were found responsible for the immunopotentiating activity of *U. tomentosa*-PC (Wagner, Kreutzkamp, et al., 1985; Wagner, Proksch, et al., 1985; Wagner, 1987b; Kreutzkamp, 1984). This research has also shown that by checking for any apparent increases in phagocytic activity (chemoluminescence test), rynchophylline, isorynchophylline, and mitraphylline are inactive (Kreutzkamp, 1984; Keplinger, 1994). Note that for isorynchophylline, this finding contradicts Wagner, Kreutzkamp, et al. (1985) and Wagner, Proksch, et al., (1985).

Among other oxindole alkaloids in *U. tomentosa* stalk bark and root (Laus et al., 1997), speciophylline (POA) stimulated granulocyte phagocytosis in vitro by 25% to 35% (Wagner, 1987a). Among the minor alkaloids that occur in the root (Laus et al., 1997), the tetracyclic indoles dihydrocorynantheine, hirsutine, and hirsuteine also stimulated granulocyte phagocytosis, by 25% to 35% (Wagner, 1987a).

In concentrations of 1 mg/mL and higher, the activity of the OAs in *U. tomentosa* approach cytotoxic levels and no immunologic activity is found in chemoluminescence from the granulocyte phagocytosis test (Wagner, Kreutzkamp, et al., 1985; Wagner, 1987a). The oxindole alkaloids in a concentration of 1% in vitro caused the granulocytes to lyse (Keplinger, 1994). The immunologically active alkaloids of cat's claw exhibited in vitro immunological activity in these tests at concentrations of 0.1-100 μg/mL granulocytes (Wagner, Kreutzkamp, et al., 1985; Keplinger, 1994). Therefore, the immunologically effective dosage is correspondingly low and the amount of root bark (*Uncaria tomentosa*-PC) to achieve a toxic dose is correspondingly high (Immodal Pharmaka, 1995).

Immunosuppression. Sandoval et al. (2000) compared the in vitro immunomodulating effects of cat's claw bark aqueous decoctions on the inhibition of tumor necrosis factor-α (TNF-α) synthesis/release. The extracts were prepared from micropulverized bark which were either freeze-dried or left in solution. Cells pretreated with either cat's claw preparation showed a significant 65% to 85% decrease in the synthesis of lipopolysaccharide-induced TNF-α synthesis ($p < 0.001$). With the freeze-dried preparation, the effect was evident from a wide range of concentrations (0.001 to 3 μg/mL; maximal inhibition 86.0% at 1.2 ng/mL) and more pronounced compared to the aqueous extract in solution (0.01 to 100 μg/mL; maximal inhibition 84.0% at 28 ng/mL). This study provides compelling preliminary evidence of a pharmacological basis to the use of cat's claw against inflammatory diseases. Using a model of NSAID-induced gastritis, Miller et al. (1999) reported that an extract of *U. tomentosa* bark inhibited TNF-α gene expression in gastric mucosa, an effect that Sandoval-Chacón et al. (1998) reported to be the result of cat's claw inhibiting the activation of nuclear factor-kappa B (NF-κB) (see Antioxidant Activity). Piscoya et al. (2001) reported inhibition of TNF-α synthesis/release from two species of cat's claw using a murine macrophage stimulated by lipopolysaccharide (LPS). Adding them before LPS stimulation, the activity of freeze-dried water extracts of *U. tomentosa* and *U. guianensis* were compared. Either extract caused a highly significant and dose-dependent reduction in levels of TNF-α and they were equally potent, and at very low concentrations of 10.2-10.9 ng/mL. The extract of *U. tomentosa* was tested for in vitro inhibition of prostaglandin E_2 (PGE_2) production using the same cell line and LPS as the inducer. The extract had no effect on basal PGE_2 levels, but significantly decreased LPS-induced increases. The dose required (10 μg/mL) was greater than that for suppression of TNF-α production.

Infectious Diseases

Viral infections. Quinovic acid glycosides derived from the root showed in vitro cytotoxic activity in vesicular stomatitis virus cells; however, in relation to a toxic dose to normal cells, the concentrations required were relatively high (Aquino et al., 1989; Cerri et al., 1988).

Cytotoxic activity (in vitro) against rhinovirus type 1B infected cells was shown from two of the quinovic acid glycosides. But again, the concentrations required to inhibit the cytopathic effect of the rhinovirus by 50% (30 and 20 μg/mL, respectively) were not that far from their maximum nontoxic concentrations (60 and 100 μg/mL, respectively) (Aquino et al., 1989).

The inhibition of herpesvirus (H. labialis and H. genitalis) was shown in vitro by a standardized root extract of *U. tomentosa*-PC. H. genitalis appeared to be more susceptible to inactivation by the extract (0.3-10 μg/mL, 65-100% inhibition) than H. labialis (1-10 μg/mL, 19-100% inhibition) (Immodal Pharmaka, 1995).

Inflammatory Response

From the bark, Wirth and Wagner (1997) isolated acetylated (–)-epicatechin and the procyanidins cinchonain 1a and 1b. Cinchonain 1b (42.5 μM/mL) inhibited 5-lipoxygenase in vitro, an important mediator of inflammatory substances, such as leukotrienes. The researchers postulated that the anti-inflammatory, antioxidative, and antiviral activities of *U. tomentosa* might be partly due to all three of these compounds acting in concert.

Aquino et al. (1991) showed that a water extract of the root bark (84 mg/kg p.o.) inhibited carrageenan-induced edema in the rat paw by 41.2%, and by 69.2% from a chloroform-methanol extract (50 mg/kg); however, the doses, corresponding to 2 g of dried root bark/kg, were extremely high. Various quinovic acid glycosides tested individually in low doses (more akin to amounts in the crude extract) showed no antiedemic activity. One quinovic acid glycoside (quinovic acid-3-β-*O*-(β-D-quinovopyranosyl)-(27 α 1)-β-D-glucopyranosyl ester) was most active, but at a dosage not achievable from the root bark decoction or extract (20 mg/kg p.o., 33% inhibition at 3 h). Individual triterpenic acids derived from the root bark, including oleanolic acid, were inactive at the same dose. A minor active constituent may have been missed in this study and could not be ruled out as more active (Aquino et al., 1991).

In the same test in rats, antiedemic activity of the alkaloid fraction of the root bark of *U. tomentosa*-PC was shown from dosages of 2-100 mg/kg p.o. (16% to 42% inhibition). Administered i.p., 10 mg/kg produced a slightly greater inhibition of edema (47%) than a comparable dose of indomethacin (9 mg/kg i.p., 43% inhibition) (Keplinger, 1982).

A significant inhibition of stress-induced ulcer formation in rats was shown following pretreatment with 3 mL of a decoction of *U. tomentosa* root bark added to drinking water. The size and number of large gastric ulcers was significantly inhibited compared to controls (Fazzi, 1989).

As part of the inflammatory response, platelet aggregation effects of cat's claw appear to remain largely unexplored. However, a major alkaloid constituent, rynchophylline, has shown in vitro inhibitory activity against platelet aggregation induced by collagen, adenosine 5'-diphosphate (ADP), and arachidonic acid (AA) (IC_{50}: 7.4, 6.7, and 7.2 μmol/L, respectively) (Chen et al., 1992).

Metabolic and Nutritional Functions

Antioxidant Activity

Piscoya et al. (2001) demonstrated that freeze-dried water extracts of the stalk barks of *U. tomentosa* and *U. guianensis* were active as antioxidants in the scavenging DPPH (α,α-diphenyl-β-picrylhydrazyl) radical. The concentration of *U. guianensis* required (13.6 μg/mL) was less than that of *U. tomentosa* (EC_{50} 21.7 μg/mL), yet the researchers considered them to be of comparable potency.

In a study by Rizzi et al. (1993), six fractions and five extracts of the chloroform-ethanol extract of the root bark of cat's claw in the Ames test, with or without the addition of 8-methoxypsoralen and treatment with UVA irradiation, showed protective activity against induced photomutagenicity. Antimutagenic activity reached 70% and a minimum of 30%. The alcoholic extract inhibited mutagenesis by 59%. By comparison, β-carotene inhibited mutagenic activity by 68%. Antimutagenic activity was also noted in a volunteer smoker instructed to drink the root bark decoction (6.5 g/day) for 15 days. Positive mutagenic activity of the subject's urine was confirmed to decrease dramatically during the ingestion of the root bark decoction, and remained at lower levels for eight days after the treatment ended. This effect was attributed to a possible antioxidant action (Rizzi et al., 1993). The cytoprotective constituents more likely involved were catechin tannins and proanthocyanidins (Montenegro de Matta et al., 1976), or a combination of constituents including the oxindole alkaloids (Stuppner et al., 1993).

The stalk bark of *U. tomentosa* has shown cytoprotective activity against oxidant-induced stress to macrophages in vitro, significantly lowering the rate of cell death (apoptosis quantified by ELISA assay) induced by peroxynitrite (Sandoval et al., 1997). In further in vitro tests of antioxidant activity, Sandoval et al. (2000) compared the effects of aqueous extracts prepared by decocting micropulverized bark and either freeze-drying the extract or leaving it in solution. Concentration-dependent inhibition of the DPPH radical was evident from simultaneous treatment of cells with either extract at low concentrations (0.1-300 µg/mL); however, the freeze-dried extract was significantly more effective ($p < 0.001$) than the simple extract, showing maximal inhibition at a far smaller concentration (EC_{50} 1.8 µg/mL versus EC_{50} 150 µg/mL, respectively). Cells treated simultaneously with the free radical and the freeze-dried water extract (10 µg/mL) and incubated together showed significantly greater preservation of cell viability compared to control cells ($p < 0.01$). When studied in cell death induced by UV-irradiation, cells pretreated with the freeze-dried cat's claw extract (1 or 10 µg/mL) showed significantly less necrosis, but no added protection against apoptosis.

Sheng, Bryngelsson, et al. (2000) administered C-MED-100 (40 or 80 mg/kg per day by gavage) or sterile tap water (controls) to female rats for 8 weeks before exposing half the rats to whole body irradiation (12 Gy). The animals were then allowed to naturally repair from the irradiation for 3 h before examination of immune enhancement. Compared to nonirradiated controls and the active treatment groups, tap water-treated controls showed significantly greater amounts of DNA single strand and double strand breaks (DSB). The animals pretreated with the cat's claw extract showed nearly complete repair of single strand breaks, and at the high dose, significant repair of DNA double strand breaks, and the effect appeared to be dose-dependent. Although the level of DSB repair from lower dose failed to reach significance, there was a clear tendency towards enhanced repair.

Desmarchelier et al. (1997) demonstrated that in vitro, methanol extracts of the stalk bark and the roots of *U. tomentosa* prevent free radical-mediated damage to DNA sugar, and antioxidant activity in the hydroperoxide-initiated chemiluminescence assay using catechin as the standard. Aqueous, decocted, and methanolic extracts of the stalk bark showed considerably greater antioxidant activity than the root in the same extract forms (10 to 1000 µg/mL). The exception was the dichloromethane extract, in which case the root extract inhibited oxidation more than the stalk bark. At the lowest dose tested (10 µg/mL), both the stalk bark and root produced 0% or pro-oxidant activity in each extract form, except for the methanolic extract of the stalk bark (22% inhibition), and in the case of root, both the methanolic and dichloromethane extract (9% and 4% inhibition, respectively).

Ostrakhovich et al. (1997) reported that an *U. tomentosa* powder (lyophilized) extract (Induchimica S.A., Peru; presumably from stalk bark) could inhibit oxidant activity in a number of oxygen free radical systems, including oxygen radical production of peritoneal macrophages in two different models. Superoxide production and xanthine oxidase was significantly inhibited from a concentration of cat's claw extract of 2-20 µg/mL. For example, at a concentration of 20 µg/mL in the xanthine-xanthine oxidase system, the extract inhibited superoxide production by over 95%, and by 60% at 10 µg/mL. The results suggest that a decrease in the activity of NADPH-oxidase was involved, and that direct inhibition of free radicals by the extract was not significant.

In further tests, Ostrakhovich et al. (1997) showed that the *U. tomentosa* extract failed to decrease hydroxyl radical formation in the Fenton reaction, but rather enhanced its production. Using rat brain homogenates to test the ability of the extract to inhibit the oxidation of fatty cells (lipid peroxidation), the average degree of "general antioxidant activity" was 80% at a concentration of 20 μg/mL and 50% at 5 μg/mL. These "strong" rates of inhibition are typical of antioxidants that inhibit the "chain process" of lipid peroxidation. Incubated with peritoneal macrophages, the extract (5 μg/mL) had no effect on free radical production in a chemoluminescent (CL) test system; significant inhibition was only found at higher concentrations of the extract (≥10 μg/mL). Further incubation tests (monitoring cytochrome c reduction in parallel with nicotinamide adenine dinucleotide phosphate (NADPH)-oxidase activity) indicated that the extract (10 and 20 μg/mL) inactivates the NADPH-oxidase system and possibly influences macrophage receptors. The cat's claw extract (5 μg/mL) still decreased superoxide production compared to the control, though not significantly, and had no effect on the activity of the NADPH-oxidase enzyme (Ostrakhovich et al., 1997).

Ostrakhovich et al. (1998) examined *U. tomentosa* extract for peroxynitrite production-inhibiting activity on polymorphonuclear (PMN) lymphocytes taken from the peripheral blood of diabetes mellitus type I patients (n = 15), and from healthy donors (n = 10). A markedly higher level of neutrophilic peroxynitrite production in the PMN lymphocytes from the type I diabetics was noted compared to those from the healthy donors. Incubation of the PMN lymphocytes from both donor groups produced comparatively different results. Peroxynitrite formation by neutrophils (stimulated with phorbolmyristate acetate, PMA) from either donor group was significantly inhibited by the cat's claw extract (5 μg/mL) in the diabetes mellitus donor (DMD) neutrophils, but not in those of the healthy donors. Peroxynitrite formation was significantly increased in the healthy donor neutrophils (10 μg/mL), yet significantly decreased in the DMD neutrophils. However, at a higher dose (20 μg/mL) the extract caused a significant decrease in peroxynitric production in both kinds of donor neutrophils, though more so in those of DMD neutrophils ($p < 0.05$ versus $p < 0.01$). The results of this study represent a significant advance toward the application of cat's claw extract in diabetes mellitus therapy.

At concentrations of 25-100 μg/mL, a water extract of the stalk bark of *U. tomentosa* did not affect the cell viability of human intestinal epithelial cells (HT29) or murine macrophages (RAW 264.7). At a relatively high concentration, however difficult if not impossible to achieve in vivo (100 μg/mL), the extract significantly decreased lipopolysaccharide-mediated nitrite formation in human intestinal epithelial cells (HT29) and in murine macrophages

(RAW 264.7). At the same concentration, the extract also caused a significant *direct* decrease in peroxynitrite and nitric oxide levels, inhibited gene expression of inducible nitric oxide synthetase (iNOS) in HT29 cells, significantly decreased peroxynitrite-induced apoptosis (DNA fragmentation) of HT 29 cells and murine macrophages, and inhibited NF-κB activation in macrophages (Sandoval-Chacón et al., 1998).

Inhibitors of apoptosis are currently of great interest as potential therapeutic agents to inhibit neurologically-degenerative processes, such as Alzheimer's and Parkinson's disease, and retinal degeneration, while activators of apoptosis are of considerable interest in the field of cancer research (Kinloch et al., 1999). NF-κB, a protein found in the cytoplasm of cells, is a transcriptional factor, which, when activated, can induce inflammatory processes in endothelial cells and is an important target of anti-inflammatory drug development. NF-κB activation can be set off by viral products, bacteria, proinflammatory cytokines, and oxidative or physical stress (Lee, 1994), and the inhibition of NF-κB glucocorticoids can turn off inducible nitric oxide expression (Sandoval-Chacón et al., 1998). By blocking improperly activated NF-κB, expression of the proinflammatory cytokine cyclooxygenase-2 (COX-2) can also be inhibited (Surh et al., 2001) (see Immunosuppression).

Neurological, Psychological, and Behavioral Functions

Neurodegenerative Disorders

Alzheimer's disease. A water-soluble fraction derived from the stalk bark of *U. tomentosa* has shown in vitro and in vivo β-amyloid inhibiting activity (Snow, 1999; Snow et al., 2000; Petersen, 1999; Cummings et al., 2000). Experiments have shown that the extract inhibits not only formation and deposition of Alzheimer's β-amyloid protein deposits, but even their growth (McCurley et al., 1998; Castillo, Snow, et al., 2001). Researchers believe that, when identified, the active amyloid-dissolving constituents isolated from the extract will represent the most active compounds ever discovered exhibiting this kind of activity. These constituents are potential therapeutic agents in the treatment of early to midstage Alzheimer's disease (inhibiting initiation and growth of amyloid fibrils), and mid- to late stages of the disease (dissolving preformed amyloid fibrils); the latter also indicating application in type II diabetes amyloidosis (McCurley et al., 1998) in which the growth of amyloid fibrils in the pancreas compromises the normal function of the islets of Langerhans (Höppener et al., 2000). Studies to date have found that the major alkaloids of cat's claw are inactive. Compared to the active extract of cat's claw, a fraction consisting of as many as seven major water-soluble constituents showed even greater inhibitory activity against in vitro Alzheimer's β-amyloid fibril growth (53.2% versus 87.3% inhibition) as well as growth in a rodent model (51.0% versus 89.2% inhibition) (Snow et al., 2000).

The initial water-soluble extract derived from the bark of *U. tomentosa* inhibited the formation of both type II diabetes and Alzheimer's disease amyloidosis in vitro, as measured by a thioflavin T fluorometry assay. Dose-dependent inhibition of β-amyloid fibril growth and formation was shown when the extract was found also to inhibit β-amyloid-β-amyloid interactions in a solid phase binding assay. In addition, thioflavin T fluorometry tests of various sources of the extract revealed a potent dose-dependent amyloid-dissolving activity against preformed Alzheimer's disease amyloid fibrils, with low doses dissolving the fibrils by ~70% in 2 h of incubation. Similarly, islet amyloid fibrils or islet amyloid polypeptide dissolved by more than 80% in the same time period from exposure to the extract (McCurley et al., 1998).

In a rat model of Alzheimer's disease β-amyloid deposition, an extract of *U. tomentosa* administered by direct infusion into rat hippocampus caused a significant 74% inhibition of β-amyloid deposition ($p < 0.01$) from a dose of 1 μL, and 87% inhibition from a dose of 10 μL, each applied for seven days. Following the treatment, the cellular architecture of hippocampal brain sections showed no obvious adverse effects. These results indicate a potential use of the extract in the diet as a preventive measure against the deposition of amyloids as part of normal aging, and in Alzheimer's disease (Snow, Castillo, et al., 1999).

The in vitro β-amyloid formation-inhibiting, growth-inhibiting, and preformed β-amyloid-dissolving activity of cat's claw extract was markedly enhanced by the addition of a standardized *Ginkgo biloba* extract (Snow, Cummings, et al., 1999; Snow, 1999). However, in further in vitro studies in which ginkgo and β-amyloid protein were incubated together, the network of β-amyloid fibrils that formed showed no disruption. The same results were found using gotu kola *(Centella asiatica)* and red ginseng *(Panax ginseng),* whereas in the presence of the cat's claw extract the cells that formed were nonfibrillar and amorphous. The X ray pattern of these cells suggested that the cat's claw extract weakened and broadened hydrogen bonding in the fibril cells, which may be one of the mechanisms by which cat's claw inhibits the formation of these fibrils and the plaques they form (Castillo et al., 2000).

Parkinson's disease. Castillo, Choi, et al. (2001) reported that the same water-soluble constituents that inhibit the growth of Alzheimer's disease β-amyloid fibrillogenesis inhibited the in vitro growth of α-synuclein fibrillogenesis which causes the formation of amyloid plaques in Parkinson's disease. A peptide fragment of α-synuclein also forms amyloidlike fibrils and was used to test the active components of cat's claw. After incubating the fragment with the cat's claw constituents for 14 days, the researchers observed a dose-dependent inhibition of fibril formation by the seventh day from every concentration tested. At a weight ratio of ten parts fragment to one part of the active cat's claw components, fibril formation was significantly inhibited by 82.7%. Even at a weight ratio of one-hundredth parts of the cat's claw components, fibril formation was inhibited by 39.4%, and the results were similar in experiments using preformed fibrils.

Neurotoxicity/Neuroprotection

Shimada et al. (1999) studied the in vitro neuroprotective effects of indole and oxindole alkaloids common to the genus *Uncaria* against glutamate-induced neural death. Although glutamate is the major CNS excitatory neurotransmitter, brain ischemia is attended with increased extracellular concentrations of glutamate in the brain. Central neuron death is mediated by glutamate in epilepsy, neurodegenerative disease, and ischemic-hypoxic diseases, and the release of excess glutamate causes glutamate receptors to become overstimulated, resulting in toxicity to neuronal cells. In the MTT assay using cultured cerebellar granule cells, Shimada and colleagues examined the protective effect of the alkaloids against glutamate-induced neuronal death. According to cell viability, the most neuroprotective activity (55.7-97.0%) was shown from the oxindole alkaloids isorhynchophylline (10^{-4}-10^{-3} M) and isocorynoxeine (56.8-74.4% inhibition at 10^{-4}-10^{-3} M). The indole alkaloids hirsutine and hirsuteine were comparatively weaker, and the oxindole alkaloid rhynchophylline was only significantly effective at a high concentration (85.2% inhibition at 10^{-3} M). The active alkaloids appeared to afford protection by inhibiting glutamate-induced $^{45}Ca^{2+}$ influx (isorhynchophylline showing a 4.7-fold and isocorynoxeine a 3.4-fold inhibition at 3×10^{-4} M). At this, hirsutine and hirsuteine showed a 4.4-fold and a 3.8-fold inhibition of $^{45}Ca^{2+}$ influx (at 3×10^{-4} M).

Individual and total alkaloids of *U. tomentosa* were tested for antiamnesia effects in male mice; however, at doses too high to be relevant to human doses, and then not by the oral route. The deficits in retention performance induced by scopolamine were shown to be significantly and dose-dependently ameliorated by pretreatment by the total alkaloids (100-200 mg/kg i.p.). The more potent individual alkaloids were rynchophylline, isorynchophylline, and isopteropodine (each 200 mg/kg i.p.), with mitraphylline or pteropodine requiring twice the dose to show significance. The researchers concluded that impairment of memory acquisition induced by scopolamine is significantly ameliorated by the total alkaloids of *U. tomentosa,* and that since they could not rule out the involvement of other individual alkaloids in the fraction, those tested were either wholly or partly responsible (Mohamed et al., 2000).

CLINICAL STUDIES

Immune Disorders; Inflammation and Disease

Cancer

Chemotherapy adjunct treatments. An open-label trial of a proprietary extract of cat's claw root bark (Immodal Pharmaka, GmbH, Austria, Krallendorn a.k.a. Savéntaro) (*Uncaria tomentosa*-PC, 20-60 mg daily) as an adjuvant with conventional treatments was reported over a period of nine years in 53 patients with tumors. All patients were reported to have less side effects from radiation and chemotherapy and increased mobility and vitality. Those with early-stage tumors remained in remission ten years later, while those with advanced tumors showed, in some cases, arrested cancer growth for several months. Preliminary results indicated promise for the adjuvant in acute myeloid leukemia, brain stem glioma, adenocarcinoma of the colon, testicular teratoma, cervical carcinoma stage IVA, relapsing melanoma, and medulloblastoma (Immodal Pharmaka, 1996).

A 12-month open-label trial therapy of the same extract at 60 mg/day as an adjuvant with conventional cancer treatments in 78 cases of brain tumors was conducted by the University of Innsbruck, Austria. The best results appeared in patients who remained in remission after treatment for some types of brain tumors (e.g., ependymoblastoma WHO II and II, astrocytoma WHO II) more than others (e.g., glioblastoma multiforme WHO IV, malignant meningioma) (Immodal Pharmaka, 1996).

Immune Disorders

HIV/AIDS. In Europe, physicians using cat's claw in the form of 4:1 standardized, hydrochloric acid extract of the root bark (Immodal Pharmaka, GmbH, Austria, Krallendorn a.k.a. Savéntaro) (*Uncaria tomentosa*-PC) have reported benefits in their patients with viral infections of HIV (Keplinger, 1992, 1993), herpes simplex, and h. zoster (Immodal Pharmaka, 1996). The patients were also taking AZT; however, the extract used was without cytotoxicity to HIV (Immodal Pharmaka, 1996). In a group of 13 HIV patients who refused all other treatments, the same standardized powder extract (total POA content, 12 mg/g) was taken voluntarily for five months (20 mg/day p.o.). Measurements of total leukocyte numbers within the group showed that in those for whom numbers were low ($< 4000/\mu L$) before taking the extract, leukocyte numbers increased, and that for those who showed high counts beforehand ($> 9000/\mu L$), numbers were lowered following the extract. There were no significant changes in T4/T8 cells ratios; however, absolute and relative lymphocyte counts showed a significant increase, and the four cases who showed 20% less than normal levels before taking the extract showed normal levels after 3.9-4.9 months of treatment (Keplinger et al., 1999).

Immune Modulation

Immunomodulation. Lamm et al. (2001) conducted a study on the potential of a stalk bark extract of *U. tomentosa* (C-Med-100) to enhance the persistence of antibody responses to a 23 valent pneumococcal vaccine (Pneumovax). Previous studies have shown that pneumococcal vaccine is effective in only 60% to 80% of elderly subjects and that pneumococcal vaccination is also considerably lower in non-Hodgkin's lymphoma patients, HIV-seropositive patients, and children. Male volunteers ($n = 23$) ages 40-60 who had not received previous pneumococcal vaccines and had no chronic disease or were taking nutritional supplements or medications were randomly assigned to two groups: one group received the cat's claw extract ($n = 11$) for 60 days at a dosage of 350 mg taken twice daily (morning and evening), and the other group did not receive the extract ($n = 12$). On day 30, all volunteers were treated with the vaccine (0.5 mL i.m.) and their pneumococcal antibody titers were measured on days 1, 30, and 60. At the two-month point, the cat's claw group showed a significant enhancement in the ratio of lymphocytes to neutrophils ($p = 0.05$), but no changes in other blood cells, including helper and suppressor T cells, monocytes, basophils, and eosinophils. No significant difference was found in antibody titers, but after testing again at five months, the cat's claw group showed no drop in pneumococcal immunity whereas the other group had significantly decreased pneumococcal antibody titers. Clinical chemistry profiles of the volunteers showed no significant changes and there were no reports of side effects attributable to the cat's claw extract.

Integumentary, Muscular, and Skeletal Disorders

Osteoporosis

Piscoya et al. (2001) examined the potential therapeutic benefit and safety of a freeze-dried water extract of cat's claw bark in patients with osteoarthritis of the knee. The extract (concentration not stated) was prepared from *Uncaria guianensis* and administered in the form of tablets. The study was designed as a prospective, multicenter, parallel trial and was randomized, double-blind, and placebo-controlled. Male patients age 45-75 years were recruited who met the criteria of symptomatic osteoarthritis of the knee of grades II-II and who experienced pain on the majority of days in the preceding month and who needed therapy with NSAIDs for the prior three months or more. In patients with persistent pain, acetaminophen was permitted during the trial. After a washout period for NSAIDs and analgesics, the subjects were randomly assigned to either a cat's claw group or a placebo group. Patients who had any serious illness, drug abuse, alcoholism, secondary osteoarthritis, or were receiving injections of glucocorticoids into the knee or using oral anticoagulants were not allowed. Capsules containing cat's claw extract or placebo were administered for four weeks at a daily dosage of 100 mg. The placebo consisted of the excipient used in the cat's extract. Pain on activity scores showed a significant decrease ($p < 0.01$) in the cat's claw group ($n = 15$) compared to those receiving placebo ($n = 30$) after the first seven days. The decrease became highly significant in favor of the cat's claw group ($p < 0.001$) during the second and last week of the trial and was equally significant in the patient assessment scores. However, there were no significant improvements in knee circumference, pain at night or at rest compared to placebo. Improvements in these parameters might be seen from a longer trial. Blood chemistry showed changes in both groups during the study and side effects reported showed no differences in form or incidence between the two groups.

Metabolic and Nutritional Disorders

Aging and Senescence; Longevity Enhancement

After finding *U. tomentosa* root bark nonmutagenic in the Ames test, and protective against photomutagenesis in vitro, Rizzi et al. (1993) tested the root bark decoction for antimutagenic activity in two healthy volunteers. Both volunteers were 35-year-old males, one of whom was a smoker for more than 15 years and smoked about a pack a day. The decoction was prepared according to "traditional medicine" by boiling the bark in water for 3 h until the volume of liquid became one-third reduced. For 15 days, the volunteers followed the instructions to drink the decoction, consuming the equivalent of about 6.5 g/day. The researchers made certain that the volunteers had not received radiation or drug treatments during the previous six months and that they were free from viral infections. It was also determined that neither subject had worked with carcinogenic or mutagenic substances and were negative in tests for tumors. Urine was collected from the volunteers before the administration of the decoction and during eight days following the last dose. The Ames test was used to determine mutagenicity of their urine in three concentrations. The smoker's urine showed mutagenic activity before the period of the decoction and a "dramatic decrease" by the end of the treatment, which continued up to eight days following the last dose. The nonsmoker's urine was negative for mutagenic activity before, during, and after the test (Rizzi et al., 1993).

Following up on this study, Leon et al. (1996) conducted a double-blind, placebo-controlled, randomized study of a freeze-dried aqueous extract of *U. tomentosa* bark to determine mutagenic or antimutagenic activity in the urine of nonsmokers and smokers. For an average of 32 days, 24 volunteers, of whom 1/2 were smokers, received placebo or the bark extract in two dosage strengths: 90 mg or 270 mg/day. Using the same test (Ames) as Rizzi and colleagues, Leon et al. (1996) determined that the urine of the nonsmokers was free from mutagenic activity upon entry to the study. On days 17 and 32 of the treatment period, they found that all those taking the bark extract also showed no mutagenic activity in their urine samples, whereas no change in mutagenic activity showed up in urine samples from those on placebo. In the smokers, the dosage of bark extract consumed showed a linear and significant correlation with the changes observed in mutagenic activity of their urine (Leon et al., 1996).

Respiratory and Pulmonary Disorders

Allergies and Asthma

Open-label pilot studies in small numbers of patients have been conducted in Europe with patients on the same extract and dosages suffering from allergic respiratory diseases (bronchial asthma, allergic rhinitis, chronic bronchitis, neurodermatisis), gastritis, and duodenal ulcers. A ten-year follow-up found no side effects and some patients reported improvement (Immodal Pharmaka, 1996).

DOSAGE

In popular herbal medicine in Peru, the dosage for the stalk bark of cat's claw in the prevention of disease is 1 cup/week of the decocted bark, or 1 cup/15 days. In treating serious diseases, the dosage is 1 L/day for 3 months or more, or until all symptoms have abated. The stalk bark is prepared by decocting approximately 28 g/L of water for a minimum of 15 min. The decoction is then taken cold, warm, or hot at any time of day and may be sweetened. Alternatively, pieces of the stalk bark are placed in a small amount of water and decocted for at least 1 h before drinking the liquid cold during the day (Jones, 1995). Extracts of the stalk bark sold in the United States and Canada have usually been standardized to contents of total oxindole alkaloids and isopteropodine without consideration of the content of TOAs. Recommended dosages of stalk bark preparations range from 100-1,000 mg/day.

Asháninka shamans traditionally prepare the root of *U. tomentosa*-PC by decoction (Keplinger et al., 1999) using 20 g root/L cold water. Researchers in Europe have replicated the traditional method as follows: placing the root bark in an enameled vessel, heat is applied for 45 min at 85°C and the liquid is removed to cool for 10 min before filtering. The decoction is then diluted 1:1 with hot water to be consumed before breakfast. The researchers suggest the following dosages: ages 12 to adult, 60 mL decoction diluted with 60 mL hot water/day, before breakfast; ages 10-12, 50 mL decoction:50 mL hot water; ages 7-9, 30 mL decoction:30 mL hot water; and ages 3-6, 20 mL decoction:20 mL hot water (Immodal Pharmaka, 1995; Keplinger et al., 1999).

Among tested proprietary extracts, a standardized, hydrochloric acid powder extract of the root, prepared with hydrolysable tannins removed (*U. tomentosa*-PC, Immodal Pharmaka, Krallendorn, a.k.a. Savéntaro), is taken as an immunoregulatory supplement in Europe (Keplinger et al., 1999; Wurm et al., 1998). The dosage used is 20 mg/day, and by patients with more serious conditions, 60 mg/day. Each 20-mg dose is standardized to contain a minimum of 260 µg POAs and a maximum 12 mg TOAs (Immodal Pharmaka, 1996). C-MED-100 (CampaMed, New York, NY) is a low molecular weight water-soluble subfraction of *U. tomentosa* stalk bark, standardized to contain 8% or more carboxyl alkyl esters. The extract is depleted of indole alkaloids to contain <0.05%, and of high molecular weight (>10,000 MW) conjugated compounds such as tannins (Sheng, Bryngelsson, et al., 2000; Sheng, Pero, et al., 2000; Pero, 2000). The daily dose is 350 mg (Sheng, Bryneglsson, et al., 2000).

SAFETY PROFILE

Contraindications

In Europe, use of the root (*U. tomentosa*-PC) and preparations thereof is not advised for infants under three years of age because of a lack of clinical data. Other contraindicated patients are those waiting to undergo bone marrow or any other organ transplants (Immodal Pharmaka, 1995).

Drug Interactions

In Europe, patients are advised to avoid the root (*U. tomentosa*-PC) or extract preparations thereof if receiving or about to receive treatment with any of the following medical interventions: any treatment using immunosuppressant agents; hyperimmunoglobulin therapy (i.v.); thymic extracts (i.v.); hormone treatments with animal peptide or protein hormones, such as insulin derived from pigs or cattle; cryoprecipitates or fresh plasma (in hemophiliacs), although standardized factor presents no problem; and passive vaccines made from animal sera which present a risk of serum reaction, although active vaccinations present no risk except for the possibility of a more severe postvaccinational reaction which may be attended with fever (Immodal Pharmaka, 1995).

A Peruvian woman, 35 years of age with systemic lupus erythematosus (SLE) of 14 years duration, was diagnosed with acute allergic interstitial nephritis following the addition of a cat's claw supplement (1 capsule, q.i.d.) to her daily immunosuppressive medications (atenolol, furosemide, metolazone, nefedipine, and prednisone, p.o.). No other supplement had been added to her regime and she presented without complaining of symptoms (Hilepo et al., 1998). The imported Peruvian product (presumably stalk bark) was purchased in Queens, New York and the label was entirely in Spanish without any warnings, precautions, ingredient statement, or dosage recommendation (Hilepo, 1998). Upon the advice of physicians, she stopped taking the cat's claw supplement. When she returned to the clinic one month later, her serum creatinine concentration had fallen to 2.7 mg/dL from a high of 3.6 mg/dL when she was on the cat's claw supplement. Her baseline reading had previously been measured at 2.0 mg/dL (Hilepo et al., 1998). Outruling the chance of an allergic reaction to the cat's claw product having been part of a SLE history, clinicians found no evidence of active lupus in her serum antibody titers, nor evidence of lupus nephritis (Hilepo, 1998). As noted, the concomitant use of cat's claw with immunosuppressants is not advised. However, the authenticity of the cat's claw product implicated here is in question owing to lack of conclusive taxonomic identification (Hilepo, 1998). Moreover, there are at least seven completely different plants in Peru that share the same common name, *uña de gato* (cat's claw) (Cabieses, 1994).

Keplinger et al. (1996), noting differences in the alkaloid pattern of the two *U. tomentosa* chemotypes, have suggested that whereas the TOAs have shown CNS activity, the pentacyclic forms show immunomodulating activity. They assert, therefore, that mixtures of the two chemotypes in therapeutic applications may lead to "unexpected side-effects" (Keplinger et al., 1996), or at least weakly active preparations. Analysis of approximately 50 different cat's claw products obtained from the United States, Peru, and Central America found up to 80% of the total alkaloid contents were TOAs (Keplinger et al., 1999).

The TOAs in Peruvian *Uncaria* (primarily rynchophylline and isorynchophylline) antagonize the immunological activity (lymphocyte proliferation regulating factor) produced by the pentacyclic alkaloids (Keplinger et al., 1999; Wurm et al., 1998). Since the most abundant TOAs in *U. tomentosa* barks are rynchophylline and isorynchophylline (Hemingway and Phillipson, 1974; Keplinger et al., 1996), they would be of main concern.

Rynchophylline has also shown a marked hypotensive effect in hypertensive rats (50 mg/kg i.g. daily for 15 days) (Chang et al., 1978). However, this amount is not readily obtainable from the bark of *U. tomentosa* (Keplinger et al., 1996).

Toxicity studies in cultured cerebellar granule cells without glutamate revealed no compromised cell viability from the oxindole alkaloids isorynchophylline, rhynchophylline, or corynoxeine, but significant reductions in cell viability from isocorynoxeine (at 10^{-3}M only) and from hirsutine and hirsuteine (10^{-3}M and 3×10^{-4}M); the same concentrations which showed inhibition of glutamate-induced $^{45}Ca^{2+}$ influx and glutamate-induced neuronal death. The weaker activity of hirsutine and hirsuteine compared to isorynchophylline and isocorynoxeine was attributed to toxicity (Shimada et al., 1999). Mimaki et al. (1997) have shown a dose-dependent and significant inhibition of glutamate-induced convulsion in mice from hirsuteine, but only from extremely high oral doses (100 and 200 mg/kg) unobtainable from the oral use of herbal extracts of *Uncaria*.

Serotonin (5-hydroxytryptamine) antagonist/agonist activity from TOAs was shown by Kanatani et al. (1985). Dihydrocorynantheine and corynantheine reduced specific binding of [^{3}H]5-hydroxytryptamine to membrane preparations from rat brain. In small concentrations in vitro, dihydrocorynantheine antagonized the contraction of guinea-pig ileum (5 doses of 10^{-5}M/200-300 g ileum), and inhibited 5-hydroxytryptamine-specific binding to rat brain membranes (IC_{50}: 0.36 M/0.7 mL membrane). Noting that compounds suspected of antagonizing 5-HT have been used in the prophylaxis of migraine headaches, Kanatani et al. (1985) raised the possibility of utilizing dihydrocorynantheine and other TOAs in the treatment of vascular headaches or migraine; however, they recognized that serotonin has a wide and diverse range of activity.

In the same 5-HT binding assay, the TOAs rynchophylline, isorynchophylline, and corynoxeine, and the indole alkaloids hirsutine and hirsuteine were inactive (Kanatani et al., 1985). Shi and colleagues (1993) have shown that from a high dose in rats of either sex, rynchophylline (200 mg/kg i.p.) dose-dependently increases the 5-HT content of the hypothalamus. However, in vitro studies with rat brain stem slices showed that rynchophylline (30 μmol/L) reduced the release of endogenous 5-HT in hypothalamus slices. For dopamine, the same in vivo dose caused brain contents to increase in the hypothalamus, brain stem, and spinal cord and to decrease in the cortex, and amygdala. Yet, the release of endogenous dopamine in rat brain slices in vitro was increased by rynchophylline in hypothalamus, brain stem, cortex and amygdala (Shi et al., 1993). In addition, a high dose of isorhynchophylline appears to exert a sedative effect, as shown by a significant decrease of total locomotor activity in mice from 60 and 100 mg/kg p.o., a finding interpreted as evidence of a central dopaminergic receptor antagonist activity (Sakakibara et al., 1999). Again, these amounts are hardly relevant to human doses of *Uncaria* extracts, unless the extract used contained largely isorynchophylline and was taken in amounts that exceeded the recommended dosage.

All five of the alkaloids studied in the 5-HT binding assay (Kanatani et al., 1985) occur in *U. tomentosa,* with highest concentrations in the tetracyclic oxindole alkaloid chemotype (TC). The indole alkaloid dihydro-corynantheine occurs in the roots of both chemotypes, although it appears to occur in much higher amounts in the TC (0.23-1.51 μg/g) than in roots of the pentacyclic oxindole alkaloid chemotype (PC) (0.01-0.05 μg/g). Indeed, in one-third of the PC samples tested, dihydrocorynantheine was absent. Minor oxindole and indole alkaloids which occur in the roots of either chemotype of *U. tomentosa* are: isocorynoxeine (0.01-0.95 mg/100 mg), hirsutine (0.03-1.0), hirsuteine (0.01-0.19), dihydrocorynantheine (0.01-1.51), and corynoxeine (0.01-0.51) (Laus et al., 1997).

Among 21 ethanolic herbal extract products sold in Canada which were tested for in vitro inhibitory activity on cytochrome P450 3A4 (CYP3A4), about 66% showed significant inhibition of CYP3A4 at concentrations of less than 10% of their full strength source preparations. Only three showed activity from a median inhibitory concentration of less than 1% "full strength": an extract of goldenseal (*Hydrastis canadensis,* 0.03% full strength) was the most potent; followed by St. John's wort (*Hypericum peforatum*) (0.04%); and third, cat's claw (*Uncaria tomentosa,* 0.79% full strength). Although this activity requires in vivo studies to be confirmed, because the P450 3A4 (CYP3A4) hepatic enzyme system is responsible for the metabolism of most drugs taken orally (Budzinski et al., 2000), cat's claw extracts may interfere with the metabolism of drugs taken concomitantly.

Pregnancy and Lactation

Use of cat's claw root (*U. tomentosa*-PC) and extract preparations is contraindicated for pregnant or lactating women (Reinhard, 1999; Immodal Pharmaka, 1995). However, the considerations for pregnancy and lactation differ and will be reviewed separately.

Cat's claw root has been traditionally used in Peru as a contraceptive and to treat menstrual irregularities. A number of studies have demonstrated hormonal effects of *U. tomentosa* extract that may interfere with fertility as well as cause miscarriage during pregnancy. Mice administered an aqueous extract of cat's claw root *(U. tomentosa)* in their drinking water (6.25 mg/kg and 25 mg/kg) showed no signs of toxicity. However, when caged with male mice, the female mice produced no offspring (Keplinger, 1982). Cat's claw stalk bark *(U. tomentosa)* has shown in vitro anti-estrogenic activity (Salazar and Jayme, 1998). Amounts equivalent to dietary doses caused a dose-dependent (100 pg/mL to 10 μg/mL) and statistically significant inhibition of progesterone production in vitro. In sexually mature female rats, cat's claw bark (2 mg/day or 20 mg/kg p.o.) reduced serum progesterone (P4) and estradiol (E2) levels by 68% and 71%, respectively (Rodriguez et al., 1998). Low progesterone states are known to reduce fertility, trigger miscarriage, and contribute to menstrual difficulties. No scientific studies of the efficacy of cat's claw as birth control or for menstrual difficulties exist, though hormonal effects in animals indicate potential efficacy. The risk of miscarriage during pregnancy must be balanced by the benefits that may be gained when *U. tomentosa* is used to treat serious illnesses.

Uncaria tomentosa is traditionally used in recovery after childbirth. Lactation almost always occurs during this period, and use of cat's claw during early lactation can be inferred. The hypoprogesteronic effect of *U. tomentosa* may not be of negative consequence to lactation because the drop in circulating progesterone after placental delivery is the main trigger for the onset of milk production. Therefore, cat's claw may even stimulate a more rapid than usual increase in milk production immediately after birth. Just as many other botanicals with phytoestrogenic activity show a galactogenic effect, *U. tomentosa* may increase milk supply through modulation of estrogen as well. For women with low milk supply due to retained placental fragments, cat's claw may be able to reverse the high estrogen and progesterone levels caused by this condition and thus increase milk supply (speculative). Indeed, the hormonal activity of cat's claw may provide a rationale for its traditional use in the postpartum period. Later in lactation, however, cat's claw may interfere with a mother's ability to become pregnant once her fertility returns. No information exists regarding cat's claw and milk entry. However, as with other substances, only very small amounts of any one constituent are expected to enter breast milk. No studies of cat's claw in lactating animals exist. No cases of adverse reactions of infants exposed to cat's claw are known.

Side Effects

In the *American Herbal Products Association's Botanical Safety Handbook,* the root of *Uncaria tomentosa* is listed as a class 4 herb, meaning that the data so far received is insufficient to provide a classification (McGuffin et al., 1997).

The root bark decoction (*U. tomentosa*-PC) may, in some patients, result in temporary constipation during the first course of ingestion. The problem is readily managed with laxatives (Immodal Pharmaka, 1995).

In Peruvian popular medicine, it is advised that ingesting too much of the stalk bark decoction results in a loose stool, a problem which can be easily remedied by consuming plenty of water and avoiding the decoction for two days (Jones, 1995).

Aggravation of acne papulosa on the shoulders of one patient with HIV was noted following therapy with a standardized powder extract of the root bark (*U. tomentosa*-PC). In patients infected with HIV and in cancer patients, however, rarely, an increase in uric acid may result from an increased lysis of tumor and virally-infected cells. In patients with tumors taking the same extract, a resultant lytic fever may persist for as long as two weeks. In patients with autoimmune diseases or tumors, intermittent constipation and/or diarrhea may occur as a result of additive lactose, both of which are readily treatable with available agents. (Keplinger, 1999; Immodal Pharmaka, 1995; Reinhard, 1999).

Special Precautions

Patients receiving large doses of chemotherapy and taking a standardized liquid extract of the root (*U. tomentosa*-PC, p.o.) have sometimes shown a dramatic fall in erythrocytes, which may be the result of increased elimination of damaged cells. The effect can be avoided by taking the extract up to two days prior to and every two to six days following chemotherapy (Immodal Pharmaka, 1995).

Toxicology

In Vitro Toxicity

The toxicity of aqueous extracts of *U. tomentosa* stalk barks was examined in vitro using bacterial and mammalian cells in culture by Santa Maria et al. (1997). The extracts prepared from stalk barks collected in northern Peru (Department of San Martin) were tested for cytotoxicity in the neutral red assay, total protein content assay, tetrazolium (MTT) assay, the Microtox assay, and in cultured ovary cells from Chinese hamsters. No toxicity of any significance was found in any of the assays with concentrations of 10-100 mg/mL (Santa Maria et al., 1997).

Mutagenicity

The root bark in the form of a lyophilisate showed no mutagenicity in the Ames test in five different strains of *Salmonella typhimurium*. Tests were conducted with the extract in concentrations of 50, 500, 1,500, and 5,000 mg/plate. Six fractions and five extracts of the chloroform-ethanol extract in the *Salmonella*/mammalian-microsome test also showed no mutagenicity. The same extracts tested in TA 102 with or without 8-methoxypsoralen and treatment with UVA irradiation produced no mutagenicity (Rizzi et al., 1993). In yeast assays for DNA damage, pteropodine and isopteropodine showed only weak activity. An ethanolic extract of *U. guianensis* bark was even weaker (Lee et al., 1999).

Toxicity in Animal Models

Acute oral toxicity. A freeze-dried aqueous extract of the root (*U. tomentosa*-PC) as a 40% suspension in tragacanth gruel (0.5%) was tested in ten mice at the maximum dose of 40 mL/kg p.o. The extract contained a POA content of 35 mg/g. Controls received aqueous gum tragacanth alone. Histological examination was made after 14 days of observation. The two mice that died showed a pallor of the liver and spleen and hemorrhage of the intestines and stomach. The surviving mice made an apparent complete recovery within five days of the treatment and showed normal gains in body weight and normal findings upon autopsy compared to the controls. The study established an acute median lethal dose (LD_{50}) of the extract in mice of greater than 16 g/kg (Reinhard, 1999; Keplinger et al., 1999).

The oral LD_{50} of C-MED-100 from a single dose in female rats was calculated to be >8 g/kg. Another commercial cat's claw preparation (water/ethanol extract containing 4% alkaloids) obtained in the United States showed an LD_{50} of >5 g/kg p.o., while a commercial bark powder product (Schuler) showed an LD_{50} of 2 g/kg p.o. (Sheng, Bryngelsson et al., 2000).

Subacute oral toxicity. An aqueous-acid extract of the root *(U. tomentosa)* containing 7.5 mg oxindole alkaloids/g showed no toxicity in rats after a daily dosage of 1 g/kg p.o. for four weeks (Reinhard, 1999). The four-week oral toxicity test was conducted in both sexes of rats according to Organization for Economic Co-operation and Development (OECD) guidelines for testing chemicals. The rats were administered an aqueous hydrochloric acid extract of the root of *U. tomentosa*-PC (total oxindole alkaloids 7.5 mg/g plus remnant sodium chloride, 300 mg from neutralization) for 28 days (1 g/kg/day p.o.). In the blood of the extract group, dosing caused a slight yet statistically significant difference in the higher percentage of lymphocytes and decreased percentage of neutrophilic granulocytes. Lymphocyte counts were still within a normal range compared to controls. In animals of both sexes in the extract-treated group, relative kidney weights were slightly greater; however, they showed no histological changes of any significance compared to the control rats. No other differences were found and there were no fatalities (Keplinger et al., 1999).

The maximum tolerable oral dose (MTD) of C-MED-100 in female rats was calculated to be >8 g/kg and there were no signs of toxicity during the two-week observation period. A commercial bark powder product (Schuler) showed an MTD of 2 g/kg p.o. without signs of toxicity, and a cat's claw extract obtained in the United States (water/ethanol extract containing 4% alkaloids) showed an MTD of 2.5-5 g/kg with diarrhea and sedation (Sheng, Bryngelsson, et al., 2000).

REFERENCES

Anonymous (1997). Cat's claw has gone from street trade's barrow to a top seller: So what is it? *Health Food Business* (Britain) (September): 18-19.

Aquino, R., De Feo, V., De Simone, F., Pizza, C., and Cirino, G. (1991). Plant metabolites: New compounds and anti-inflammatory activity of *Uncaria tomentosa*. *Journal of Natural Products* 54: 453-459.

Aquino, R., De Simone, F., Pizza, C., Conti, C., and Stein, M.L. (1989). Plant metabolites: Structure and in vitro antiviral activity of quinovic acid glycosides from *Uncaria tomentosa* and *Guettarda platypoda*. *Journal of Natural Products* 52: 679-685.

Aquino, R., De Simone, F., Vincieri, F.F., Pizza, C., and Gacs-Baitz, E. (1990). New polyhydroxylated triterpenes from *Uncaria tomentosa*. *Journal of Natural Products* 53: 559-564.

Aquino, R., De Tommasi, N., De Simone, F., and Pizza, C. (1997). Triterpenes and quinovic acid glycosides from *Uncaria tomentosa*. *Phytochemistry* 45: 1035-1040.

Budzinski, J.W., Foster, B.C., Vandenhoek, S., and Arnason, J.T. (2000). An in vitro evaluation of human cytochrome P450 3A4 inhibition by selected commercial herbal extracts and tinctures. *Phytomedicine* 7: 273-282.

Cabieses, F. (1994). *The Saga of Cat's Claw*. Lima, Peru: Via Lactea Editores.

Castillo, G.M., Choi, P.Y., Cumings, J.A., and Snow, A.D. (2001). Inhibition of Parkinson's disease alpha-synuclein fibrillogenesis by PTI-777. *Society for Neuroscience Abstracts* 27: 608 (abstract).

Castillo, G.M., Kirschner, D.A., Yee, A.G., and Snow, A.D. (2000). Electron microscopy and X-ray diffraction studies further confirm the efficacy of PTI-00703TM (cat's claw derivative) as a potent inhibitor of Alzheimer's Beta-amyloid protein fibrillogenesis. World Alzheimer Congress 2000, Washington, DC, July 9-13, 2000. Abstract of oral presentation.

Castillo, G., Snow, A.D., and DeSantis, D.A. (2001). Compositions for treating Alzheimer's disease and other amyloidoses. United States Patent 6,262,994 B1, July 24, 2001.

Cerri, R., Aquino, R., De Simone, F., and Pizza, C. (1988). New quinovic acid glycosides from *Uncaria tomentosa*. *Journal of Natural Products* 51: 257-261.

Chang, T.H., Li, H.T., Li, Y., Wang, Y.F., Wu, L., and Li, T.H. (1978). Hypotensive effect of *Uncaria rynchophylla* total alkaloids and rynchophylline. *National Medical Journal of China* 58: 408-411, in *Chemical Abstracts* 92 (1980): 191363c.

Chen, C.X., Jin, R.M., Li, Y.K., Zhong, J., Yue, L., Chen, S.C., and Zhou, J.Y. (1992). Inhibitory effect of rynchophylline on platelet aggregation and thrombosis. *Acta Pharmacologica Sinica* 13: 126-130.

Cummings, J.A., Castillo, G.M., Choi, P.Y., and Snow, A.D. (2000). Disruption of pre-deposited Alzheimer's Aβ 1-42 fibrils by PTI-00703 (cat's claw derivative) in a rodent model of Aβ fibrillogenesis. World Alzheimer Congress 2000, Washington, DC, July 9-13, 2000.

De Feo, V. (1992). Medicinal and magical plants in the northern Peruvian Andes. *Fitoterapia* 63: 417-440.

de Jong, W., Melnyk, M., Lozano, L.A., Rosales, M., and Garcia, M. (1999). *Uña de Gato: Fate and Future of a Peruvian Forest Resource.* Occasional Paper No. 22. Bogor, Indonesia: Center for International Forestry Research.

De Ugaz, O.L. (1995). Professor of Chemistry, Pontifica Universidade Catolica del Peru, Lima, Peru, personal communication with Kenneth Jones, August 15, 1995.

Desmarchelier, C., Mongelli, E., Coussio, J., and Ciccia, G. (1997). Evaluation of the in vitro antioxidant activity in extracts of *Uncaria tomentosa* (Willd.) DC. *Phytotherapy Research* 11: 254-256.

Duke, J.A. and Vasquez, R. (1994). *Amazonian Ethnobotanical Dictionary.* Boca Raton, FL: CRC Press.

Fazzi, M.A.C. (1989). "Evaluation de la *Uncaria tomentosa* (uña de gato) en la prevencion de ulceras gastricas de stress producidas experimentalmente en rats." [Evaluation of *Uncaria tomentosa* (uña de gato) in the prevention of gastric ulcers of stress experimentally produced in rats]. (Dissertation of the Faculty of Medicine, University Peruana Cayetano Heredia, Lima, Peru) 18 pp.

Hemingway, S.R. and Phillipson, J.D. (1974). Alkaloids from S. American species of *Uncaria* (Rubiaceae). *Journal of Pharmacy and Pharmacology* 26(Suppl.): 113P.

Hilepo, J.N. (1998). Personal communication with Kenneth Jones, September, 1998.

Hilepo, J.N., Bellucci, A.G., and Mossey, R.T. (1998). Acute renal failure caused by "cat's claw" herbal remedy in a patient with systemic lupus erythematosus. *Nephron* 77: 361 (letter).

Holdsworth, D. and Mahana, P. (1983). Traditional medicinal plants of the Huon Peninsula Morobe Province, Papua New Guinea. *International Journal of Crude Drug Research* 21: 121-133.

Höppener, J.W.M., Ahrén, B., and Lips, C.J.M. (2000). Islet amyloid and type 2 diabetes mellitus. *New England Journal of Medicine* 343 (August 10): 411-419.

Huang, K.C. (1993). *The Pharmacology of Chinese Herbs.* Boca Raton, FL: CRC Press, pp. 137-138.

Immodal Pharmaka (1995). *Krallendorn®, Uncaria tomentosa* (Willd.) DC *Root Extract: Information for Physicians and Dispensing Chemists,* Third Revised Edition. Volders, Austria: Immodal Pharmaka GmbH, pp. 1-20.

Immodal Pharmaka (1996). *Krallendorn®, Uncaria tomentosa* (Willd.) DC *mod. pent. Root Extract: Report on Experiences with Probands.* Volders/Tirol, Austria: Immodal Pharmaka GmbH, pp. 1-20.

Irvine, F.R. (1961). *Woody Plants of Ghana.* Oxford University Press, pp. 715-716.

Jones, K. (1995). *Cat's Claw: Healing Vine of Peru.* Seattle, WA: Sylvan Press, Inc.

Jovel, E.M., Cabanillas, J., and Towers, G.H.N. (1996). An ethnobotanical study of the traditional medicine of the Mestizo people of Suni Miraño, Loreto, Peru. *Journal of Ethnopharmacology* 53: 149-156.

Kanatani, H., Kohda, H., Yamasaki, K., Hotta, I., Nakata, Y., Segawa, T., Yamanaka, E., Aimi, N., and Sakai, S. (1985). The active principles of the branchlet and hook of *Uncaria sinensis* Oliv. examined with a 5-hydroxytryptamine receptor binding assay. *Journal of Pharmacy and Pharmacology* 37: 401-404.

Keplinger, J. (1999). Letter to Kenneth Jones, Feb. 26, 1999.

Keplinger, K. (1982). Composition allowing for modifying the growth of living cells, preparation and utilization of such a composition. PCT International Application WO 82/01130, April 15.

Keplinger, K. (1994). Oxindole alkaloids having properties stimulating the immunologic system and preparation containing same. United States Patent 5,302,611, April 12.

Keplinger, K., Laus, G., Wurm, M., Dierich, M.P., and Teppner, H. (1999). *Uncaria tomentosa* (Willd.) DC.—Ethnomedical use and new pharmacological, toxicological and botanical results. *Journal of Ethnopharmacology* 64: 23-34.

Keplinger, K., Wurm, M., and Laus, G. (1996). *Uncaria tomentosa* (Willd.) DC., two natural modifications. *2nd International Congress on Phytomedicine,* September 11-14.

Keplinger, U.M. (1992). Einfluss von krallendornextract auf retrovirale infektioned [Influence of cat's claw extract upon retroviral infection]. *Zürcher AIDS Kongress,* Zurich, Switzerland, October 16 and 17, program and abstracts.

Keplinger, U.M. (1993). Therapy of HIV-infected individuals in the pathological categories CDC A1 and CDC B2 with a preparation containing IMM-207. IV. *Österreichischer AIDS-Kongress,* Vienna, Austria, September 17 and 18, abstracts: 45.

Kinloch, R.A., Treherne, J.M., Furness, L.M., and Hajimohamadreza, I. (1999). The pharmacology of apoptosis. *Trends in Pharmacological Sciences* 20: 35-42.

Kitajima, M., Hashimoto, K., Yokoya, M., Takayama, H., and Aimi, N. (2000). Two new 19-hydroxyursolic acid-type triterpenes from Peruvian "Una de Gato" *(Uncaria tomentosa). Tetrahedron* 56: 547-552.

Kitajima, M., Hashimoto, K., Yokoya, M., Takayama, H., Aimi, N., and Sakai, S.I. (2000). A new gluco indole alkaloid, 3, 4-dehydro-5-carboxystrictosidine, from Peruvian una de gato *(Uncaria tomentosa). Chemical and Pharmaeutical Bulletin* 48(10): 1410-1412.

Kreutzkamp, B. (1984). "Niedermolekulare inhalstoffe mit immunstimulierenden eigenschaften aus *Uncaria tomentosa, Okoubaka aubrevillei* und anderen drogen" [Low molecular weight constituents with immunostimulating activity from *Uncaria tomentosa, Okoubaka aubrevillei* and other drugs]. (Dissertation of the Faculty of Chemistry and Pharmacy of Ludwig Maximilians University, Munich, May 1984).

Lamm, S., Sheng, Y., and Pero, R.W. (2001). Persistent response to pneumococcal vaccine in individuals supplemented with a novel water soluble extract of *Uncaria tomentosa*, C-Med-100®. *Phytomedicine* 8: 267-274.

Laus, G., Brossner, D., and Keplinger, K. (1997). Alkaloids of Peruvian *Uncaria tomentosa*. *Phytochemistry* 45: 855-860.

Laus, G., Brossner, D., Senn, G., and Wurst, K. (1996). Analysis of the kinetics of isomerization of spiro oxindole alkaloids. *Journal of the Chemical Society, Perkin Transactions* 2: 1931-1936.

Laus, G. and Keplinger, D. (1994). Separation of stereoisomeric oxindole alkaloids from *Uncaria tomentosa* by high performance liquid chromatography. *Journal of Chromatography* A 662: 243-249.

Laus, G. and Keplinger, K. (1997). [Radix *Uncaria tomentosa* (Willd.) DC.—A monographic description]. *Zeitschrift für Phytotherapie* 18: 122-126.

Laus, G., Keplinger, K., Wurm, M., and Dierich, M.P. (1998). Pharmacological activities of two chemotypes of *Uncaria tomentosa* (Willd.) DC. *46th Annual Congress of the Society for Medicinal Plant Research*, Vienna, Austria, 1998, poster presentation.

Lavault, M., Moretti, C., and Bruneton, J. (1983). Alcaloïdes de l'*Uncaria guianensis*. [Alkaloids of *Uncaria guianensis*] *Planta Medica* 47: 244-245.

Lee, J.C. (1994). Transcription factor NF-κB: An emerging regulator of inflammation. *Annual Reports in Medicinal Chemistry* 29: 236-244.

Lee, K.K., Zhou, B.N., Kingston, D.G.I., Vaisberg, A.J., and Hammond, G.B. (1999). Bioactive indole alkaloids from the bark of *Uncaria guianensis*. *Planta Medica* 65: 759.

Lemaire, I., Assinewe, V., Cano, P., Awang, D.V.C., and Arnason, J.T. (1999). Stimulation of interleukin-1 and -6 production in alveolar macrophages by the neotropical liana, *Uncaria tomentosa* (uña de gato). *Journal of Ethnopharmacology* 64: 109-115.

Leon, F.R., Ortiz, N., Atunez de Mayalo, A., Namisato, T., and Monge, R. (1996). Antimutagenic activity of a freeze-dried aqueous extract of *Uncaria tomentosa* in smokers and non-smokers. *Abstracts from the 3rd European Colloquium on Ethnopharmacology [and] 1st International Conference on Anthropology and History of Health and Disease*, Genoa, Italy, May 29-June 2, 1996. Genoa, Italy: Erga edizioni, p. 255, poster.

McCurley, D., Castillo, G.M., and Snow, A.D. (1998). Therapeutic implications of PTI-00703: A natural plant extract that is a potent dissolver of Alzheimer's disease amyloid. *Neurobiology of Aging* 19(Suppl.): S256 (abstract).

McGuffin, M., Hobbs, C., Upton, R., and Goldberg, A. (Eds.) (1997). *American Herbal Products Association Botanical Safety Handbook*. Boca Raton, FL: CRC Press, p. 119.

Miller, M.J.S., Zhang, X.J., Charbonnet, R.M., Clark, D.A., and Sandoval, M. (1999). The anti-inflammatory actions of the herbal medicine, cat's claw, are due to a suppression of NF-κB activation and inhibition of gene expression. *Pediatric Research* 45: 114A (abstract).

Milliken, W. and Albert, B. (1996). The use of medicinal plants by the Yanomami Indians of Brazil. *Economic Botany* 50: 10-25.

Mimaki, Y., Toshimizu, N., Yamada, K., and Sashida, Y. (1997). [Anti-convulsion effects of choto-san and chotoko *(Uncariae Uncis cam Ramlus)* in mice, and identification of the active principles]. *Yakugaku Zasshi* 117: 1011-1021 (Japanese with English summary).

Mohamed, A.F., Matsumoto, K., Tabata, K., Takayama, H., Kitajima, M., and Watanabe, H. (2000). Effects of *Uncaria tomentosa* total alkaloid and its components on experimental amnesia in mice: Elucidation using the passive avoidance test. *Journal of Pharmacy and Pharmacology* 52: 1553-1561.

Montenegro de Matta, S., Delle Monache, F., Ferrari, F., and Marini-Bettolo, G.B. (1976). Alkaloids and procyanidins of an *Uncaria* sp. from Peru. *Il Farmaco Edizione Scientifica* 31: 527-535.

Muhammad, I., Dunbar, C.C., Khan, R.A., Ganzera, M., and Khan, I.A. (2001). Investigation of uña de gato I. 7-Deoxyloganic acid and 15N NMR spectroscopic studies on pentacyclic oxindole alkaloids from *Uncaria tomentosa. Phytochemistry* 57: 781-785.

Oliver-Bever, B. (1986). *Medicinal Plants in Tropical West Africa.* Cambridge, England: Cambridge University Press, p. 115.

Ostendorf, F.W. (1962). Nuttige planten en sierplanten in Suriname [Useful and ornamental plants in Suriname]. *Landbouwproefstation Suriname Bulletin* (79): 199-200.

Ostrakhovich, E.A., Getmanskaya, N.V., and Durnev, A.D. (1998). Effects of *Uncaria tomentosa* extract on the peroxynitrite production by polymorphonuclear leukocytes of peripheral blood in healthy donors and diabetes mellitus patients. *Pharmaceutical Chemistry Journal* 32: 543-545.

Ostrakhovich, E.A., Mikhal'chik, E.V., Getmanskaya, N.V., and Durnev, A.D. (1997). Antioxidant activity of the extract from *Uncaria tomentosa. Pharmaceutical Chemistry Journal* 31: 326-329.

Peluso, G., La Cara, F., and De Feo, V. (1993). Effetto antiproliferativo su cellule tumorali di estratti e metaboliti da *Uncaria tomentosa.* Studi in vitro sulla loro azione su DNA polimerasi [Antiproliferative effect on tumor cells treated with metabolites of *Uncaria tomentosa.* An in vitro investigation of their activity towards DNA polymerase] *II Congreso Italo-Peruano de Etnomedicina,* Andina, Lima, Peru, October 27-30, abstracts, pp. 21-22.

Pero, R.W. (2000). Method of preparation and composition of a water soluble extract of the plant species *Uncaria.* United States Patent 6,039, 949, March 21, 2000.

Perry, L.M. and Metzger, J. (1980). *Medicinal Plants of East and Southeast Asia and Uses.* Cambridge, MA: The MIT Press, p. 359.

Petersen, A.F. (1999). Alzheimer's research advance: Structure causing enhancement of Aβ fibril formation is identified. *Genetic Engineering News* 19: 1, 20.

Phillipson, J.D., Hemingway, S.R., and Ridsdale, C.E. (1978). Alkaloids of *Uncaria.* Part V. Their occurrence and chemotaxonomy. *Journal of Natural Products* 41: 503-570.

Piscoya, J., Rodriguez, Z., Bustamante, S.A., Okuhama, N.N., Miller, M.J.S., and Sandoval, M. (2001). Efficacy and safety of freeze-dried cat's claw in osteoarthritis of the knee: Mechanisms of action of the species *Uncaria guianensis. Inflammation Research* 50: 442-448.

Reinhard, K.H. (1999). *Uncaria tomentosa* (Willd.) DC.: Cat's claw, *uña de gato* or savéntaro. *The Journal of Alternative and Complementary Medicine* 5: 143-151.

Reynolds, J.E.F. (Ed.) (1996). *Martindale. The Extra Pharmacopoeia,* Twenty-First Edition. London: Royal Pharmaceutical Society, p. 1687.

Ridsdale, C.E. (1978). A revision of *Mitragyna* and *Uncaria* (Rubiaceae). *Blumea* 24: 43-100.

Riva, L., Coradini, D., Di Fronzo G., De Feo, V., De Tommasi, N., De Simone, F., and Pizza, C. (2001). The antiproliferative effects of *Uncaria tomentosa* extracts and fractions on the growth of breast cancer cell line. *Anticancer Research* 21(4A):2457-2461.

Rizzi, R., Re, F., Bianchi, A., De Feo, V., de Simone, F., Bianchi, L., and Stivala, L.A. (1993). Mutagenic and antimutagenic activities of *Uncaria tomentosa* and its extracts. *Journal of Ethnopharmacology* 38: 63-77.

Rodriguez, H., Massey, P.J., Rodriguez, K., Pedigo, E.C., Keenan, J.A., Harris, G., Warikoo, P., and Chen, T.T. (1998). Inhibition of steroid production by a nutrition supplement "una de gato," or "cat's claw." *Biology of Reproduction* 58(Suppl. 1): 136, abstract 208.

Sakakibara, I., Terabayashi, S., Kubo, M., Higuchi, M., Komatsu, Y., Okada, M., Taki, K., and Kamei, J. (1999). Effect on locomotion of indole alkaloids from the hooks of *Uncaria* plants. *Phytomedicine* 6: 163-168.

Salazar, E.L. and Jayme, V. (1998). Depletion of specific binding sites for estrogen receptor by *Uncaria tomentosa. Proceedings of the Western Pharmacology Society* 41: 123-124.

Sandoval, M., Charbonnet, R.M., Okuhama, N.N., Roberts, J., Krenova, Z., Trentacosti, A.M., and Miller, M.J.S. (2000). Cat's claw inhibits TNF-α production and scavenges free radicals: Role in cytoprotection. *Free Radical Biology and Medicine* 29: 71-78.

Sandoval, M., Mannick, E.E., Mishra, J., Sadowska-Krowicka, H., Clark, D.A., and Miller, M.J.S. (1997). Cat's claw *(Uncaria tomentosa)* protects against oxidative stress and indomethicin-induced intestinal inflammation. *Gastroenterology* 112: A1091 (abstract).

Sandoval-Chacón, M., Thompson, J.H., Zhang, X.J., Liu, X., Mannick, E.E., Sadowska-Krowicka, H., Charbonnet, R.M., Clark, D.A., and Miller, M.J. (1998). Anti-inflammatory actions of cat's claw: The role of NF-B. *Alimentary Pharmacology and Therapeutics* 12: 1279-1289.

Santa Maria, A., Lopez, A., Diaz, M.M., Alban, J., Galan de Mera, A., Vicente Orellana, J.A., and Pozuelo, J.M. (1997). Evaluation of the toxicity of *Uncaria tomentosa* by bioassays in vitro. *Journal of Ethnopharmacology* 57: 183-187.

Schultes, R.E. and Raffauf, R.E. (1990). *The Healing Forest: Medicinal and Toxic Plants of Northwest Amazonia.* Portland, OR: Dioscorides Press, p. 401.

Senatore, A., Cataldo, A., Iaccarino, F.P., and Elberti, M.G. (1989). Ricerche fitochimiche e biologiche sull *Uncaria tomentosa.* [Phytochemical and biological study of *Uncaria tomentosa*] *Bollettino Societa di Italiano Biologia Sperimentale* (Napoli) 65: 517-520.

Sharma, H.K., Chhangte, L., and Dolui, A.K. (2001). Traditional medicinal plants in Mizoram, India. *Fitoterapia* 72: 146-161.

Sheng, Y., Bryngelsson, C., and Pero, R.W. (2000). Enhanced DNA repair, immune function and reduced toxicity of C-MED™, a novel aqueous extract from *Uncaria tomentosa. Journal of Ethnopharmacology* 69: 115-126.

Sheng, Y., Pero, R.W., Ammir, A., and Bryngelsson, C. (1998). Induction of apoptosis and inhibition of proliferation in human tumor cells treated with extracts of *Uncaria tomentosa. Anticancer Research* 18: 3363-3368.

Sheng, Y., Pero, R.W., and Wagner, H. (2000). Treatment of chemotherapy-induced leukopenia in a rat model with aqueous extract from *Uncaria tomentosa. Phytomedicine* 7: 137-143.

Shi, J.S., Huang, B., Wu, Q., Ren, R.X., and Xie, X.L. (1993). Effects of rynchophylline on motor activity of mice and serotonin and dopamine in rat brain. *Acta Pharmacologica Sinica* 14: 114-117.

Shimada, Y., Goto, H., Itoh, T., Sakakibara, I., Kubo, M., Sasaki, H., and Terasawa, K. (1999). Evaluation of the protective effects of alkaloids isolated from the hooks and stems of *Uncaria sinensis* on glutamate-induced neuronal death in cultured cerebellar granule cells from rats. *Journal of Pharmacy and Pharmacology* 51: 715-722.

Snow, A.D. (1999). Personal communication with Kenneth Jones, May, 1999.

Snow, A.D., Castillo, G.M., Cummings, J.A., Vrablic, A.S., and DeSantis, D.A. (1999). Neurosharp™: A new dietary supplement containing PTI-00703 for the prevention and treatment of brain amyloidosis associated with Alzheimer's disease and aging. *The FASEB Journal* 13: A145 (abstract 152.6).

Snow, A.D., Choi, P.Y., Cummings, J.A., Wood, S., Kirschner, D.A., and Castillo, G.M. (2000). Isolation and testing of the amyloid-inhibiting ingredients derived from the natural Beta-amyloid protein fibrillogenesis inhibitor PTI-00703TM. 30th Annual Meeting Society for Neuroscience, New Orleans, LO, November 4-9, 2000, Abstracts. *Society for Neuroscience* 26(Part 1): abstract 299.3.

Snow, A.D., Cummings, J.A., Castillo, G.M., Vrablic, A.S., and DeSantis, D.A. (1999). Further efficacy of PT-00703: A dietary supplement which causes a dose-dependent inhibition of Alzheimer's disease amyloid deposition in a rodent model. *The FASEB Journal* 13: A145 (abstract 152.5).

Standley, P.C. (1930). Flora of Costa Rica. *Field Museum of Natural History,* Botanical Series 18 (Part 4): 1379.

Stuppner, H.A., Sturm, S., Geisen, G., Zillian, U., and Konwalinka, G. (1993). A differential sensitivity of oxindole alkaloids to normal and leukemic cell lines. *Planta Medica* 59(Suppl.): A583.

Surh, Y.J., Chun, K.S., Cha, H.H., Han, S.S., Keum, Y.S., Park, K.K., and Lee, S.S. (2001). Molecular mechanisms underlying chemopreventive activities of anti-inflammatory phytochemicals: Down-regulation of COX-2 and iNOS through suppression of NF-κB activation. *Mutation Research, Fundamental and Molecular Mechanisms of Mutagenesis* 480-481: 243-268.

Teppner, H., Keplinger, K., and Wetschnig, W. (1984). Karyosystematic von *Uncaria tomentosa* und *U. guianensis* (Rubiaceae–Cinchoneae). [Karyosystematics of *Uncaria tomentosa* and *U. guianensis* (Rubiaceae-Cinchoneae. (Botanical studies from Pozuzo, Peru, I.)]. *Phyton* (Austria) 24: 125-134.

Tu, G., Fang, Q., Guo, J., Yuan, S., Chen, C., Chen, J., Chen, Z., Cheng, S., Jin, R., Li, M., et al. (Eds.) (1992). *Pharmacopoeia of the People's Republic of China.* Guangzhou, China: Guangdong Science and Technology Press, p. 138.

Uphof, J.C. Th. (1968). *Dictionary of Economic Plants,* Second Edition. New York: Verlag von J. Cramer, p. 534.

Wagner, H. (1987a). Immunostimulants from higher plants (recent advances). In Hostettmann, K. and Lea, P.J. (Eds.), *Biologically Active Natural Products.* Annual Proceedings of the Phytochemical Society of Europe, 27. Oxford, England: Claredon Press/Oxford University Press, pp. 127-141.

Wagner, H. (1987b). Krallendorn-tee, eine zusatztherapie bei krebs und polyarthritis? [Cat's claw tea, a supplementary therapy for cancer and polyarthritis?] *Forschrift für Phytotherapie* (July): 86.

Wagner, H., Kreutzkamp, B., and Jurcic, K. (1985). Die alkaloide von *Uncaria tomentosa* und ihre phagozytose-steigernde wirkung [The alkaloids of *Uncaria tomentosa* and their phagocytosis-stimulating action] *Planta Medica* 51: 419-423.

Wagner, H., Proksch, A., Vollmar, A., Kreutzkamp, B., and Bauer, J. (1985). In-vitro-phagozytose-stimulierung durch isolierte pflanzenstoffe gemessen im phagozytose-chemolumineszenz-(CL)-modell. [In vitro phagocytosis stimulation by isolated plant materials in a chemoluminescence-phagocytosis model]. *Planta Medica* 51: 139-144.

Wirth, C. and Wagner, H. (1997). Pharmacologically active procyanidines from the bark of *Uncaria tomentosa*. *Phytomedicine* 4: 265-266.

Woodson, R.E. and Schery, R.W. (1980). Flora of Panama part IX family 179. Rubiaceae—Part II. *Annals of the Missouri Botanical Garden* 67: 257-522.

Wurm, M., Kacani, L., Laus, G., Keplinger, K., and Dierich, MP. (1998). Pentacyclic oxindole alkaloids from *Uncaria tomentosa* induce human endothelial cells to release a lymphocyte-proliferation-regulating factor. *Planta Medica* 64: 701-704.

Yano, S., Horiuchi, H., Horie, S., Aimi, N., Sakai, S.I., and Watanabe, K. (1991). Ca^{2+} channel blocking effects of hirsutine, an indole alkaloid from *Uncaria* genus, in the isolated rat aorta. *Planta Medica* 57: 403-405.

Yepez, A.M., De Ugaz, O.L., Carmen, M., Alvarez, A., De Feo, V., Aquino, R., De Simone, F., and Pizza, C. (1991). Quinovic acid glycosides from *Uncaria guianensis*. *Phytochemistry* 30: 1635-1637.

Zavala Carrillo, C.A. and Zevallos Pollito, P.A. (1996). *Taxonomía, Distrubución Geográfica y Status del Género Uncaria en el Peru: Uña de Gato* [Taxonomy, Geographic Distribution and Status the Genus *Uncaria* of Peru: Cat's Claw]. Lima, Peru: Universidade Nacional Agraria La Molina, Facultad de Ciecncias Forestales.

Zhu, Y.P. (1998). *Chinese Materia Medica: Chemistry, Pharmacology and Applications*. Amsterdam, The Netherlands: Harwood Academic, pp. 525-527.

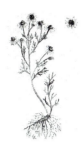

Chamomile

BOTANICAL DATA

Classification and Nomenclature

Scientific name: *Matricaria recutita* L. (formerly *Chamomilla recutita* [L.] Rauschert; *Matricaria chamomilla* [L.]); other recognized species: *Anthemis nobilis* (Roman chamomile, camomile) (Heneka, 1993)

Family name: Asteraceae (Compositae)

Common names: chamomille, German chamomile, camomile, Matricaria, Matricaria flos, Hungarian chamomile flowers (Bradley, 1992), wild camomile, bitter chamomile, Hippocrates chamomile, scented mayweed, sweet false chamomile (Heneka, 1993)

Description

Indigenous to most of Europe and Western Asia, *Matricaria* is naturalized in the United States, Australia, and Britain. Described as grayish-green and downy, *Matricaria recutita* is an annual herbaceous plant with an erect stem, alternate leaves (mostly sessile), and small-headed inflorescences, with white ray flowers attached around a hollow, conical yellow receptacle (like that of daisies). In Europe, the plant grows wild to a height of 60 to 100 cm in meadows, roadsides, fields, hedgerows, and on mountain slopes, and prefers a temperature of 7-26°C (Heneka, 1993; Grieve, 1980).

HISTORY AND TRADITIONAL USES

Chamomile was so revered by the Egyptians for its ability to cure malarial symptoms that they dedicated the plant to their many gods. In England, chamomile was used and grown for many centuries. The Greeks named it *kamai* (ground-apple), and the Spanish, who made sherries flavored with the plant, named it *manzanilla* (little apple), because of the strong, yet agreeable apple-like odor given off by the herb (Grieve, 1980).

The flowers of *Matricaria recutita* are aromatic, bitter-tasting, carminative, tonic, and sedative. Among its many traditional uses, the flowers have long been taken as a nervine sedative and gastrointestinal tonic. In the form of a tea, the herb was used as an anticonvulsant for teething children, and for earaches, nerve pain, and stomach ailments in children (Grieve, 1980). During the 12th century in Europe, an oil infusion of the fresh plant or dried flowers was used to treat rashes of the head. In the 1500s it was recommended by European herbalists for what may have been acne and pimples, as it was taken to "purge the head and to empty it of superfluous humour and other grosse matter," including mouth sores (Heneka, 1993, p. 34). Also in this period, it was regarded for painful diseases of the liver. A century or so later in Europe, it was used as a "comfort to the brain," and it was at this time that the famous 17th century herbalist Nicholas Culpeper grew the plant in herb gardens of London, where Camomile Street is named in his memory. Culpeper knew the herb as a diaphoretic and used it for pain, melancholy (depression), inflammatory conditions of the bowels, and phlegm. He also noted its usefulness in diseases of the liver or spleen, for swellings, weariness and strained muscles, colic, stones, and menstruation (Heneka, 1993). Other European traditional uses include: ocular discomfort or irritation, epigastric distention, belching, flatulence, poor digestion or appetite, and a sore or hoarse throat (Bradley, 1992). In Latin America today, an after-dinner tea of chamomile is a common beverage (Duke, 1985).

The fragrant essential oil of chamomile is used in perfumes, soaps, creams, detergents and shampoos, and in baked goods, candies, ice creams, puddings, beverages, and liqueurs, such as benedictine, vermouths, and bitters (Duke, 1985; Mann and Staba, 1986). The part used medicinally today is the flower heads (Reichling and Beiderbeck, 1991), whether fresh or dried (Heneka, 1993). In Belgium, the flower head is permitted for use as a "traditional" digestive aid, topical soothing agent, and stomatological (mouth) agent (De Smet et al., 1993).

CHEMISTRY

Many active compounds are known in *Matricaria recutita;* although some are more active than others, flavonoids and essential oils are considered the most active (Heneka, 1993). At least four chemotypes of the plant are known and distinguished according to their production of bisabolol or bisabolonoxide A (Franz and Wickel, 1979; Das et al., 1999).

Carbohydrates

Polysaccharides

Three water-soluble polysaccharide fractions have been identified, which contain a fructan polysaccharide of an inulin type (3.5 kDa), several rhamnogalacturonan type pectins (11 kd, 83 kDa, and 300 kDa), and a high molecular weight 4-*O*-methylglucuronoxylan of 340 kDa (Fuller et al., 1991, 1993).

Lipid Compounds

Oils

Farnesol is a fragrant constituent of the essential oil of chamomile. Farnesol is similar in odor to angelica seeds and linden flowers and is added to perfumes to impart a harmony and enhance floral scents. Borneol lends a pine scent and (–)-α-bisabolol is used as a fixative in perfumes (Mann and Staba, 1986).

The major constituents of the essential oil are: α-bisabololoxide B, farnesene, α-bisabololoxide A, *cis*-en-yn-dicycloether, chamazulene, α-bisabolol, and spathulenol (Becker et al., 1982). The major constituents according to high pressure liquid chromatography (HPLC) analysis are en-yn-dicycloethers (31.9%), followed by *cis*-α-bisabolol (21.1%), chamazulene (13.7%), (*E*)-β-farnesene (12.1%), *cis*-α-bisabololoxide A (7.3%), and *cis*-α-bisabololoxide B (5.4%) (Repcak et al., 1999).

Chamazulene gives the essential oil of chamomile flowers (0.4% to 1% dry weight) its characteristic blue coloration (Reichling and Beiderbeck, 1991), and is the constituent by which the quality of the essential oil is measured (Gasic et al., 1983). The essential oil is obtained in higher yields from frozen flowers than from any drying process (Carle et al., 1989). In the bisabolol chemotype, the content of (–)-α-bisabolol in the essential oil has been shown to vary from 15% to 30% (Carle et al., 1990) and as much as 50% (Isaac, 1979). However, recent calibrated HPLC analysis found that, contrary to gas chromatography (GC) analysis which showed (–)-α-bisabolol in the amount of 36.3%, the amount was only 21.1%. Previous GC methods for analysis of the essential oil appear to have miscalculated contents of en-yn-dicycloethers, thereby allowing other constituents to appear in higher amounts than they occur (Repcak et al., 1999). The essential oil is sometimes adulterated with the identical terpene derived from a cheaper, more abundant source in the Brazilian tree *Vanillosmopsis erythropappa* (Asteraceae), which contains as much as 3% essential oil. Nearly the entire content of this oil is (–)-α-bisabolol (Carle et al., 1990).

Organic Acids

In small amounts, phenolic acids are found in the flower heads, although not in other parts of *M. recutita,* and include caffeic acid, anisic acid, syringic acid, and vanillic acid (Reichling et al., 1979).

Phenolic Compounds

Flavonoids

Along with the flowers themselves, the flavonoid derivatives apigenin and apigenin glucoside are used in hair dyes to impart a yellow coloration (Mann and Staba, 1986). The florets contain considerable amounts of flavonoids, especially apigenin 7-*O*-glucoside and various acylated derivatives (Maier et al., 1993), of which free apigenin was determined to be an enzymatically produced postharvest by-product (Schreiber et al., 1990; Maier et al., 1991). The average ratio of apigenin to apigenin 7-glycoside was found at 1:20 (Schreiber et al., 1990). Along with its glucosides, apigenin is the most abundant flavonoid in the florets and occurs in quantities varying from 2.46 mg% to 4.43 mg% (Redaelli et al., 1981a). Another study found total apigenin glucosides in the florets in quantities of 7% to 9% and free apigenin in quantities of 0.3% to 0.5% (Redaelli et al., 1980). Total free apigenin in commercial hydroalcoholic extracts of *M. recutita* was found to vary from 0.91 to 14.10 mg/100 mL, and total apigenin from 23.17 to 70.65 mg/100 mL (Redaelli et al., 1981a).

Various monoacetates of apigenin 7-*O*-glucoside (Carle et al., 1992; Redaelli et al., 1980) and diacetates also occur in the flowers (Redaelli et al., 1982). In the flowers of Egyptian plants, highly methylated flavonoid-aglycones were measured. They mostly consisted of derivatives of quercetagetin (6-methoxy-quercetin): axillarin, chrysoeriol, chrysosplenol, eupatoletin, eupalitin, isorhamnetin, jaceidin, and spinacetin (Exner et al., 1981).

Coumarins

The main coumarins in the flowers of *M. recutita* are herniarin and umbelliferone, which occur in a ratio of about 5:1, respectively. Quantitatively, their amounts in commercial chamomile extracts represent about 10% of the apigenin content, or on average 10-15 mg/100 mL and 2-3 mg/100 mL, respectively (Redaelli et al., 1981b). Ceska et al. (1992) analyzed the coumarin content of chamomile from various brands of commercial tea bags, dried flowers, oil of chamomile, and a chamomile product (Kamillosan) imported from Germany. Total coumarin content varied widely in the tea bag material from concentrations of 371.5 to 1102.4 mg/g (dry weight). Herniarin content ranged from 321.3 to 916.0 mg/g (dry weight) while umbelliferone content in the same material ranged from 16.9 to 289.4 mg/g (dry weight). The amounts of herniarin and umbelliferone per tea bag in hot water extracts were determined as 381.6 to 1295.0 mg/bag and 22.7 to 258.1 mg/bag, respectively. The content of coumarins in the imported hydroalcoholic extract (Kamillosan) was herniarin 93.1 mg/mL and umbelliferone 41.8 mg/mL (Ceska et al., 1992).

Terpenoid Compounds

Sesquiterpenes

The primary medicinally active constituents of *M. recutita* are the (–)-α-bisabololoxides A, B, and C, (–)-α-bisabolol, (–)-α-bisabolonoxide, and the sesquiterpene lactone matricine. Other sesquiterpenes in the flower heads of *M. recutita* are: chamaviolene, calamene, cadinene, α-cubebene, and α-muurolene, spathulenol, *trans*-β- and *trans*-α-farnesene, and the sesquiterpene hydrocarbon chamazulene, produced during steam distillation of the flower heads from the matricine content (Reichling and Beiderbeck, 1991).

Reichling et al. (1979) examined various parts of the plant, finding that while all tissues contained sesquiterpenoids, there were quantitative differences from one part to another (flowers, herb, tumors, and root).

Other Constituents

Various other constituents in the flower heads of *Matricaria recutita* are: *cis*/trans-en-in-dicycloether (polyine) (Gasic et al., 1983); salicin, arbutin, narigenin 7-*O*-glucoside, luteolin 5-*O*-glucoside, various *p*-nitrophenyl compounds (-β-D-glucoside, -β-D-galactoside, -β-D-fucoside, and a-nitrophenyl-β-D-glucoside (Maier et al., 1993), and anthecotulid (37-120 mg/g) (Hausen et al., 1984). More common constituents include thiamine (Mann and Staba, 1986), niacin (14.9 mg/100 g dry weight), sugars (fructose, glucose, and galactose, 9%), starch (4%) (Pedersen, 1994), choline (up to 0.3%) (Bradley, 1992), ascorbic acid, and various polyphenols (quercetin, rutin, geraniol, gallic acid tannin, catechin tannin, caprylic acid, kaempferol, thujone) and fatty acids (oleic acid, linoleic acid, palmitic acid, sinapic acid) (Mann and Staba, 1986). Ahmad and Misra (1997) isolated oleanolic acid, β-sitosterol, and β-sitosterol glucoside from the flowers. Mucilages in *M. recutita* are mostly found in the ovaries and make up to 10% of the dry weight. The mucilage consists of various complex carbohydrates, including fructose, arabinose, xylose, glucose, galactose, rhamnose, galacturonic acid, and glucosamine (Carle and Issac, 1985).

An extensive review on *C. recutita* constituents can be found in Mann and Staba (1986).

THERAPEUTIC APPLICATIONS

The vast majority of known contemporary therapeutic applications of *M. recutita* are cited by Bradley (1992) and Mann and Staba (1986). Among them are: mucosal infections (mouthwash and dilute extracts), cutaneous infections (topical extracts and preparations), wounds and sores, eczema, flaky, dry or irritated skin, psoriasis, and use as a skin wash and in cosmetics. Internal conditions treated with *M. recutita* include: minor digestive problems, flatulence, dental afflictions, cystitis, colic, and fevers (Mann and Staba, 1986). In contemporary Europe, uses include mild infantile insomnia, peptic ulcer, upper respiratory tract irritations (inhalation), itchy skin, chapped skin, and gastrointestinal spasms or inflammatory conditions, including belching, sore throat, hoarse throat, and insect bites (Bradley, 1992).

Chamomile flower *(M. recutita)* is approved in Germany for use externally in the treatment of bacterial skin diseases, and inflammations involving the mucous and skin membrane, which include uses for the gums and oral cavity; and for use in baths and as an irrigant for the treatment of anogenital inflammations. For internal use, the German health authority has approved the species for use in treating inflammatory diseases that affect the gastrointestinal tract and for gastrointestinal spasms (Blumenthal, 1998).

PRECLINICAL STUDIES

Immune Functions; Inflammation and Disease

Cancer

Chemopreventive activity. The major flavonoid of chamomile flowers, apigenin (Redaelli et al., 1981a), has shown considerable chemopreventive activity in vitro (Hirano et al., 1989; Wei et al., 1990); so much so that it was suggested as a good candidate as a cancer chemopreventive agent and for development as an antitumor drug (Sato et al., 1994). One of the most important mechanisms involved may be the inhibition of angiogenesis, in which smooth muscle cells and endothelial cells are believed to play an important role. In vitro studies of apigenin in these types of cells found the proliferation and migration of endothelial cells respectively inhibited by 74% and 48% and that apigenin also inhibited capillary formation. Apigenin (5 µg/mL) inhibited the formation of capillary-like structures by 70%. The mechanism of endothelial cell inhibition was shown to involve blockage of the cell cycle in the G_2/M phase as a consequence of retinoblastoma protein of the hyperphosphorylated form. The growth of vascular smooth muscle cells, in contrast, was strongly stimulated by apigenin (5 µg/mL), an effect attributed to reduced expression of inhibitory proteins in smooth muscle cells (cyclin-dependent kinase inhibitors p21 and p27) and subsequent stimulation of the cell cycle (Trochon et al., 2000). Sato et al. (1994) reported that apigenin inhibited the in vitro growth of a rat neuronal tumor cell line (B104) by arresting cell cycle progression at the G^2/M phase, an action also reported from genistein.

Apigenin was shown to potently inhibit the growth of human thyroid carcinoma cell lines, including anaplastic (UCLA RO-81A-1), follicular (UCLA RO-82W-1), papillary (UCLA NPA-87-1), and thyroid carcinomas (Yin et al., 1999a, 1999b). Inhibition of the anaplastic cell line was observed from a concentration of 12.5-50 μM apigenin which resulted in programmed cell death (apoptosis). Apigenin also inhibited anchorage-independent and dependent growth of the thyroid cancer cells, signal transduction pathways which allow these cancer cells to grow and survive (Yin et al., 1999a). The mechanism of inhibition was shown to involve attenuation of the phosphorylation of Erk mitogen-activated protein (MAP) kinase and epidermal growth factor receptor tyrosine phosphorylation (Yin et al., 1999b). Apigenin also showed potent growth inhibitory activity in the human breast carcinoma cells, MDA-MB-468 and MCF-7 (IC_{50} 8.9 μM/mL and 7.8 μM/mL, respectively). The mechanisms involved were shown to be identical or similar to those of apigenin against breast carcinoma cells. The inhibition of Erk MAP kinase activation and phosphorylation in the MDA-MB-468 cell line was both time- and dose-dependent and apigenin also potently inhibited CDK1 kinase activity. In the MCF-7 cell line, apigenin caused a marked reduction in Rb phosphorylation (Yin et al., 2001). From a higher concentration, apigenin (100 μm/mL) also suppressed the in vitro proliferation of androgen-independent human prostate tumor cells (PC-3 cell line) by 70% (Knowles et al., 2000).

Promising results are reported on the chemopreventive activities of apigenin against chemically-induced skin tumors in mice (Wei et al., 1990). Because topical application of apigenin also significantly inhibited the formation of ultraviolet B-induced skin tumor formation in the skin of mice, the potential of the flavonoid as a topical chemopreventive/sunscreen agent has been the subject of intensive research into the mechanisms involved (Lepley et al., 1996; Lepley and Pelling, 1997; McVean et al., 2000; Trochon et al., 2000). Moreover, apigenin and other flavones of chamomile flowers were found to penetrate the deeper layers of skin of female volunteers when applied topically in aqueous alcoholic solutions saturated with the individual flavones (Merfort et al., 1994). Apigenin proved highly active as a growth inhibitor of cultured human choroidal melanoma cells (spindle-shape OCM-1 cell line), inhibiting growth by about 90% from a concentration of 28 μM/mL. The inhibitory mechanisms involved are at least partly attributable to the induction of G_2/M cell cycle arrest as a consequence of impaired dephosphorylation of the kinase CDK1 on Tyr15 residue. However, the induction of apoptosis by apigenin in this cell line was not observed (Casagrande and Darbon, 2001).

Immune Functions

Immunopotentiation. Wagner et al. (1985) found heteroglycan polysaccharides in *M. recutita* that enhanced phagocytosis in mice in the chemoluminescence model. Increases in phagocytic activity were greater than those of a polysaccharide derived from *Echinacea purpurea* in all doses tested. The maximum increase of 64% was observed at a concentration of 10^{-3} mg/mL. Higher concentrations showed less activity, although at 0.1 mg/mL phagocytosis was still increased by 48%.

Infectious Diseases

Fungal infections. Mares et al. (1993) and Szalontai et al. (1976) reported antifungal activity from chamomile. Mares and colleagues showed that infusions of *M. recutita* exhibit an antifungal activity against the dermatophytic fungus *Microsporum cookei* following UVA irradiation. Inhibition of the fungus was comparable to that of the coumarin derivative constituent herniarin, which was significantly fungistatic without the addition of UVA irradiation and highly fungistatic with the irradiation. Umbelliferone was weakly active at all doses tested, even following UVA irradiation. It was concluded that the antidermatophytic activity of chamomile aqueous preparations (in vitro) were due to a combined action of UVA and herniarin and that the fungistatic activity of the chamomile constituent coumarin umbelliferone was unconfirmed (Mares et al., 1993).

Microbial Infections. Extracts of *M. recutita* inhibit the growth of Gram-positive microorganisms (Aggag and Yousef, 1972; Yousef and Tawil, 1980). A hydroalcoholic extract of *M. recutita* and a commercial hydroalcoholic extract (Kamillosan) showed a weak inhibitory activity in vitro in *Escherichia coli* (Ceska et al., 1992). However, in the salt aggregation test (used to examine the hydrophobicity/aggregative ability of bacterial cell walls as a measure of their ability to adhere to cells), an aqueous extract of wild chamomile was found to completely block the aggregative property of 40 strains of *E. coli*. A higher number of aggregative strains of *E. coli* were found in unhealthy versus healthy organisms, including humans, and the ability of the bacteria to stick to mucosa or mucous membranes increased the likelihood of their initiating a pathogenic process (Turi et al., 1997).

Inflammatory Response

In a study by Miller et al. (1996), provoked histamine release from rat mast cells was inhibited by constituents of the essential oil of *M. recutita,* with en-in-dicyloether appearing considerably more active than others.

However, *M. recutita* has shown no inhibitory activity against local edema induced by bradykinin, serotonin, or histamine injections (Breinlich and Scharnagel, 1968). The essential oil of *M. recutita* (p.o.) showed equipotent activity to bisabolol in the cotton pellet granuloma test in rats, but no activity in the carrageenan edema test in rat paws. In the same study, azulene showed a lower oral ED_{50} (850 mg/kg) in the carrageenan edema test than either guaiazulene (1,100 mg/kg) or bisabolol (2,200 /mg/kg); however, all were close to equipotent in the cotton pellet granuloma test (Mann and Staba, 1986).

Although both chamazulene (7-ethyl-1,4-dimethylazulene) and prochamazulene have shown anti-inflammatory activity in vivo, only chamazulene showed significant in vitro inhibition of leukotriene B_4 formation (IC_{50} 15 mM). In addition, chamazulene (IC_{50} approx. 2 mM), but not prochamazulene, blocked peroxidation of arachidonic acid and decreased the formation of 5-lipoxygenase products (IC_{50} approx. 10 mM). Safayhi et al. (1994) concluded that since 5-lipoxygenase, the key enzyme for leukotrienes, which function in a variety of inflammatory processes, is inhibited by chamazulene, the constituent may contribute to the anti-inflammatory and antiphlogistic activity of chamomile through antioxidant activity. The quantity of chamazulene in a commercial ethanolic extract (54 mM) was much lower than the amount (315 mM) found in a propylene glycol extract of chamomile (Safayhi et al., 1994).

Topically applied to mice using the croton oil test, hydroalcoholic extracts of *M. recutita* flowers have shown significant antiedema activity, similar in potency to the nonsteroidal agent benzydamine (Tubaro et al., 1984). The wide use of chamomile formulations in topical applications prompted Della Loggia et al. (1990) to study the anti-inflammatory activity of various chamomile preparations. In the croton oil-induced ear inflammation model, 42% (v/v) hydroalcohol preparations of fresh and dried flowers were compared for anti-inflammatory activity with the essential oil, and the main compounds isolated from the hydroalcoholic preparations of *M. recutita* (apigenin, bisabolol, chamazulene, and matricine). The extract made from the fresh flowers showed 40% more inhibitory activity than the extract of dried flowers (31.6 % versus 23.7%, respectively). Although significant, they were only mildly active, for the fresh flower extract attained the same level of activity as the reference anti-inflammatory compound (benzydamine). The essential oil showed no significant inhibitory activity (6.6%). Apigenin showed 10 times the activity of matricine, and chamazulene 10 times less activity than matricine (Della Loggia et al., 1990). Apigenin at 2 mg/ear inhibited TPA (tetradecanoylphorbol-13-acetate)-induced edema of the mouse ear by 75% (Yasukawa et al., 1989).

A significant antiedemic (antiphlogistic) effect was shown with (-)-α-bisabolol in rats, which also promoted granulation and epithelization in burns of guinea pigs (Isaac, 1979). In rat models of yeast-induced fever and adjuvant arthritis, and in UV-induced erythema in guinea pigs, the same compound showed significant antiedemic (antiphlogistic) activity (Jakovlev et al., 1979).

Topically applied, polysaccharides of *M. recutita* significantly inhibited edema in mice in the croton oil ear test. However, the anti-inflammatory activity of even the most active polysaccharide (PS1, administered simultaneously or after croton oil) could only be considered mild (75 mg/ear, 33% inhibition before and 0% after) by comparison to the trihydroxyflavone apigenin (30 mg/ear, 38% before and 37% after) (Fuller et al., 1993).

Integumentary, Muscular, and Skeletal Functions

Dermatitis

Maiche et al. (1991) reported that chamomile has been used as a means of alleviating radiation burns of the skin without proof of efficacy. Using a standardized extract of chamomile flower heads (Kamillosan, AP Medical AB, Stockholm, Sweden), Maiche and colleagues compared its effects to almond ointment which had been used routinely at their clinic as a means of protecting the skin from radiation burns. The controlled, "physician-blind," randomized study involved the random assignment of 50 female patients (ages 30-79) to receive almond ointment or chamomile cream who had undergone surgery for localized breast cancer. Patients were instructed to gently apply the preparations to the area above and below their operation scars, b.i.d., 30 min before radiation (2 Gy five times/week up to 50 Gy) and again prior to bedtime, during their course of radiotherapy. Two patients discontinued the therapy owing to personal reasons, leaving 48 for evaluation. The results showed that according to statistical analysis, skin reactions were not significantly different in the two treatment groups and that neither treatment could prevent the reactions. The researchers added that while all the patients developed grade one erythema, in the chamomile group, changes in the skin seemed to show a tendency to appear later and there were fewer patients with grade two reactions compared to the almond ointment group (7 versus 13, respectively). Pain and itching were uncommon and equal in occurrence in the two groups and the majority of patients preferred the chamomile cream over the almond ointment because it rapidly absorbed and left no stains.

Topical application of a standardized chamomile extract preparation (50 mg α-bisabolol and 3 mg chamazulene) was investigated in 14 healthy adult male patients after they underwent dermabrasion with a Derma III abrasion instrument (1.5 mm depth) of the upper and lower arm for tattoo removal. The double-blind study involved applying chamomile dressings t.i.d., 2 h per application, until attaining a complete drying of the wounded skin surface. The placebo consisted of the same chamomile with odor intact and main active substances removed by precipitation. According to physician assessment, the active preparation decreased the drying process of weeping wounds significantly faster (30%) than the placebo by day 14, while on day four onwards wound healing (epithelization) became obviously more pronounced in the active chamomile group. By day eight, the difference compared to placebo was close to 50% (Glowania et al., 1987). Similar results were reported by patients using chamomile topically in dressings applied to stasis dermatitis. The preparation also contained corticosteroids, antihistamine, and calcium. A slight analgesic effect was noted in addition to deodorant, anti-inflammatory, and cooling effects (Mann and Staba, 1986).

Aertgeerts et al. (1985) conducted a bilateral, 21-28-day comparative study of chamomile cream (Kamillosan, ethanolic extract of the flowers, 2 g/100 g cream) versus three anti-inflammatory agents: two steroidal preparations (0.25% hydrocortisone salve and a 0.75% fluocortin butyl ester cream), and a nonsteroidal salve consisting of 5% bufexamac. The patients (n = 161) had been treated initially with 0.1% difluocortolone valerate (salve/cream) for neurodermatitis consisting of inflammatory dermatoses on the lower legs, hands, and forearms (e.g., irritative cumulative contact dermatitis, atopic endogenous eczema, seborrhial eczema). The results showed that the chamomile cream was about as equally effective when compared to the 0.25% hydrocortisone salve, and superior to either of the other two treatments.

Muscular Functions

Chamomile oil and bisabololoxides A and B have all shown papaverine-like, dose-dependent spasmolytic activity in isolated smooth muscles. However, (–)-α-bisabolol appeared equipotent to papaverine and twice as potent as bisabololoxides A and B. Among other constituents of *M. recutita,* the flavone apigenin (5,7,4'-trihydroxyflavone) appeared to be a more active antispasmodic than luteolin, patuletin, quercetin, apigenin 7-glucoside, or the coumarins herniarin and umbelliferone, and showed greater activity in vitro than papaverine. The *cis*-en-in-ether showed spasmolytic activity, but not dose-dependently (Achterrath-Tuckermann et al., 1980). However, when compared to ten other constituents of chamomile, which showed weak smooth muscle-relaxing activity, Isaac (1980) found the most potent smooth muscle relaxant by far was apigenin. The second most active was (–)-α-bisabolol. Given the release of apigenin through intestinal flavonoid hydrolysis, the apigenin 7-glycoside and its various glycoside derivatives are considered as prodrugs in chamomile (Schreiber et al., 1990).

Hydroalcoholic extracts of *M. recutita* tested in guinea pig ileum against the spasmodic effects of histamine and acetylcholine significantly decreased the induced contractions. They were less potent than that of a normal human therapeutic dosage of atropine, but were nonetheless significant (Achterrath-Tuckermann et al., 1980).

Extracts of *M. recutita* have been found to enhance the muscle tone of the uterus (Shipochliev, 1981).

Digestive, Hepatic, and Gastrointestinal Functions

Gastric Functions

Indomethacin-, ethanol-, heat coagulation-, acetic acid-, or stress-induced ulcers were inhibited by $(-)$-α-bisabolol. Ethanol-induced ulcers were inhibited by a commercial hydroalcoholic extract of *M. recutita* (Szelenyi et al., 1979). In vitro, $(-)$-α-bisabolol, azulene, and a total extract of *M. recutita* have shown antipeptic activity (Thiemer et al., 1972; Isaac and Thiemer, 1975).

Pharmacokinetics

Heilmann et al. (1993) studied adsorption and cutaneous penetration of chamomile flavonoids in healthy female volunteers. Saturated 20% alcohol solutions of chamomile flavonoids were applied to the upper arms of the volunteers using glass chambers filled with the solution. Decreases in contents were measured every 7 h and the amount of flavonoids that penetrated the dermis was calculated. The greatest flux was found from apigenin, while luteolin was second. A steady state was noted after 3 h, which indicated penetration of the flavonoids through deeper layers of skin.

Neurological, Psychological, and Behavioral Functions

Neurotoxicity/Neuroprotection

The major flavonoid of chamomile, apigenin, was shown to inhibit the in vitro neurotoxicity of amyloid β protein (Aβ), a neurotoxin associated with the development of Alzheimer's disease. Apigenin (50 μM) decreased the rate of cell death of cortical neuronal cells by 49%. Another flavonoid, quercetin, was found to potentiate the effect of apigenin whereas quercetin alone (1-50 μM) failed to inhibit Aβ-induced cell death (Wang et al., 2001).

Psychological and Behavioral Functions

Anxiety and stress response. Della Loggia et al. (1982) reported a mild hypnogenic effect from chamomile extracts and a central nervous system-depressive action. Anxiolytic effects of dried Argentine *M. recutita* flowers and branchlets were studied in mice (i.p.) by Viola et al. (1995). In addition to anxiolytic effects (3 mg/kg), they found slight sedative effects, but only from a high dose (30 mg/kg i.p.). Through activity-guided fractionation, apigenin was isolated as the more active constituent of chamomile and found to be a ligand for central benzodiazepine receptors, although it was without muscle-relaxant or anticonvulsant activity. Free apigenin was found in greater concentrations in Argentine chamomile plants than in those of any other country of origin. However, apigenin cannot be the only constituent in chamomile infusions with these effects. Furthermore, chrysin, which is derived from *Passiflora coerulea,* behaved similarly, and when administered in a comparable dose to apigenin (1 mg/kg i.p.) exhibited anxiolytic effects (Viola et al., 1995).

CLINICAL STUDIES

Digestive, Hepatic, and Gastrointestinal Disorders

Buccal Health

Fidler et al. (1996) performed a phase III, double-blind, placebo-controlled prospective trial of chamomile following data from a pilot study suggesting that a mouthwash of the herb might ameliorate stomatitis caused by 5-fluorouracil-based chemotherapy treatments, which are dose-limited primarily because of this side effect. Because cryotherapy was shown to reduce the incidence of stomatitis, the patients (n = 164) were randomized to receive 30 min of cryotherapy in addition to a chamomile mouthwash (ASTA Medica Incorporated, Hackensack, NJ). The dosage was 30 drops of chamomile concentrate/100 mL water, swished around in the mouth for 1 min/wash until 100 mL, t.i.d. for 14 days, or an "identical-appearing placebo" mouthwash. These treatments began from the start of the first five-day treatment cycle with 5-fluorouracil. Cryotherapy consisted of swishing ice chips around in the mouth for 5 min prior to each dose of chemotherapy. The severity of stomatitis was evaluated from 135 patients who provided sufficient data to analyze. The results showed that while no toxicity could be ascribed to the chamomile mouthwash, any benefit it provided was small and not significant compared to the placebo mouthwash. Curiously, the results of a gender-based subset analysis suggested that "chamomile might be beneficial for males and detrimental for females" using the mouthwash during 5-fluorouracil-based chemotherapy (Fidler et al., 1996, p. 524). Other than chance, the researchers could offer no "biologically plausible explanation" for the gender difference (Fidler et al., 1996, p. 524).

Carl and Emrich (1991) conducted a comparative uncontrolled clinical study of a chamomile oral rinse (chamomile flower preparation, Kamillosan Liquidum, Asta Pharma A.G., Frankfurt, Germany) in 78 patients (sex and age not mentioned) who had received chemotherapy for head and neck cancers and 20 about to receive radiation therapy for same. Among those being administered chemotherapy, 16 received the chamomile oral rinse (10-15 drops/100 mL warm water used to rinse the mouth "vigorously," ≥ t.i.d.) while they underwent their second repeated cycle of chemotherapy, and 32 received the oral rinse after developing mucositis. Of these, five developed grade one, 13 grade two, and 14 grade three mucositis. The chamomile mouth rinse seemed to help. Those with grade three mucositis achieved a grade one and zero condition after an average of five to seven days, with a "marked improvement" evident after three days, and every patient claimed relief from discomfort was "immediate." Among those with grade two mucositis, it took three to five days for their condition to revert to grades one and zero, and of those with grade one mucositis there was no further deterioration after they used the oral rinse. The other 46 patients receiving chemotherapy showed no signs of clinical mucositis while receiving the chamomile rinse; however, two who received leucovorin and 5-fluorouracil combined later presented with grade three mucositis, one with a moderate grade two musositis, and seven with grade 1 mucositis. Of the 16 patients who received the chamomile oral rinse while they underwent repeated cycles of their therapy, four already showed a grade three mucositis, nine grade two, and three grade one. When on their second cycle they began to use the chamomile rinse on the same day, 15 "remained free of clinically noticeable tissue changes" and only one patient developed grade one mucositis affecting the tongue (Carl and Emrich, 1991, p. 365). In total, Carl and Emrich (1991) found 78% of those who received the chamomile rinse while receiving chemotherapy showed no noticeable signs of mucositis (Carl and Emrich, 1991).

Carl and Emrich (1991) reported that of the 20 patients about to receive radiation therapy, one (5%) developed grade three mucositis after receiving 5800 cGy of radiation, and after a level of 4000-5000 cGy, 13 (65%) developed grade two mucositis, and six (35%) grade one. Whereas these grades were maintained throughout the course of radiotherapy, the researchers point out that compared to patients who had received the same amounts of radiation and standard oral care using a rinse consisting of 3% hydrogen peroxide, saline, and 5% sodium bicarbonate, the results with chamomile appeared considerably better. On the standard oral care solution, grade two mucositis developed after less radiation (about 2000 to 3000 cGy) and in the majority there was a rapid progression to grade three mucositis (Carl and Emrich, 1991).

In another study, cutaneous and mucosal infections of the mouth were treated in a double-blind clinical trial of *M. recutita,* with saline or water as the control. Patients used a mouth wash with dilute extracts of chamomile five to six times/day, alternating with saline. With the exception of patients with glossodynia, the effect of the extract was astringent and cooling (Nasemann, 1975).

Gastric Disorders

Infantile colic. In a prospective randomized, double-blind, placebo-controlled study, Weizman et al. (1993) examined the effect of chamomile-based tea (Calma-Bebi, Bonomelli, Dolzago, Italy) in the treatment of infantile colic. The tea consisted of an instant powder containing extracts of chamomile, vervain *(Verbena officinalis)*, licorice *(Glycyrrhiza glabra)*, fennel *(Foeniculum vulgare)*, lemon balm *(Melissa officinalis)*, glucose, and natural flavors; the latter two ingredients serving as the placebo. Seventy-two healthy term infants (ages two to eight weeks) were administered either placebo or the tea (no more than 150 mL/dose, t.i.d. times seven), and diaries recording the effects were maintained by the infant families, however unobjective they may have been. Significant results were found in the chamomile-based tea group compared to placebo in the colic improvement score and the percentage of infants with colic eliminated. No significant differences were found versus placebo in the number of tea administrations/day, the volume of tea consumed, or the number of night awakenings. No adverse effects were noticed in either treatment group.

Respiratory and Pulmonary Functions

Respiratory Infections

Saller et al. (1990) used a chamomile alcoholic extract as an inhalant in a placebo-controlled, randomized trial in 60 outpatients with the common cold. Patients were randomly assigned to a control group to inhale a steam containing a 35% alcohol solution, while three groups of patients were assigned to ten minute steam inhalation of solutions containing three progressively higher doses of the chamomile extract (13, 26, and 39 mL/L water). A towel over the head allowed the steam to be confined. Starting immediately prior to inhalations, the patients were instructed to give their estimated extent of symptoms, again after every 15 minutes of the first hour, and then hourly up to the fifth hour. Significant differences were found among all the groups. The reduction in symptoms (self-reported) was pronounced and dose-dependent. Middle and upper respiratory tract symptoms were relieved the most, and no side effects in any of the groups were reported. Onset of action appeared after 15 minutes and reached a maximum at 0.5-2 h. Analogue scores for each of the respective groups at the end of the trial were: 32 (control), 41 (13 mL), 62 (26 mL), and 106 (39 mL). As many as 40% of those in the 39 mL group reported experiencing a mild dizziness at the start of treatment which, however, was self-limiting.

DOSAGE

The *British Herbal Compendium* (Bradley, 1992) gives the oral dosage of *M. recutita* dried flower heads as 2-4 g, t.i.d. The tincture is given in the dosage of 1-4 mL, t.i.d. External use of infusions are recognized as containing 3% to 10% of chamomile, or an equivalent extract (1:1, 45% ethanol) or tincture (1:5, 45% ethanol). For internal use, the German Commission E monograph on *M. recutita* recommends one cup of freshly brewed flower head tea between meals, t.i.d. to q.i.d. Brewing instructions recommend 3 g/150 mL hot water steeped for 5-10 min and filtered by a tea strainer before drinking. The inhalate of chamomile is prepared with 1-2 tablespoons of flower heads/150 mL hot water, and the tea for gargle or rinse (several times daily) is allowed in mucosal inflammations of the mouth and throat. For external applications, 3% to 10% infusions or semisolid preparations are allowed for compresses and rinses. In the form of a bath additive, 50 g/10 L water is allowed (Bradley, 1992).

Extracts of *C. recutita* could be standardized to any one or more of a number of active constituents, including the flavonoids luteoline and apigenine, bisabolols, matricine, essential oils, en-indicycloether, polysaccharides, and chamazulene. The most active antispasmodic and anti-inflammatory constituents are mostly found in the volatile oil and consist of the sesquiterpenes (–)-α-bisabololoxides A and B and (–)-α-bisabolol, and matricine (prochamazulene), while coumarins and flavonoids contribute to the spasmolytic activity (Robbers et al., 1996). The commonly used standard is a minimum of 1% apigenin plus 0.5% essential oil of chamomile. For anxiety or nervousness, dosages of 400 mg standardized extract in capsule form have been used, one to four times/day (Flynn and Roest, 1995).

SAFETY PROFILE

In Sweden, *C. recutita* is classified as a natural product and foodstuff, while in Germany the flower head is allowed for oral use and as an herbal tea for oral or inhalation uses with the provision that it not be applied "near the eye" (De Smet et al., 1993). The use of chamomile tea as an eyewash by sensitive patients has been associated with angioedema of the eyelids (allergic conjunctivitis) (Subiza et al., 1990).

Contraindications

The German Commission E and the *British Compendium* list *C. recutita* as having no known contraindications (Blumenthal et al., 1998, Bradley, 1992).

Drug Interactions

None known.

Pregnancy and Lactation

None known.

Side Effects

The German Commission E states that chamomile has no known side effects (Blumenthal, et al., 1998). The *British Compendium* lists *M. recutita* as having the "extremely rare" side effect of contact allergy (Bradley, 1992). In a study of subjects with known or suspected allergies, only two out of 25 showed any allergic reaction to chamomile. In these individuals, a cross-reactivity was found between chamomile and other members of the Asteraceae (Hausen et al., 1984). On the skin of humans, after a 48-h closed patch test (4% chamomile oils in petrolatum), there were no signs of irritation (Mann and Staba, 1986).

A case of contact dermatitis was reported in a female florist who reacted to the petals and leaves of *M. recutita*. She tested more strongly positive to alcoholic extracts of the plant and to chamomile teas and a chamomile lotion and ointment (Van Ketel, 1982). In another case, within a few minutes after sipping chamomile tea, a woman with previously diagnosed hay fever from ragweed experienced stomach cramps, throat constriction, and a thickening of the tongue, followed by diffuse pruritus, angioedema of the eyes and lips, and a sensation in her ears. After ingesting a capsule of diphenhydramine followed by a steroid injection, her symptoms gradually dissipated over 2 h and by the next morning she was well again. Following a scratch test with chamomile tea, she reacted with a substantial wheal-and-flare accompanied with pseudopod formation. Subsequent testing of 15 patients with allergy to ragweed found five patients with positive reactions to the tea. It was therefore recommended that patients with allergies to ragweed be cautioned about exposure to chamomile (Benner and Lee, 1973). A coumarin (herniarin) with photosensitizing capability in chamomile has been postulated as a likely allergen involved in reactions to the plant (Ceska et al., 1992).

Special Precautions

Overdosage of chamomile may result in emesis (Osol and Farrar, 1950; Wood and Bache, 1845) and flaccidity of the stomach muscles (Mann and Staba, 1986).

The Ministries of Pharmacy and Medications of the government of France cautions that chamomile should not be used for symptoms that persist more than two days, and that it should only be used for minor problems. They also caution that it should not be used for irritations accompanied by pus, nor when there are sharp pains or in problems following injury of direct impact (Bradley, 1992). This precaution stems from the popular European folk use of chamomile tea as an eyewash to treat ocular reactions, including conjunctivitis. A study in seven patients diagnosed with hay fever found that two developed eyelid angioedema after using chamomile tea as an eyewash. When conjunctival provocations were performed using an extract of the chamomile tea, all seven patients tested positive, as they all did to skin prick tests with the extract and pollen extracts of mugwort *(Artemisia vulgaris)* or chamomile *(M. chamomilla = M. recutita);* however, when taken orally by the patients, the tea extract failed to elicit any symptoms. Sera from the patients revealed IgE activity developed in response to the three test preparations and in an ELISA inhibition study, researchers observed a cross-reactivity from the preparations. However, in all seven cases, IgE activity was absorbed by the chamomile pollen. In 100 hay fever control patients subjected to conjunctival and skin prick tests, 15 showed a positive immediate response in the skin test to mugwort pollen, eight of whom also showed a positive response to chamomile pollen. Of the latter, five also tested positive to the chamomile tea, and of these patients only two showed immediate positive skin responses to chamomile pollen, mugwort pollen, and a positive conjunctival response to chamomile tea. In another study, it was concluded that the use of chamomile tea as an eyewash was capable of inducing conjunctivitis and that the offending allergens were pollens of the plant contained in the tea (Subiza et al., 1990). A similar case of eyelid angioedema following topical application of chamomile tea to the eyelids of an atopic patient was reported by Foti et al. (2000).

Individuals with allergies to ragweed have long been cautioned about exposure to chamomile (Casterline, 1980; Benner and Lee, 1973). An eight-year-old boy with a history of bronchial asthma and hay fever caused by pollen of mugwort, olive, and grass experienced a severe anaphylactic reaction after the first time he ingested chamomile tea (prepared by infusion). In the ELISA-inhibition study, tests showed a cross-reactivity between the tea extract and pollens of *M. chamomilla (= M. recutita),* mugwort *(Artemisia vulgaris),* and giant ragweed *(Ambrosia trifida).* The patient also showed an immediate reaction to both a positive transfer and a skin test using an extract of the tea and by way of an ELISA technique, specific IgE antibodies (antichamomile-pollen and antichamomile-tea IgE). The anaphylactic symptoms were likely mediated by an IgE mechanism and the patient likely cross-reacted to the chamomile pollen because he was already sensitized to mugwort pollen. Two other cases occurred in which anaphylactic reactions following the ingestion of "chamomile" tea were suspected to have resulted from cross-reactivity between chamomile and ragweed (Subiza et al., 1989).

Anaphylactic reaction to an enema containing an extract of chamomile flowers (Kamillosan) administered during labor was reported in a 35-year-old woman without a history of atopy. The patient developed septic fever and died, despite administration of antibiotics for three weeks. Preceding her demise, skin prick responses to glycerol contained in the enema, latex, inhalant allergens, and birch pollen extracts were all negative, while the response to the chamomile extract was positive. Using RAST testing, researchers detected specific IgE for chamomile and then analyzed the IgE of the patient for reactivity. IgE binding to allergens of 17 kd in the extract preparation and to chamomile led to the identification of homologues of a birch pollen allergen, Bet v 1, having the same weight. IgE of the patient recognized the Bet v 1 homologues which were subsequently found in minute amounts in the chamomile extract used in the enema. Although RAST results were negative for the homologue and amounts in the chamomile extract were minute, the authors concluded that they were enough to set off anaphylaxis and that this might have owed to the large area of the colonic mucosa exposed to the extract during administration of the enema (Jensen-Jarolim et al., 1998).

In another study, the sensitizing capacity of *M. recutita* in guinea pigs was found to be low. The constituent anthecotulid (sesquiterpene lactone) is a known skin allergen, but in *M. recutita* the concentration is extremely low and was not expected to cause allergic reactions (Hausen et al., 1984). A popular chamomile skin cream (Kamillosan) is reported to be devoid of the allergen (Jablonska and Rudzki, 1996). An exhaustive examination of *M. recutita* for allergic reactions resulted in the conclusion that such reactions were "unequivocally" extremely rare (Hausen et al., 1984). Since then, case reports of allergic reactions continue to be reported, however rarely (Subiza et al., 1989, 1990; Jensen-Jarolim et al., 1998; Rodriguez-Serna et al., 1998; Foti et al., 2000). Historically, allergic reactions involving Roman chamomile *(Anthemis nobilis)* or the related, adulterant species, dog chamomile *(Anthemis cotula),* are more common and have obfuscated case reports of reactions to chamomile *(M. recutita)* (Hausen et al., 1984).

Toxicology

Mutagenicity

In the Ames test, an extract of chamomile flowers prepared with boiling water produced a relatively high degree of mutagenicity (Yamamoto et al., 1982), an effect which may have been the result of photoactivation of coumarins in the extract (Ceska et al., 1992).

Toxicity in Animal Models

Long-term oral toxicity from *M. recutita* extracts p.o. in rats and dogs was not found; nor were there any changes in prenatal development of puppies or teratogenic effects in rats from long-term administration of *M. recutita*. A three-week cutaneous application of *M. recutita* on rabbits produced no signs of toxicity. In guinea pigs, daily administration of *M. recutita* extracts by inhalation for three weeks produced no toxicity (Mann and Staba, 1986).

The application of the essential oil of *M. recutita* in rabbits produced an oral LD_{50} of greater than 5 g/kg. When applied topically on the backs of hairless mice, the undiluted oil produced no signs of toxicity. When applied to the abraded or normal skin of rabbits for 24 h, the undiluted oil produced only limited irritation (Mann and Staba, 1986).

REFERENCES

Achterrath-Tuckermann, U., Kunde, R., Flaskamp, E., Isaac, O., and Thiemer, K. (1980). Pharmacologische untersuchungen von kamillen-inhaltsstoffen. V. Untersuchungen uber die spasmolytische wirkung von kamillen-inhaltsstoffen und von Kamillosan® am isolierten meerschweinchen-ileum [Pharmacological investigations with compounds of chamomile. V. Investigations on the spasmolytic effect of compounds of chamomile and Kamillosan® on the isolated guinea pig ileum]. *Planta Medica* 39: 38-50.

Aertgeerts, P., Albring, M., Klaschka, F., Nasemann, T., Patzelt-Wenczler, R., Rauhut, K., and Weigl, B. (1985). Verfleichende prüfung von Kamillosan® creme gegenüber steroidalen (0.25% hydrocortison, 0.75% fluocortinbutylester) und nuichtsteroidalen (5% bufexamac) externa in der erhaltungstherapie von ekzemerkrankungen [Comparison of Kamillosan® cream (2 g ethanolic extract from Chamomile flowers in 100 g cream) versus steroidal (0.25% hydrocortisone, 0.75% fluocortin butyl ester) and non-steroidal (5% bufexamac) dermatics in the maintenance therapy of eczema]. *Zeitschrift fur Hautkrankheiten* 60: 270-277.

Aggag, M.E. and Yousef, R.T. (1972). Antimicrobial activity of chamomile oil. *Planta Medica* 22: 140-144.

Ahmad, A. and Misra, L.N. (1997). Isolation of herniarin and other constituents from *Matricaria chamomilla* flowers. *International Journal of Pharmacognosy* 35: 121-125.

Becker, H., Reichling, J., and Hsieh, W.C. (1982). Water-free solvent system for droplet counter-current chromatography and its suitability for the separation of non-polar substances. *Journal of Chromatography* 237: 307-310.

Benner, M.H. and Lee, H.J. (1973). Anaphylactic reaction to chamomile tea. *Journal of Allergy and Clinical Immunology* 52: 307-308.

Blumenthal, M. (1998). The German Commission E monograph system for phyto-medicines: A model for regulatory reform in the United States. In Lawson, L.D. and Bauer, R. (Eds.), *Phytomedicines of Europe: Chemistry and Biological Activity* (pp. 30-36). ACS Symposium Series 691. Washington, DC: American Chemical Society.

Blumenthal, M., Busse, W.R., Goldberg, A., Gruenwald, J., Hall, T., Riggins, C.W., and Rister, R.S. (Eds.) (1998). *The Complete German Commission E Monographs*. Austin, TX: American Botanical Council, p. 107.

Bradley, P.R. (Ed.) (1992). *British Herbal Compendium, 1*. Bournemouth, Dorset, England: British Herbal Medicine Association, pp. 154-157.

Breinlich, J. and Scharnagel, K. (1968). Pharmakologische eigenschaften des en-in-dicycloether aus *Matricaria chamomilla* [Pharmacological properties of the en-in-dicyloether from *Matricaria chamomilla*. Study of the anti-inflammatory, anti-anaphylactic, spasmolytic and bacteriostatic activity]. *Arzneimittel-Forschung/Drug Research* 18: 429-431.

Carl, W. and Emrich, L.S. (1991). Management of oral mucositis during local radiation and systematic chemotherapy: A study of 98 patients. *The Journal of Prosthetic Dentistry* 66: 361-369.

Carle, R., Dolle, B., Müller, W., and Baumeister, U. (1992). Thermospray liquid chromatography-mass spectrometry (TSP LC-MS) analysis of acetylated apigenin 7-glucosides from *Chamomilla recutita*. *Planta Medica* 58(Suppl.): A686-A687.

Carle, R., Dolle, B., and Reinhard, E. (1989). A new approach to the production of chamomile extracts. *Planta Medica* 55: 540-543.

Carle, R., Fleischhauer, I., Beyer, J., and Reinhard, E. (1990). Studies on the origin of (–)-α-bisabol and chamazulene in chamomile preparations; part I. Investigations by isotope ratio mass spectrometry (IRMS). *Planta Medica* 56: 456-460.

Carle, R. and Isaac, O. (1985). Fortschritte in der kamillenforschung in den jahren 1974 bis 1984 [Progress in the research of chamomile in the years 1974 to 1984]. *Deutsche Apotheker Zeitung* 125(Suppl. 1): 2-8.

Casagrande, F. and Darbon, J. (2001). Effects of structurally related flavonoids on cell cycle progression of human melanoma cells: Regulation of cyclin-dependent kinases CDK2 and CDK1. *Biochemical Pharmacology* 61(10): 1205-1215.

Casterline, C.L. (1980). Allergy to Chamomile tea. *Journal of the American Medical Association* 244: 330-331 (letter).

Ceska, O., Chaudhary, S.K., Warrington, P.J., and Ashwood-Smith, M.J. (1992). Coumarins of chamomile, *Chamomilla recutita*. *Fitoterapia* 63: 387-394.

Das, M., Kumar, S., Mallavarapu, G.R., and Ramesh, S. (1999). Composition of the essential oils of the flowers of three accessions of *Chamomilla recutita* (L.) Rausch. *Journal of Essential Oil Research* 11: 615-618.

De Smet, P.A.G.M., Keller, K., Hänsel, R., and Chandler, R.F. (Eds.) (1993). *Adverse Effects of Herbal Drugs, 2*. New York: Springer-Verlag, p. 55.

Della Loggia, R., Carle, R., Sosa, S., and Tubaro, A. (1990). Evaluation of the anti-inflammatory activity of chamomile preparations. *Planta Medica* 56: 657-658.

Della Loggia, R., Traversa, V., Scarcia, V., and Tubaro, V. (1982). Depressive effects of *Chamomilla recutita* (L.) Rausch, tubular flowers, on central nervous system in mice. *Pharmacological Research Communications* 14: 153-162.

Duke, J.A. (1985). *CRC Handbook of Medicinal Herbs.* Boca Raton, FL: CRC Press, pp. 297-298.

Exner, J., Reichling, J., Cole, T.C.H., and Becker, H. (1981). Methylated flavonoidaglycones from "Matricariae Flos." *Planta Medica* 41: 198-199.

Fidler, P., Loprinzi, C.L., O'Fallon, J.R., Leitch, J.M., Lee, J.K., Hayes, D.L., Novotny, P., Clemens-Schutjer, D., Bartel, J., and Michalak, J.C. (1996). Prospective evaluation of a chamomile mouthwash for prevention of 5-FU-induced oral mucositis. *Cancer* 77: 522-525.

Flynn, R. and Roest, M. (1995). *Your Guide to Standardized Herbal Products.* Prescott, AZ: One World Press, pp. 14-15.

Foti, C., Nettis, E., Panebianco, R., Cassano, N., Diaferio, A., and Pia, D.P. (2000). Contact urticaria from *Matricaria chamomilla. Contact Dermatitis* 42: 360-361.

Franz, C. and Wickel, I. (1979). The composition of essential oil in crossing- and self-progenies of *Matricaria chamomilla* L. *Planta Medica* 36: 281-282.

Fuller, E., Blaschek, W., and Franz, G. (1991). Characterization of water-soluble polysaccharides from chamomile flowers. *Planta Medica* 57(Suppl. 2): A40.

Fuller, E., Sosa, S., Tubaro, A., Franz, G., and Della Loggia, R. (1993). Anti-inflammatory activity of *Chamomilla* polysaccharides. *Planta Medica* 59(Suppl.): A666-A667.

Gasic, O., Lukic, V., and Nikolic, A. (1983). Chemical study of *Matricaria chamomilla* L. - II. *Fitoterapia* 54: 51-55.

Glowania, H.J., Raulin, C., and Swoboda, M. (1987). Wirkung der kamille der wundheilung—eine klinische doppelblindstudie [The effect of chamomile on wound healing—a controlled clinical experimental double-blind trial]. *Zeitschrift für Hautkrankheiten* 62: 1262, 1267-1271.

Grieve, M. (1980). *A Modern Herbal.* New York: Penguin Books, pp. 185-188.

Hausen, B.M., Busker, E., and Carle, R. (1984). [The sensitizing capacity of Compositae plants VII. Experimental investigations with extracts and compounds of *Chamomilla recutita* (L.) Rauschert and *Anthemis cotula* L.]. *Planta Medica* 50: 229-234.

Heilmann, J., Merfort, I., Hagedorn, U., and Lippold, B.C. (1993). In vivo skin penetration studies of chamomile flowers. *Planta Medica* 59 (Suppl.): A638.

Heneka, N. (1993). *Chamomilla recutita. Australian Journal of Medical Herbalism* 5: 33-39.

Hirano, T., Oka, K., and Akiba, M. (1989). Anti-proliferative effects of synthetic and naturally occurring flavonoids on tumor cells of the human breast-carcinoma line, ZR-75-1. *Research Communications in Chemical Pathology and Pharmacology* 64: 69-78.

Isaac, O. (1979). Pharmakologische untersuchungen von kamillen-inhaltsstoffen. I. Zur pharmakologie des $(-)$-α-bisabolols und der bisabololoxide (ubersicht)

[Pharmacological investigations with compounds of chamomile. I. On the pharmacology of (–)-α-bisabolol oxides (review)]. *Planta Medica* 35: 118-124.

Isaac, O. (1980). Chamomile therapy-experimentation and verification. *Deutsche Apotheker Zeitung* 120: 567-570.

Isaac, O. and Thiemer, K. (1975). Biochemical studies on camomile components. III: *In vitro* studies about the antipeptic activity of (–)-bisabolol. *Arzneimittel-Forschung/Drug Research* 25: 1352-1354.

Jablonska, S. and Rudzki, E. (1996). [Kamillosan™ concentrate—a non-allergizng camomile extract]. *Zeitschrift fur Hautkrankheiten* 71: 542-546.

Jakovlev, V., Isaac, O., Thiemer, K., and Kunde, R. (1979). Pharmacological investigations with compounds of chamomille. II. New investigations on the antiphlogistic effects of (–)-α-bisabolol and bisabolol oxides. *Planta Medica* 35: 125-140.

Jensen-Jarolim, E., Reider, N., Fritsch, R., and Breiteneder, H. (1998). Fatal outcome of anaphylaxis to chamomile-containing enema during labor. *Journal of Allergy and Clinical Immunology* 102: 1041-1042.

Knowles, L.M., Zigrossi, D.A., Tauber, R.A., Hightower, C., and Milner, J.A. (2000). Flavonoids suppress androgen-independent human prostate tumor proliferation. *Nutrition and Cancer* 38: 116-122.

Lepley, D.M., Li, B., Birt, D.F., and Pelling, J.C. (1996). The chemopreventive flavonoid apigenin induces G_2/M arrest in keratinocytes. *Carcinogenesis* 17: 2367-2375.

Lepley, D.M. and Pelling, J.C. (1997). Induction of p21/WAF1 and G_1 cell-cycle arrest by the chemopreventive agent apigenin. *Molecular Carcinogenesis* 19: 74-82.

Maiche, A.G., Grohn, P., and Maki-Hokkonen, H. (1991). Effect of chamomile cream and almond ointment on acute radiation skin reaction. *Acta Oncologica* 30: 395-396 (letter).

Maier, R., Carle, R., Kreis, W., and Reinhard, E. (1993). Purification and characterization of a flavone 7-*O*-glucoside-specific glucosidase from ligulate florets of *Chamomilla recutita*. *Planta Medica* 59: 436-441.

Maier, R., Kreis, W., Carle, R., and Reinhard, E. (1991). Partial purification and substrate specificity of a β-glucosidase from *Chamomilla recutita*. *Planta Medica* 57(Suppl. 2): A84-A85.

Mann, C. and Staba, E.J. (1986). The chemistry, pharmacology, and commercial formulations of chamomile. In Cracker, L.E. and Simon, J.E. (Eds.), *Herbs, Spices, and Medicinal Plants: Advances in Botany, Horticulture, and Pharmacology* (pp. 235-280). 1. Phoenix, AZ: Oryx Press.

Mares, D., Romagnoli, C., and Bruni, A. (1993). Antidermatophytic activity of herniarin in preparations of *Chamomilla recutita* (L.) Rauschert. *Plantes Médicinales et Phytothérapie* 26: 91-100.

McVean, M., Xiao, H., Isobe, K.I., and Pelling, J.C. (2000). Increase in wild-type p 53 stability and transactivational activity by the chemopreventive agent apigenin in keratinocytes. *Carcinogenesis* 21: 633-639.

Merfort, I., Helimann, J., Hagedorn-Leweke, U., and Lippold, B.C. (1994). In vivo skin penetration studies of chamomile flowers. *Pharmazie* 49: 509-511.

Nasemann, T. (1975). [Kamillosan therapy in dermatology]. *Zeitschrift für Allegemeinmedizin* 51: 1105-1106.

Osol, A. and Farrar, G.E. (1950). *The Dispensatory of the United States of America.* Philadelphia, PA: J.B. Lippincott Co., p. 2075.

Pedersen, M. (1994). *Nutritional Herbology.* Warsaw, IN: Wendell W. Whitman Co., pp. 67-69.

Redaelli, C., Formentini, L., and Santaniello, E. (1980). Apigenin 7-glucoside and its 2''- and 6''-acetates from ligulate flowers of *Matricaria chamomilla. Phytochemistry* 19: 985-986.

Redaelli, C., Formentini, L., and Santaniello, E. (1981a). HPLC determination of coumarins in *Matricaria chamomilla. Planta Medica* 43: 412-413.

Redaelli, C., Formentini, L., and Santaniello, E. (1981b). Reversed-phase high-performance liquid chromatography analysis of apigenin and its glucosides in flowers of *Matricaria chamomilla* and chamomile extracts. *Planta Medica* 42: 288-292.

Redaelli, C., Formentini, L., and Santaniello, E. (1982). Apigenin 7-glucoside diacetates in ligulate flowers of *Matricaria chamomilla. Phytochemistry* 21: 1828-1830.

Reichling, J. and Beiderbeck, R. (1991). *Chamomilla recutita* (L.) Rauschert (Camomile): In vitro culture and the production of secondary metabolites. In Bajaj, Y.P.S. (Ed.), *Biotechnology in Agriculture and Forestry, 15. Medicinal and Aromatic Plants,* III (pp. 156-175). Berlin, Germany: Springer-Verlag.

Reichling, J., Beiderbeck, R., and Becker, H. (1979). Vergleichende untersuchungen über sekundäre inhaltstoffe bei pflanzen-tumoren, blüte, kraut und wurzel von *Matricaria chamomilla* L. [Comparative studies on secondary products from tumors, flowers, herb and roots of *Matricaria chamomilla* L.]. *Planta Medica* 36: 322-332.

Repcak, M., Imrich, J., and Garcar, J. (1999). Quantitative evaluation of the main sesquiterpenes and polyacetylenes of *Chamomilla recutita* essential oil by high-performance liquid chromatography. *Phytochemical Analysis* 10: 335-338.

Robbers, J.E., Speedie, M.K., and Tyler, V.E. (1996). *Pharmacognosy and Pharmacobiotechnology.* Baltimore, MD: Williams and Wilkins, p. 87.

Rodriguez-Serna, M., Sánchez-Motilla, J.M., Ramón, R., and Aliaga, A. (1998). Allergic and systemic contact dermatitis from *Matricaria chamomilla* tea. *Contact Dermatitis* 39: 192-193.

Safayhi, H., Sabieraj, J., Sailer, E.R., and Ammon, H.P. (1994). Chamazulene: An antioxidant-type inhibitor of leukotriene B_4 formation. *Planta Medica* 60: 410-413.

Saller, R., Beschorner, M., Hellenbrecht, M., and Bühring, M. (1990). Dose-dependency of symptomatic relief of complaints by chamomile steam inhalation in patients with common cold. *European Journal of Pharmacology* 183: 728-729.

Sato, F., Matsukawa, Y., Matsumoto, K., Nishino, H., and Sakai, T. (1994). Apigenin induces morphological differentiation and G_2/M arrest in rat neuronal cells. *Biochemical and Biophysical Research Communications* 204: 578-584.

Schreiber, A., Carle, R., and Reinhard, E. (1990). On the accumulation of apigenin in chamomile flowers. *Planta Medica* 56: 179-181.

Shipochliev, T. (1981). Extracts from a group of medicinal plants enhancing uterine tonus. *Veterinarno-Meditsinski Nauki* 18: 94-98.

Subiza, J., Subiza, J.L., Alonso, M., Hinojosa, M., Garcia, R., Jerez, M., and Subiza, E. (1990). Allergic conjunctivitis to chamomile tea. *Annals of Allergy* 65: 127-132.

Subiza, J., Subiza, J.L., Hinojosa, M., Garcia, R., Jerez, M., Valdivieso, R., and Subiza, E. (1989). Anaphylactic reaction after the ingestion of chamomile tea: A study of cross-reactivity with other composite pollens. *Journal of Allergy and Clinical Immunology* 84: 353-358.

Szalontai, M., Verzar, P.G., and Florian, E. (1976). Data on the antifungal effect of the biologically active components of *Matricaria chamomilla* L. *Acta Pharmaceutica Hungarica* 46: 232-247.

Szelenyi, I., Isaac, O., and Thiemer, K. (1979). Pharmakologische untersuchungen von kamillen-inhaltsstoffen. III. Tier experimentelle untersuchungen uber die ulkusprotektive wirkung der kamille [Pharmacological experiments with compounds of chamomile. III. Experimental studies of the ulcer-protective effect of chamomile]. *Planta Medica* 35: 218-227.

Thiemer, K., Stadler, R., and Isaac, O. (1972). [Biochemical study on camomile ingredients. I. Antipeptic activity of camomile extract and 1,4-dimethyl-7-isopropylazulene sulfoacidic sodium]. *Arzneimittel-Forschung/Drug Research* 22: 1086-1087.

Trochon, V., Blot, E., Cymbalista, F., Engelmann, C., Tang, R.P., Thomaidis, A., Vasse, M., Soria, J., Lu, H., and Soria, C. (2000). Apigenin inhibits endothelial-cell proliferation in G_2/M phase whereas it stimulates smooth-muscle cells by inhibiting P21 and P27 expression. *International Journal of Cancer* 85(5): 691-696.

Tubaro, A., Zilli, C., Redaelli, C., and Della Loggia, R. (1984). Evaluation of anti-inflammatory activity of a chamomile extract after topical application. *Planta Medica* 51: 359.

Turi, M., Turi, E., Koljalg, S., and Mikelsaar, M. (1997). Influence of aqueous extracts of medicinal plants on surface hydrophobicity of *Escherichia coli* strains of different origin. *Acta Pathologica, Microbiologica et Immunologica Scandinavica* 105: 956-962.

Van Ketel, W.G. (1982). Allergy to *Matricaria chamomilla*. *Contact Dermatitis* 8: 143.

Viola, H., Wasowski, C., Levi de Stein, M., Wolfman, C., Silveira, R., Dajas, F., Medina, J.H., and Paladini, A.C. (1995). Apigenin, a component of *Matricaria recutita* flowers, is a central benzodiazepine receptors-ligand with anxiolytic effects. *Planta Medica* 61: 213-216.

Wagner, H., Proksch, A., Vollmar, A., Kreutzkamp, B., and Bauer, J. (1985). In vitro phagocytosis stimulation by isolated plant materials measured in the phagocytosis-chemoluminescence (CL) model. *Planta Medica* 44: 139-144.

Wang, C.N., Chi, C.W., Lin, Y.L., Chen, C.F., and Shiao, Y.J. (2001). The neuroprotective effects of phytoestrogens on amyloid beta protein-induced toxicity are mediated by abrogating the activation of caspase cascade in rat cortical neurons. *Journal of Biological Chemistry* 276: 5287-5295.

Wei, H., Tye, L., Bresnick, E., and Birt, D.F. (1990). Inhibitory effect of apigenin, a plant flavonoid, on epidermal ornithine decarboxylase and skin tumor promotion in mice. *Cancer Research* 50: 499-502.

Weizman, Z., Alkrinawi, S., Goldfarb, D., and Bitran, C. (1993). Efficacy of herbal tea preparation in infantile colic. *The Journal of Pediatrics* 122: 650-652.

Wood, G.B. and Bache, F. (1845). *The Dispensatory of the United States of America,* Sixth Edition. Philadelphia, PA: Grigg and Elliot, p. 1368.

Yamamoto, H., Mizutani, T., and Nomura, H. (1982). Studies on the mutagenicity of crude drug extracts. I. *Yakugaku Zasshi* 102: 596-601.

Yasukawa, K., Takido, M., Takeuchi, M., and Nakagawa, S. (1989). Effect of chemical constituents from plants on 12-*O*-tetradecanoylphorbol-13-acetate-induced inflammation in mice. *Chemical and Pharmaceutical Bulletin* 37: 1071-1073.

Yin, F., Giuliano, A.E., Law, R.E., and Van Herle, A.J. (2001). Apigenin inhibits growth and induces G_2/M arrest by modulating cyclin-CDK regulators and ERK MAP kinase activation in breast carcinoma cells. *Anticancer Research* 21(1A): 413-240.

Yin, F., Giuliano, A.E., and Van Herle, A.J. (1999a). Growth inhibitory effects of flavonoids in human thyroid cancer cell lines. *Thyroid* 9: 369-376.

Yin, F., Giuliano, A.E., and Van Herle, A.J. (1999b). Signal pathways involved in apigenin inhibition of growth and induction of apoptosis of human anaplastic thyroid cancer cells (ARO). *Anticancer Research* 19: 4297-4303.

Yousef, R.T. and Tawil, G.G. (1980). Antimicrobial activity of volatile oils. *Pharmazie* 35: 698-701.

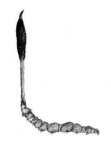

Cordyceps

BOTANICAL DATA

Classification and Nomenclature

Scientific name: *Cordyceps sinensis* (Berk.) Sacc. Link

Family name: Claviceptaceae (Ascomycetes)

Common names: cordyceps, caterpillar fungus (English), dong zhong chang cao, dongchongxiacao, zhongcao, chongcao (China), semitake (Japan)

Description

The stroma (fruit body) appears above the ground in summer as a dark brownish-black blade, approximately 3-6 cm long by about 0.4-0.7 cm thick. *Cordyceps sinensis* is parasitic on the larvae of moths, especially bat moths (*Hepialis* species). The larvae are colonized by the fungus until the inner body is filled with mycelium. The remaining form of the caterpillar is retained, including the dried outermost skin. The stroma, which grows out from the top of the caterpillar larva, is characterized by the Latin name, *Cordyceps,* because of its swollen head. *Cordyceps sinensis* grows at altitudes of 3,000 meters or more in the cold, grassy, alpine marshlands of mountainous regions in China in the provinces of Sichuan, the autonomous region of Tibet, northwest Yunnan, Gansu, Hubei, Zhejiang, Shanxi, Guizhou, and Qinghai. Elsewhere, *C. sinensis* grows in Japan, Australia, New Zealand, Canada, the United States, Mexico, Russia, Norway, the Netherlands, Italy, Kenya, Tanzania, and Ghana (Pegler et al., 1994; Grey and Barker, 1993; Zang et al., 1990; Ying et al., 1987; Yue et al., 1995).

Recent advances in the cultivation of cordyceps in China have resulted in a number of aseptic mycelial products which are grown in culture from strains derived from the wild fungus in its teleomorphic (sexual) stage as imperfect, conidial (anamorphic stage) forms. These imperfect forms, of which there are now at least ten, are given different Latin binomials to distinguish them from the natural wild form, *Cordyceps sinensis*. The two most intensively studied of these mycelial strains in China are named *Paecilomyces hepiali* Chen (strain Cs-4) and *Cephalosporium sinensis* (Zhu et al., 1998a, 1998b; Yin and Tang, 1995). Otherwise known as anamorphs of *C. sinensis*, these and other species isolated from the fruiting body were also considered to be the anamorph of *C. sinensis*, based on chemical and morphological analyses of the mycelia. Yet, until very recently, they remained without clearly defined links to their teleomorphic or sexual stage, making identification of mycelial strains of *C. sinensis* a major problem. A genetic method to find the identities of fungal isolates to establish their connection to the wild form of cordyceps was reported by Chen et al. (2001). Based on a comparative analysis of internal transcriber spacer regions of nuclear ribosomal DNA of various proposed strains of anamorphs (e.g., *Cephalosporium* sp., *Hirsutella sinensis, Paecilomyces* sp. *Stachybotrys* sp., *Tolypocladium sinensis*) and those of *C. sinensis*, it was determined that the anamorph is *Hirsutella sinensis*, rather than *Paecilomyces sinensis*. Therefore, *C. sinensis* and *H. sinensis* are "different life cycle stages of same taxa," or put another way, a "teleomorph-anamorph pair" (Chen et al., 2001, pp. 604-605). In addition, when researchers isolated *H. sinensis* from fresh fruiting bodies of *C. sinensis*, they found optimum growth at 15-20°C and growth inhibited at 25°C, a characteristic probably related to the high altitudes at which *C. sinensis* thrives. However, in the laboratory it was generally at higher temperatures that *Tolypocladium* sp. and *Paecilomyces* sp. were repeatedly isolated from *C. sinensis* as the anamorph, indicating that temperature plays a decisive role in the ability to obtain the correct anamorph. Moreover, results suggest that any species other than *H. sinensis* are either inhabitants (epiphytic) of the caterpillar or larvae, or endoparasitic (Chen et al., 2001). Therefore, use of the term "cordyceps" in association with anamorphs other than *H. sinensis* is a misnomer.

Among wild specimens, *C. sinensis* shows a high degree of genetic variation. Of 29 samples collected in the eastern extension of the Qinghai-Tibet plateau at 3,800-4,600 m elevation, populations from northern, southern, and middle regions of the plateau showed an average genetic variation of 49% between populations and an average of 51% genetic variation within the region of collection. None of the samples showed identical DNA patterns in the random amplified polymorphic DNA technique (RAPD); however, the genetic patterns suggest a general geographic separation between the populations at the three regions of the plateau, and that these populations are subspecies rather than different species of *C. sinensis*. The samples also showed differences when compared to the "type specimen" kept at the Herbarium of the Royal Botanic Garden, Kew, England, suggesting that the "type specimen" may therefore not be the best standard for *C. sinensis*. Only those specimens collected in the northern region of the plateau matched the type specimen in the size of their ascus and ascospore (one-celled segment). Otherwise, the ascus of *C. sinensis* measures 220-280 × 13 μm and the ascospore is filiform, breaking into a one-celled only slightly narrow part consisting of a spore measuring 9-15 × 4-5 μm. The ascus of the type specimen measures 160-240 × 5.2-6.5 (120 μm) and the ascospore 120-190 × 0.6-1.3 μm (Chen et al., 1999). In addition to the future possibility of distinguishing geographic origins and quality of specimens, the RAPD technique may also be useful for the identification of counterfeit *C. sinensis* (Cheng et al., 1998). Among them are various other species of cordyceps (e.g., *C. militaris, C. barnesii, C. shanxiensis,* and *C. liangshanensis* (Tang and Eisenbrand, 1992)

HISTORY AND TRADITIONAL USES

The common name in China, *dongchongxiacao,* meaning summer-plant-winter-worm, can be traced to a belief in ancient China that the embodiment of the fungus returned to an insect in winter if it was not picked in summer when it transformed into a blade of grass (Lloyd, 1918). The wild fungus (attached to the naturally myceliated larvae of caterpillars) is sold as a medicine or food in small bundles tied with thread. Its use as a food and a medicine in the Orient has continued for millennia. In China, cordyceps is eaten in soups (Pegler et al., 1994; Chamberlain, 1996) and cooked with meats, including pork, seafood, and poultry (Zhu et al., 1998a). When cooked with duck (8.85 g) and administered to elderly patients recovering from illness, the effect is said to be equal to that of 50 g of ginseng (Ying et al., 1987; Liu and Bau, 1980). When cooked with pork, cordyceps (15-30 g) is used to treat impotence and anemia (Yen, 1992). Boiled together with pork, it has been used to cure opium dependence and as an antidote for opium poisoning. Added to chicken and pork, it has been used as a tonic and mild stimulant by "convalescent persons" to rapidly restore them "to health and strength" (Gist Gee, 1918, p. 767). Recently, cordyceps has been used as part of a dietary supplement regime by Chinese athletes (Gordon, 1993; Creadon and Dam, 1996).

Traditionally, the powdered fungus is mixed with other tonic herbal medicines such as ginseng, or it may be boiled and taken as a tea, or soaked in alcohol for a tincture. It is mainly used to treat low energy following serious illness and as a strengthening tonic. Other traditional uses include the treatment of cough, anemia, tuberculosis, lower back pain, impotence, infertility, irregular menstruation, night sweats, and senile weakness (Pegler et al., 1994). It continues to be used as a tranquilizer or sedative in traditional Chinese medicine (TCM) (Ying et al., 1987; Liu and Bau, 1980; Guo, 1986), although compared to Western drug standards these effects are inherently mild. Cordyceps is also taken in TCM to keep the lungs fit, strengthen the kidneys, build up the bone marrow, reduce phlegm, and to stop hemorrhages (Ying et al., 1987; Liu and Bau, 1980).

The use of cordyceps in the West can be traced to a Chinese pharmacy in Denver, Colorado in the early 1900s, and probably other Chinese apothecaries in the United States of the day (Lloyd, 1918). In France during the eighteenth century, a Jesuit priest described its use for the treatment of debility and fatigue, noting that it was only used by the wealthy and among members of the imperial palace in China who could afford the rare and costly medicine (Pereira, 1843). Wild cordyceps remains rare and costly and is currently endangered from overharvesting.

CHEMISTRY

Carbohydrates

Polysaccharides

Polysaccharides from cordyceps have shown various activities: immunostimulating (polysaccharide I) (Zang et al., 1985), antileukemic (polysaccharide fraction-conditioned medium) (Chen et al., 1997), and radioprotective/antitumor (polysaccharide I) (Zang et al., 1985).

Nitrogenous Compounds

Nucleotides and Nucleosides

C. sinensis contains various nucleosides including adenosine, uracil, uridine, guanine, and guanosine (Shiao et al., 1994). There are conflicting reports of the occurrence of 2-' and 3'-deoxyadenosine (cordycepin). Whereas Chen and Chu (1996) reported its presence, Shiao et al. (1994) reported its absence in the fruiting body.

Evidence suggests that adenosine may not occur in the larval part of wild *C. sinensis,* whereas hypoxanthine, inosine, thymine, thymidine, and uridine occur in both fungal and larval parts (Leung et al., 2000). Nucleosides in cordyceps, such as adenosine, inhibit platelet aggregation (Ikumoto et al., 1991; Shiao et al., 1994). Other studies have shown calcium antagonist and inotropic activity (Furuya et al., 1983). Electrophoretic analyses of a dozen cordyceps samples collected from four provinces in China found nucleosides greatly varied in content and some samples held none (Li et al., 2001a).

Other Constituents

Cordyceps sinensis also contains: galactomannans (Miyazaki et al., 1977; Kiho et al., 1986); polyamines (spermine, spermidine, homospermidine, putrescine, 1,3-diaminopropane) (Zhu and Masaru, 1993); various uncommon cyclic dipeptides, minerals, vitamins (B_1, B_2, B_{12}, E and K); all of the essential amino acids (Huang et al., 1991; Xu et al., 1992; Guo, 1986; Tao, 1995; Xia et al., 1985); glutamic acid, *L*-tryptophan, *L*-arginine, and lysine (Zhang et al., 1991); d-mannitol, ergosterol, ergosterol derivatives, alkaloids, fatty acids (mainly oleic, linoleic, palmitic, and stearic acids) (Shiao et al., 1989), and sterols (Kadota et al., 1986) (see Figure 1).

THERAPEUTIC APPLICATIONS

Cordyceps is currently used as a traditional medicine (see History and Traditional Uses) and in research on the treatment of chronic nephritis, sexual hypofunction, arrhythmia, tinnitus (Tang and Eisenbrand, 1992), gastric spasm, gastric atony, consumptive cough, spontaneous sweating, and as a tonic for convalescing patients (Chang and But, 1986).

PRECLINICAL STUDIES

Genitourinary and Renal Functions

Renal Toxicity

Several studies in China have shown that cordyceps can prevent gentamicin-induced nephrotoxicity in animals. Cordyceps ameliorated deterioration of tubule metabolism and ion transport (Tian et al., 1991a), promoted DNA synthesis of kidney cells, lessened urinary β-*N*-acetylglucosaminidase (NAGase) and lysosyme levels, and delayed proteinuria (Tian et al., 1991b; Tian, Yang et al., 1991).

Lin et al. (1999) developed an animal model of Berger's disease (immunoglobulin A nephropathy model) to investigate constituents of cordyceps as potential treatments for the disease. Starting with in vitro tests, three fractions of a methanolic extract of dried and powdered cordyceps were isolated and showed inhibitory effects against IL-1- and IL-6-induced proliferation of cultured human mesangial (HMC) cells. F2, the most potent fraction, was administered for seven consecutive days by gastric tube as 0%, 0.5%, and 1% of the normal diet to three respective groups of female mice, all with experimental Berger's disease. Mice in the 1% F2 group showed a significant decrease in hematuria, proteinuria, mesangial cell proliferation, mesangial expansion, and the immunoflorescent intensity of complement 3 (C3) and IgA

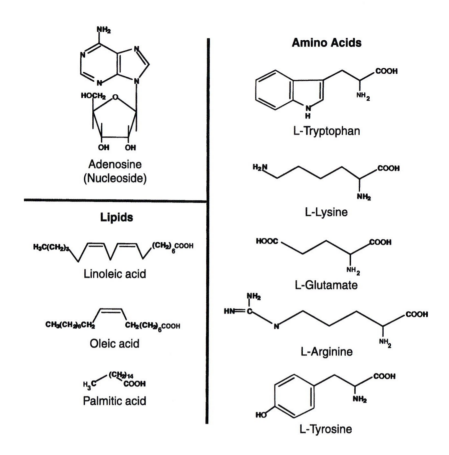

FIGURE 1. Major Small Molecular Weight Constituents of *Cordyceps sinensis*

of the mesangial area. In an acute toxicity test of F2 as 2% of the normal diet in Institute of Cancer Research mice, no differences were found compared to mice not fed F2 in cholesterol level, body weight, or liver enzyme levels (ALT and AST). The only significant differences were that the F2 group showed an increased content of liver cytochrome P-450 and an increase in the ratio of liver weight to body weight (each $p < 0.001$). However, the toxicity of F2 was judged to be low. These differences were ascribed to the model of Berger's disease, adding that after treatment with F2 there was a significant decrease in the liver/body weight ratio compared to mice not treated with F2. Furthermore, it was believed that the increase in cytochrome P-450 was indicative of a benefit in the animal model.

Lin et al. (1999) used the previous activity-guided fraction methods to isolate an active compound from F2 in the form of H1-A—an ergosterol-like compound with a molecular weight of 410 reportedly devoid of gluco-corticoid receptor-binding ability (Yang et al., 1999; Lin et al., 1999)—that reached detectable levels in the blood of mice fed F2. The authors report that H1-A showed no mutagenicity in the Ames test and exhibited similar acute toxicity in mice to that of F2 in the same test. Neither substance exhibited cytotoxic activity as measured by the MTT assay, cellular lactate dehydro-genase release (72 h incubation), and tryptan blue incorporation (Lin et al., 1999).

Immune Functions; Inflammation and Disease

Cancer

Antiproliferative activity. A hot-water extract of the dried, cultured fruit bodies in the form of a freeze-dried powder (Xinhui Xinhan Artificial Cordyceps Factory, Guangdong, China) was studied in female mice for activity against spontaneous metastases of B16 melanoma (B16M) and drug-resistant Lewis lung carcinoma (dr-LLC). For tests against dr-LLC, the cordyceps powder extract was administered after dissolving in water (100 mg/kg p.o. daily) one week prior to tumor induction and for 20 days after, and for B16 melanoma, 7 days prior and 26 days after (100 and 200 mg/kg p.o. daily). Tests were also made with cordycepin (3'-deoxy-adenosine), an antitumor constituent identified in *C. sinensis*. Significant differences were found in decreased liver weights in the B16M mice treated with the higher dosage of cordyceps compared to untreated controls ($p < 0.01$), and in the dr-LLC mice treated with cordyceps compared to the control ($p < 0.05$). Livers of the cordyceps-treated dr-LLC mice (100 mg/kg p.o.) showed significantly fewer metastatic foci compared to the control mice ($p < 0.05$). The same test was not made for the B16 mice. At 200 mg/kg p.o., cordyceps reduced the weights of primary tumors in the dr-LLC mice by 20% and the B16M mice by 47% compared to the control mice. However, owing to a wide variation in the control values these reductions were not statistically significant (Nakamura et al., 1999).

Testing the same water extract at 10 μg/mL for direct in vitro antitumor activity, researchers found dr-LLC cells decreased by 96% after 96 h. From the same dose after 48 h, B16M cells decreased by 62% and by 85% after 96 h compared to controls. The antitumor constituent cordycepin (10-1,000 ng/mL) showed no direct cytotoxicity against either tumor in vitro compared to control cells, despite having previously shown in vitro cytotoxic activity on human lymphoblasts (WI-L2), human kerotinocytes, hamster fibroblasts, and HIV-infected cells (Nakamura et al., 1999). Because not all analyses have detected cordycepin in *C. sinensis* (Shiao et al., 1994), its occurrence in this species is controversial and calls into question the identity of the species of cordyceps fruit bodies actually cultured.

Immune Functions

Immunopotentiation. A biphasic action was found in mice administered a freeze-dried ethanol extract of the fruit body (50-300 mg/kg i.p. 5 times/ day). Erythroid and fibroblast colony-forming units in their bone marrow were significantly increased from 100, 150, and 200 mg/kg doses, but higher and lower doses were ineffective. The extract suppressed the colony forming units in vitro at 300 µg/mL, but increased them at 150 and 200 µg/mL. In mice administered the natural anticancer agent harringtonine, a three-day pretreatment with the extract (150 mg/kg i.p.) significantly reversed decreases in colony-forming units caused by the agent (Li et al., 1993). At high doses in mice (3 g and 5 g/kg i.p.), an extract of the cordyceps fruit body increased natural killer (NK) cell activity, prevented cyclophosphamide-induced suppression of NK cell activity, increased human NK cell activity in vitro, and significantly reduced (after pretreatment) the incidence of mouse melanoma (Xu et al., 1992). Prior to and after implantation of mouse lymphoma, treatment with an extract of the fruit body (50 mg/kg p.o.) caused a significant prolongation of survival time, an additive antitumor effect with cyclophosphamide, and enhanced B cell activity. The treatment also ameliorated cyclophosphamide-induced suppression of B cell activity (in IgG and IgM antibody-producing cells), and caused a fourfold increase in macrophage chemotactic activity compared to baseline. In lymphoma-bearing mice challenged with *Salmonella enteritidis,* the extract in the same dosage allowed mice to live 2.48 times longer than controls (Yamaguchi et al., 1990).

Immunosuppression. The majority of immunological studies on cordyceps have shown immunopotentiating activity. However, immunosuppressive fractions of the fruit bodies were shown to inhibit tumor necrosis factor-α (TNF-α), interleukin-2 (IL-2), and NK cell activity (Kuo et al., 1996). In a lupus animal model, cordyceps (100 mg/kg p.o. in mouse chow/day) significantly prolonged the survival time of the animals and significantly inhibited production of anti-ds DNA antibodies. In preliminary studies in patients with systemic lupus erythematosus (SLE), cordyceps fruit body extract ameliorated defective production of IL-2 (Chen et al., 1993).

Yang et al. (1999) investigated the effects of a purified constituent of cordyceps, an ergosterol-like compound named H1A, in autoimmune MRL lrp/lrp mice, which commonly serve as a mouse model of SLE. Autoimmune disease progression in mice administered H1A (40 mg/kg/day p.o. for eight weeks) was significantly ameliorated compared to controls. Compared to controls, significant differences were found in the progressively decreased production of IgG anti-ds-DNA ($p < 0.005$), decreased lymphadenopathy ($p < 0.05$), delayed progression of proteinuria ($p < 0.005$), and improvement of kidney function ($p < 0.05$). Upon histological examination, mice that received H1A showed less mesangial proliferation in their kidneys, albeit without a significant change in the deposition of immune complex. Life span of the H1A-treated mice was also superior to the controls (100% versus 66.6%, respectively).

Inflammatory Response

Kuo et al. (2001) investigated in vitro immunomodulatory effects of methanolic extracts of the dried fruit body of cordyceps on antigen-stimulated inflammatory responses of human bronchoaveolar lavage fluids (BALF). Lipopolysaccharide (LPS) was chosen as the antigen since LPS is found in organic dusts and has previously been shown to induce inflammatory cytokines and an accumulation of macrophages and neutrophils in the BALF of humans. BALF was obtained from five healthy males (ages 22 to 38) who had never smoked, had no history of pulmonary disease, and were taking no medications. The extracts of the fruit body suppressed LPS-induced proliferation of BALF cells, producing 92% inhibition at a concentration of 200 µg/mL. At the same concentration, a related fungus (Cordyceps cicadae) showed an inhibition rate of only $1.89 \pm 2.0\%$. Contrary to *C. sinensis,* this species is without reports of benefits against asthma. After screening for the same activity using 15 subfractions of the methanolic extract of the fruit body of *C. sinensis,* fraction CS-19-22 (IC_{50} 10.9 ± 1.2 µg/mL) was selected for further investigation. After showing no adverse effects on the viability of BALF cells in vitro, CS-19-22 was investigated for inhibitory activity on inflammatory cytokines in relation to their inhibition of LPS-stimulated proliferation of BALF cells. In short, CS-19-22 significantly suppressed the production of some cytokines (at 100 µg/mL, completely blocking the production of TNF-α, IL-1β, IL-6, and IL-8), and although it decreased the production of IL-10, it also significantly stimulated the production of both gamma interferon (INF-γ) and IL-12 (by about 75% and 159%, respectively). It was then determined that this fraction affected the production of IL-12, INF-γ, and IL-10 by modulating their gene expression. However preliminary these results, the inhibition of cytokine proliferation from LPS-activated BALF cells by CS-19-22 could involve several immunomodulatory mechanisms which are currently the subject of ongoing studies, including characterization of the active fraction (Kuo et al., 2001).

Metabolic and Nutritional Functions

Antioxidant Activity

Water extracts prepared from dried, natural cordyceps were examined for antioxidant activity in three different assays. In the xanthine oxidase assay, the extract prepared from cordyceps obtained from the regions in Tibet (IC_{50} 0.08 mg/mL) or Sichuan were more potent than samples collected from the regions of Yunnan (IC_{50} 0.24 mg/mL) or Qinghai. In the induction of hemolysis assay, water extract of samples from Sichuan and Tibet were also the most potent. For all samples tested the IC_{50}s varied from 1.5 to 2.0 mg/mL. In the lipid microsomal lipid peroxidation assay (Fe-induced), the results were poor, showing less than 20% inhibition of oxidation and an extrapolated IC_{50} of 5 mg/mL. Although the antioxidant constituents of cordyceps remain to be elucidated, polysaccharides are at least partly responsible (Li et al., 2001b), while the adenosine content has been ruled out (Li et al., 2001a).

CLINICAL STUDIES

Genitourinary and Renal Disorders

Renal Disorders

Cordyceps is widely regarded as a premier "kidney tonic" in TCM, and there are indications that it may be of use in the treatment of Berger's disease (IgA nephropathy) (Lin et al., 1996).

Xu et al. (1995) reported the successful use of cordyceps (3 g/day) in a placebo-controlled study in 69 kidney-transplanted patients. Twelve weeks after organ transplantation, matched patients receiving cyclosporine (5 mg/kg per day for 15 days) were randomly assigned to a placebo group or a cordyceps group. Over the course of 15 days, the cordyceps plus cyclosporine group showed an increasingly significant decrease in nephrotoxicity compared to the cyclosporine plus placebo group—in blood urea nitrogen (BUN), N-acetylglucosamine (NAG), and serum creatinine (SCr)—which indicated that cordyceps had exerted a protective effect against toxic effects of cyclosporine in these patients (Xu et al., 1995).

A randomized, placebo-controlled trial of cordyceps in 21 elderly patients receiving amikacin sulfate found less nephrotoxicity (β-microglobulin and urinary NAGase) compared to the placebo group (Bao et al., 1994). A double-blind, placebo-controlled study in 52 elderly and young respiratory disease patients with no history of renal diseases found that cordyceps significantly protected against gentamicin-nephrotoxicity, which was pronounced in the placebo group (Li and Zheng, 1992). A comparative clinical study of cordyceps (3-5 g/day) was conducted in 51 patients with chronic renal failure. For the 28 who received cordyceps, a significant increase in renal function and T-lymphocyte subsets occurred, including the T helper cell ratio (T4/T8 cells) compared to the control group (Guan et al., 1992).

DOSAGE

Wild cordyceps is traditionally taken in a dosage of 5-10 g/day (Yen, 1992). Liu and Bau (1980) state that 3-9 g can be taken for sedative and invigorating effects, sexual impotence, debility following illness, anemia, night sweats, cough, and excessive tiredness, and that 15 g steamed with chicken can be taken as a tonic.

SAFETY PROFILE

Contraindications

According to TCM, cordyceps is contraindicated in cases of bleeding (Yen, 1992).

Drug Interactions

No information is available on drug interactions with *Cordyceps sinensis;* however, due to the content of adenosine in the fungus (Shiao et al., 1994), the inhibition of platelet aggregation (Hammerschmidt, 1980) may affect patients on blood-thinning and antithrombotic medications. Because of the application of cordyceps as a substitute for immunosuppressant medication in organ transplanted patients (Lin et al., 1996), individuals taking corticosteroids should consult with their physician before use of cordyceps products because of possible additive effects which may require a lower dosage of corticosteroids.

Pregnancy and Lactation

No information is available on the safety of cordyceps for pregnant or lactating women, or breast feeding infants.

Side Effects

No reports of side effects were found.

Special Precautions

Cases of lead poisoning from contaminated batches of wild cordyceps (Wu et al., 1996) suggest caution without proper mineral analysis.

Toxicology

Toxicity in Animal Models

Cordyceps sinensis in a dose of 30-50 g/kg i.p. in mice caused death in every mouse. At 5 g/kg i.p. some mice perished. Administered s.c. or i.v., a boiled extract and an alcohol extract were nontoxic (Chang and But, 1986). At a dosage of 80 g/kg p.o. for seven days and longer, no deaths occurred in mice. No mutagenic activity was found in the Ames test in strains of *Salmonella typhimurium* and no teratogenic activity was found in animal studies (Zhu et al., 1998b).

REFERENCES

Bao, Z.D., Wu, Z.G., and Zheng, F. (1994). [Amelioration of aminoglycoside nephrotoxicity by *Cordyceps sinensis* in old patients]. *Chinese Journal of Integrated Medicine* 14: 259, 271-273.

Chamberlain, M. (1996). Ethnomycological experiences in South West China. *Mycologist* 10 (4): 173-176.

Chang, H.M. and But, P.P.H. (Eds.) (1986). *Pharmacology and Applications of Chinese Materia Medica,* 1. Philadelphia, PA: World Scientific, pp. 410-413.

Chen, J.R., Yen, J.H., Lin, C.C., Tsai, W.J., Liu, W.J., Tsai, J.J., Lin, S.F., and Liu, H.W. (1993). The effects of Chinese herbs on improving survival and inhibiting anti-ds DNA antibody production in lupus mice. *American Journal of Chinese Medicine* 21: 257-262.

Chen, S.Z. and Chu, J.Z. (1996). [NMR and IR studies on the characterization of cordycepin and 2´deoxyadenosine]. *Zhongguo Kangshengsu Zazhi* 21: 9-12.

Chen, Y.J., Shiao, M.S., Lee, S.S., and Wang, S.Y. (1997). Effect of *Cordyceps sinensis* on the proliferation and differentiation of human leukemic U937 cells. *Life Sciences* 60: 2349-2359.

Chen, Y.Q., Wang, N., Qu, L., Li, T., and Zhang, W. (2001). Determination of the anamorph of *Cordyceps sinensis* inferred from the analysis of the ribosomal DNA internal transcribed spacers and 5.8S rDNA. *Biochemical Systematics and Ecology* 29: 597-607.

Chen, Y., Zhang, Y.P., Yang, Y., and Yang, D. (1999). Genetic diversity and taxonomic implication of *Cordyceps sinensis* as revealed by RAPD markers. *Biochemical Genetics* 37: 201-213.

Cheng, K.T., Su, C.H., Chang, H.C., and Huang, J.Y. (1998). Differentiation of genuines and counterfeits of *Cordyceps* species using random amplified polymorphic DNA. *Planta Medica* 64: 451-453.

Creadon, M. and Dam, J. (1996). "Drink up." *Time* (August 19): 55.

Furuya, T., Hirotani, M., and Matsuzawa, M. (1983). N^6-(2-hydroxyethyl) adenosine, a biologically active compound from cultured mycelia of *Cordyceps* and *Isaria* species. *Phytochemistry* 22: 2509-2512.

Gist Gee, N. (1918). Notes on *Cordyceps sinensis*. *Mycological Notes* 54: 767-768.

Gordon, D. (1993). "The rumored dope on Beijing's women." *Newsweek* (September 27): 63.

Grey, P. and Barker, R. (1993). *Cordyceps* or plant eats animal! *The Victorian Naturalist* 110: 98-107.

Guan, Y.J., Hu, G., Hou, M., Jiang, H., Wang, X., and Zhang, C. (1992). [Effect of *Cordyceps sinensis* on T-lymphocyte subsets in chronic renal failure]. *Chinese Journal of Integrated Medicine* 12: 323, 338-339.

Guo, Y.Z. (1986). [Medicinal chemistry, pharmacology and clinical applications of fermented mycelia of *Cordyceps sinensis* and JinShuBao capsule]. *Journal of Modern Diagnostics and Therapeutics* (1): 60-65.

Hammerschmidt, D.E. (1980). Szechwan purpura. *New England Journal of Medicine* 302: 1191-1193.

Huang, Q., Li, D., Liang, J., Liao, S., and Liang, S. (1991). [Weak polar chemical components in *Cordyceps*]. *Journal of Chinese Medical Materials* 14: 33-34.

Ikumoto, T., Sasaki, S., Namba, H., Toyama, R., Moritoki, H., and Mouri, T. (1991). [Physiologically active compounds in the extracts from tochukaso and cultured mycelia of *Cordyceps* and *Isaria*]. *Yakugaku Zasshi* 111: 504-509.

Kadota, S., Shima, T., and Kikuchi, T. (1986). [Steroidal components of "I-Tiam-Hong" and *Cordyceps sinensis*. Separation and identification by high-performance liquid chromatography]. *Yakugaku Zasshi* 106: 1092-1097.

Kiho, T., Tabata, H., Ukai, S., and Hara, C. (1986). A minor protein-containing galactomannan from a sodium carbonate extract of *Cordyceps sinensis*. *Carbohydrate Research* 156: 189-197.

Kuo, Y.C., Tsai, W.J., Shiao, M.S., Chen, C.F., and Lin, C.Y. (1996). *Cordyceps sinensis* as an immunomodulatory agent. *American Journal of Chinese Medicine* 24: 111-125.

Kuo, Y.C., Tsai, W.J., Wang, J.Y., Chang, S.C., Lin, C.Y., and Shiao, M.S. (2001). Regulation of bronchoalveolar lavage fluids cell function by the immunomodulatory agents from *Cordyceps sinensis*. *Life Sciences* 68: 1067-1082.

Leung, A.K., Gong, F., and Chau, F. (2000). Analysis of the water soluble constituents of *Cordyceps sinensis* with heuristic evolving latent projections. *Analytical Letters* 33: 3195-3211.

Li, L.S. and Zheng, F. (1992). Clinical protection of aminoglycoside nephrotoxicity by *Cordyceps sinensis* (CS). *Journal of the American Society of Nephrology* 3: 726 (abstract 24P).

Li, S.P., Li, P., Dong, T.T., and Tsim, K.W. (2001a). Determination of nucleosides in natural *Cordyceps sinensis* and cultured *Cordyceps* mycelia by capillary electrophoresis. *Electrophoresis* 22: 144-150.

Li, S.P., Li, P., Dong, T.T.X., and Tsim, K.W.K. (2001b). Anti-oxidation activity of different types of natural *Cordyceps sinensis* and cultured *Cordyceps* mycelia. *Phytomedicine* 8: 207-212.

Li, Y., Chen, G.Z., and Jiang, D.Z. (1993). Combined traditional Chinese and Western medicine: Effect of *Cordyceps sinensis* on erythropoiesis in mouse bone marrow. *Chinese Medical Journal* 106: 313-316.

Lin, C.Y., Ku, F.M., Kuo, Y.C., Chen, C.F., Chen, W.P., Chen, A., and Shiao, M.S. (1999). Inhibition of activated human mesangial cell proliferation by the natural product of *Cordyceps sinensis* (H1-A): An implication for treatment of IgA mesangial nephropathy. *Journal of Laboratory and Clinical Medicine* 133: 55-63.

Lin, C.Y., Shiao, M.S., and Wang, Z.N. (1996). Active fractions of *Cordyceps sinensis* and method of isolation thereof. United States Patent 5,582,828, December 10.

Liu, B. and Bau, Y.S. (1980). *Fungi Pharmacopoeia (Sinica)*. Oakland, CA: The Kinoko Co., pp. 14-21.

Lloyd, C.G. (1918). *Cordyceps sinensis,* from N. Gist Gee, China. *Mycological Notes* 54: 766-767.

Miyazaki, T., Oikawa, N., and Yamada, H. (1977). Studies on fungal polysaccharides. XX. Galactomannan of *Cordyceps sinensis. Chemical and Pharmaceutical Bulletin* 25: 3324-3328.

Nakamura, K., Yamaguchi, Y., Kagota, S., Kwon, Y.M., Shinozuka, K., and Kunitomo, M. (1999). Inhibitory effect of *Cordyceps sinensis* on spontaneous liver metastasis of Lewis lung carcinoma and B16 melanoma cells in syngeneic mice. *The Japanese Journal of Pharmacology* 79: 335-341.

Pegler, D.N., Yao, Y.J., and Li, Y. (1994). The Chinese 'Caterpillar Fungus.' *Mycologist* 8 (part 1): 3-5.

Pereira, J. (1843). Summer-plant-winter-worm. *New York Journal of Medicine* 1: 128-132.

Shiao, M.S., Lin, L.J., Lien, C.Y., Tzean, S.S., and Lee, K.R. (1989). Natural products in Cordyceps. *Proceedings of the National Science Council, Republic of China* 13 (Part A): 382-387.

Shiao, M.S., Wang, Z.N., Lin, L.J., Lien, J.Y., and Wang, J.J. (1994). Profiles of nucleosides and nitrogen bases in Chinese medicinal fungus *Cordyceps sinensis* and related species. *Botanical Bulletin of Academia Sinica* 35: 261-267.

Tang, W. and Eisenbrand, G. (1992). *Chinese Drugs of Plant Origin*. Berlin, Germany: Springer-Verlag, pp. 373-376.

Tao, Z.H. (1995). [From *Cordyceps sinensis* and better than *Cordyceps sinensis*]. *Journal of Administration of Traditional Chinese Medicine* 5(Suppl.): 20-21.

Tian, J., Chen, X.M., and Li, L.S. (1991a). Effects of *Cordyceps sinensis* on renal cortical Na-K-ATPase activity and calcium content in gentamicin nephrotoxic rats. *Journal of the American Society of Nephrology* 2: 670 (abstract).

Tian, J., Chen, X.M., and Li, L.S. (1991b). Use of *Cordyceps sinensis* in gentamicin induced ARF: A preliminary animal experimentation and observation of cell culture. *Journal of the American Society of Nephrology* 2: 670 (abstract 83P).

Tian, J., Yang, J.Y., and Li, L.S. (1991). Observation of effects of *Cordyceps sinensis* in isolated perfused kidney of gentamicin nephrotoxic rats. *Journal of the American Society of Nephrology* 2: 671 (abstract).

Wu, T.N., Yang, K.C., Wang, C.M., Lai, J.S., Ko, K.N., Chang, P.Y., and Liou, S.H. (1996). Lead poisoning caused by contaminated *Cordyceps,* a Chinese herbal medicine: Two case reports. *The Science of the Total Environment* 182: 193-195.

Xia, Y.C., Yang, M., and Chen, S.M. (1985). [Measurement of trace elements in *Cordyceps sinensis* and its mycelia]. *Research for Patent Traditional Chinese Medicine* 10: 29-30.

Xu, F., Huang, J.B., Jiang, L., Xu, J., and Mi, J. (1995). Amelioration of cyclosporin nephrotoxicity by *Cordyceps sinensis* in kidney-transplanted recipients. *Nephrology, Dialysis, Transplantation* 10: 142-143 (letter).

Xu, R.H., Peng, X.E., Chen, G.Z., and Chen, G.L. (1992). Effects of *Cordyceps sinensis* on natural killer activity and colony formation of B16 melanoma. *Chinese Medical Journal* 105: 97-101.

Yamaguchi, N., Yoshida, J., Ren, L.J., Chen, H., Miyazawa, Y., Fujii, Y., Huang, Y.X., Takamura, S., Suzuki, S., Koshimura S., et al. (1990). Augmentation of various immune reactivities of tumor-bearing hosts with an extract of *Cordyceps sinensis*. *Biotherapy* 2: 199-205.

Yang, L.Y., Chen, A., Kuo, Y.C., and Lin, C.Y. (1999). Efficacy of a pure compound H1-A extracted from *Cordyceps sinensis* on autoimmune disease of MRL lpr/lpr mice. *Journal of Laboratory and Clinical Medicine* 134: 492-500.

Yen, K.Y. (1992). *The Illustrated Chinese Materia Medica Crude and Prepared.* Taipei, Taiwan: SMC Publishing, Inc., p. 223.

Yin, D.H. and Tang, X.M. (1995). [Progresses of cultivation research of *Cordyceps sinensis* in China]. *China Journal of Chinese Materia Medica* 20: 707-709.

Ying, J., Mao, X., Ma, Q., Zong, Y., and Wen, H. (1987). *Icones of Medicinal Fungi from China*. Beijing: Science Press.

Yue, D., Feng, X., Liu, H., and Bao, T.T. (1995). [*Cordyceps sinensis*. In Institute of Materia Medica (Ed.), *Advanced Study for Traditional Chinese Herbal Medicine,* 1] (pp. 91-113), Beijing: Medical University and China Peking Union Medical University Press.

Zang, M., Yang, D.R., and Li, C.D. (1990). A new taxon in the genus *Cordyceps* from China. *Mycotaxon* 37: 57-62.

Zang, Q., He, G., Zheng, Z., Zeng, Z., Xu, J., Liu, J., Wang, S., Huang, J., Du, D., Zeng, Q., et al. (1985). Pharmacological action of the polysaccharide from Cordyceps *(Cordyceps sinensis)*. *Zhongcaoyao* 16: 306-311. In *Chemical Abstracts* 103: 205581g.

Zhang, S.S., Zhang, D.S., Zhu, T.J., and Chen, X.Y. (1991). A pharmacological analysis of the amino acid components of *Cordyceps sinensis* (Berk.) Sacc. *Acta Pharmaceutica Sinica* 26: 326-330.

Zhang, Z. and Xia, S.S. (1990). *Cordyceps sinensis*-I as an immunosuppressant in heterotopic heart allograft model in rats. *Journal of Tongji Medical University* 10: 100-103.

Zhu, C.L. and Masaru, A. (1993). [Analysis of polyamines in Chinese caterpillar fungus]. *Chinese Traditional and Herbal Drugs* 24: 71-72, 110.

Zhu, J.S., Halpern, G.M., and Jones, K. (1998a). The scientific rediscovery of an ancient Chinese herbal medicine: *Cordyceps sinensis*. Part I. *The Journal of Alternative and Complementary Medicine* 4: 289-303.

Zhu, J.S., Halpern, G.M., and Jones, K. (1998b). The scientific rediscovery of an ancient Chinese herbal medicine: *Cordyceps sinensis*. Part II. *The Journal of Alternative and Complementary Medicine* 4: 429-457.

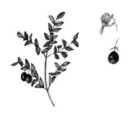

Cranberry

BOTANICAL DATA

Classification and Nomenclature

Scientific name: *Vaccinium macrocarpon* Aiton (synonym: *O. macrocarpus*)

Family name: Ericaceae

Common names: cranberry, American cranberry, trailing swamp cranberry (Tyler, 1994)

Description

The name *Vaccinium* derives from the Latin for pustule; *macrocarpon* means large-fruited. *Oxycoccos* means acidic (oxy) round-berry (coccus); *quadripetalus* refers to the flower's four petals (Coombes, 1985). American cranberry (*V. macrocarpon* Ait.) is native to eastern North America (Uphof, 1968) whereas *V. oxycoccos* L. is native to northern Europe, northern Asia, and North America (Bailey and Bailey, 1976). It grows wild in bogs and muskegs in eastern Canada in Labrador and in the Pacific Northwest of Canada and the United States. It also occurs in Eurasia and Iceland (Marles et al., 2000).

American cranberry *(V. macrocarpon)* is a small, mat-forming, evergreen, creeping shrub natively found in swamps and acid bogs in a range from North Carolina to Minnesota and north to Newfoundland (Bailey and Bailey, 1976). The red fruits measure 12-20 mm wide, whereas those of the European cranberry measure 6-8 mm wide (Vaughan and Geissler, 1997). The leaves are 1.9 cm in length, elliptical-oblong with whitish undersides. The pink flowers (0.8 cm long) occur in clusters (Bailey and Bailey, 1976). Cultivars are grown commercially in Canada, England, and the United States. Related species include *V. oxycoccos* L. (small cranberry or European cranberry), *V. erythrocarpum* Michx. (southern mountain cranberry), *V. vitis* (lowbush cranberry), and *V. corymbosum* (highbush cranberry) (Vaughan and Geissler, 1997).

HISTORY AND TRADITIONAL USES

Recorded knowledge of cranberry use in North America dates back to 1621 when Pilgrims are said to have eaten them during the first Thanksgiving. In 1864 during the Civil War, cranberry sauce became a Thanksgiving dinner staple when Ulysses S. Grant ordered that it be served to his troops. New England sailors favored the berries when they found that those who ate them were unaffected by scurvy (Castleman, 1991). In Canada, the Cree and the Déné Indians of Alberta eat the berries of mountain cranberry (*V. vitis-idaea* L ssp. *minus* [Lodd.] Hulten) for the relief of a "bad fever" in the spring. Otherwise, the berries are eaten to cleanse the stomach, and in treating bladder problems a decoction of the stems and roots is drunk. Canadian Indians have used the berries of *V. oxycoccus* for food (Marles et al., 2000), as have American Indians. The Ojibwás have used this species to prepare tea to treat nausea in persons who were slightly ill (Vogel, 1970). A tea made from the branches of the American cranberry was used by the Montagnais to treat pleurisy (Moerman, 1998).

German chemists in the 1840s discovered that eating cranberries produced urine containing hippuric acid, a bacteriostatic metabolite of benzoic acid. Around 1900, researchers in the United States theorized that acidified urine caused by a continual intake of cranberries could inhibit urinary tract infections (UTIs). Women have long used cranberry juice steadily since then to prevent recurrences of UTIs (Castleman, 1991). Although doubts arose regarding the effect of cranberry on the acidity of urine (Sobota, 1984; Castleman, 1991; Leaver, 1996), recent evidence indicates that cranberry fruit works by preventing *Escherichia coli* associated with UTIs from adhering to the lining of the urinary tract (Ofek et al., 1991; Avorn et al., 1994; Ahuja et al., 1998; Foo et al., 2000).

Cranberries are available in the form of dried fruit, frozen berries, juice (e.g., cranberry juice cocktail at 25% concentration), fresh berries, dehydrated berry juice concentrate in capsules, dry powdered cranberries in capsules, berry tea, and sweetened or unsweetened berry concentrate. In the United States, cranberries are regulated as GRAS (generally recognized as safe) (Duke, 1992; Pedersen, 1994).

CHEMISTRY

Organic Acids

Cranberries contain the following organic acids: citric, quinic, benzoic, malic, glucoronic, parascorbic, ursolic, and oleanolic acid (Cardellina and Meinwald, 1980; Croteau and Fagerson, 1971). Undiluted cranberry juice cocktail was found to contain quantities of quinic acid (1.11-1.62%), malic acid (0.75-1.14%), citric acid (0.94-1.30%), and benzoic acid (0.020%) (Coppola et al., 1978).

Parasorbic acid, an antimicrobial lactone, has been isolated from whole plant extracts of *Vaccinium macrocarpon*. Parasorbic acid was found to inhibit seed germination and plant growth, and was surmised to afford the plant some protection from fungal attack. Parasorbic acid had previously been reported only from the fruit of the mountain ash (*Sorbus aucuparia*, family Rosaceae) (Cardellina and Meinwald, 1980).

Phenolic Compounds

Polyphenolics

Deubert (1978) extracted total anthocyanins from fresh cranberry fruit in the amount of 17.8 mg/100 g fruit. Camire and Clydesdale (1979) confirmed the identities of the following four major and two minor anthocyanins in commercial cranberry juice: peonidin-3-arabinoside, cyanidin-3-arabinoside, peonidin-3-galactoside, cyanidin-3-galactoside, peonidin-3-monoglucoside, and cyanidin-3-monoglucoside, respectively. From an ethyl acetate extract of the ripe berries, Foo et al. (2000) identified procyanidin B2, procyanidin A2, and 3 proanthocyanidin trimers composed of A-type interflavonoid linkages: e.g., epicatechin-(4β→8, 2β→O→7)-epicatechin.

Terpenoid Compounds

Triterpenic compounds constitute 50% of the wax (0.21% of cranberries by fresh weight). The waxy cuticle also contains long-chain alcohols, esters, and hydrocarbons. Aldehydes make up a considerable portion (14.3%) of the aliphatic waxes. Among the unsaturated fatty acids found in the wax are linolenic, linoleic, and oleic acids, which also make up most of the seed lipids (Croteau and Fagerson, 1971). Ursolic and linolenic acids were identified from cranberry pomace and from the cuticle wax by Croteau and Fagerson (1971) who confirmed the presence of β-sitosterol, stigmasterol, as well as β-amyrin and β-amyrin.

Other Constituents

Cranberries, or unadulterated cranberry juice, contain glucose (3.1%), fructose (1%), anthocyanins, catechin, triterpenoids, carbohydrates, small amounts of protein, fiber, and vitamin C (Zafriri et al., 1989). Raw cranberry fruits contain (per 100 g) vitamin C (13.5 mg), protein (0.4 g), fat (0.2 g), dietary fiber (1.2 g), iron (0.2 mg), sodium (1 mg), potassium (71 mg), calcium (7 mg), calories (49), and carbohydrates (12.7 g total) (Kuzminski, 1996). The seed oil contains 33% linolenic acid and tocotrienols (1.73 g/kg) composed of delta-isomers (50 mg/kg), α-isomers (180 mg/kg), and γ-tocotrienols (1.5 g/kg) (Nawar, 2001).

THERAPEUTIC APPLICATIONS

Cranberry juice and extracts have mainly been used therapeutically in chronic or acute UTIs, cystitis, kidney infections (Werbach and Murray, 1994; Nazarko, 1995), as a urinary deodorant (Rogers, 1991), and for adjusting urinary pH (Jackson and Hicks, 1997).

PRECLINICAL STUDIES

Cardiovascular and Circulatory Functions

Peripheral Vascular Functions

Maher et al. (2000) demonstrated a vasodilatory activity from cranberry juice in isolated rat aortae. Against phenylephrine-induced contractions, endothelium-intact aortae showed a more pronounced vasodilatory effect (56.7% relaxation) from cranberry juice (1:100 dilution in vitro) than endothelium-free aortae (8.9% relaxation). Using standard tests, there was evidence to suggest that the relaxant effect of cranberry juice was nitric oxide-dependent. Although these effects were comparable to those of wines and Concord grape juice at 1:100 dilution, in unpublished experiments employing the aortae of spontaneously hypertensive rats, vasodilatory effects were found from cranberry juice at dilutions as low as 1:5,000.

Immune Functions; Inflammation and Disease

Cancer

Chemopreventive activity. Kapadia et al. (1996) tested the antitumor-promoting effect of cranberries using the TPA-induced Epstein-Barr virus early antigen assay. At various concentrations, the berry extract was found to be less active than short bell pepper and red onion skin extracts, but more active than long red bell pepper extract.

Bomser et al. (1996) tested cranberry fruit extract for in vitro induction of the cell-protective Phase II xenobiotic detoxification enzyme quinone reductase. They also tested the berry extract for inhibition of ornithine decarboxylase (ODC) induction, the rate-limiting enzyme involved in the synthesis of polyamines (TPA-induced ornithine decarboxylase assay). Carcinogenesis was induced by the tumor promoter TPA (phorbol 12-myristate 13-acetate). The ethyl acetate extract, but not the crude extract, proanthocyanidin or anthocyanin fraction of the fruit was active as a quinone reductase (QR) inducer. The crude extract showed activity as an inhibitor of ornithine decarboxylase (IC_{50} 7.0 µg/well), with most of the activity found in the polymeric proanthocyanidin fraction (IC_{50} 6.0 µg/well). The researchers concluded that cranberries are potential inhibitors of cancers caused by chemical carcinogens (Bomser et al., 1996).

Fungal infections. Swartz and Medrek (1968) attempted to determine the nature of cranberry's alleged antifungal activity after prescribing an ointment (Vaccinol) which consisted of cranberry as the major ingredient. It was allegedly "surprisingly effective" against certain dermatoses. Using cranberry juice (Ocean Spray) adjusted to a pH that would allow fungi to grow, they sterilized the juice and added it to cultures of various fungi, including *Candida albicans*. At a 40% concentration, the juice caused complete growth inhibition of the following species of dermatophytic fungi: *Epidermophyton floccosum, Microsporum audouinii, M. canis, M. gypseum, Trichophyton rubrum,* and *T. schoenleinii.* However, no growth inhibition was found with *Candida albicans.*

Infectious Diseases

Microbial infections. Attachment appendages known as fimbriae allow *E. coli* to adhere and remain in the urinary tract where they can cause pyelonephritis and cystitis (Ofek et al., 1996). Tests of cranberry juice show that bacterial fimbriae can be irreversibly and totally inhibited by cranberry juice. The juice tested (Ocean Spray) was sugar- and preservative-free and the concentration (25%) consistent with that of most commercial cranberry juices. Researchers concluded that this effect may reduce the severity and duration of UTIs. The best use for cranberry juice at present is that of a preventive agent, as well as being used in combination with antibiotics following a diagnosis of UTI (Ahuja et al., 1998).

Studies showed that at least two inhibitors of lectin-mediated adherence of uropathogens to eucaryotic cells, detected in both blueberries and cranberries, appear to prevent *E. coli* colonization in the gut and in the bladder (Zafriri et al., 1989). It was later determined by Ofek et al. (1996) that cranberry juice contains at least two compounds thought to inhibit the adhesing substance of *E. coli* known as adhesin. The first, fructose, a constituent of all juices, inhibits mannose-specific fimbrial adhesin; and the second, an unidentified high molecular weight polymeric compound with characteristics of a proanthocyanidin inhibits adhesins associated with pyelonephritogenic strains of *E. coli*. Howell et al. (1998) identified proanthocyanidins as the active antiadhesive compounds in cranberries, which showed activity at amounts of 10-50 µg/mL in vitro. Foo et al. (2000) elucidated three proanthocyanidin trimers from an ethyl acetate extract of the ripe fruits of a common cultivar of cranberry (Early Black) which showed activity against the adhering ability of *E. coli* isolated from the urinary tract. The assay employed required that the substance suppressed agglutination of P-fimbriated *E. coli* (urine isolates from human UTI patients) to latex beads coated with synthetic P receptor analogue and agglutination to human red blood cells. The active constituents were identified as epicatechin-(4β→8, 2β→O→7)-epicatechin, epicatechin-(4β→8, 2β→O→7)-epicatechin-(4β→8)-epicatechin, and epicatechin-(4β→8)-epicatechin-(4β→8, 2β→O→7)-epicatechin.

Schmidt and Sobota (1988) tested cranberry against various Gram-negative pathogens *(Proteus, Klebsiella,* and *Pseudomonas)* associated with UTIs, including 63 isolates of *E. coli* obtained from hospitalized patients diagnosed with UTIs. Incubation experiments using cranberry cocktail juice and the undiluted expressed juice of fresh cranberries in human uroepithelial cells revealed that urinary isolates were significantly more (300%) adherent than nonurinary isolates; cranberry juice selectively inhibited strongly adhering isolates from urine, but not the adherence of nonurinary isolates. Adherence of all isolates from urine and uroepithelial cells collected from subjects following ingestion of cranberry juice cocktail (12 oz) was significantly decreased. A further demonstration showed that seconds after adding cranberry juice cocktail to uroepithelial cells having attached *E. coli,* adherence of the bacteria decreased. After 5 min, 70% of the adhering bacteria were removed. Cranberry juice cocktail had the least antiadherence effect on pre-attached bacteria. It appeared to bind tighter to bacteria cell surface receptors than to bacteria already attached to epithelial cells. In addition, when one of the strongest adhering *E. coli* isolates was preincubated with cranberry juice cocktail, the mean reduction in adherence was 93.5%, but when the same bacterial isolate was incubated with epithelial cells, the reduction in adherence was only 41.6%. This observation was also demonstrated with *Pseudomonas* and *Proteus* isolates.

Sobota (1984) demonstrated that cranberry juice cocktail could be diluted 1:30 and still significantly inhibit adherence of *E. coli* to uroepithelial and buccal cells. This finding conflicted with earlier studies showing that higher concentrations of cranberry juice product was required to be effective.

Sobota (1984) showed that cranberry juice was a potent inhibitor of bacterial adherence in uroepithelial cells, but that it appeared to lack any bactericidal effect. He reported that cranberry juice inhibited adherence of *E. coli* in over 60% of the strains tested. Further tests revealed that active factors in the juice could survive normal metabolic degradative processes and accumulate in the urine. Factors in cranberry juice also inhibited *E. coli* adherence to buccal cells, which suggests that cranberry juice or products of the berry may be beneficial in the treatment of other infections involving bacterial adherence. Weiss et al. (1998) reported that an uncharacterized high molecular weight substance isolated from cranberry juice inhibited interspecies coaggregation in vitro of many of the bacteria known to form dental plaque. Cranberry juice was also active in completely reversing the coaggregation between the plaque bacteria *Fusobacterium nucleatum* PK1594 and *Streptococcus oralis* H1. In addition, Burger et al. (2000) isolated a high molecular mass constituent from the berry juice which inhibited in vitro adhesion of *Helicobacter pylori* strains (17874, BZMC-25, and EHL-65) to human gastric mucus (IC_{50} 37-305 $\mu g/mL^{-1}$). Because the high molecular substance (unidentified) inhibited the sialic acid-specific adhesion of clinical strains of *H. pylori* strains to erythrocytes and to human gastric mucus, it was suggested that cranberry juice may also inhibit adhesion of the ulcer bug to new sites in the stomach (Weiss et al., 1998).

Urine becomes bacteriostatic at a pH of about 5.0, and at this pH most UTIs are prevented (Kinney and Blount, 1979; Moen, 1962). However, cranberry juice preparations have not shown consistent acidification of the urine of patients (Tsukada et al., 1994; Kinney and Blount, 1979), nor have they always sufficiently inhibited bacterial growth (Nazarko, 1995). Although cranberry juice may not be bactericidal (Avorn et al., 1994; Sobota, 1984), patients with urological infections caused by *Pseudomonas aeruginosa* receiving the antibiotic novobiocin and cranberry juice showed an increase in the acidity of their urine that was believed to cause a significant increase in activity in vitro of novobiocin against *P. aeruginosa*, *Proteus,* and *Staphylococci* (Chernomordik and Vasilenko, 1981).

Metabolic and Nutritional Functions

Antioxidant Activity

Wilson et al. (1998) reported that cranberries significantly inhibited the in vitro modification of LDL cholesterol (low-density lipoprotein) by free radicals using a cupric sulfate and air exposure assay. The inhibition of LDL oxidation by Concord grape juice at dilutions less than or similar to those of the cranberry extract was only found with juice containing a polyphenolic content twice that of the cranberry extract, indicating that cranberries may have twice the potency of Concord grape juice (Wilson et al., 1998). In further studies, Wilson et al. (1999) reported that cranberry juice possesses "a true and potent" antioxidant activity (rather being due to the action of flavonoids chelating oxidants), as evidenced in human LDL (obtained from 9 h-fasted, nonsmokers, ages 25-35 years, who had not consumed antioxidant supplements during the two weeks prior to LDL collection). This became evident as the juice of cranberries in high dilution (1:10,000 parts) produced a significant inhibition of not only metal initiated (cupric ion-initiated) oxidation of human LDL, but of oxidation induced by a nonmetal initiator (2,2'-azobis-amidinopropane, or AAPH-initiated oxidation) at a dilution of 1:5,000 parts (each $p < 0.05$). Through a capacity to bind to metal, flavonoids may exhibit antioxidant activity by just removing ions of copper. Therefore, the inhibition by cranberry juice of LDL oxidation produced by a nonmetal initiator confirms that cranberry is a true antioxidant.

Wang and Jiao (2000) compared the in vitro radical scavenging capacities of berries (seeds removed) harvested at commercial maturity from five different cultivars of cranberry against four types of radicals: hydroxyl radicals, hydrogen peroxide, superoxide radicals, and singlet oxygen. Compared to the cultivars Ben Lear, Cropper, Franklin, and Howes, Early Black was the clear winner showing the highest antioxidant and scavenging capacity against all four reactive oxygen species. The differences in antioxidant and radical scavenging activities of the cultivars were significant ($p < 0.05$). However, when the antioxidant and radical scavenging activities of various cultivars of small berry crops (cranberries, blueberries, blackberries, strawberries, and raspberries) were compared, "Hull Thornless" blackberries and "Earliglow" strawberries showed the most activity overall while the activity of the cranberry cultivars was fairly comparable to cultivars of raspberries and blueberries.

Wang and Stretch (2001) examined the oxygen radical absorbance capacity (ORAC) of the fruit from ten different cultivars of cranberry (Ben Lear, Cropper, Crowley, Early Black, Franklin, Howes, Pilgrim, Stevens, and Wilcox). They also examined the effect of storage temperature on antioxidant capacity and on contents of anthocyanins and total phenolics. Mean ORAC values obtained from averages of all results of the particular cultivar at different storage temperatures (0°C to 20°C) showed that the highest were those of the Early Black and Crowley cultivars (16.8 and 15.3 µmol trolox equivalents/g, respectively). However, in mean ORAC values obtained at harvest, Early Black (14.1) was followed by Franklin (12.7) and then Crowley (11.9). ORAC values, levels of total phenolic contents, and anthocyanin contents showed significant increases during storage. After three months of storage, increases in ORAC values were highest in fruits at 15°C storage, and in all of the cultivars, ORAC values were positively related to contents of total phenolics and to anthocyanin contents at the different storage temperatures.

CLINICAL STUDIES

Immune Disorders; Inflammation and Disease

Infectious Diseases

Microbial infections. Clinical trials of cranberry preparations in the treatment of UTIs are to date lacking. The handful of trials on cranberry in the prevention of UTIs are judged as poor and have been attended by high numbers of dropouts (20% to 55%), likely owing to objection to the taste of cranberry juice (Jepson et al., 2000). Other reviewers have suggested that the evidence from the clinical trials to date suggests that cranberry is possibly beneficial in the prevention of UTIs and although the benefits demonstrated over placebo are small, a three-arm placebo-controlled trial may have cleared up the question of efficacy (Lowe and Fagelman, 2001). Examples of the studies on cranberry against bacterial infections of the urinary tract are briefly reviewed as follows.

In an open, randomized, controlled trial incorporating a twelve-month follow-up, Kontiokari et al. (2001) compared the UTI-preventive effects of a cranberry-lingonberry juice concentrate (Maija, Marli, Finland) to a *Lactobacillus* GG drink (Gefilus, Valio, Finland) in 150 women diagnosed with UTIs caused by *Escherichia coli* and who were not using antimicrobials as a prophylactic treatment (Kontiokari et al., 2001). Lingonberry, also known as mountain cranberry (*Vaccinium vitis-idaea* L.), is sometimes used as substitute for cranberry in jams and jellies and has recently become domesticated (Vaughan and Geissler, 1997). Both beverages were commercially available and were used only occasionally by any of the participants prior to the trial. Participants were instructed to take the cranberry-lingonberry concentrate, which contained more cranberry than lingonberry (7.5 g/ and 1.7 g/50 mL water, respectively), diluted in 200 mL water and not to add sugar. The dosage was 50 mL concentrate/day for six months. Another group received the *Lactobacillus* GG beverage (4×10^{10} colony forming units/100 mL) with the instruction to drink 100 mL/day five days per week for 12 months. A third group of participants served as the open control and received no intervention for UTIs. All participants were recruited at a university and consisted of students and staff and all had received successful treatment for the first UTI with antimicrobials. Urine samples were then obtained from participants reporting subsequent symptoms suggesting UTI. Urine cultures of $\geq 10^5$ cfu/mL served as positive events. The researchers used a study endpoint of first recurrence of UTI and judged a reduction in occurrence to 10% as of clinical importance.

The rate of recurrence in Finnish women was shown in a previous study to be $\geq 30\%$, with 78% of recurrent UTI episodes caused by *E. coli* (Kontiokari et al., 2001 citing Ikäheimo et al., 1996). Unfortunately, the manufacturer of the cranberry juice ceased production, which stopped recruitment before the trial was completed. However, meaningful comparative data was still obtained. The cranberry-lingonberry group showed a significant reduction in the occurrence of UTIs compared to the control group at both 6 months and 12 months ($p = 0.014$ and $p = 0.052$, respectively). Only 12 of these women had a recurrence of UTIs at 12 months, compared to 21 in the *Lactobacillus* GG group and 19 in the controls. It was calculated that the cranberry-lingonberry group had a reduction in the absolute risk of UTI recurrence of 20% versus the control group. The UTI was caused by *E. coli* in 80% of cases. With the exception of complaints concerning the bitter taste of the cranberry-lingonberry juice, no adverse effects were reported (Kontiokari et al., 2001).

Habash et al. (1999) studied the effect of three substances used to reduce the chance of UTI (cranberry supplement, ascorbic acid, and increased water consumption) on changes to the surface tension of urine—the higher the surface tension the less likely uropathogens would adhere to cell walls. The use of ascorbic acid to acidify urine and the increased consumption of water which reduces nutrients and salts utilized by bacteria are believed to decrease the number of microbes in patients during urological procedures. Ten healthy male volunteers were recruited to serve as controls, and the other groups were: cranberry supplement users (CranActin, Solaray, U.S.A., 400 mg t.i.d. × 2), ascorbic acid users (500 mg b.i.d. × 2), and water consumers. Urine collected on the day following the last treatment dose showed that the water treatment produced a significantly lower protein content than provided by either the cranberry supplement or the ascorbic acid; and the cranberry supplement or increased water consumption resulted in urine with higher surface tensions compared to either the control or the ascorbic acid treatment. Uropathogenic organisms showed good adhering activity to silicone rubber used in urinary tract catheterization when normal human urine was present. For *Enterococcus faecalis,* adhering ability in the presence of urine from ascorbic acid or cranberry supplementation became slightly lower, yet showed a tenfold higher adhesion rate in urine from the excess water supplementation. Because the tannins in cranberry are metabolized, the resulting compounds that might be responsible for the antiadhering activity remain unknown. It was also pointed out that the risk of colonization by *Enterococci* was not reduced by the use of the cranberry supplement, and that after 4 h the urine from any of the supplements showed no difference in the number of adherent microorganisms. In conclusion, ascorbic acid and cranberry supplementation offered some protection against uropathogenic colonization.

Schlager et al. (1999) conducted a double-blind, placebo-controlled crossover trial on the prophylactic effect of cranberry juice on symptomatic UTI and rates of bacteriuria in children diagnosed with neurogenic bladder caused by myelomeningocele. All the patients were receiving clean intermittent catheterization (CIC) and any therapies they received from their physician were allowed to continue. Fifteen children were enrolled (ages 2 to 18) and in each of two treatment periods lasting three months, they randomly received a daily two-ounce drink of cranberry juice concentrate (Ocean Spray) or placebo. The dosage was equal to 300 mL of cranberry juice cocktail used in a previous study in elderly women (Schlager et al., 1999) albeit, with a lower incidence of bacteriuria (Avorn et al., 1994). After three months, patients were crossed over to receive the alternate juice concentrate or placebo. The participants were told not to consume any other cranberry or blueberry products for the duration of the study. Urine samples were collected weekly during routine CIC for determination of bacteriuria (10^4 colony-forming units of pathogen/mL urine obtained by bladder catheterization). Symptomatic UTI was defined as bacteriuria accompanied with abdominal pain, fever, change in odor or color of urine, or change in the pattern of continence. The results showed no significant difference in the acidification of urine, which was uncommon in patients during the placebo or cranberry periods, and that UTIs occurred in the same number of patients in each treatment period, regardless of which treatment they received first. The rate of bacteriuria in these patients was 70% and was unaltered by their drinking a cranberry juice concentrate. The form of cranberry used was a concentrate and because a juice would have provided greater fluid intake and hence an increased washout effect, it might have produced positive results.

Walker et al. (1997) reported results of a randomized, double-blind, crossover, placebo-controlled clinical trial in 19 women (ages 28-44) with a history of recurring UTIs. The initial UTIs were treated with a course of standard antibiotic therapy for ten days, with or without cranberry. Patients then continued with either placebo powder or cranberry solids (CranActin, 400 mg) in the form of an encapsulated nutritional supplement for six months, crossing over at three months. Both groups were crossed over at three months to receive the opposite capsules for the final three months. Among the ten subjects who completed the study, a total of 21 UTIs occurred during the trial, six during the time when they were taking the cranberry supplement, and 15 during the period they were taking placebo. Walker and colleagues concluded that the cranberry supplement was effective as a prophylactic in the treatment of women with a history of recurrent UTIs.

In a double crossover study, Jackson and Hicks (1997) studied the effects of cranberry in 21 elderly men (mean age 73) who had a history of or risk factors for UTIs, such as stroke and the use of catheters. The subjects drank a moderate dose of commercial cranberry juice (concentration 25%) during each of their three daily meals (709.8 mL/day). Urinary pH showed a significantly lower value during the seven days when they received the juice, but not during no-juice periods. Patients and staff reported a decrease in urine odor, less constipation, and decreased incontinence and no adverse effects (Jackson and Hicks, 1997).

Avorn et al. (1994) conducted a six-month, placebo-controlled, double-blind trial, in which they administered 300 mL daily of a commercially available, low-calorie cranberry juice cocktail to 153 elderly women. In vitro tests showed that the juice inhibited adhesion of *E. coli* to uroepithelial cells. Significant differences between the groups were found after the first 30 days. Bacteriuria with pyuria was found in 28.1% of the urine samples from the group administered the placebo beverage, compared to 15.0% of those given the cranberry juice cocktail.

A study of unmarried female university students (ages 18-39) in the United States (Foxman et al., 1995) found an increased risk of UTIs associated with increased frequency of vaginal intercourse. The risk of UTI doubled among those who had sex with the same partner for less than one year compared to a year or more. The researchers then conducted a study of first-time UTI frequency and cranberry juice consumption in this population in which they compared the risk of developing UTIs in 86 subjects taking the juice versus 288 control subjects. The risk of UTI increased in association with carbonated soft drink intake, whereas habitual cranberry juice intake appeared to protect against UTI occurrence. Regular consumption of cranberry juice may have lowered the risk of UTIs in these young women. However, because a placebo-control group was not included, the results were inconclusive.

Metabolic and Nutritional Disorders

Antioxidant Activity

Pedersen et al. (2000) investigated the potential of a commercial cranberry juice (Ocean Spray, UK, Cranberry Classic) to increase the plasma antioxidant capacity in nine healthy female volunteers (ages 23-41) and compared the effects to those of organic blueberry juice (Beutelsbacher, Germany). None of the volunteers had taken mineral or vitamin supplements for at least three weeks prior to the start of the tests. The beverages were administered after an overnight fast in a dose of 500 mL and effects were compared to a sucrose control (9% w/v in water) containing a content of sugar similar to that of the juices. The beverages were drunk in a period of 10 min. Antioxidant capacity of plasma was measured by electronic spin resonance (ESR) spectroscopy according to the ability to reduce potassium nitrosodisulphonate and Fe(III)-2,46 Tri(2-pyridly)-s-triazine. Despite a close to threefold greater content of total phenol (gallic acid equivalents) in the blueberry juice, and twice the FRAP value (ferric reducing antioxidant potential) of the cranberry juice, only the cranberry juice produced a significant increase ($p < 0.001$) in antioxidant capacity in the plasma of the volunteers. It reached a maximum after 60-120 min and resulted in a significant increase ($p < 0.001$) in plasma vitamin C of 30%. (The vitamin C content of the cranberry juice was 1.5 mM and the blueberry juice was 0 mM.) It was calculated that 86-89% of the increase in plasma antioxidant capacity at 120 min after the cranberry juice was ingested was due to vitamin C and that the role of phenolics was minor. Among the three treatments, amounts of phenolics excreted in urine 4 h after ingestion of the beverages were not significantly different; however, the increase in total phenol in the plasma after ingestion of the cranberry juice reached some significance ($p < 0.05$), whereas no such effect was found from the other beverages. The possibility that a longer period than 4 h might have been necessary for the plasma phenol content to increase after ingestion of the blueberry juice could not be discounted.

DOSAGE

Pedersen (1994) gives typical daily dosages for the fresh fruit as 1/2 cup and the dried fruit as 15 mL (1 tbsp). Tyler (1994) notes that the dosage of cranberry juice cocktail recommended for prevention of UTIs is 90 mL (approximately 1/3 being pure juice) or 3 fl oz. The dosage is increased in the treatment of UTIs to between 12 and 32 fl oz, or 390-960 mL. The dried berry powder in capsules is reported as being equivalent to 90 mL of the berry juice cocktail per six capsules, which is the generally recommended amount for use in preventing UTIs (Tyler, 1994). Also, 45 g (1.5 oz) of frozen or fresh cranberries is equivalent to 90 mL (3 fl oz) of the berry cocktail (Tyler, 1994). A survey of "cranberry juices" sold in the United States found that the contents of cranberry juice varied from 25% to 30% (*Consumer Reports,* 2001).

In the United States, extracts and powder concentrates of cranberries have been standardized according to total organic acids. They may also be standardized to polyphenolic contents as gallic acid equivalents to estimate total polyphenol contents. As gallic acid equivalents, the polyphenolic contents of cranberry extract would mostly consist of anthocyanidins and flavonols (Wilson et al., 1998). Following the work of Bomser et al. (1996) and Foo et al. (2000), proanthocyanidin content may be another consideration for standardization of cranberry extracts.

Hughes and Lawson (1989) analyzed the contents of total and individual organic acids in cranberry juice cocktail and compared them to two cranberry powder extract products sold in the United States as food supplements. In one commercial powder extract (Murdock Pharmaceuticals, Inc.), they found higher quantities of total organic acids (1.49 g versus 1.03 g) than they detected in cranberry juice cocktail (Ocean Spray). Twelve capsules of this powder extract (6.9 g) was equivalent in amounts of total organic acids to 6 oz of cranberry juice cocktail. With the exception of benzoic acid (0.02 g versus 0.001 g), quantities of individual organic acids found in 6 oz of the cranberry juice cocktail were also less than those found in the powder extract (6.9 g): citric acid (0.28 g versus 0.46 g), malic acid (0.30 g versus 0.53 g), and quinic acid (0.45 g versus 0.50 g).

SAFETY PROFILE

Contraindications

Because of the propensity of uric acid and oxalate stones to form in urine that is more acidic and the relatively high content of oxalates in cranberries (Howe and Bates, 1987), it has been suggested that intake of cranberry juice be limited to no more than one liter per day to avoid possible aggravation in patients with existing stones (Rogers, 1991; Leaver, 1996). Paradoxically, cranberries were once used empirically for the treatment of urinary stones (Kahn et al., 1967).

A case report of recurrent kidney stones in a 47-year-old male patient with a distant history of calcium oxalate nephrolithiasis who had taken cranberry concentration tablets twice daily for a period of six months was reported by Terris et al. (2001). The patient presented to an emergency clinic with severe renal colic and hematuria. Tests revealed large stones in his kidneys and a creatine level of 2.1 mg/dL. Six years earlier he passed two small urinary calculi and since then was well and without stones since his last follow-up 12 months earlier. Treatment consisted of extracorporeal shock wave lithotripsy combined with endoscopic removal of the stones which were subsequently found to contain calcium oxalate. Since discontinuing the tablets, stones did not recur and his disease did not progress. It was calculated that if taken twice daily, tablets of cranberry concentrate could increase the normal dietary intake of calcium oxalate in North Americans and Europeans by 142% (Terris et al., 2001).

Prompted by this case, Terris et al. (2001) conducted a pilot study to examine the urinary content of five healthy volunteers (three men and two women, ages 26-37) after a seven-day ingestion of cranberry concentrate tablets taken at a dosage recommended by the manufacturer (both undisclosed) while they maintained their usual diets. Urinary components were measured for the risk of stone development using UroRisk analysis (Mission Pharmacal, San Antonio, TX), which, in addition to urine pH, measures total excretion of creatine, calcium, sodium, potassium, magnesium, citrate, uric acid, and oxalate, and both uric acid supersaturation and calcium oxalate supersaturation. Compared to baseline readings of 24-h urine, the results showed a statistically significant ($p < 0.01$) increase in urinary oxalate excretion in all the volunteers, which ranged from 34.2% to 45.5% (average 43.4%). The greatest increase was found in a subject with a family history of kidney stones. An increase of 10% over normal is known to result in calcium oxalate crystallization and the increase in volunteers was similar to levels obtained in normal volunteers in dietary oxalate loading studies. Calcium oxalate supersaturation also increased in volunteers by an average of 50.7%, while urine volume, pH, citrate and uric acid levels showed no increase and uric acid supersaturation fell by a mean of 33.7%. Although other components of kidney stones showed some increase (calcium, phosphorus, and significantly, sodium), this was attended by significant increases in urinary levels of potassium (average 67.5%) and magnesium (average 47.3%), which inhibit stone formation. A number of caveats were given to these results, including the small number of subjects, the short intake period, and the relatively high urinary calcium levels and urine output of the volunteers, which may have rendered them poorly representative of the population at large "and/or stone-forming individuals" (Terris et al., 2001, p. 28). This study has been criticized for not measuring intakes of calcium and vitamin C, both contributors to urinary oxalates, and for failing to measure the actual content of oxalates in the tablets (Leahy et al., 2001). In a previous study in nonstone-forming people, however, cranberry juice had a negligible effect on urinary oxalates (Finch et al., 1981). Until more is known of the risk of concentrated cranberry supplements to kidney stone patients, these individuals may want to increase their daily water intake to 48 oz or more, as is suggested for patients with UTIs (Hughes and Lawson, 1989).

Drug Interactions

When taken in combination with vitamin C, cranberry juice reduced urine pH levels in patients with multiple sclerosis more than orange juice combined with ascorbic acid (Schultz, 1984). Cranberry juice taken in combination with methenamine mandelate may increase the antibacterial effect of this agent and of other drugs used to treat UTIs, which are affected by adjusted pH, such as tetracycline, cycloserine, and novobiocin (Chernomordik and Vasilenko, 1981).

The ingestion of cranberry juice by elderly patients being treated with omeprazole may increase absorption of protein-bound vitamin B_{12} (Saltzman et al., 1994).

Pregnancy and Lactation

No contraindications for the use of cranberry juice or extracts by breast-feeding mothers or pregnant women are known. Use of cranberry juice or extracts by breastfeeding mothers and pregnant women is not expected to have any adverse effects. Cranberries are a common food.

Side Effects

Taken at the suggested dosages, side effects from cranberry are unknown.

Special Precautions

Sweetened cranberry preparations should be used with caution by diabetics.

The ingestion of unreasonable amounts of cranberry juice (3-4 L per day) may result in diarrhea and other GI symptoms (Kinney and Blount, 1979; Sobota, 1984).

REFERENCES

Ahuja, S., Kaack, B., and Roberts, J. (1998). Loss of fimbrial adhesion with the addition of *Vaccinium macrocarpon* to the growth medium of P-fimbriated *Escherichia coli. Journal of Urology* 159: 559-562.

Avorn, J., Monane, M., Gurwitz, J.H., Glynn, R.J., Choodnovskiy, I., and Lipsitz, L.A. (1994). Reduction of bacteriuria and pyuria after ingestion of cranberry juice. *Journal of the American Medical Association* 271: 751-754.

Bailey, L.H. and Bailey, E.Z. (1976). *Hortus Third.* New York: Macmillan General reference, p. 1142.

Bomser, J., Madhavi, D.L., Singletary, K., and Smith, M.A.L. (1996). In vitro anticancer activity of fruit extracts from *Vaccinium* species. *Planta Medica* 62: 212-216.

Burger, O., Ofek, I., Tabak, M., Weiss, E.I., Sharon, N., and Neeman, I. (2000). A high molecular mass constituent of cranberry juice inhibits *Helicobacter pylori* adhesion to human gastric mucus. *FEMS Immunology and Medical Microbiology* 29: 295-301.

Camire, A.L. and Clydesdale, F.M. (1979). High-pressure liquid chromatography of cranberry anthocyanins. *Journal of Food Science* 44: 926-927.

Cardellina, J.H. and Meinwald, J. (1980). Isolation of parascorbic acid from the cranberry plant, *Vaccinium macrocarpon. Phytochemistry* 19: 2199-2200.

Castleman, M. (1991). *The Healing Herbs.* Emmaus, PA: Rodale Press, pp. 141-142.

Chernomordik, A.B. and Vasilenko, E.G. (1981). [Increased activity of novobiocin and widening of its antimicrobial spectrum]. *Antibiotiki* 26: 456-460.

Coombes, A.J. (1985). *Dictionary of Plant Names.* Portland, OR: Timber Press.

Coppola, E.D., Conrad, E.C., and Cotter, R. (1978). High pressure liquid chromatographic determination of major organic acids in cranberry juice. *Journal of the Association of Analytical Chemists* 61: 1490-1492.

Croteau, R. and Fagerson, I.S. (1971). The chemical composition of the cuticular wax of cranberry. *Phytochemistry* 10: 3239-3245.

Deubert, K.H. (1978). A rapid method for the extraction and quantitation of total anthocyanin of cranberry fruit. *Journal of Agricultural and Food Chemistry* 26: 1452-1453.

Duke, J.A. (1992). *Handbook of Phytochemical Constituents of GRAS Herbs and Other Economic Plants.* Boca Raton, FL: CRC Press.

Finch, A.M., Kasidas, G.P., and Rose, G.A. (1981). Urine composition in normal subjects after oral ingestion of oxalate-rich foods. *Clinical Science* 60: 411-418.

Foo, L.Y., Lu, Y., Howell, A.B., and Vorsa, N. (2000). A-type proanthocyanidin trimers from cranberry that inhibit adherence of uropathogenic P-fimbriated *Escherichia coli. Journal of Natural Products* 63: 1225-1228.

Foxman, B., Geiger, A.M., Palin, K., Gillespie, B., and Koopman, J.S. (1995). First-time urinary tract infection and sexual behavior. *Epidemiology* 6: 162-168.

"Go ahead: Find the cranberry." (2001). *Consumer Reports,* June, 8-9.

Habash, M.B., Van der Mei, H.C., Busscher, H.J., and Reid, G. (1999). The effect of water, ascorbic acid, and cranberry derived supplementation on human urine and uropathogen adhesion to silicone rubber. *Canadian Journal of Microbiology* 45: 691-694.

Howe, S.M. and Bates, P. (1987). The cranberry juice cure: Fact or fiction? *AUAA Journal* (July-September): 13-16.

Howell, A.B., Vorsa, N., Marderosian, A.D., and Foo, L.Y. (1998). Inhibition of the adherence of P-fimbriated *Escherichia coli* to uroepithelial-cell surfaces by proanthocyanidin extracts from cranberries. *New England Journal of Medicine* 339: 1085-1086 (letter).

Hughes, B.G. and Lawson, L.D. (1989). Nutritional content of cranberry products. *American Journal of Hospital Pharmacy* 46: 1129.

Ikäheimo, R., Siitonen, A., Heiskanen, T., Kärkkänen, U., Kuosmanen, P., Lipponen, R., and Makela, P.H. (1996). Recurrence of urinary tract infection in a primary care setting: Analysis of a 1-year follow-up of 179 women. *Clinical Infectious Diseases* 22: 91-99.

Jackson, B. and Hicks, L.E. (1997). Effect of cranberry juice on urinary pH in older adults. *Home Healthcare Nurse* 15: 199-202.

Jepson, R.G., Mihaljevic, L., and Craig, J. (2000). Cranberries for treating urinary tract infections (Cochrane Review). In: *The Cochrane Library* (4). Oxford, England: Update Software. <http://www.update-software.com/cochrane/>.

Kahn, H.D., Panariello, V.A., Saeli, J., Sampson, J.R., and Schwartz, E. (1967). Effect of cranberry juice on urine. *Journal of the American Dietetic Association* 51: 251-254.

Kapadia, G.J., Tokuda, H., Konoshima, T., and Nishino, H. (1996). Chemoprevention of lung and skin cancer by *Beta vulgaris* (beet) root extract. *Cancer Letters* 100: 211-214.

Kinney, A.B. and Blount, M. (1979). Effect of cranberry juice on urinary pH. *Nursing Research* 28: 287-290.

Kontiokari, T., Sundqvist, K., Nuutinen, M., Pokka, T., Koskela, M., and Uhari, M. (2001). Randomized trial of cranberry-lingonberry juice and *Lactobacillus* GG drink for the prevention of urinary tract infections in women. *British Medical Journal* 322: 1-5.

Kuzminski, L.N. (1996). Cranberry juice and urinary tract infections: Is there a beneficial relationship? *Nutrition Reviews* 54(Suppl.): S87-S90.

Leahy, M., Roderick, R., and Brilliant, K. (2001). The cranberry—Promising health benefits, old and new. *Nutrition Today* 36: 254-265.

Leaver, R.B. (1996). Cranberry juice. *Professional Nurse* 11: 525-526.

Lowe, F.C. and Fagelman, E. (2001). Cranberry juice and urinary tract infections: What is the evidence? *Urology* 57: 407-413.

Maher, M.A., Mataczynski, H., Stefaniak, H.M., and Wilson, T. (2000). Cranberry juice induces nitric oxide-dependent vasodilation in vitro and its infusion transiently reduces blood pressure in anesthetized rats. *Journal of Medicinal Food* 3: 141-147.

Marles, R.J., Clavelle, C., Monteleone, L., Tays, N., and Burns, D. (2000). *Aboriginal Plant Use in Canada's Northwest Boreal Forest*. Vancouver, B.C., Canada: University of British Columbia Press, pp. 184-186.

Moen, D.V. (1962). Observations on the effectiveness of cranberry juice in urinary infections. *Wisconsin Medical Journal* 61: 282.

Moerman, D.E. (1998). *Native American Ethnobotany*. Portland, OR: Timber Press, p. 583.

Nawar, W.W. (2001). Tocotrienols and Omega-3 fatty acids in cranberry seed oil. *FASEB Journal* 15: A985 (abstract 754.6).

Nazarko, L. (1995). The therapeutic uses of cranberry juice. *Nursing Standard* 9: 33-35.

Ofek, I., Goldhar, J., and Sharon, N. (1996). Anti-*Escherichia coli* adhesin activity of cranberry and blueberry juices. *Advances in Experimental Medicine and Biology* 408: 179-183.

Ofek, I., Goldhar, J., Zafirii, D., Lis, H., Adar, R., and Sharon, N. (1991). Anti-*Escherichia coli* adhesin activity of cranberry and blueberry juices. *New England Journal of Medicine* 324: 1599 (letter).

Pedersen, C.B., Kyle, J., Jenkinson, A.M., Gardner, P.T., McPhail, D.B., and Duthie, G.G. (2000). Effects of blueberry and cranberry juice consumption on the plasma antioxidant capacity of healthy female volunteers. *European Journal of Clinical Nutrition* 54: 405-408.

Pedersen, M. (1994). *Nutritional Herbology: A Reference Guide to Herbs*. Warsaw, IN: Wendell W. Whitman Co.

Rogers, J. (1991). Pass the cranberry juice. *Nursing Times* 87: 36-37.

Schlager, T.A., Andersen, S., Trudell, J., and Hendley, J.O. (1999). Effect of cranberry juice on bacteriuria in children with neurogenic bladder receiving intermittent catheterization. *Journal of Pediatrics* 135: 698-702.

Schmidt, D.R. and Sobota, A.E. (1988). An examination of the anti-adherence activity of cranberry juice on urinary and nonurinary bacterial isolates. *Microbios* 55: 173-181.

Schultz, A. (1984). Efficacy of cranberry juice and ascorbic acid in acidifying the urine in multiple sclerosis patients. *Journal of Community Health Nursing* 1: 159-169.

Sobota, A.E. (1984). Inhibition of bacterial adherence by cranberry juice: Potential use for the treatment of urinary tract infections. *Journal of Urology* 131: 1013-1016.

Swartz, J.H. and Medrek, T.F. (1968). Antifungal properties of cranberry juice. *Applied Microbiology* 16: 1524-1527.

Terris, M.K., Issa, M.M., and Tacker, J.R. (2001). Dietary supplementation with cranberry concentrate tablets may increase the risk of nephrolithiasis. *Urology* 57: 26-29.

Tsukada, K., Tokunaga, K., Iwama, T., Mishima, Y., Tazawa, K., and Fujimaki, M. (1994). Cranberry juice and its impact on peristomal skin conditions for urostomy patients. *Ostomy/Wound Management* 40: 60-62, 64, 66-68.

Tyler, V.E. (1994). *Herbs of Choice: The Therapeutic Use of Phytomedicinals.* Binghamton, NY: The Haworth Press, Inc., pp. 80-81.

Uphof, J.C. (1968). *Dictionary of Economic Plants,* Second Edition. New York: Verlag von J. Cramer, pp. 537-538.

Vaughan, J.G. and Geissler, C. (1997). *The New Oxford Book of Food Plants.* New York: Oxford University Press, p. 88.

Vogel, V.J. (1970). *American Indian Medicine.* Norman, OK: University of Oklahoma Press, p. 296.

Walker, E.B., Barney, D.P., Mickelsen, J.N., Walton, R.J., and Mickelson, R.A. Jr. (1997). Cranberry concentrate: UTI prophylaxis. *Journal of Family Practice* 45: 167-168 (letter).

Wang, S.Y. and Jiao, H. (2000). Scavenging capacity of berry crops on superoxide radicals, hydrogen peroxide, hydroxyl radicals, and singlet oxygen. *Journal of Agricultural and Food Chemistry* 48: 5677-5684.

Wang, S.Y. and Stretch, A.W. (2001). Antioxidant capacity in cranberry is influenced by cultivar and storage temperature. *Journal of Agricultural and Food Chemistry* 49: 969-974.

Weiss, E.I., Lev-Dor, R., Kashamn, Y., Goldhar, J., Sharon, N., and Oftek, I. (1998). Inhibiting interspecies coaggregation of plaque bacteria with a cranberry juice constituent. *Journal of the American Dental Association* 129: 1719-1723.

Werbach, M.R. and Murray, M.T. (1994). *Botanical Influences on Illness: A Sourcebook of Clinical Research.* Tarzana, CA: Third Line Press.

Wilson, T., Porcari, J.P., and Harbin, D. (1998). Cranberry extract inhibits low density lipoprotein oxidation. *Life Sciences* 62: 381-386.

Wilson, T., Porcari, J.P., and Maher, M.A. (1999). Cranberry juice inhibits metal and non-metal initiated oxidation of human low density lipoproteins. *Journal of Nutraceuticals, Functional and Medical Foods* 2: 5-14.

Zafriri, D., Ofek, I., Adar, R., Pocino, M., and Sharon, N. (1989). Inhibitory activity of cranberry juice on adherence of Type 1 and Type P fimbriated *E. coli* to eucaryotic cells. *Antimicrobial Agents and Chemotherapy* 33: 92-98.

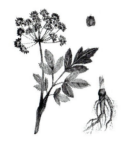

Dong Quai

BOTANICAL DATA

Classification and Nomenclature

Scientific name: *Angelica sinensis* (Oliv.) Diels.; synonym: *A. polymorpha* Maxim. var. *sinensis* Oliv.

Family name: Apiaceae

Common names: dang quei, tang-kuei (China), dong quai (westernization); *Angelicae radix* (the root of *Angelica sinensis*). The common Chinese name, dang quei, means literally "state of return," referring to its restorative powers

Description

The many *Angelica* species belong to the Apiaceae (formerly called the Umbelliferae), or parsley family, and are distributed worldwide. Dong quai *(Angelica sinensis)* is a common, fragrant perennial herb which grows in mainland China, Korea, and Japan. It has a strong scent, between that of celery and licorice. It grows naturally at high altitude on cold, damp mountain slopes in rich, deep soil. The stem is glabrous, smooth, and purplish, with light linear striations, growing about 0.5-1 m high. Inferior leaves are tripinnate; superior leaves are often simply pinnate. Leaf segments are oval and dentate. The petiole is 3-11 cm long, prominently sheathed, and bracts are rudimentary. The flower is a multiflorous umbel, 10-14 of which may radiate above the plant's foliage on slender pedicels. Each umbel has 12-36 flowers on stems up to 1.5 cm long. Flowers are white with five petals, blooming in June and July. The fruit is borne in July and August as bipartite carpophores. The carpels are flat and slightly winged, with two seeds (Dobelis et al.; 1986, Zhu, 1987).

Dong quai are harvested after two to three years of cultivation (Foster and Yue, 1992). The roots are dug out in the fall, cleaned, and dried in semi-shade without the stems. Because the roots are rich in volatile oils, they must be stored in airtight containers (Zhu, 1987).

HISTORY AND TRADITIONAL USES

Dong quai is said to appear more frequently in traditional Chinese medi-cine (TCM) prescriptions than any other drug except licorice, is as widely respected as ginseng, and has been used in China for at least 2,000 years. It has long been regarded as a valuable remedy in the treatment of menstrual and puerperal disorders and of sterility in women, though it is also used in a variety of other conditions. Lei Gong's *Treatise on Preparation of Materia Medica* (588 A.D.) says about dong quai:

> Its taste is bitter-sweet and spicy, it is warming to the body, and it is non-poisonous. The root is used medicinally as a strengthener of the heart, lung, and liver meridians; it is a tonic of the blood and promotes blood circulation; it regulates the menstrual cycle and stops menstrual pain; it lubricates the bowel . . . . Almost all Chinese families have used dong quai for generations as a 'tonic and spice,' and particularly in treating women's disorders (Zhu, 1987, p. 117). For that reason it has been popularly referred to as the "female ginseng." (Murray, 1995)

The drug was introduced into Western medicine in 1899 by Merck in the form of a liquid extract sold under the name of Eumenol, and later in the form of Eumenol tablets. These preparations were recommended in the treatment of menstrual disorders, and the results obtained were reported to be favorable (Belford-Courtney, 1993).

Dong quai is regarded by most Asian, European, and American herbal-ists as a wonder herb for the female system. Contemporary Chinese theories of TCM maintain that the different parts of the dong quai root are responsi-ble for different effects: the head of the root to stop bleeding, the body or middle of the root for a tonic to regulate blood and alleviate pain, and the tail portion to eliminate blood stasis. Acupuncturists who also practice Chinese herbalism are reported to have successfully used a fluid extraction of dong quai injected into acupuncture points for a number of ailments, and to allevi-ate pain (Zhu, 1987). dong quai has also been used in traditional medicine for treating glaucoma (Yoshihiro, 1985), and as a diuretic (Hsu et al., 1986); the latter possibly due to a 40% sucrose content (Zhu, 1987).

In China, several species of *Angelica* are officially recognized, each hav-ing different methods of preparation and indications for use. Traditionally, *A. sinensis* is gathered in late autumn, allowed to slightly dry before being tied in small bundles, and then smoke-dried. After being cleaned and washed to soften it thoroughly, slices of the root are dried at low temperature or sun-dried. When the root slices are stir-fried in wine until dried, they are indicated for stimulating menstrual discharge and activating the circulation. Otherwise, the root slices are indicated in menstrual disorders, amenorrhea, dysmenorrhea, anemia accompanied with palpitation and dizziness, sores, boils, carbuncles, traumatic injuries, rheumatoid arthritis, and constipation (Tu et al., 1992).

CHEMISTRY

Carbohydrates

Polysaccharides

An acidic polysaccharide of low molecular weight (about 3,000) composed of 4.73% protein was identified in the root by Choy et al. (1994). Others have reported lower (82 to 670 MW) (Cho et al., 2000) and higher molecular weight polysaccharides (av. 65,765 and 85,000 MW) in dong quai (Chen et al., 2001). Polysaccharide fractions in oriental *Angelica* species contain widely varying amounts of hexose, uronic acid, protein, and an array of seven sugars (Yamada et al., 1984).

Lipid Compounds

Oils

The root of dong quai contains 0.4-0.7% volatile oil comprised of angelicide, ferulic acid, butylidene phthalide, *n*-valerophenone-*O*-carboxylic acid, dihydrophthalic anhydride, carvacrol, safrol, isosafrol, sesquiterpenes, β-cadinene, *n*-dodecanol, *n*-tetradecanol, *n*-butylpthalic acid, (Zhu, 1987, 1998), choline (989 μg/g) (Yamasaki et al., 1994), carvacrol, cadinene, *n*-dodecanol, *n*-teradecanol, *n*-tetradecane (Awang, 1999), scopeletin, vanillic acid, facarinol, falcarinolone, falcarindiol, and nubelliferone (Mei et al., 1991). Ligustilide makes up 45% of the oil (Zhu, 1998).

All parts of the *Angelica* plant contain the volatile active constituents, with the leaves and branching roots containing the most (Sheu et al., 1987).

Organic Acids

Organic acids found in the plant include nicotinic, folic, folinic (Awang, 1999), and vanillic acid (Mei et al., 1991). Contents of ferulic acid are twice as high in methanolic extracts compared to water extracts (Wang et al., 1999).

Phenolic Compounds

Angelica species are rich in coumarins which occur throughout the plant (Leung and Foster, 1996). Among them are nubelliferone (Mei et al., 1991), angelol, angelicone, angelicide, bergapten, butylphthalide, butylidenephthalide, imperatorin, ligustilide, osthol, osthenol, oxypeuedanin, safrole, and isosafrole (Awang, 1999). The content of ligustilide is 53 times higher in methanolic extracts compared to water extracts (Wang et al., 1999). The root contains the phthalide Z-ligustilide as its main component (Zschocke et al., 1998), along with at least 23 other phthalide derivatives. These compounds are considered active constituents in *A. sinensis* and are found in a number of other prominent Chinese medicinal herbs of the Apiaceae family (Lin et al., 1998; Zschocke et al., 1998).

Other Constituents

Other constituents include β-sitosterol, vitamin E, vitamin B_{12} (0.25-40 mg/100g), vitamin A, and related substances (0.0675%), sucrose (40%), uracil, adenine, folinic acid (Zhu, 1987), biotin, pantothenic acid (Awang, 1999), scopoletin (Mei et al., 1991), and coniferyl ferulate (Lin et al., 1998).

THERAPEUTIC APPLICATIONS

Dong quai is most renowned for its ancient and widespread use in balancing female reproductive processes. It is favored in TCM to treat such conditions as dysmenorrhea, amenorrhea, metorrhagia, menopausal symptoms (especially hot flashes), and to assure a healthy pregnancy and easy delivery (Murray, 1995). However, others warn that care should be taken in its administration to pregnant women (Northrup, 1995).

PRECLINICAL STUDIES

Endocrine and Hormonal Functions

Reproductive Hormone Interactions

Both inhibitory and stimulating actions on the uterus have been shown with dong quai. The contractive and excitatory component is thought to be a water- and alcohol-soluble, nonvolatile oil, whereas the relaxing, inhibitory component is considered to be a volatile oil with a high boiling point. The volatile oil found in the root relaxes the uterus by antagonizing the action of epinephrine, pituitrin, or histamine. The excitatory effect can cause contractions if there is intrauterine pressure; hence its use in childbirth (Hsu et al., 1986; Bensky et al., 1986; Willard, 1991; Belford-Courtney, 1993).

Liu et al. (2001) tested the in vitro estrogenic activity of a methanolic extract of the root using dong quai plants cultivated at the University of Illinois. Evidence of estrogenic activity was absent in a test of the extract for alkaline phosphate-inducing activity and in estrogen-positive endometrial carcinoma (Ishikawa) cells, and the extract was only weakly active at inducing up-regulation of progesterone receptor mRNA. At binding to human recombinant estrogen receptors types alpha and beta, the extract was inactive, and at stimulating the expression of an estrogen-inducible gene (presenelin-2) in a line of estradiol-responsive breast cancer cells (S-30) the extract exhibited only weak activity. No cytotoxicity was found from the extract in either type of cells.

The Japanese *A. acutiloba* has demonstrated uterine tonic activity, causing an initial increase in uterine contraction, followed by relaxation. When administered to mice as part of their daily feed it resulted in increased uterine weight, markedly increased DNA content of the uterus and liver, and increased glucose utilization by the liver and uterus (Yoshihiro, 1985). Similar results were reported by Eagon et al. (1997) and Eagon (1999) with an alcoholic extract of dong quai root administered for three weeks as part of a liquid diet in ovariectomized rats (at one-third the human dose equivalent): decreased uterine *c-myc* mRNA levels, increased uterine weight, and an increase in hepatic ceruloplasmin mRNA levels.

Ozaki and Ma (1990) administered a constituent of dong quai and ferulic acid in high doses (300 and 1,000 mg/kg p.o.) to adult female virgin rats in the estrous phase of the estrous cycle to examine its effects on spontaneous movement of the uterus. A maximal inhibition of uterine contractions of approximately 30% was found from the lower dose, with contractions returning to original levels after 45 min and 60 min in the case of the higher dose.

In another study testing for estrogenicity, an alcoholic extract of dong quai as part of a standard liquid diet in ovariectomized rats administered for three weeks at 1/3 the human dose equivalent increased uterine weight while decreasing uterine *c-myc* mRNA expression levels, which are otherwise increased by estrogen (Eagon et al., 1997; Eagon, 1999). Using a competitive estrogen receptor binding assay with radiolabeled estradiol, Eagon et al. (1997) reported inhibition of estradiol binding to estrogen receptors in vitro from the extract as significant and dose-dependent. Dong quai also increased levels of hepatic ceruloplasmin mRNA, indicating an increased hepatic estrogenic response.

Immune Functions; Inflammation and Disease

Cancer

Antiproliferative activity. The in vitro growth-inhibiting activity of an extract of dong quai roots was tested in T47-D breast cancer cells, an estrogen-

and progesterone-positive cell line. At a concentration of 1.0%, growth of the cells was inhibited by 78%; however, lower concentrations were ineffective (Dixon-Shanies and Shaikh, 1999).

Immune Functions

Immunomodulation. Choy et al. (1994) reported strong antitumor activity in Ehrlich ascites tumor-bearing female mice administered a low molecular weight polysaccharide (F-2pc-A) isolated from the root of *A. sinensis.* Tumor growth was inhibited by 98% from a dose of 0.4 mg/kg i.p. for five days. The researchers also showed that in mice (2-4 mg/kg i.v.), the polysaccharide increased natural killer cell activity and exhibited in vitro immunostimulating activity in the form of lymphocyte proliferation.

Immunosuppression. Individuals who are sensitive to a variety of environmental substances (pollen, dust, animal dander, food, etc.) produce antibodies of the IgE class at levels three to ten times greater than normal. An aqueous extract of *A. sinensis* root has been shown in TCM and clinical studies to inhibit the production of IgE antibodies in a selective manner, so that a strong suppression of both primary and secondary reaginic responses occur. *A. polymorpha* var. *sinensis* Diels. (= *A. sinensis*) root extract administered i.p. to mice at dilutions of 1:3 to 1:160 of the original extract (soluble material, 210 mg/mL,) and orally at dilutions of 1:3 to 1:100 of an original extract (soluble material, 100 mg/mL), significantly inhibited the production of IgE antibodies in a selective manner, but not that of IgG. Extracts of the roots inhibited the release of IgE mediators, which when combined with antigen can cause syndromes of atopy (Sung et al., 1982).

Infectious Diseases

Microbial infections. Decoctions of the root of Chinese *Angelica* have been shown to inhibit the growth of a number of bacteria, both Gram-positive and Gram-negative (Hsu et al., 1986; Bensky et al., 1986; Willard, 1991). Dong quai inhibited the growth of Gram-positive bacteria such as *B. typhi, B. comma,* hemolytic *Streptococcus* type A and B, and *Corynebacterium diphtheriae,* and Gram-negative bacteria such as *Escherichia coli* (Zhu, 1987). According to Murray (1995), extracts of Japanese *Angelica* exhibit no antibacterial action. This inconsistency could be due to different essential oil concentrations of the extracts used in the studies.

Inflammatory Response

Platelet aggregation (a diagnostic attribute of the condition in TCM called "stagnant blood") was inhibited in vitro by the combined action of the components of *Angelica acutiloba*. A correlation was noted between ligustilide content and antiplatelet aggregation activity (Shimizu et al., 1991). Ferulic acid in dong quai also inhibits platelet aggregation. It retards platelet release of 5-HT (5-hydroxytryptamine) and ADP (adenosine diphosphate) which can cause platelets to aggregate, resulting in obstructed blood flow (Zhu, 1987).

An extract of the roots consisting of 95% polysaccharides was examined for protective effect against indomethacin- and ethanol-induced ulcer formation in male rats compared to pretreatment with the anti-inflammatory prostaglandin E_2 (PGE_2). Against ethanol-induced ulcer formation, rats pretreated with the polysaccharide-rich extract (10 or 30 mg/kg i.p.) showed significantly less damage to the gastric mucosa compared to controls. The effect was dose-dependent and the higher dose was comparable in effect to that of PGE_2 (each $p < 0.001$). Either dose of the extract significantly ameliorated the increase in myeloperoxidase (MPO) activity of the gastric mucosa compared to controls; the higher dose of the extract was comparable to that of PGE_2; however, the lower dose provided more significant inhibition of MPO than the higher dose ($p < 0.001$ versus $p < 0.01$). Against indomethicin-induced ulcers, the lower dose provided significant protection against the formation of lesions in the duodenum and antrum, but not from those in the small intestine. The higher dose produced significant protection against lesion formation in all these areas and reduced damage to other areas of the gastric mucosa of the small intestine. Even 6 h after indomethacin, the 30 mg dose caused a significant reduction in the number of lesions formed in the duodenum and antrum (Cho et al., 2000).

In vitro studies which were conducted to elucidate the protective effect exhibited by the extract have shown that when incubated with experimentally-wounded, normal rat epigastric mucosal cells (RGM-1), the extract caused a dose-dependent and significant acceleration of normal RGM-1 cells to the wound area at doses of 2, 10, and 50 μg/mL, but not at 250 μg/mL. At 24 h the size of the wounds were treated with 50μg/mL reduced to about half the size of controls and at 36 h they healed to become one-third the size of the controls. As to what was causing the acceleration in wound repair, further experiments showed that in normal RGM-1 cells the extract caused a dose-dependent and significant increase in [3H]-thymidine incorporation (with a peak increase in DNA synthesis from 2 μg/mL after 5 h) and that at the lowest dose it caused epidermal growth factor gene (EGF mRNA) expression to nearly double (Ye et al., 2001).

Metabolic and Nutritional Functions

A four-week diet of 5% raw root (mixed with food) is reported to have enhanced the metabolism of mice which showed improved oxygen utilization in the liver, and enhanced glutamic acid and cysteine oxidation (Hsu et al., 1986; Bensky et al., 1986; Willard, 1991).

Neurological, Psychological, and Behavioral Functions

Receptor- and Neurotransmitter-Mediated Functions

In China, dong quai is frequently injected into acupuncture points to inhibit pain (Hsu, 1986; Bensky et al., 1986; Willard, 1991).

Reproductive Functions

Infertility (Female)

Dong quai has shown no effect, positive or negative, on the fertility of mice (Matsui, et al., 1967).

Sexual Dysfunctions (Female)

In a feeding study, dong quai at 5% of the diet was found to increase the sexual activity of female mice (Zhu, 1987).

Hypertension

In animal studies, a 40% hot water extract of dong quai (2 mL/kg p.o.) was shown to lower blood pressure and dilate blood vessels (Yoshihiro, 1985). The hypotensive activity of dong quai in anaesthetized animals may be due to the release of chemical transmitters that excite acetylcholine and histamine receptors, causing dilation of peripheral blood vessels (Hsu et al., 1986; Bensky et al., 1986; Willard, 1991).

CLINICAL STUDIES

Immune Disorders; Inflammation and Disease

Inflammatory Response

Terasawa et al. (1985) tested decoctions made from two species of *Angelica (A. sinensis* and *A. acutiloba)* upon whole blood viscosity and core temperatures in human subjects. Essential oils present in both decoctions contained ligustilide as a major component; however, their HPLC profiles differed with the decoction of *A. acutiloba* containing almost tenfold the amount of ligustilide as *A. sinensis*. No distinct difference in their effect on the circulation in subjects was detected after oral administration at doses of 1 mL/kg. *A. acutiloba* appeared to produce an abnormal increase in the core temperature in some subjects. Both decoctions decreased whole blood viscosity for approximately 3 h after administration, an effect of longer duration with *A. acutiloba*. It was concluded that neither ligustilide nor essential oils directly participate in decreasing whole blood viscosity. The core temperature variations in contraindicative and indicative patients (in terms of TCM treatment of "stagnant blood") were considered significant. This illustrates a well-known empirical concept on the properties of crude drugs in TCM; namely, that a drug induces two different types of responses (the indicative and the contraindicative), depending on the physical conditions of the patients. Terasawa et al. (1985) concluded that commercially available *Angelica,* which is derived from different plant species, differs not only in the contents of ligustilide and essential oils, but also in clinical effects.

Reproductive Disorders

Menopause

A 24-week, double-blind, randomized placebo-controlled clinical trial of dong quai (4.5 g/day) was conducted by Hirata et al. (1997) in 71 American, postmenopausal, mostly Caucasian women who suffered from hot flashes. The incidence of hot flashes decreased in the dong quai group from 47/week to 35/week, and from 33/week to 27.5/week in the placebo control group, an insignificant difference. An equivocal Kupperman Menopausal Index score of 25% reduction in menopausal symptoms in both groups was compounded with the finding that changes in endometrial thickness had increased by the same amount in both treatment groups by 1/3 that normally found with increased estrogen. The number claiming good to excellent control of hot flashes in the active treatment group (33%) was also not significantly different from that of the placebo group (29%). It was concluded that "Dong quai does not produce estrogen-like responses in endometrial thickness or in vaginal maturation," and was no more effective than a placebo in providing relief from menopausal symptoms (Hirata et al., 1997, p. 985).

Zava et al. (1998) tested human saliva for estrogenic content following the ingestion of dong quai by women volunteers. Estradiol levels were found consistently very low which suggested that dong quai may suppress the synthesis of estradiol. From a 50% ethanol/water extract, in vitro tests for estrogenic and estrogen receptor binding showed that the bioactivity was very low.

DOSAGE

In China, the official dosage is 4.5-9 g (Tu et al., 1992). Several authorities have summarized different dosages and preparations for dong quai:

Powdered root: 1-2 g three times/day, or as tea
Tincture (1:5): 4 mL (1 tsp)
Fluid extract: 1 mL (1/4 tsp) (Murray, 1995)

10-40 drops of tincture, one to three times/day (Northrup, 1995)
3-30 g/day as tea or in capsules (Willard, 1991)

Zhu (1987) summarizes the Chinese uses and dosages of dong quai extracts for intravenous and arterial injection, as well as for injection into acupuncture points. There appears to be no consensus on standardization of dong quai extracts; both the lipid-soluble and the water-soluble fractions have shown activities in a variety of assays, and it is likely that these activities result from interactions between a number of active compounds.

SAFETY PROFILE

Dong quai is generally considered safe; however, because it contains photoreactive substances (coumarins), overexposure to sunlight should be avoided (Murray, 1995).

Forty patients injected with *A. sinensis* (25% solution i.v. at 200-240 mL/day for 15-30 days) for the treatment of severe ischemic apoplexy are reported to have shown no significant side effects (Mei et al., 1991).

No information was found on overdosage from dong quai.

Contraindications

TCM recommends that dong quai not be taken in cases of

1. diarrhea caused by weak digestion;
2. hemorrhagic disease;
3. hypermenorrhea;
4. first trimester of pregnancy;
5. spontaneous abortion; and
6. during flu or cold.

Some practitioners claim that *A. sinensis* should not be used during menstruation (Yoshihiro, 1985).

Drug Interactions

Furocoumarins in *A. sinensis* may potentiate existing anticoagulant medications if consumed in doses exceeding amounts normally consumed in foods. Individuals on anticoagulant medications should consult their physician before using this plant (Newall et al., 1996; Lo et al., 1995).

Only weak inhibition of cytochrome P450 3A (CYP3A) was found from a decoction and an ethanolic infusion of tang-kuei *(Angelica sinensis),* indicating that interactions with many types of drugs used in Western medicine are not likely. The inhibitory activity of a decoction or ethanolic infusion of *Angelica acutiloba* was marginal, and for each herb the activity seen corresponded with the content of the coumarin compound imperatorin, according to HPLC (Guo et al., 2001).

An oft-cited case report of an apparent drug interaction of a dong quai product with warfarin concerned a 46-year-old woman who at the time was taking other heart medications (digoxin and furosemide). When her international normalization ratio (INR) rose to 4.05, a battery of tests failed to uncover the cause. After a 24 h discontinuation of the warfarin (5 mg/day), she resumed the dosage and made an appointment for a follow-up visit scheduled for one week later. When she returned four weeks later and her INR was 4.09, she claimed not to have taken anything besides her prescribed medications, nor had she been ill or made changes to her diet. The only thing she had taken was dong quai for the treatment of perimenopausal symptoms at the suggestion of an herbalist. Although she had taken the herb in tablet form for the past four weeks (Nature's Way, 565 mg, one to two times/day), she forgot to mention it. She was then instructed to stop the warfarin for a day and resume it the next day while discontinuing the dong quai. After two weeks, her INR was 3.41 and after another two weeks, 2.48 (Page and Lawrence, 1999). Based on the possibility of the herb acting as an inhibitor of cyclooxygenase (COX) this case was rated as a "likely" drug interaction with tang-kuei (Fugh-Berman and Ernst, 2001). Another case involving warfarin and tang-kuei in which the patient displayed extensive bruising and showed an INR of 10 (Ellis and Stephens, 1999) was rated as a "possible" drug interaction, again, based on the possibility of COX-inhibitory activity of the herb (Fugh-Berman and Ernst, 2001). However, because a search of the literature found this activity reported only from a dichloromethane extract of the roots of *Angelica pubescens* f. *biserrata* (Liu et al., 1998), COX inhibition remains to be established as the cause of the side effects temporally associated with tang-kuei.

Pregnancy and Lactation

Dong quai may stimulate bleeding and some warn against its use during menstruation or pregnancy (Northrup, 1995). Brinker (1998) lists tang-kuei as contraindicated in pregnancy due to its action as an emmenagogue. On the other hand, Duke (1985) and others report that in China, tang-kuei is widely used "to assure a healthy pregnancy and easy delivery" (Duke, 1985, p. 44), due to its tonifying effect on the uterus. The *American Herbal Products Association's Botanical Safety Handbook* (McGuffin et al., 1997) classifies tang-kuei as an herb not to be taken during pregnancy though it should be noted that no contraindications during pregnancy were found in a review of Chinese herbal references. Both inhibitory and stimulating actions on the uterus have been shown with tang-kuei. Current research with tang-kuei indicates only very weak, if any, estrogenic activity (see Reproductive Hormone Interactions).

Use of tang-kuei during the postpartum period is common in many Asian cultures. Traditionally, the dried roots are simmered in specially prepared soups that often also contain stock made with bones, green vegetables, and other special foods and herbs deemed helpful to the new mother. Such practice infers use of the herb during early lactation. The *American Herbal Products Association's Botanical Safety Handbook* (McGuffin et al., 1997) does not identify any safety concerns during lactation, which coincides with TCM's lack of adverse reports or warnings up to this time. One anecdotal report (Nambiar et al., 1999) has been published involving a mother and three-week-old baby in which the Chinese-Malaysian mother had been consuming a soup containing what was believed to be tang-kuei. The mother presented to the ER with acute onset of headache, weakness, light-headedness, and vomiting. She was found to have hypertension (195/85) though she had been normotensive and normoglycemic during her uneventful and term delivery. Symptoms developed after two days of consuming the soup twice a day. The dose of tang-kuei used could not be ascertained. The patient denied consuming any other herbs or medicinals. The mother became normotensive within 12 h. The next day, an examination of the infant revealed a probably elevated systolic blood pressure: 115/69 and 117/63 in the left leg and arm, respectively, which normalized within 48 h. During that time, breast feeding was withheld. Hypotension, but not hypertension, is an observed response to tang-kuei in animals (see Therapeutic Applications: Hyptertension). No other reports of adverse effects associated with tang-kuei use during lactation are known (see Side Effects for more details).

Side Effects

Because dong quai may stimulate bleeding, some practitioners warn against its use during menstruation or pregnancy. There are no clinical studies to verify this, but in cases of hemorrhage or heavy bleeding it may exacerbate the problem (Northrup, 1995).

All species of dong quai have a high saccharide content, with the result that ingestion typically produces a rise in blood sugar (Yoshihiro, 1985).

A report of hypertension in a mother and her breast-fed infant after the mother consumed a soup containing dong quai may be the only case of its kind ever reported. Indeed, the investigators found no previous reports of hypertension from dong quai. Medical records showed that the 32-year-old Chinese-Malaysian mother was previously normoglycemic and normotensive and that her term delivery was uneventful. Yet she presented at the emergency clinic with weakness, headaches of acute onset, vomiting, and lightheadedness and showed a BP reading of 195/85 mm Hg, repeatedly. She claimed not to have taken anything unusual or herbal recently except for two servings that day of a traditional Malaysian soup that her recently arrived mother had prepared using pieces of the root obtained in Malaysia. A CT scan of her head revealed nothing unusual and within 12 h she became normotensive. On the day after this event, she took her three-week-old son to a pediatrician to check his BP since he was being breast-fed. His BP was also elevated and then over the next 48 h normalized while she withheld further breast-feeding. Although the dose of root she had taken was not assessable, to their credit, the investigators managed to obtain dong quai from the same shop in Malaysia as the root used to make the soup. A pharmacy specializing in Chinese medicine in the United States confirmed that it was dong quai. Furthermore, analyses were done on the root slices which were compared to a sample of granular dong quai root product obtained in the United States in capsule form (Nature's Way). No differences in identity were found (Nambiar et al., 1999). Whether this was an allergic reaction or the result of contamination isn't known and wasn't mentioned by the investigators; nor were other ingredients in the soup.

Special Precautions

The furocoumarins psoralen and bergapten can induce photosensitization, resulting in potentially severe photodermatitis. Episodes have generally been confined to direct dermal contact from persons collecting plants of the family Umbelliferae; although some persons may be affected by taking dong quai medicinally (Murray, 1995).

Safrole, found in the essential oil of dong quai, has been identified as a carcinogen. Duke (1985) warns of its toxicity without further instruction.

Traditional Chinese medicine practitioners warn against using dong quai in cases of "cold deficient" diarrhea (Willard, 1991).

Toxicology

Mutagenicity

No mutagenic activity was found from a methanol/water extract of the root in a modified Ames test with *Salmonella typhimurium* in the absence or presence of rat liver *S*-9 Mix (Yamamoto et al., 1982).

Toxicity in Animal Models

The oral median lethal dose of the extract of dong quai in mice is 30-90 g/kg (Zhu, 1998).

Rats fed a diet containing 5% *A. sinensis* for 105 days showed no abnormal growth and hepatic oxidization of glutamic acid was enhanced (Mei et al., 1991).

Lo et al. (1995) found the mean prothrombin time significantly lowered in rabbits administered a single dose of warfarin (2 mg/kg s.c) three days after coadministration of a high dosage of *A. sinensis* in the form of a water extract (2 g/kg p.o. b.i.d. for three days). This effect was not found in rabbits that received the same dosage of *A. sinensis* extract alone. When warfarin concentrations were at a steady state, mean prothrombin values showed a significant increase after administration of *A. sinensis* extract, and 2 of 6 rabbits died on the second day following the coadministered substances. Although no significant differences were found in the average plasma warfarin steady state concentration following administration of *A. sinensis* extract, Lo et al. (1995) concluded that patients receiving chronic treatment with warfarin should be precautioned about self-medicating with *A. sinensis*.

Dong quai has shown no effect, positive or negative, on the fertility of mice (Matsui et al., 1967). The alkaloid tetramethylpyrazine, found in the Chinese herb *Ligusticum wallachii* Franch, was shown to be synergistic with ferulic acid from dong quai at inhibiting uterine contractions in virgin female rats when administered i.v. (Ozaki and Ma, 1990).

REFERENCES

Awang, D.V.C. (1999). Dong quai. *Canadian Pharmaceutical Journal* 132: 38-41.

Belford-Courtney, R. (1993). Comparison of Chinese and Western uses of *Angelica sinensis*. *Australian Journal of Medical Herbalism* 5: 87-91.

Bensky, D., Gamble, A., and Kaptchuk, T. (1986). *Chinese Herbal Medicine: Materia Medica*. Seattle, WA: Eastland Press, pp. 474-476.

Brinker, F. (1998). *Herb Contraindications and Drug Interactions*. Sandy, OR: Eclectic Medical Publications, pp. 173-175.

Chen, R., Wang, H., Xu, H., Xu, G., and Chang, L. (2001). [Isolation, purification and determination of polysaccharides X-C-3-III and X-C-3-IV from *Angelica sinensis* (Oliv) Diels]. *Zhong Yao Cai* 24: 36-37.

Cho, C.H., Mei, Q.B., Shang, P., Lee, S.S., So, H.L., Guo, X., and Li, Y. (2000). Study of the gastrointestinal protective effects of polysaccharides from *Angelica sinensis* in rats. *Planta Medica* 66(4): 348-351.

Choy, Y.M., Leung, K.N., Cho, C.S., Wong, C.K., and Pang, P.K.T. (1994). Immunopharmacological studies of low molecular weight polysaccharide from *Angelica sinensis*. *American Journal of Chinese Medicine* 22: 137-145.

Dixon-Shanies, D. and Shaikh, N. (1999). Growth inhibition of human breast cancer cells by herbs and phytoestrogens. *Oncology Reports* 6: 1383-1387.

Dobelis, I.N., Dwyer, J., and Rattray, D. (Eds.) (1986). *Magic and Medicine of Plants*. New York: Reader's Digest International.

Duke, J.A. (1985). *CRC Handbook of Medicinal Herbs*. Boca Raton, FL: CRC Press, p. 44.

Eagon, C.L., Elm, M.S., Teepe, A.G., and Eagon, P.K. (1997). Medicinal botanicals: Estrogenicity in rat uterus and liver. *Proceedings of the American Association for Cancer Research* 38: 293 (abstract).

Eagon, P. (1999). Personal communication with Kenneth Jones, August 23, 1999.

Ellis, G.R. and Stephens, M.R. (1999). Untitled. *British Medical Journal* 319: 650.

Foster, S. and Yue, C. (1992). *Herbal Emissaries: Bringing Chinese Herbs to the West.* Rochester, VT: Healing Arts Press, p. 71.

Fugh-Berman, A. and Ernst, E. (2001). Herb-drug interactions: Review and assessment of report reliability. *British Journal of Clinical Pharmacology* 52: 587-595.

Guo, L.Q., Taniguchi, M., Chen, Q.Y., Baba, K., and Yamazoe, Y. (2001). Inhibitory potential of herbal medicines on human cytochrome P450-mediated oxidation: Properties of umbelliferous or citrus crude drugs and their relative prescriptions. *Japanese Journal of Pharmacology* 85: 399-408.

Hirata, J.D., Swiersz, L.M., Zell, B., Small, R., and Ettinger, B. (1997). Does dong quai have estrogenic effects in postmenopausal women? A double-blind, placebo-controlled trial. *Fertility and Sterility* 68: 981-986.

Hsu, H.Y., Chen, Y.P., Shen, S.J., Hsu, C.S., Chen, C.C., and Chang, H.C. (Eds.) (1986). *Oriental Materia Medica: A Concise Guide.* Long Beach, CA: Oriental Healing Arts Institute, pp. 540-542.

Leung, A. Y. and Foster, S. (1996). *Encyclopedia of Common Natural Ingredients Used in Food, Drugs, and Cosmetics,* Second Edition. New York: John Wiley and Sons, pp. 32-34.

Lin, L.Z., He, X.G., Lian, L.Z., King, W., and Elliot, J. (1998). Liquid chromatographic-electrospray mass spectrometric study of the phthalides of *Angelica sinensis* and chemical changes of Z-ligustilide. *Journal of Chromatography* 810: 71-79.

Liu, J., Burdette, J.E., Xu, H., Gu, C., van Breemen, R.B., Bhat, K.P., Booth, N., Constantinou, A.I., Pezzuto, J.M., Fong, H.H., et al. (2001). Evaluation of estrogenic activity of plant extracts for the potential treatment of menopausal symptoms. *Journal of Agricultural and Food Chemistry* 49: 2472-2479.

Liu, J.H., Zschocke, S., Reininger, E., and Bauer, R. (1998). Inhibitory effects of *Angelica pubescens* f. *biserrata* on 5-lipoxygenase and cyclooxygenase. *Planta Medica* 64: 525-529.

Lo, A.C.T., Chan, K., Yeung, J.H.K., and Woo, K.S. (1995). Danggui *(Angelica sinensis)* affects the pharmacodynamics but not the pharmacokinetics of warfarin rabbits. *European Journal of Drug Metabolism and Pharmacokinetics* 20: 55-60.

Matsui, A.S., Rogers, J., Woo, Y.K., and Cutting, W.C. (1967). Effects of some natural products on fertility in mice. *Medicina et Pharmacologia Experimentalis. International Journal of Experimental Medicine* 16: 414-424.

McGuffin, M., Hobbs, C., Upton, R., and Goldberg, A. (1997). *American Herbal Products Association's Botanical Safety Handbook.* Boca Raton, FL: CRC Press, p. 11.

Mei, Q.B., Tao, J.Y., and Cui, B. (1991). Advances in the pharmacological studies of radix *Angelica sinensis* (Oliv) Diels (Chinese danggui). *Chinese Medical Journal* 104: 776-781.

Murray, M.T. (1995). *The Healing Power of Herbs*. New York: Prima Publishing, pp. 43-49.

Nambiar, S., Schwartz, R.H., and Constantino, A. (1999). Hypertension in mother and baby linked to ingestion of Chinese herbal medicine. *Western Journal of Medicine* 171: 152 (letter).

Newall, C.A., Anderson, L.A., and Phillipson, J.D. (1996). *Herbal Medicine. A Guide for Health Care Professionals*. London: The Pharmaceutical Press, pp. 28-29.

Northrup, C. (1995). *Meno Times*. San Rafael, CA: The Menopause Center, Fall.

Ozaki, Y. and Ma, J.P. (1990). Inhibitory effects of tetramethylpyrazine and ferulic acid on spontaneous movement of rat uterus *in situ*. *Chemical and Pharmaceutical Bulletin* 38: 1620-1623.

Page, R.L. and Lawrence, J.D. (1999). Potentiation of warfarin by dong quai. *Pharmacotherapy* 19: 870-876.

Sheu, S.J., Ho, Y.S., Chen, Y.P., and Hsu, H.Y. (1987). Analysis and processing of Chinese herbal drugs, VI. The study of *Angelicae radix*. *Planta Medica* 53: 377-378.

Shimizu, M., Matsuzawa, T., Suzuki, S., Yoshizaki, M., and Morita, N. (1991). Evaluation of *Angelicae radix* (Touki) by the inhibitory effect on platelet aggregation. *Chemical and Pharmaceutical Bulletin* 39: 2046-2048.

Sung, C.P., Baker, A.P., Holden, D.A., Smith, W.J., and Chakrin, L.W. (1982). Effect of extracts of *Angelica polymorpha* on reaginic antibody production. *Journal of Natural Products* 45: 398-406.

Terasawa, K., Imadaya, A., Tosa, H., Mitsuma, T., Toriizuke, K., Takeda, K., Mikage, M., Hattori, M., and Namba, T. (1985). Chemical and clinical evaluation of crude drugs derived from *Angelica acutilobae* and *A. sinensis*. *Fitoterapia* 56: 201-208.

Tu, G., Fang, Q., Guo, J., Yuan, S., Chen, C., Chen, J., Chen, Z., Cheng, S., Jin, R., Li, M., et al. (Eds.) (1992). *Pharmacopoeia of the People's Republic of China*. Guangzhou, China: Guangdong Science and Technology Press, p. 150.

Wang, H., Kong, L., and Zhang, Y. (1999). Screening and analysis of biologically active compounds in *Angelica sinensis* by molecular biochromatography. *Chromatographia* 50: 439-445.

Willard, T. (1991). *The Wild Rose Scientific Herbal*. Calgary, Alberta, Canada: Wild Rose College of Natural Healing.

Yamada, H., Kiyohara, H., Cyong, J.C., Kojima, Y., Kumazawa, Y., and Otsuka, Y. (1984). Studies on polysaccharides from *Angelica acutiloba*. Part 1. Fractionation and biological properties of polysaccharides. *Planta Medica* 50: 163-167.

Yamamoto, H., Mizutani, T., and Nomura, H. (1982). Studies on the mutagenicity of crude drug extracts. I. *Yakugaku Zasshi* 102: 596-601.

Yamasaki, K., Kikuoka, M., Nishi, H., Kokusenya, Y., Miyamoto, T., Matsuo, M., and Sato, T. (1994). Contents of lecithin and choline in crude drugs. *Chemical and Pharmaceutical Bulletin* 42: 105-107.

Ye, Y.N., Koo, M.W., Li, Y., Matsui, H., and Cho, C.H. (2001). *Angelica sinensis* modulates migration and proliferation of gastric epithelial cells. *Life Sciences* 68: 961-968.

Yoshihiro, K. (1985). The physiological actions of tang-kuei and cnidium. *Bulletin of the Oriental Healing Arts Institute of USA* 10: 269-278.

Zava, D.T., Dollbaum, C.M., and Blen, M. (1998). Estrogen and progestin bio-activity of foods, herbs, and spices. *Proceedings of the Society for Experimental Biology and Medicine* 217: 369-378.

Zhu, D.P. (1987). Dong quai. *American Journal of Chinese Medicine* 15: 117-125.

Zhu, Y.P. (1998). *Chinese Materia Medica: Chemistry, Pharmacology and Applications*. Amsterdam, The Netherlands: Harwood Academic, pp. 579-583.

Zschocke, S., Liu, J.H., Stuppner, H., and Bauer, R. (1998). Comparative study of roots of *Angelica sinensis* and related Umbelliferous drugs by thin layer chromatography, high-performance liquid chromatography, and liquid chromatography-mass spectrometry. *Phytochemical Analysis* 9: 283-290.

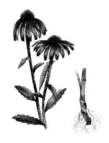

Echinacea

BOTANICAL DATA

Classification and Nomenclature

Scientific name: *Echinacea purpurea* (L.) Moench, *Echinacea angustifolia* DC var. *angustifolia, Echinacea angustifolia* DC var. *strigosa* McGregor, and *Echinacea pallida* (Nutt.) Nutt.

Family name: Asteraceae (Compositae)

Common names: echinacea; *E. angustifolia:* narrow-leaved purple coneflower, black sampson, snake root; *E. purpurea:* purple coneflower; *E. pallida:* pale purple coneflower. Other common names applied to one or more species include: American coneflower, black Susan, comb flower, hedgehog, Indian head, Kansas snakeroot, Missouri snakeroot, scurvy root (Foster, 1991)

Description

Echinacea species are native to North America and are distributed throughout the eastern and central United States and southern Canada. Three *Echinacea* species, as noted, are commercially important sources of phytopharmaceuticals and other medicinal preparations. The most widely accepted taxonomic interpretation of the genus is found in McGregor (1968), under which there are nine species and two varieties. Formerly considered a variety of *Echinacea pallida, E. angustifolia* and *E. purpurea* are treated as separate species by McGregor on the basis of morphological criteria, cultivation and hybridization experiments, and cytological features (Foster, 1991). In the future, however, the name *E. purpurea* (L.) Moench could be revised to *E. serotina* (Nutt.) DC. (Binns et al., 2001a,b). Studies on commercial preparations of *E. angustifolia* published before 1987 may therefore be those of *E. pallida*, or other common adulterants, such as *Parthenium integrifolium* (Bradley, 1992; Hobbs, 1989).

HISTORY AND TRADITIONAL USES

Echinacea is a true Native American medicinal plant, and was used for a variety of medicinal purposes by American Indian tribes including the Cheyenne (sore mouth and gums); Choctaw (coughs, dyspepsia), Comanche (toothache, sore throat); Crow (colds, toothache, colic); Dakota (inflammation, bowel complaints, sepsis, tonsillitis, hydrophobia, toothache, snakebite; headache and distemper in horses); Delaware (gonorrhea); Hidatsa (stimulant); Kiowa (coughs, sore throat); Meskwaki (stomach cramps, fits); Omaha (septic diseases, stings); Omaha-Ponca (eyewash, hair comb); Pawnee (rattlesnake bites) and Winnebago (anesthetic) (Hobbs, 1989).

Echinacea first entered mainstream herbal medicine in 1870 when H.C.F. Meyer, a German lay healer, introduced "Meyer's Blood Purifier." It was an extract containing echinacea, among other constituents, and was widely touted as a cure-all. Anecdotal reports of efficacy in the treatment of snakebites, typhus, diphtheria, and other infections attracted the attention of ninteenth century eclectic physicians, particularly John King, author of the *American Dispensatory* (1852), and the pharmacist and writer John Uri Lloyd. Echinacea was introduced into eclectic medical practices in 1887 and remained a popular remedy used by eclectic physicians for the following 50 years. In the 1920s, echinacea was sold to medical practitioners in the United States more extensively than any other herb, and from 1950 to 1991, over 200 studies were published on the chemistry, pharmacology, and clinical application of echinacea (Foster, 1991). It was estimated that at least 150 studies remained unpublished (Hobbs, 1989). Echinacea is used today in dozens of preparations in European phytomedicine, and is an ingredient, along with pot marigold *(Calendula officinalis)* and wormwood *(Artemisia absinthium),* of the antiseptic liniment Absorbine Jr. (Awang and Kindack, 1991).

CHEMISTRY

Echinacea species contain a great variety of chemical components which contribute to their activity. Some of the constituents are unique to one species, while others occur in two or more of the commercially important species. Seven classes of secondary compounds are considered important to the therapeutic actions of echinacea, and these have received the most intensive study (Bauer and Wagner, 1991) (see Figure 1).

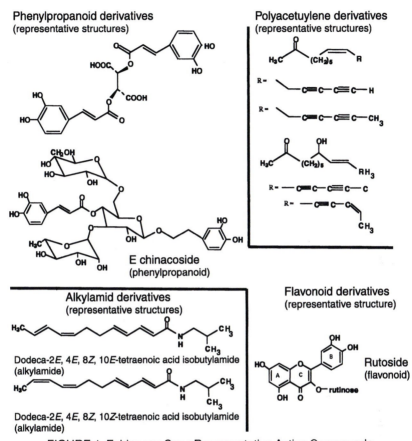

Phenylpropanoid derivatives
(representative structures)

E chinacoside
(phenylpropanoid)

Polyacetuylene derivatives
(representative structures)

Alkylamid derivatives
(representative structures)

Dodeca-2*E*, 4*E*, 8*Z*, 10*E*-tetraenoic acid isobutylamide
(alkylamide)

Dodeca-2*E*, 4*E*, 8*Z*, 10*Z*-tetraenoic acid isobutylamide
(alkylamide)

Flavonoid derivatives
(representative structure)

Rutoside
(flavonoid)

FIGURE 1. Echinacea Spp.: Representative Active Compounds

Caffeic Acid Derivatives

Caffeic acid derivatives reported from *Echinacea* species include echin-acoside, verbascoside, des-rhamnosylverbascoside and 6-*O*-caffeoylechin-acoside, cynarin, cichoric acid, caftaric, chlorogenic and isochlorogenic ac-ids, and others (Bauer and Wagner, 1991). Cichoric acid was identified as the main phenolic compound in the tops (mean 2.02%) and roots (mean 2.27%) of *E. purpurea* and showed much higher mean concentrations in summer than autumn. The main phenolic in the roots of *E. pallida* (August) and *E. angustifolia* (May) was identified as echinacoside (mean 0.34% and 1.04%, respectively). Cynarin was found in *E. angustifolia* roots at a mean concentration of 0.12%, whereas only trace amounts were found in the roots or tops of the two other species (Perry et al., 2001).

Flavonoids

Rutoside is the major flavonoid found in the leaves of *Echinacea angustifolia, E. pallida,* and *E. purpurea.* In addition, the following flavonoids have been reported, and occur as both the aglycones and as conjugates with various sugars: luteolin, kaempferol, quercetin, quercetagetin, apigenin, and isorhamnetin. The flavonoid content of the leaves, calculated as quercetin, has been estimated at 0.48% for *E. purpurea* and 0.38% for *E. angustifolia* (Bauer and Wagner, 1991).

Essential Oil

All three commercially important *Echinacea* species contain varying amounts of essential oils in the roots, leaves, flowers, and other aerial parts. Concentrations of total essential oil vary widely from species to species. Typical concentrations for fresh materials range from 0.05-0.48%, and in dried materials from <0.1% to 1.25%, depending on the plant part (Bauer and Wagner, 1991).

Essential oil components common to the three most investigated species *(Echinacea angustifolia, E. pallida,* and *E. purpurea)* include borneol, bornylacetate, pentadeca-8-ene-2-one, germacrene D, caryophyllene, caryophyllene epoxide, and palmitic acid. In addition to these constituents, volatile components have been identified that are unique to each species (Bauer and Wagner, 1991).

Polyacetylenes

Polyacetylenes are widespread in the Asteraceae family, and Schulte et al. (1967) determined the structures of 5 compounds in the series found in *Echinacea.* An additional eight were partially elucidated. The main constituents were determined as trideca-1-en-3,5,7,9,10-pentayne and ponticaepoxide, present in *Echinacea purpurea* and *E. angustifolia.* A total polyace content of 2 mg% of the fresh roots was reported and it was observed that the content decreased markedly during long-term storage of the ground root; four commercial samples of echinacea preparations contained no detectable polyacetylenes.

Alkylamides

Natural alkylamides (or alkamides) are abundant in *Echinacea* species, as well as other members of the Compositae tribes, *Anthemideae* and *Heliantheae.* The first alkylamide isolated from *Echinacea,* echinacein (dodeca-(2E,6Z,8E,10E)-tetraenoic acid), was reported in the roots of *E. angustifolia* (0.01%) and *E. pallida* (0.001%). Numerous other alkylamides have since been identified by Bauer et al. (1989) in *E. purpurea* and *E. angustifolia* (Bauer, 1998). Determination of the major alkylamides showed that they accumulate primarily in the roots and inflorescences, with the highest content being found in the roots of *E. angustifolia* (0.009-0.15%); by contrast, *E. pallida* roots contain very low levels, and *E. purpurea* roots contain 0.004-0.039% (Bauer and Remiger, 1989). In a more extensive determination, Perry et al. (1997) found the major alkylamides in 1.5-year-old *E. purpurea* at highest levels (mean 14.1 mg/g) in the vegetative stems, with lesser amounts in the rhizome (mean 5.7 mg/g), flower (mean 2.7 mg/g), and root (mean 1.7 mg/g). The higher levels of alkylamides in the New Zealand-grown samples of *E. purpurea,* compared to earlier determinations of the species by Bauer and Remiger (1989), may be due to losses upon storage or differences in growing areas. Alkylamides are also present in other *Echinacea* species (Bauer and Remiger, 1989) and are susceptible to temperature-related degradation during storage of root material (Perry et al., 2000; Wills and Stuart, 2000; Livesey et al., 1999).

Alkaloids

Early reports of an "alkaloid" in *Echinacea* species were subsequently shown to be due to the presence of betaine *(Echinacea angustifolia)* and/or glycine betaine *(E. purpurea).* Traces of the pyrrolizidine alkaloids (0.006% in dried materials) tussilagine and isotussilagine, were reported in both *E. purpurea* and *E. angustifolia.* According to structure/activity studies, a 1,2-unsaturated necine ring system is necessary for pyrrolizidine alkaloids to be hepatotoxic. Since neither of the pyrrolizidines from *Echinacea* have this structure, there is little risk of liver damage for consumers (Bauer and Wagner, 1991).

Polysaccharides

Polysaccharides have been implicated as one of the primary classes of immunostimulatory compounds in *Echinacea* species. Two immunostimulatory polysaccharides, PS I and PS II, were isolated from the aerial parts of *Echinacea purpurea.* Structural studies revealed PS I to be a 4-*O*-methyl-glucuronoarabinoxylan with an average molecular weight (MW) of 35 kDa, while PS II is an acidic arabinorhamnogalactan of 50 kDa. A xyloglucan (79 kDa) was also isolated from the leaves and stems of *E. purpurea.* None of these are identical to a pectinlike polysaccharide, isolated from the expressed juice, which possessed only weak immunostimulatory activity (Bauer and Wagner, 1991). The immunostimulatory polysaccharides of *Echinacea* species can be produced in cell cultures of *E. purpurea* on an industrial scale (Bauer and Wagner, 1991). In the pressed juice of *E. purpurea,* Classen et al. (2000) identified a high-molecular weight arabinogalactan-protein ("Echinacea AGP" with estimated weight 1.2×10^6 Da) which showed a number of great similarities to arabinogalactan-proteins isolated from apple juice and grape juice.

Echinacea also contains fructose and fructan polymers. Giger et al. (1989) reported that the total fructosan content of *Echinacea purpurea* increased during the winter, whereas this process occurred later in the season in *E. angustifolia.* The fructan content of the aerial parts of *E. purpurea* was ten times less than that of the roots, and the leaves and stems of *E. angustifolia* contained practically none. Homeopathic tinctures were also found to contain fructans (Giger et al., 1989).

Other Constituents

Other constituents reported from echinacea species include reducing sugars, phytosterols, a series of n-alkanes (see Essential Oil) and inorganic constituents (potassium, calcium, magnesium, iron (III), aluminum, sulphate, carbonate, chloride, and silicate). Ascorbic acid has been found in the leaves of *Echinacea purpurea* (0.214% of dry weight). Sitosterol, myristic, and linoleic acid were detected in *E. angustifolia.* Cyanidin glycosides have been isolated from the flowers of *E. purpurea* and *E. pallida.* Three glycoproteins (MW 17, 21, and 30 kDa) were isolated from *E. angustifolia* (Bauer and Wagner, 1991).

The sesquiterpene esters, echinadiol-, echinaxanthol-, and dihydroxynardolcinnamate, originally described by Bauer et al. (1986) as constituents of *Echinacea purpurea* roots, are in fact derived from the adulterant, *Parthenium integrifolium,* which was mistakenly processed at the time when adulteration by this species was common in commercial echinacea products (Bauer et al., 1987).

THERAPEUTIC APPLICATIONS

In Germany, echinacea root products must state on the label that they are used to help the body resist common cold infections affecting the throat, nasal passages, and head. When required, these uses do not exclude concomitant use of chemotherapeutic drugs or antibiotics, which may be necessary (Bradley, 1992). The German Commission E on herbal medicines lists indications for the fresh-pressed juice of *Echinacea purpurea* (aerial parts) in supportive therapy to treat colds, chronic infections of the respiratory tract, and of the lower urinary tract (Blumenthal, 1998). It is interesting to note that at least 14 early studies of echinacea in Germany reported benefits in urogenital diseases, two of which concerned prostatitis (Hobbs, 1989). The

German Commission E also lists *E. pallida* root tinctures as a supportive therapy in the treatment of common coldlike infections (Bauer, 1998).

In the *British Herbal Compendium* (1992), a companion to the *British Herbal Pharmacopoeia* Volume 1, echinacea is indicated in the treatment of chronic bacterial and viral infections, skin complaints, furunculosis, and mild septicemia. Other included uses are the prophylaxis of influenza and colds (Bradley, 1992).

PRECLINICAL STUDIES

Immune Functions; Inflammation and Disease

Cancer

Antiproliferative activity. The antitumor effects of echinacea are related to its general immunopotentiating actions and specifically to its activation of macrophages (Bauer and Wagner, 1991; Steinmüller et al., 1993); however, (Z)-1,8-pentadecadiene, a component of *E. angustifolia* and *E. pallida* root, possesses significant in vitro antitumor effects (Voaden and Jacobson, 1972).

Immune Functions

Immunopotentiation. Although some controversy exists about which of the constituents of echinacea contribute to immunostimulatory activity (Rininger et al., 2000; Witthohn et al., 2000; South and Exon, 2001; Goel et al., 2002), there is a consensus that the lipophilic alkylamides, as well as the polar caffeic acid derivative, cichoric acid, probably make the primary contribution to the activity of alcoholic extracts. In addition to these constituents, polysaccharides are implicated in the activity of the expressed juice of aerial parts of *E. purpurea* (Echinacin) (Witthohn et al., 2000) and aqueous extracts, and in the response to the powdered whole drug. However, only low concentrations of polysaccharides are found in the expressed juice, and they are different in composition to those in the extract of the aerial parts (Bauer and Wagner, 1991).

Echinacea appears to enhance cell-mediated immunity by activating T lymphocytes and NK cells. The polysaccharides of echinacea are reported to bind to the surface of T cells, inducing interferon and other immunopotentiating substances. The result is enhanced T cell replication, increased macrophage activity, antibody binding, and an increase in the numbers of circulating neutrophils which phagocytize bacteria, viruses, tumor cells, and particulates. This nonspecific immune stimulation also stimulates NK cells, a type of white blood cell important in the destruction of tumor cells and virus-infected cells (Bauer and Wagner, 1991).

Low concentrations (0.012 μg/mL) of the unpurified fresh-pressed juice of *E. purpurea* aboveground parts (Echina-Fresh), as well as the dried juice cultured with normal human peripheral blood macrophages, significantly increased production of IL-10, IL-6, IL-1, and TNF-α (Burger et al., 1997).

Brokos et al. (1999) reported a greater in vitro stimulation of human white blood cells from a standardized sap preparation than from a standardized extract of *E. purpurea* (Herbapol, Kleka, Poland). Compared to the extract, the sap elevated the mitotic indices of human lymphocytes about 200% more effectively. T helper (CD4) cells showed no difference in frequency compared to the control, but T suppressor (CD8) cells were found to decrease from the echinacea preparations by about 20% to 25%, although only significantly from the sap. B lymphocytes showed a decrease of about 25% from either preparation, and NK cells increased in number by 30% to 90% from the sap, and by 5% to 30% from the extract. Free radical generation by nonstimulated, resting granulocytes (a measure of activation) was enhanced by the sap, whereas the extract caused a marked inhibition of free radical generation (by 25% at the highest concentration tested). In stimulated granulocytes, the sap caused free radical generation to markedly decrease (by 20% at the highest concentration tested), whereas the extract had no effect. At the lowest concentration, the extract rather enhanced free radical generation, although only by 10%. It was concluded that the sap caused potentially more beneficial effects compared to the extract. The results were interpreted as an indication that the sap may serve as an immunostimulant on resting human granulocytes when they are starting to act against foreign cells, while at the same time it may limit the damage to cells (free radical inhibition) at times when granulocytes are battling foreign cells.

Echinacea polysaccharides activate macrophages, a type of white blood cell which engulfs foreign particles, including bacteria and cellular debris. The polysaccharides enhance phagocytosis and induce macrophages to produce immune-potentiating compounds (cytokines), including interferon, TNF, and ILs. The stimulation of macrophages is one of the primary mechanisms responsible for the immune-potentiating actions of the echinacea polysaccharides. The alkylamides and caffeic acid derivatives also contribute to macrophage activation. Since the alkylamides yield the most potent macrophage-stimulating action, it is likely that these compounds are responsible for the activity of alcoholic extracts, which contain little or no polysaccharide (Bauer and Wagner, 1991).

Root extracts of echinacea have shown greater phagocytic stimulating activity in mice (1.66 mg/100 g p.o., t.i.d. for two days) in the carbon clearance and granulocyte smear tests than the aerial portion, in the order *E. purpurea* > *E. angustifolia* > *E. pallida* (Bauer et al., 1989, 1988; Bauer and Wagner, 1991). Also, alcoholic extracts were more active than aqueous extracts of the aerial parts (Bauer et al., 1989). Alcoholic extracts of the roots of echinacea in the same dosages and tests showed phagocytic stimulating activity in the order of *E. purpurea* > *E. angustifolia* or *E. pallida* (Bauer et al., 1988), and all these extracts caused phagocytosis to increase by 20% to 30%, which corresponded well with in vivo results (Bauer and Wagner, 1991).

Rehman et al. (1999) examined the effect of an *E. angustifolia* root extract (Eclectic Institute, Sandy, OR) on antigen-specific immunity in male rats; specifically on immunoglobulins G and M. Antibodies were elicited by repeated exposure of the rats to keyhole limpet hemocyanin (KLH) antigen and the control group was treated with vehicle (ethanol). The echinacea group received 1 g/mL in ethanol per liter of drinking water, and normal drinking water was also provided. Between the two groups, no significant difference in water consumption was found. Compared to the control group, the echinacea-treated rats showed significantly higher production levels of IgG antibodies (anti-KLH), which showed a rapid increase in the first seven days and reached significance on day 7. Even with a booster shot of the antigen on day 14, IgG levels remained high in the echinacea group, and were significantly higher than the control group when checked on days 21, 24, and 27. On day 31, at which point the control group attained their maximum levels of anti-KLH IgG titers, the difference was no longer significant. As for IgM, no significant difference compared to the levels in the control group was evident, although there was a trend towards higher levels in the echinacea group. In further studies of immunomodulatory medicinal plants, attention should be given to time-dependent effects in the assessment of immune functions to identify the times at which the plant produces maximal results (Rehman et al., 1999). IgG makes up about 75% of the immunoglobulin in the serum of normal adults and can cross the human placenta. IgG protects newborns in their first months out of the womb, and patients with a selective IgG deficiency suffer from recurrent infections of the respiratory tract. Selective IgM deficiency is also associated with susceptibility to recurrent respiratory infections (Stites et al., 1994).

In a detailed study, Currier and Miller (2000) examined the effect of a proprietary extract of *E. purpurea* root (Phyto Adrien Gagnon, Sante Naturelle, LaPrairie, Quebec, Canada) on NK cell function and production in aging male mice (15-16 months old). The extract was added to mouse chow to provide a dose of 0.45 mg/day for 14 days. The addition of the extract had no effect on the quantity of chow consumed compared to controls fed plain chow. Results were compared to the effects of a ten-day, bidaily treatment with thyroxin i.p., a known NK cell stimulant. Thyroxin treatment resulted in a significant elevation in the cytolytic function of NK cells compared to untreated controls; however, bone marrow production of NK cells, and subsequently numbers of NK cells in the spleen, were not significantly affected and there was no significant effect on other hemopoietic and immune cells lineages in either the bone marrow or spleen. Practically the opposite results were found in the aging mice that fed on the echinacea-supplemented feed, with both function and number of NK cells significantly increased and reaching levels comparable to those of young, adult mice. The increase in their number in bone marrow compared to plain chow-fed aging mice was highly significant ($p < 0.004$), in part because the level was undetectable in the control group, as is the norm in aging mice. Subsequently, the echinacea group showed 30% more NK cells in their spleens compared to the control group, and the total absolute level of their activity was 20% higher than those of the controls. Cytolytic activity of the NK cell also showed a significant increase ($p < 0.03$-0.001), indicating increased function. However, just as the result with thyroxin, no significant effect was found on other hemopoietic and immune cells lineages in either the bone marrow or spleen.

As are part of the first line of immunological defense of the body against virus-infected and tumor cells, the stimulation of monocytes and NK cells by echinacea represents a chemopreventive action. Surgical interventions and stress in rats have been shown to cause a significant suppression of NK cell activity which resulted in a greater incidence of death from mammary tumors and leukemia as a result of decreased host resistance (Ben-Eliyahu et al., 1999).

Infectious Diseases

Fungal infections. Monocytes and granulocytes collected from healthy human donors were treated in vitro with a liquid extract (22% alcohol) of the fresh blossoms of *E. purpurea* to test the ability of the herb to increase phagocytosis of *Candida albicans*. Phagocytic activity of both immune cell populations was significantly increased against *C. albicans* by 30% to 45% (Wildfeuer and Mayerhofer, 1994).

Möse (1983) used the blood from 12 men (ages 21-24) following their treatment with the fresh expressed juice of *E. purpurea* aerial parts (Echinacin, 2 mL/day i.m. for four consecutive days). In vitro granulocytic phagocytosis of *Candida albicans* increased from 20% to 30% at the start to nearly 50% on days three or four of the treatment.

Roesler et al. (1991) used purified polysaccharides derived from large-scale cultures of *E. purpurea* plant cells to test the ability of mouse-derived immunological cells to inhibit *Candida albicans*. These were two neutral fucogalactoxyloglucans of mean MW 10,000 and 25,000 and one acidic arabinogalactan of mean MW 75,000 in a ratio of two parts xyloglucans to one of arabinogalactan. Kupffer cells preincubated with the mixture of polysaccharides (0.2 mg/mL) were then incubated with *C. albicans*. Macrophages activated by the polysaccharides (1:10 parts growth medium) inhibited the growth of the yeast cells by approximately 70%. Following coincubation with the polysaccharides (1 mg/mL), macrophage release of reactive oxygen intermediates (free radicals) was increased by approximately 270%. Roesler et al. showed that the polysaccharide mixture administered 24 h prior to, at infection, and 24 h postinfection (0.2 mg i.v.) protected mice infected with a lethal dose of *C. albicans.* Colony-forming units (CFUs) of *C. albicans* were reduced to 5% of the number found in yeast-infected, untreated control mice; however, when administered 18 h following infection, there was little if any reduction in the growth of *C. albicans* by the polysaccharide treatment (Roesler et al., 1991).

Steinmüller et al. (1993) conducted similar studies in immunodeficient mice. Treatment with the polysaccharide mixture (0.2 mg i.v. on the same day, 24 and 48 h following *C. albicans* infection) in cyclophosphamide-treated mice (200 mg/kg, three days prior to infection) resulted in a 36.9 to 80% reduction in CFUs of *C. albicans* in their kidneys. Cyclosporine-induced immunodeficiency in mice was ameliorated following treatment with the same dose of polysaccharides. Challenged with *C. albicans,* their kidneys showed about 80% less CFUs.

Binns et al. (2000) examined the ability of *n*-hexane extracts of *E. purpurea* to inhibit the growth of *Saccharomyces cerevisiae* and clinical and nonpathogenic strains and species of *Candida* after exposure to near UV light. Near UV-mediated growth inhibition of the pathogenic fungi was found from locally purchased products, including a tincture of *E. purpurea* root, a tincture containing roots of *E. purpurea* and *E. angustifolia* in equal parts, and a tincture made up of 5% root mother tincture and 95% herb mother tincture (each in 55% ethanol). However, an echinacea tea and an extract prepared from the tops of the plant (inflorescences, stems, and leaves) was inactive. Greatest near UV-mediated inhibition of fungal growth was exhibited by an *n*-hexane extract prepared from fresh *E. purpurea* and *E. pallida* roots, which were significantly more active that *n*-hexane extracts prepared from the tops of these species. Compared to all the other preparations tested, the *n*-hexane extract of *E. purpurea* root was the most active, with phototoxicity evident in 12 isolates of the fungi and in eight showing light-independent growth inhibition. The extract of the inflorescence was active against seven isolates and light-independently against two. The difference was attributed to types and amounts of acetylenic compounds in the different plant parts. Active constituents in the form of polyacetylenic compounds were isolated from *n*-hexane extracts of the root and tops of *E. purpurea.* Preliminary results against *S. cerevisiae* revealed three photoactive polyacetylenes, the most significantly active ($p = 0.065$) being dodeca-2*E*,4*E*,8*E*,10*E*/*Z*-tetranoic acid isobutylamide (536 ppm and 1123 ppm in the root and inflorescence, respectively), and undeca-2*E*,4*Z*-diene-8,10-diynoic isobutylamide ($p = 0.116$), which was the most abundant (7.57% and 1.45% of the inflorescence and root, respectively).

Microbial infections. Echinacea has some mild antimicrobial activity which is attributed primarily to echinacoside, a caffeic acid derivative (Stoll et al., 1950). Echinacoside occurs in the roots (0.3% to 1.3% mg/g, dry weight) and flowers (0.1% to 1%) of *Echinacea angustifolia,* and in the roots of *E. pallida* (0.4% to 1.4% mg/g dry weight), but not in *E. purpurea* (Bauer and Wagner, 1991). Echinacoside has shown in vitro activity against the growth of *Staphylococcus aureus,* against which a concentration of 6 mg was found about as potent as one unit of penicillin (Stoll et al., 1950). Polyacetylene compounds from the roots of *E. angustifolia* and *E. purpurea* have shown strong inhibitory activity in vitro against *Pseudomonas aeruginosa* and *Escherichia* (Schulte et al., 1967). *Echinacea pupurea* in a diluted concentration of 1:1,000 totally inhibited growth of *Epidermophyton interdigitale* (Jung and Schröeder, 1954), a pathogen that causes athlete's foot.

Viral infections. Alcoholic and aqueous extracts of echinacea inhibit some viruses in cell culture, including influenza, herpes, and vesicular stomatitis viruses (Wacker and Hilbig, 1978; May and Wiluhn, 1978). The aqueous extract of *E. angustifolia* root showed no activity against poliovirus type 1, influenza A_2, or herpes simplex type 2 (HSV2), but that of *E. purpurea* was moderately active against HSV2 and influenza A_2 (May and Willuhn, 1978). *Echinacea purpurea* root extract was reported to be more potent than those of *E. angustifolia* or *E. pallida* at increasing host resistance and in stimulating macrophages, production of IL-1, IL-6, TNF-α, and $INF_{a,b}$ in vivo and in vitro, and at exhibiting antiviral activity against influenza A (Hong Kong) and herpes simplex virus 1 in vitro (Bodinet et al., 1993).

Wacker and Hilbig (1978) reported that both aqueous and methanolic extracts of echinacea (20 mg/mL) were active against viral cytopathogenicity following incubation of cells with the extracts (*E. purpurea* roots). They found mouse fibroblasts became 50-80% resistant to the viruses for 24 h or more, and that the resistance was absent at 48 h. In the presence of hyaluronidase, however, mammalian cells incubated with extracts of *E. purpurea* showed no resistance to the viruses (Wacker and Hilbig, 1978).

Some components, such as caffeic acid derivatives, may block viral receptors on the cell surface (Bauer and Wagner, 1991). In addition to caffeic acid, the caffeic acid derivative echinacoside, and chicoric acid, a tartaric acid derivative, derived from the flowers and leaves of *E. pallida,* were reported to show in vitro virustatic and antiviral activity against vesicular stomatitis virus (VSv) (Cheminat et al., 1988). In other cases, the inhibition of hyaluronidase is the likely antiviral mechanism; the viral inhibitory actions of echinacea extracts in vitro are diminished when hyaluronidase is added to the cell cultures (Bauer and Wagner, 1991). Antihyaluronidase activity was shown from the caffeoyl conjugates caftaric and cichoric acids isolated from *E. angustifolia* roots (Maffei Facino et al., 1993).

Wacker and Hilbig (1978) also showed that the fresh juice of the whole plant *(E. purpurea)* was 30% more effective against the cytopathogenicity of VSv, influenza, and herpes viruses than the aqueous or the methanolic extracts. No additional juice or extracts were required for virustatic activity once the fibroblast cells had been cultured with them. Hydrochloric acid diminished the virustatic activity of the active parts of the extracts; however, at a concentration of 25 mg/mL, temperatures of 60-80°C for two h had little effect (Wacker and Hilbig, 1978; Hobbs, 1989).

Glycoprotein-rich fractions of *E. purpurea* roots administered to mice (i.v.) have shown significant immunomodulating activity, resulting in the release of cytokines interleukin-1 (IL-1) and tumor necrosis factor-α (TNF-α). The addition of the glycoprotein-rich fractions to mouse spleen cells in culture produced significant amounts of interferon α,β, which showed activity against vesicular stomatitis virus. Tested for direct antiviral activity in a herpes simplex plaque-reduction assay, the glycoprotein-rich fractions reduced 80% of plaques. Using the same assay, the ultrafiltered root extract of *E. purpurea* also showed direct activity against herpes simplex, reducing plaque formation by 100%, but only from a minimum high concentration of 200 mg/mL (Bodinet and Beuscher, 1991).

See et al. (1997) treated peripheral blood mononuclear cells from 20 normal subjects, 20 AIDS patients, and 20 chronic fatigue syndrome (CFS) patients with extracts of fresh *E. purpurea* (characterized according to the presence of alkylamides) in increasing concentrations. The extract (≥ 0.1 mg/mL) significantly increased natural killer (NK) cell function (K562-cell test), with each progressive increase in concentration of the extract (0.001 mg/mL to 100 mg/mL), regardless of the subject blood sample, compared to untreated cells. Cellular immune functionality of NK function was also shown using a T cell line infected with human herpesvirus 6 (HHV-6). The reactivation of this virus was suggested by others to possibly play a role in the pathogenesis of both AIDS and CFS. See and colleagues also reported a significant increase in antibody-dependent cellular cytotoxicity (ADCC) of *E. purpurea* extract-treated peripheral blood mononuclear cells against HHV-6 in the same concentrations used to test NK cell functionality; again, regardless of the subject blood sample. However, Möse (1983) found no effect on NK cell function (K562-cell test) in the blood from healthy males following a four-day treatment with Echinacin (2 mL/day, i.m.).

Inflammatory Response

Anti-inflammatory activities of echinacea extracts have been attributed to direct inhibition of hyaluronidase (Bauer and Wagner, 1991). An *n*-hexane extract of *E. angustifolia* roots inhibited 5-lipoxygenase by 81.8% (11.5 μg/mL) and cyclooxygenase by 62.4% (50 μg/mL). The inhibitory activities could be partly attributed to a mixture of alkamides isolated from the dried root; however, they showed less potency than the whole extract of the root (Müller-Jakic et al., 1994). Topically applied polysaccharide fractions and alkylamide fractions have displayed anti-inflammatory activity in the rat paw edema model, and the alkylamides strongly inhibited arachidonic acid metabolism in vitro (Bauer and Wagner, 1991).

Tubaro et al. (1987) administered the polysaccharide fraction of *E. angustifolia* roots (i.v.) to rats one hour before carrageenan-induced paw edema. A dosage of 50 mg/kg inhibited edema by 64.6%, and 89.7% with double the dose. In the Croton oil-induced edema model, swelling of the rat ear was significantly reduced by the polysaccharide fraction applied topically. In this model, the polysaccharide fraction (450 mg/ear, 96.3% inhibition) was approximately 50% as potent as indomethacin. It was determined that in the Croton oil ear test, high molecular weight polysaccharides in the fraction were more active than lower weight polysaccharides.

Integumentary, Muscular, and Skeletal Functions

Connective Tissue Functions

In Europe, topical preparations containing echinacea have a wide range of application in the treatment of skin problems. Research has indicated that they may also be potentially useful in the prevention of UV-induced skin damage. For example, in micromole amounts in vitro, echinacoside has shown a protective effect against free radical-induced degradation of collagen (Maffei Facino et al., 1995). In vitro studies using a mouse fibroblast populated collagen lattice as a model of wound healing demonstrated that ethanolic extracts of the aboveground parts of *E. purpurea* were more active than the root (Zoutewelle and van Wijk, 1990).

The fresh pressed juice of *Echinacea purpurea,* as well as the polysaccharide components, were shown to promote tissue regeneration in mice (Bauer and Wagner, 1991), an action most likely related to the ability of echinacea to stabilize hyaluronic acid and stimulate fibroblasts.

Hyaluronic acid, also known as kinetin, is a matrix of high molecular weight mucopolysaccharides, consisting principally of glutaminic acid and acetylglucosamine, which surrounds healthy cells, prevents the penetration of pathogenic organisms, and regulates the exchange of fluid and matter between the cells, including vascular cells and other tissues. Certain pathogenic bacteria *(Staphylococci, Pneumococci, Clostridium)* secrete an enzyme, hyaluronidase, which depolymerizes the polysaccharides of hyaluronic acid, enabling the pathogen to penetrate the cells (Bonadeo et al., 1971; Hobbs, 1989). An uncharacterized polysaccharide, echinacin B, is thought to form a complex with hyaluronic acid, thereby increasing resistance to hyaluronidase attack and leading to increased hyaluronic acid production, fibrosis, and the infiltration of fibroblasts necessary for wound healing (Bonadeo et al., 1971).

CLINICAL STUDIES

A number of controlled clinical trials have been conducted with echinacea species for various indications. Some of the key studies are summarized as follows. Although in European phytotherapy standardized preparations of echinacea extract are commonly given via injection (i.m., i.v., s.c.), preponderant evidence suggests that oral administration is also effective.

Immune Disorders; Inflammation and Disease

Immune Modulation

Melchart et al. (1994) provided a systematic review of controlled clinical trials in which echinacea was used as an immunomodulator. Out of 26 trials, 19 concerned the efficacy of echinacea against infections; four investigated the chance of reducing side effects of cancer therapies; and three concerned the modulation of immune system cells. Although 30 of the 34 primary researchers claimed that the treatments provided greater efficacy compared to the control groups, Melchart and colleagues determined that most of the studies scored low on quality of methodology. Only eight studies received a score of over 50% of the maximum score points possible. Melchart and colleagues concluded that while the clinical evidence available clearly shows that preparations containing echinacea can be effective as immunomodulators, insufficient evidence exists to recommend individual preparations for therapeutic use and what proper doses to give in specific conditions. They also cited the need for further, well-designed clinical studies to resolve these issues.

Jurcic et al. (1989) administered an ethanolic extract of *E. purpurea* root (30 drops p.o. t.i.d.) to a treatment group of 12 healthy males for five consecutive days and compared immunological changes to a placebo group of 12 men. Compared to readings taken at the start, granulocytic phagocytosis (modified Brandt test) on day five showed a maximal increase of 120% in the echinacea group. Granulocytic phagocytosis increased in the placebo group maximally by 30% compared to initial activity levels. Cessation of treatment in the echinacea group resulted in a gradual decrease in phagocytosis over three days to normal levels. Immunoglubulin and leukocyte levels, as well as the erythrocyte sedimentation rate, showed no change from their normal ranges. The treatment was well-tolerated by all participants. In this study, oral administration resulted in a considerably higher rate of immune stimulation than from parenteral administration (Jurcic et al., 1989).

Immunoprotection. In a study on the counteraction of exercise-induced immunosuppression, Berg et al. (1998) examined the immunoprotective effects of an *E. purpurea* extract (Madaus AG, Cologne, Germany, Echinacin EC31) in a double-blind, placebo-controlled, parallel group study. The extract was used as a pre-exercise treatment in 42 male triathletes (ages 18-47) while they underwent regular competitive sprint training. Randomized into three treatment groups using a double-dummy technique, the athletes received the extract (120 drops or 8 mL t.i.d. 28 days), a magnesium supplement (Madaus AG, Biomagnesin, t.i.d. for 28 days, equivalent to 43 mg magnesium), or placebo (flavored tablets and flavored drops of ethanol). The results showed that although the magnesium supplement-treated group responded much as the placebo-treated subjects, the echinacea-treated subjects showed a significantly enhanced exercised-induced decrease in levels of soluble IL-2 receptor (sIL-2R), a significantly greater exercise-induced increase in urine levels of IL-6, and a significantly greater exercise-induced increase in cortisol concentrations (but not one hour after the competition exercise). In addition, whereas three of the subjects in the magnesium group and four in the placebo group developed upper respiratory tract infections, previously known to be associated with strenuous exercise, there were no such cases in the echinacea group. The most consistently reported cytokine responses in athletes from exhaustive or strenuous exercise were increases in the release of IL-6 and sIL-2R, and IL-6 in the acute phase response to injury or infection. The absence of a significant decrease in NK cells in the echinacea groups suggested a counteraction of the effect of cortisol on these cells. Adverse effects were only reported in the placebo and magnesium groups who collectively lost 37 days of training time as a result, not counting two subjects who lost all of their training time due to upper respiratory tract infection. It was concluded that the results of this pilot study need to be validated by further clinical trials to confirm the findings.

Infectious Diseases

Microbial infections. In providing an assessment of randomized trials of echinacea in the treatment of upper respiratory tract infections (URTIs), Barrett (2000) examined six double-blind, randomized, placebo-controlled trials of formulations tested for the prevention of URTIs from 1981-2000. Only one trial (Forth and Beuscher, 1981) found a clear benefit rather than a trend of benefit; however, the preparation consisted of other herbs in addition to *Echinacea* species and other substances, as did another trial reporting only a trend of benefit. In the ten trials Barrett examined that tested formulations of echinacea for the treatment of URTIs (1984-1999), seven reported benefits, one reported no benefit, and in two only a trend of benefit was reported. All were double-blind, randomized, placebo-controlled trials. However, three used products containing other species of herbs besides *Echinacea*.

Only four trials reporting clear benefits used echinacea extracts alone. In seven of the treatment trials, Barrett noted three major faults: (1) whether subjects thought they were receiving placebo or test preparation not reported; (2) concealment and allocation procedures not adequately described; and (3) their lack of "objective, validated measures" (Barrett, 2000, p. 213).

Giles et al. (2000) reviewed trials of echinacea in the treatment of the common cold spanning the years 1961-1997. Twelve trials during this period reported benefits as did five since 1997. In their evaluation, Giles and colleagues concluded that all of these trials contained design flaws which rendered the results unclear and the efficacy of echinacea in the treatment of the common cold inconclusive.

The following summaries of placebo-controlled, double-blind studies on echinacea preparations in the treatment or prevention of the common cold serve to illustrate the recent history of clinical research on echinacea. For details of the methodologies employed in these trials the reader will need to consult the references cited.

A comparative study of four different echinacea preparations was conducted by Brinkeborn et al. (1999) in 246 healthy adult volunteers who easily caught colds. The preparations were compared in a randomized, placebo-controlled, double-blind trial in which patients were randomly assigned to groups given different treatments:

1. An *E. purpurea* crude extract consisting of 5% root and 95% above-ground parts (Echinaforce, 6.78 mg/tablet, two tablets t.i.d.)
2. The latter crude extract in higher concentration (48.27 mg/tablet, two tablets t.i.d.)
3. A "special" crude extract of the root (*E. purpurea,* 29.60 mg/tablet, two tablets t.i.d.)
4. Placebo

Patients were instructed to take their medication at the prescribed dosage immediately after noticing the earliest symptoms of the common cold and until they felt "healthy." The medicating period was not to exceed seven days. An index of 12 symptom complaints recorded by the patients and the attending physicians was used to evaluate the results. According to physician records of the 12 symptom complaints, the "special" root extract was no better than placebo in reducing symptoms (by 44.8% and 29.3%, respectively), whereas the concentrated and simple extract were each significantly effective, ameliorating symptoms of the common cold by 64.3% and 62.7%, respectively. In reducing symptoms, the concentrated extract showed somewhat better per protocol results than the simple extract according to the symptom record of the patients (55.9% versus 50.6%), and the patient and physician judgements of efficacy. Overall, the physicians judged the echinacea preparations to be 70% effective, while the patients judged them as 80% effective. Adverse events were noted for 13% of the patient population which were not significantly greater in the placebo group. Only in one case (mild and transient nausea) was the event definitely or likely due to treatment. Brinkeborn and colleagues concluded that the concentrated and simple crude extracts of echinacea were equally effective and low-risk alternatives to the medications available for treating symptoms of the common cold.

Grimm and Müller (1999) reported no significant decrease in respiratory infection or colds and their severity and duration in patients receiving a fluid extract of *E. purpurea* (Madaus AG, 4 mL twice daily for eight weeks) compared to placebo. The placebo-controlled, double-blind, randomized study was conducted in 109 patients who had more than three colds or upper respiratory tract infections in the twelve months prior to the trial. The liquid extract, described as the fresh expressed juice of whole flowering *E. purpurea* without the roots, contained alcohol (22%) and was described as indistinguishable from the placebo in flavor, color, and appearance. Their analysis of the data found 65% in the echinacea group developed one or more colds or respiratory infections during the eight-week treatment period, compared to 74% in the placebo group. Illness duration in the placebo group was 6.5 days and in the echinacea group 4.5 days. Half of those in the echinacea group stated at the end of the follow-up portion of the trial that they preferred to continue taking the extract they had received, compared to 43% of those on placebo stating the same. Adverse effects were reported in 20% of the echinacea group and in 13% of the placebo group. In the echinacea group, there were four reports of central nervous system symptoms, four of gastrointestinal complaints, and one report each for eczema, an increase in hair loss, and an increased urge to micturate. In the placebo group, there was one patient with the latter complaint, none with central nervous system symptoms (aggressive tendency, tiredness, headache, dizziness, somnolence), and the same number with gastrointestinal complaints. Seven patients dropped out of the trial before its completion owing to complaints of either side effects, the taste of the medication, or for no stated reason (four in the echinacea group and three in the placebo group). Other adverse effects were matched in each of the groups and all side effects reported were reversible and mild. Certain limitations of the trial were cited, including lack of prior proof that the placebo was indistinguishable from the active preparation, a study size too small to detect moderate and small differences in severity of respiratory infections and colds, and unknown effects of the alcohol in the preparations on patient symptoms (Grimm and Müller, 1999).

A double-blind, placebo-controlled randomized trial of echinacea (root extract of *E. angustifolia, E. purpurea,* or placebo) by Melchart et al. (1998) found no significant difference in results compared to placebo with either plant extract taken five days/week for 12 weeks as a prophylactic treatment for upper respiratory tract infections. This trial was flawed, however, by the fact that participants ($n = 302$) were able to guess correctly that they were receiving echinacea in 53% of cases versus 22% who guessed wrong and 25% who felt they could not make a guess. Coupled with the fact that 45% of the participants reported previous use of echinacea, as Melchart et al. (1998) pointed out, this trial emphasizes the need for a suitably indistinguishable echinacea placebo to obtain meaningful data.

Hoheisel et al. (1997) used a product made from the expressed juice of the aboveground parts of *E. purpurea* (Echinagard) in a double-blind, placebo-controlled clinical trial in 120 adult patients who presented with the first signs of common cold symptoms. All patients had experienced at least three respiratory infections during the six months leading up to the trial. The dosage was 20 drops of juice or placebo in half a glass of water every 2 h on day one, followed by 20 drops three times daily for no longer than the next ten days. After randomly assigning patients to placebo and *E. purpurea* groups, 50% of the patients were found to have a "real" cold (36 on placebo and 24 on *E. purpurea*). Although the other half showed less severity of symptoms, they were still experiencing the first indications of the common cold. All 120 patients completed the study and recorded their subjective symptoms in addition to undergoing interviews with an attending physician concerning the course of their illness and individual symptoms. The median amount of time required before patients improved was zero days for the *E. purpurea* group and five days for the placebo group, a highly significant ($p < 0.0001$) difference. Among those in the subgroup of patients with "real" colds, the time to improvement was four days versus eight days in the placebo group. In the subgroup, those on *E. purpurea* drops discontinued the treatment after a median time of six days versus ten days in the placebo drops group. Curiously, there were no reported side effects in either treatment group (Hoheisel et al., 1997).

Dorn et al. (1997) entered 160 adult patients into a placebo-controlled, double-blind clinical study of *E. pallida* root liquid extract (uncharacterized) who had a symptom score meeting their criteria for upper respiratory tract infection: sufficient symptoms of headache, sore throat, sweating, burning sensation in the eyes, tearing, weakness, earache, and pain in the extremities. Patients were randomly assigned to a placebo group (42 males and 38 females) and a treatment group (39 females and 41 males) who would take 90 drops (900 mg) of the medications daily for eight to ten days. At nine to ten days, the score for overall symptoms of upper respiratory tract infection were significantly better for the *E. pallida* group ($p < 0.0004$) compared to placebo. Symptoms and signs of infection diminished rapidly in the echinacea group compared to the placebo group and correlated with neutrophil and lymphocyte count changes. Four major symptoms in the *E. pallida* extract-treated group significantly decreased compared to the placebo group ($p <$

0.0001): headache, pain in the arms and legs, and weakness. Compared to the corresponding placebo groups with bacterial and viral infections, patients treated with *E. pallida* extract showed a significantly shortened length of illness (by 3.2 days), and among those with viral infections echinacea significantly shortened the length of illness (by 3.8 days) (each $p > 0.0001$) (Dorn et al., 1997).

In a placebo-controlled, double-blind study in 160 patients of either sex suffering from upper respiratory tract infections, Bräunig and Knick (1993) evaluated the response to a standardized *E. pallida* preparation (Pascotox 100, 90 drops/day, equivalent to 900 mg extract). Response criteria was based on reduction of flulike symptoms and a reduction in the duration of the disease. Duration of the disease was significantly reduced (from 13 to 9.8 days) in patients with chiefly bacterial infections, and in those with chiefly viral infections (from 13 to 9.1 days). Strongest effects were seen in those with chiefly viral infections after eight to ten days of treatment and improvements in clinical symptoms corresponded well with the reduced duration of the disease. The relative percentage of lymphocytes in patients with viral infections and the relative percentage of granular leukocytes in those with bacterial infections, which were elevated in response to the infections, were, however, only slightly reduced.

Schöneberger (1992) studied the freshly pressed juice of *E. purpurea* aerial parts (Echinacin 4 mL, twice daily for eight weeks) in 108 patients (ages 13-84) during the winter season, and compared the results to a placebo-control group in a double-blind method. Patients were selected for the study on the basis of an increased susceptibility to colds; specifically, those who experienced a minimum of three cold-related infections during the winter before, whether pneumonia, catarrh, bronchitis, pharyngitis, tracheitis, tonsillitis, sinusitis, rhinitis, or lymphadenitis. The results showed that 35.2% of the patients receiving echinacea remained without infections versus 25.9% of the placebo group. The average length of time until contracting first infections in the echinacea group was 40 days versus 25 days in the placebo group. Infections in the echinacea group were of minor occurrence in 78%, and in the placebo group in 68% of patients. In total, the placebo group experienced 35 infections whereas the echinacea group had 23. By comparison, this amounted to 36% more subjects who were free from infections in the echinacea group versus the placebo group. Infections in the echinacea group were of lesser duration than in the placebo group (155 versus 279 days), and on average appeared to be less severe and resolved more quickly than for those on placebo (5.34 days versus 7.54 days). The periods between infections were, by comparison, longer in the echinacea group and they also experienced fewer lower respiratory tract infections (e.g., bronchitis). Infections in the placebo group were more severe in those who showed evidence of a weakened immune system (low ratio of T cells, T4/T8 ratio <1.5) and the same participants also showed the most benefit from echinacea.

Viral infections. Bräunig et al. (1992) conducted a double-blind, placebo-controlled trial with *Echinacea purpurea* root liquid extract in 180 patient volunteers (ages 18-60) with influenza-like infections of less than three days duration. Results were compared using an unstandardized liquid extract (1:5 ethanol; 50% volume %) of *E. purpurea* and a standardized liquid extract, in two dosages: 450 mg (90 drops or two dropperfuls) of root extract/dose and 900 mg (180 drops or four dropperfuls) per dose. Standardization was made to both hydrophilic (chicoric acid and other caffeic acid derivatives) and lipophilic constituents (isobutylamides). The placebo group received drops of a colored mixture of water and ethanol. Bräunig and colleagues reported highly significant differences between each of the study groups and dosages on days three to four ($p < 0.05$) and eight to ten ($p < 0.0001$) of the treatment period. The unstandardized extract group and the group receiving the low dose of standardized extract showed no significant improvement compared to the placebo group. However, the patients taking the high dose of standardized extract showed a significant reduction of flulike symptoms at three to four days, and in the clinical rating of the seriousness of their disease. Compared to the other groups and to pretreatment symptoms, the flulike symptoms included: nasal inflammation, sneezing, nasal secretions, stuffed nasal passages, low energy/weakness, muscle/limb pains, sore eyes/tearing, frontal headache/hot head/head pressure, sore throat, difficulty swallowing, earaches, swollen lymph glands, and sweating/chills. At eight to ten days of treatment with the high dose standardized extract, tongue coating was also significantly improved compared to the other groups ($p < 0.0001$). The investigators also noted that in those subjects with a strictly viral infection (influenza), granulocyte levels increased faster than in subjects with bacterially-related disease (colds).

Vonau and colleagues (2001) conducted a prospective, double-blind, placebo-controlled, crossover trial of a commercially available echinacea product (Echinaforce, 5% root and 95% upper plant parts of *E. purpurea* extract) in 50 patients (26 women and 24 men ages 22-72) diagnosed with recurrent genital herpes, proven by culture or serology for herpes simplex type 2 antibodies. The study was performed over a period of 12 months with patients receiving tablets containing the extract (800 mg b.i.d.) or placebo for six months before being switched over to the opposite treatment. Exclusion criteria included the use of acyclovir or similar drugs, pregnancy, renal or liver disease, intolerance to lactose (part of the echinacea preparation), severe forms of cardiovascular disease, and immunosuppression. Nineteen patients dropped out of the trial: four because of adverse events consisting mostly of diarrhea, eight for unknown reasons, and the remaining patients because of pregnancy or plans to conceive, and time constrictions. Based on

23 patients who returned a questionnaire, five claimed to feel better while on placebo versus twelve who felt better while taking the extract. Another six patients felt no difference whether they were taking placebo or the extract. Tests of immunological changes showed no significant difference in counts of CD4 cells and neutrophils in the two study groups, nor was there a statistically significant change in the frequency of genital herpes.

Fungal infections. In an open-label comparative study, Coeugniet and Kühnast (1986) used the fresh expressed juice of echinacea (Echinacin) as an adjuvant immunotherapy in a ten-week treatment of 203 women with recurrent vaginal candidiasis. It was used in combination with a locally applied antimycotic (econazol nitrate cream) alone, or in addition to the extract administered s.c., i.v., i.m., or p.o. The condition recurred in 60.5% of the patients using antimycotic cream alone. With the antimycotic cream plus i.v. echinacea (2 mL/week), recurrence was reduced to 15%, and to 5% in the i.m. echinacea group. With the antimycotic plus s.c. echinacea (2 mL/week), the rate of recurrence was 15%, and 16.7% for the group taking echinacea p.o. (3 mL/day) in addition to the antimycotic. A cutaneous test for cell-mediated immunity of the patients (Multitest Merieux) showed that within two weeks, normalization of immunity reached statistical significance in all the patients receiving echinacea, whether administered p.o. ($p < 0.05$) or parenterally ($p < 0.01$) (Coeugniet and Kühnast, 1986).

Integumentary, Muscular, and Skeletal Disorders

Skin Disorders

Echinacea is reputed to enhance wound healing. In a large five-month uncontrolled clinical study involving 4,598 patients, a salve prepared from the juice of the aerial portion of *E. purpurea* was reported to produce an 85% overall success rate in the treatment of the following inflammatory skin conditions: abscesses, wounds, folliculitis, burns, eczema, Herpes simplex, and varicose ulcers of the leg (Bauer and Wagner, 1991).

DOSAGE

Because of the existence of many different types of echinacea preparations, and the presence in various preparations of more than one immunologically active class of constituents, firm recommendations regarding dosage are difficult to make. In a recent review, Wagner (1997) advised that for oral administration the best response is obtained from allopathically prepared alcoholic tinctures or homeopathic mother tinctures, up to a dilution of D2. Tinctures are taken in doses of 30 to 40 drops, t.i.d. to q.i.d. for a period of at least five to six days at the onset of acute infections. Wagner added that for prophylaxis, longer treatment times (4-6 weeks), including short intervals (4-5 days) of nontreatment, provide better results than continuous treatment.

The *British Herbal Compendium* recommends a dosage of 1 g of dried root *(E. angustifolia),* or 2-5 mL of a 1:5, 45% ethanol tincture, t.i.d. (Bradley, 1992). The German Commission E states that oral use of *E. purpurea* herb (i.e., aboveground parts) should not exceed 6 weeks (De Smet et al., 1993).

Commercial extracts of *E. angustifolia* and *E. purpurea* sold in the United States have commonly been standardized to contain echinacosides and 4-sesquiterpene esters (Flynn and Roest, 1995). More recently, Bauer (1998) suggested that the active substances in echinacea which may be best utilized as standards are caffeic acid derivatives, such as echinacoside and cichoric acid, and other substances, especially polysaccharides, glycoproteins, alkamides, and polyacetylenes. In an analysis of six commercial *E. purpurea* expressed juice preparations, Bauer (1999) found that alkamide concentration ranged from 0.1-1.8 mg/mL, and cichoric acid ranged from 0.0-0.4%.

SAFETY PROFILE

At recommended doses little or no toxicity is associated with the use of echinacea. Fresh-pressed juice of *E. purpurea* (aerial parts) is sometimes given by injection in European phytotherapy (i.m., s.c., and i.v. routes) and this can result in a slight fever (elevation of temperature of 0.5 to 1 degree). This response is interpreted as a reflection of the immune-stimulating action, viz., the secretion of interferon and IL-1 by activated macrophages (Mengs et al., 1991).

Contraindications

According to McGuffin et al. (1997), the use of *Echinacea* species is contraindicated in cases of progressive systemic diseases (e.g., AIDS, tuberculosis, diabetes), or systemic diseases in which an autoimmune component is known or suspected, including multiple sclerosis, leukemia, lupus erythematosus, collagenosis, and other connective tissue diseases. De Smet et al. (1993) note that the German Commission E specifies contraindications for the use of *E. purpurea* herb in progressive systemic diseases including MS and TB, and in pregnancy and patients with an "inclination to hypersensitivity." The German authority gives no contraindications for the root of *E. angustifolia,* which is permitted for use in the form of an herbal tea.

Opinions differ as to whether echinacea extracts should be contraindicated in AIDS patients or not (Berger, 1993). Some researchers have theorized that HIV triggers autoimmune responses which may be responsible for many of the symptoms of AIDS, because the cell coating of HIV resembles CD4 receptors that are found on normal cells. If AIDS does include an autoimmune component, then echinacea should probably be avoided by AIDS patients, or at least only taken for acute infections and for less than ten days.

Drug Interactions

None known.

Pregnancy and Lactation

Pregnant and lactating women are advised to consult their physicians prior to using any medication, however, the German Commission E monograph on E. pallida "root" suggests that there are no effects on pregnancy or lactation (Blumenthal et al., 1998). The Commission E states that parenteral use of E. purpurea herb (i.e., aboveground parts) is contraindicated in pregnancy (De Smet et al., 1993).

Gallo et al. (2000) conducted a prospective pregnancy outcome study in 206 Canadian women who were already using echinacea products. In this study the first of its kind, the outcome of pregnancy was compared to a matched control group of 206 women not using echinacea products. Among the 198 respondents who had live births, the products used consisted of E. angustifolia and E. purpurea, either in the form of tinctures (by 38%; five to ten drops/day to a maximum of 30 drops/day) or tablets and capsules (by 58%; 250-1000 mg/day). One respondent used E. pallida (form not stated) and for this and the other species, plant parts used in the manufacture of the products were not reported. Even at a maximum dose of 30 drops/day of the tincture products (= approx. 1 mL alcohol/day), it was determined that it was unlikely that the alcohol content (25% to 48%) had any effect on the outcomes of pregnancy, given that the normal duration of use of echinacea products stated by the participants was short, continuous periods of five to seven days. The time of use of echinacea products by the 206 women enrolled in the study was largely during the first trimester of pregnancy (54%). Only 8% used echinacea during all trimesters. The results of the study showed that statistically, there were no differences between pregnancy outcome in the echinacea users compared to the control group, whether in the number of spontaneous abortions, therapeutic abortions, live births, delivery methods (cesarean or vaginal), or major malformations. Nor were any statistically significant differences between the study groups found in fetal stress, birth weight, gestational age, or maternal weight gain. Of interest is the fact that 81% of the participants reported that their upper respiratory tract ailments were improved from the use of echinacea.

Side Effects

The German Commission E notes no adverse reactions from oral use of *E. purpurea* "herb" and a worsening of symptoms in diabetics after parenteral use. From parenteral use, they received reports of acute allergic reactions and of dose-dependent nausea, vomiting, and fever (De Smet et al., 1993).

An eleven-year-old girl with diabetes since the age of two was given echinacea during the cold and flu season. She developed unexplained high blood sugar readings for a period of months, despite a steady increase in insulin levels. A return to normal insulin dosage was possible after discontinuing echinacea. An authority on herbal medicines suggested that since bacterial and viral infections are associated with the release of stress hormones such as cortisol, norepinephrine, and epinephrine, they may have caused glucose control to be compromised (Finlay, 1999).

Isolated cases of allergic responses to echinacea have occurred. Skin patch testing of an echinacea-containing (10% tincture) ointment resulted in two cases out of 1,032 who reacted positively; however, due to the presence of additive materials in the preparation used, a false-positive reaction in those two cases could not be ruled out (Bruynzeel et al., 1992). In Germany, during the period from 1989-1995, out of 13 cases of putative side effects from oral *E. purpurea* fresh-pressed juice (Echinacin) reported, only four cases—all allergic skin reactions—could be considered as causally resulting from the treatment (Parnham, 1996).

A case of anaphylaxis in a woman with atopy (allergy) was reported as likely due to the ingestion of echinacea (*E. angustifolia* whole plant and *E. purpurea* root extract), even though she had been taking other dietary supplements as well. Radioallergosorbent (RAST) testing by skin prick test of other atopy patients found that echinacea-binding IgE antibodies occurred in 19% (Mullins, 1998).

In Australia, two years earlier, it was estimated that as many as 5% of atopy patients were taking echinacea on a regular basis. In the RAST test for echinacea-binding IgE, 20% of stored sera samples showed a "moderate to strong reactivity" (Mullins, 1998). From July 1996 to November 1998 in Australia, there were 37 reports of "suspected adverse reactions in association" with echinacea. Twenty-one of these reports concerned allergiclike reactions in patients ages 3-58. In 19 of these cases, echinacea was the sole suspect, and onset of symptoms occurred within three days from the start of treatment. In 12 cases, patients had a medical history of hay fever/conjunctivitis/allergic rhinitis and/or asthma. In 21 of the cases, the allergiclike effects consisted of angioedema ($n = 3$), bronchospasm ($n = 9$), chest pain ($n = 4$), dyspnea ($n = 8$), and urticaria ($n = 5$) (Anonymous, 1999).

In Canada, recurrent erythema nodosum in a 41-year-old man with a history of allergy was associated (causally or temporally) with routine self-medication with echinacea for influenzalike illnesses over a period of 18 months. He was taking St. John's wort for depression, and for his allergies, loratadine whenever needed. The appearance of tender nodules followed a prodrome consisting of headache, fever, malaise, sore throat, arthralgias, and myalgias which lasted several days and up to two weeks. Each episode of erythema nodosum was preceded by his use of echinacea and responded to treatment with prednisone alone or in combination with erythromycin. After he discontinued use of echinacea the episodes failed to return after a 12-month follow-up (Soon and Crawford, 2001).

Special Precautions

None known.

Toxicology

Mutagenicity

Tests of *E. purpurea* have shown no mutagenicity or carcinogenicity (Wagner, 1997; Mengs et al., 1991).

Toxicity in Animal Models

The LD_{50} of fresh-pressed *E. purpurea* juice in mice has been measured at 50 mL/kg i.v. (Bauer and Wagner, 1991). The polysaccharides from the aerial portions of *E. purpurea* showed an LD_{50} of 1,000 to 2,500 mg/kg i.p. in mice. Chronic administration of the fresh-pressed juice (*E. purpurea* aerial parts) to rats at doses many times the human therapeutic dose produced no evidence of toxic effects. Acute and subacute toxicity studies in rats found no significant toxicity from oral dosing up to 15 g/kg and 8 g/kg, respectively (Mengs et al., 1991).

REFERENCES

Anonymous (1999). Allergic reactions with echinacea. *Australian Adverse Reactions Bulletin* 18: 3.

Awang, D.V.C. and Kindack, D.G. (1991). Echinacea. *Canadian Pharmaceutical Journal* 124: 512-516.

Barrett, B. (2000). Echinacea for upper respiratory tract infection: An assessment of randomized trials. *Healthnotes Review of Complementary and Integrative Medicine* 7: 211-218.

Bauer, R. (1998). Echinacea: Biological effects and active principles. In Lawson, L.D. and Bauer, R. (Eds.), *Phytomedicines of Europe: Chemistry and Biological Activity*, ACS Symposium Series 691 (pp. 140-157). Washington, DC: American Chemical Society.

Bauer, R. (1999). Standardization of *Echinacea purpurea* expressed juice with reference to chicoric acid and alkamides. *Journal of Herbs, Spices and Medicinal Plants* 6: 51-62.

Bauer, R., Jurcic, K., Puhlmann, J., and Wagner, H. (1988). Immunologische invivo und in-vitro-untersuchungen mit Echinacea-extrakten [Immunological in vivo and in vitro examinations of Echinacea extracts]. *Arzneimittel-Forschung/ Drug Research* 38: 276-281.

Bauer, R., Kahn, I.A., and Wagner, H. (1986). [Echinacea drugs. Standardization with HPLC and TLC]. *Deutsche Apotheker Zeitung* 126: 1065-1070.

Bauer, R. and Remiger, P. (1989). TLC and HPLC analysis of alkylamides in *Echinacea* drugs. *Planta Medica* 55: 367-371.

Bauer, R., Remiger, P., Jurcic, K., and Wagner, H. (1989). [Influence of Echinacea extracts on phagocytic activity]. *Zeitschrift fur Phytotherapie* 10: 43-48.

Bauer, R. and Wagner, H. (1991). Echinacea species as potential immunostimulatory drugs. In Farnsworth, N.R. and Wagner, H. (Eds.), *Economic and Medicinal Plant Research,* 5 (pp. 253-321). New York: Academic Press.

Bauer, R., Wray, V., and Wagner, H. (1987). The chemical discrimination of *Echinacea angustifolia* and *E. pallida*. *Pharmaceutisch Weekblad Scientific* 9: 220.

Ben-Eliyahu, S., Page, G.G., Yirmiya, R., and Shakar, G. (1999). Evidence that stress and surgical interventions promote tumor development by suppressing natural killer cell activity. *International Journal of Cancer* 80: 880-888.

Berg, A., Northoff, H., Konig, D. Weinstock, C., Grathwohl, D., Parnham, M.J., Stuhlfauth, I., and Keul, J. (1998). Influence of Echinacin (EC31) treatment on the exercise-induced immune response in athletes. *Journal of Clinical Research* 1: 367-380.

Berger, P. (1993). Is echinacea contraindicated in HIV infection? *Medical Herbalism* 5 (Spring).

Binns, S.E., Baum, B.R., and Arnason, J.T. (2001a). Proposal to conserve the name *Rudbeckia purpurea* (Asteraceae) with a conserved type. *Taxon* 50:1199-1120 .

Binns, S.E., Baum, B.R., and Arnason, J.T. (2001b). Typification of *Echinacea purpurea* (L.) Moench (Heliantheae: Asteraceae) and its implications for the correct naming of two *Echinacea* taxa. *Taxon* 50: 1169-1175.

Binns, S.E., Purgina, B., Bergeron, C., Smith, M.L., Ball, L., Baum, B.R., and Arnason, J.T. (2000). Light-mediated antifungal activity of *Echinacea* extracts. *Planta Medica* 66: 241-244.

Blumenthal, M. (1998). The German Commission E monograph system for phytomedicines: A model for regulatory reform in the United States. In Lawson, L.D. and Bauer, R. (Eds.), *Phytomedicines of Europe: Chemistry and Biological Ac-*

tivity, ACS Symposium Series 691 (pp. 30-43). Washington, DC: American Chemical Society.

Bodinet, C. and Beuscher, N. (1991). Antiviral and immunological activity of glycoproteins from *Echinacea purpurea* radix. *Planta Medica* 57(Suppl. 2): A33-A34 (poster).

Bodinet, C., Willigmann, I., and Beuscher, N. (1993). Host-resistance increasing activity of root extracts from *Echinacea* species. *Planta Medica* 59(Suppl.): A672 (abstract).

Bonadeo, I.G., Botazzi, G., and Lavazza, M. (1971). Echinacin B, an active polysaccharide from Echinacea. *Revista Italiana Essenzea-Profumi-Piante Officinale Armoi-Saponi-Cosmetici-Aerosol* 53: 281-295.

Bradley, P. (Ed.) (1992). *British Herbal Compendium,* 1. Bournemouth, Dorset, England: British Herbal Medicine Association.

Bräunig, B., Dorn, M., and Knick, E. (1992). *Echinacea purpurea* radix: zur starking der körpereigenen abwehr bei grippalen infekten [*Echinacea purpurea* radix therapy for the enhancement of the body's own immune defense mechanisms in influenza-like symptoms]. *Zeitschrift für Phytotherapie* 13: 7-13.

Bräunig, B. and Knick, E. (1993). Therapeutische erfahrungen mit *Echinaceae pallidae* bei grippalen infekten [Therapeutical experiences with *Echinacea pallida* for influenza-like infections]. *Naturheilpraxis* 1: 72-75.

Brinkeborn, R.M., Shah, D.V., and Degenring, F.H. (1999). Echinaforce® and other *Echinacea* fresh plant preparations in the treatment of the common cold. A randomized, placebo-controlled, double-blind clinical trial. *Phytomedicine* 6: 1-5.

Brokos, B., Gasiorowski, K., and Noculak-Palczewska, A. (1999). Stimulation of human lymphocytes and granulocytes in vitro by extract and sap from *Echinacea purpurea* L. *Bulletin of the Polish Academy of Sciences, Biological Sciences* 47: 35-41.

Bruynzeel, D.P., Van Ketel, W.G., Young, E., van Joost, T., and Smeenk, G. (1992). Contact sensitization by alternative topical medicaments containing plant extracts. *Contact Dermatitis* 27: 278-279.

Burger, R.A., Torres, A.R., Warren, R.P., Caldwell, V.D., and Hughes, B.G. (1997). Echinacea-induced cytokine production by human macrophages. *International Journal of Immunopharmacology* 19: 371-379.

Cheminat, A., Zawatzky, R., Becker, H., and Brouillard, R. (1988). Caffeoyl conjugates from *Echinacea* species: Structures and biological activity. *Phytochemistry* 27: 2787-2794.

Classen, B., Witthohn, K., and Blaschek, W. (2000). Characterization of an arabinogalactan-protein isolated from pressed juice of *Echinacea purpurea* by precipitation with the β-glucosyl Yariv reagent. *Carbohydrate Research* 327: 497-504.

Coeugniet, E.G. and Kühnast, R. (1986). Rezidivierende candidiasis: adjuvante immuntherapie mit verschiedenen Echinacin®-darreichungsformen [Recurrent candidiasis: adjuvant immunotherapy with different formulations of Echinacin®]. *Therapiewoche* (Munich) 36: 3352-3358.

Currier, N.L. and Miller, S.C. (2000). Natural killer cells from aging mice treated with extracts from *Echinacea purpurea* are quantitatively and functionally rejuvenated. *Experimental Gerontology* 35: 627-639.

De Smet, P.A.G.M., Keller, K., Hänsel, R., and Chandler (Eds.) (1993). *Adverse Effects of Herbal Drugs,* 2. New York: Springer-Verlag, p. 39.

Dorn, M., Knick, E., and Lewith, G. (1997). Placebo-controlled, double-blind study of *Echinacea pallidae* radix in upper respiratory tract infections. *Complementary Therapies in Medicine* 5: 40-42.

Finlay, P. (1999). Echinacea troubles. *Diabetes Forecast* 52 (April): 15-16.

Flynn, R. and Roest, M. (1995). *Your Guide to Standardized Herbal Products.* Prescott, AZ: One World Press, pp. 20-21.

Forth, H. and Beuscher, N. (1981). [The influence of Esberitox on the frequency of minor colds]. *Zeitschrift fur Allgemeinmedizin* 57: 2272-2275.

Foster, S. (1991). *Echinacea: Nature's Immune Enhancer.* Rochester, VT: Healing Arts Press.

Gallo, M., Sarkar, M., Au, W., Pietrzak, K., Comas, B., Smith, M., Jaeger, T.V., Einerson, A., and Koren, G. (2000). Pregnancy outcome following exposure to echinacea: A prospective controlled study. *Archives of Internal Medicine* 160: 3141-3143.

Giger, E., Keller, F., and Baumann, T.W. (1989). Fructans in Echinacea and in its phytotherapeutic preparations. *Planta Medica* 55: 638.

Giles, J.T., Palat III, C.T., Chien, S.H., Chang, Z.G., and Kennedy, D.T. (2000). Evaluation of echinacea for treatment of the common cold. *Pharmacotherapy* 20: 690-697.

Goel, V., Chang, C., Slama, J.V., Barton, R., Bauer, R., Gahler, R., and Basu, T.K. (2002). Alkylamides of *Echinacea purpurea* stimulate alveolar macrophage function in normal rats. *International Immunopharmacology* 2: 381-387.

Grimm, W. and Müller, H.H. (1999). A randomized controlled trial of the effect of fluid extract of *Echinacea purpurea* on the incidence and severity of colds and respiratory infections. *American Journal of Medicine* 106: 138-143.

Hobbs, C. (1989). *The Echinacea Handbook.* Sandy, OR: Eclectic Medical Publications.

Hoheisel, O., Sandberg, M., Bertram, S., Bulitta, M., and Schäfer, M. (1997). Echinagard treatment shortens the course of the common cold: A double-blind, placebo-controlled clinical trial. *European Journal of Clinical Research* 9: 261-268.

Jung, H.D. and Shröeder, H. (1954). Zur antimykotischen wirksamkeit pflanzlicher extrakte [On the antimycotic activity of plant extracts]. *Archiv für Dermatologie und Syphilis* 197: 130-144.

Jurcic, K., Melchart, D., Holzmann, M., Martin, P., Bauer, R., Doenicke, A., and Wagner, H. (1989). Zwei probandenstudien zur stimulierung der granulozytenphagozytose durch echinaceaextraktthaltige präparate [Two studies on the stimulation of the phagocytosis of granulocytes by drug preparations containing extracts of echinacea in healthy volunteers]. *Zeitschrift für Phytotherapie* 10: 67-70.

Livesey, J., Awang, D.V.C., Arnason, J.T., Letchamo, W., Barrett, M., and Penny-royal, G. (1999). Effect of temperature on stability of marker constituents in *Echinacea purpurea* root formulations. *Phytomedicine* 6: 347-349.

Maffei Facino, R., Carini, M., Aldini, G., Marinello, C., Arlandini, E., Franzoi, L., Co-lombo, M., Pietta, P., and Mauri, P. (1993). Direct characterization of caffeoyl esters with antihyaluronidase activity in crude extracts from *Echinacea angustifolia* roots by fast atom bombardment tandem mass spectrometry. *Il Farmaco* 48: 1447-1461.

Maffei Facino, R., Carini, M., Aldini, G., Saibene, L., Pietta, P., and Mauri, P. (1995). Echinacoside and caffeoyl conjugates protect collagen from free radical-induced degradation: A potential use of echinacea extracts in the prevention of skin photodamage. *Planta Medica* 61: 510-514.

May, G. and Willuhn, G. (1978). Antivirale wirkung wäßriger pflanzenextrakte in gewebekulturen [Antiviral activity of aqueous extracts from medicinal plants in tissue cultures]. *Arzneimittel-Forschung/Drug Research* 28: 1-7.

McGregor, R.L. (1968). The taxonomy of the genus *Echinacea* (Compositae). *University of Kansas Science Bulletin* 48: 113-142.

McGuffin, M., Hobbs, C., Upton, R., and Goldberg, A. (Eds.) (1997). *American Herbal Products Association's Botanical Safety Handbook*. Boca Raton, FL: CRC Press, pp. 43-44.

Melchart, D., Linde, K., Worku, F., Bauer, R., and Wagner, H. (1994). Immuno-modulation with echinacea—A systematic review of controlled clinical trials. *Phytomedicine* 1: 245-254.

Melchart, D., Walther, E., Linde, K., Brandmaier, R., and Lersch, C. (1998). Echinacea root extracts for the prevention of upper respiratory tract infections. *Archives of Family Medicine* 7: 541-545.

Mengs, U., Clare, C.B., and Poiley, J.A. (1991). Toxicity of *Echinacea purpurea*. *Arzneimittel-Forschung/Drug Research* 41: 1076-1081.

Möse, J.R. (1983). Zur wirkung von Echinacin auf phagozytoseaktivität und natural killer cells [Effect of Echinacin on phagocytosis and natural killer cells]. *Med Welt* 34: 1463-1467.

Müller-Jakic, B., Breu, W., Pröbstle, A., Redl, K., Greger, H., and Bauer, R. (1994). *In vitro* inhibition of cyclooxygenase and 5-lipoxygenase by alkamides from *Echinacea* and *Achillea* species. *Planta Medica* 60: 37-40.

Mullins, R.J. (1998). Echinacea-associated anaphylaxis. *Medical Journal of Australia* 168: 170-171.

Parnham, M.J. (1996). Benefit-risk assessment of the squeezed sap of the purple coneflower *(Echinacea purpurea)* for long-term oral immunostimulation. *Phytomedicine* 3: 95-102.

Perry, N.B., Burgess, E.J., and Glennie, V.L. (2001). *Echinacea* standardization: Analytical methods for phenolic compounds and typical levels in medicinal species. *Journal of Agricultural and Food Chemistry* 49: 1702-1706.

Perry, N.B., van Klink, J.W., Burgess, E.J., and Parmenter, G.A. (1997). Alkamide levels in *Echinacea purpurea:* A rapid analytical method revealing differences among roots, rhizomes, stems, leaves and flowers. *Planta Medica* 63: 58-62.

Perry, N.B., van Klink, J.W., Burgess, E.J., and Parmenter, G.A. (2000). Alkamide levels in *Echinacea purpurea:* Effects of processing, drying and storage. *Planta Medica* 66: 54-56.

Rehman, J., Dillow, J.M., Carter, S.M., Chou, J., Le, B., and Maisel, A.S. (1999). Increased production of antigen-specific immunoglobulins G and M following in vivo treatment with the medicinal plants *Echinacea angustifolia* and *Hydrastis canadensis. Immunology Letters* 68: 391-395.

Rininger, J.A., Kickner, S., Chigurupati, P., McLean, A., and Franck, Z. (2000). Immunopharmacological activity of *Echinacea* preparations following simulated digestion on murine macrophages and human peripheral blood mononuclear cells. *Journal of Leukocyte Biology* 68: 503-510.

Roesler, J., Steinmüller, C., Kiderlen, A., Emmendörffer, A., Wagner, H., and Lohmann-Mathes, M.L. (1991). Application of purified polysaccharides from cell cultures of the plant *Echinacea purpurea* to mice mediates protection against systemic infections with *Listeria monocytogenes* and *Candida albicans. International Journal of Immunopharmacology* 13: 27-37.

Schöneberger, D. (1992). [The influence of immunostimulating effects of pressed juice from *Echinacea purpurea* on the course and severity of colds. Results of a double-blind study]. *Forum Immunologie* 8: 2-12.

Schulte, K.E., Ruecker, G., and Perlick, J. (1967). Das vorkommen von polyacetylenverbindungen in *Echinacea purpurea* Mnch. und *Echinacea angustifolia* DC. [The presence of polyacetylene compounds in *Echinacea purpurea* Mnch. and *E. angustifolia* DC.]. *Arzneimittel-Forschung/Drug Research* 17: 825-829.

See, D.M., Broumand, N., Sahl, L., and Tilles, J.G. (1997). *In vitro* effects of Echinacea and ginseng on natural killer and antibody-dependent cell cytotoxicity in healthy subjects and chronic fatigue syndrome or acquired immunodeficiency syndrome patients. *Immunopharmacology* 35: 229-235.

Soon, S.L. and Crawford, R.I. (2001). Recurrent erythema nodosum associated with echinacea herbal therapy. *Journal of the American Academy of Dermatology* 44: 298-299.

South, E.H. and Exon, J.H. (2001). Multiple immune functions in rats fed echinacea extract. *Immunopharmacology and Immunotoxicology* 23: 411-421.

Steinmüller, C., Roesler, J., Gröttrup, E., Franke, G., Wagner, H., and Lohmann-Mathes, M.L. (1993). Polysaccharides isolated from plant cell cultures of *Echinacea purpurea* enhance the resistance of immunosuppressed mice against systemic infections with *Candida albicans* and *Listeria monocytogenes. International Journal of Immunopharmacology* 15: 605-614.

Stites, D.P., Terr, A.I., and Parslow, T.G. (Eds.) (1994). *Basic and Clinical Immunology,* Eighth Edition. Norwalk, CT: Appleton and Lange.

Stoll, A., Renz, J. and Brack, A. (1950). Isolierung und konstitution des echinacosids, eines glykosids aus den wurzeln von *Echinacea angustifolia* DC. [Isolation and constitution of echinosides and glycosides of the roots of *Echinacea angustifolia* DC.]. *Helvetica Chimica Acta* 33: 1877-1893.

Tubaro, A., Tragni, E., Del Negro, P., Galli, C.L., and Della Logia, R. (1987). Anti-inflammatory activity of a polysaccharide fraction of *Echinacea angustifolia*. *Journal of Pharmacy and Pharmacology* 39: 567-569.

Voaden, D. J. and Jacobson, M. (1972). Tumor inhibitors. 3. Identification and synthesis of an oncolytic hydrocarbon from American coneflower roots. *Journal of Medicinal Chemistry* 15: 619-623.

Vonau, B., Chard, S., Mandalia, S., Wilkinson, D., and Barton, S.E. (2001). Does the extract of the plant *Echinacea purpurea* influence the clinical course of recurrent genital herpes? *International Journal of STD and AIDS* 12: 154-158.

Wacker, A. and Hilbig, W. (1978). Virushemmung mit *Echinacea purpurea* [Virus inhibition by *Echinacea purpurea*]. *Planta Medica* 33: 89-102.

Wagner, H. (1997). Herbal immunostimulants for the prophylaxis and therapy of colds and influenza. *The European Journal of Herbal Medicine* 3: 22-20.

Wildfeuer, A. and Mayerhofer, D. (1994). Untersuchung des einflusses von phytopräparaten auf zelluläre funktionen der körpereigenen abwehr [Study on the influence of phytopreparations on the cellular function of body defense]. *Arzneimittel-Forschung/Drug Research* 44: 361-366.

Wills, R.B.H. and Stuart, D.L. (2000). Effect of handling and storage on alkylamides and cichoric acid in *Echinacea purpurea*. *Journal of the Science of Food and Agriculture* 80: 1402-1406.

Witthohn, K., Schwarz, T., and Odenthal, K.P. (2000). Phagocytosis is less influenced by low molecular weight substances of *Echinacea purpurea* herb's pressed juice. In Third International Congress on Phytomedicine, October 11-13, 2000, Munich, Germany, Abstracts. *Phytomedicine* 7(Suppl. II): 31 (abstract SL-59).

Zoutewelle, G. and van Wijk, R. (1990). Effects of *Echinacea purpurea* extracts on fibroblast populated collagen lattice contraction. *Phytotherapy Research* 4: 77-81.

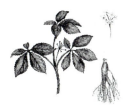

Eleuthero

BOTANICAL DATA

Classification and Nomenclature

Scientific name: *Eleutherococcus senticosus* (Rupr. and Maxim.) Maxim.; alternate binomials formerly used: *Acanthopanax senticosus* Harms., *Hedera senticosa* (no authority cited)

Family name: Araliaceae

Common names: eleuthero, eleutherococc, spiny eleutherococc, touch-me-not, devil's shrub, wild pepper, devil's bush, ciwujia, wujiapi (bark) (China), shigoka (Japan), Siberian ginseng (U.S. commerce)

Description

Eleuthero *(Eleutherococcus senticosus)* belongs to the same family (Araliaceae) as *Panax ginseng* C.A. Meyer, but the root is woody rather than fleshy ("seng"). The shrub is a perennial deciduous plant with prickly stems that attains a height of 2.4-4.5 m. It has gray or grayish-brown bark and numerous thin thorns. The dark green palmate leaves with hairy veins appear on a short stalk (7.6-12.7 cm in length) and have long petioles. The flowers are globular, umbrella-shaped, 3.8 cm wide, with bisexual, male and female flowers borne on separate plants; male flowers are purplish, while female flowers are yellowish. The fruit is a black, oval berry which measures 1.3 cm in diameter when ripe (Li, 2001).

Eleuthero senticosus commonly grows at elevations of 800 m above sea level in forests of broad-leaved species, or mixed broadleaf and spruce and cedar forests, and is most abundant in the Primorsk and Khabrarosvk Districts of the former Soviet Union; however, its range extends to the Middle Amur region in the north, Sakhalin Island, and Japan in the east, and Korea and the Chinese provinces of Hopei and Shansi in the south. This range of distribution corresponds closely with the range of *Panax ginseng,* for which it is often substituted (Li, 2001; Foster and Yue, 1992).

HISTORY AND TRADITIONAL USES

In traditional Chinese medicine (TCM), eleuthero is used as a preventive medicine and tonic in the belief that it will increase longevity, improve general health, improve the appetite, and restore memory. Specific uses of the herb in TCM include treatments for bronchitis, chronic lung ailments, hypertension, hypercholesterolemia, impotence, low blood oxygen, stress (Chang and But, 1986), kidney and lower back pain, rheumatoid arthritis, poor appetite, and as a diuretic (Foster and Yue, 1992).

Until recently, eleuthero received little attention from Western pharmacologists. As a result, most of the clinical studies, in vivo and in vitro evaluations, and phytochemical investigations have been published in Soviet journals.

Eleuthero was subjected to intensive scientific study in the late 1950s by Soviet pharmacologists looking for an "adaptogen" that could be used as an inexpensive substitute for ginseng (*Panax ginseng* C.A. Meyer). The term adaptogen was introduced by N.V. Lazarev in 1947 to describe the action of dibazole (2-benzylbenzimadazole), which was claimed to increase "nonspecific" resistance of an organism to adverse influences (Brekhman and Dardymov, 1969). Brekhman defined "adaptogen" as a substance that (1) must be innocuous and cause minimal physiological disturbances in an organism; (2) must have a nonspecific action (i.e., it should increase resistance to adverse influences by a variety of physical, chemical, and biochemical factors); and (3) usually has a normalizing action regardless of the direction of the pathologic state. Under this definition, many herbs traditionally regarded as "tonics" could be considered adaptogens. For a recent review of herbal adaptogens, see Wagner et al., 1992 (available from the American Botanical Council in English translation). Davydov and Krikorian (2000) reviewed the pharmacological literature on eleuthero and concluded that while the term adaptogen could just as well be applied to substances with anticancerogenic, choleretic, hypocholesterolemic, hypoglycemic, or immunomodulatory actions, in its classical definition, an adaptogen is similar to contemporary concepts of what constitutes the "placebo effect." Because of the vague nature of the term, they recommended that the use of the term "adaptogen" in association with eleuthero be dropped.

CHEMISTRY

Farnsworth et al. (1985) remark that no unusual compounds or compound types characteristic only of eleuthero have been isolated in appreciable amounts from this plant. Kurkin et al. (1991) identified the most abundant compounds in the root of eleuthero as chlorogenic acid, lignans, and other phenylpropanoids.

Most of the phytochemical work on eleuthero has focused on the characterization of "eleutherosides," a term which is, in some respects, regarded as a deliberate misnomer intended to emphasize some correspondence to the ginsenosides or panaxosides of *Panax* species. However, the eleutherosides are chemically distinct from these classes of compounds (Tyler, 1998).

Carbohydrates

Polysaccharides

Various polysaccharides have been detected in eleuthero (Shen et al., 1991; Fang et al., 1985), including glycans (eleutherans A to G) (Hikino et al., 1986).

Phenolic Compounds

Lignans

From the roots of eleuthero, Makarieva et al. (1997) isolated and identified the lignans (–)-syringaresinol-4-*O*-β-D-glucopyranoside, meso-seco-isolariciresinol, and several others.

Polyphenolics

A series of eleutherosides designated from A to M has been identified by various groups since studies were initiated in 1965. In many cases, they proved to be known compounds which had been previously characterized in other plant species; in other cases the eleutherosides were incompletely characterized (Farnsworth et al., 1985). For example, eleutheroside B was previously already known as syringin, eleutheroside D as syringaresinol diglucoside, and eleutheroside B1 as isofraxidin glucoside (Kurkin et al., 1991).

Terpenoid Compounds

Triterpenes

The root contains oleanic acid (the aglycone of eleutherosides I-M). Eleutherosides I, K, L, and M are oleanic acid derivatives. Senticosides A-F are a series of oleanic acid derivatives with uncharacterized glycone moieties which were isolated from the leaves of *E. senticosus* (Farnsworth et al., 1985).

Other Constituents

Eleuthero contains various constituents, most of which are widely distributed in many species. These include free sugars, sitosterol (the aglycone of eleutheroside A), vitamin E, β-carotene, (–)syringaresinol (lignan), and the phenylpropanoids caffeic acid, caffeic acid ethyl ester, coniferyl alcohol, coniferyl acetaldehyde, and sinapyl alcohol (the latter the aglycone of eleutheroside B) (Farnsworth et al., 1985), syringic acid, isofraxidin glucoside (eleutheroside B1), *p*-hydroxybenzoic acid, vanillic acid, vanillin, chlorogenic acid, and ferulic acid (Kurkin et al., 1991).

THERAPEUTIC APPLICATIONS

Voluminous Russian literature describes clinical studies on the adaptogenic uses of eleuthero extracts in healthy subjects, as well as its prophylactic and curative uses for a variety of disorders. This work has been summarized by Farnsworth et al. (1985). Russian clinical studies in over 2,000 healthy subjects indicate that eleuthero can: (1) increase human ability to withstand adverse physical conditions; (2) increase mental alertness and work output; and, (3) improve the quality of work output and athletic performance. Eleuthero also appears to have some adaptogenic properties in the treatment of various mental disturbances. Extracts have been shown to increase the sense of well-being in patients suffering from various psychological complaints, including insomnia, hypochondria, and depression. Modulation of biogenic amine neurotransmitters such as epinephrine, serotonin, and dopamine may be the mechanism responsible for its putative normalizing influence on psychological states and brain activity (Farnsworth et al., 1985).

Russian clinicians also evaluated the applications of eleuthero extracts in various disease states. Extracts have been administered to over 2,200 human subjects with a variety of diseases including angina, hypertension, hypotension, acute pyelonephritis, various neuroses, acute craniocerebral trauma, rheumatic heart disease, chronic bronchitis, and cancer. However, in the vast majority of these studies, sufficient controls to allow an evaluation of the efficacy of eleuthero in any condition are lacking (Farnsworth et al., 1985).

Pizzorno and Murray (1993) summarized the pharmacological activities attributed to eleuthero extracts by Russian studies in animals, the majority of which found "normalizing" activities which are consistent with the classification of eleuthero as an adaptogen. Their research demonstrated that the same extract can cause opposite effects, depending on the pathological or metabolic dysfunction treated.

PRECLINICAL STUDIES

Endocrine and Hormonal Functions

Pearce et al. (1982) reported that in vitro, a liquid extract of the roots (Medexport, USSR) bound to receptors of progestin, modestly to estrogen receptors, and highly to receptors of glucocorticoid and mineralcorticoid, but not to androgen receptors. Farnsworth et al. (1985) cited two Russian studies reporting that a diluted (1:1) extract of the root (5 mL/kg per day i.p. × 30) administered to immature male mice greatly increased the weight of seminal vesicles and the prostate by 70% and 118%, respectively. The root extract administered to immature rats (1 mL/kg i.p.) was reported to show an "anabolic effect" equivalent to testosterone (6 mg/kg i.m.). Another group reported estrogenic activity in immature female mice.

Immune Functions; Inflammation and Disease

Cancer

Chemopreventive activity. Farnsworth et al. (1985) recounted Russian studies showing that when administered to rodents, eleuthero extracts delayed the growth of transplanted tumors, delayed or prevented metastasis, prevented or delayed spontaneous mammary tumor development and spontaneous leukemia, and delayed chemically-induced or spontaneous tumors in mice. Guinea pigs administered an extract of eleuthero showed an increased tolerance to the toxic effects of the antibiotic rubromycin C.

Fang et al. (1985) reported that when administered to mice (100 mg/kg i.p.), a β-1,4 heteroxylan and a crude polysaccharide fraction of the roots caused significant antitoxic effects ($p < 0.01$) against the white blood cell-decreasing activity of cyclophosphamide and the liver toxicity of thioacetamide.

Chemotherapy adjunct treatments. Studies in which eleuthero extracts were administered concomitantly with antitumor agents (e.g., thio-TEPA, 6-mercaptopurine, cyclophosphan, ethymidine, benzo-TEPA, and sarcolysin) found both a decrease in their toxicity and improved antitumor effects. Tissue hypoxic effects due to malonic acid and hemic hypoxia induced in mice by $NaNO_2$ or CO_2 decreased with administration of eleuthero extracts (Farnsworth et al., 1985).

Immune Functions

Immunopotentiation. A β-1,4 heteroxylan and a crude polysaccharide fraction of the roots were reported by Fang et al. (1985) to show potent immunological activity, increasing phagocytosis by 30% in two immunological systems. Shen et al. (1991) reported that a polysaccharide derived from the roots (yield 0.5%) caused diverse immunological activity in mice (100 mg/kg i.p.), significantly increasing IgM antibody activity in vitro, phagocytic activity in vivo, and the rate of lymphocyte transformation in vitro. The polysaccharide fraction (100 mg/kg i.p.) significantly increased the phagocytic index and spleen cell counts (each $p < 0.01$), and at a higher dose (200 mg/kg i.p.) caused a significant inhibition of tumor growth (Ehrlich carcinoma and sarcoma 180, each $p < 0.05$). In guinea pigs (40 mg/kg i.p. every second day), the polysaccharide fraction exhibited protective effects against tubercular bacillus infection; however, quantitative measurements of TB colonies in the lungs revealed that only intramuscular injections significantly lowered their numbers. A single swollen lumbar lymph node was found in the polysaccharide-treated animals, compared to 11/13 of the saline-treated group. An equal number in the control group showed skin reactions when challenged with old tuberculin (i.v.), whereas the polysaccharide group showed these reactions in only 4/16 cases with considerably ameliorated skin responses (Shen et al., 1991).

Metabolic and Nutritional Functions

Antidiabetic Activity

Rabbits administered the root extract (1 mL/kg p.o. daily for 30 days) were reported to show an increase in serum glucose levels of 17% (Farnsworth et al., 1985). However, Hikino et al. (1986) reported that a water extract of the root (10 mg/kg i.p.) produced significant hypoglycemic activity in alloxan-induced hyperglycemic mice at 7 and 24 h postadministration (65% and 78% of control, respectively). They isolated six dose-dependently active glycans as eleutherans A-F and G. Among them, eleutheran G showed the most potency: plasma glucose decreased to 50% of control from 10 mg/kg i.p. after 7 h ($p < 0.01$). Eleutherosides were also reported to exert a preventive effect against alloxan-induced diabetes in rats (Dardymov et al., 1978).

Performance Enhancement

In cold-water swimming trials in male mice, Lewis et al. (1983) found no significant increase in physical stamina or longevity, either from a commercial extract of eleuthero root prepared as an infusion (wuchaseng infusion with sugar), or a sugar-free infusion administered ad libitum in distilled water (306.96 mg/day and 239 mg/kg p.o., respectively), whether for 38, 46, or 96 days. The group administered the commercial root extract with sugar showed significant signs of abuse and fighting after 46 and 96 days of ingestion, while the simple infusion group showed none. Martinez and Staba (1984) reported similar results in male rats subjected to a swimming test after administration of the saponin fraction of the root (50 mg/kg p.o.). In both cases, these results were in contrast to those reported by Russian researchers (Farnsworth et al., 1985) who administered extracts of the root to rodents intraperitoneally. For example, a root extract (1.0 mL/kg i.p.) increased the swimming duration in mice, and the total eleutheroside fraction administered to rats (5 mg/kg i.p.) caused a partial reversal of the decrease in levels of muscle adenosine triphosphate (ATP), pyruvic acid, lactic acid, glycogen, and creatine phosphate, and administered orally to rats (2.5 mg/kg p.o.), ameliorated the increase in adrenal weight caused by prolonged stress.

Using an aqueous extract of the stem bark, Nishibe et al. (1990) examined the effect of eleuthero on prolonged swimming stress in male rats. Administered in a high dosage (500 mg/kg p.o. daily for 25 days), the stem bark extract significantly increased the swimming time to exhaustion ($p < 0.05$) from the fifteenth day of treatment. HPLC analysis of the extract revealed two major phenolic compounds, which were also major constituents of the methanolic extract: compound A, (+)-syringaresinol-di-O-β-D-glucoside, and compound B, chlorogenic acid. Two groups of rats administered compounds A and B separately in high dosages (50 mg/kg p.o.) for 22 days and subjected to the same swimming test on day 8 showed a significant increase in swimming time to exhaustion compared to the control in the case of compound A ($p < 0.01$), but not from compound B.

In a comparative study of antistress or adaptogenic herbs, Singh et al. (1991) administered an extract of eleuthero to mice (Adaptation Energy Institute of Biology, Vladivostok, USSR, 70% alcoholic extract of the dried, powdered root, 10, 20, and 30 mg/kg p.o. for six days) prior to subjecting them to a swimming endurance test. At all three doses, the eleuthero group showed significant increases in the swimming duration (30%, 49%, and 60%, respectively, each $p < 0.001$) compared to the control group. The increases were not as great as those from an extract of holy basil *(Ocimum sanctum),* but in each dose they were much superior to those of an extract of ginseng prepared in the same strength (dried powdered roots of *Panax ginseng* C.A. Meyer, Pharmaton, Lugano, Switzerland). Increases in adrenal weights resulting from the stress of the swimming test were significantly ameliorated by all three extracts, with eleuthero preventing the increases by 39.7%, 71.7%, and 90.9% from the respective doses. Again, the results were not as great as those from the basil extract and were superior to those of ginseng, although statistically, they were all of equal significance. The stress-induced decrease in adrenal levels of vitamin C were ameliorated far more significantly by eleuthero than ginseng, although not as much as by the basil extract and then only at the two higher doses (63% and 82%, respectively). However, against immobilization stress-induced ulcer development in rats, eleuthero was superior to the other two extracts, producing a highly significant rate of inhibition at all doses (33.33%, 73.33%, and 93.33%, respectively).

Fujikawa et al. (1996) studied the effect of a methanol extract of the stem bark harvested in the Hakkaido region, Japan on cold water stress-induced ulcer formation in male rats. A dose-dependent and significant protective effect was found from the extract dissolved in water (50 mg/kg p.o. for 14 days), which resulted in an ulcer inhibition rate of 41.2%. An n-butanol extract used in the same test at a higher dose (100 mg/kg p.o.) produced a greater rate of inhibition compared to the controls (61.1%, $p < 0.01$) than any other forms of stem bark extract (ether, chloroform, and aqueous residue). Like Nishibe et al. (1990), these researchers also tested the two major compounds of the stem bark, which were evident in the n-butanol extract. Syringaresinol-di-O-β-D-glucoside (50 mg/kg per day p.o. for 14 days) produced more significant ulcer-inhibiting activity (51.3%) than chlorogenic acid (21.4%) versus the control ($p < 0.01$ and $p < 0.05$, respectively).

Neurological, Psychological, and Behavioral Functions

Psychological and Behavioral Functions

Sleep disturbances. A freeze-dried water extract of the root administered to mice reduced sleep latency and increased sleep duration following hexobarbital (100 mg/kg i.p.) in both chronic dosing and acute dosing schedules. Results from acute dosing, one hour after a single dose of a root extract (40 mg/kg i.p.), showed that the duration of hexobarbital-induced sleep was significantly prolonged ($p < 0.005$). At four times the dose (160 mg/kg i.p.), sleep latency was significantly reduced by 47% ($p < 0.01$) and sleep duration was significantly prolonged by close to 200% ($p < 0.005$). In the chronic study, one hour after the fifth day of treatment with the extract (80 mg/kg i.p. daily), mice showed a significant increase in sleep duration ($p < 0.0005$), but not 24 h after four days of the same daily dosing. In vitro tests of hexobarbital metabolism in mouse liver preparations (S-9 microsomal enzyme) found a significant inhibition from the root extract at 100 μg/mL, leading the researchers to conclude that the inhibition of liver enzymes may be responsible for the prolonged sedative activity in the hexobarbital-treated mice (Medon et al., 1984).

Receptor- and Neurotransmitter-Mediated Functions

Farnsworth et al. (1985) recounted research showing that brain, urine, and adrenal gland levels of biogenic amines increased in rats after administration of the root extract of eleuthero (1 mL/kg p.o. daily). Winterhoff et al.

(1993) assumed that the antistress activity of eleuthero was mediated by the pituitary-adrenal system and endeavored to demonstrate this in male rats with extracts of the root (eleutheroside B at 0.6% and E at 1%). Injection of an aqueous extract (3 mg/kg i.p.) in the morning produced a significant increase in corticosterone levels after two h ($p < 0.01$), but produced no change in ACTH levels and caused a less pronounced increase when injected in the evening. In humans the reverse is true, with highest susceptibility of the pituitary occurring in the afternoon versus and highest reactivity of the adrenals in the morning. Following a subchronic treatment of the rats with the aqueous extract (100 and 500 mg/kg by gavage daily for seven weeks), significant amelioration of stress-induced (by injection of saline) increase of adrenocorticotropic hormone (ACTH) was found from a high single high dose (500 mg/kg p.o., $p < 0.05$), and by injection a low dose of the ethanolic extract (3 mg/kg i.p., $p < 0.01$); however, a single dose of the aqueous extract at 100 mg/kg p.o. was ineffective. Winterhoff and colleagues concluded that the subchronic treatment had reduced the reactivity of the pituitary-adrenal system to the stress. In further tests of the subchronically treated rats administered either 100 or 500 mg/kg p.o. daily, improvement was found in passive-avoidance behavior, learning, and reduced anxiety versus the controls. (Toxic effects of the seven-week treatment were absent in body and organ weights compared to the controls.) Further supporting their supposition of a pituitary-adrenal-related antistress action of eleuthero, in vitro exposure of rat primary pituitary cell cultures to the aqueous extract (0.1 g/mL) caused a significant increase in ACTH secretion ($p < 0.05$). Further studies are suggested to clarify the changes in central neurotransmitters that may precede effects on the pituitary-adrenal system or adapation reaction.

Yamazaki et al. (1994) reported that (+)-syringaresinol glucosides isolated from the root exhibited a significant neurite outgrowth-stimulating effect in PC12h cells in vitro, adding that the nerve-growth factorlike effect of the traditionally "restorative" herbal medicine was an intriguing coincidence.

CLINICAL STUDIES

Immune Disorders; Inflammation and Disease

Immunomodulation

Cellular immune response. In a double-blind study, the immunomodulating effects of an eleuthero extract was evaluated in 36 healthy volunteers. Subjects received 10 mL of a standardized ethanolic extract, or an ethanol placebo, t.i.d. for four weeks. At the end of the treatment period, the extract group showed marked increases in the number of immunocompetent cells, especially of T lymphocytes, but also of cytotoxic and natural killer (NK) cells, and there was a general increase in T lymphocyte activation. In addition, during a six-month observation period there were no side effects from the extract (Bohn et al., 1987).

Metabolic and Nutritional Disorders

Aging and Senescence; Longevity Enhancement

In a placebo-controlled study, Rovesti (1981) reported that compared to a face creme made with *Panax ginseng* extract (3%), and to a placebo face creme, a methanolic extract of eleuthero root (90%) as 3% of a facial creme applied for 30 days (2 g/day) to the skin of ten women (ages 30-40) produced superior results, with improvements in skin hydration, wrinkling, and sebum secretion.

Performance and Endurance Enhancement

Dowling et al. (1996) conducted an eight-week randomized double-blind, placebo-controlled trial of eleuthero (NutraPharm Incorporated, 3.4 mL/day of a 30% to 34% ethanolic extract characterized as containing eleutherosides B and E) on submaximal and maximal exercise performance in 20 distance runners (4 females and 16 males ages 29-45), all highly trained. No significant differences compared to placebo were found in oxygen uptake (VO_2), oxygen minute ventilation (V_E), or their ratio (measurement of the ventilatory equivalent for the amount of oxygen uptake, V_E/VO_2), the respiratory exchange ratio, the Tmax test, metabolic measurements, serum lactate levels, or the rating of perceived exertion test (psychological).

A randomized placebo-controlled study of eleuthero (uncharacterized, 1 g/day each morning for six weeks) in 15 male and 15 female athletes by McNaughton et al. (1989) found pectoral strength significantly improved by an average of 13% ($p < 0.05$), and quadriceps strength improved by an average of 15% ($p < 0.05$) versus placebo. However, another group taking *Panax ginseng* (uncharacterized, 1 g/day each morning for six weeks) showed clearly superior results, with significant improvement compared to placebo in maximal oxygen uptake (VO_2max) ($p < 0.01$), recovery time ($p < 0.05$), quadriceps strength (average 18%, $p < 0.05$), and pectoral strength (average 22%, $p < 0.01$).

DOSAGE

Eleuthero is generally taken in doses of 150-200 mg/day of a 10:1 standardized root extract containing 0.8% eleutherosides B and E. Most of the clinical studies have used a 33% ethanol extract of the root. Doses ranged from 2-16 mL, one to three times daily for up to 60 consecutive days (Pizzorno and Murray, 1993).

The *British Herbal Compendium* (Bradley, 1992) provides the dosage recommendations of 2-3 g of dried root or the equivalent as a tincture. The *Compendium* advises that eleuthero extracts should not be taken continuously for long periods, and recommends a four-week continuous usage followed by an eight-week interval. Regulatory guidelines from other EC (European Community) countries are similar (Bradley, 1992). The German Commission E gives the daily dosage for eleuthero as 2-3 g of the root or equivalent preparations and specifies its use as a tonic for treating convalescing persons and those with debility of fatigue or individuals experiencing a decline in their work capacity and ability to concentrate (Blumenthal et al., 1998).

SAFETY PROFILE

In Russian studies of eleuthero in over 2,100 healthy subjects, no side effects were documented (Newall et al., 1996). In clinical studies of a 33% ethanol extract of the root administered orally (0.5-6.0 mL one to three times daily) to over 2,200 unhealthy individuals in Russia of both sexes (ages 19-60), what side effects were reported were extremely few. For example, from high dosages of the extract in rheumatic heart disease patients, 2/55 reported elevations in blood pressure, headaches, palpitations, and pericardial pain. Patients with atherosclerosis treated with the extract were reported in two clinical studies to have shown only "some incidence" of tachycardia, insomnia, hypertonia, extrasystole, and heart rhythm shifts (Farnsworth et al., 1985).

Contraindications

The German Commission E states that use of the root is contraindicated in hypertension (De Smet et al., 1993). In two clinical studies in Russia, researchers recommended that persons with blood pressure over 180/90 mm Hg not take the root extract (Farnsworth et al., 1985). Others have cautioned that individuals with febrile states, hypertonic crisis, rheumatic heart disease, or myocardial infarctions should avoid the use of eleuthero (Anonymous, 1996).

Drug Interactions

Siberian ginseng may interact with cardiac, hypoglycemic, and hypo/hypertensive medications. Persons taking any medication requiring medical supervision should consult their physicians prior to use of eleuthero.

Eleuthero products have been substituted/contaminated with silk vine *(Periploca sepium),* a Chinese medicinal plant containing cardiac glycosides (Awang, 1991a, 1991b). In Canada, Koren et al. (1990) reported a case of neoandrogenization after prolonged use of an eleuthero product (Jamieson, Windsor, Ontario, Canada, 650 mg b.i.d. for 18 months). In this case, a 30-year-old female had taken double the dosage recommended by the manufacturer to treat herself for mood swings and irritability. She continued to take the product during nine months of pregnancy and two weeks of breast-feeding. The baby boy was born with red and swollen nipples, enlarged testes, thick, black pubic hair, and hair covering the whole area of the forehead. Yet, tests for androgen production showed nothing out of the ordinary. The mother also noted thicker and increased pubic, facial, and head hair in herself, along with premature uterine contractions during the late stages of her pregnancy (Koren et al., 1990). The product was subsequently shown to be devoid of eleutherosides, but contained compounds characteristic of *Periploca* (Awang, 1991a,b). Although the factors responsible for the neoandrogenization and the mother's apparent androgenization remain unknown, silk vine is highly suspected.

In another case, an apparently serious drug interaction from a product purporting to be eleuthero was reported in Canada when an elderly man with atrial fibrillation receiving long-term treatment with digoxin showed highly elevated serum levels of the drug during times when he ingested an eleuthero product. Although he had no symptomatic complaints, the high levels persisted when he was taken off digoxin. All common reasons for the elevated levels were eliminated. Analysis of the eleuthero product revealed no digoxin, but the researchers failed to test for eleutherosides to authenticate the product (McRae, 1996). Contamination/substitution of eleuthero with Chinese silk vine *(Periploca sepium)* remains the most likely cause, especially since this plant contains cardiac glycosides (Awang, 1996a,b). However, there is also the possibility that eleuthero interferes with drug metabolizing enzymes of the liver, as indicted by in vitro studies using recombinant human cytochrome P450 isoforms. In these studies, water extracts of the dried and powdered root and ethanol extracts of eleuthero obtained from commercial extracts both inhibited CY1A2 and CYP3A4 isozymes. The water extracts were less potent than the commercial ethanol extracts, producing IC_{50}s of 40-150 μg/mL and 0.12-21 μg/mL, respectively. In contrast, eleutherosides B and E showed no activity on five different recombinant isozymes (Harkey et al., 2001).

Pregnancy and Lactation

The German Commission E monograph on eleuthero does not contraindicate for pregnancy or lactation (Blumenthal et al., 1998). Studies of pregnant animals given eleuthero showed no adverse effects on fetuses. Administration of eleuthero to animals starting in pregnancy and continuing for their course of lactation showed no adverse effects (see Toxicology: Toxicology in Animal Models). Feeding studies of eleuthero in pregnant rats, minks, lambs, and rabbits have shown no evidence of teratogenic effects on the fetuses, or adverse effects on the mothers or offspring compared to controls. In one study, a 10% extract was fed to pregnant minks (10 mL/kg) and their offspring from the first day of lactation until the pups were 45 days old. No adverse effects on the mothers or pups were observed (Farnsworth et al., 1985). No reports of adverse effects during pregnancy or lactation in humans are known.

Side Effects

Documented side effects from eleuthero are rare. They include languor or drowsiness immediately after ingestion, which may be a result of a hypoglycemic effect of the extract. Side effects observed after prolonged use of higher doses include insomnia, irritability, melancholy, and anxiety. Individuals with rheumatic heart disease have reported side effects including pericardial pain, headaches, palpitations, and elevations in blood pressure (Pizzorno and Murray, 1993).

Special Precautions

See Contraindications.

Toxicology

Toxicity in Animal Models

Feeding studies of eleuthero in pregnant rats, minks, lambs, and rabbits have shown no evidence of teratogenic effects on the fetuses, or adverse effects on the mothers or offspring compared to controls. In one study, a 10% extract was fed to pregnant minks (10 mL/kg) and to the offspring of these animals from the first day of lactation until the pups were 45 days old. No adverse effects on the mothers or pups were observed (Farnsworth et al., 1985).

No pathologic, histologic, or cytotoxic changes were observed in livers, brains, and kidneys of mice that ingested infusions of eleuthero for up to 96 days; however, evidence of significant aggressive behavior (abuse and fighting) was seen in mice from a commercial extract infusion containing sugar (Lewis et al., 1983). Rats administered 5 mL/kg of a 33% ethanol extract of eleuthero for 320 days showed no toxic manifestations or deaths after 800 days from birth. A freeze-dried, aqueous extract of eleuthero failed to produce death in mice at oral doses of 3 g/kg (Farnsworth et al., 1985).

The acute LD_{50} of a 70% alcohol extract of the dried powdered roots in mice is reported to be $3,880 \pm 74$ mg/kg (Singh et al., 1991).

REFERENCES

Anonymous (1996). Eleutherococcus. *Lawrence Review of Natural Products* (May).

Awang, D.V.C. (1991a). Maternal use of ginseng and neonatal androgenization. *Journal of the American Medical Association* 265: 1829.

Awang, D.V.C. (1991b). Maternal use of ginseng and neonatal androgenization. *Journal of the American Medical Association* 266: 363.

Awang, D.V.C. (1996a). Eleuthero. *Canadian Pharmaceutical Journal* 129: 52-54.

Awang, D.V.C. (1996b). Siberian ginseng toxicity may be case of mistaken identity. *Canadian Medical Association Journal* 155: 1237.

Blumenthal, M., Busse, W.R., Goldberg, A., Gruenwald, J., Hall, T., Riggins, C.W. and Rister, R.S. (Eds.) (1998). *The Complete German Commission E Monographs.* Austin, TX: American Botanical Council, pp. 124-125.

Bohn, B., Nebe, C.T., and Birr, C. (1987). Flow cytometric studies with *Eleutherococcus senticosus* extract as an immunomodulatory agent. *Arzneimittel-Forschung/Drug Research* 37: 1193-1196.

Bradley, P.R. (Ed.) (1992). *British Herbal Compendium,* 1. Bournemouth, Dorset, England: British Herbal Medicine Association, pp. 89-91.

Brekhman, I.I. and Dardymov, I.V. (1969). New substances of plant origin which increase nonspecific resistance. *Annual Review of Pharmacology* 4: 419-430.

Chang, H.M. and But, P. P. (Eds.) (1986). *Pharmacology and Applications of Chinese Materia Medica,* 1. Hong Kong: World Scientific.

Dardymov, I.V., Khasina, E.I., and Bezdetko, G.N. (1978). [Insulin-like action of eleutherosides from the roots of *Eleutherococcus senticosus*]. *Rastitel'nye Resursy* 14: 86-89. In *Chemical Abstracts* 88: 115363e.

Davydov, M. and Krikorian, A.D. (2000). *Eleutherococcus senticosus* (Rupr. & Maxim.) Maxim. (Araliaceae) as an adaptogen: A closer look. *Journal of Ethnopharmacology* 72(3): 345-393.

De Smet, P.A.G.M., Keller, K., Hänsel, R., and Chandler (Eds.) (1993). *Adverse Effects of Herbal Drugs,* 2. New York: Springer-Verlag, p. 39.

Dowling, E.A., Rendondo, D.R., and Branch, J.D. (1996). Effect of *Eleutherococcus senticosus* on submaximal and maximal exercise performance. *Medicine and Science in Sports and Medicine* 28: 482-489.

Fang, J.N., Proksch, A., and Wagner, H. (1985). Immunologically active polysaccharides of *Acanthopanax senticosus. Phytochemistry* 24: 2619-2622.

Farnsworth, N.R., Kinghorn, A.D., Soejarto, D.D., and Waller, D.P. (1985). Siberian ginseng *(Eleutherococcus senticosus):* Current status as an adaptogen. In Wagner, H., Hikino, H., and Farnsworth, N.R. (Eds.), *Economic and Medicinal Plant Research,* 1 (pp. 155-215). New York: Academic Press.

Foster, S. and Yue, C. (1992). *Herbal Emissaries: Bringing Chinese Herbs to the West*. Rochester, VT: Healing Arts Press, pp. 23-29.

Fujikawa, T., Yamaguchi, A., Morita, I., Takeda, H., and Nishibe, S. (1996). Protective effects of *Acanthopanax senticosus* Harms from Hokkaido and its components of gastric ulcer on restrained cold water stressed rats. *Biological and Pharmaceutical Bulletin* 19: 1227-1230.

Harkey, M.R., Henderson, G.L., Zhou, L., Sakai, S., and Gershwin, M.E. (2001). Effects of Siberian ginseng *(Eleutherococcus senticosus)* on c-DNA-expressed P450 drug metabolizing enzymes. *Alternative Therapies in Health and Medicine* 7: S14 (abstract).

Hikino, H., Takahashi, M., Otake, K., and Konno, C. (1986). Isolation and hypoglycemic activity of eleutherans A, B, C, D, E, F and G: Glycans of *Eleutherococcus senticosus* roots. *Journal of Natural Products* 49: 293-297.

Koren, G., Randor, S., Martin, S., and Danneman, D. (1990). Maternal ginseng use associated with androgenization. *Journal of the American Medical Association* 264: 2866.

Kurkin, V.A., Zapesochnaya, G.G., and Bandyshev, V.V. (1991). Phenolic compounds of *Eleutherococcus senticosus*. *Chemistry of Natural Compounds* 27: 755-756.

Lewis, W.H., Zenger, V.E., and Lynch, R.G. (1983). No adaptogenic response of mice to ginseng and *Eleutherococcus* infusions. *Journal of Ethnopharmacology* 8: 209-214.

Li, T.S.C. (2001). Siberian ginseng. *HortTechnology* 11(1): 79-85.

Makarieva, T.N., Dmitrenok, A.S., Stonik, V.A., Patel, A.V., and Canfield, L.M. (1997). Lignans from *Eleutherococcus senticosus* (Siberian ginseng). *Pharmaceutical Sciences* 3: 525-527.

Martinez, B. and Staba, E.J. (1984). The physiological effects of *Aralia, Panax* and *Eleutherococcus* on exercised rats. *Japanese Journal of Pharmacology* 35: 79-85.

McNaughton, L., Egan, G., and Caelli, G. (1989). A comparison of Chinese and Russian ginseng as ergogenic aids to improve various facets of physical fitness. *International Clinical Nutrition Review* 9: 32-35.

McRae, S. (1996). Elevated serum digoxin levels in a patient taking digoxin and Siberian ginseng. *Canadian Medical Association Journal* 155: 293-295.

Medon, P.J., Ferguson, P.W., and Watson, C.F. (1984). Effects of *Eleutherococcus senticosus* extracts on hexobarbital metabolism in vivo and in vitro. *Journal of Ethnopharmacology* 10: 235-241.

Newall, C.A., Anderson, L.A., and Phillipson, J.D. (1996). *Herbal Medicines: A Guide for Health Care Professionals*. London: The Pharmaceutical Press, pp. 141-144.

Nishibe, S., Knoshita, H., Takeda, H., and Okano, G. (1990). Phenolic compounds from stem bark of *Acanthopanax senticosus* and their pharmacological effect in chronic swimming stressed rats. *Chemical and Pharmaceutical Bulletin* 38: 1763-1765.

Pearce, P.Y., Zois, I., Wynne, K.N., and Funder, J.W. (1982). *Panax ginseng* and *Eleutherococcus senticosus* extracts—In vitro studies on binding to steroid receptors. *Endocrinologica Japonica* 29: 567-573.

Pizzorno, J.E. and Murray, M.T. (1993). *A Textbook of Natural Medicine*. Seattle, WA: Bastyr College Publications.

Rovesti, P. (1981). Azione cosmetologica dell'*Eleutherococcus senticosus* Maxim. [Cosmetological action of *Eleutherococcus senticosus* Maxim.]. *Revista Italiana E.P.P.O.S.* 63: 75-78. In *Chemical Abstracts* 1981, 95:12567q.

Shen, M.L., Zhai, S.K., Chen, H.L., Luo, Y.D., Tu, G.R., and Ou, D.W. (1991). Immunopharmacological effects of polysaccharides from *Acanthopanax senticosus* on experimental animals. *International Journal of Immunopharmacology* 13: 549-554.

Singh, N., Verma, P., Mishra, N., and Nath, R.A. (1991). A comparative evaluation of some anti-stress agents of plant origin. *Indian Journal of Pharmacology* 23: 99-103.

Tyler, V.E. (1998). Importance of European phytomedicinals in the American market: An overview. In Lawson, L.D. and Bauer, R. (Eds.), *Phytomedicines of Europe: Chemistry and Biological Activity* (pp. 2-12). Washington, DC: American Chemical Society.

Wagner, H., Nörr, H., and Winterhoff, H. (1992). Drugs with adaptogenic effects for strengthening the powers of resistance. *Zeitschrift für Phytotherapie* 13: 42-54 (translated by C. Hobbs and S. Coble; available from the American Botanical Council, Austin, TX).

Winterhoff, H., Meisel, M.L., Vahlensieck, U., Nörr, H., and Wagner, H. (1993). Interference of *Eleutherococcus senticosus* extract with LHRH and LH stimulation ("in vitro"). *Pharmaceutical and Pharmacological Letters* 3: 95-98.

Yamazaki, M., Hirota, K., Chiba, K., and Mohri, T. (1994). Promotion of neuronal differentiation of PC12h cells by natural lignans and iridoids. *Biological and Pharmaceutical Bulletin* 17: 1604-1608.

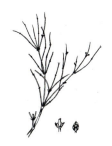

BOTANICAL DATA

Classification and Nomenclature

Scientific name: *Ephedra sinica* Stapf, *E. equisetina* Bunge, *E. intermedia* Schrenk et C.A. Meyer

Family name: Ephedraceae

Common names: Ma huang (má-huáng), *Ephedrae herba,* herbaceous *Ephedra* (tsao ma huang), field ma huang (tien ma huang) *(E. sinica),* horsetail *Ephedra* (mu tsei ma huang), mountain *Ephedra* (shan ma huang), wood *Ephedra* (mu ma huang) *(E. equisetina),* and intermediate *Ephedra* (chung ma huang) *(E. intermedia)* (Hu, 1969). Ma huang refers to the dried herbaceous stem of the three official species in China, while ma huang gen refers to the dried rhizomes and roots of *E. sinica* and *E. intermedia* (Tu et al., 1992). However, Herba Ephedrae, mao (Japan), ma huang gen (ma huang root) (China), and ma kon (*Ephedra* root) (Japan) refer to all three species (Zhu, 1998). Ephedra is the common English name. Unless otherwise indicated in this chapter, ma huang or ephedra refers to the aerial parts of the three official *Ephedra* species in China.

Description

Numbering about 50 species worldwide, *Ephedra* is found in such diverse areas as Central, South and North America, Afghanistan, Pakistan, Mediterranean Europe, north and central Europe, and Russia, including Siberia (Price, 1996; Stevenson, 1993). The common Chinese name, ma huang, is said to derive from the yellow color (huang) and the numbing action (ma) of the plant (Zhu, 1998), described as "numbing" to the tongue (Hsu et al., 1986). Only the three species listed previously are official in the

Pharmacopoeias of China and Japan (Tu et al., 1992; Kondo et al., 1999); however, *E. distachya* L., *E. gerardiana* Wall. ex Stapf., and other species of *Ephedra* are currently identified in commerce (Liu et al., 1993; Blumenthal, 1998; McGuffin et al., 1997; Kondo et al., 1999).

In dry highland areas, on hilly slopes, mountain fields, and dry river beds, *E. sinica* occurs in northeastern China in the provinces of Liaoning and Jilin and in the north in the provinces of Shaanxi, Shanxi, Hebei, Henan, and Inner Mongolia. *Ephedra sinica* grows to a height of 20-40 cm and is described as a nearly leafless perennial herbaceous shrub with a slender woody main stem and erect aerial stems which are used medicinally (Hu, 1969). The plant is infrequently branched (1-2 mm in diameter), cylindrical, and very pale green to yellowish-green in color. The easily broken stems are light and when fractured show a reddish-brown pith and a greenish-yellow edge. Their odor is slightly aromatic and their taste is slightly bitter and astringent. The leaves are described as scaly (Tu et al., 1992), membranaceus and sheathlike, acutely triangular, with half connate basal leaves surrounding nodes. A brownish-red pith shows through the broken surface of the slender internodes (1-1.5 mm in diameter and 2.5-5 cm in length). It flowers in May with conelike inflorescences. In July, the mature plant develops red, berrylike seeds (Hu, 1969).

Ephedra equisetina occurs in the provinces of Xinjiang and western Sichuan, in the northwest in Gansu, and in the north in Shaanxi, Shanxi, Hebei, and Inner Mongolia. *Ephedra equisetina* is a small erect shrub growing 30-50 cm in height commonly found on cliffs. It has a coarse woody stem and the internodes (1-1.5 mm in diameter and 1.5-2.5 cm long) of green stem are short and slender (Hu, 1969). It is described as being frequently branched (1-1.5 mm in diameter), and smooth to the touch. The upper part is grayish-white, short-triangular, and the base of the plant has a brownish-red or brownish-black color. The leaves are membranaceus, scaly, small (1-2 mm long) (Tu et al., 1992), opposite, short, and triangular with obtuse lobes which are usually brown. Female flowers are solitary, sessile, and narrowly ellipsoid with bracts in three to four pairs. It flowers in June and July. When the seed matures in August and September the flowers appear fleshy, berrylike, and red.

Ephedra intermedia occurs in Xinjiang, Ningxia, Tibet, Qinghai, Shandong, Shaanxi, Shanxi, Gansu, Hebei, Liaoning, and Inner Mongolia. *Ephedra intermedia* is a shrub found in desert sandy areas. It grows to a height of 1 m with stout, erect aerial shoots of a brown color which often appear as if covered with a white powder (Hu, 1969). The plant is described as being frequently branched (1.5-3 mm in diameter) and rough (Tu et al., 1992). The internodes are at least 2 mm in diameter and 3-6 cm long. When young, the leaves are acute. They occur on the same point on the axis, the basal leaves are two-thirds united, and the apical part is deltoid. The flower bracts and leaves occur in whorls. The oblong female flowers (1.5-2.5 mm long) are spiral, and occur in a whorl when three, and opposite on the node when two. When the seeds (two-three) are mature (about 5 mm in length) the flowers appear red and look as if they are covered with a white powder (Hu, 1969).

The dried roots and rhizomes of *E. sinica* and *E. intermedia* are described as slightly curved and cylindrical, 8-25 cm in length, and 0.5-1.5 cm in diameter with longitudinal scars and wrinkles and an easily removable rough outer bark. They are odorless, have a slightly bitter taste, and externally are grayish- or reddish-brown. Their texture is light, fragile, and hard. The powdered root and rhizome contain crystals of calcium oxalate (Tu et al., 1992). After collection in late autumn the plant parts are dried in the sun (Tu et al., 1992) or shade (Zhu, 1998).

HISTORY AND TRADITIONAL USES

Ma huang has a long history of use in China where it first appears in the *Shen Nong Ben Cao Jing* (about 3100 B.C.) as *long sha* (dragon sand). Here, ma huang is described as a bitter and warm herb, nontoxic, used to treat malaria, headache, and as a cough suppressant (Yang, 1997). In traditional Chinese and Japanese medicine, the aerial part is typically stir-fried in honey and combined with other botanicals for the treatment of bronchial asthma (Yuan et al., 1998), cough, edema in acute nephritis, to induce diuresis or perspiration, and symptoms of the common cold (Tu et al., 1992). The inner bark of *Ephedra sinica* is used in an ancient traditional formula to treat viral infections, influenza, sore throat, fever, chills, headache, polyarthralgia, and cervical muscle tension (Shiraki et al., 1999). Although the entire plant has been used, the root is said to have the opposite effects of the aerial part (Hu, 1969). This observation appears to be born out in contemporary studies which show that whereas the aerial parts are diaphoretic and increase blood pressure, the root is hypotensive and is used topically in powdered form to stop excessive sweating (Zhu, 1998; Tu et al., 1992). Although the stems are officially used as a diuretic in China (Tu et al., 1992), in Western medicine the main alkaloid constituents, ephedrine and pseudoephedrine, were at one time used to treat urinary incontinence (Reynolds, 1996). Following the isolation of ephedrine from ma huang in 1885 (Holmstedt, 1991), and of pseudoephedrine from *E. vulgaris* by Merck in 1893 (Chen and Schmidt, 1924), ma huang has been associated with both drugs (Robbers and Tyler, 1999).

Other members of the genus used medicinally that also contain ephedrine alkaloids include the Indian species called "asmania" (*E. gerardiana* Wall.). For the treatment of asthma, preparations include a decoction, alcoholic extract or tincture of the dried root, and an alcoholic extract of the dried and powdered twigs of *E. gerardiana* and *E. intermedia* (imported from Tibet). The decoction is used to improve digestion, and in the treatment of syphilis and acute articular and muscular rheumatism. The berry juice has been used in the treatment of disturbances of the respiratory passage (Nadkarni, 1976). In Iraqi folk medicine, *E. foliata* is used for the relief of asthma and cough (Alwan et al., 1986). In the area of the Khyber Pass in Afghanistan, the locals boil *E. pachyclada* in milk to prepare an aphrodisiac beverage (Stark, 1980). The U.S. species commonly known as Mormon tea (*E. nevadensis* S. Wats.) contains little or no alkaloids (Robbers and Tyler, 1999; Nadkarni, 1976).

The potency of ephedrine as a central nervous system stimulant was recognized by the Japanese armed forces during World War II when ephedrine was called *philopon* (love of work) and administered by injection to kamikaze pilots. Following the War, military supplies of ephedrine made their way to the black market which led to a major epidemic of ephedrine abuse in many of the larger cities in Japan. Abusers called the drug *hirapon* which they self-administered by injection (Karch, 2000).

Ephedrine was introduced for the treatment of bronchial asthma in children in the 1920s (Munns and Aldrich, 1927; Miller, 1925) when its comparatively far more persistent and gradual action replaced the use of adrenaline which could not be administered orally (Kalix, 1991). As a bronchodilator, ephedrine has since been largely superseded by more preferred and more selective β_2-adrenergic agents (e.g., salbutamol) used in the treatment of asthma. Ephedrine is a sympathomimetic agent primarily used today as a nasal decongestant administered orally, by spray, topically, or as nasal drops in numerous over-the-counter preparations (Reynolds, 1996). Other less preferred uses of ephedrine (oral route) include chronic urticaria (Bierman and Pearlman, 1988), diabetic neuropathic edema, nocturnal eneuresis, and motion sickness. The constituent pseudoephedrine has a similar and weaker action compared to ephedrine and is taken orally for symptomatic relief of nasal congestion. The nasal decongestant phenylpropanolamine or (±)-norephedrine is a synthetic isomer of the alkaloid constituent (–)-norephedrine (Reynolds, 1996). Until a recent ban of phenylpropanolamine due to a risk of hemorrhagic stroke (FDA, 2000; Kernan et al., 2000), it was widely used in a diversity of cold and sinus products (e.g., Dimetapp, Contac Severe Cold and Flu, Sinutab, Triaminic Oral Infant Drops, Vicks DayQuil), and as an appetite suppressant (Dexatrim) (Reynolds, 1996).

The only other major use of ephedrine is in weight loss. This application followed the accidental discovery by a Danish physician in 1972 of weight loss in asthmatic patients from a combination of ephedrine, caffeine, and phenobarbital (Malchow-Møller et al., 1981). Today, *E. sinica* and ephedrine continue to be studied for the treatment of obesity, often in combination with caffeine, aspirin, or other substances (Woodgate and Conquer, 2001;

Boozer et al., 2001; Martinet et al., 1999; Astrup, Breum et al., 1992; Krieger et al., 1990; Dulloo and Miller, 1987). Both the safety and efficacy of this application is controversial, as is the popular use of ma huang or ephedrine for energy enhancement (Blumenthal and King, 1995; Sprague et al., 1998; Fugh-Berman and Allina, 2000; Bedard, 2000; Clarkson and Thompson, 1997; Nightingale, 1996).

Ma huang is currently listed in the pharmacopoeias of China, Japan, and Germany (Reynolds, 1996). In 1955, *Ephedra* was listed as an official drug in the United States. With the subsequent availability of synthetic ephedrine and ephedrine-type alkaloids in the United States, clinical use of the herb was abandoned (Betz et al., 1997).

CHEMISTRY

Nitrogenous Compounds

Alkaloids

The major alkaloids in the aerial parts of the main medicinal Chinese *Ephedra* species *(E. sinica, E. intermedia,* and *E. equisetina)* are (–)-ephedrine and (+)-pseudoephedrine. Other closely related alkaloids occurring in trace amounts are (–)-norephedrine, (+)-norpseudoephedrine, (–)-methylephedrine, and (+)-methylpseudoephedrine (Zhang et al., 1988; Zhu, 1998). Ephedroxane, an analogue of ephedrine, occurs in trace amounts in the main species of *Ephedra* and in some but not all species in China and Japan. Highest concentration (0.0021% by dry weight) was found in *E. equisetina* from Japan (Konno et al., 1979). The presence of (+)-ephedrine or other chiral isomers indicates adulteration with synthetic alkaloids (Betz et al., 1997; Flurer et al., 1995). In the crude herb *("Ephedrae herba"),* tetramethylpyrazine (ligustrazine) occurs in minute amounts (ca. 0.2 mg/g) (Kun et al., 2000), and in higher amounts in stir-fried and honey-cured ma huang (Leung and Foster, 1996). Ephedrine is absent in *Ephedra* species of North and South America. Pseudoephedrine may occur in these species, but only in minute amounts, if at all (Caveney et al., 2001).

Norpseudoephedrine or cathine also occurs in khat (*Catha edulis* Forsk., Celastraceae) in which it is the main alkaloid. Khat is a stimulant plant used in Africa and some Arabian countries (Kalix, 1991). Ephedrine is also reported to occur in *Sida cordifolia* L. (Malvaceae) (Nadkarni, 1976; Franzotti et al., 2000), in minute amounts in the tubers of *Pinellia ternata* (Thunb.) Breitenbach (Araceae) (Oshio et al., 1978; Moriyasu et al., 1984), and in the leaves of the English yew (*Taxus baccata* L.; Taxaceae) (Lewis and Elvin-Lewis, 1977) in *Hamelia patens* (Chaudhuri and Thakur, 1991); *Roemeria refracta* DC., and *Aconitum napellus* L. (Smith, 1977). Tetramethylpyrazine also occurs in the Chinese medicinal plants *Ligusticum wallachii* (Pang et al., 1996), and *Cnidium monnieri* (Watanabe, 1997), as well as cocoa beans *(Theobroma cocao)* (Sanagi et al., 1997).

According to the Chinese pharmacopoeia, the aerial part or stem contains no less than 0.8% alkaloids, calculated as ephedrine (Tu et al., 1992). In a survey of 12 Chinese species of *Ephedra* grown in 24 districts, wild *E. sinica* showed higher levels of alkaloids compared to a cultivated sample (Zhang et al., 1989). Most of the alkaloid content is in the green stems (Hu, 1969) and greatly varies with geographical origin (Zhang et al., 1989; Nadkarni, 1976), soil pH, genetic factors (Kondo et al., 1999), and the seasons, the content being highest in the autumn when the plant matures (Hu, 1969). In northern India, highest alkaloid levels were found in the green stems of *E. gerardiana* during the autumn (October-November); however, the Chinese *Ephedra* have shown a higher alkaloid content than either *E. gerardiana* or the European *E. vulgaris* (Nadkarni, 1976).

The yields of total alkaloid, ephedrine, and pseudoephedrine in the official species of Chinese medicine are: *E. sinica* (0.48-1.38%; 55-78% ephedrine, and 12-23% pseudoephedrine); *E. intermedia* (1.05-1.56%; 12-31% ephedrine, and 59-75% pseudoephedrine); and *E. equisetina* (2.09-2.43%; 53-58% ephedrine, and 19-27% pseudoephedrine) (Zhu, 1998). Among 22 commercial samples of ma huang sold in Taiwan *(E. sinica, E. intermedia, E. equisetina,* and *E. distachya),* higher amounts of alkaloids were found in the internodes and thin stems. Alkaloid content varied from 0.536% to 2.308% (Liu et al., 1993).

The proportions of the various alkaloids also show variation depending on the species (Zhu, 1998; Zhang et al., 1988, 1989; Nadkarni, 1976). Among Chinese species, *E. intermedia* and *E. lomatolepsis* may be unique in that they show a higher ratio of pseudoephedrine to ephedrine compared to other species which show a higher ratio of ephedrine:pseudoephedrine (Zhang et al., 1989). This difference may be useful in distinguishing the species (Sheu, 1997; Liu et al., 1993). In addition, the methylephedrine content was found to be higher in *E. sinica* from northeastern China and in *E. intermedia* var. *tibetica* from Tibet (Zhang et al., 1989).

The roots contain the spermine-type alkaloids ephedradines A, B, C, and D (Hikino, Ogata et al., 1982; Tamada, Endo, Hikino et al., 1979; Tamada, Endo, and Hikino, 1979; Konno et al., 1980). They also contain the alkaloids maokonine (Tamada et al., 1978) and the imidazole alkaloid feruloylhistamine (Hikino, Ogata, and Konno 1983; Hikono et al., 1984).

Miscellaneous Nitrogenous Compounds

Maokonine (*l*-tyrosine betaine) was isolated from the roots of Japanese *Ephedra mao-kon* (Tamada et al., 1978).

Organic Acids

Aerial parts contain cinnamic acid, vanillic acid, *p*-coumaric acid, benzoic acid, *p*-hydroxybenzoic acid, and protocatechuic acid (Zhu, 1998).

Phenolic Compounds

Flavonoids

The roots contain the biflavanols mahuannin A, B, C, and D (Hikino, Shimoyama et al., 1982; Kasahara et al., 1983; Kasahara and Hikino, 1983) and the flavonflavanol, ephedrannin A (Hikino, Takahashi et al., 1982).

Tannins

The aerial parts contain (–)-epicatechin, and (–)-epigallocatechin (Takechi et al., 1985), catechin, gallocatechin (Zhu, 1998).

Other Constituents

Mixed Volatile Oils

Terpenoids constitute 38.9% of the volatile oil (Miyazawa et al., 1997). Others include myrcene, β-terpinol, tetramethylpyrazine, and terpinol-4-ol (Zhu, 1998; Miyazawa et al., 1997). At 31.64%, the main constituent of the essential oil of *E. sinica* dried stems was *l*-α-terpinol. In the dried stems of *E. intermedia* and *E. equisetina,* the main constituents of the essential oil were reported to be 1,4-cineole (12.80%) and hexadecanoic acid (26.22%), respectively (Ji et al., 1997).

THERAPEUTIC APPLICATIONS

Uses of the aerial part of ma huang in Chinese medicine include diuretic ("easing the excretion of urine"), the treatment of colds, pain throughout the body, painful joints, swelling of the ankles, shortness of breath, fevers with an absence of sweating, typhoid (Hu, 1969), high fever (Hsu, 1973), and acute nephritis (Ling et al., 1995). For such problems, ma huang is traditionally used in combination with other medicinal plants. In the treatment of the common cold or flu, for example, ma huang is combined with licorice root, cinnamon bark, and apricot seed (Chang and But, 1987).

In the Chinese pharmacopoeia, only honey-processed ma huang is officially used for the following: as a diuretic; for the relief of cough and asthma; the treatment of bronchial asthma; edema in cases of acute nephritis; and the common cold when attended by mild fever, stuffy and running nose, chills, headache, and an absence of sweating (Tu et al., 1992). Commonly referred to as roasted ma huang (Huntley and Ernst, 2000), honey-processed ma huang is traditionally prepared by mixing honey in boiled water which is added to the softened, cut and air-dried stems and mixed. The mixture is then placed into a cauldron and roasted by turning. When all the water is evaporated and the honey has lost its stickiness, the mixture is taken out and allowed to cool (Hu, 1969; Tu et al., 1992). The powdered, dried root and rhizome *(E. sinica and E. intermedia)* is used externally in the treatment of weak patients to check excessive sweating, spontaneous sweating, and night sweating (Tu et al., 1992; Hu, 1969).

Despite the main traditional Chinese uses of ma huang in the treatment of colds, the relief of cough and bronchial asthma, and as a diuretic (Hu, 1969; Tu et al., 1992)—typically combined with other medicinal plants (Chang and But, 1987; Zou et al., 1996; Yuan et al., 1998)—by far its main use in the West has been in weight management formulas, typically combined with caffeine or caffeine-containing botanicals. Ma huang has also been used in the West for bodybuilding, as an energy booster, and as a recreational drug (Fugh-Berman and Allina, 2000). Due to reports of serious side effects, the use of *Ephedra* in dietary supplements in the United States is controversial (Seckman, 2000; Fugh-Berman and Allina, 2000) (see Safety Profile).

PRECLINICAL STUDIES

Cardiovascular and Circulatory Functions

Hypertension

Tannin fractions of ma huang *("Ephedrae Herba")* were shown to non-competitively inhibit angiotensin-converting enzyme (ACE) activity with I_{50} concentrations of 1.9 mg/mL and 4.5 mg/mL. However, the activity was much less than that of captopril (Inokuchi et al., 1985).

A minor constituent of the roots of *Ephedra* used in Japan, an alkaloid named maokonine (*l*-tyrosine betaine; 7.05 mg/kg of dried roots), was reported to show mildly hypertensive activity in anesthetized rats which was comparable to that of ephedrine, an effect reportedly opposite to that of the root extract itself (Tamada et al., 1978; Tamada, Endo and Hikino, 1979). However, hypotensive activity of the root (crude methanol extract, 2 g/kg i.v.) (Tamada, Endo, Hikino, et al., 1979), along with the various alkaloids, including ephedradines A, B, C, and D (Hikino, Ogata et al., 1982; Hikino, Shimoyama, et al., 1982; Hikino, Takahashi, et al. 1982; Hikino, Ogata, Konno, et al. 1983; Tamada, Endo, Hikino, et al., 1979; Tamada, Endo, and Hikino, 1979; Konno et al., 1980), and feruloylhistamine (Hikino, Ogata, and Konno, 1983; Hikino et al., 1984), and bisflavanols (mahuannins A, B, C, and D) (Hikino, Shimoyama, et al., 1982; Kasahara et al., 1983; Kasahara and Hikino, 1983) to which hypotensive activity of the root is attributed, derives from intravenous administrations which may not be representative of orally administered preparations or constituents.

Peripheral Vascular Functions

A water extract of ma huang administered to rats (75-300 mg/kg p.o.) exhibited a dose-dependent diaphoretic effect (Zhu, 1998). Ephedrine at oral doses of 2-8 mg/kg in male rats caused significant increases in respiratory dry heat loss. At doses of 4 or 8 mg/kg, significant respiratory evaporative water loss was demonstrated. However, significant dry heat loss or evaporative water loss from the body surface was not found from any of these doses (Yuan et al., 1999, 1998).

Digestive, Hepatic, and Gastrointestinal Functions

Gastric Functions

The alkaloid feruloylhistamine, a minor constituent of the roots of ma huang, exhibited potent inhibiting activity in vitro against the enzyme histidine decarboxylase (IC_{50}: 1.4×10^{-5} M), indicating that it may decrease or suppress ulcer formation since the enzyme is involved in the formation of histamine which in turn increases the output of gastric acid (Hikino et al., 1984). A comparison of the in vitro inhibiting activity of *Ephedra* alkaloids (ephedrine, pseudoephedrine, ephadroxane, and pseudoephedroxane) against histamine-induced contraction of isolated guinea pig ileum showed that by comparison to the control (diphenhydramine), ephedrine and pseudoephedrine were the more active alkaloids (Hikino et al., 1985).

Hepatic Functions

Feruloylhistamine significantly inhibited the in vitro cytotoxicity of galactosamine on cultured rat hepatocytes at a concentration of 0.1 mg/mL, and of carbon tetrachloride at a concentration of 1.0 mg/mL (Hikino et al., 1984).

Endocrine and Hormonal Functions

Adrenal Functions

Ephedrine and pseudoephedrine are classified as indirect-acting sympathetic nervous system stimulants. Mimicking the effects of adrenaline, they are adrenergic sympathomimetic compounds, an action shared with amphetamine and phenylpropanolamine (Reynolds, 1996). Involvement of adrenoreceptor β_3 may be responsible for 40% of the thermogenesis induced by ephedrine chloride with the possible involvement of all three β-adrenoreceptor subtypes; β_1 and β_2-adrenoreceptors (β_1- and β_2-ARs) accounting for 60% of the increase in energy expenditure caused by ephedrine (Liu et al., 1995). However, this theory is refuted by in vitro studies. At concentrations considerably greater than what is achieved in plasma from oral ($\pm$)-ephedrine at a dose of 50 mg, these studies showed no binding of ($\pm$)-ephedrine to human β_3-ARs and relatively weak binding (partial agonist activity) to human β_1- and β_2-ARs. Based on these results, it is postulated that the metabolic effects of ephedrine must largely be due to direct actions on β_1-ARs and/or β_2-ARs. In addition, the chance that these effects are being mediated indirectly on all 3 β-ARs "through the release of noradrenaline" is unlikely since urinary noradrenaline showed a significant decrease in volunteers taking oral ephedrine (50 mg thrice daily) in a short-term, placebo-controlled study (see Clinical Studies) (Shannon et al., 1999).

Carbohydrate Metabolism; Antidiabetic Activity

Xiu et al. (2001) examined the effect of a water extract of *Ephedra sinica* *("Ephedrae herba")* in mice with diabetes induced by streptozotocin (STZ). The extract was prepared by boiling the crude herb in water (10 g/600 mL water) until the volume reached 350 mL. They also tested the crude alkaloid fraction of the herb and *l*-ephedrine (each 0.62 mg/kg p.o. in the drinking water at a dosage equal to the alkaloid fraction of the crude herb). STZ-diabetic mice administered the water extract in diluted form for five weeks (equivalent to the crude herb at a dosage of 1.4 g/kg) showed a decrease in blood glucose on the third day ($p < 0.1$) and a significant decrease by day 14 compared to controls ($p < 0.01$), a result also found in the mice administered the crude alkaloid fraction ($p < 0.05$). Those administered ephedrine showed a significant decrease in blood glucose on day three ($p < 0.05$), but not after day six. Body weight of the control animals receiving water decreased as the experiment continued whereas by day six those receiving the water extract in their drinking water showed an increased body weight compared to the controls, as did the ephedrine-treated group on day 14. Those treated with the alkaloid fraction showed a higher body weight on day six compared to controls, but by day 12 it was equal to or less than the control group. Histological examination of the pancreas of the animals revealed atrophied islets of Langerhans in the control group, but in the groups that received the water extract, existence of alkaloid fraction or ephedrine was evidence of regeneration of the islets, which reached significance compared to the controls in the groups that received either the water extract or ephedrine in their drinking water (each $p < 0.05$). However, when the proportion of total islet tissue was measured relative to the pancreas as a whole, the improvements in all three groups reached significance, with those in the ephedrine group showing the greatest improvement ($p < 0.01$), followed by the water extract and alkaloid groups (each $p < 0.05$). The researchers concluded that the active hypoglycemic component of the herb is ephedrine and that it may be capable of not only regenerating atrophic islets, but also of restoring insulin secretion.

Genitourinary and Renal Functions

Renal Toxicity

Yokozawa et al. (1995) used an animal model of renal failure (adenine-induced) to investigate the potential of *Ephedra distachya* L. *("Ephedrae Herba")* to reduce uremic toxins. Groups of male rats with renal failure were administered a 1:10 w/v water extract of the stems (prepared by boiling in water for 60 min) or one of three fractions of the herb: a nonphenolic fraction (fraction 1), a lower molecular weight phenolic fraction containing flavonoids (fraction 2), or a fraction containing a mixture of largely condensed tannins or catechins (fraction 3). According to changes in serum contents of urea nitrogen (Urea-N), creatine (Cr), methylguanidine (MG), and guanidinosuccinic acid (GSA), the group that received the water extract showed a significant decrease in all the uremic toxins with the highest dosage (120 mg/kg per day). At the lowest daily dosage (30 mg/kg) only MG showed a significant decrease whereas at twice that amount Urea-N, MG, and GSA were significantly decreased compared to controls administered water only. The fractions, which were administered at doses of one-tenth to about one-twentieth of the herb extract, produced dissimilar results. Levels of uremic toxins in the rats that received the various fractions showed the following: fraction 1 at oral doses of 2.5 and 5 mg/kg per day was not much better than the control; fraction 2 (flavonoid fraction) at a dose of 5 mg significantly decreased only MG and Urea-N; and fraction 3, consisting of catechin tannins, caused significant decreases in Urea-N, MG, and GSA at 2.5 mg and of all the uremic toxins at a dose of 5 mg.

Immune Functions; Inflammation and Disease

Cancer

Carcinogenicity/mutagenicity. An anticarcinogenic effect using a water extract of *E. sinica* (1.25 g/L water, freely available in the drinking water, 6.5 mg/50 weeks) was tested on benzo[*a*]pyrene-induced tumors in male F344/DuCrj rats. Tumor incidence was reduced by 20%, which was not significant compared to the untreated control group (Horikawa et al., 1994).

The in vitro antimutagenic activity of a water extract of *E. sinica* (1.25 g/L water) was examined in an assay using *Salmonella typhimurium* TA98. At a concentration of 1 mg, the extract inhibited the mutagenicity of the carcinogen benzo[*a*]pyrene by 91%, and the mutagenicity of the environmental mutagens, 3,9-dinitrofluoranthene, and 1,6-dinitropyrene, by 52% and 32%, respectively (Horikawa et al., 1994).

Immune Functions

Immune modulation. In vitro experiments using a crude extract of ma huang *(E. sinica)* and a water extract prepared by boiling the dried leaves have shown anticomplement activity. This activity might help to explain the traditional use of ma huang in the treatment of acute nephritis and other autoimmune diseases (e.g., autoimmune thyroid disease, systemic lupus erythematosus, and rheumatoid arthritis). When administered to rats for five days (5 mg/day p.o.), an uncharacterized complement-inhibiting component of the water extract of the dried leaves (calculated as approximately 250 mg/kg of dried leaves) inhibited alternative pathway activity by 25% and the classical complement pathway by 30% without causing any apparent side effects or weight loss. Inhibition of the classical pathway reached statistical significance, but inhibition of the alternative pathway fell just short of significance. In vitro tests using sera from rabbits, guinea pigs, rats, and pigs also showed that the complement-inhibiting component inhibited the classical pathway. Using human sera, the component acted more efficiently with 50-80 µg/mL inhibiting the classical pathway by 50%. Complete inhibition of complement in human serum in vitro was found from a concentration of 400 µg/mL, which was comparable to that of other natural inhibitors of complement (e.g., heparins). The components of complement inhibited were determined to be C9 in the terminal pathway and C2 in the classical pathway. Preliminary efforts to characterize the active component revealed a high molecular weight polyanionic carbohydrate (Ling et al., 1995).

In an in vitro screening study of medicinal plants used in Korea to treat inflammatory diseases, a total methanolic extract of ma huang *(E. sinica)* inhibited the induction of CINC (cytokine-induced neutrophil chemoattractant, a member of the interleukin-8 family of cytokines). In lipopolysaccharide-activated peritoneal macrophages of rats, CINC was inhibited by 20%, which was less than that produced by prednisolone (36%) in the same assay, yet more potent than aspirin (0%), ibuprofen (0%), indomethicin (3%), or ketoprofen (4%). IL-8 is involved in a number of inflammatory diseases (e.g., psoriasis, pulmonary thrombosis) and is found in high concentrations in the patients with rheumatoid arthritis (Lee et al., 1995).

Infectious Diseases

Microbial infections. A decoction of ma huang is reported to have inhibited the growth or a number of pathogenic microorganisms: *Bacillus anthracis,*

Corynebacterium diptheriae, Salmonella typhi, Shigella dysenteriae, Staphylococcus aureus, and *Pseudomonas aeruginosa* (Chang and But, 1987).

Viral infections. A decoction of ma huang is reported to have inhibited the in vitro growth of type A Asian influenza virus (MIC: 2 mg/mL). The essential oil was also active (Chang and But, 1987). The in vitro concentration-dependent inhibition of influenza A/PR/8/34 virus in Madin-Darby canine kidney cells by a freeze-dried water extract of "*Ephedrae herba*" (400 μg/mL) was demonstrated from noncytotoxic doses of the extract (MTT assay). The yield of virus was reduced by greater than 50% if the cells were treated within five to ten min postinfection, but not later than 15 min. Inhibition of the virus was shown to be the result of inhibitory activity on acidification of lysosomes and endosomes. A tannin-deficient preparation of the extract was ineffective, suggesting that tannin is one of the active constituents, possibly condensed tannins or catechins (Mantani et al.,1999; Takechi et al., 1985).

Inflammatory Response

Kim et al. (1997) reported anti-inflammatory activity from a methanolic extract of *E. sinica* (200 mg/kg p.o. per day) in a model of arthritis in rats (hind paw swelling induced by injection of heat-killed *Mycobacterium butyricum* into the right hind paw). Secondary arthritic swelling following an acute primary swelling phase was significantly inhibited by the extract, suggesting an antiarthritic potential.

Konno et al. (1979) isolated an analogue of ephedrine known as ephedroxane as an anti-inflammatory principle of *E. intermedia,* which was found in trace amounts and displayed only weak activity. Ephedroxane was subsequently found in some species *(E. distachya, E. equisetina, E. sinica,* and *E. gerardiana)* but not other species of *Ephedra* from China and Japan (Konno et al., 1979).

Hikino et al. (1980) demonstrated anti-inflammatory activity from a crude methanolic extract of *E. intermedia* obtained as a commercial preparation from China. In the fertile egg method using chick embryos, the formation of granulated tissue was inhibited by 37% from 2.5 mg of extract/disc. Since ephedroxane was known to be only weakly active, the effects of other alkaloids were examined. In mice, no anti-inflammatory activity was evident from (–)-ephedrine using the Whittle's method, even from a dose of 50 mg/kg which was equivalent to 5 g of the crude herb if the ephedrine content was 1%. Therefore, the extract was fractionated to separate the active parts from the basic portion which were only found in the Whittle method. Two anti-inflammatory compounds were then isolated as ephedroxane and (+)-pseudoephedrine. A comparison of the anti-inflammatory activity of ephedrine analogues on acetic acid-induced capillary permeability in mice revealed no significant activity from ephedrine and highest activity from pseudoephedrine. The same analogues tested on carrageenan-induced swelling of the hind paw in mice revealed dose-dependent inhibition of hind paw swelling from ephedrine at 200 mg/kg p.o. and from pseudoephedrine at 100 and 200 mg/kg p.o., which were significant compared to phenylbutazone. At the same doses, neither (–)-methylephedrine or (+)-methylpseudoephedrine inhibited swelling. Given that ephedroxane occurs in minute amounts, if at all, in ma huang, Hikino et al. (1980) concluded that pseudoephedrine is the main anti-inflammatory constituent of the aerial parts of the herb.

Upon further investigation, Kasahara et al. (1985) found that as pretreatments, ephedroxane, pseudoephedroxane, ephedrine, and pseudoephedrine each dose-dependently inhibited acute edema induced by various agents in the hind paws of both adrenalectomized and sham-operated mice. The agents used were serotonin, carrageenan, bradykinin, and histamine. Because the anti-inflammatory activity in both groups of mice was much the same, it was concluded that their anti-inflammatory effects were not related to adrenal gland activity. Against the biosynthesis of prostaglandin E_1 (PGE_1) by activated peritoneal macrophages, each of the alkaloids (1.0 mg/mL) incubated with the macrophages showed significant activity in vitro compared to the untreated control, but none were as potent as aspirin. The most potent was pseudoephedrine (92.1% inhibition), while the others were of comparable potency with 78.9% inhibition from ephedrine. Against PGE_1-induced hind paw swelling in mice, pseudoephedrine and ephedrine as pretreatments (50-200 mg/kg p.o.) were more potent that either ephedroxane or pseudoephedroxane at the same dosages. Because the alkaloids also caused dose-dependent inhibition of hind paw edema induced by the other mediators, Kasahara and colleagues concluded that the alkaloids exhibit their anti-inflammatory activity at the exudative stage. However, it became evident that the anti-inflammatory activity of the alkaloids at least partially involved the sympathetic nervous system (SNS). For instance, in mice pretreated with resperine, decreased anti-inflammatory effects were observed from administration of either alkaloid. In mice pretreated with propanolol (s.c.) plus the alkaloids (200 mg/kg p.o.), anti-inflammatory activity increased. Furthermore, it was concluded that the anti-inflammatory effect of pseudoephedrine (and ephedroxane) was not mediated by the central nervous system. When these were administered (100 mg/kg p.o.) at the same time as morphine (100 mg/kg s.c.) (against carrageenan-induced edema) the action of morphine was increased. Although several mechanisms appear to be involved in the anti-inflammatory activity of these alkaloids, the inhibition of PGE_1 biosynthesis appeared to be especially significant (Kasahara et al., 1985).

Metabolic and Nutritional Functions

Aging and Senescence; Longevity Enhancement

Antioxidant activity. At a high dose (1,500 mg/kg i.p.), a crude ethanolic extract of *E. sinica* (5:1) caused a significant 112.9% augmentation of SOD (superoxide dismutase) activity in the blood plasma of mice. However, oral administration of the extract (1,500 or 2,000 mg/kg) produced insignificant increases in SOD activity. Xanthine oxidase activity, which increases superoxide, was inhibited by the extract by 56% (Yoshizaki et al., 1996).

Obesity and Weight Loss. The potential use of ephedrine as an antiobesity drug has been the subject of numerous studies in rodents. As a sympathomimetic agent (an indirect acting norepinephrine-release enhancer) that activates brown adipose tissue thermogenesis in animal models of obesity (Arch et al., 1982), ephedrine has shown potent activity. Ephedrine is a more potent thermogenic in animals than its congeners pseudoephedrine or phenylpropanolamine. Low doses of ephedrine activate brown tissue thermogenesis in animals through enhancing norepinephrine release by the sympathetic nervous system (Dulloo et al., 1991). Studies have shown that the effect is enhanced when ephedrine is combined with methylxanthines such as caffeine, or with aspirin (Dulloo et al., 1991; Dulloo and Miller, 1986). For example, ephedrine alone (1 g/kg of diet for six weeks) caused a reduction in body weight of 16% in monosodium glutamate-induced obese mice. By itself, caffeine in the diet caused little antiobesity effects; however, when combined with ephedrine (1 g/kg plus caffeine, 3.63 g/kg of the diet), the body composition of the mice normalized to that of lean mice, with levels of fat, protein, and weight all similar (Dulloo and Miller, 1986).

A significant decrease in the body weight of mildly to moderately obese monkeys was reported from the combination of ephedrine (6 mg) and caffeine (50 mg) administered orally t.i.d. for eight weeks. Compared to lean monkeys treated with the combination, most of the weight loss was in body fat which was reduced by 19%. Curiously, food intake showed a decrease only in the obese monkeys while nighttime energy expenditure was significantly increased in both groups (by 24% in the lean group and 21% in the obese group) (Ramsey et al., 1998).

Pharmacokinetics

Oral doses of ephedrine undergo rapid and complete absorption from the gastrointestinal tract within 2-2.5 h, and within 24 h is largely eliminated through urinary excretion with 55-75% in unchanged form and the reminder in the form of metabolites (as norephedrine, 8-20%, as 1-phenylpropan-1,2-diol, and as hippuric and benzoic acid, 4-13% of the oral dose). Distribution of ephedrine throughout the body is extensive and rapid, and it can be found in the brain, spleen, liver, kidneys, and lungs. The pharmacokinetics of pseudoephedrine are similar to those of ephedrine and phenylpropano-lamine (Wilkinson and Beckett, 1968; Kanfer et al., 1993; Warot et al., 2000; Dollery, 1991).

Neurological, Psychological, and Behavioral Functions

Receptor- and Neurotransmitter-Mediated Functions

Reports of benefits in patients with myasthenia gravis treated with ephedrine in the 1930s and a more recent subjective beneficial response reported by patients with congenital myasthenic syndromes receiving the alkaloid, led Sieb and Engel (1993) to examine the potential effects of (–)-ephedrine hydrochloride on neuromuscular transmission. Using canine intercostal muscle tissue, the kinetics of ephedrine on acetylcholine channel conductance were measured with microelectrodes. Results failed to show how ephedrine might be of benefit to patients with myasthenia gravis or other disorders characterized by abnormal neuromuscular transmission. Neuromuscular transmission in vitro was not effected by a concentration of ephedrine (5×10^{-7} M) equal to the approximate peak serum concentration in humans after a single oral dose of 25 mg ephedrine; however, the possibility of delayed effects on synaptic function which were not detectable in the particular experiments could not be ruled out.

Respiratory and Pulmonary Functions

Allergies and Asthma

The reputation of ma huang in the treatment of bronchial asthma is largely attributed to ephedrine. Due to β_2-adrenoreceptor-agonist activity, ephedrine (hydrochloride or sulfate) relaxes bronchial smooth muscles which increases liquification of mucus, in turn, leading to an expectorant effect (Robbers and Tyler, 1999). Similarly, ephedrine sulfate (25 mg t.i.d.) has been used in the treatment of hiccups (Rakel, 2000). Due to side effects, the use of ephedrine compounds for bronchodilation in the treatment of asthma was abandoned in favor of more specific β_2-agonists (Robbers and Tyler, 1999; Reynolds, 1996).

As a decongestant, ephedrine acts primarily through the release of catecholamines through stimulation of the sympathetic nervous system. Norepinephrine is released, which binds to and activates both the α_1 and α_2 adrenergic receptors. Activation of the α_2-adrenergic receptors, which show high concentration in precapillary arterioles, induces smooth muscle constriction by way of an increase in calcium ion influx, in turn causing blood flow to capillaries in the nasal mucosa to diminish, which in turn reduces the excess fluids that cause nasal congestion. Similarly, the activation of α_1-drenergic receptors causes blood volume reaching the mucosa to be reduced, leading to decreased congestion in the nasal passages. Due to CNS-stimulant properties, ephedrine was removed from oral decongestant formulas (Johnson and Hricik, 1993).

Apart from the bronchodilating effect of ephedrine, the use of ma huang in the treatment of asthma in TCM may be partly attributable to tetramethylpyrazine, caryophyllene, and *l*-α-terpinol which are found in higher concentrations in stir-fried and honey-cured ma huang than the simple dried form (Leung and Foster, 1996). Tetramethylpyrazine is believed to play an important role in the use of ma huang against asthma (Kun et al., 2000). A potent pulmonary vasorelaxing activity may be explained by its action as a calcium antagonist (Pang et al., 1996).

Bronchial Functions

Ma huang is reported to produce a relaxant effect on bronchial smooth muscles. It exhibits a weaker action compared to epinephrine, but it is more prolonged. Dilation of bronchial smooth muscles was demonstrated from methylephedrine, pseudoephedrine, or ephedrine in bronchi and lung tissue in vitro, and in dogs administered acetylcholine or histamine. The latter two ma huang alkaloids abrogated the induced increase in respiratory tract resistance (Chang and But, 1987).

Antitussive activity was demonstrated in mice administered a water-soluble extract of *E. sinica* (ED_{50}: 134-227.5 mg/kg p.o.). The total alkaloid concentration of the extract was 5.13%, with ephedrine (4.23%) and pseudoephedrine (0.69%) constituting the main alkaloids (Shoji and Kisara, 1975).

Respiratory Infections

Ephedrine hydrochloride (15-30 mg/day) is approved for use in Canada for the symptomatic relief of nasal congestion resulting from various infections of the upper respiratory tract (Gillis et al., 1999). Pseudoephedrine (hydrochloride or sulfate) is also used for the symptomatic relief of nasal congestion, usually in oral doses of 60 mg t.i.d. or q.i.d. (Reynolds, 1996).

CLINICAL STUDIES

Endocrine and Hormonal Disorders

Adrenal Functions

In a double-blind, randomized, placebo-controlled, crossover study in ten "normal," nonsmoking volunteers (ages 26-34), Shannon et al. (1999)

reported a significant decrease in urinary noradrenaline with (±)-ephedrine (50 mg t.i.d.) during a 24 h study period compared to placebo ($p < 0.05$). This effect was found despite a lack of significant change in urinary adrenaline.

In a randomized, double-blind, placebo-controlled, crossover design clinical study in ten obese subjects who received a six-week very low-calorie diet program (1,965 kJ) prior to ephedrine administration, Pasquali et al. (1992) reported no significant effects on 24 h urinary levels of noradrenaline, adrenaline (or dopamine) from either *L*-(–)-ephedrine (50 mg t.i.d. for two weeks), the diet, or their combination.

Thyroid and Parathyroid Functions

Treatment of ten obese subjects with ephedrine (50 mg t.i.d. for two weeks) in a randomized, double-blind, placebo-controlled, crossover design clinical study resulted in significant prevention of a further decrease in the serum triodothyronine/thyroxine ratio and their serum trio-iodothyronine levels after the subjects maintained a six-week very low-calorie diet (1,965 kJ) (Pasquali et al., 1992).

Metabolism and Nutrient Utilization

A single-blind, placebo-controlled crossover design trial in nine healthy male volunteers (ages 21-28) found that (–)-ephedrine chloride (30 mg/day with 200 mL tap water for five days) caused a significant increase in basal metabolic rate (thermogenesis) whereas 20 mg was ineffective. Compared to baseline, the increase in energy expenditure from the 30 mg dose was 6.6% which remained significantly higher compared to placebo ($p < 0.01$). Yet, no significant mean difference was found in the respiratory quotient compared to placebo and an increase in systolic blood pressure showed a mean of only 8 mmHg in the ephedrine chloride group. Treatment with ephedrine chloride also caused a significant increase in plasma glucose levels which then stayed elevated throughout the trial. Noting that increases in plasma glucose were reported in previous studies of ephedrine, it was postulated that the effect may have been due to an increase in hepatic glucose production and output through involvement of both α- and β-adrenoreceptors (Liu et al., 1995).

Chronic administration of ephedrine (50 mg p.o. t.i.d. for two weeks) in obese subjects during the second to fifth weeks of a six-week diet very low in calories (1,965 kJ) was compared to placebo in a randomized, double-blind, crossover design trial in ten subjects. Daily urinary nitrogen excretion was significantly lowered by ephedrine compared to placebo. Ephedrine also caused a significant prevention of the decrease in the resting metabolic rate (fasting resting) as measured by changes in oxygen consumption, and significantly increased the 24 h urinary levels of homovanillic and vanillyl-mandelic acids, raising them to pretreatment values after they were significantly decreased by the very low-calorie diet. No reports of side effects were reported (Pasquali et al., 1992).

Obesity and Weight Loss

In humans, ephedrine is reported to increase the metabolic rate by about 10%, increase the oxidation of lipids, and stimulate thermogenesis by 20-30% (1 mg/kg p.o.) (Astrup, 1986). However, despite a number of trials, evidence that ma huang or ephedrine alone cause any significant amount of weight loss compared to placebo in humans is lacking. Indeed, the majority of human studies failed to find significant weight loss from ephedrine compared to placebo (Pasquali and Casimirri, 1993; Toubro et al., 1993; Pasquali et al., 1992, 1985; Astrup, Toubro et al., 1992; Astrup et al., 1985, 1995).

Performance and Endurance Enhancement

Evidence in support of ephedrine as a performance-enhancing agent is lacking (Clarkson and Thompson, 1997). The short-term effect of ephedrine on energy expenditure was examined in a double-blind, randomized, placebo-controlled, crossover study in ten "normal," nonsmoking volunteers (ages 26-34). Incorporating two periods of crossover, the study used a force platform and calorimeter to measure 24 h mechanical work and energy expenditure on a minute-by-minute basis during two 24 h periods at which times subjects received placebo or ephedrine (50 mg t.i.d.). No significant difference was found in the amount of mechanical work performed compared to placebo, yet the mean amount of energy expenditure was significantly greater in the subjects during the periods in which they received ephedrine ($p < 0.05$). Energy expenditure with ephedrine showed the greatest increase compared to placebo (7.3% greater; $p < 0.005$) during the night, an effect found in every subject. However, basal metabolic rate at baseline compared to placebo or ephedrine compared to placebo was not significantly different, nor was the composition of the diet and caloric intake. The increase amounted to 314 kJ/day, calculated as equivalent to a single 14 min walk on pavement or a single slice of white bread. It was further calculated that if the increase in energy expenditure was sustained for one year the amount of weight loss would be 3 kg. Seven of the subjects reported one or more side effects while taking ephedrine (decreased appetite, a stronger or increased heartbeat, and difficulty sleeping), while in the placebo group two subjects complained of side effects (one reported difficulty sleeping and a pounding heart and the other reported decreased appetite and reported palpitations for brief time) (Shannon et al., 1999).

Neurological, Psychological, and Behavioral Disorders

Receptor- and Neurotransmitter-Mediated Functions

The effect of ephedrine sulfate on physiological and subjective sexual arousal was examined in a placebo-controlled, double-blind, randomized crossover protocol trial in 20 women (ages 19-44). None of the participants had used medications except for birth control pills during the preceding six months and none had a history of being treated for sexual dysfunction, depression, or high or low blood pressure. Tests showed that all the women were normative in their range of sexual experience and functioning. Capsules containing either ephedrine sulfate (50 mg) or placebo were taken orally with water before each experiment, 24 h before which subjects were requested to abstain from alcohol and caffeine and strenuous physical activity. Measurement of physiological arousal was conducted using a vaginal photoplethysmograph combined with viewing of erotic and nonerotic films, while psychological arousal was measured using a questionnaire. Compared to placebo during the viewing of the erotic films, ephedrine sulfate produced a significant increase in the vaginal pulse amplitude in 17 of the subjects. Heart rate scores were also significantly greater from ephedrine compared to placebo, but only during the viewing of the erotic films. Yet subjective ratings to physical or mental sexual arousal showed no significant difference between the treatment groups. It was speculated that ephedrine may have caused increased "physiological sexual responding" in women who are sexually functional by boosting their increased level of sexual arousal (Meston and Heiman, 1998).

Pharmacokinetics

The pharmacokinetics of an encapsulated ma huang *(E. sinica)* powder product were examined in six normotensive, nonsmoking volunteers (ages 23-40) who ingested four 375 mg capsules of the product (actual range 368-411 mg/capsule) with a light breakfast and again nine h later with the evening meal. Analysis of the product revealed that for every four capsules the subjects ingested they received a mean dose of 19.4 mg ephedrine, 4.9 mg pseudoephedrine, and 1.2 methylephedrine. Results were compared to a 20 mg immediate-release tablet of ephedrine and an ephedrine solution. These showed that absorption of ephedrine was significantly slower from the herbal product, which showed an absorption rate constant of 0.49 versus 1.73 for the tablets and 2.35 for the solution. The respective times to reach maximum concentrations were 3.90, 1.69, and 1.81 h. However, among the products, according to maximum plasma concentrations, lag time, and the area under the concentration-time curve, the extent and onset of absorption of ephedrine was not much different (White et al., 1997).

Similar conclusions were made by Gurley, Gardner et al. (1998) who conducted a randomized, crossover study in ten healthy volunteers (ages 22-40) administered each of three different dietary supplement products (two capsules or tablets/dose) containing various constituents besides ma huang, although all contained kola nut *(Cola nitida)* and guaraná *(Paullinia cupana),* sources of caffeine. Mean quantities of ephedrine/dose form in the three products were 23.6, 25.6, and 27 mg. Pharmacokinetics were compared to results from single ingestion of 50.5 mg of ephedrine hydrochloride in capsule form which was taken by the subjects in one of the four phases of the study. A seven-day washout phase attended each of the product ingestion periods. The pharmacokinetics of the botanical sources of ephedrine showed no significant difference compared to conventional ephedrine in a capsule. The exception was one product in tablet form which showed a significantly slower absorption rate constant and area under the curve (AUC) (ng/h) compared to the capsule of ephedrine hydrochloride. All of the subjects reported minor side effects which were typical of the ephedrine alkaloids and included anxiety, loss of appetite, headache, tachycardia, insomnia, and irritability. Compared to the results of White et al. (1997), it was surmised that because the k_a values were much larger in this study, gastrointestinal absorption of ephedrine may have been occurring at a faster rate when coadministered with botanicals, although no evidence that the extent of absorption was any greater was found. Which botanical was responsible for the increased rate of absorption of ephedrine was not apparent (Gurley, Gardner, et al., 1998).

Respiratory and Pulmonary Disorders

Allergies and Asthma

In the Chinese traditional treatment of asthma and bronchial asthma, ma huang is combined with other herbal medicines (Fratkin, 1986; Chang and But, 1987; Naeser, 1996; Huntley and Ernst, 2000). Clinical studies on the use of ma huang alone in the treatment of asthma, bronchial asthma, or allergies are lacking. Chang and But (1987) mention a study in 20 children with bronchial asthma treated with a decoction of "roasted" ma huang and equal parts sugar. The results were reported to be satisfactory.

As for ephedrine, in a placebo-controlled, double-blind study of 16 asthmatic children ages 7-13 who were already receiving theophylline, Tinkelman and Avner (1977) reported good results from ephedrine sulfate (25 mg p.o. t.i.d.). Because ephedrine is a relatively weak bronchodilator and its use was limited to mild cases of asthma (Bierman and Pearlman, 1988), it has since largely been abandoned in favor of safer, more effective and more selective β_2-adrenergic agonists (Nelson, 1995; Reynolds, 1996).

Bronchial Disorders

See Allergies and Asthma.

DOSAGE

The dosage of ma huang used in Chinese medicine varies from 1.5-9 g (Tu et al., 1992), and depends on the condition being treated. The general dosage is 5-6 g with a smaller dose for debilitated patients (2-5 g), and a higher dosage of the purpose of increasing diaphoresis or the treatment of asthma (Hsu et al., 1986). In the treatment of night sweating and spontaneous sweating, 3-9 g of the dried and powdered root is dabbed on the body (Tu et al., 1992; Hsu et al., 1986).

The German Commission E gives the single dosage of ma huang for adults as a corresponding amount of herb for 15-30 mg total alkaloids (calculated as ephedrine). Using the same calculation, the maximum daily dosage for adults is 300 mg total alkaloids, and the dosage for children over age six is 0.5 mg total ma huang alkaloids/kg body weight with a maximum daily dosage of 2 mg/kg. The only use given is mild bronchospasms in respiratory tract diseases (Blumenthal, 1998). The American Herbal Products Association recommends that the daily dosage of total ma huang alkaloids be limited to 100 mg in four divided doses of not more than 25 mg (Ephedra Education Council, 2000).

SAFETY PROFILE

Contraindications

Ma huang is contraindicated in anorexia, bulimia (McGuffin et al., 1997), anxiety, restlessness, glaucoma, thyrotoxicosis, pheochromocytoma, impaired cerebral circulation, high blood pressure, and in cases of adenoma of the prostate attended by an accumulation of residual urine (Blumenthal, 1998).

Drug Interactions

The government of Canada (Health Canada) issued a health advisory in 2001 warning the public not to use ephedra or ephedrine in combination with caffeine "and other stimulants" because "ephedrine may cause serious, possibly fatal, adverse effects" when combined with such ingredients (Health Canada, 2001, p. 30).

The German Commission E warns of the following drug interactions with ma huang: MAO inhibitors, secale (ergot) alkaloid derivatives, oxytocin, cardiac glycosides, halothane, and guanethidine (Blumenthal, 1998). Butcher's broom *(Ruscus aculaetus)* may potentiate the actions of ephedrine/ma huang due to its activation of noradrenaline release and postjunctional α_1 and α_2-adrenergic receptors (Cappelli et al., 1988; Marcelon et al., 1983). The combination of caffeine and ephedrine is suspected of potentiating cardiac effects, placing some individuals at risk of cardiovascular symptoms (e.g., hypertension, tachycardia, palpitations, stroke, and seizures) (Michaelis et al., 1987). Although the reasons for individual susceptibility remain to be determined (Haller and Benowitz, 2000), hypothetically, they may involve adrenoreceptor polymorphisms (Büscher et al., 1999).

In an analysis of the alkaloid contents of 20 commercially available ma huang-containing dietary supplements sold in the United States, Gurley et al. (2000) found that 4 of 20 products contained substantial levels of "potent CNS stimulants": (+)-norpseudoephedrine (2 of 20 products, range 0.38 ± 0.06 to 0.42 ± 0.02 mg/dosage unit); (–)-methylephedrine (2 of 20 products, range 2.58 ± 0.27 to 2.71 ± 0.11 mg/dosage unit); and (+)-pseudoephedrine (4 of 20 products, range 3.37 ± 0.96 to 9.45 ± 0.64 mg/dosage unit). The main concern is that in these relatively high concentrations, these highly CNS-active alkaloids could pose serious problems when combined with caffeine or even the component (–)-ephedrine. Both (–)-methylephedrine and (+)-norpseudoephedrine have a high potential for abuse and are linked with neurological toxicities. (+)-Norpseudoephedrine is a Schedule IV controlled substance not permitted by the FDA in nonprescription drugs. Furthermore, evidence suggests that stimulant effects similar to those produced by methamphetamine may result from mixtures containing (–)-methylephedrine and caffeine. These concerns are compounded by the fact that in 55% of the products tested, a greater than 20% variation in label claims of alkaloid content (0% to 154%) compared to actual amounts was found. In addition, 55% of the products claimed contents of two other stimulants (caffeine and synephrine) (Gurley et al., 2000). In an earlier analysis of nine commercially available *Ephedra*-containing dietary supplements, Gurley, Wang et al. (1998) found that the ma huang alkaloid content varied from 1.23 to 23.5 mg/unit and that one product showed a lot to lot variation in ephedrine content of 137%.

An analysis of the adverse event reports concerning supplements containing ephedra alkaloids reported to the FDA was performed by Cantox Health Sciences International (Cantox, 2000). Based on the information in the FDA's database (Special Nutritionals/Adverse Event Monitoring System), they were only able to make "a qualitative evaluation of trends" and concluded as follows:

> The non-life threatening adverse events that were reported were attributable to the pharmacological actions of ephedra, and none of the seri-

ous adverse events could be directly (causally) related to the use of
ephedra-containing products. However, it is logical that specific factors such as pre-existing medical conditions (e.g., cardiovascular problems) or concomitant use of sympathomimetic agents (e.g., caffeine)
could lead to serious adverse effects and the use of these types of products (including dietary supplements containing ephedra or other stimulants) should be avoided. (Cantox, 2000, p. 64)

Haller and Benowitz (2000) conducted an independent review of 140 reports received by the FDA of adverse effects in individuals using supplements containing ma huang alkaloids. Symptom recurrence after reintro-
duction of the alkaloids or cases in which symptom onset corresponded with
known peak plasma concentration and duration of ephedrine effects, were
critical in defining adverse events as being "definitely" related to ma huang
alkaloid-containing dietary supplements. Cases were judged as "probably"
related to the used of ma huang-containing dietary supplements when most
of the evidence supported a link, but at least one aspect was unknown (e.g.,
time of last dose) or an inconsistent aspect of the evidence (e.g., "low reported dose") could be considered minor. Cases evaluated as "possibly" related to the use of ma huang-containing dietary supplements were those in
which the association was pharmacologically plausible, but could equally
be due to unrelated factors. In all, 31% of the cases were considered as being
probably or definitely related to ma huang-containing supplements (PODR)
and 31% as possibly related. Among the PODR cases, the majority of adverse events were cardiovascular: hypertension, 21%; tachycardia, palpitations or both, 17%; cardiac arrest or "sudden death," 10%; arrhythmia, 6%;
and myocardial infarction, 4%. Adverse events involving the CNS which
were PODR to the use of ma huang-containing supplements consisted of
stroke (8%), seizure (2%), and transient ischemic attack (2%). In the three
cases PODR to ma huang alkaloids in which the outcome was death, the
daily amounts of ma huang alkaloids taken were 60 mg for seven months,
36 mg/day for one week, and 20 mg/day for one year (Haller and Benowitz,
2000).

Among the PODR cases, Haller and Benowitz (2000) provide some details of seven cases in which the outcome was permanent disability. In two
cases, the adverse event was hemorrhagic stroke and the estimated daily
dose of ma huang alkaloids was unknown. In one case, a male age 39, had
taken a product claiming to contain 415 mg ma huang alkaloids plus
guaraná (a source of caffeine) per serving. In the other case, a male age 47
had taken a product containing ma huang alkaloids for a period of three
weeks. Details on the contents of the product were not provided. In another
case of permanent disability, a healthy female age 35 had taken an estimated
dosage of ma huang alkaloids of 45 mg/day for one week. According to the
label, this product also contained caffeine (40 mg/capsule). The daily sug-

gested dosage was one capsule three times daily with meals. She was not taking medications of any kind. Permanent disability resulted from a sub-arachnoid hemorrhage. The range of estimated ma huang alkaloid dosages in the cases of permanent disability was 20 to 66 mg/day and the durations of use ranged from one day to one year. Most, if not all, of the ma huang-containing supplements used in these cases also contained caffeine. Additional amounts of caffeine may have been ingested in soft drinks, coffee, and tea, and because caffeine facilitates the release of catecholamines, (like ephedrine), the combination could have led "to increased stimulation of the central nervous system and cardiovascular system" (Haller and Benowitz, 2000, p. 1837).

Hutchins (2001) reviewed 22 of the reports received by the FDA in which the outcome was death. He concluded that the pathological or clinical features of the adverse events reported to the FDA were inconsistent and showed that it was unlikely that the contributing or causative factors in these deaths were ephedrine-type alkaloids. Among these reports were eight of those evaluated by Haller and Benowitz (2000). He notes that in the list of PODR adverse events, Haller and Benowitz failed to include important concurrent or preexisting conditions of three of the patients, one each with hypertension, chest pain, and severe coronary artery disease. Among other omissions by Haller and Benowitz was that of a premature infant who actually died from necrotizing enterocolitis rather than an adverse event, related, however temporally, to an ephedrine-containing substance (Hutchins, 2001). In reply, Haller and Benowitz (2001) restated that while admittedly uncommon, adverse events related to ma huang have a greater chance of occurring in vulnerable persons, especially those with "unrecognized cardiovascular disease" (p. 1096). As for the individual cases, they noted that in some of the cases the data provided by the FDA was not exactly the same as the information that Hutchins cited. In the case of the infant death, they note that the cause was presumed to be premature delivery, an event which may have been induced by an ephedrine-containing dietary supplements. In closing, Haller and Benowitz (2001) point out the need for a case-control study of dietary supplements containing ephedrine alkaloids similar to the recently published large-scale study on phenylpropanolamine on the risk of hemorrhagic stroke (Hemorrhagic Stroke Project).

As other cases of temporally associated adverse reactions to ma huang alkaloid-containing dietary supplements continue to appear in the literature (Traub et al., 2001; Borum, 2001; Kockler et al., 2001), the following case reports are summarized as examples of the difficulty inherent in evaluating the safety of ma huang in the absence of large-scale case-control studies.

Psychotic episodes associated with products containing ma huang in combination with various other substances may have been the result of ingredient interactions in susceptible individuals. Two such possible cases were reported by the Naval Medical Center in San Diego, California, but in only one case were the ingredients given and then without specifics: "two Ma huang-containing dietary supplements, together with ginseng, DHEA (dehydroepiandrosterone), creatine monohydrate, and copious amounts of coffee" for a period of "several months." A computed tomography scan of the patient's head and a physical examination found nothing abnormal and the patient, a 20-year-old male, had no previous history of psychiatric illness. After discontinuation of the supplements for three months following initial treatment with haloperidol and olanzapine (antipsychotics), and benztropine (anticholinergic), and follow-up treatment with antipsychotics, the patient's mental state returned to normal and he resumed duty (Jacobs and Hirsch, 2000).

A randomized, double-blind, placebo-controlled trial in 32 adult males in their twenties found that ephedrine (s.c.) potentiated the analgesic effects of morphine (s.c.) in the treatment of postoperative pain. The analgesic effect of 10 mg morphine compared to ephedrine 25 mg plus morphine 5 mg was not significantly different. These results were confirmed in Swiss albino mice (n = 240, of both sexes) (Tekol et al., 1994).

In a detailed case report, Zaacks et al. (1999) concluded that for a male patient age 39 with a two-year history of hypertension who developed hypersensitivity myocarditis, the cause was suspected to be use of a ma huang extract, both because of the temporal nature of the disease and the ability of ephedrine to cause vasculitis. Ma huang was taken by the patient over a period of three months in the form of a dietary supplement reported to contain 7 mg ephedrine alkaloids/tablet. At the dosage claimed by the patient, he ingested 7-21 mg of ephedrine alkaloids twice a day in addition to his regular medications (furosemide and pravastatin). The case is complicated by the fact that other complex dietary supplements were taken at the same time. The tablets containing ma huang extract contained, among other substances, yerba maté, providing approximately 10 mg caffeine/tablet, papain, an ingredient labeled "Herbs," and several other natural products. In addition, he was taking four other complex dietary supplement formulas, one of which also contained caffeine). In total, the patient was taking over 70 different natural products in addition to furosemide and pravastatin. Sympathomimetics associated with myocarditis are primarily L-norepinephrine, phenylpropanolamine, and cocaine. Although none of the other ingredients in the supplements taken by the patient were known to be associated with hypersensitivity myocarditis (Zaacks et al., 1999), given the complexity of ingredients in the formulas, a drug interaction with the patient's regular medications was still a distinct possibility. Serious consideration must also be given to the content of caffeine in the regimen since it is also a sympathomimetic and has been shown to intensify the myocardial effects of ephedrine (and catecholamines) by increasing the levels of cyclic adenosine monophosphate (Theoharides, 1997).

A product containing a combination of caffeine and ephedrine was temporally linked to the death of a healthy 23-year-old male. The dosage was estimated to be 15 mg caffeine plus 25 mg ephedrine alkaloids from "ma huang extract" once or twice daily for a period of over six months. Autopsy revealed a "patchy myocardial necrosis"; however, there was no sign of myocarditis (Theoharides, 1997). In reviewing this case, Theoharides (1997) called attention to reports of ephedrine-induced cardiomyopathy in patients who consumed small, repeated doses of the alkaloid or used ephedrine over prolonged periods. These case reports indicate that sustained use may result in focal myocardial necrosis and cardiac hypertrophy (Theoharides, 1997).

The combination of ephedrine and caffeine has been clinically studied in obese patients, and in a number of these trials it produced side effects (Cantox, 2000). A six-month, randomized, placebo-controlled, double-blind study of ephedrine/caffeine (20 mg/200 mg three times daily) in 180 obese patients on a special diet (4.2 MJ/day) found that side effects of dizziness, tremor, and insomnia were transient and that after the eighth week of treatment they reached levels found in the placebo group. Only three patients withdrew from the trial due specifically to side effects. Subjects in the ephedrine/caffeine group showed a significantly greater mean amount of weight loss compared to placebo (16.6 kg versus 13.2 kg, respectively) (Astrup, Breum et al., 1992). The combination of caffeine (20 mg/dose) and ephedrine (10 mg/dose), as provided by plant extracts of kola nut and *Ephedra* standardized to those compounds, may have caused a significant rise in peak 45-minute oxygen consumption in obese subjects (Greenway et al., 2000). In a trial of ephedrine/caffeine compared to placebo in obese subjects, Astrup, Toubro et al. (1992) estimated that 75% of weight loss was due to appetite suppression with resultant caloric intake being decreased, and 20% was due to an increase in oxygen consumption.

In some trials, side effects associated with the combination of ephedrine and caffeine may be obfuscated by additional ingredients in the formulation. As a case in point, Boozer et al. (2001) conducted an eight-week, randomized, double-blind, placebo-controlled trial on the safety and efficacy of a dietary supplement tablet on weight loss in 48 overweight men and women ages 25-55 who were weight stable for at least three months preceding evaluation for entry to the trial. According to the label, the test product consisted of ma huang (12 mg) and guaraná (40 mg), plus the following: chromium picolinate (75 µg), magnesium protein chelate (75 mg), vitamin E (6 IU), and 586 mg made up of undisclosed amounts of "bee pollen; ginseng (root); ginger (root); damiana (leaf); sarsaparilla (root); goldenseal (aerial part); nettles (leaf); bovine complex; gotu kola; lecithin; spirulina algae; royal jelly; and other ingredients (binders). . . ." (Boozer et al., 2001, p. 324). HPLC analysis of the product revealed on average 50.0 mg/tablet (47.0-55.1 mg) caffeine which was higher than the label amount of "Guarana"

(40 mg). The analysis also showed that the label amount of "Ma Huang" (12 mg/tablet) closely matched the detected amount of ephedrine total alkaloids (12.2-13.4 mg; av. 12.9 mg), an amount far in excess of what 12 mg of the herb ma huang would provide. The amount of ephedrine in the tablets (9.7-11.7 mg; av. 10.5 mg) was not disclosed on the label. Whereas the authors state that the patients received 240 mg/day caffeine and 72 mg/day ephedrine alkaloids, they actually received an average of 300 mg/day caffeine and 77.4 mg/day ma huang alkaloids, plus 3.5 g/day of other ingredients. Regardless, the incidence of "symptoms" reported by the active treatment group compared to placebo showed greatest differences in the occurrence of insomnia (13 reports versus 9), dry mouth (11 versus 4), and headache (7 versus 4). Whereas no subjects dropped out of the placebo group (25%) for reasons of side effects potentially related to treatment, before the first follow-up visit or after week two, all but two of the dropouts in the active treatment group (23%) were removed for those reasons (i.e., elevated BP, palpitations without or without chest pain, increased palpitations, increased BP, or extreme irritability). For those remaining in the trial, weight loss (600 g to 7.4 kg) and fat loss (0% to 5.1%) were significant compared to placebo (Boozer et al., 2001). Given the long list of ingredients in the active formula, associating side effects with interactions between ma huang or caffeine alone is practically impossible.

A 15-week, double-blind, multicenter trial in 103 obese patients on a special diet (5 MJ/day) compared the weight loss and side effects of dexfenfluramine (15 mg twice daily) to those of ephedrine/caffeine (20 mg/ 200 mg, three times daily). Mean heart rate was increased in the ephedrine/caffeine group compared to baseline at week 15 by 1.1 ± 11.6 beats/ minute. Mean weight loss after 15 weeks in the ephedrine/caffeine group was 9.0 ± 5.3 kg which was not significantly different compared to the dexfenfluramine group (6.9 ± 4.3 kg). Complaints of side effects were reported by 43% of the dexfenfluramine group and by 54% of the ephedrine/caffeine group. These were most prevalent during the first four weeks of treatment, and mostly consisted of agitation and insomnia, and rapidly subsided after the first seven days of treatment. Gastrointestinal side effects were significantly more frequent in the dexfenfluramine group whereas CNS side effects were significantly more common in the ephedrine/caffeine group. Six of the 40 patients in the ephedrine/caffeine group were withdrawn from the trial due to side effects of tremor, syncope, and palpitations ($n = 1$), abdominal pains and vomiting ($n = 2$), and insomnia, vertigo, and nausea ($n = 3$). One patient in the ephedrine/caffeine group died "due to fatal gastric bleeding in combination with alcohol intoxication." The event was not likely due to ephedrine/caffeine and no cases of hemorrhage or gastrointestinal bleeding had previously been reported from the combination in Denmark, where for the previous two years until the trial, over 9.6 million doses of ephedrine/caffeine had been used and only 86 adverse drug reactions from the combination were reported (Breum et al., 1994). Gastrointestinal bleeding was also reported in a toxicity study of ma huang in mice (see Toxicity in Animal Models).

Pregnancy and Lactation

Recommendations regarding ephedra use during pregnancy or lactation vary. The American Herbal Products Association recommends that pregnant or nursing women seek the advice of a physician or other health care practitioner before using ma huang (McGuffin et al., 1997). The German Commission E monograph does not contraindicate for pregnancy or lactation, and provides a pediatric dose maximum of 2 mg of total ephedra alkaloids per kg per day (Blumenthal et al., 1998). As considerations for early versus late pregnancy and lacatation differ, they will be discussed separately.

The use of sympathomimetic drugs during pregnancy is implicated in the development of human fetal cardiovascular abnormalities (Park et al., 1990). First trimester use of sympathomimetic drugs has been found to be associated with minor malformations, inguinal hernia, and clubfoot (Briggs et al., 1990). The use of pseudoephedrine-containing drugs during pregnancy has been associated with the development in children of gastroschisis (Werler et al., 1992; Torfs et al., 1996).

Two cases of malformed offspring from mothers taking sympathomimetic drugs during pregnancy were reported by Gilbert-Barness and Drut (2000). In case one, a 23-year-old mother had taken two tablets of Primatene 4 times daily to control her asthma. The drug contained ephedrine, theophylline, and phenobarbital. Use began before pregnancy and continued until the sixth month of gestation. The child developed severe skeletal defects of the arms and hands, with one hand having only three fingers. In the other case, the use of Triaminic, a similar agent containing pseudoephedrine, phenylephrine, and phenylpropanolamine, began before pregnancy and was maintained throughout the first trimester. The child was born with severely defective upper and lower limbs. Birth defects, including limb defects, were also reported in pregnant rabbits administered low and high doses of Primatene. Defects of the body wall are already known to be associated with limb anomalies and human epidemiological studies have found an association between the use of ephedrine during the first trimester of pregnancy and the development of abdominal wall defects (Gilbert-Barness and Drut, 2000). On the other hand, ephedrine is routinely used to treat or prevent maternal hypotension during labor (Hale, 2000). It is known to enter freely into fetal circulation, causing changes to the fetal heart rate (Briggs et al., 1990). However, the risks:benefit ratio dictates its use because other agents available to raise blood pressure, specifically dopamine, decrease uterine blood flow.

Briggs et al., (1990) report a single case of an adverse effect on a three-month old, breast-feeding infant when the mother consumed a long-acting preparation of d-isoephedrine (120 mg), a congener of ephedrine, combined with dexbrompheniramine (6 mg). The baby developed irritability, and excessive crying and sleep disturbances after the mother had taken this dose twice a day for one to two days. These symptoms resolved within 12 hours after breast-feeding was stopped. On principle, single-ingredient, short-acting drug products used in a minimal dose are preferred during lactation. Long-acting preparations maximize a baby's exposure through breast milk. Use of pseudoephedrine products during lactation is associated with reports of decreased milk supply, although no human studies have been conducted (Anderson, 2000). Anderson describes possible mechanisms of action including decreased serum prolactin and decreased suckling-induced oxytocin release which are known effects of alpha-adrenergic agents such as pseudoephedrine. A possible decrease in blood flow to the breasts is also mentioned. The American Academy of Pediatrics' current recommendations regarding pseudoephedrine note the lack of adverse effects in breast-feeding infants while noting that it concentrates in milk (American Academy of Pediatrics, 2001). Anderson (2000) points out that potential impact on milk supply is an overlooked aspect of pharmacological recommendations. He describes clinical use of pseudoephedrine to treat oversupply (30 mg t.i.d. to q.i.d.), and as an aid to weaning (60 mg t.i.d. to q.i.d.). He warns against its use for mothers of newborns whose lactation is not as yet well-established, and for mothers experiencing milk supply difficulties. During late lactation, when a milk supply decrease would be less "devastating," small dose, short-term use may be more acceptable, although alternatives are urged (Anderson, 2000).

Rapid weight loss can become an important goal for many postpartum women in Western culture. Use of ephedra/caffeine combination products would be expected to cause irritability and sleep disturbances in infants and may contribute to dehydration in breast-feeding women; caffeine alone is known to have these effects. Anderson (2000) documents lower milk supply with use of ephedra products. Some mothers have chosen to use such products despite learning the potential negative effects on the child or to their milk supply. One mother stated that she would wean her child if necessary to use the weight loss product (personal communication, Humphrey). Lowering the dose of ephedra and ephedra/caffeine products may at least minimize these negative effects and is definitely preferable to total abrupt weaning.

Side Effects

The German Commission E lists the following side effects from ma huang: tachycardia, motor restlessness, irritability, insomnia, "disturbances of urination," nausea, and vomiting. Under "higher dosage," the Commission lists the development of dependency, a "drastic increase in blood pressure," and cardiac arrhythmia (Blumenthal, 1998, p. 125).

A recent extensive toxicological review on the safety of *Ephedra* and ephedrine alkaloids concluded that for "a generally healthy population," a dosage of ephedrine alkaloids of 90 mg (in *Ephedra*) per day, in three divided doses, would likely present no adverse effects. This amount represents the upper limit dosage established by the review which was based on the National Academy of Sciences Upper Limit Model for nutrients (Cantox, 2000). In establishing this safe upper limit, it was specified that it "does not apply to specific groups of persons" and is conditional upon label instructions that inform the consumer to "check with their healthcare provider about taking the product; direct the consumer to split the daily dose into at least three parts, so that no dose exceeds 30 mg; the product is intended for use for not more than 6 months; and provide information to facilitate postmarket monitoring" (Cantox, 2000, p. 2). The upper limit dosage was determined based on 19 published studies of ephedrine and/or ma huang in obese adults which were evaluated as being of sufficient extent and quality to be included in the critical dataset. In addition, for a generally healthy adult population, an identical dosage would serve as the "No Adverse Effect Level" of ephedrine ("in an herbal ephedra supplement") (Cantox, 2000, p. 1).

White et al. (1997) examined the effect of ma huang (375 mg/capsule) on ambulatory blood pressure and heart rate in 12 normotensive, healthy, nonsmoking adults (six males, six females, ages 23-40). In phase I of the study, ambulatory BP was measured every 15 minutes from 7 a.m. to 8 p.m. In phase II, the first dose of four capsules was taken with a light breakfast of juice and bagel and the second was taken 9 h later with an evening meal. Caffeine intake was monitored to ensure that the amounts ingested (undisclosed) were consistent from the control to the treatment phase. HPLC analysis of the ma huang product revealed a low variability of ephedrine alkaloids from one capsule to the next. The mean amounts of ephedrine alkaloids detected in a four-capsule dose were: ephedrine 19.4 mg, pseudoephedrine 4.9 mg, and methylephedrine 1.2 mg. In percent amounts per capsule, these concentrations were 1.24% ephedrine, 0.313% pseudoephedrine, and 0.08% methylephedrine, which were found to be in accordance with amounts previously reported for the species by Zhang et al. (1989). Although no side effects were reported by any of the 12 participants, including palpitations and tachycardia, in 6 there was a significant increase ($p < 0.05$) in the mean 12 h heart rate compared to baseline (78 ± 6 beats/ minute compared to 89 ± 9), in three the increase didn't reach statistical significance, and in the remaining three there was no change. When 3 h data was compared from each phase of the study, the mean 3 h heart rate (hours 8-11) showed a significant increase in six participants (72 ± 10 compared to 81 ± 14). At the same time, four showed a significant increase in systolic BP and two a significant decrease in diastolic BP. The effects on BP from the ma huang product were clinically insignificant. As for the variance of effects on BP in the participants, a plausible explanation may be that the amount of ephedrine contained in the encapsulated herbal product was too low to cause significant changes in every participant.

A placebo-controlled, double-blind, double-dummy, crossover study on the cardiovascular effects and abuse liability potential of ephedrine hydrochloride in healthy male Caucasians ($n = 16$) found that an oral dose of 50 mg was sufficient to cause a "substantial increase in blood pressure and orthostatic hypotension" (Berlin et al., 2001, p. 447). The increases in blood pressure were comparable to those observed by White et al. (1997) in subjects administered ma huang. A long-lasting drop in systolic BP in subjects in the standing position (mean maximal drop, 14 ± 10 mmHg) was not compensated. The absence of a counterbalancing increase in the heart rate led the investigators to conclude that such an effect may have deleterious clinical consequences in subjects when engaging in sports. At this dose, subjects reported palpitations and feeling less tired. Evidence of abuse liability in the subjects was not found. However, all the subjects were without any history of drug dependence. It was concluded that the central nervous system, cardiovascular, and abuse liability of ephedrine needs to be studied in large, community-based populations (Berlin et al., 2001).

In a randomized, double-blind, placebo-controlled trial lasting three months, Pasquali et al. (1985) administered ephedrine hydrochloride p.o. to obese male and female patients on calorie-restricted diets (1,000 kcal/day and 1,200 kcal/day, respectively). The dosages were 25 mg (group II) or 50 mg (group III) three times daily in tablet form. Group I received placebo. As in most if not all other trials involving ephedrine, patients were excluded if they had hypertension, diabetes, heart, kidney, or liver diseases. Of the initial 62 patients recruited, ten dropped out due to side effects (four from group II, four from group III, and two from group I), mainly of headache, agitation, insomnia, and constipation. One patient from group II and one from group III dropped out because of cutaneous erythema, a condition which quickly reversed after discontinuation of the drug. Due to noncompliance of patients, only 46 completed a minimum of four weeks' treatment, 13 in group II, 17 in group III, and the rest on placebo (group I). In group III the pulse rate showed a significant increase compared to placebo, but this was not the case for group II. A significantly greater incidence of side effects was found in group III compared to placebo, but not in group II compared to placebo. The reported side effects were: insomnia, headache, weakness, constipation, giddiness, palpitation, and tremor. No significant amount of weight loss was found compared to placebo.

A woman initially diagnosed with congestive cardiomyopathy of unknown cause was subsequently treated by a psychiatrist when it was learned that she had abused ephedrine-containing drugs for the last ten years to counteract depression and chronic fatigue and because the agents provided her with a "feeling of well-being" and "gave her energy" (To et al., 1980, p. 36). Over the ten years, she had progressed from Ephedrobarbital (30 mg ephedrine hydrochloride plus 15 mg phenobarbital/tablet) to 10-30 tablets of Tababsan/day (15 mg ephedrine HCL plus 30 mg theobromine and 60 mg salicylamide/tablet) and later used three bottles of Phensedyl elixir/day (180 mg ephedrine HCL, 225 mg codeine phosphate and 90 mg promethazine HCL/bottle) (To et al., 1980).

Case reports of ephedrine-induced psychosis have been reported in the literature since the 1930s and appear to be the result of high daily doses (Whitehouse and Duncan, 1987). However, cases of ephedrine psychosis have been associated with doses of 144-300 mg/day (Roxanas and Spalding, 1977). Psychotic episodes associated with ma huang alone appear to be rare and are due to abusively high doses, or are particular to individuals with a history of psychiatric problems (Jacobs and Hirsch, 2000). After an extensive search of the medical literature, only one case report was found which attributed a psychotic episode to an uncharacterized substance described as ma huang (Capwell, 1995). The patient, a 45-year-old man with no history of substance abuse or psychiatric problems, had been taking a supplement labeled "Ma huang" for weight loss in increasing doses (not specified) over a period of several weeks when the psychotic episode occurred. A physical exam and laboratory tests found hypertension, and the patient had no medical problems of a serious nature and was not taking any prescription or OTC drugs. The reporting physician noted the possibility of a family history of bipolar depression in the patient's father (Capwell, 1995) which may have predisposed the patient to the psychotic episode.

Special Precautions

Based on the pharmacokinetics of ephedrine in humans, and its known adverse effects on the cardiovascular system, patients taking ephedra are cautioned to discontinue its use at least 24 h before surgery (Ang-Lee et al., 2001).

Allergic reactions to oral doses of ephedrine, while extremely rare, have appeared in the form of dermatitis (Villas Martinez et al., 1993; Audicana et al., 1991).

Due to the possibilities of addiction and tachyphylaxis, the German Commission E recommends that preparations of "Ephedra" be taken only on a short-term basis. The Commission notes that preparations containing ephedrine are listed among addictive substances by the German Sports Association and by the International Olympic Committee (Blumenthal, 1998).

In a placebo-controlled, double-blind study, ephedrine in a single dose of 50 mg reached maximum plasma concentration significantly sooner and was significantly more rapidly absorbed when taken in a sauna, relative humidity 30-50%, temperature 80-100(C) (Vanakoski et al., 1993).

Herbal supplements containing ma huang and drugs containing ephedrine or pseudoephedrine should be kept away from pets (Means, 1999; Ooms et al., 2001).

Toxicology

In Vitro Toxicity

Using MTT colorimetry, Lee et al. (2000) examined the cytotoxic effects of various ma huang extracts prepared from the "whole herb" on human hepatoblastoma cells (HepG2) and various animal cell lines. The extracts were prepared using various methods, such as grinding, extracting once or twice, and boiling for 30 min or 2 h (20 g/200 mL distilled water at 20ºC). Apparently, no effort was made to determine the species of *Ephedra* employed; Lee and colleagues obtained the ma huang from local vendors in the Hupei Province in China. The presence of ephedrine alkaloids, determined by HPLC, provided the only proof that the material used was *Ephedra*. Today, ma huang is traditionally prepared in China from the branches and stems; however, the Chinese grind the "whole herb of ma huang into powdered form" (Lee et al., 2000, p. 425), which would indicate that they include the underground parts of the plant. Citing several authorities on ancient Chinese medicine and older authoritative texts, Lee and colleagues note that ma huang was used in whole-plant form and extracted for a longer time than other herbs in a formula. In the past, herbs were only extracted once before use whereas today it is common practice to extract them twice and then combine the individual extracts. As expected, the 2 h boiling time of powdered material yielded the greatest amounts of total ephedrine alkaloids (0.902% of the plant material), whereas only a portion of the alkaloids were extracted after 30 min of boiling. Also, most of the alkaloid content was liberated in the first extraction. The difference in total alkaloid content between boiling the material once or twice was within 15%. Taken together, this indicated that if boiled for a longer period (2 h), even the unground herb would yield comparable amounts of ephedrine alkaloids. The only notable in vitro cytotoxicity was seen in mouse neuroblastoma cells (Neuro-2a) which indicated that neuronal cells may be sensitive to toxic principles in ma huang extracts. Of all the cell lines tested, ma huang extracts produced the lowest IC_{50} (concentration that inhibited cell viability by 50%) in Neuro-2a cells. Also noteworthy was the fact that both ephedrine and the extracts prepared by first grinding the herb to powder produced significantly lower IC_{50}s compared to extracts prepared in the more traditional way from unground material, as indicated in five cell lines: two types of human α-adrenergic receptors (L-α-2A and L-α-1b cells), rat β3 adrenergic receptors (CHO-β3), human hepatoblastoma cells (HepG2), and mouse neuroblastoma cells (Neuro-2a). However, the ephedrine contents of the various extracts could not be responsible for all of the cytotoxicity detected, indicating the presence of other toxins (Lee et al., 2000).

Although these other toxins have yet to be identified in ma huang, kynurenates (chemically related to quinoline-2-carboxylic acids), found in other species of *Ephedra,* are potential sources of toxicity with potent antimicrobial activity (Al-Khalil et al., 1998; Caveney et al., 2001). Kynurenates have also shown potent inhibitory activity against glutamatergic neurotransmission (Leeson et al., 1992). In addition to kynurenates, cyclopropyl amino acids (carboxycyclopropylglycines) have been isolated from some *Ephedra* species (Caveney et al., 1996, 2001) and, like kyurenates, could also occur in ma huang. Some cyclopropyl amino acids are central nervous system (CNS) toxins (Kawai et al., 1992). Others are of interest as potential new drugs for the treatment of CNS disorders (Conn and Pin, 1997).

Mutagenicity

Hilliard et al. (1998) reported the absence of in vitro chromosomal aberrations and little toxicity from ephedrine in Chinese hamster ovary cells. Yamamoto et al. (1982) reported the absence of mutagenic effects from a crude "methanol or water" extract of *"Ephedrae Herba"* in the Ames test modified by the use of *Salmonella typhimurium* TA98 and TA100 in the absence or presence of rat liver S-9 mix.

Using a water extract of *E. sinica* prepared by boiling the finely powdered herb in water for 90 min, Yin et al. (1991) reported an absence of mutagenicity in the Ames test (modified by the use of *Salmonella typhimurium* TA98 and TA100 in the absence or presence of rat liver S-9 mix), and in chromosomal and micronucleus assays in mice of either sex administered the extract i.p.

Toxicity in Animal Models

In a study on the subacute oral toxicity of a concentrated extract of ma huang (9% wt/wt *l*-ephedrine) in male and female BALB/c mice, a dose of 2 g/kg per day p.o. (by gavage) for two weeks was reported to be well-tolerated in both sexes; however, at this dose there was evidence of gastrointestinal bleeding which was more pronounced from the LD_{50} dose of 4 g/kg p.o. At either dose, liver weights were not significantly different compared to controls. The oral LD_{50} of ephedrine in the form of the extract administered to these mice was calculated to be 360 mg/kg twice daily.

Based on these results, the oral LD_{50} of the extract for a human weighing 70 kg would be 23.3 g twice daily and that of ephedrine as provided by the extract would be 2.1 g twice daily (Law et al., 1996).

The acute oral LD_{50} of a water extract of ma huang in male ICR mice was determined to be approximately 5,300 mg/kg. The extract was prepared by heating the dried herb in distilled water (1:20) at 100°C for 1 h to produce a filtrate which was freeze-dried for use in the experiments. The alkaloid content of the extract was determined by HPLC to contain 2.27% ephedrine, 2.14% pseudoephedrine, and 0.057% norephedrine. Thus, the acute oral lethal dose contained 120 mg ephedrine and 113 mg pseudoephedrine. On the basis of the volume of extract obtained, the LD_{50} of the crude herb was calculated to be approximately 2,400 mg/kg (Minematsu et al., 1991). In an earlier study by Shoji and Kisara (1975), a freeze-dried water extract of *E. sinica* produced an acute oral LD_{50} in mice of $\geq 8,000$ mg/kg. Minematsu et al. (1991) hypothesized that the difference may have been attributable to the comparatively higher ratio of ephedrine to pseudoephedrine in the extract (4.23% ephedrine and 0.69% pseudoephedrine), a difference possibly due to the species of *Ephedra* employed (Zhu, 1998). In addition, Shoji and Kisara (1975) reported an acute i.p. LD_{50} in mice of 620 mg/kg from a freeze-dried water extract of *E. sinica*. They calculated that the total alkaloid concentration of the extract was 5.13% with ephedrine (4.23%) and pseudoephedrine (0.69%) constituting the main alkaloids. Similar p.o. and i.p. LD_{50}s are cited by Zhu (1998) for a water extract of *Ephedra* in mice at 7,800 mg/kg and 650 mg/kg, respectively.

The acute oral LD_{50} of ephedrine hydrochloride (as free base) in male ICR mice was found by Minematsu et al. (1991) to be approximately 520 mg/kg. Compared to the water extract, symptoms of toxicity, although much the same, were more intense and onset of death was markedly faster from ephedrine with twice the number of animals perishing after 8 h. A major difference in signs of toxicity was that unlike the mice administered the water extract (4,000 mg/kg p.o.), those receiving ephedrine hydrochloride (as free base, 520 mg/kg p.o.) showed a significant decrease in water intake, food intake, and body weight gain. Histopathological examination revealed that in both groups changes in organs were mostly seen in the kidneys and hearts. However, unlike those receiving ephedrine, the myocardium of the mice administered the water extract showed no degenerative lesions. Based on these differences, it was concluded that the toxicity of the water extract of ma huang was not solely attributable to ephedrine alkaloids (Minematsu et al., 1991). The same conclusion was arrived at by Lee et al. (2000) after an in vitro cytotoxicity assessment of *Ephedra* extracts (see In Vitro Toxicity).

Alwan et al. (1986) showed that "under physiological conditions," carcinogenic nitrosamines (*N*-nitrosoephedrine and *N*-nitrosopseudoephedrine) are formed when small amounts of sodium nitrate and ephedrine or pseudoephedrine are present together (e.g., 25 mg ephedrine and 50 mg nitrate). Using sodium nitrate (1 g/300 mL), nitrosation of a decoction and an alcoholic extract prepared from an Iraqi species of *Ephedra (E. foliata)* yielded related nitrosamines under physiological conditions (1 h at 37°C and pH 2). The alcoholic extract produced a higher yield of nitrosamines than the decoction (8.3 mg/100 g versus 0.77 mg/100 g of green plant parts dry weight, respectively). The LD_{50} of *N*-nitrosephedrine in mice was reported to be 392 mg/kg from a single i.p. injection and the dose to induce metastasizing liver cell carcinoma was 600 mg/kg in total. Yet given the significant amounts of nitrosamines formed from the plant extracts, the potential risk of nitrosamine formation from ephedrine can be extended to "extracts of the plant commonly used in folk medicine" (Alwan et al., 1986, p. 226).

The teratogenicity of ephedrine in the developing chick heart was examined alone and in combination with exposure to forskolin. Ephedrine alone caused a frequency of 8% malformed embryos from a concentration of 0.5 µmol and 26% from exposure to 5 µmol. At a concentration of 1 nmol, forskolin caused no significant increase in the frequency of cardiac malformations; however, when combined with the doses of ephedrine, even this amount caused the frequency of malformed embryos to increase to 47-72% (Nishikawa et al., 1991).

Adult male rats administered ephedrine hydrochloride (*l*-ephedrine, four doses of 25 mg/kg s.c.) developed degenerated cells in the forebrain if the body temperature was at or above 40.0°C (104°F). Below this temperature, there were no signs of degeneration (Bowyer et al., 2001). The calculated plasma levels of ephedrine resulting from the treatment (0.3-1.2 µM) were comparable to those found in humans (0.08-0.7 µM) who developed neurotoxicity from taking ma huang alkaloids (Bowyer et al., 2001 citing Haller and Benowitz, 2000).

REFERENCES

Al-Khalil, S., Alkofahi, A., El-Eisawa, D., and Al-Shibib, A. (1998). Transtorine, a new quinoline alkaloid from *Ephedra transitoria*. *Journal of Natural Products* 61: 262-263.

Alwan, S.M., Al-Hindawi, M.K., Abdul-Rahman, S.K., and Al-Sarraj, S. (1986). Production of nitrosamines from ephedrine, pseudoephedrine, and extracts of *Ephedra foliata* under physiological conditions. *Cancer Letters* 31: 221-226.

American Academy of Pediatrics Committee on Drugs (2001). The transfer of drugs and other chemicals into human milk. *Pediatrics* 108: 776-789.

Anderson, P.O. (2000). Decongestants and milk production. *Journal of Human Lactation* 16: 294.

Ang-Lee, M.K., Moss, J., and Yuan, C.S. (2001). Herbal medicines and perioperative care. *Journal of the American Medical Association* 286: 208-216.

Arch, J.R.S., Ainsworth, A.T., and Cawthorne, M.A. (1982). Thermogenic and anorectic effects of ephedrine and congeners in mice and rats. *Life Sciences* 30: 1817-1826.

Astrup, A. (1986). Thermogenesis in human brown adipose tissue and skeletal muscle induced by sympathomimetic stimulation. *Acta Endocrinologica* 112(Suppl. 278): 7-33.

Astrup, A., Breum, L., and Toubro, S. (1995). Pharmacological and clinical studies of ephedrine and other thermogenic agonists. *Obesity Research* 3(Suppl. 4): 537S-540S.

Astrup, A., Breum, L., Toubro, S., Hein, P., and Quaade, F. (1992). The effect and safety of an ephedrine/caffeine compound and placebo in obese subjects on an energy restricted diet: A double blind trial. *International Journal of Obesity* 16: 269-277.

Astrup, A., Lundsgaard, C., Madsen, J., and Christensen, N.J. (1985). Enhanced thermogenic responsiveness during chronic ephedrine treatment in man. *American Journal of Clinical Nutrition* 42: 83-94.

Astrup, A., Toubro, S., Christensen, N.J., and Quaade, F. (1992). Pharmacology of thermogenic drugs. *American Journal of Clinical Nutrition* 55(Suppl.): 246S-248S.

Audicana, M., Urrutia, I., Echechipia, S., Munoz, D., and De Corres, L.F. (1991). Sensitization to ephedrine in oral anticatarrhal drugs. *Contact Dermatitis* 24(3): 223.

Bedard, M. (2000). Ma huang. Is it a safe product? *Canadian Pharmaceutical Journal* 133 (November): 38-39.

Berlin, I., Warot, D., Aymard, G., Acquaviva, E., Legrand, M., Labarthe, B., Peyron, I., Diquet, B., and Lechat, P. (2001). Pharmacodynamics and pharmacokinetics of single nasal (5 mg and 10 mg) and oral (50 mg) doses of ephedrine in healthy subjects. *European Journal of Clinical Pharmacology* 57: 447-455.

Betz, J.M., Gay, M.L., Mossoba, M.M., Adams, S., and Portz, B.S. (1997). Chiral gas chromatographic determination of ephedrine-type alkaloids in dietary supplements containing *má huáng*. *Journal of AOAC International* 80: 303-315.

Bierman, C.W. and Pearlman, D.S. (Eds.) (1988). *Allergic Diseases from Infancy to Adulthood,* Second Edition. Philadelphia, PA: W.B. Saunders Company, pp. 258, 421, and 589.

Blumenthal, M., Busse, W.R., Goldberg, A., Gruenwald, J., Hall, T., Riggins, C.W., and Rister, R.S. (Eds.) (1998). *The Complete German Commission E Monographs.* Austin, TX: American Botanical Council, pp. 125-126.

Blumenthal, M. and King, P. (1995). Ma huang: Ancient herb, modern medicine, regulatory dilemma. *HerbalGram* 34: 22-27, 42-43, 56-57.

Boozer, C.N., Nasser, J.A., Heymsfield, S.B., Wang, V., Chen, G., and Solomon, J.L. (2001). An herbal supplement containing ma huang-guarana for weight loss: A randomized, double-blind trial. *International Journal of Obesity Research* 25: 316-324.

Borum, M.L. (2001). Fulminant exacerbation of autoimmune hepatitis after the use of ma huang. *American Journal of Gastroenterology* 96: 1654-1655.

Bowyer, J.F., Hopins, K.J., Jakab, R., and Ferguson, S.A. (2001). L-ephedrine-induced neurodegeneration in the parietal cortex and thalamus of the rat is dependent on hyperthermia and can be altered by the process of in vivo brain microdialysis. *Toxicology Letters* 2001; 125: 151-166.

Breum, L., Pedersen, J.K., AhlstrØm, F., and Frimodt-Moller, J. (1994). Comparison of an ephedrine/caffeine combination and dexfenfluramine in the treatment of obesity: A double-blind multi-centre trial in general practice. *International Journal of Obesity* 18: 99-103.

Briggs, G.G., Freeman, R.K., and Yaffe, S.J. (1990). *Drugs in Pregnancy and Lactation,* Third Edition. Baltimore, MD: Williams and Wilkins.

Büscher, R., Herrmann, V., and Insel, P.A. (1999). Human adrenoreceptor polymorphisms: Evolving recognition of clinical importance. *Trends in Pharmacological Sciences* 20: 94-99.

Cantox (2000). *Safety Assessment and Determination of a Tolerable Upper Limit for Ephedra.* Mississauga, ON, Canada: Cantox Health Sciences International. Accessed January 3, 2001 at <http://www.crnusa.org/CRNantoxreportindex.html>.

Cappelli, R., Nicora, M., and Di Perri, T. (1988). Use of *Ruscus aculeatus* in venous disease. *Drugs Under Experimental and Clinical Research* 14: 277-283.

Capwell, R.R. (1995). Ephedrine-induced mania from a herbal diet supplement. *American Journal of Psychiatry* 152: 647 (letter).

Caveney, S., Charlet, D.A., Freitag, H., Mair-Stolte, M., and Starratt, A.N. (2001). New observations on the secondary chemistry of world *Ephedra* (Ephedraceae). *American Journal of Botany* 88: 1199-1208.

Caveney, S., McLean, H.M., Watson, I., and Starratt, A.N. (1996). Affinity of an insect Na$^+$-dependent glutamate transporter for plant-derived cyclic substrates. *Insect Biochemistry and Molecular Biology* 26: 1027-1036.

Chang, H.M. and But, P.P.H. (Eds.) (1987). *Pharmacology and Applications of Chinese Materia Medica,* 2. Singapore: World Scientific, pp. 1119-1124.

Chaudhuryi, P.K. and Thakur, R.S. (1991). *Hamelia patents:* A new source of ephedrine. *Planta Medica* 57: 199.

Chen, K.K. and Schmidt, C.F. (1924). The action of ephedrine, an alkaloid from ma huang. *Proceedings of the Society for Experimental Biology and Medicine* 21: 351-354.

Clarkson, P.M. and Thompson, H.S. (1997). Drugs and sport: Research findings and limitations. *Sports Medicine* 24: 366-384.

Conn, P.J. and Pin, J.P. (1997). Pharmacology and functions of metabotropic glutamate receptors. *Annual Review of Pharmacology and Toxicology* 37: 205-237.

Dollery, C. (1991). *Therapeutic Drugs.* New York: Churchill Livingstone, pp. 26-29, 92-93, 297-299.

Dulloo, A.G. and Miller, D.S. (1986). The thermogenic properties of ephedrine/ methylxanthine mixtures: Animal studies. *American Journal of Clinical Nutrition* 43: 388-394.

Dulloo, A.G. and Miller, D.S. (1987). Aspirin as a promoter of ephedrine-induced thermogenesis: Potential use in the treatment of obesity. *American Journal of Clinical Nutrition* 45: 564-569.

Dulloo, A.G., Seydoux, J., and Girardier, L. (1991). Peripheral mechanisms of thermogenesis induced by ephedrine and caffeine in brown adipose tissue. *International Journal of Obesity* 15: 317-326.

Ephedra Education Council (2000). *Scientific and Medical Experts Support Current National Standards for Ephedra* [press release]. Washington, DC: Ephedra Education Council, August 7. Accessed May 2, 2001 at: <http://www. ephedrafacts.com/august7.htm>.

FDA (2000). Food and Drug Administration Public Health Advisory. Subject: Phenylpropanolamine. Washington DC: FDA/Center for Drug Evaluation and Research, November 6; accessed January 6, 2001 at: <http://www.fda.gov/ cder/drug/infopage/ppa/advisory.htm>.

Flurer, C.L., Lin, L.A., Satzger, R.D., and Wolnik, K.A. (1995). Determination of ephedrine compounds in nutritional supplements by cyclodextrin-modified capillary electrophoresis. *Journal of Chromatography* B 669: 133-139.

Franzotti, E.M., Santos, C.V., Rodrigues, H.M., Mourao, R.H., Andrade, M.R., and Antoniolli, A.R. (2000). Anti-inflammatory, analgesic activity and acute toxicity of *Sida cordifolia* L. (malva-branca). *Journal of Ethnopharmacology* 72: 273-277.

Fratkin, J. (1986). *Chinese Herbal Patent Formulas: A Practical Guide.* Boulder, CO: Shya Publications, pp. 62, 67, and 266.

Fugh-Berman, A. and Allina, A. (2000). Ephedra for weight loss. *Alternative Therapies in Women's Health* 2 (November): 81-84.

Gilbert-Barness, E. and Drut, R.M. (2000). Association of sympathomimetic drugs with malformations. *Veterinary and Human Toxicology* 42: 168-171.

Gillis, M.C., Welbanks, L., Bergeron, D., Cormier-Boyd, M., Hachborn, F., Jovaisas, B., Pagotto, S., and Repchinsky, C. (Eds.) (1999). *CPS: Compendium of Pharmaceuticals and Specialities,* Thirty-Fourth Edition. Ottawa, ON, Canada: Canadian Pharmacists Association, pp. 603-604.

Greenway, F.L., Raum, W.J., and DeLany, J.P. (2000). The effect of an herbal dietary supplement containing ephedrine and caffeine on oxygen consumption in humans. *Journal of Alternative and Complimentary Medicine* 6: 553-555.

Gurley, B.J., Gardner, S.F., and Hubbard, M.A. (2000). Content versus label claims in ephedra-containing dietary supplements. *American Journal of Health-System Pharmacists* 57: 963-969.

Gurley, B.J., Gardner, S.F., White, L.M., and Wang, P. (1998). Ephedrine pharmacokinetics after the ingestion of nutritional supplements containing *Ephedra sinica* (ma huang). *Therapeutic Drug Monitoring* 20: 439-445.

Gurley, B.J., Wang, P., and Gardner, S.F. (1998). Ephedrine-type alkaloid content of nutritional supplements containing *Ephedra sinica* (ma huang) as determined by high performance liquid chromatography. *Journal of Pharmaceutical Sciences* 87: 1547-1553.

Hale, T. (2000). *Medications and Mother's Milk*. Amarillo, TX: Pharmasoft Medical Publications, pp. 298-299.

Haller, C.A. and Benowitz, N.L. (2000). Adverse cardiovascular and central nervous system events associated with dietary supplements containing *Ephedra* alkaloids. *New England Journal of Medicine* 343: 1833-1838.

Haller, C.A. and Benowitz, N.L. (2001). Letter to the editor in reply to Hutchins, G.M. *New England Journal of Medicine* 344 (April 5): 1096-1097.

Health Canada (2001). Advisory. Advisory not to use products containing Ephedra or ephedrine. Ottawa, Ontario: Health Canada, June 14. Accessed June 15, 2001 at: <http://www.hcsc.gc.ca/english/archives/warnings/2001/2001_67e.htm>.

Hikino, H., Kiso, Y., Ogata, M., Konno, C., Aisaka, K., Kubota, H., Hirose, N., and Ishihara, T. (1984). Pharmacological actions of analogues of feruloylhistamine, an imidazole alkaloid of *Ephedra* roots. *Planta Medica* 50: 478-480.

Hikino, H., Konno, C., Takata, H., Konno, C., Aisaka, K., Kubota, H., Hirose, N., and Ishihara, T. (1980). Anti-inflammatory principle of *Ephedra* herbs. *Chemical and Pharmaceutical Bulletin* 28: 2900-2904.

Hikino, H., Ogata, K., Kasahara, Y., and Konno, C. (1985). Pharmacology of ephedroxanes. *Journal of Ethnopharmacology* 13: 175-191.

Hikino, H., Ogata, M., and Konno, C. (1982). Structure of ephedradine D, a hypotensive principle of *Ephedra* roots. *Heterocycles* 14: 155-158.

Hikino, H., Ogata, M., and Konno, C. (1983). Structure of feruloylhistamine, a hypotensive principle of *Ephedra* roots. *Planta Medica* 48: 108-110.

Hikino, H., Ogata, K., Konno, C., and Sato, S. (1983). Hypotensive actions of ephedradines, macrocyclic spermine alkaloids of *Ephedra* roots. *Planta Medica* 48: 290-293.

Hikino, H., Shimoyama, N., Kasahara, Y., Takahasi, M., and Konno, C. (1982). Structures of mahuannin A and B, hypotensive principles of *Ephedra* roots. *Heterocycles* 19: 1381-1384.

Hikino, H., Takahashi, M., and Konno, C. (1982). Structure of ephedrannin A, a hypotensive principle of *Ephedra* roots. *Tetrahedron Letters* 23: 673-676.

Hilliard, C.A., Armstrong, M.J., Bradt, C.I., Hill, R.B., Greenwood, S.K., and Galloway, S.M. (1998). Chromosome aberrations *in vitro* related to cytotoxicity of nonmutagenic chemicals and metabolic poisons. *Environmental and Molecular Mutagenesis* 31: 316-326.

Holmstedt, B. (1991). Historical perspective and future of ethnopharmacology. *Journal of Ethnopharmacology* 32: 7-24.

Horikawa, H., Mohri, T., Tanaka, Y., and Tokiwa, H. (1994). Moderate inhibition of mutagenicity and carcinogenicity of benzo[*a*]pyrene, 1,6-dinitropyrene and 3,9-dinitrofluoranthese by Chinese medicinal herbs. *Mutagenesis* 9: 523-526.

Hsu, C. (1973). [Puerperal mastitis treated with Fructus Gleditsiae: Report of 43 cases]. *Chinese Medical Journal* 11: 685-686 (English abstract).

Hsu, H.Y., Chen, Y.P., Shen, S.J., Hsu, C.S., Chen, C.C., and Chang, H.C. (Eds.) (1986). *Oriental Materia Medica: A Concise Guide*. Long Beach, CA: Oriental Healing Arts Institute, pp. 52-53, 606-607.

Hu, S.Y. (1969). *Ephedra* (ma-huang) in the new Chinese materia medica. *Economic Botany* 23: 346-351.

Humphrey, S. (2001). Sheila Humphrey, RN, BSc, ICBLC, personal communication with INPR, September.

Huntley, A. and Ernst, E. (2000). Herbal medicines for asthma: A systematic review. *Thorax* 55: 925-929.

Hutchins, G.M. (2001). Letter to the editor. *New England Journal of Medicine* 344 (April 5).

Inokuchi, J.I., Okabe, H., Yamauchi, T., Nagamatsu, A., Nonaka, G.I., and Nishioka, I. (1985). Inhibitors of angiotensin-converting enzyme in crude drugs. II. *Chemical and Pharmaceutical Bulletin* 33: 264-269.

Jacobs, K.M. and Hirsch, K.A. (2000). Psychiatric complications of ma huang. *Psychosomatics* 41: 58-62.

Ji, L.X.Z., Pan, G., and Yang, G. (1997). [GC-MS analysis of constituent of essential oils from stems of *Ephedra sinica* Stapf., *E. intermedia* Schrenk et C.A. Mey. and *E. equisetina* Bge]. *Zhongguo Zhongyao Zazhi* 22: 489-492, 512 (English abstract).

Johnson, D.A. and Hricik, J.G. (1993). The pharmacology of α-adrenergic decongestants. *Pharmacotherapy* 13(6 Part 2; Suppl.): 110S-115S.

Kalix, P. (1991). The pharmacology of psychoactive alkaloids from *Ephedra* and *Catha. Journal of Ethnopharmacology* 32: 201-208.

Kanfer, I., Dowse, R., and Vuma, V. (1993). Pharmacokinetics of oral decongestants. *Pharmacotherapy* 13(6 Part 2; Suppl.): 116S-128S.

Karch, S.B. (2000). Ma huang and the *Ephedra* alkaloids. In Cupp, M.J. (Ed.), *Toxicology and Clinical Pharmacology of Herbal Products* (pp. 11-30). Totowa, NJ: Humana Press.

Kasahara, Y. and Hikino, H. (1983). Structure of mahuannin D, a hypotensive principle of *Ephedra* roots. *Heterocycles* 20: 1953-1956.

Kasahara, Y., Hikino, H., Tsurufuji, S., Watanabe, M., and Ohuchi, K. (1985). Antiinflammatory actions of ephedrines in acute inflammations. *Planta Medica* 51: 325-331.

Kasahara, Y., Shimoyama, N., Konno, C., and Hikino, H. (1983). Structure of mahuannin C, a hypotensive principle of *Ephedra* roots. *Heterocycles* 20: 1741-1744.

Kawai, M., Horikawa, Y., Ishiwara, T., Shimamoto, K., and Ohfune, Y. (1992). 2-(Carboxycyclopropyl) glycines: Binding, neurotoxicity and induction of intracellular Ca^{++} increase. *European Journal of Pharmacology* 211: 195-202.

Kernan, W.N., Viscoli, C.M., Brass, L.M., Broderick, J.P., Brott, T., Feldmann, E., Morgenstern, L.B., Wilterdink, J.L., and Horwitz, R.I. (2000). Phenylpropanolamine and the risk of hemorrhagic stroke. *New England Journal of Medicine* 343: 1826-1832.

Kim, S.Y., Son, K.H., Chang, H.W., Kang, S.S., and Kim, H.P. (1997). Inhibitory effects of plant extracts on adjuvant-induced arthritis. *Archives of Pharmacal Research* (Seoul) 20: 313-317.

Kockler, D.R., McCarthy, M.W., and Lawson, C.L. (2001). Seizure activity and unresponsiveness after hydroxycut ingestion. *Pharmacotherapy* 21: 647-651.

Kondo, N., Mikage, M., and Idaka, K. (1999). Medico-botanical studies of *Ephedra* plants from the Himalayan region, part III. Causative factors of variation of alkaloid content in herbal stems. *Shoyakugaku Zasshi [Natural Medicines]* 53: 194-200.

Konno, C., Taguchi, T., Tamada, M., and Hikino, H. (1979). Ephedroxane, antiinflammatory principle of *Ephedra* herbs. *Phytochemistry* 18: 697-698.

Konno, C., Tamada, M., Endo, K., and Hikino, H. (1980). Structure of ephedradine C, a hypertensive principle of *Ephedra* roots. *Heterocycles* 14: 295-298.

Krieger, D.R., Daly, P.A., Dulloo, A.G., Ransil, B.J., Young, J.B., and Landsberg, L. (1990). Ephedrine, caffeine and aspirin promote weight loss in obese subjects. *Transactions of the Association of American Physicians* 103: 307-312.

Kun, L., Li, H., and Ding, M. (2000). Analysis of tetramethylpyrazine in *Ephedrae herba* by gas chromatography-mass spectrometry and high-performance liquid chromatography. *Journal of Chromatography* A 878: 147-152.

Law, M.Y., Pedersen, G.H., Hennen, W.J., McCausland, C.W., and Sidwell, R.W. (1996). Subacute toxicity study of ma-huang in mice. *Fundamental and Applied Toxicology* 30(1, Part 2): 111 (abstract 566).

Lee, G.I., Ha, J.Y., Min, K.R., Nakagawa, H., Tsurufuji, S., Chang, I.M., and Kim, Y. (1995). Inhibitory effects of Oriental herbal medicines on IL-8 induction in lipopolysaccharide-activated rat macrophages. *Planta Medica* 61: 26-30.

Lee, M.K., Cheng, B.W., Che, C.T., and Hsieh, D.P. (2000). Cytotoxicity assessment of ma-huang *(Ephedra)* under different conditions of preparation. *Toxicological Sciences* 56(2): 424-430.

Leeson, P.D., Baker, R., Carling, R.W., Curtis, N.R., Moore, K.W., Williams, B.J., Foster, A.C., Donald, A.E., Kemp, J.A., and Marshall, G.R. (1992). Kynurenic acid derivatives: Structure-activity relationships for excitatory amino acid antagonism and identification of potent and selective antagonists at the glycine site on the N-methyl-D-aspartate receptor. *Journal of Medicinal Chemistry* 34: 1243-1252.

Leung, A.Y. and Foster, S. (1996). *Encyclopedia of Common Natural Ingredients,* Second Edition. New York: John Wiley and Sons, pp. 227-229.

Lewis, W.H. and Elvin-Lewis, M.P.F. (1977). *Medical Botany: Plants Affecting Man's Health.* New York: John Wiley and Sons.

Ling, M., Piddlesden, S.J., and Morgan, B.P. (1995). A component of the medicinal herb *Ephedra* blocks activation in the classical and alternative pathways of complement. *Clinical and Experimental Immunology* 102: 582-588.

Liu, Y.L., Toubro, S., Astrup, A., and Stock, M.J. (1995). Contribution of β_3-adrenoreceptor activation to ephedrine-induced thermogenesis in humans. *International Journal of Obesity* 19: 678-685.

Liu, Y.M., Sheu, S.J., Chiou, S.H., Chang, H.C., and Chen, Y.P. (1993). A comparative study on commercial samples of Ephedrae Herba. *Planta Medica* 59: 376-378.

Malchow-MØller, A., Larsen, S., Hey, H., Stokholm, K.H., Juhl, E., and Quaade, F. (1981). Ephedrine as an anorectic: The story of the "Elsinore pill." *International Journal Obesity* 5: 183-187.

Mantani, N., Andoh, T., Kawamata, H., Terasawa, K., and Ochiai, H. (1999). Inhibitory effect of *Ephedrae herba,* an Oriental traditional medicine, on the growth of influenza A/PR/8 virus in MDCK cells. *Antiviral Research* 44: 193-200.

Marcelon, G., Verbeuren, T.J., Lauressergues, H., and Vanhoutte, P.M. (1983). Effect of *Ruscus aculeatus* on isolated canine cutaneous veins. *General Pharmacology* 14: 103-106.

Martinet, A., Hostettman, K., and Schutz, Y. (1999). Thermogenic effects of commercially available plant preparations aimed at treating human obesity. *Phytomedicine* 6: 231-238.

McGuffin, M., Hobbs, C., Upton, R., and Goldberg, A. (Eds.) (1997). *American Herbal Products Association's Botanical Safety Handbook.* Boca Raton, FL: CRC Press, pp. 45-46.

Means, C. (1999). Ma huang: All natural but not always innocuous. *Veterinary Medicine* 94: 511-512.

Meston, C.M. and Heiman, J.R. (1998). Ephedrine-activated physiological arousal in women. *Archives of General Psychiatry* 55: 652-656.

Michaelis, R.C., Holloway, F.A., Bird, C.C., and Huerta, P.L. (1987). Interactions between stimulants: Effects on DRL performance and lethality in rats. *Pharmacology, Biochemistry and Behavior* 27: 299-306.

Miller, T.G. (1925). A consideration of the clinical value of ephedrine. *American Journal of Medical Science* 170: 157-181.

Minematsu, S., Kobayashi, Y., Kobayashi, N., Fujii, Y., Aburada, M., and Yamashita, M. (1991). Acute *Ephedrae Herba* and ephedrine poisoning in mice. *Chudoku Kenkyu [Japanese Journal of Toxicology]* 4: 143-149.

Miyazawa, M., Minamino, Y., and Kameoka, H. (1997). Volatile components of *Ephedra sinica. Flavour and Fragrance Journal* 12: 15-17.

Moriyasu, M., Endo, M., Kanazawa, R., Hasimoto, Y., Kato, A., and Mixuno, M. (1984). High-performance liquid chromatography determination of organic substances by metal chelate derivatization. III. Analysis of *Ephedra* bases. *Chemical and Pharmaceutical Bulletin* 32: 744-747.

Munns, G. and Aldrich, C. (1927). Ephedrine in the treatment of bronchial asthma in children. *Journal of the American Medical Association* 88: 1233.

Nadkarni, K.M. (1976). *Indian Materia Medica,* Volume 1. Bombay, India: Popular Prakashan Private Ltd., pp. 486-503.

Naeser, M.A. (1996). *Outline Guide to Chinese Herbal Patent Medicines in Pill Form,* Second Edition. Boston, MA: Boston Chinese Medicine, pp. 74, 75, and 96.

Nelson, H.S. (1995). β-Adrenergic bronchodilators. *New England Journal of Medicine* 333: 499-506.

Nightingale, S.L. (1996). Adverse events associated with ephedrine-containing products—Texas, December 1993-September 1995. *Journal of the American Medical Association* 276 (December 4): 1711-1712.

Nishikawa, T., Kasajima, T., and Kanai, T. (1991). Potentiating effects of forskolin on the cardiovascular teratogenicity of ephedrine in chick embryos. *Toxicology Letters* 56: 145-150.

Ooms, T.G., Khan, S.A., and Means, C. (2001). Suspected caffeine and ephedrine toxicosis resulting from ingestion of an herbal supplement containing guarana and ma huang in dogs: 47 cases (1997-1999). *Journal of the American Veterinary Medical Association* 218: 225-229.

Oshio, H., Tsukui, M., and Matsuoka, T. (1978). Isolation of *l*-ephedrine from "Pinelliae Tuber." *Chemical and Pharmaceutical Bulletin* 26: 2096-2097.

Pang, P.K.T., Shan, J.J., and Chui, K.W. (1996). Tetramethylpyrazine, a calcium antagonist. *Planta Medica* 62: 431-435.

Park, J.M., Schmer, V., and Myers, T.L. (1990). Cardiovascular anomalies associated with prenatal exposure to theophylline. *Southern Medical Journal* 83: 1487-1488.

Pasquali, R., Baraldi, G., Cesari, M.P., Melchionda, N., Zamboni, M., Stefanini, C., and Raitano, A. (1985). A controlled trial using ephedrine in the treatment of obesity. *International Journal of Obesity* 9: 93-98.

Pasquali, R. and Casimirri, F. (1993). Clinical aspects of ephedrine in the treatment of obesity. *International Journal of Obesity* 17(Suppl. 1): S65-S68.

Pasquali, R., Casimirri, F., Melchionda, N., Grossi, G., Bortoluzzi, L., Morselli Labate, A.M., Stefanini, C., and Raitano, A. (1992). The effects of chronic administration of ephedrine during very-low-calorie diets on energy expenditure, protein metabolism and hormone levels in obese subjects. *Clinical Science* 82: 85-92.

Price, R.A. (1996). Systematics of the Gnetales: A review of morphological and molecular evidence. *International Journal of Plant Science* 157(Suppl. 6): S40-S49.

Rakel, R.E. (Ed.) (2000). *Conn's Current Therapy.* Philadelphia, PA: W.B. Saunders Company, p. 14.

Ramsey, J.J., Colman, R.J., Swick, A.G., and Kenmitz, J.W. (1998). Energy expenditure, body composition, and glucose metabolism in lean and obese rhesus monkeys treated with ephedrine and caffeine. *American Journal of Clinical Nutrition* 68: 42-51.

Reynolds, J.E.F. (Ed.) (1996). *Martindale. The Extra Pharmacopoeia,* Twenty-First Edition. London: Royal Pharmaceutical Society, pp. 1575-1577, 1588-1589.

Robbers, J.E. and Tyler, V.E. (1999). *Tyler's Herbs of Choice: The Therapeutic Use of Phytomedicinals.* Binghamton, NY: The Haworth Press, pp. 112-116.

Roxanas, M.G. and Spalding, J. (1977). Ephedrine abuse psychosis. *Medical Journal of Australia* 2: 639-640.

Sanagi, M.M., Hung, W.P., and Yasir, S.M. (1997). Supercritical fluid extraction of pyrazines in roasted cocoa beans. Effect of pod storage period. *Journal of Chromatography* A 785: 361-367.

Seckman, D. (2000). Comments from the Ephedra hearings. *Nutritional Outlook* (October) 3: 26.

Shannon, J.R., Gottesdiener, K., Jordan, J., Chen, K., Flattery, S., Larson, P.J., Candelore, M.R., Gertz, B., Robertson, D., and Sun, M. (1999). Acute effect of ephedrine on 24-hr energy balance. *Clinical Science* 96: 483-491.

Sheu, S.J. (1997). Identification by chemical analysis of the botanical sources of commercial samples of Chinese herbal drugs. *Journal of Food and Drug Analysis* 5: 285-294.

Shiraki, K., Kurokawa, M., Imakita, M., Sato, H., Yamamura, J.I., Li, Z.H., and Kageyama, S. (1999). Efficacy of kakkon-to, a traditional herbal medicine, against *Herpes simplex* virus type 1 and influenza infection in mice. In Watanabe, H. and Shibuya, T. (Eds.), *Pharmacological Research on Traditional Herbal Medicines* (pp. 197-217). Amsterdam, the Netherlands: Harwood Academic.

Shoji, T. and Kisara, K. (1975). [Pharmacological studies of crude drugs showing antitussive and expectorant activity (Report 1)—The combined effects of some crude drugs in antitussive activity and acute toxicity.] *Oyo Yakuri [Pharmacokinetics]* 10: 407-415.

Sieb, J.P. and Engel, A.G. (1993). Ephedrine: Effects on neuromuscular transmission. *Brain Research* 623: 167-171.

Smith, T.A. (1977). Phenethylamine and related compounds in plants. *Phytochemistry* 16: 9-18.

Sprague, J.E., Harrod, A.D., and Teconchuk, A.L. (1998). The pharmacology and abuse potential of ephedrine. *Pharmacy Times* 64 (May): 72-80.

Stark, R. (1980). *The Book of Aphrodisiacs.* Toronto, ON, Canada: Methuen, p. 36.

Stevenson, D.W. (1993). Ephedraceae. In: Flora of North America Editorial Committee (Eds.), *Flora of North America,* vol. 2, pp. 428-434. New York: Oxford University Press.

Takechi, M., Tanaka, Y., Takehara, M., Nonaka, G.I., and Nishioka, I. (1985). Structure and antiherpetic activity among the tannins. *Phytochemistry* 24: 2245-2250.

Tamada, M., Endo, K., and Hikino, H. (1978). Maokonine, hypertensive principle of *Ephedra* roots. *Planta Medica* 34: 291-293.

Tamada, M., Endo, K., and Hikino, H. (1979). Structure of ephedradine B, a hypotensive principle of *Ephedra* roots. *Heterocycles* 12: 783-786.

Tamada, M., Endo, K., Hikino, H., and Kabuto, C. (1979). Structure of ephedradine A, a hypotensive principle of *Ephedra* roots. *Tetrahedron Letters* 10: 873-876.

Tekol, Y., Tercan, E., and Esmaoglu, A. (1994). Ephedrine enhances analgesic effect of morphine. *Acta Anaesthesiologica Scandinavica* 38: 396-397.

Theoharides, T.C. (1997). Sudden death of healthy college student related to ephedrine toxicity from ma huang-containing drink. *Journal of Clinical Psychopharmacology* 17: 437-439 (letter).

Tinkelman, D.G. and Avner, S.E. (1977). Ephedrine therapy in asthmatic children: Clinical tolerance and absence of side effects. *Journal of the American Medical Association* 237: 553-557.

To, L.B., Sangster, J.F., Rampling, D., and Cammens, I. (1980). Ephedrine-induced cardiomyopathy. *Medical Journal of Australia* 2: 35-36.

Torfs, C.P., Katz, E.A., Bateson, T.F., Lam, P.K., and Curry, C.J. (1996). Maternal medication and environmental exposures as risk factors for gastroschisis. *Teratology* 54: 84-92.

Toubro, S., Astrup, A.V., Breum, L., and Quaade, F. (1993). Safety and efficacy of long-term treatment with ephedrine, caffeine and an ephedrine/caffeine mixture. *International Journal of Obesity* 17(Suppl. 1): S69-S72.

Traub, S.J., Hoyek, W., and Hoffman, R.S. (2001). Letter to the editor. *New England Journal of Medicine* 344 (April 5): 1096.

Tu, G., Fang, Q., Guo, J., Yuan, S., Chen, C., Chen, J., Chen, Z., Cheng, S., Jin, R., Li, M., et al. (Eds.) (1992). *Pharmacopoeia of the People's Republic of China,* English Edition. Guangzhou, China: Guangdong Science and Technology Press, pp. 99-100, 159-160.

Vanakoski, J., Strömberg, C., and Seppälä, T. (1993). Effects of a sauna on the pharmacokinetics and pharmacodynamics of midazolam and ephedrine in healthy young women. *European Journal of Clinical Pharmacology* 45: 377-381.

Villas Martinez, F., Badas, A.J., Garmendia Goitia, J.F., and Aguirre, I. (1993). Generalized dermatitis due to oral ephedrine. *Contact Dermatitis* 29(4): 215-216.

Warot, D., Berlin, I., Aymard, G., Acquviva, E., Legrand, M., Labarthe, B., Diquet, B., and Lechat, P.H. (2000). Comparative pharmacodynamics and pharmacokinetics of oral and intranasal ephedrine. *Fundamental and Clinical Pharmacology* 14: 237-297 (abstract).

Watanabe, H. (1997). Candidates for cognitive enhancer extracted from medicinal plants: Paeoniflorin and tetramethylpyrazine. *Behavioural Brain Research* 83: 135-141.

Werler, M.M., Mitchell, A.A., and Shapiro, S. (1992). First trimester maternal medication use in relation to gastroschisis. *Teratology* 45: 361-367.

White, L.M., Gardner, S.F., Gurley, B.J., Marx, M.A., Wang, P.L., and Estes, M. (1997). Pharmacokinetics and cardiovascular effects of ma-huang *(Ephedra sinica)* in normotensive adults. *Journal of Clinical Pharmacology* 37: 116-122.

Whitehouse, A.M. and Duncan, J.M. (1987). Ephedrine psychosis rediscovered. *British Journal of Psychiatry* 150: 258-261.

Wilkinson, G.R., and Beckett, A.H. (1968). Absorption, metabolism and excretion of ephedrine in man. II. Pharmacokinetics. *Journal of Pharmaceutical Sciences* 57: 1933-1938.

Woodgate, D.E. and Conquer, J.A. (2001). Double-blind study evaluating the effects of a novel herbal supplement on weight loss in overweight adults. *FASEB Journal* 15: A302 (abstract 254.9).

Xiu, L.M., Miura, A.B., Yamamoto, K., Kobayashi, T., Song, Q.H., Kitamura, H., Cyong, J.C. (2001). Pancreatic islet regeneration by ephedrine in mice streptozotocin-induced diabetes. *American Journal of American Medicine* 29: 493-500.

Yamamoto, H., Mizutani, T., and Nomura, H. (1982). Studies on the mutagenicity of crude drug extracts. I. *Yakugaku Zasshi* 102: 596-601 (in Japanese with English abstract and tables).

Yang, S.Z. (1997). *The Divine Farmer's Materia Medica: A Translation of the Shen Nong Ben Cao Jing*. Boulder, CO: Blue Poppy Press, Inc., pp. x, 51-52.

Yin, X.J., Liu, D.X., Wang, H., and Zhou, Y. (1991). A study on the mutagenicity of 102 raw pharmaceuticals used in Chinese traditional medicine. *Mutation Research* 260: 73-82.

Yokozawa, T., Fujioka, K., Oura, H., Tanaka, T., Nonaka, G., and Nishioka, I. (1995). Decrease in uraemic toxins, a newly found beneficial effect of Ephedrae Herba. *Phytotherapy Research* 9: 382-384.

Yoshizaki, F., Komatsu, T., Inoue, K., Kanari, R., Ando, T., and Hisamichi, S. (1996). Survey of crude drugs effective in eliminating superoxides in blood plasma of mice. *International Journal of Pharmacognosy* 34: 277-282.

Yuan, D., Komatsu, K.I., Cui, Z., and Kano, Y. (1999). Pharmacological properties of traditional medicines. XXV. Effects of ephedrine, amygdalin, glycyrrhizin, gypsum and their combinations on body temperature and body fluid. *Biological and Pharmaceutical Bulletin* 22: 165-171.

Yuan, D., Komatsu, K., Tani, H., Cui, Z., and Kano, Y. (1998). Pharmacological properties of traditional medicines. XXIV. Classification of anti-asthmatics based on constitutional predispositions. *Biological and Pharmaceutical Bulletin* 21: 1169-1173.

Zaacks, S.M., Klein, L., Tan, C.D., Rodriguez, E.R., and Leikin, J.B. (1999). Hypersensitivity myocarditis associated with ephedra use. *Journal of Toxicology (Clinical Toxicology)* 37: 485-489.

Zhang, J., Tian, Z., and Lou, Z.C. (1988). Simultaneous determination of six alkaloids in Ephedrae Herba by high performance liquid chromatography. *Planta Medica* 54: 69-70.

Zhang, J.S., Tian, Z., and Lou, Z.C. (1989). [Quality of evaluation of twelve species of Chinese *Ephedra*, ma huang]. *Acta Pharmaceutica Sinica* 24: 865-871 (English abstract).

Zhu, Y.P. (1998). *Chinese Materia Medica: Chemistry, Pharmacology and Applications*. Amsterdam, the Netherlands: Harwood Academic, pp. 45-51, 661-662.

Zou, J.P., Gu, F.Q., and Liao, W.J. (1996). [Clinical study on treating asthma of cold type with Wenyang Tonglulo mixture]. *Chung Kuo Ching Hsi I Chieh Ho Tsa Chih* 16: 529-532.

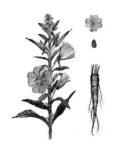

Evening Primrose Oil

BOTANICAL DATA

Classification and Nomenclature

Scientific name: *Oenothera biennis* L.

Family name: Onagraceae

Common names: Evening primrose, scabish, king's cure-all, night-willow herb, German rampion (Foster, 1995)

Description

Oenothera biennis L. is a large wildflower native to North America but is not a true primrose. Rather, it belongs to the family Onagraceae (also called the Evening Primrose family), which also includes the fireweeds and fuchsias. It is a biennial that grows to approximately 2.4 m tall and flowers in the second season (as with many perennials). In both North America and Europe, *Oenothera biennis* has escaped cultivation and has naturalized into the environment (Foster, 1995).

HISTORY AND TRADITIONAL USES

Evening primrose has been traditionally used by a variety of peoples. Because all parts of the plant are edible, the Native Americans of Utah and Nevada ate the seeds. The young leaves may also be used raw in salads, or cooked with several changes in water to get rid of the bitterness. The English settlers took the seeds to the British Isles where they were then grown by both English and German gardeners for their roots, which have a nutlike flavor and resemble rampion *(Campanula rapunculs)* in taste (hence the common name "German rampion"). The seeds have also been used as a substitute for poppy seeds because of their similar appearance (Foster, 1995).

Native Americans used evening primrose as a poultice for bruises (Ojibway) and to take off weight (Cherokee). European medicinal use began in the eighteenth century. The leaves and roots were used externally by the Shakers to promote healing of wounds, and as the ingredients of a tea used to treat upset stomach (Foster, 1995).

Although the evening primrose plant does not produce a large amount of seeds when compared to other oilseed crops, it is preferred to other sources of γ-linolenic acid (GLA) because it is easy to produce and harbors little or no α-linolenic acid (Hudson, 1984). A crossbred commercial variety yields an oil with 72% *cis*-linoleic acid and 9% GLA (Liberti, 1983). The seeds are mainly produced in the United States, Europe, Israel, and New Zealand (Gunstone et al., 1986; Schweain, 1997).

CHEMISTRY

Lipid Compounds

Fats

Evening primrose oil (EPO) is of special interest because of its characteristically large amount of GLA (all *cis*- 6:9:12-octadecatrienoic acid, also designated 18:3-ω6), which is a precursor of prostaglandin E_1 (Hudson, 1984). Although borage seed oil contains higher amounts of GLA (see appendix), EPO is touted as having the most clinical significance, producing the most beneficial effects on the formation of GLA metabolites (Awang, 1990).

The fatty acids in EPO are reported by Hudson (1984) to be 65-80% linoleic and 7-14% of γ-linolenic, with no α-linolenic acid (ALA). However, Awang (1990) gives the profile as 5-6% palmitic, 1-2% stearic, 8-12% oleic, 70-79% linoleic, 0.1-0.4% α-linolenic, 8-12% γ-linolenic, and 1-1.5% >C20. Everett, Greenough et al. (1988) explain that the content of γ-linolenic acid in seeds of wild varieties widely varies, from 2-16% of total fatty acids. A commonly used proprietary product uses a strain of the seeds containing 70-73% linoleic acid and 8.5-9.0% γ-linolenic acid.

A note on nomenclature: a simple shorthand notation, often used to describe the different essential fatty acids, is important to understand when reviewing the research on EPO. The notation 18:2n-6 is linoleic acid, 18:3n-3 is α-linoleic acid, and 18:3n-6 is γ-linoleic acid. The first number (18) is the number of carbon atoms in the molecule, the second (after the colon) is the number of double bonds (unsaturations), and the last number (after the "n-")

identifies the series to which the fatty acid belongs: either ω6 (*n*-6) or ω3 (*n*-3) (Horrobin, 1990).

Other sources of EFAs are given in the appendix at the end of this chapter.

Other Constituents

Evening primrose seed contains approximately 15% protein, 24% oil, and 43% cellulose plus lignin (Hudson, 1984). The roots contain gallic acid, maslinic acid, oleanolic acid, tetramethylellagic acid, and 2, 7, 8-trimethylgallic acid (Shukla et al., 1999).

THERAPEUTIC APPLICATIONS

Deficiency in dietary EFAs has been shown in animal studies to cause eczemalike lesions, hair loss, poor immune function, poor connective tissue synthesis (demonstrated by poor wound healing), infertility (especially in males), fatty degeneration of the liver, renal lesions, lack of normal water balance, and degeneration of the exocrine glands (lacrimal, salivary). Illnesses that share similar symptoms suggest that EFA deficiency, either as a result of poor dietary intake or inability to metabolize sufficient amounts of EFAs, may cause many health problems. In theory, the GLA provided by EPO may be converted in the body to the prostaglandin precursor dihomo-GLA (DGLA) and be useful to people with either a metabolic inability to convert *cis*-linoleic acid to GLA, or with low dietary intake of *cis*-linoleic acid (Schweain, 1997). Although prostaglandins (PGs) and other metabolites of arachidonic acid are mediators of inflammation, some prostaglandins have also shown anti-inflammatory properties. It is believed that supplementation with EFAs may promote a more "healthy balance" of prostaglandins by increasing the levels of "good" prostaglandins and minimizing the "bad" (Jantti et al., 1985).

Factors thought to interfere with metabolism of ω-6 fatty acids are aging, diabetes, high alcohol intake, high fat diets, certain vitamin and mineral deficiencies (especially zinc, vitamin C, vitamin B6, and niacin), hormones, high cholesterol levels, and viral infections. The conversion process from linoleic acid (LA) to GLA is rate-limiting, with only a relatively small amount of dietary LA converted to GLA by Δ-6-desaturase (Schweain, 1997). It is thought that this enzyme is the rate-limiting step in linoleic acid metabolism, and may be inhibited by several factors, such as protein restriction, fasting, premedication, anesthesia, and several other nutritional or hormonal alterations involved with the stress reaction (Traitler et al., 1984).

PRECLINICAL STUDIES

Digestive, Hepatic, and Gastrointestinal Functions

Gastric Functions

EPO has been shown to prevent alcohol-induced gastric erosion in rats. The amount of prevention was shown to be similar to cyclic somatostatin (Diel, 1985). Compared to rats fed a standard rat chow supplemented with corn oil, rats on the same diet supplemented with EPO (10 mL/kg p.o.) showed significantly less gastric ulcer formation. EPO produced a significant inhibition of gastric ulcer formation against the effects of aspirin and phenylbutazone, and inhibition of intraluminal bleeding (Al-Shabanah, 1997).

Cardiovascular and Circulatory Functions

Cholesterol and Lipid Metabolism

The cholesterol-lowering effects of EPO have been studied in various animals. De La Cruz et al. (1997) found that rabbits on a high-cholesterol diet showed significant reduced levels of cholesterol when a high amount of EPO (15%) supplemented the diet. Total cholesterol was reduced by 25%, triglyceride levels were inhibited by 51%, while high density lipoprotein (HDL) cholesterol levels rose by 64%.

Fukushima et al. (1997) reported that in a 13-week feeding study, rats fed a cholesterol-enriched diet containing 10% EPO from a wild plant (14% GLA) or 10% EPO (Efamol, 9% GLA) showed significantly lower levels of serum total cholesterol, VLDL, IDL, and LDL than rats on the same diet supplemented with either palm oil, soybean oil (8% ALA and about 51% LA content), safflower oil (75% LA), or bio-GLA derived from mold (about 23% GLA). It was concluded that EPO inhibits increasing levels of cholesterol in a diet containing excess cholesterol.

As supplements in cholesterol-enriched diets administered to rats for six weeks, an equal amount of EPO (10% and 20%) produced lower levels of liver cholesterol than palm oil, soybean oil, sunflower oil, or high-oleic acid safflower oil. Serum levels of total cholesterol, very low density lipoprotein (VLDL), intermediate density lipoprotein (IDL), and low density lipoprotein (LDL) were also significantly lower in the EPO group compared to the other groups. Yet among the groups there were no significant differences in total bile acid and fecal neutral steroid concentrations. The EPO used in this study contained approximately 14% GLA and about 71% LA (Fukushima et al., 1997).

Hypertension

Engler (1993) reported that spontaneously hypertensive rats fed diets containing GLA-rich oils (EPO, borage, black current, sesame, and fungal oil) showed significant reductions in blood pressure (BP), despite great differences in the fatty acid composition of the various oils, and no significant differences in body weights. Engler noted that EPO showed the highest BP-lowering activity although the GLA content was the lowest among the oils tested.

Mills et al. (1989) found BP elevations in response to chronic social isolation stress ameliorated in rats fed a fat-free diet plus 10% of calories as EPO (Efamol). No increase in BP in the stressed rats on EPO was detected whereas increased BP was found in stressed rats that received fish oil, sunflower oil, or canola oil. The researchers found no significant change in the heart rate of stressed rats in the EPO group, yet significant increases were shown in the stressed rats receiving sunflower oil, fish oil, or canola oil. Urinary epinephrine and norepinephrine increases in the stressed rats were not found in those receiving either fish oil, canola oil, or EPO. These results suggest that the amelioration of increased BP in rats on EPO may have some relation to modulation of stress-induced catecholamine responses.

Immune Functions; Inflammation and Disease

Cancer

Chemopreventive activity. Animal studies have shown positive results from supplementation of EPO in the prevention of mammary adenocarcinoma. In one study, EPO (50-400 mL/day) inhibited R323OAC mammary adenocarcinoma in female rats, whereas pure γ-linolenic supplementation had no effect (Karmali et al., 1984, 1985).

In vitro studies have shown that with the addition of GLA cells reversed from a cancerous state to normal. In almost all cancer cells studied there is an intracellular deficiency of the Δ-6-desaturase enzyme. Hypothetically, the loss of this enzyme provides a block in the metabolism of linoleic acid through the $\omega 6$ fatty acid metabolism pathway, and this leads to abnormalities in thromboxane A_2 activity, disturbed calcium homeostasis, and decreased cyclic AMP synthesis (Booyens and Katzeff, 1983).

Immune Functions

Immunosuppression. In animal models, EFAs (*n*-6 EFAs) have been shown to suppress cell-mediated immune responses, including lymphocyte proliferation (Jeffery et al., 1996). This pharmacological activity has several applications, including that of organ transplantation (Mertin et al., 1985; Watson et al., 1988).

Metabolic and Nutritional Functions

Antioxidant Activity

An ethanolic extract of the aboveground parts of evening primrose (150 mg/L) produced a higher antioxidant activity than butylated hydroxy anisole (8 mg/L), as measured by the decoloration of a β-carotene emulsion. A synergistic action was observed from the addition of citric acid (Budincevic et al., 1995). In various models of antioxidant activity including the β-carotene assay, the freeze-dried, defatted seed prepared as a methanol/water (9:1) extract was comparable in potency to that of butylated hydroxy toluene (BHT) (Birch et al., 2001). Using the β-carotene assay, Shahidi et al. (1997) found strongest antioxidant activity from fractions of an ethanolic extract of EPO (Efamol) containing a high concentration of total phenolics. Rahbeeni et al. (2000) reported that normal cells of female mice administered EPO (10 μL/day p.o. by gavage) for two weeks prior to and four weeks after radiation treatment of tumors (rhabdomyosarcoma) showed reduced sensitivity to the treatment as evidenced by a reduction in moist desquamation. However, EPO treatment had no effect on the response of the tumor cells to radiation, nor did it alter the fatty acid content or blood flow of tumors.

Nutrient Utilization

Supplementation with EFAs, including EPO, has been shown to ameliorate zinc deficiency. Male rats subjected to a zinc-deficient diet and administered a daily supplement of safflower or olive oil (250 μL s.c.) developed postural defects, alopecia, keratosis, dermal lesions, and bleeding of the nose and paws. For the rats given a daily supplement of EPO (250 μL s.c.), growth was restored to half that of controls on a normal diet, postural abnormalities were absent, and they showed only a few dermal lesions (Cunnane and Horrobin, 1980). The gross effects of a deficiency of either zinc or dihomo-γ-linolenic acid are very similar in quality, suggesting a close physiologic relationship thought to be related to prostaglandin synthesis from the metabolism of essential fatty acids (Cunnane and Horrobin, 1980).

Performance Enhancement

Kaur and Kulkarni (1998) investigated the potential antifatigue effects of EPO in a study of albino mice using the forced swimming-induced immobility model to induce chronic fatigue. EPO was administered for 7 days, 30 min before each forced swimming (10 mL/kg p.o.). Compared to the untreated control group, results from the EPO group were highly significant ($p < 0.001$) and even superior to effects obtained from the administration of the antidepressant fluoxetine (10 mg/kg i.p.). The authors hypothesized that EPO may be useful in the treatment of chronic fatigue syndrome.

Respiratory and Pulmonary Functions

Allergies and Asthma

In a 21-week, double-blind, placebo-controlled, crossover study in 35 dogs, Scarff and Lloyd (1992) reported significant results from EPO as a dietary supplement (150 mg/kg b.i.d.) in the treatment of canine nonseasonal atopic dermatitis.

CLINICAL STUDIES

Cardiovascular and Circulatory Disorders

Effects on Cholesterol and Lipid Metabolism

Abraham et al. (1990) studied the effects of EPO supplementation (Efamol) on changes in serum lipids and fatty acid composition of adipose tissue in 29 apparently healthy men (ages 35-54), each of whom showed low levels of adipose tissue dihomo-γ-linolenic acid (DGLA). The double-blind, placebo-controlled trial examined the effects of EPO at 10, 20, or 30 mL/day. The study was prompted by the finding of a strong association between occult coronary heart disease and low levels of DGLA in adipose tissue. The results showed a highly significant increase of 2.2 kg mean body weight in the group receiving EPO at 30 mL/day, but not in the other groups. At 20 and 30 mL/day, EPO caused a significant increase in levels of adipose tissue DGLA whereas despite a high content of linoleic acid, safflower oil (placebo) had no effect.

Boberg et al. (1986) compared the lipid lowering effects of EPO (Efamol, 4 g/day) supplementation to a concentrated marine oil supplement rich in Omega-3 fatty acids (MaxEPA, 10 g/day) in patients diagnosed with hypertriglyceridemia. The 16-week, double-blind, placebo-controlled, crossover study involved 27 patients of both sexes (ages 39-71). Olive oil served as the placebo. All of the patients had been on a diet designed to lower lipid levels. No changes were found in body weight, blood pressure, serum insulin levels, or fasting blood glucose levels in either of the treatment groups. In the marine oil group, Boberg and colleagues found a significant decrease in triglyceride concentrations of 30%, whereas those receiving EPO showed no change of any significance. No significant change in platelet aggregation was found in either treatment group. The lack of lipid-lowering by EPO in the study may have resulted because the patients had already been adhering to a linoleic acid-rich diet, which may also have beneficially affected platelet aggregation rates.

Horrobin (1982) reviewed several clinical studies which measured the effect of EPO on plasma cholesterol levels. In studies using a mean daily dose of 3.8 g of EPO (Efamol), the majority of patients showed a decrease in serum cholesterol of 0.84 mmol/L or 30.4 mg/100 mL. The decrease in cholesterol levels produced by EPO was calculated to be 163 times greater than that produced by LA, without decreasing the amount of saturated fats in the diet (Horrobin, 1982).

Raynaud's syndrome. Due to the reported success of using vasodilating antiplatelet prostaglandins, prostaglandin E_1 (PGE_1) and prostacyclin (PGI_2) in the treatment of Raynaud's Phenomenon (RP), EPO was tested in 21 patients with Raynaud's syndrome (RS). For eight weeks, 11 received EPO and ten received placebo. Six of the 11 RS patients claimed a definite benefit from the treatment, two others felt moderate improvement in symptoms, and three experienced no benefit at all (Belch et al., 1985).

Endocrine and Hormonal Disorders

Diabetes

In a preliminary, double-blind, randomized, placebo-controlled study, 22 patients with diabetic neuropathy were given either EPO (Efamol, 4 g/day p.o. in 500 mg capsules) or placebo for 6 months. The parameters measured included nerve conduction and thermal thresholds in all measured variables. Significant improvements were found compared to placebo in motor nerve conduction and sensory nerve action potentials, whereas symptoms in the placebo group worsened; however, while significant improvements were found in the heat threshold values of ankle measurements, no significant difference compared to placebo was evident in wrist measurements of cold thresholds (Jamal et al., 1986).

A randomized, double-blind, placebo-controlled trial of EPO (EF4, identical to Epogam) in 111 patients with mild diabetic neuropathy ran for a full year. Patients received an identical appearing and tasting placebo (liquid paraffin) or the EPO at a dosage of six capsules twice daily, providing 480 mg/day of GLA. Before the end of the 12-month treatment period, 84 patients remained. Among those who dropped out due to adverse effects, the only treatment-related cases were two in each group who experienced nausea or vomiting. The results showed that in 5/6 neurological assessments and in 8/10 neurophysiological assessments, the improvements in the EPO group were superior to placebo. In 13 of these assessments, the results were significantly better than placebo, including: muscle strength of the arms, tendon reflexes of the arms and legs, sensation in the arms and legs, cold threshold of the wrists, and heat threshold of the ankles. The EPO was also well-tolerated and no clinically adverse events were found that could be attributed to the active treatment (Keen et al., 1993).

Immune Disorders; Inflammation and Disease

Cancer

Cancer treatment. EPO was given to six patients suffering from histologically diagnosed primary liver cell cancer. Half showed clinical improvement and reduction in tumor size (Booyens et al., 1984). Van der Merwe et al. (1987) reported various apparent benefits of oral EPO (Efamol G, 9-18 g/day) in 21 cancer patients with untreatable malignancies (hepatocellular carcinoma, malignant mesothelioma, cerebral astrocytoma, breast adenocarcinoma, renal clear cell carcinoma, cerebellar epdendymoma, esophageal adenocarcinoma, bronchogenic carcinoma, and gastric adenocarcinoma). The case reports gave indications of subjective improvements in the majority of patients and in many cases there were objective signs of improvements, including measured tumor mass reductions and X-ray evidence. These effects appeared to be due to γ-linolenic acid rather than LA, and more double-blind clinical trials to evaluate the treatment further should be conducted (Van der Merwe et al., 1987).

Kenny et al. (2000) conducted a study on the effects of GLA in 38 elderly breast cancer patients aged over 70 who were administered tamoxifen plus GLA (2.8 g/day in eight capsules) compared to matched controls (*n* = 47) receiving tamoxifen (20 mg/day) alone. The patients were diagnosed with stage I-II breast cancer. Response to treatment was achieved significantly sooner in the GLA plus tamoxifen group compared to those treated with tamoxifen alone (*p* = 0.010). GLA was well-tolerated (without major side effects requiring cessation of treatment), and while the expression of estrogen receptor of tumors at the six-week and six-month biopsy was significantly reduced in both treatment groups, those receiving GLA plus tamoxifen showed a greater reduction at both times (*p* = 0.026 and *p* = 0.019, respectively). Although further studies of GLA in the treatment of breast cancer are required, in the treatment of endocrine-sensitive breast cancer, it serves as a useful adjunct to the main treatment with tamoxifen. Despite the high dose of GLA, the most common side effect was a loose stool (*n* = 13).

Immune Disorders

Autoimmune disorders. Hansen et al. (1983) conducted a study involving administration of Efamol and Efavit or placebo in 20 patients with active rheumatoid arthritis. A 12-week treatment showed no clinical significance. However, Leventhal et al. (1993), using 1.4 g/day of γ-linolenic acid supplied in borage seed oil, reported good results in a 24-week, randomized, double-blind, placebo-controlled trial in 37 patients diagnosed with rheumatoid arthritis. In the active treatment group, scores were reduced for swollen joints by 41% and for tender joints by 45%, while their number was reduced by 36%. The clinical improvement compared to placebo was overall significantly greater in the patients administered γ-linolenic acid ($p < 0.05$), whereas the placebo group showed no improvement or a worsening of their symptoms.

Sjögren's syndrome involves dry eyes with diminished or absent tear and salivary secretion, rheumatoid arthritis, and positive RA factor. Manthorpe et al. (1984) examined the effect of Efamol (1,500 mg twice daily) versus placebo in 36 patients with Sjögren's syndrome in a randomized, double-blind, crossover, placebo-controlled study. The Schirmer-I-test showed significant improvement, while measurements of break up time, van Bijsterveld score, cornea sensitivity, tear-lysozyme and nuclear chromatin in conjunctival epithelial cells failed to reach clinical significance. However, the researchers concluded that the only treatments available for Sjögren's syndrome that were better than placebo were bromhexine and Efamol (Manthorpe et al., 1984).

Immune Modulation

Cellular Immune Response

The effect of a moderate dose of GLA on the cellular immune function of healthy Caucasian volunteers ($n = 46$) aged 55-71 years was examined in a randomized, placebo-controlled, double-blind, parallel study. An oil blend providing GLA or placebo was administered at a dosage of 700 mg/day in capsules, three taken before each of three daily meals for 12 weeks. The results showed that after 12 weeks the only noticeable effect on the cellular immune system from the moderate dosage of GLA in these volunteers was a decrease in lymphocytes proliferation; the mean decrease was up to 61% which was significantly lower than baseline and compared to placebo. At week 16 after a four-week washout, the increase in the stimulation index was still not as high as baseline values (Thies et al., 2001).

Integumentary, Muscular, and Skeletal Disorders

Dermatitis

A parallel, double-blind, placebo-controlled trial of EPO (Epogam) in the treatment of hand dermatitis was conducted with 39 outpatients, all diagnosed with chronic dermatitis (greater than one year in duration), but otherwise in good health. The active treatment group ($n = 20$) received EPO at a dosage of 12 × 500 mg capsules/day and were provided GLA 600 mg/day for 16 weeks. Administered at the same dosage, the placebo group ($n = 19$) received capsules containing 500 mg of sunflower oil. Patient evaluations were conducted during an eight-week washout period after the treatment period. Topical steroid cream was allowed in limited, monitored amounts and then only in the form of a semipotent group III formulation. The use of emollients was not restricted. Improvements compared to baseline showed no significant differences in the EPO group compared to the placebo group, although both groups showed statistically significant improvements compared to baseline in cracking, dryness, itch, edema, redness, and vesiculation (Whitaker et al., 1996). Similar results were reported by Hederos and Berg (1996) in a double-blind, placebo-controlled parallel group study of EPO (Epogam) in the treatment of eczema in children diagnosed with atopic dermatitis and asthma.

Muscular Disorders

Charcot-Marie-Tooth disease (CMT) is a hereditary neuropathy characterized by abnormal peripheral myelination in which the muscles of the feet deteriorate. A trial involving 18 patients with CMT was conducted to test the observation that CMT patients may have defective or unbalanced fatty acid metabolism. A three-month period in which placebo and vitamin E was given was followed by one year of supplementation with vitamin E and EFAs (Efamol). The altered serum and nerve phospholipid levels after the one year trial suggested a defect in EFA metabolism, but administration of EFAs did not reverse the deficiency. After the placebo period in which vitamin E was also given, a significant increase in neuropsychological tests and improvements in strength, sensation, and total disability scores was noted. It was postulated that vitamin E may have caused these effects through membrane stabilization (Williams et al., 1986).

Respiratory and Pulmonary Disorders

Allergies and Asthma

A preliminary randomized double-blind, crossover trial in 1981 indicated benefits from EPO in children (1 g twice daily) and adults (2 g twice daily) with atopic eczema (Lovell et al., 1981). Since then, a number of trials conducted in Europe on the benefits of EPO in atopic eczema have largely reported positive results. The basis for these trials was a noted dysfunction in atopic eczema patients of the Δ-6-desaturase enzyme which was proposed to be a major factor in the disease since the fatty acid profile of patients with the disease showed lower plasma levels of GLA, arachidonic acid (AA), and DGLA, along with a higher than normal *cis*-linolenic acid level (Kerscher and Korting, 1992). By 1989, four controlled trials using a parallel design found that patients treated with EPO showed highly significant improvements, including less scaling, dryness, inflammation, and severity of overall symptoms; however, five trials using a crossover design showed no improvements other than less itchy skin (Morse et al., 1989). Nonetheless, when measurements of plasma phospholipid profiles were conducted, a positive correlation was found between the improvement of eczema and increased levels of AA and DGLA (Kerscher and Korting, 1992).

Biagi et al. (1994) examined the effect of EPO (Epogam, Serle, United Kingdom) in children diagnosed with abnormal IgE-mediated immunological responses and on atopic dermatitis. The randomized, double-blind, placebo-controlled trial in 48 children (ages 2.2-8.5 years) employed a placebo made of olive oil (490 mg) and vitamin E (10 mg) (500 mg/kg per day), which was compared to results obtained from a low-dose mixed treatment of 50% placebo and 50% EPO capsules, and a high-dose single treatment of EPO (500 mg/kg per day). One group of the children were nonallergic patients ($n = 25$). For a 15 kg child, this amounted to taking 15×500 mg capsules/day. After an eight-week treatment period, the results showed that compared to placebo, the low-dose group was little improved ($p < 0.077$), while the high-dose group showed clear improvements ($p < 0.046$). Compared to the other groups, the high-dose group showed significant elevations in erythrocyte membrane $\omega 6$ fatty acids, and in the $\omega 6/\omega 3$ ratio. This was the only group that showed a significant increase in DGLA, a precursor of anti-inflammatory prostaglandins. However, microviscosity of the erythrocytes showed no evidence of change in any of the groups and no adverse events were found.

Schalin-Karrila et al. (1987) conducted a 12-week, randomized, double-blind, placebo-controlled trial in 25 atopic eczema patients (ages 19-31, both sexes) who were allowed to use topical steroid creams as needed. The patients who received EPO (Efamol, 2 g twice daily) showed significant improvements in skin dryness, itchiness, inflammation grade, amount of the total skin area affected with eczema (reduced by 30-50%), and in the overall severity of their symptoms compared to placebo (liquid paraffin). Patients in the EPO group who continued to use topical steroid creams during the trial used 60% less. The DGLA level in the EPO group showed a significant increase, becoming significantly greater than that of healthy individuals by the end of the trial. However, EPO caused no change in levels of arachidonic acid, plasma concentrations of prostaglandin E_1, 6-keto-prostaglandin $F_{1\alpha}$, or thromboxane B_2 (TXB_2), and the quantity of TXB_2 released during clotting (Schalin-Karrila et al., 1987).

In Italy, Bordoni et al. (1987) studied the effects of EPO (Efamol) in 24 young children (ages two to four, both sexes) with atopic eczema in a randomized, double-blind, placebo-controlled, parallel trial. The placebo (olive oil) or EPO were taken orally by the children in a dosage of 3 g/day (six capsules/day) for four weeks. The only concurrent medications were continuing treatment with weak topical steroids and emollients. The results of EPO treatment were significant compared to placebo ($p < 0.01$). Both groups showed a significant increase in plasma arachidonic acid compared to baseline, with a more significant increase in the EPO group ($p < 0.01$). Compared to the placebo group, and to their baseline reading, the EPO group also showed results consistent with the theory of an EFA-desaturation defect in this disease: a significant decrease in the plasma ratio of linoleic acid:arachidonic acid (18:2/20:4), and a significant increase in DGLA (20:3 *n*-6). The researchers surmised that the superior results of their trial compared to others may have been due to the higher dosage of EPO used, or to the fact that the Italian diet is known to provide lower concentrations of saturated fat, or to both factors.

A placebo-controlled, randomized crossover study was conducted to assess the therapeutic effect of EPO versus placebo in 50 patients with atopic dermatitis. After 24 weeks, the therapeutic benefit judged by both patients and physicians was found to be independently significant (Wright and Burton, 1982). Manku and Horrobin (1982) analyzed the plasma of the 50 patients being concurrently studied by Wright and Burton (1982). The biochemical findings indicated a defect in the Δ-6-desaturase enzyme in the atopic patients. They also confirmed the clinical observations made by Wright and Burton (1982).

Neurological, Psychological, and Behavioral Disorders

Psychological and Behavioral Disorders

Alcoholism and chemical dependence. A preliminary trial on the effect of EPO or placebo was conducted in 24 patients hospitalized for alcohol withdrawal syndrome. Although the numbers of patients involved were small, it appeared that Efamol reduced the symptoms of tenseness and the need for diazepam (Glen et al., 1987).

Attention deficit hyperactivity disorder. A number of case studies were detailed on hyperactive children given Efamol and Efavit. Among the observed improvements in their health and hyperactivity were attention span, self-confidence, eczema, and abnormal sleeping patterns (Colquhoun and Bunday, 1981). However, a randomized, double-blind, placebo-controlled, crossover trial with over 90 hyperkinetic children ages 5-15 administered EPO as a supplement found no change in general behavior, obedience, or restlessness from EPO versus placebo (safflower oil) (Gibson, 1985).

Pharmacokinetics

In a study of 39 breast-feeding women, an EPO supplement (Efamol, 2 capsules 2 times/day 3 days prior to expected menstrual period) or placebo was administered for 8 months starting between the second and sixth month of lactation. Total fat and EFA contents of the milk declined in the placebo group but rose in the group receiving EPO (Cant et al., 1991).

Reproductive Disorders

Mastalgia

A survey of differential responses to drug therapy for mastalgia in 291 patients was conducted using danazol, bromocriptine, and EPO. Beneficial responses to drug therapy were found in 70% of women with cyclical mastalgia using danazol, 47% using bromocriptine, and 45% using EPO. In patients with noncyclical mastalgia, the respective percentages of treatment success were 31%, 20%, and 27%. The use of EPO to treat mastalgia was well-accepted by patients due to the lack of side effects (2%) and the reluctance to use other, hormonally oriented drugs. Drawbacks were relapse rate, which had not been tested, and the cost of treatment (Pye et al., 1985).

Pashby et al. (1981) conducted a randomized, double-blind, crossover study examining the effect of EPO or placebo in 73 patients with cyclic or noncyclic mastalgia. After three months, pain and tenderness were significantly decreased in the active treatment group. The use of EPO may help to reduce breast pain and tenderness in both types of mastalgia patients, especially in the noncyclical form, and may be useful as a first line of therapy for mastalgia.

Menstrual Disorders

Premenstrual syndrome. In 1994, a critical review of clinical studies on EPO against PMS (or premenstrual dysphoric disorder) concluded that while several studies showed benefits, a preponderance of well-designed clinical trials showed no benefits at all compared to placebo (Williams and Casper, 1994). Similar conclusions were arrived at by Budeiri et al. (1996) who found that a lack of consistent scoring and consistent response criteria precluded a meta-analysis. On the basis of current evidence however, Budeiri et al. (1996) concluded that EPO is of "little if any value in PMS" and that larger studies are needed to uncover what small effects there may be (p. 67).

Cotterell et al. (1990) conducted a double-blind, placebo-controlled, randomized, crossover design trial on EPO (Efamol, 500 mg/day) in 40 women diagnosed with food-intolerant irritable bowel syndrome. The subjects experienced the symptoms of IBS only just before and during the first few days of the menstrual period. The treatment was followed for three cycles with a washout period at the fourth cycle. The placebo was encapsulated olive oil (500 mg/day). Of those in the active group ($n = 19$), 53% reported an improvement in symptoms in one of the phases, whereas no improvement was noted from the placebo group ($n = 17$). Improvement was seen in most cases in the second month of EPO, and in some no improvement was apparent until the third and last month of EPO administration. Through blood analysis, fatty acid abnormalities detected at the beginning of treatment were found to have significantly improved in the EPO group (Cotterell et al., 1990).

DOSAGE

The dosage of EPO depends on the condition in question. Based on an EPO product standardized to contain 8% GLA in the treatment of mastalgia, the recommended dose is 3-4 g/day. In the treatment of atopic eczema the recommended daily dosage is 2-4 g/day for children and 6-8 g/day for adults (Newall et al., 1996). In most of the studies performed with EPO to date, the dose used was 3-6 g/day containing at least 9% γ-linolenic acid (Horrobin, 1992). The highest dose normally recommended for humans is approximately 0.25 mL/kg/day (Everett, Greenough et al., 1988).

SAFETY PROFILE

In clinical studies involving some 4,000 patients, no side effects have been reported that were significantly greater than those from placebo (Kruger et al., 1998).

The endogenous production of GLA in the normal adult is estimated to be about 2-20 mg/kg per day, and the daily intake of a breast-fed human infant is estimated at 20-80 mg/kg per day. In consideration of the toxicology studies, and these estimates, it has been termed "unlikely" that doses of less than 100 mg/kg per day would produce any toxicity. In addition, about 500,000 prescriptions of one-month supplies of EPO have been dispensed in the United Kingdom by the National Health Service for the treatment of atopic eczema or breast pain. Reports of adverse drug reactions have been far lower than for most drugs, and there appears to be no pattern of side effects related to GLA consumption (Horrobin, 1992).

Contraindications

EPO is cautioned against in schizophrenics and patients receiving phenothiazines and other epileptogenic drugs since it has the potential to render apparent previously undiagnosed temporal lobe epilepsy (Newall et al., 1996).

Drug Interactions

No drug interactions are known.

Shuster (1996) reported a case of nocturnal seizures in a 45-year-old woman after she took EPO in addition to separate bottled herbal products of black cohosh and vitex *(Vitex agnus-castus)* for about four months. The seizures appeared to be of the general tonic-clonic type and ceased upon her discontinuation of the herbs (Shuster, 1996).

Pregnancy and Lactation

Midwives have been known to use EPO to hasten ripening of the cervix to shorten labor time and to lessen the likelihood of postdate pregnancies. However, research suggests that EPO neither shortens gestation nor causes the length of labor to decrease. Dove and Johnson (1999) conducted a two-group retrospective study comparing the effect of EPO in 54 women who had used EPO orally during their first pregnancy to 54 women who had taken none. A reference control group consisted of women previously registered for care at a birthing center and all three groups were well-matched according to extensive criteria. The dosage of EPO prescribed was 500 mg t.i.d. for one week starting at 37 weeks gestation, and then 500 mg/day to the time of labor. A valid analysis of variance for length of labor could not be conducted as the test assumption of equal group variance was not met. The control groups showed a greater variation in the five-minute Apgar score compared to the EPO group ($p = 0.007$) while the EPO group showed a greater variance in length of labor. In a descriptive analysis, compared to the control groups, women in the EPO group showed a significantly greater variation in the length of labor ($p = 0.002$), a 9% greater risk of a protracted active phase of labor. Labor time in the EPO group lasted an average of three hours longer than the control group. The EPO group also showed a tendency for prolonged membrane rupture time, arrest of descent, and a need for oxytocin augmentation. Birth weights were somewhat larger in the EPO group (by 156 g on average), although this probably had little effect on the outcomes of the study. Dove and Johnson (1999) conclude that despite the limitations of the study, EPO showed no benefit in terms of decreasing the overall length of labor or in lessening adverse outcomes of labor. They called for larger studies of EPO on pregnancy and of topical use of the oil administered a few weeks before delivery.

Evidence suggests that EPO supplementation can aid in preventing mastalgia (Pashby et al., 1981; Pye et al., 1985). However, these studies were done with nonlactating women suffering breast tenderness specifically related to the menstrual cycle (the term mastalgia is rarely encountered in lactation literature). As breast pain can have many causes in breast-feeding women, these findings cannot be used to indicate a role for EPO specifically during lactation. Successful use of EPO to relieve menstrual cycle-related breast pain in breast-feeding women has been informally reported (personal communication, Humphrey, 2001). Maternal EPO supplementation during breast-feeding can raise the essential fatty acid content of breast milk (Cant et al., 1991). The nutritional necessity of routine supplementation of essential fatty acids or their metabolites during lactation has not been established. On the other hand, there are no cases of adverse reactions to EPO supplementation during lactation (personal communication, Humphrey, 2001). The *American Herbal Products Association's Botanical Safety Handbook* (McGuffin et al., 1997) lists no contraindication during lactation.

Side Effects

None known (Burnham, 1997).

Special Precautions

In women who were previously obese, a dosage of 2 g/day of GLA was found to increase their serum phospholipid content of arachidonate. Since research has shown that a build up of tissue arachidonate might lead to the promotion of immunosuppression, inflammation, and thrombosis, Phinney (1994) cautions that patients and physicians should become alert to this possibility; advice considered prudent in the case of long-term GLA supplementation. However, several patients with synovitis are reported to have experienced a worsening of symptoms following withdrawal of GLA supplementation (Phinney, 1994).

Toxicology

Toxicity in Animal Models

Results in a chronic toxicity study of Efamol EPO ($\geq$ 2.5 mL/kg per day by gavage for 53 weeks) in male and female Sprague-Dawley rats ($n = 100$ of each sex) were compared to controls administered the same dosages of corn oil with vitamin E (2.7% by volume) added to equal the amount found in Efamol and an untreated control group. Female rats in two of the EPO groups (0.3 and 2.5 mL/kg per day) showed a marginal increase in potassium levels compared to controls ($p < 0.05$), and male rats in the 2.5 mL/kg per day group showed a higher incidence of testicular softening or shrinkage ($n = 6/25$) compared to controls ($n = 2/25$). Otherwise, the results showed no significant differences that could be attributed to EPO compared to controls whether in histopathology of major and minor organs, hematology, urinalysis, ophthalmological examination, or clinical chemistry. With the exception of changes in potassium levels and testicular changes, the same results were found in beagle dogs administered Efamol EPO ($\geq$ 5.0 mL/kg per day p.o. for 52 weeks) compared to corn oil plus the added vitamin E. The researchers concluded that Efamol EPO in amounts higher than those likely to be taken as a dietary supplement by humans are just as safe as corn oil (Everett, Greenough et al., 1988).

A study in rats fed a diet supplemented with EPO (Efamol) as 3% of caloric intake found no significant difference between control animals on normal feed alone, either in litter size, survival of litters, birth weight and postnatal growth rate of litters, or prostaglandin E_2 concentrations of the fetal membrane, placenta, or uterine wall (Leaver et al., 1986).

Efamol EPO was examined for carcinogenic effects in a study involving 500 Sprague-Dawley rats of either sex. For a period of 104 weeks, the rats were fed a normal diet and either EPO (≥ 2.5 mL/kg per day by gavage), corn oil (2.5 mL/kg per day by gavage) with vitamin E added in the amount found in the Efamol EPO (2.7% by volume), or no dietary supplement. The same conditions and treatment were administered to 500 CD-1 mice of either sex for 78 weeks. The results showed no significant differences in tumor incidence in animals receiving the oils versus untreated controls. Although there was a tendency towards fewer tumors in the male animals treated with the oils, it failed to reach statistical significance. Also, no adverse effects were found that could be attributed to Efamol EPO (Everett, Perry et al., 1988).

APPENDIX: ADDITIONAL INFORMATION ON EFAS

TABLE 1. Other Sources of EFAs

Sources of EFAs		% Essential Fatty Acids		
Family	Species	γ-linolenic (GLA)	α-linolenic (ALA)	linoleic (LA)
Boraginaceae	*Adelocaryum coelestinum*	12.41[1]	4.71[1]	14.11[1]
Boraginaceae	*Alkanna froedinii*	9.9[1]	27.1[1]	26.3[1]
Boraginaceae	*Alkanna orientalis*	12.4[1]	31.7[1]	26.1[1]
Boraginaceae	*Amsinckia intermedia*	8.2[1]	17.4[1]	13.3[1]
Boraginaceae	*Amsinckia lunaris*	8.9[1]	12.2[1]	13.4[1]
Boraginaceae	*Anchusa strigosa*	7.4[1]	trace[1]	38.0[1]
Boraginaceae	*Borago officinalis* (borage)	20-26[2]	0.1-2[2]	34-39[2]
Boraginaceae	*Brunnera orientalis*	15.4[1]	8.8[1]	27.1[1]
Boraginaceae	*Cryptantha grayi*	6.2[1]	33.8[1]	21.4[1]
Boraginaceae	*Cynoglossum nervosum*	7.8[1]	7.0[1]	21.7[1]
Boraginaceae	*Ecbium glomeratum*	6.6[1]	44.6[1]	15.3[1]

Sources of EFAs		% Essential Fatty Acids		
Family	Species	γ-linolenic (GLA)	α-linolenic (ALA)	linoleic (LA)
Boraginaceae	*Hackelia floribunda*	6.4[1]	13.8[1]	15.5[1]
Boraginaceae	*Nonnea macrosperma*	13.1[1]	9.0[1]	34.4[1]
Boraginaceae	*Pectocarya platycarpa*	15.2[1]	19.9[1]	17.9[1]
Boraginaceae	*Trichodesma zeylanicum*	4.3[1]	24.3[1]	20.5[1]
Cannabaceae	*Humulus lupulus* (hops seed)	0.34[3]	No data found	No data found
Cannabaceae	*Cannabis sativa* (hemp seed)	1-6[4]	15-25[4]	50-70[4]
Onagraceae	*Oenothera agrillicolla*	6.7[1]	0.1[1]	69.4[1]
Onagraceae	*O. biennis* (evening primrose)	8-12[2]	0.1-0.4[2]	70-79[2]
Onagraceae	*O. brevipes*	0	0.1[1]	78.2[1]
Onagraceae	*O. cardiophylla*	0	0.2[1]	77.7[1]
Onagraceae	*O. clavaeformis*	0	0.1[1]	84.1[1]
Onagraceae	*O. depressa*	6.3[1]	0.2[1]	69.8[1]
Onagraceae	*O. drummondii*	0.5[1]	No data found	76.2[1]
Onagraceae	*O. elata*	6.7[1]	0.4[1]	73.3[1]
Onagraceae	*O. grandiflora*	9.3[1]	0.2[1]	67.4[1]
Onagraceae	*O. hookeri*	7.0[1]	0.2[1]	74.0[1]
Onagraceae	*O. laciniata*	3.9[1]	0.1[1]	77.4[1]
Onagraceae	*O. lamarckiana*	8.2[1]	0.2[1]	62.2[1]
Onagraceae	*O. leptocarpa*	0	0.4[1]	82.8[1]
Onagraceae	*O. missouriensis*	0	0.2[1]	71.5[1]
Onagraceae	*O. odorata*	1.7[1]	0.1[1]	70.5[1]
Onagraceae	*O. parviflora*	7.1[1]	0.3[1]	70.9[1]
Onagraceae	*O. rhombipetala*	6.1[1]	0.1[1]	75.0[1]
Onagraceae	*O. rosea*	0	0.4[1]	77.9[1]

TABLE 1 *(continued)*

Sources of EFAs		% Essential Fatty Acids		
Family	Species	γ-linolenic (GLA)	α-linolenic (ALA)	linoleic (LA)
Onagraceae	*O. serrulata*	1.2[1]	0.2[1]	68.3[1]
Onagraceae	*O. stricta*	1.9[1]	0.3[1]	75.8[1]
Onagraceae	*O. strigosa*	7.0[1]	0.2[1]	72.6[1]
Onagraceae	*O. tetragona*	5.9[1]	0.3[1]	73.9[1]
Scrophulariaceae	*Scrophularia canina*	4.5[1]	trace[1]	55.9[1]
Scrophulariaceae	*S. grayana*	3.8[1]	0.5[1]	71.0[1]
Scrophulariaceae	*S. koraiensis*	3.7[1]	0.1[1]	70.5[1]
Scrophulariaceae	*S. lanceolata*	8.0[1]	0.5[1]	66.0[1]
Scrophulariaceae	*S. marilandica*	9.6[1]	0.6[1]	62.6[1]
Scrophulariaceae	*S. michoniana*	3.5[1]		55.8[1]
Saxifragaceae	*Ribes alpinum*	8.9[1]	22.0[1]	39.0[1]
Saxifragaceae	*R. inebrians*	3.4[1]	26.4[1]	40.4[1]
Saxifragaceae	*R. montigenum*	3.7[1]	28.9[1]	32.5[1]
Saxifragaceae	*R. nigrum*	14-19[2]	12-15[2]	45-50[2]
Saxifragaceae	*R. orientale*	1.9[1]	19.6[1]	49.1[1]
Saxifragaceae	*R. rubrum* (red currant seeds)	4-63	No data found	No data found
Saxifragaceae	*R. uva crispa* (gooseberry seeds)	10-12[3]	No data found	No data found

Sources: (1) Wolf et al., 1983; (2) Awang, 1990; (3) Traitler et al., 1984; (4) Deferne and Pate, 1996.

Note: Of the species surveyed by Wolf et al. (1983), five *(Alkanna froedinii, Alkanna orientalis, Adelocryum coelestinum, Brunnera orientalis,* and *Nonnea macrosperma)* were found to be richer sources of GLA than evening primrose. One example is *Nonnea macrosperma* seeds, which contain 38.6% oil comprised of 13.1% GLA, which represents a total of 5.1% of the seed. In addition, many members of the Boraginaceae and *Ribes* species also contain large amounts of octadecatetraenoic acid (a metabolite of Omega-3 EFA metabolism).

TABLE 2. Major Physiological Effects of Certain Essential Fatty Acids*

EFA common name	Chemical Notation**	Function
General fatty acids Omega-6	n-6	According to Horrobin, the n-6 EFAs have at least four roles: "a. modulation of membrane structure; b. the formation of short-lived local regulating molecules such as prostaglandins (PGs) and leukotrienes (LT); c. the control of the water impermeability of the skin and possibly the permeability of other membranes such as the gastrointestinal tract and the blood-brain barrier; d. the regulation of cholesterol transport and cholesterol synthesis."[2]
Linoleic acid (LA)	18:2n-6	This fatty acid requires conversion by Delta-6-desaturase enzyme in order to exert its full range of biological activity.[1] Increased LA intake may result in lowered plasma cholesterol levels.[3]
Gamma-linolenic acid (GLA)	18:3n-6	GLA may reduce the development of atherosclerosis and its sequelae,[1] reduces tumor cell growth and viability (may have potential for future cancer therapy),[1] may be able to reduce the effects of alcohol withdrawal symptoms,[1] may protect the liver from alcohol damage,[1] may be of benefit in PMS,[1] may be able to improve tear production in sicca and Sjögren's syndromes,[1] and may be beneficial to the conditions and complications of diabetes, obesity, schizophrenia, and some other psychiatric disorders.[1]
Dihomo-gamma-linolenic acid (DGLA)	20:3n-6	DGLA is the precursor of the 1 series prostaglandins, which play many "beneficial" roles in the body, especially in preventing cardiovascular disease since it inhibits platelet aggregation.[4] DGLA may reduce the development of atherosclerosis and its sequelae,[1] it may be able to reduce the effects of alcohol withdrawal symptoms,[1] and it may be of benefit in PMS.[1]
Arachidonic acid (AA)	20:4n-6	AA is the precursor of the 2 series prostaglandins, also called the "bad" prostaglandins because they promote platelet aggregation; therefore, high amounts of AA may lead to hardening of the arteries, heart disease, and strokes.[4] AA reduces tumor cell growth and viability, may have potential in future cancer therapy,[1] and may protect the liver from alcohol damage.[1]
General fatty acids Omega-3	n-3	Although the Omega-3 oils play important biological roles, Horrobin (1992) contends that they are not as important as the Omega-6 oils. One reason for this belief is that it has been difficult to demonstrate biological "deficiency" due to only the omega-3 oils. It seems that the Omega-3 oils are preferentially metabolized in the body.[2]

TABLE 2 *(continued)*

EFA common name	Chemical Notation**	Function
Alpha-linolenic (ALA)	18:3n-3	ALA requires conversion by Delta-6-desaturase enzyme in order to exert its full range of biological activity.[1]
Eicosapentaenoic (EPA)	20:5n-3	EPS is the precursor for the 3 series prostaglandins, also called the "good" prostaglandins because both 1 and 3 series inhibit platelet aggregation.[4]
Docosahexaenoic (DHA)	22:6n-3	DHA reduces tumor cell growth and viability, however weakly.[1]

Sources: (1) Willis and Smith, 1989; (2) Horrobin, 1992; (3) Horrobin, 1982; (4) Horrobin, 1980.

*Absolute amounts or administration of the essential fatty acids may be poor ways of understanding the physiological effects of EFAs. The ratios of intake, or total "EFA pool" in the body may be more relevant to the amounts and types of prostaglandins formed and the overall therapeutic effects of EFA administration and synthesis.[4]

**See note in "Chemistry" section for explanation of the chemical notation of essential fatty acids.

REFERENCES

Abraham, R.D., Riemersma, R.A., Elton, R.A., Macintyre, C., and Oliver, M.F. (1990). Effects of safflower oil and evening primrose oil in men with a low dihomo-γ-linolenic level. *Atherosclerosis* 81: 199-208.

Al-Shabanah, O.A. (1997). Effect of evening primrose oil on gastric ulceration and secretion induced by various ulcerogenic and necrotizing agents in rats. *Food and Chemical Toxicology* 35: 769-775.

Awang, D.V.C. (1990). Herbal medicine: Borage. *Canadian Pharmaceutical Journal* 123: 121-126.

Belch, J.J., Shaw, B., O'Dowd, A., Saniabadi, A., Leiberman, P., Sturrock, R.D., and Forbes, C.D. (1985). Evening primrose oil (Efamol) in the treatment of Raynaud's phenomenon: A double blind study. *Thrombosis and Haemostasis* 54(2):490-494.

Biagi, P.L., Bordoni, A., Hrelia, S., Celadon, M., Ricci, G.P., Cannella, V., Patrizi, A., Specchia, F., and Masi, M. (1994). The effect of gamma-linolenic acid on clinical status, red cell fatty acid composition and membrane microviscosity in infants with atopic dermatitis. *Drugs in Experimental and Clinical Research* 20: 77-84.

Birch, A.E., Fenner, G.P., Watkins, R., and Boyd, L.C. (2001). Antioxidant properties of evening primrose seed extracts. *Journal of Agricultural and Food Chemistry* 49: 4502-4507.

Boberg, M., Vessby, B., and Selinus, I. (1986). Effects of dietary supplementation with *n*-6 and *n*-3 long-chain polyunsaturated fatty acids on serum lipoproteins and platelet function in hypertriglyceridaemic patients. *Acta Medica Scandinavica* 220: 153-160.

Booyens, J., Engelbrecht, P., Roux, S., Louwrens, C.C., Van der Merwe, C.F., and Katzeff, I.E. (1984). Some effects of the essential fatty acids linoleic acid and Alpha-linolenic acid and of their metabolites Gamma-linolenic acid, arachidonic acid, eicosapentaenoic acid, docosahexaenoic acid and of prostaglandins A_1 and E_1 on the proliferation of human osteogenic sarcoma cells in culture. *Prostaglandins, Leukotrienes and Medicine* 15: 15-33.

Booyens, J. and Katzeff, I.E. (1983). Cancer: A simple metabolic disease? *Medical Hypotheses* 12: 195-201.

Bordoni, A., Biagi, B.L., Massi, M., Ricci, G., Fanelli, C., Patrizi, A., and Ceccolini, E. (1987). Evening primrose oil (Efamol) in the treatment of children with atopic eczema. *Drugs in Experimental and Clinical Research* 14: 291-297.

Budeiri, D., Po, A.L.W., and Doran, J.C. (1996). Is evening primrose oil of value in the treatment of premenstrual syndrome? *Controlled Clinical Trials* 17: 60-68.

Budincevic, M., Vrbaski, Z., Turkulov, J., and Dimic, E. (1995). Antioxidant activity of *Oenothera biennis* L. *Fat Science Technology* 97: 277-280.

Cant, A., Shay, J., and Horrobin, D.F. (1991). The effect of maternal supplementation with linoleic and Gamma-linolenic acids on the composition and content of human milk: A placebo-controlled trial. *Journal of Nutrition Science and Vitaminology* (Tokyo) 37: 573-579.

Colquhoun, I. and Bunday, S. (1981). A lack of essential fatty acids as a possible cause of hyperactivity in children. *Medical Hypotheses* 7: 673-679.

Cotterell, J.C., Lee, A.J., and Hunter, J.O. (1990). Double-blind cross-over trial of evening primrose oil in women with menstrually-related irritable bowel syndrome. In Horrobin, D.F. (Ed.), *Omega-6 Essential Fatty Acids: Pathophysiology and Roles in Clinical Medicine* (pp. 421-426). New York: Wiley-Liss.

Cunnane, S.C. and Horrobin, D.F. (1980). Parenteral linoleic and Gamma-linolenic acids ameliorate the gross effects of zinc deficiency (40920). *Proceedings of the Society for Experimental Biology and Medicine* 164: 583-588.

Deferne, J.L. and Pate, D.E. (1996). Hemp seed oil: A source of valuable essential fatty acids. *Journal of the International Hemp Association* 3: 1, 4-7.

De La Cruz, J.P., Martin-Romero, M., Carmona, J.A., Villalobos, M.A., and Sanchez De La Cuesta, F. (1997). Effect of evening primrose oil on platelet aggregation in rabbits fed an atherogenic diet. *Thrombosis Research* 87: 141-149.

Diel, F. (1985). Effects of somatostatin and Gamma-linolenic acid (Efamol) on the ethanol induced hemorrhagic gastric erosion in the rat. *Digestive Diseases and Sciences* 30: 373.

Dove, D. and Johnson, P. (1999). Oral evening primrose oil: Its effect on length of pregnancy and selected intrapartum outcomes in low-risk nulliparous women. *Journal of Nurse-Midwifery* 44: 320-324.

Engler, M.M. (1993). Comparative study of diets enriched with evening primrose, black current, borage or fungal oils on blood pressure and pressor responses in spontaneously hypertensive rats. *Prostaglandins Leukotrienes and Essential Fatty Acids* 49: 809-814.

Everett, D.J., Greenough, R.J., Perry, C.J., MacDonald, P., and Bayliss, P. (1988). Chronic toxicity studies of Efamol evening primrose oil in rats and dogs. *Medical Science Research* 16: 863-864.

Everett, D.J., Perry, C.J., and Bayliss, P. (1988). Carcinogenicity studies of Efamol evening primrose oil in rats and mice. *Medical Science Research* 16: 865-866.

Foster, S. (1995). Evening primrose: An important treatment for essential fatty acid deficiency. *The Herb Companion* 8 (October/November): 65-66.

Fukushima, M., Matsuda, T., Yamagishi, K., and Nakano, M. (1997). Comparative hypocholesterolemic effects of six dietary oils in cholesterol-fed rats after long-term feeding. *Lipids* 32: 1069-1074.

Gibson, R.A. (1985). The effect of dietary supplementation with evening primrose oil of hyperkinetic children. *Proceedings of the Nutrition Society of Australia* 10: 196 (abstract).

Glen, I., Skinner, F., Glen, E., and MacDonell, L. (1987). The role of essential fatty acids in alcohol dependence and tissue damage. *Alcoholism, Clinical and Experimental Research* 11: 37-41.

Gunstone, F.D., Harwood, J.L., and Padley, F.B. (1986). *The Lipid Handbook*. London: Chapman and Hall.

Hansen, T.M., Lerche, A., Kassis, V., Lorenzen, I., and Sondergaard, J. (1983). Treatment of rheumatoid arthritis with prostaglandin E_1 precursors *cis*-linoleic acid and Gamma-linolenic acid. *Scandinavian Journal of Rheumatology* 12: 85-88.

Hederos, C.A. and Berg, A. (1996). Epogam evening primrose oil treatment in atopic dermatitis and asthma. *Archives of Disease in Childhood* 75: 494-497.

Horrobin, D.F. (1980). A new concept of lifestyle-related cardiovascular disease: The importance of interactions between cholesterol, essential fatty acids, and prostaglandin E_1 and thromboxane A_2. *Medical Hypotheses* 6: 785-800.

Horrobin, D.F. (1982). The lowering of plasma cholesterol levels by essential fatty acids. In Horrobin, D.F. (Ed.), *Clinical Uses of Essential Fatty Acids* (pp. 86-96). London: Eden Press, Inc.

Horrobin, D.F. (1990). Gamma-linolenic acid: An intermediate in essential fatty acid metabolism with potential as an ethical pharmaceutical and as a food. *Review of Contemporary Pharmacotherapy* 1: 1-45.

Horrobin, D.F. (1992). Nutritional and medical importance of Gamma-linolenic acid. *Progress in Lipid Research* 31: 163-194.

Hudson, B.J.F. (1984). Evening primrose (*Oenothera* spp.) oil and seed. *Journal of the American Oil Chemists' Society* 61: 540-543.

Humphrey, S. (2001). Sheila Humphrey, RN, BSc, ICBLC, personal communication with INPR, September.

Jamal, G.A., Carmichael, H., and Weir, A.I. (1986). Gamma-linolenic acid in diabetic neuropathy. *Lancet* 1 (May 10): 1098.

Jantti, J., Isomaki, H., Laitinen, O., Nikkari, T., Seppala, E., and Vapaatalo, H. (1985). Linoleic acid treatment in inflammatory arthritis. *International Journal of Clinical Pharmacology, Therapy, and Toxicology* 23: 89-91.

Jeffery, N.M., Yaqoob, P., Wiggins, D., Gibbons, G.F., Newsholme, E.A., and Calder, P.C. (1996). Characterization of lipoprotein composition in rats fed different dietary lipids and of the effects of lipoproteins upon lymphocyte proliferation. *Journal of Nutritional Biochemistry* 7: 282-292.

Karmali, R. A., Marsh, J., and Fuchs, C. (1984). Effect of Omega-3 fatty acids on growth of a rat mammary tumor. *Journal of the National Cancer Institute* 73: 457-461.

Karmali, R.A., Marsh, J. and Fuchs, C. (1985). Effects of dietary enrichment with Gamma-linolenic acid upon growth of the R3230AC mammary adenocarcinoma. *Journal of Nutrition, Growth and Cancer* 2: 41-51.

Kaur, G. and Kulkarni, S.K. (1998). Reversal of forced swimming-induced chronic fatigue in mice by antidepressant and herbal psychotropic drugs. *Indian Drugs* 35: 771-777.

Keen, H., Payan, J., Allawi, J., Walker, J., Jamal, G.A., Weir, A.I., Henderson, L.M., Bissessar, E.A., Watkins, P.J., Sampson, M., et al. (1993). Treatment of diabetic neuropathy with γ-linolenic acid. *Diabetes Care* 16: 8-15.

Kenny, F.S., Pinder, S.E., and Robertson, J.F.R. (2000). Gamma linolenic acid with tamoxifen as primary therapy in breast cancer. *International Journal of Cancer* 85: 643-648.

Kerscher, M.J. and Korting, H.C. (1992). Treatment of atopic eczema with evening primrose oil: Rationale and clinical results. *Clinical Investigator* 70: 167-171.

Kruger, M.C., Coetzer, H., de Winter, R., Gericke, G., and van Papendorp, D.H. (1998). Calcium, Gamma-linolenic acid and eicosapentaenoic acid supplementation in senile osteoporosis. *Aging: Clinical and Experimental Research* 10: 385-394.

Leaver, H.A., Lytton, F.D., Dyson, H., Watson, M.L., and Mellor, D.J. (1986). The effect of dietary ω3 and ω6 polyunsaturated fatty acids on gestation, parturition and prostaglandin E_2 in intrauterine tissues and the kidney. *Progress in Lipid Research* 25: 143-146.

Leventhal, L.J., Boyce, E.G., and Zurier, R.B. (1993). Treatment of rheumatoid arthritis with Gammalinolenic acid. *Annals of Internal Medicine* 119: 867-873.

Liberti, L.E. (1983). Evening primrose oil. *The Lawrence Review of Natural Products* 4 (October): 1-4.

Lovell, C.R., Burton, J.L., and Horrobin, D.F. (1981). Treatment of atopic eczema with evening primrose oil. *Lancet* 1 (January 31): 278 (letter).

Manku, M.S. and Horrobin, D.F. (1982). Essential fatty acid levels in the plasma of patients with atopic eczema. In Horrobin, D.F. (Ed.), *Clinical Uses of Essential Fatty Acids* (pp. 81-88). London: Eden Press, Inc.

Manthorpe, R., Petersen, S., and Prause, J.U. (1984). Primary Sjögren's syndrome treated with Efamol/Efavit. *Rheumatology International* 4: 165-167.

McGuffin, M., Hobbs, C., Upton, R., and Goldberg, A. (1997). *American Herbal Products Association's Botanical Safety Handbook*. Boca Raton, FL: CRC Press.

Mertin, J., Stackpoole, A., and Shumway, S. (1985). Nutrition and immunity: The immunoregulatory effect of *n*-6 essential fatty acids is mediated through prostaglandin E. *International Archives of Allergy and Applied Immunology* 77: 390-395.

Mills, D.E., Ward, R.P., and Huang, Y.S. (1989). Effects of *n*-3 and *n*-6 fatty acid supplementation on cardiovascular and endocrine responses to stress in the rat. *Nutrition Research* 9: 405-414.

Morse, P.F., Horrobin, D.F., Manku, M.S., Stewart, J.C., Allen, R., Littlewood, S., Wright, S., Burton, J., Gould, D.J., Holt, P.J., et al. (1989). Meta-analysis of placebo controlled studies of the efficacy of Epogam in the treatment of atopic eczema. Relationship between plasma essential fatty acid changes and clinical response. *British Journal of Dermatology* 121: 75-90.

Newall, C.A., Anderson, L.A., and Phillipson, J.D. (1996). *Herbal Medicines: A Guide for Health-Care Professionals*. London: The Pharmaceutical Press, pp. 110-113.

Pashby, N.L., Mansel, R.E., Hughes, L.E., Hanslip, J., and Preece, J.P. (1981). A clinical trial of evening primrose oil in mastalgia. *British Journal of Surgery* 68: 801 (abstract).

Phinney, S. (1994). Potential risk of prolonged Gamma-linolenic acid use. *Annals of Internal Medicine* 120: 629 (letter and response of Zurier, R.B.).

Pye, J.K., Mansel, R.E., and Hughes, L.E. (1985). Clinical experience of drug treatments for mastalgia. *Lancet* 2 (August 17): 373-377.

Rahbeeni, F., Hendrikse, A.S., Smuts, C.M., Gelderblom, W.C.A., Abel, S., and Blekkenhorst, G.H. (2000). The effect of evening primrose oil on the radiation response and blood flow of mouse normal and tumour tissue. *International Journal of Radiation Biology* 76(6): 871-877.

Scarff, D.H. and Lloyd, D.H. (1992). Double blind, placebo-controlled, crossover study of evening primrose oil in the treatment of canine atopy. *Veterinary Record* 131: 97-99.

Schalin-Karrila, M., Mattila, L., Jansen, C.T., and Uotila, P. (1987). Evening primrose oil in the treatment of atopic eczema: Effect on clinical status, plasma phospholipid fatty acids and circulating blood prostaglandins. *British Journal of Dermatology* 117: 11-19.

Schweain, S.L. (Ed.) (1997). Oil of evening primrose (OEP) (EPO). *The Review of Natural Products* (August): 1-3.

Shahidi, F., Amarowicz, R., He, Y., and Wettasinghe, M. (1997). Antioxidant activity of phenolic extracts of evening primrose *(Oenothera biennis):* A preliminary study. *Journal of Food Lipids* 4: 75-86.

Shukla, Y.N., Srivastava, A., and Kumar, S. (1999). Aryl, lipid and triterpenoid constituents from *Oenothera biennis. Indian Journal of Chemistry* 38B: 705- 708.

Shuster, J. (1996). ISMP adverse drug reactions. *Hospital Pharmacy* 31: 1553- 1554.

Thies, F., Nebe-von-Caron, G., Powell, J.R., Yaqoob, P., Newsholme, E.A., and Calder, P.C. (2001). Dietary supplementation with γ-linolenic acid or fish oil decreases T lymphocyte proliferation in healthy older humans. *Journal of Nutrition* 131: 1918-1927.

Traitler, H., Winter, H., Richli, U., and Ingenbleek, Y. (1984). Characterization of Gamma-linolenic acid in *Ribes* seed. *Lipids* 19: 923-928.

Van der Merwe, C.F., Booyens, J., and Katzeff, I.E. (1987). Oral Gamma-linolenic acid in 21 patients with untreatable malignancy: An ongoing pilot open clinical trial. *British Journal of Clinical Practice* 41: 907-915.

Watson, J., Godfrey, D., Stimson, W.H., Belch, J.J., and Sturrock, R.D. (1988). The therapeutic effects of dietary fatty acid supplementation in the autoimmune disease of the MRL-mp-1pr/1pr mouse. *International Journal of Immunopharmacology* 10: 467-471.

Whitaker, D.K., Cilliers, J., and De Beer, C. (1996). Evening primrose oil (Epogam) in the treatment of chronic hand dermatitis: Disappointing therapeutic results. *Dermatology* 193: 115-120.

Williams, K. and Casper, R. (1994). Primrose oil in the treatment of premenstrual dysphoric disorder: Is the bloom off the rose? *Psychiatric Annals* 24: 255-258.

Williams, L.L., O'Dougherty, M.M., Wright, F.S., Bobulski, R.J., and Horrocks, L.A. (1986). Dietary essential fatty acids, vitamin E, and Charcot-Marie-Tooth disease. *Neurology* 36: 1200-1205.

Willis, A.L. and Smith, D.L. (1989). Dihomo-gamma-linolenic and gamma-linolenic acids in health and disease. *Current Topics in Nutrition and Disease* 22: 39-108.

Wolf, R.B., Kleinman, R., and England, R.E. (1983). New sources of Gamma-linolenic acid. *Journal of the American Oil Chemists' Society* 68: 1858-1860.

Wright, S. and Burton, J.L. (1982). A placebo-controlled trial of the effects of Efamol® (evening primrose oil) on atopic eczema and blood lipids. In Horrobin, D.F. (Ed.), *Clinical Uses of Essential Fatty Acids* (pp. 73-79). London: Eden Press, Inc.

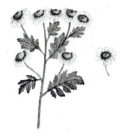

Feverfew

BOTANICAL DATA

Classification and Nomenclature

Scientific name: *Tanacetum parthenium* (L.) Schultz Bip.; synonyms: *Matricaria parthenium* L., *Chrysanthemum parthenium* (L.) Bernh., *Leucanthemum parthenium* (L.) Gren. & Godron, *Pyrethrum parthenium* L. Sm.

Family name: Asteraceae (Compositae)

Common names: Feverfew, featherfew, featherfoil, midsummer daisy, bachelor's buttons, flirtwort, vetter-voo, feather-fully, mutterkraut (German), parthenium (Greek)

Description

Feverfew is presently recognized by taxonomists under the binomial *Tanacetum parthenium,* but it has undergone numerous nomenclatural revisions since it was first classified as *Matricaria parthenoides* by Linnaeus in the early 1800s. Subsequently, it was reclassified as a species of *Chrysanthemum* (*C. parthenium*), but has most recently been placed in the genus *Tanacetum,* which it shares with the common tansy, *Tanacetum vulgare.* There are three or four recognized horticultural varieties of feverfew itself, including *T. parthenium* var. *crispum,* and *T. parthenium* var. *aureum.* There are also several recognized forms of "wild" feverfew. One (silverball), has two or more rows of white ray flowers, another has no white ray flowers, and one has only a single row of white ray flowers. The latter has been recommended as best suited for medicinal purposes (Leung and Foster, 1996; Hobbs, 1989), although Awang (1993) disputed this, pointing out that the highest level of parthenolide, the then putative active principle of feverfew, had been found in a species tentatively identified as *T. parthenium* forma *flosculosum,* which has no ray florets.

Feverfew, a member of the daisy family (Asteraceae), is a bushy, leafy perennial, about 0.3-0.9 m tall with nearly hairless, alternate, deeply lobed leaves. The flowers are borne in open terminal clusters, about 1.9 cm in diameter, with a single row of white rays and a yellow center containing disk flowers. Feverfew, thought to be native to the mountains of the Balkan peninsula, has been cultivated for centuries throughout Europe, and now occurs as a cultivated or escaped plant in eastern North America and Central and South America (Hobbs, 1989; Leung and Foster, 1996).

HISTORY AND TRADITIONAL USES

The use of feverfew in traditional medicine dates back to Dioscorides (1st century A.D.) who recommended it "for inflammations and hot swellings." Gerard's Herbal (1633) recommended it "for them that are giddie in the head" (Hobbs, 1989, p. 28), which may be a reference to headaches or melancholia. He also recommended feverfew to treat malarial fevers. The 18th century herbalist John Hill noted the use of feverfew for "the worst headache" (Hobbs, 1989, p. 28), possibly a reference to migraine. Culpeper, author of one of the earliest and most practical herbals (1649), recommended feverfew to women as a general strengthener of the womb and noted that it "is very effectual for all pains in the head" (Hobbs, 1989, p. 28). Other authorities also recommend feverfew for female complaints, especially as an emmenagogue. Other traditional uses include the fresh, flowering heads as an insect repellant, and as a tincture for the relief of pain and swelling due to insect bites (Hobbs, 1989).

Feverfew is not used in traditional Chinese medicine (TCM), but several species of the closely related genus *Chrysanthemum* are valued in TCM for treating various "hot" conditions, including inflammations, influenza, headaches, and as a sedative (Hobbs, 1989).

CHEMISTRY

Phenolic Compounds

Flavonoids

In the seeds, flowers and leaves as the major flavonoid component, Williams et al. (1999) have identified the flavonol santin (6-hydroxykaempferol 3,6,4'-trimethyl ether), previously thought to be a new compound with a different structure (tanetin) (Williams et al., 1995). The main water-soluble flavonoid constituents of feverfew leaf and flower have been identified as santin, quercetagetin 3,6,3'-trimethyl ether (assumed structure), querce-tagetin 3,6,4'-trimethyl ether (assumed structure), quercetagetin 3,6-dimethyl ether, 6-hydroxykaempferol 3,6-dimethyl ether, and chrysoeriol 7-glucuronide. Other water-soluble flavonoids in feverfew are apigenin, apigenin 7-glucuronide, luteolin 7-glucuronide, luteolin 7-glucoside (leaf and flower), apigenin 7-diglucouronide, apigenin 7-glucosylglucuronide, luteolin, chrysoeriol, and quercetin 7-glucuronide (flower) (Williams et al., 1999).

Terpenoid Compounds

Monoterpenes

In the aerial parts, monoterpenes, including 7 alpha-pinene derivatives, bornyl acetate and bornyl angelate have been identified (Bohlmann and Zdero, 1982). The main constituents of the essential oil derived from samples of Belgian, Dutch, English, and Egyptian feverfew buds, flowers, and leaves, are camphor (> 25%) and chrysanthenyl acetate (> 10%) (Hendriks et al., 1996).

Sesquiterpenes

The antimigraine activity of feverfew has consistently been assumed to be due to the content of sesquiterpene lactones, of which parthenolide is the major component of the European type. Parthenolide comprises 85% of the total sesquiterpenes in that type of feverfew in which concentrations reported in the aerial portions of the plant range from absent to 1.82% (Bohlmann and Zdero, 1982; Heptinstall et al., 1992; Cutlan et al., 2000). The presence of an α-methylene-lactone or unsaturated lactone moiety in the molecule has been associated with biological activity. A study by Groenewegen and Heptinstall (1990) on the antisecretory compounds in *Tanacetum* concluded that all of the active compounds contained this structural feature. Five active lactones containing this structure were identified in the dried leaves: parthenolide, canin, seco-tanaparthenolide, artecanin, and 3-(-hydroxyparthenolide). All are classed as germacranolide-type sesquiterpenes. Other sesquiterpene lactones and related sesquiterpenes isolated from the aerial parts of feverfew include canin (Hewlett et al., 1996), bicyclogermacrene, santamarine, chrysartemin A, chrysartemin B, chrysanthemonin, partholide, chrysanthemolide, reynosin, and magnolialide (Hobbs, 1989; Bohlmann and Zdero, 1982).

At least three sesquiterpene lactone chemotypes of feverfew have been identified (Awang, 1989). Mexican-grown feverfew contains no parthenolide and the sesquiterpene content is dominated by the eudesmanolides santamarin and reynosin, with lesser amounts of the guaianolides canin and artecanin. Parthenolide was not detected in Yugoslavian-grown feverfew; only eudesmano-lides were detected. A trace amount of reynosin (parthenolide:reynosin = 200:1) was detected in Belgian feverfew. Awang (1989) states that it is likely that some constituents are artifacts, the result either of degradation during extraction, or the use of chlorinated solvents as in the case of the "chlorinated sesquiterpenes" reported by Wagner et al. (1988).

Nonlactone type terpenes, including camphor, beta-farnesene and germacrene D have been identified in the aerial parts (Bohlmann and Zdero, 1982).

Steroids

Sitosterol and stigmasterol, both widespread plant sterols, have been identified in the foliage (Banthorpe and Brown, 1989).

Other Constituents

Murch et al. (1997) reported the occurrence of N-acetyl-5-methoxytryptamine in (melatonin) in the leaves at up to 2.45 μg/g, which was still lower than amounts detected in the flowers of St. John's wort (4.39 μg/g) or *Scutellaria baicalensis* (7.11 μg/g).

THERAPEUTIC APPLICATIONS

Antispasmodic, antiaggregatory, antisecretory, and anti-inflammatory properties of feverfew extract suggest that it may be efficacious for disorders in which inflammatory and contractile responses are significant features.

PRECLINICAL STUDIES

Feverfew displays a spectrum of pharmacological actions that are indicative of probable mechanisms underlying its anti-inflammatory and antimigraine properties. Many of these are related to its influences on arachidonate metabolism and platelet functions.

Cardiovascular and Circulatory Functions

Vascular Smooth Muscle Activity

Barsby et al. (1993) found in vitro results suggesting that marked differences exist between the pharmacological potency of dried and fresh feverfew, which may be related to lactone content. They reported that a parthenolide-free chloroform extract of commercially available dried and powdered feverfew leaf showed no inhibitory activity of rabbit aortic ring contractile responses, but caused sustained and strong contractions of aortic smooth muscle. Because the dried-leaf extract showed a reversible spasmogenic action, they concluded that this was not a toxic action. The loss of lactones in the dried leaves was presumed to be due to prolonged storage or a result from protein breakdown reactions. Ketanserin, a 5-HT$_2$ receptor antagonist, failed to antagonize the contractions, whereas a methanolic extract of the fresh leaves time- and dose-dependently inhibited aortic ring contractile responses to every receptor-acting agonist tested to date. Therefore, the spasmogenic action of the dried-leaf extract did not appear to be 5-HT$_2$ receptor-mediated.

Barsby et al. (1991) reported that chloroform extracts of "fresh" feverfew leaves irreversibly inhibited the contraction of isolated rings of rabbit aorta induced by 5-HT and other smooth-muscle contractile agonists, including phenylephrine, U46619, and angiotensin. Because all of these agonists mediate smooth muscle contraction by independent receptor systems, the results indicated that fresh feverfew inhibits contraction nonspecifically, possibly by interference with "postreceptor contractile mechanisms." Adding the extract to precontracted rings resulted, gradually, in a loss of precontracted muscle tone. Barsby and colleagues obtained similar results by the addition of purified parthenolide, but the effect was not observed in commercial preparations of dried feverfew leaves found devoid of parthenolide, or other sesquiterpene α-methylene butyrolactones. The potentially toxic, irreversible response could have resulted from an additional reaction between the active lactones and essential sulfhydryl groups in vascular smooth muscle proteins.

Immune Functions; Inflammation and Disease

Cancer

Antiproliferative activity. From up to 72 h exposure, parthenolide caused in vitro concentration-dependent, reversible cytostatic activity against human lymphoma TK6 (2.5 μM) and mouse fibrosarcoma MN-11 (2.5 μM). Tumor growth ceased at 3.0-3.5 μM in these tumor cell lines from a 48 h exposure without any difference in tumor cell numbers. The cytostatic activity was postulated as being due to inhibition of protein kinases. At a higher concentration and shorter exposure time (5 μM at 24 h), parthenolide caused cytotoxic activity in both tumor cells lines, and was extensively cytotoxic at higher concentrations (15 μM at 24 h and 10 μM at 48 h exposure) (Ross et al., 1999).

Cytotoxicity. In a breast cancer cell line (MDA-MB-231), parthenolide increased sensitivity of the cells to paclitaxel while decreasing the binding activity of constitutive NF-κB DNA. Parthenolide inhibited in vitro growth of the breast cancer cells (IC_{50} 2 μM) and showed more than an additive inhibitory effect when combined with paclitaxel. In another nonestrogen-dependent breast cancer cell line (HBL100), parthenolide ($IC_{50} < 0.1$ μM) exhibited a synergistic effect when combined with paclitaxel (~0.8 μM) at lower growth-inhibitory concentrations than exhibited by either agent alone (0.8 μM and 10 nM, respectively) (Patel et al., 2000).

Heblich et al. (1997) reported a likely cytotoxic action from the presence of cinnamoyl-dihydroxynardol, a sesquiterpene ester, in a chloroform extract of feverfew. The sesquiterpene ester inhibited part of the voltage-dependent potassium current in undifferentiated NG108-15 (mouse neuroblastoma × rat glioma hybrid) cells.

O'Neill et al. (1987) rationalized that some cytotoxic effect on overactive lymphocytes and macrophages could explain feverfew's amelioration of the symptoms of arthritis. They reported that feverfew extracts and parthenolide could inhibit DNA synthesis in peripheral mononuclear cells and that they inhibited interleukin-2-induced proliferation of lymphoblasts. The extracts also inhibited prostaglandin E_2 production by synovial cells. This mechanism could possibly explain some of the anti-inflammatory effects of feverfew.

Immune Functions

Immunomodulation. Brown et al. (1997) studied the effect of feverfew leaf extracts containing various concentrations of parthenolide in a whole blood human polymorphonuclear leukocyte (PMNL) cellular chemiluminescence test. Oxidative burst was reduced by all the leaf extracts in a parthenolide concentration-dependent manner with the most inhibition from the greatest parthenolide concentration. However, the activity found was consistently more than what could be predicted if parthenolide was regarded as the only active constituent. This was apparent in the relative activity and relative parthenolide concentrations of the acetone-ethanol extract (1.3 ± 0.2% parthenolide by dry leaf weight) compared to the phosphate buffered saline extract (0.5 ± 0.1% parthenolide by dry leaf weight), which showed the same bioactivity value. Brown and colleagues concluded, therefore, that in addition to parthenolide, yet-to-be determined metabolites, probably of solubility similar to that of parthenolide, are involved in the inhibitory activity found in the human PMNL assay.

Williamson et al. (1988) reported that a chloroform/methanol (1.5 mL/3.5mL) extract of dried feverfew leaves showed a dose-dependent inhibition of the in vitro phagocytosis against *Candida guilliermondii*. The extract showed inhibitory activity against neutrophil phagocytosis of *C. guilliermondii* at 25 μL. At 100 μL, 50% of the neutrophils showed no phagocytosis (engulfing) of *C. guilliermondii*. Intracellular killing of *C. guilliermondii,* however, was not inhibited by the extract, even at 180 μL compared to the normal rate of the control. Williamson et al. (1988) note that the concentrations which markedly inhibited phagocytosis in vitro are the same as those found by Heptinstall et al. (1985) to inhibit the excretion of blood platelet and PMNL granule constituents. Williamson and colleagues commented that together, these actions lend credence to the use of feverfew against inflammatory states. They also suggested that future clinical trials of feverfew should examine patients' neutrophil function ex vivo to determine whether such an impairment in neutrophil phagocytic ability attends oral ingestion of the herb.

Infectious Diseases

Microbial infections. A 45% and a 90% ethanol extract of feverfew dry leaves prepared from plants collected at the flowering stage showed antimicrobial activity against different microorganisms. Gram-negative species showed far less sensitivity to the extracts than Gram-positive species. The 45% ethanol extract had no effect on Gram-negative species whereas the 90% ethanol extract inhibited the growth of *Serratia* sp., *Proteus mirabilis, P. morganii, P. rettgeri,* and *Escherichia coli*. Both extracts were equally potent against *Trychophyton mentagrophytes,* whereas against *Candida albicans* the 90% ethanol extract (90 EE) was about 40% more active. The 45% ethanol extract (45 EE) was completely ineffective against *C. kruzei* and *C. tropicalis,* for which the [90EE] displayed both microbicidal and inhibitory activity. The 90 EE showed twice the inhibitory potency of the 45 EE against *Staphylococcus haemolyticus* and *S. aureus;* equal activity against *Sarcina flava* and *Bacillus pumilus;* 10% less potency against *B. subtilis;* and whereas the 90 EE showed no microbicidal activity against *B. subtilis,* the 45 EE did from a 100% concentration (Kalodera et al., 1996).

Inflammatory Response

The increased expression of intercellular adhesion molecule-1 (ICAM-1) by fibroblasts in the synovial fluid of rheumatoid arthritis patients is believed to be part of the pathogenesis of the disease. Using cultured synovial fibroblasts from rheumatoid arthritis patients, Piela-Smith and Liu (2001) examined the in vitro effects of parthenolide and various herbal products for their ability to inhibit the expression of proinflammatory cellular adhesion molecules. The commercial herbal products they tested all consisted of dry feverfew leaf *(Tanacetum parthenium),* feverfew extract prepared from whole feverfew plants, ginger *(Zingiber officinale),* devil's claw *(Harpagophytum procumbens),* alfalfa *(Medicago sativa),* and a liquid herbal formula ("arthritis relief medication") (Piela-Smith and Liu, 2001, p. 90) composed of black cohosh *(Cimicifuga racemosa),* poison ivy *(Rhus toxicodendron),* honeybee *(Apis mellifica),* wind flower *(Pulsatila nigricans),* and bittersweet *(Dulcamara).* The extract and the liquid formula were simply diluted in 70% ethanol and the dried herbs were prepared as 70% ethanol extracts which were diluted before adding them to cultures of the synovial fibroblasts. Induction of ICAM-1 by the cytokine interleukin-1 (IL-1) was inhibited by the feverfew extract, but not by devil's claw, alfalfa, ginger, or the herbal formula. The feverfew extract inhibited the increased expression of ICAM-1 by 80% and produced near complete inhibition from a 1:40 dilution. Higher dilutions were less effective. Longer incubation times had no effect on the inhibitory activity of the feverfew extract. Subsequent tests showed that the feverfew extract could also inhibit the increased expression of ICAM-1 induced by other cytokines, including tumor necrosis factor (TNF), and interferon-gamma (IFN-γ). In tests using IL-1-stimulated ICAM-1 expression, the inhibitory effect of the feverfew extract was shown to be reversible. Parthenolide also exhibited dose-dependent inhibition of ICAM-1 expression stimulated by either IL-1 or TNF. At a concentration of 2.0 mg/mL, parthenolide caused ICAM-1 levels to fall below those of unstimulated cells and still exhibited inhibitory activity at a concentration of 50 ng/mL. Further tests revealed that pretreatment with either parthenolide or the feverfew extract correlated with decreased functional T cell adhesion to the synovial fibroblasts stimulated by TNF. Either substance also inhibited other adhesion molecules related to inflammatory processes and expressed by synovial fibroblasts, including LFA-3 and VCAM-1.

The intracellular transcription factor nuclear factor κB (NF-κB) activates many of the genes operating in processes of inflammation, including upregulation of ICAM-1. In vitro studies have shown that parthenolide inhibits the activation of NF-κB by binding to and inhibiting the IkB kinase complex (IKK) which is composed of catalytic subunits (e.g., IKKα and IKKβ) (Hehner et al., 1999). Production of the proinflammatory cytokine interleukin-12 (IL-12) by lipopolysaccharide-activated macrophages was significantly ($p < 0.01$) inhibited by parthenolide (0.25 μM), partly by down-regulating the activation of NF-kB and its binding to the gene transcriptional factor, p40-κB (Kang et al., 2001). Parthenolide was found to directly and specifically inhibit IKKB and when modified, lost this ability. Applied topically to the ears of mice at the same time as an inflammatory agent phorbol myristate acetate (PMA), the unmodified form caused swelling to be reduced whereas the modified form caused little anti-inflammatory activity compared to the PMA-treated controls (Kwok et al., 2001).

In high doses, parthenolide as a 30 min pretreatment caused a dose-dependent inhibition of the formation of ethanol-induced ulcers in rats (e.g., 87% inhibition at 100 mg/kg p.o.). As a 24 h pretreatment, parthenolide (100 mg/kg p.o.) inhibited ethanol-induced ulcers in rats by 39% ($p < 0.05$). Complete restoration of mucosal suphydryl content to normal and 91% protection of the gastric mucosa was only achieved from a much higher dosage (400 mg/kg p.o.) (Tournier et al., 1999).

Jain and Kulkarni (1999) demonstrated that an ethanolic extract of feverfew (Dabur Research Foundation, New Delhi, India; parthenolide content 0.856%) exhibited significant dose-dependent anti-inflammatory activity (carrageenan-induced paw edema) and antinociceptive activity in mice and rats (acetic acid writhing test and the tail-flick test, respectively) when administered in oral doses of 10, 20, 40, and 60 mg/kg. The pain threshold was significantly raised from 10 mg/kg p.o., but only lasted 5 min versus at least 15 and 20 min with the 20 to 60 mg/kg doses, respectively. From higher doses (40 and 60 mg/kg p.o.), no signs of altered behavior, potentiation of pentobarbitone-induced (45 mg/kg i.p.) sleep time and onset of sleep, nor alterations in locomotor activity compared to diazepam (2 mg/kg) could be found in mice, and the rectal temperature of rats remained unchanged. Parthenolide (Aldrich, 1 and 2 mg/kg i.p.) also exhibited antinociceptive and anti-inflammatory effects. Naloxone (1 mg/kg i.p.) failed to reverse the antinociceptive effects of either feverfew preparation, indicating that the action is not mediated by opiate receptors. Both the antinociceptive and anti-inflammatory activities of the feverfew extract and parthenolide were shown to be comparable to the nonsteroidal anti-inflammatory drug nimesulide (2 mg/kg) (a selective cyclooxygenase-2 inhibitor), although parthenolide was superior against rat paw edema.

Flavonol-containing extracts of feverfew seeds and leaves are reported to have shown potent antinociceptive activity in mice, and santin (previously identified as tanetin) (in vitro) potent inhibitory activity in rat peritoneal leukocytes against the generation of eicosanoids, including 5-lipoxygenase (IC50: 11 μM) and cyclooxygenase (IC50: 6-11 μM) (Hoult et al., 1995). At 40 μM tanetin (revised as santin) (Williams et al., 1999), prostaglandin E_2 generation was inhibited by approximately 85%; thromboxane B_2 generation by 97% (Williams et al., 1995)—approximately equal to indomethicin at 5 μM (Hoult et al., 1995)—and leukotriene B_4 generation by 86%. However, tanetin (revised as santin) (Williams et al., 1999) showed no inhibition of nitric oxide synthase (Williams et al., 1995). The most potent cyclooxygenase (thromboxane B_2)-inhibiting flavonoids from feverfew leaf are quercetagetin 3,6,3'-trimethyl ether (assumed structure) (IC_{50}: 22 μm), santin (IC_{50}: 27 μM), and 6-hydroxykaempferol 3,6-dimethyl ether (IC_{50}: 182 μM). The 5-lipoxygenase (leukotriene B4)-inhibiting flavonoids are santin (IC_{50}: 58 μM), quercetagetin 3,6,3'-trimethyl ether (assumed structure) (IC_{50}: 167 μM), and 6-hydroxykaempferol 3,6-dimethyl ether (IC_{50}: 182 μM) (Williams et al., 1999).

Hwang et al. (1996) demonstrated that parthenolide could inhibit the in vitro expression of pro-inflammatory cytokines (IL-1 and TNF-α; IC_{50}: 0.1 μM/mL) in stimulated alveolar macrophages, and COX-2 expression (parthenolide IC_{50}: 0.2 μM/mL); the latter correlated with suppression of protein tyrosine phosphorylation. The researchers noted the possibility of utilizing some sesquiterpene lactones in the treatment of septic shock and diseases attended with acute inflammation. PTK (protein-tyrosinase kinase) inhibitors are also of interest as potential anticancer agents.

Hewlett et al. (1996) found that the platelet aggregation-inhibitory activity of the sesquiterpene lactone constituent canin showed close to half the potency of parthenolide as measured in the same test used by Groenewegen and Heptinstall (1990). Groenewegen and Heptinstall compared the effects of parthenolide and a crude feverfew extract on 5-HT secretion from human platelets and on platelet aggregation induced by a number of aggregatory stimulants in platelet-rich plasma. Parthenolide and the extract showed similar effects on both parameters, suggesting that the actions of the crude extract are mainly due to parthenolide. Differences were found, however, in the actions of both the extract and parthenolide on 5-HT release and aggregation induced by various stimulants. The inhibition of collagen-induced 5-HT release could be overcome by increasing the concentration of collagen; however, the inhibition of 5-HT release induced by the phorbol ester myristate acetate (PMA) could not be overcome by increasing the concentration of PMA. Similar results were observed for the thromboxane mimetic U46619. In subsequent experiments, it was shown that parthenolide and feverfew extract both inhibited 5-HT secretion and platelet aggregation to similar degrees in response to adrenaline or arachidonic acid. Neither parthenolide nor the extract inhibited the aggregation induced by PMA to a significant degree, but both inhibited the PMA-induced secretion of 5-HT. PMA is known to activate protein kinase C in the cell, and this, in turn, is thought to play a role in stimulating secretion from intracellular storage granules.

The flavonol constituent tanetin (revised as santin) (Williams et al., 1999) was shown to potently inhibit the 5-lipooxygenase and cyclooxygenase pathways activated by calcium ionophore A23187 (Williams et al., 1995); however, the whole leaf extract did not (Heptinstall et al., 1985). Heptinstall et al. (1985) reported that extracts of dried feverfew leaves (chloroform/methanol and extraction directly in McEwen's buffer) inhibited the release of 5-hydroxytryptamine (5-HT, or serotonin) from platelets and PMNLs induced by various aggregating agents, including ADP, adrenaline, sodium arachidonate, collagen, and U46619, a thromboxane mimetic. Platelet aggregation was inhibited, but thromboxane synthesis was not. The extracts also inhibited the release of vitamin B_{12} binding protein from PMNs, induced by the secretogogues formyl-methionyl-leucyl-phenylalanine, sodium arachidonate, and zymosan-activated serum, but did not inhibit the secretion from PMNs, as later found by Groenewegen and Heptinstall (1990), or platelets induced by the calcium ionophore A23187. This pattern was different from that obtained with other inhibitors of platelet aggregation.

Pugh and Sambo (1988), working from a chlorophyll-free extract of fresh feverfew leaves, isolated chrysanthenyl acetate, michefuscalide, and parthenolide as active constituents showing in vitro inhibitory action against prostaglandin synthetase-mediated production of PGE_2 from arachidonic acid. The respective IC_{50} concentrations were 2.76, 3.70, and 2.73 µg/mL.

Capasso (1986) tested the effects of an aqueous extract of feverfew on the metabolism of arachidonic acid in both the cyclooxygenase and lipoxygenase pathways. Rat peritoneal cells were incubated in the presence of varying concentrations of feverfew extract, followed by further incubation with calcium ionophore and arachidonate. Formation of both cyclooxygenase products (PGE_2, $PGS_{1\alpha}$, $PGF_{2\alpha}$, PG_D, thromboxane B_2, 6-keto $PGF_{1\alpha}$) and lipoxygenase products (5-HETE and LTB_4) was inhibited in a concentration-dependent manner. These results contrast with those of Makheja and Bailey (1982), who found no evidence of direct cyclooxygenase inhibition in the feverfew extracts which they assayed.

Makheja and Bailey (1982) found that feverfew extracts were able to inhibit aggregation of human platelets induced by adenosine diphosphate (ADP), collagen, and thrombin, but not by arachidonic acid. Synthesis of thromboxane B_2 from arachidonate was not inhibited by an extract of feverfew, indicating that feverfew does not inhibit cyclooxygenase, a key enzyme mediating prostaglandin synthesis. However, the extract was able to inhibit dose-dependently the activity of a purified platelet phospholipase A_2 fraction, at concentrations about 10% of those required to inhibit platelet aggregation. These results suggest that substances in the extract interfere with the initial step of thromboxane synthesis, namely, the phospholipase A_2-mediated release of the arachidonic acid substrate from platelet phospholipids, stimulated by aggregatory agents. Since arachidonic acid is the precursor of both prostaglandins and leukotrienes, these results might explain some of the diverse pharmacological actions attributed to feverfew (Makheja and Bailey, 1982). These contrasting results suggest the need to reexamine these activities using more accurate methods of analysis, and further exploration of differences in the chemical makeup of the plants being examined.

Neurological, Psychological, and Behavioral Functions

Receptor- and Neurotransmitter-Mediated Functions

Awang (1998) notes that feverfew leaf from parthenolide-free sesquiterpene lactone chemotypes has yet to be clinically tested for the prevention of migraine and that the mitigation of migraine symptoms by the inhibition of serotonin-release by parthenolide remains to be established. Weber et al. (1997), using rabbit and rat brain cloned 5-HT_{2A} receptors, determined that parthenolide can displace [^{3}H]ketanserin from these receptors, which suggests that parthenolide may act as a low-affinity antagonist at these receptors. Weber and colleagues concluded that because the affinity for 5-HT$_{2A}$ receptors is mild, this mechanism is not likely to offer an encompassing explanation of parthenolide's action, and that other compounds in feverfew most likely contribute, through diverse mechanisms, to the medicinal activity of the herb. (Above 2% ethanol, they observed a concentration-dependent inhibition of 5-HT$_{2A}$ receptors; therefore, levels were kept below this amount.)

Excess serotonin (5-HT) release from platelets has been implicated as one of the primary mechanisms in the pathogenesis of migraine, which offers an attractive hypothesis for migraine prophylaxis from feverfew, parthenolide, and related sesquiterpenes; they may interfere with 5-HT storage, release, or interactions with serotonin receptors. The rat fundus has been used to investigate the effects of 5-HT and 5-HT antagonists and agonists on the contractile response of tissues, which is mediated by 5-HT$_{2B}$ receptors located on the surface of fundus smooth muscle cells. The isolated fundus system was used by Béjar (1996) to study the effects of parthenolide and the indirect acting serotonergic agents dextroamphetamine (DA) and fenfluramine (F) on 5-HT-mediated processes. Parthenolide did not show direct 5-HT agonist or antagonist effects at any of the concentrations used. However, it did noncompetitively antagonize the 5-HT-mediated contractile responses elicited by DA and F. The results were consistent with the hypothesis that parthenolide selectively inhibits the release of 5-HT from neuronal vesicles in the neurons of fundal tissue.

Marles et al. (1992) used an in vitro 5-HT release-inhibition assay (bovine platelet assay) to test various species of *Tanacetum* grown from seeds obtained from various parts of Europe and one from Guatemala. They reported a significant correlation between parthenolide content and serotonin release. Other members of the same plant family (Asteraceae) and other sesquiterpene lactones were also found to be active. It is interesting to note, however, that two species of *Tanacetum* containing no parthenolide showed greater potency than the most extensively and clinically researched feverfew (*T. parthenium* from University of Nottingham, England).

Respiratory and Pulmonary Functions

Allergies and Asthma

Hayes and Foreman (1987) reported that extracts of feverfew produced a dose-dependent inhibition of histamine release from rat mast cells stimulated with anti-IgE or the calcium ionophore A23187. Feverfew extract inhibited histamine release induced by the anti-IgE response when added to the cells simultaneously with IgE. The inhibitory response was reduced slightly by preincubation with the cells prior to the addition of antibody. Addition of extracellular glucose to the medium had no effect on inhibition, indicating that compounds in feverfew do not act as mitochondrial poisons that interfere with oxidative phosphorylation.

CLINICAL STUDIES

Neurological, Psychological, and Behavioral Disorders

Psychological and Behavioral Disorders

Headaches/migraine. Ernst and Pittler (2000) updated a previous systematic review of randomized, placebo-controlled, double-blind trials on feverfew (Vogler et al., 1998), concluding that while only six trials met their criteria, four clearly showed that feverfew was superior to placebo as a preventive for migraine, and efficacy had yet to be firmly established. Vogler et al. (1998), in a review of the small number of double-blind, placebo-controlled, randomized clinical trials on feverfew for migraine prophylaxis, arrived at similar conclusions, commenting that although the majority of studies to date favor feverfew over placebo, the efficacy of feverfew in preventing migraine had yet to be established "beyond reasonable doubt." With a common outcome measurement lacking in these trials, Vogler and colleagues abandoned a meta-analysis. Due to what was felt to be a lack of quality in what randomized controlled trials exist, Vogler and colleagues concluded that while the data "imply that dried feverfew preparations might be effective . . . the evidence is far from compelling" (p. 707). They called for more clinical trials using larger numbers of subjects and a greater variety of feverfew extracts which would include parthenolide-free chemotypes.

Palevitch et al. (1997) used the dried leaf of feverfew in a double-blind, placebo-controlled study in 57 migraine sufferers (ages 9-65) who had not taken the herb previously, 43% of whom had experienced over ten episodes of migraines every month. The plant was grown in Israel from seeds obtained from the Netherlands and each 100 mg of dried leaf was standardized to contain 0.2 mg parthenolide. The leaves were harvested at flowering onset, washed with water, and then soaked in sodium hypochloride for 10 min as a means of reducing bacteria. Drying was carried out for an undisclosed period in a stove (45°C) and the leaves were stored at 4°C for an undisclosed period of time before use in the trial. Phase one of the study involved group A ($n = 30$) and group B ($n = 27$) all of whom received feverfew in capsules (200 mg/day for 60 days). In the second phase, group A continued with feverfew while group B was given placebo (dried parsley leaves) for 30 days. Then the groups were crossed over in the fourth month. Patient evaluation was determined in a scaled numerical self-assessment of pain, and clinical assessment was made on the basis of pain intensity, frequency, and symptoms associated with migraine (e.g., noise, sensitivity to light, nausea, vomiting). At the end of the first phase, all of the patients taking feverfew for 60 days showed a highly significant improvement compared to pretreatment levels ($p < 0.001$), as reported in the reduction of pain intensity and symptom severity, including nausea and vomiting, and sensitivity to noise and light. At the end of the second phase, the placebo group B showed a significant decline in pain intensity, and migraine symptoms significantly worsened compared to group A, except for sensitivity to noise. At the end of the fourth month (phase three), group A (crossed over to placebo) showed significantly worse symptoms and pain levels, compared to group B, who had been crossed over to receive feverfew for 30 days. No adverse effects were reported and the results offer evidence that feverfew leaf taken prophylactically can provide substantial relief from the symptoms commonly associated with migraine and the intensity of migraine pain (Palevitch et al., 1997).

De Weerdt et al. (1996) conducted a randomized, placebo-controlled, double-blind crossover study in 50 migraine patients who had not previously used feverfew. The feverfew preparation in this study consisted of a powdered extract (dried hydroalcoholic extract of feverfew on microcrystalline cellulose) containing 0.5 mg parthenolide. Patients received one capsule per day (143 mg) or placebo (dried chlorophyll extract), without a washout period before being crossed over. Although 44 out of the 50 patients completed the nine-month study, no significant differences between the placebo group and the patients given feverfew were found. The researchers questioned whether the lower content of chrysanthenyl acetate (0.017%) in the preparation compared to 0.25% in the dried leaf material may have affected the outcome, since the compound has shown prostaglandin synthetase-inhibiting activity (De Weerdt et al., 1996 citing Pugh and Sambo, 1988) and may contribute analgesic activity. No mention of adverse effects was made by any of the patients.

Awang (1998) stresses that the trial results of De Weerdt et al. (1996) raise serious doubts about the parthenolide-serotonin hypothesis of migraine prophylaxis by feverfew. He points out (Awang, 1997) that the negative results raise several issues that should be addressed in future studies, emphasizing that at present, the only variety of feverfew shown to be efficacious is from Nottingham, England, with a single row of white ray florets, which was used in the clinical trials of Murphy et al. (1988). Awang suggests that additional clinical studies using various chemotypes of feverfew, including parthenolide-free varieties, could help to resolve this issue (Awang, 1997); an opinion later expressed by Vogler et al. (1998) in their systematic review of the clinical trials on feverfew to date.

In recognizing a prevailing lack of clinical evidence to support the efficacy of feverfew as a migraine prophylaxis, Kuritzky et al. (1994) conducted a randomized, double-blind, crossover study in 20 patients ages 18 to 60 diagnosed with migraine. For two months, patients received 100 mg of feverfew or placebo while measurements were obtained of changes in their serotonin uptake and activity in platelet-rich plasma. The results showed that at the dosage used, feverfew was ineffective as a migraine prophylaxis and there was no effect on either serotonin activity or uptake by platelets. Furthermore, platelets were not activated in either treated or untreated patients.

Murphy et al. (1988) assessed the efficacy of feverfew leaf in 60 patients (ages 24-72) in a randomized, double-blind, placebo-controlled, crossover study without an intervening washout period. Patients received dried feverfew leaf (70 to 114 mg/day; average 82 mg/day) containing an average of 2.19 μmol parthenolide or placebo each day for four months, following a one-month, single-blind, placebo run-in period. The feverfew leaf was collected from cultivated plants throughout the year except at flowering. Before encapsulation, the leaves were washed in cold water and soaked in sodium hypochlorite for 10 min. They were blot-dried and placed in a drying cabinet at 37ºC for four days before storage at 4ºC for a maximum of five months. In vitro inhibition of 5-HT release from human platelets using chloroform extracts of the leaves was tested before encapsulation of the dried and powdered leaves. Capsules ranged in weight from 70 to 114 mg and contained the equivalent of 2.19 μM parthenolide each. The placebo was dried cabbage leaves devoid of 5-HT release-inhibitory activity. A weakness of the trial was that 18 of the patients had tried feverfew previously and 11 of them believed it was "helpful." Among 59 patients who completed the study, there was a 24% reduction in the number of migraine attacks, but no change in the duration of individual attacks. There was a nonsignificant trend toward milder headaches in the feverfew group, and a significant reduction in the nausea and vomiting that accompany attacks. Sixty-eight working days were lost due to migraines among the treated group versus 76 days among the placebo group. Global assessments of efficacy showed that feverfew was better than placebo; 36% of all feverfew periods were graded as "much better" for migraine, and only 1% as "much worse." This was compared with placebo values of 21% and 10%, respectively. Although still "blind" to therapy following the study, 59% of patients reported that the feverfew period was more effective versus only 24% who chose the placebo period as being more effective. Incidences of adverse effects amounted to 36 in the placebo group versus 28 in the feverfew group. The most common adverse effects reported were mouth ulcers (placebo = 16; feverfew = 10), indigestion (placebo = 2; feverfew = 4), and heartburn (3 in each group).

Johnson et al. (1985) conducted a double-blind, placebo-controlled comparison study in 17 patients who had been daily consuming ("usually with food") one to four small, "raw" feverfew leaves (about 60 mg) for migraine prevention for several months or more. Eight patients received capsules containing freeze-dried feverfew leaf powder (25 mg, b.i.d.; parthenolide content not stated), and the others received a color- and odor-matched placebo (chlorophyll) in a double-blind fashion. The leaf material, harvested in September at Chelsea Physic Garden, London, England, consisted of five leaflets (mean weight 25.7 mg) per capsule. Acute attacks of migraine were treated with patients' usual medications or soluble aspirin. Patients given placebo experienced a significant increase in the severity and frequency of headaches, nausea, and vomiting, while those who continued taking feverfew showed no such changes. Side effects reported in the feverfew group included one patient each with slightly heavier menstrual flow, palpitations, and abdominal pain (colic). The placebo group reported 19 incidences of adverse events, and the majority were nervousness and tension ($n = 5$).

Johnson et al. (1985) suggests that feverfew may prophylactically ameliorate migraine attacks. However, the change in frequency of migraine attacks in the feverfew group was not changed. Further studies are indicated, using formulations controlled for sesquiterpene lactone content, and in patients who have not previously self-medicated with feverfew.

Immune Disorders; Inflammation and Disease

Autoimmune Disorders

Arthritic. In a prospective placebo-controlled, double-blind study (Pattrick et al., 1989), 41 female patients age 65 and under with symptomatic rheumatoid arthritis received either dried feverfew leaf (70-86 mg, equivalent to 2-3 µM parthenolide) or placebo capsules once daily for six weeks, while maintaining their medications and analgesics and NSAIDs (nonsteroidal anti-inflammatory drugs). Some were also administered steroid injections and all were assessed as having "inadequately controlled" symptoms of inflammatory joint disorder. At six weeks, no differences were found between the treatment and placebo group, with the exception of grip strength, which was increased compared to the initial value in the treatment and placebo group. Serum IgG concentrations were elevated compared to baseline in the feverfew group, but no other differences between the two groups were apparent. The researchers speculated that higher doses may be required to treat chronic arthritis symptoms, and that since both feverfew and NSAIDs interfere with arachidonate-mediated inflammation processes, it was possible that concurrent treatment with NSAIDs could have interfered with the activity of feverfew—even though the combined use of the herb is common among patients taking conventional medications. Pattrick and colleagues concluded that additional clinical trials with more effective controls for these variables are needed to determine the efficacy of feverfew in arthritic conditions, a use known from folk medicine.

Immunomodulation

Cellular immune response. The effect of a moderate dose of GLA on the cellular immune function of healthy Caucasian volunteers ($n = 46$) ages 55-71 years were examined in a randomized, placebo-controlled, double-blind parallel study. An oil blend providing GLA or placebo was administered at a dosage of 700 mg/day in capsules, three taken before each of three daily meals for 12 weeks. The results showed that after 12 weeks the only noticeable effect on the cellular immune system from the moderate dosage of GLA in these volunteers was a decrease in lymphocytes proliferation; the mean decrease was up to 61% which was significantly lower than baseline and compared to placebo. At week 16, after a four-week washout, the increase in the stimulation index was still not as high as baseline values (Thies et al., 2001).

DOSAGE

Most clinical studies have used dosages ranging from 25-82 mg/day of dried leaf. Foster (1995) suggests a daily dose of 125 mg leaf, assuming a parthenolide content of 0.2%. The *British Herbal Compendium* (Bradley, 1992) recommends a daily dose of the dried herb of 50-200 mg/day. In the form of a tincture (1:5, 25% alcohol), a dose of 5-20 drops is recommended. For acute attacks of migraine, or for rheumatoid arthritis, larger doses of up to 1-2 g/day may be required.

Based on clinical evidence and current understanding of the probable pharmacological mechanisms responsible for the actions of feverfew, the Health Protection Branch (HPB) of Canada approved the primary therapeutic application for this herb in the prophylactic treatment of migraines. The HPB requires that dried leaf products of feverfew contain at least 0.2% parthenolide, a concentration based upon levels (average 0.42%) found in leaf samples of a feverfew chemotype grown in Chelsea Physic Garden in London, England, which Johnson et al. (1985) used in a clinical trial (Heptinstall and Awang, 1998). However, the amount of 0.2% parthenolide was only intended to be one of two identity criteria for the species following analysis of a wide collection *T. parthenium* obtained from Chelsea Physic Garden; the other being the certification of the plant botanically (Awang, 1998). Heptinstall (1997) notes that the majority of commercial feverfew products analyzed (18/22) do not contain parthenolide in amounts close to that of material used in clinical trials of migraine prophylaxis. Many (10/22) contain considerably smaller concentrations or none at all (8/22) (Heptinstall, 1997). The finding of no migraine-preventive activity in one well-controlled trial of an alcoholic extract of feverfew that *did* contain parthenolide (0.5 mg/capsule) (De Weerdt et al., 1996) suggests that as yet unidentified active constituents are not extracted or affected by the extraction method used.

Parthenolide content varies from about 10-20 mg per entire plant, depending on the growth stage. The flower heads alone can contain over 10 mg/g, and while air-drying feverfew at ambient temperature does not diminish the parthenolide content, there are strains of the herb that contain no parthenolide (Hendriks et al., 1997).

SAFETY PROFILE

Contraindications

Feverfew is contraindicated in individuals with known hypersensitivity to other members of the Asteraceae, such as ragweed, chamomile, echinacea, and yarrow. It should not be used by those who develop a rash on contact with the plant (Hausen and Osmundsen, 1983; Newall et al., 1996). Allergic reactions following oral ingestion have not been documented (Newall et al., 1996). The principle allergic components of feverfew are parthenolide and other sesquiterpene lactones (Goulden and Wilkinson, 1998).

Drug Interactions

No adverse drug interactions have been documented. However, in view of feverfew's probable mechanisms of action related to inhibition of platelet aggregation and prostaglandin biosynthesis, there is a possibility of interactions with aspirin or other anticoagulant medications.

Pregnancy and Lactation

The German Commission E has not developed a monograph for feverfew. The *American Herbal Products Association's Botanical Safety Handbook* cautions against its use during pregnancy without further details (McGuffin et al., 1997). Duke (1985) states that feverfew has been reported as an abortifacient, emmenagogue, and used for dysmenorrhea and during parturition. Newall et al. (1996) contraindicates use during pregnancy, refering to documentation of feverfew causing abortion in cattle, and of having induced uterine contractions in full-term pregnant women.

Newall et al. (1996) do not discuss feverfew use during lactation. The *American Herbal Products Association's Botanical Safety Handbook* (McGuffin et al., 1997) did not classify feverfew to be of concern during lactation. No adverse reports during lactation are known. Observed pregnancy-disruptive effects seen in animals (Newall et al., 1996) could indicate that some constituents are able to influence reproductive hormones and thus lactation. However, amounts consumed by cattle are far in excess of human dosages. There is no known ethnobotanical record of galactogogue use. Use of feverfew versus other pharmaceutical agents should include the risk of use versus the severity of potential side effects for all treatment options.

Side Effects

No major adverse effects have been reported and chronic use is well-tolerated (Werbach and Murray, 1994; Ernst and Pittler, 2000). According to the *British Herbal Compendium,* contact allergy is rare, and in two clinical trials there were more side effects reported from the placebo groups than from those administered feverfew. Gastric upsets and mouth ulcerations have only occasionally been observed (Bradley, 1992), except in people who chew the leaves in which the incidence of a surveyed population of users was reported to be 11.3% (Awang, 1998). However, in a randomized, double-blind, placebo-controlled, crossover trial of feverfew in migraine sufferers ($n = 59$), more patients experienced mouth ulcerations while on the placebo (n = 16) than did those on encapsulated dried leaves ($n = 10$). The placebo was dried cabbage leaves (Murphy et al., 1988).

A survey of 300 feverfew leaf users found that 18% claimed adverse events, including mouth ulcers (11.3%), and reports that the leaf often caused their lips to swell, sometimes a loss of taste sensation, and "more wide-spread inflammation of the oral mucosa and tongue" (Johnson et al., 1985, p. 572). However, Murphy et al. (1988) found 16 patients in their placebo group versus only 10 in the feverfew group who reported mouth ulcerations. Johnson et al. (1985) also mentioned one patient in a another study (not cited) who experienced mouth ulcerations when taking feverfew tablets. The ulcerations resolved when the patient was unwittingly taking a placebo and returned when the patient was blindly switched back to feverfew tablets. The matter of mouth ulcerations from feverfew, whether as an allergic reaction or not, remains unresolved.

Adverse effects from feverfew have usually been mild and reversible. The most frequently reported are gastrointestinal symptoms and mouth ulcerations, which are also the most commonly experienced by long-time users of the herb (Vogler et al., 1998). Adverse effects noted in clinical trials include the following: mouth ulcers, dry and sore tongue, swollen lips and mouth with loss of taste, unpleasant and bitter taste, abdominal pain and indigestion, diarrhea, flatulence, nausea and vomiting, and hypersensitivity reactions (Ernst and Pittler, 2000).

In long-time users, a "postfeverfew syndrome" has been described, associated with discontinuance of prophylactic doses (Johnson et al., 1985). The syndrome, reported by about 10% of 164 feverfew users, was characterized by "moderate to severe aches, pains, and stiffness in joints and muscles together with central nervous symptoms of anxiety and poor sleep" (Johnson et al., 1985, p. 572).

Special Precautions

The essential oil is toxic and should be avoided (Duke, 1985). The fresh leaf has shown potentially toxic activity on smooth muscles ex vivo (Barsby et al., 1991). Because the herb may inhibit clotting, a female patient (age 27) about to undergo an operation was refused when it was learned that she had been taking feverfew during the previous six months. The patient's partial prothromboplastin (PTT) and prothrombin time showed readings of 28.4 and 15.3, respectively. Since the prothrombin time was abnormal (normal time = 11.0 to 13.0 seconds) and the PTT was so high (normal range = 21.0 to 3.0 seconds), the patient was advised to cease the feverfew supplement for a time until her values returned to normal, at which time the operation would be rescheduled (Murphy, 1999).

Individuals who are allergic to plants of the Compositae family have shown a high rate of positive reactions to feverfew in skin patch tests. Among 129 Compositae-allergic individuals, 81% reacted to feverfew, 77% to tansy *(Tanecetum vulgare),* 64% to wild German chamomile *(Chamomilla recutita),* 41% to milfoil *(Achillea millefolium),* and 23% to arnica *(Arnica Montana).* Among 74 chrysanthemum-allergic individuals, 95% reacted positively to patch tests using feverfew, 89% to tansy, and 85% to parthenolide. However, 41% of chrysanthemum-negative individuals also tested positive to feverfew (Paulsen et al., 2001).

Toxicology

Mutagenicity

A study of 30 female chronic users of feverfew who had consumed the herb daily for over 11 months found no differences in the frequency of chromosomal aberrations or the frequency of sister chromatid exchange compared with a matched set of nonusers. Detailed hematological analysis of 60 feverfew users, some of whom had used the herb for more than one year, did not show any significant differences from controls (Johnson et al., 1987; Anderson et al., 1988).

Toxicity in Animal Models

LD_{50} values for feverfew have not been established. No adverse effects have been reported in rats and guinea pigs receiving 100-150 times the human daily dose (Baldwin, 1987).

REFERENCES

Anderson, D., Jenkinson, P.C., Dewdney, R.S., Blowers, S.D., Johnson, E.S., and Kadam, N.P. (1988). Chromosomal aberrations and sister chromatid exchanges in lymphocytes and urine mutagenicity of migraine patients: A comparison of chronic feverfew users and matched non-users. *Human Toxicology* 7: 145-152.

Awang, D.V.C. (1989). *Proceedings of the 57th annual congress of the French-Canadian Association for the Advancement of Science*, May 15-19, University of Quebec at Montreal. Chicoutimi, Quebec: Laboratoire d'Analyse et de Séparation des Essences Vegetales, pp. 1-24.

Awang, D.V.C. (1993). Feverfew fever: A headache for the consumer. *HerbalGram* 29: 34-36, 66.

Awang, D.V.C. (1997). Dutch feverfew trial has negative outcome: The promise of and problem with standardized botanical extracts. *HerbalGram* 41: 16-17.

Awang, D.V.C. (1998). Prescribing therapeutic feverfew (*Tanacetum parthenium* (L.) Schultz Bip., syn. *Chrysanthemum parthenium* (L.) Bernh.). *Integrative Medicine* 1: 11-13.

Baldwin, C.A. (1987). What pharmacists should know about feverfew. *Pharmaceutical Journal* 239: 237-238.

Banthorpe, D.V. and Brown, D.G. (1989). Two unexpected coumarin derivatives from tissue cultures of Compositae species. *Phytochemistry* 28: 3003-3007.

Barsby, R., Salan, U., Knight, D.W., and Hoult, J.R. (1991). Irreversible inhibition of vascular activity by feverfew. *Lancet* 338: 1015 (letter).

Barsby, R., Salan, U., Knight, D.W., and Hoult, J.R. (1993). Feverfew and vascular smooth muscle: Extracts from fresh and dried plants show opposing pharmacological profiles, dependent upon sesquiterpene lactone content. *Planta Medica* 59: 20-25.

Béjar, E. (1996). Parthenolide inhibits the contractile responses of rat stomach fundus to fenfluramine and dextroamphetamine but not serotonin. *Journal of Ethnopharmacology* 50: 1-12.

Bohlmann, F. and Zdero, C. (1982). Sesquiterpene lactones and other constituents from *Tanacetum parthenium*. *Phytochemistry* 21: 2543-2549.

Bradley, P.R. (Ed.) (1992). *British Herbal Compendium, 1*. Bournemouth, Dorset, England: British Herbal Medicine Association, pp. 96-98.

Brown, A.M.G., Edwards, C.M., Davey, M.R., Power, J.B., and Lowe, K.C. (1997). Pharmacological activity of feverfew [*Tanacetum parthenium* (L.) Scultz-Bip.]: Assessment by inhibition of human polymorphonuclear leukocyte chemiluminescence in vitro. *Journal of Pharmacy and Pharmacology* 49: 558-561.

Capasso, F. (1986). The effect of aqueous extract of *Tanacetum parthenium* on arachidonic acid metabolism by rat peritoneal leukocytes. *Journal of Pharmacy and Pharmacology* 38: 71-72.

Cutlan, A.R., Bonilla, L.E., Simon, J.E., and Erwin, J.E. (2000). Intra-specific variability of feverfew: Correlations between parthenolide, morphological traits and seed origin. *Planta Medica* 66: 612-617.

De Weerdt, C.J., Bootsma, H.P.R., and Hendriks, H. (1996). Herbal medicines in migraine prevention. *Phytomedicine* 3: 225-230.

Duke, J.A. (1985). *Handbook of Medicinal Herbs.* Boca Raton, FL: CRC Press, p. 118.

Ernst, E. and Pittler, M.H. (2000). The efficacy and safety of feverfew (*Tanacetum parthenium* L.): An update of a systematic review. *Public Health Nutrition* 3(4A): 509-514.

Foster, S. (1995). Feverfew: When the head hurts. *Alternative and Complementary Therapies* 1 (September-October): 335-337.

Goulden, V. and Wilkinson, S.M. (1998). Patch testing for Compositae allergy. *British Journal of Dermatology* 138: 1018-1021.

Groenewegen, W.A. and Heptinstall, S. (1990). A comparison of the effects of an extract of feverfew and parthenolide, a component of feverfew, on human platelet activity in vitro. *Journal of Pharmacy and Pharmacology* 42: 553-557.

Hausen, B.M. and Osmundsen, P.E. (1983). Contact allergy to parthenolide in *Tanacetum parthenium* (L.) Schultz-Bip. (Feverfew, Asteraceae) and cross-reactions to related sesquiterpene lactone containing Compositae species. *Acta Dermato-Venereologica* (Stockholm) 63: 308-314.

Hayes, N.A. and Foreman, J.C. (1987). The activity of compounds extracted from feverfew on histamine release from rat mast cells. *Journal of Pharmacy and Pharmacology* 39: 466-470.

Heblich, F., Barsby, R.W.J., Houghton, P.J., and McFadzean, I. (1997). Actions of cinnamoyl-dihydroxynardol (CDN), a sesquiterpene ester extracted from the herb feverfew, on the voltage-dependent outward potassium current of mouse neuroblastoma × rat glioma hybrid (NG108-15) cells. *Journal of Physiology* 501.P: 24P-25P.

Hehner, S.P., Hofmann, T.G., Droge, W., Schmitz, M.L. (1999). The anti-inflammatory sesquiterpene lactone parthenolide inhibits NF-κB by targeting the IκB kinase complex. *Journal of Immunology* 163: 5617-5623.

Hendriks, H., Anderson-Wildeboer, Y., Engels, G., Bos, R., and Woerdenbag, H.J (1997). The content of parthenolide and its yield per plant during the growth of *Tanacetum parthenium. Planta Medica* 63: 356-359.

Hendriks, H., Bos, R., and Woerdenbag, H.J. (1996). The essential oil of *Tanacetum parthenium* (L.) Schultz-Bip. *Flavour and Fragrance Journal* 11: 367-371.

Heptinstall, S. (1997). Feverfew *(Tanacetum parthenium):* Biological and therapeutic activity. *Journal of Pharmacy and Pharmacology* 49(Suppl. 4): 33.

Heptinstall, S. and Awang, D.V.C. (1998). Feverfew: A review of its history, its biological and medicinal properties, and the status of commercial preparations of the herb. In Lawson, L.D. and Bauer, R. (Eds.), *Phytomedicines of Europe:*

Chemistry and Biological Activity (pp. 158-175). ACS Symposium Series 691. Washington, DC: American Chemical Society.

Heptinstall, S., Awang, D.V.C., Dawson, B.A., Kindack, D., Knight, D.W., and May, J. (1992). Parthenolide content and bioactivity of feverfew [*Tanacetum parthenium* (L.) Schultz-Bip.]. Estimation of commercial and authenticated feverfew products. *Journal of Pharmacy and Pharmacology* 44: 391-395.

Heptinstall, S., Williamson, L., White, A., and Mitchell, J.R. (1985). Extracts of feverfew inhibit granule secretion in blood platelets and polymorphonuclear leucocytes. *Lancet* 1 (May 11): 1071-1074.

Hewlett, M.J., Begley, M.J., Antoinette Groenwegen, W., Heptinstall, S., Knight, D.W., May, J., Salan, U., and Toplis, D. (1996). Sesquiterpene lactones from feverfew, *Tanacetum parthenium:* Isolation, structural revision, activity against human blood platelet function and implications for migraine therapy. *Journal of the Chemical Society, Perkin Transactions* 1: 1979-1986.

Hobbs, C. (1989). Feverfew—*Tanacetum parthenium*. *HerbalGram* 20: 26-35.

Hoult, J.R.S., Pang, L.H., Bland-Ward, P.A., Forder, R.A., Williams, C.A., and Harborne, J.B. (1995). Inhibition of leukocyte 5-lipoxygenase and cyclooxygenase but not constitutive nitric oxide synthase by tanetin, a novel flavonol derived from feverfew, *Tanacetum parthenium*. *Pharmaceutical Sciences* 1: 71-74.

Hwang, D., Fischer, N.H., Jang, B.C., Tak, H., Kim, J.K., and Lee, W. (1996). Inhibition of the expression of inducible cyclooxygenase and pro-inflammatory cytokines by sesquiterpene lactones in macrophages correlates with the inhibition of MAP kinases. *Biochemical and Biophysical Research Communications* 226: 810-818.

Jain, N.K. and Kulkarni, S.K. (1999). Antinociceptive and anti-inflammatory effects of *Tanacetum parthenium* L. extract in mice and rats. *Journal of Ethnopharmacology* 68: 251-259.

Johnson, E.S., Kadam, N.P., Anderson, D., Jenkinson, P.C., Dewdney, R.S., and Blowers, S.D. (1987). Investigation of possible genotoxic effects of feverfew in migraine patients. *Human Toxicology* 6: 533-534.

Johnson, E.S., Kadam, N.P., Hylands, D.M., and Hylands, P.J. (1985). Efficacy of feverfew as prophylactic treatment of migraine. *British Medical Journal* 291: 569-573.

Kalodera, Z., Pepeljnjak, S., and Petrak, T. (1996). The antimicrobial activity of *Tanacetum parthenium* extract. *Pharmazie* 51: 995-996.

Kang, B.Y., Chung, S.W., and Kim, T.S. (2001). Inhibition of interleukin-12 production in lipopolysaccharide-activated mouse macrophages by parthenolide, a predominant sesquiterpene lactone in *Tanacetum parthenium:* Involvement of nuclear factor-κB. *Immunology Letters* 77: 159-163.

Kuritzky, A., Elhacham, Y., Yerushalmi, Z., and Hering, R. (1994). Feverfew in the treatment of migraine: Its effect on serotonin uptake and platelet activity. *Neurology* 44(Suppl. 2): A201 (abstract 293P).

Kwok, B.H.B., Koh, B., Ndubuisi, M.I., Elofsson, M., and Crews, C.M. (2001). The anti-inflammatory natural product parthenolide from the medicinal herb feverfew directly binds to and inhibits IκB kinase. *Chemistry and Biology* 8: 759-766.

Leung, A.Y. and Foster, S. (1996). *Encyclopedia of Common Natural Ingredients Used in Foods, Drugs, and Cosmetics.* New York: John Wiley and Sons.

Makheja, A.J. and Bailey, J.M. (1982). A platelet phospholipase inhibitor from the medicinal herb feverfew *(Tanacetum parthenium). Prostaglandins, Leukotrienes and Medicine* 8: 653-660.

Marles, R.J., Kaminski, J., Aranson, T., Pazos-Sanou, L., Heptinstall, S., Fischer, N.H., Crompton, C.W., Kindack, D.G., and Awang, D.V.C. (1992). A bioassay for inhibition of serotonin release from bovine platelets. *Journal of Natural Products* 55: 1044-1056.

McGuffin, M., Hobbs, C., Upton, R., and Goldberg, A. (1997). *American Herbal Products Association's Botanical Safety Handbook.* Boca Raton, FL: CRC Press.

Murch, S.J., Simmons, C.B., and Saxena, P.K. (1997). Melatonin in feverfew and other medicinal plants. *Lancet* 350 (November 29): 1598-1599.

Murphy, J.J., Heptinstall, S., and Mitchell, J.R.A. (1988). Randomized double-blind, placebo-controlled trial of feverfew in migraine prevention. *Lancet* (July 23): 189-192.

Murphy, L.M. (1999). Preoperative considerations with herbal medicines. *Association of Operating Room Nurses Journal* 69: 173-183.

Newall, C.A., Anderson, L.A., and Phillipson, J.D. (1996). *Herbal Medicines: A Guide for Health Care Professionals.* London: The Pharmaceutical Press, pp. 119-121.

O'Neill, L.A.J., Barrett, L.M., and Lewis, G.P. (1987). Extracts of feverfew inhibit mitogen induced human peripheral blood mononuclear cell proliferation and cytokine mediated responses: A cytotoxic effect. *British Journal of Clinical Pharmacy* 23: 81-83.

Palevitch, D., Earon, G., and Carasso, R. (1997). Feverfew *(Tanacetum parthenium)* as a prophylactic treatment for migraine: A double-blind placebo-controlled study. *Phytotherapy Research* 11: 508-511.

Patel, N.M., Nozaki, S., Shortle, N.H., Bhat-Nakshatri, P., Newton, T.R., Rice, S., Gelfanov, V., Boswell, S.H., Goulet Jr., R.J., Sledge, G.W., et al. (2000). Paclitaxel sensitivity of breast cancer cells with constitutively active NF-κB is enhanced by IκBα super-repressor and parthenolide. *Oncogene* 19: 4159-4169.

Pattrick, M., Heptinstall, S., and Doherty, M. (1989). Feverfew in rheumatoid arthritis: A double-blind, placebo-controlled study. *Annals of the Rheumatic Diseases* 48: 547-549.

Paulsen, E., Andersen, K.E., and Hausen, B.M. (2001). Sensitization and cross-reaction patterns in Danish Compositae-allergic patients. *Contact Dermatitis* 45: 197-204.

Piela-Smith, T., and Liu, X. (2001). Feverfew extracts and the sesquiterpene lactone parthenolide inhibit intracellular adhesion molecule-1 expression in human synovial fibroblasts. *Cellular Immunology* 209: 89-96.

Pugh, W.J. and Sambo, K. (1988). Prostaglandin synthetase inhibitors in feverfew. *Journal of Pharmacy and Pharmacology* 40: 743-745.

Ross, J.J., Arnason, J.T., and Birnboim, H.C. (1999). Low concentrations of the feverfew component parthenolide inhibit in vitro growth of tumor lines in a cytostatic fashion. *Planta Medica* 65: 126-129.

Thies, F., Nebe-von-Caron, G., Powell, J.R., Yaqoob, P., Newsholme, E.A., and Calder, P.C. (2001). Dietary supplementation with γ-linolenic acid or fish oil decreases T lymphocyte proliferation in healthy older humans. *Journal of Nutrition* 131: 1918-1927.

Tournier, H., Schinella, G., De Balsa, E.M., Buschiazzo, H., Manez, S., and de Buschiazzo, P.M. (1999). Effect of the chloroform extract of *Tanacetum vulgare* and one of its active principles, parthenolide, on experimental gastric ulcer in rats. *Journal of Pharmacy and Pharmacology* 51: 215-219.

Vogler, B.K., Pittler, M.H., and Ernst, E. (1998). Feverfew as a preventive treatment for migraine: A systematic review. *Cephalalgia* 18: 704-708.

Wagner, H., Fessler, B., Lotter, H., and Wray, V. (1988). A new chlorine-containing sesquiterpenoid lactone from *Chrysanthemum parthenium*. *Planta Medica* 54: 171-172.

Weber, J.T., O'Conner, M.F., Hayataka, K., Colson, N., Medora, R., Russo, E.B., and Parker, K.K. (1997). Activity of parthenolide at $5HT_{2A}$ receptors. *Journal of Natural Products* 60: 651-653.

Werbach, M.R. and Murray, M.T. (1994). *Botanical Influences on Illness*. Tarzana, CA: Third Line Press.

Williams, C.A., Harborne, J.B., Geiger, H., and Hoult, J.R. (1999). The flavonoids of *Tanacetum parthenium* and *T. vulgare* and their anti-inflammatory properties. *Phytochemistry* 51: 417-423.

Williams, C.A., Hoult, J.R.S., Harborne, J.B., Greenham, J., and Eagles, J.A. (1995). A biologically active lipophilic flavonol from *Tanacetum parthenium*. *Phytochemistry* 38: 267-270.

Williamson, L.M., Harvey, D.M., Sheppard, K.J., and Fletcher, J. (1988). Effect of feverfew on phagocytosis of *Candida guilliermondii* by neutrophils. *Inflammation* 12: 11-16.

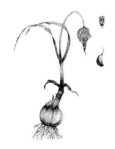

Garlic

BOTANICAL DATA

Scientific name: *Allium sativum* L.

Family name: Liliaceae

Common names: garlic, ajo, allium, stinking rose

Description

More than 700 species of *Allium* are known (Mabberley, 1990); the genus includes chives *(A. schoenoprasum),* leeks *(A. ampeloprasum* and other spp.), shallots *(A. ascalonicum,* probably a cultigen of *A. cepa),* and common onions (cultigens of *A. cepa).*

HISTORY AND TRADITIONAL USES

The Latin name *Allium* may have been derived from the Celtic word "al" which means smarting or burning (Hahn, 1996). The name "garlic" comes from the Celtic "gar," a lance, referring to its leaves, and "leek," a succulent plant (Nagourney, 1998).

Garlic is a common food plant used in all parts of the world. Modern garlic probably originated from a wild ancestor in Central Asia. One of the oldest of cultivated plants, garlic has been cultivated for more than 5,000 years. It has been valued as a flavoring, a food, and as a medicine. In addition to its well-recognized medicinal properties, it is often the strong odor of garlic that gives rise to its notoriety. As early as 3200 B.C., Egyptians wrote about garlic as an important crop and King Tutankhaman's tomb was found to contain garlic cloves. Greek laborers, while building the Cheops pyramid around 2900 B.C., lived mainly on onions and garlic, as noted by the Greek historian Herodotus. Confucius, around 500 B.C., mentioned that to reek of garlic was considered improper. Marco Polo noted that the Chinese consumed raw liver in garlic sauce. As early as the sixth century B.C., the medicinal uses of garlic were described in India, although the eating of garlic was considered a loathsome practice. The Romans used garlic for many purposes. Roman noblemen gave garlic to their soldiers and laborers, and Roman gladiators were known to eat garlic before combat (Ensminger et al., 1994).

Pedersen (1994) notes mystical stories of garlic through the ages. In a Moslem tradition, garlic is said to have sprung up from under the foot of Satan as he stepped out of the Garden of Eden after Adam's expulsion. In Scandinavian lore, a mythical female named Hulda Talle-Maja was tricked into revealing the powerful properties of garlic, which she used to keep a bull from wandering off at night. Jain and Apitz-Castro (1994) recount tales of the vampire-repellant effects of garlic.

The uses of garlic in traditional or folk medicine include the treatment of colds, coughs, chronic bronchitis, earache, toothache, high blood pressure, arteriosclerosis, dandruff, and hysteria. As a cold infusion, juice, or as a tincture, garlic has also been used to treat cancers. As a tea, syrup, tincture, other preparations, or as fresh cloves, garlic has been used to treat fever, flu symptoms, sinus congestion, shortness of breath, stomachache, headache, rheumatism, gout, hypertension, ulcers, pinworms, and snakebites. Native Americans and the Chinese used garlic as a remedy for earaches, scurvy, and flatulence (Hahn, 1996; Rivlin, 2001). The Chinese also used garlic in the treatment of diarrhea, dysentery, diphtheria, pulmonary tuberculosis, bloody urine, whooping cough, hepatitis, typhoid, tracheoma, scalp ringworm, hypersensitive teeth, and vaginal trichomoniasis (Leung and Foster, 1996).

CHEMISTRY

Fresh garlic contains minute amounts of vitamins, minerals, and trace elements. Germanium and selenium, two trace elements thought to have antitumor activities, are found in detectable amounts. The genus *Allium* contains abundant amounts of sulfur compounds (Lawson, 1996), which are primarily responsible for its therapeutic and biological activities (Abdullah et al., 1988). Many sulfur-containing compounds are intrinsically unstable and change or interconvert with enzymatic action or heat. Garlic contains enzymes such as alliinase, peroxidase, and myrosinase which can act on sulfur-containing substrates upon the crushing or maceration of the garlic cloves. Because these enzymes can be degraded or inactivated by alkali, heat, and sometimes stomach acids, the chemical composition of garlic and garlic products may vary widely, depending on cooking or processing treatments.

Fresh garlic cloves contain 0.1-0.36% volatile oils, the majority of which are allicin (diallyldisulfide-S-oxide), diallyl thiosulfinate, allylpropyl disulfide, diallyl disulfide, and diallyl trisulfide. Other lesser components contained in the volatile oils include dimethyl sulfide, dimethyl disulfide, dimethyl trisulfide, allyl methyl sulfide, and 2,3,4-trithiapentane. Recent studies suggest that diallyl trisulfide is the major component of freshly distilled garlic oils (Leung and Foster, 1996). Other constituents of the volatile oils are monoterpenoids, citral, geraniol, linalool, and α- and β-phellandrene (Leung and Foster, 1996).

Other constituents include alliin (S-allyl-L-cysteine sulfoxide), S-methyl-L-cysteine sulfoxide, enzymes (alliinase, peroxidase, and myrosinase), ajoenes (E,Z-ajoene, E,Z-methyl-ajoene, dimethylajoene), protein (16.8% dry wt.), vitamins, minerals, and amino acids (Leung and Foster, 1996). Homogenized garlic extract has been found to contain prostaglandins A_2 and F_{1a} (Leung and Foster, 1996).

First isolated in the 1940s, allicin is the source of the pungent odor of garlic. Allicin is produced by the action of the enzyme alliinase on alliin, is further converted into sulfides, and although stable to dilute acids, is decomposed by alkali and heat (Leung and Foster, 1996).

Garlic preparations vary in composition. Diallyl sulfide and other allyl sulfides are found exclusively in distilled garlic oil. Thiosulfinates, e.g., allicin, are released only from garlic cloves and garlic powder products, and vinyl dithiins and ajoenes are detected only in garlic macerated in vegetable oil (Leung and Foster, 1996).

Impact of Processing

Koch and Lawson (1996) reviewed and summarized some of the changes that can occur to the constituents of garlic through cooking and other processing treatments. Cooking denatures proteins and therefore inactivates enzymes in the process (Koch and Lawson, 1996). Allinase, the major protein in garlic, is the enzyme which converts alliin into allicin. Recent research suggests that its identity is closer to being a glycoprotein which contains mannose residues (Krest and Keusgen, 1999). Allicin produces the characteristic odor of garlic and possesses many biological actions, e.g., lipid-lowering and antithrombotic effects (Koch and Lawson, 1996).

Boiling whole garlic can completely inactivate alliinase, although approximately 1% of alliin is converted to allicin prior to inactivation. Boiling will also hydrolyze about 12% of the γ-glutamyl cysteines to S-1-propenyl cysteine and the bioactive S-allylcysteine (Koch and Lawson, 1996).

Crushing garlic transforms most of the cysteine sulfoxides into thiosulfinates. Heating crushed garlic at boiling temperature in a closed container completely converts thiosulfinates into diallyl trisulfide and other sulfides. Boiling in an open container, however, evaporates 97% of the sulfides but retains 7% of the thiosulfinates. Crushed garlic stir-fried in hot soybean oil retains about 16% of the sulfides, but destroys all the allicin. Microwaving at 650 watts (single whole cloves of garlic weighing 5-6 g) inactivates alliinase completely in 30 seconds, with methyl-specific alliinase inactivated in 15 seconds (Koch and Lawson, 1996).

The formation of volatile flavor components by various cooking treatments such as oil-frying, boiling, and microwaving has been studied. Sixteen volatile compounds were identified for boiled garlic, while 40-60 compounds were identified for other methods (Koch and Lawson, 1996).

Investigations by Weber et al. (1992) have shown that allinase is completely and irreversibly inhibited by stomach acid due to its inability to form allicin or other thiosulfinates below pH 3.6.

THERAPEUTIC APPLICATIONS

Garlic is often reported to be a cure-all for diseases common in modern Western civilization. Diseases and conditions such as hyperlipemia, hypertension, heavy-metal disorders, and various infections are reported to have been successfully treated with garlic (Abdullah et al., 1988). Table 1 summarizes the major classes of therapeutic activity that have been identified for garlic and lists the constituents most likely implicated.

PRECLINICAL STUDIES

Cardiovascular and Circulatory Functions

Arrhythmia

Evidence of antiarrhythmic effects of garlic has been reported by Martin et al. (1994) after animal and in vitro studies. The results suggest that garlic dialysate has a significant antiarrhythmic effect in both ventricular and supraventricular arrhythmias and that the effect resulted from calcium modulation.

Cholesterol and Lipid Metabolism

The fact that the sulfur-containing constituents of garlic are readily transformed due to enzymatic processes, heat, or other treatments, bears importantly on the potential therapeutic effects, or lack of effects, of various garlic extracts and preparations. For instance, a recent study in the *Journal of the American Medical Association* (Berthold et al., 1998) received much attention because in a double-blind, placebo-controlled, crossover study in 25 patients, those receiving garlic oil over a period of 12 weeks failed to display significantly lower plasma levels of cholesterol compared to the pla-

TABLE 1. Actions of Active Constituents

Therapeutic Action	Active Constituents
Lipid- and cholesterol-lowering	Allicin, possibly S-allyl cysteine and other compounds
Hypotensive	Apparently not allicin; responsible compounds are unknown
Antithrombotic	Allicin, ajoene
Antibiotic and antifungal	Allicin and related thiosulfinates, ajoene
Anticancer	Allicin-derived compounds (probably not allicin since cooked garlic is active), S-allyl cysteine, diallyl sulfide, and possibly other unidentified compounds
Antioxidant	Allicin, allicin-derived sulfides at low concentrations; glutamylcysteines, S-allyl-cysteines at higher concentrations
Immunomodulatory	Multiple compounds; allicin-derived oils and allicin-depleted extracts are both active; possibly also protein constituents
Hypoglycemic	Allicin
Liver-protective	Allicin, S-methylmercaptocysteine, S-allylmercaptocysteine, diallyl sulfide, and others

Source: Koch and Lawson, 1996.

cebo group. Although this study has been touted as "debunking" the putative cholesterolemic properties of garlic, a closer examination of the known chemical composition of garlic oil reveals that the garlic oil in the study contained primarily sulfides, but no significant quantities of allicin, the constituent most closely linked to hypocholesterolemic activity (see Table 1). Failing to utilize an allicin-containing preparation has rendered this much publicized study fundamentally flawed.

Numerous studies have established a consensus that garlic is effective in lowering serum cholesterol; however, the mechanism of action is not yet completely understood. Garlic appears to affect liver enzymes involved in lipogenesis (Yeh and Yeh, 1994). Oral supplementation with garlic extracts may also facilitate mobilization of tissue lipids into circulation (Lau, 1989). It has been suggested that organic tellurium compounds, present in high concentrations in fresh garlic, may block cholesterol formation by inhibiting squalene epoxide, the penultimate enzyme in the biosynthetic pathway to cholesterol (Larner, 1994). Other garlic compounds (e.g., *S*-allyl cysteine sulfoxide) may also be implicated in the cholesterol-lowering actions (Sheela and Augusti, 1995). Exactly which compounds in garlic are mainly responsible for this action is not presently known.

Hypertension

The exact mechanism of action of garlic on blood pressure is not known. However, garlic juice has been shown to exert a direct relaxant effect on isolated smooth and cardiac muscle, suggesting a likely mechanism for its antihypertensive effects (Aqel et al., 1991). Others have found evidence suggesting that garlic prevents hypertension by activating the production of nitric oxide (NO). Rats chronically administered the NO synthase inhibitor L-NAME (N^ω-nitro-L-arginine-methyl-ester) as part of their diet developed arterial hypertension, whereas rats administered the same amount of the inhibitor plus 2% of their diet as dried garlic did not. (Systolic blood pressure remained the same in control and garlic-fed rats.) Urinary excretion of NO metabolism end products (nitrite and nitrate) increased in the garlic-fed rats more than any of the others. In the group receiving L-NAME, they were significantly lower than that of control rats, and in the garlic plus L-NAME group the levels were the same as those of the control rats. The researchers concluded that the hypertension induced by L-NAME was blocked by the ability of garlic to antagonize L-NAME inhibition of NO (Pedraza-Chaverri et al., 1998).

Thrombosis, Hemostasis, and Embolism

In vitro and animal studies have supported most of the clinical findings of the cardioprotective effects of garlic (Ali et al., 2000). For instance, Orekhov et al. (1995) found that garlic extract added to cell cultures of smooth muscle cells derived from human aortic atherosclerotic plaques of heart attack victims lowered levels of cholesterol and cholesterol esters and inhibited atherosclerotic cell proliferative activity, suggesting that garlic possesses direct antiatherosclerotic effects at the arterial cell level. Another group studied the effect of ajoene, one of the sulfur compounds from garlic, on platelet deposition in isolated pig aortic subendothelia (Apitz-Castro et al., 1992). In an assay that mimicked interaction of blood with deeply injured vessel walls, at physiologically relevant shear rates, ajoene inhibited platelet-dependent thrombus formation, and this action was related to a concomitant inhibition of fibrinogen binding.

Efendy et al. (1997) found that an aged garlic extract (AGE) (Wakunaga Pharmaceutical Co., Ltd., Hiroshima, Japan, Kyolic) could directly inhibit the proliferation of smooth muscle in vitro. On experimentally induced atherosclerosis in rabbits, those fed the same AGE showed 20% less cholesterol than other groups. A group fed a standard diet supplemented with 1% cholesterol showed a high degree of fatty streak lesions on the surface of the thoracic aorta, whereas rabbits on the same dietary regimen supplemented with AGE showed approximately 64% less. The size of neointima in this group was half that of the 1% cholesterol group which also showed lipid-filled lesions not found in the AGE group.

Immune Functions; Inflammation and Disease

Cancer

Antiproliferative activity. Lamm and Riggs (2001) reported that aged garlic extract administered in the drinking water (500 mg/mL) of mice with bladder cancer caused a significant increase in the rate of survival ($p < 0.048$) and inhibition of tumor volume ($p < 0.001$). The researchers attributed the antitumor effect of garlic to enhancement of the immune system. Ip et al. (1996) found that selenium-enriched garlic administered to rats could inhibit early-stage mammary carcinogenesis but not the late stage. Other studies have emphasized the significance of dietary synergism in cancer chemoprevention. For example, Schaffer et al. (1997) reported that a combination of dietary garlic powder and selenium was more effective than either dietary adjunct alone in preventing the induced formation of adducts in mammary epithelial cells of the rat. Dietary concentrations of sodium selenite required to reduce adduct formation by 50% were increasingly lowered with increasing amounts of garlic in the diet. However, in animal studies Ip and Lisk (1995) presented evidence suggesting that the tumor-inhibiting activity of high-selenium garlic primarily depends on the greater amount of selenium available from the garlic, rather than the garlic itself.

Allicin has shown tumor-inhibiting effects in mice (Reuter, 1995). Besides allicin, other constituents of garlic have shown activity (Dirsch et al., 1998; Pinto et al., 1997). The proliferation of human prostate carcinoma (LNCaP) cells was significantly inhibited in vitro by the AGE water-soluble constituent *S*-allylmercaptocysteine (SAMC). Notably, the inhibition persisted following removal of the media. Tumor growth compared to the control at seven days postexposure to SAMC was inhibited by 79%. In the same test, oil-soluble constituents of AGE, diallylsulfide and diallyldisulfide, also inhibited tumor growth by highly significant amounts (80% and 85%, respectively). The researchers postulated that the inhibition of the human prostate cancer cells in vitro by SAMC may be due to inhibition of ornithine decarboxylase activity, an enzyme that allows initiation of polyamine biosynthesis which leads to cell division (Pinto et al., 1997).

Chemopreventive activity. Binding of metabolites formed through bioactivation of DMBA (7,12-dimethylbenz[a]anthracene) to the epithelial

DNA of mammary cells resulted in an increase of mammary tumor incidence (Liu et al., 1992). Rats administered DMBA that were fed a diet containing peeled and crushed garlic (700 mg in corn oil three times/week p.o. by gavage) showed significantly (64%) less DMBA-induced DNA adducts compared to corn oil-fed controls. Heating the garlic in a microwave oven (600 watts) for 30 seconds resulted in only slightly less anticarcinogenic activity, while heating for 60 seconds resulted in a complete absence of protective activity. However, if the peeled and crushed garlic was allowed to stand for 10 min at room temperature prior to microwave heating for 60 seconds, the protective effect was intact.

Similar results were obtained using a convection oven (45 min at 176°C). Microwave heating for 30 seconds resulted in a 90% loss of alliinase enzyme activity and 60 seconds treatment abolished the activity of the enzyme. In tests using the garlic constituents alliin, SAC (*S*-allyl cysteine), and DADS (diallyl disulfide), only the latter two inhibited DMBA-DNA binding which resulted in 47% and 51% less DMBA-induced DNA adduct formation, respectively. In conclusion, the method of processing garlic has a major impact on its activity, with the active allyl sulfur compounds dependent on the time alliinase activity is given to act and the amount of alliinase activity available. This is because the release of alliinase from the crushing or chapping of garlic results in the rapid conversion of alliin to the chemopreventive allicin, which in turn is converted to DADS, diallyl disulfide, ajoene and other sulfur compounds (Song and Milner, 1999).

Rats challenged with the carcinogen benzo[*a*]pyrene and fed powdered garlic as 0.1%, 0.5%, and 1% of their standard diet for four weeks, showed significantly less urinary mutagens at all concentrations of garlic ($p < 0.001$). Researchers also found that the addition of garlic caused a significant stimulation of cancer chemopreventive substances in the lung and microsomes of the liver (quinone reductase and liver glutathione-*S*-transferase) at each concentration of garlic (Polasa and Krishnaswamy, 1997). Mice of both sexes administered the mutagenic toxin, sodium arsenite, and fed garlic clove paste in an amount based on a daily human intake equivalent (6 g/60 kg), showed significantly less chromosomal aberrations in their bone marrow (Choudhury et al., 1997).

Dimethylhydrazine (DMH) is a potent necrogenic hepatocarcinogen that alkylates hepatocellular DNA. In experiments with rats subjected to partial hepatectomy (to stimulate liver cell proliferation) and exposure to DMH, Hayes et al. (1987) found that pretreatment with diallyl sulfide (25-100 mg/kg i.g.) completely prevented liver necrosis initiated by the toxin, reduced levels of enzymatic markers for liver damage in hepatocytes, and substantially reduced the binding of [^{14}C]-DMH to DNA in cultured liver cells. According to the researchers, DMH probably inhibited hepatocarcinogenicity by reducing the promoting influences of postnecrotic regeneration, rather than by preventing initiation of the process.

Garlic was shown to have a protective effect against experimental heavy metal intoxication in rats (Reuter, 1995). The mechanism of action appears to be that garlic extracts protect the membranes of red blood cells against heavy metal ions by binding to the metal ions and excreting the heavy metal sulfur complexes. Binding capacity of garlic has been determined for mercury, lead, organic mercury compounds, cadmium, and zinc (Reuter, 1995).

Cytotoxicity. A major constituent of crushed garlic, ajoene, has recently been shown to induce apoptosis (programmed cell death) of human leukemic (HL-60) cells in vitro. Exposure of the cells to ajoene caused the cells to undergo DNA fragmentation in a dose-dependent manner. Concentrations of ajoene above 5 μM caused a significant increase in the concentration of apoptotic cells (Dirsch et al., 1998). Ajoene also caused a dose-dependent induction of apoptosis in the peripheral mononuclear blood cells (PMBC) of a patient with chronic leukemia and exhibited similar apoptotic potency in the patient's leukemia cells in vitro as previously found in the HL-60 cells. Yet, in PMBC from healthy human donors, apoptosis was not induced by ajoene. Ajoene was also ineffective at inducing apoptosis in human neuroblastoma cells (SH-SY5Y), colon carcinoma cells (DLD-1), squamous carcinoma cells (A431), and in 200 human carcinoma cell lines. In addition, Dirsch and colleagues showed that in HL-60 cells, ajoene could stimulate the production of reactive oxygen species (free radicals), and activate nuclear translocation of NF-κB, a transcriptional factor involved in signaling apoptotic processes. They concluded that the results support the argument for consuming garlic as a means of cancer treatment and prevention (Dirsch et al., 1998).

Siegers, Steffen et al. (1999) reported no significant in vitro antitumor activity from garlic powder (Lichtwer Pharma, Berlin) against human colon carcinoma (Caco-2) or human hepatoma (HepG2) cells, nor from an AGE (Lichtwer, Berlin, Kyolic) with an enriched alliin content (8-10% L(+)-alliin, a.k.a. *S*-allyl-*L*-cysteine sulfoxide). However, the garlic extract plus garlic powder at 10% of the preparation significantly inhibited the growth of both tumor cell types in a concentration-dependent manner. The researchers theorized that the breakdown products of alliin (e.g., polysulphides or allicin) were the more likely active constituents, whereby allinase, provided by the garlic powder but devoid in the extract, may have facilitated the release of the active breakdown products (Siegers, Steffen et al., 1999). The processing of garlic powder can significantly alter alliinase; however, even though enzyme activity becomes lower in the process, it remains intact enough to facilitate the conversion of alliin to allicin (Krest and Keusgen, 1999). When Siegers, Steffen et al. (1999) also tested the two garlic preparations against human lymphatic leukemia cells (CCRF CEM), they found significant growth-inhibitory activity from either preparation ($\geq$ 30 μg/mL), but in this instance they found no increased activity from their combination (Siegers, Steffen et al., 1999).

Immune Functions

Immunopotentiation. Garlic administration may enhance immune function (Kyo, Uda, Kasuga, et al., 1999). Although the therapeutic actions of garlic extracts have been mostly attributed to low-molecular weight constituents such as the sulfur-containing compounds, evidence suggests that higher molecular weight components of the protein fraction may contribute to an immunostimulatory effect. Hirao et al. (1987) reported that F-4, a protein fraction isolated from aged garlic extract (AGE) (Wakunaga Pharmaceutical Co., Ltd., Japan) strongly stimulated macrophages, as measured by elevated glucose utilization and stimulation of cytostatic action on co-cultured P815 tumor cells. The fraction also stimulated lymphocyte proliferation in cultured spleen cells and, from intraperitoneal administration in vivo, was active in the carbon clearance test, a measure of macrophage activation. Kyo et al. (1998) showed that the increase in NK (natural killer) cell activity from oral administration of AGE in tumor-bearing mice was just as potent as PSK (a natural polysaccharide immunomodulator used clinically in Japan) (Kureha Chemical Co., Ltd.) and comparatively more effective at stimulating T cell functions.

Immunoprotection. The effect aged garlic extract (AGE, 0.1% *S*-allyl-cysteine) on the amelioration of immune suppression was examined in an animal model of psychological stress-induced immune suppression. Compared to unstressed male mice, those subjected to psychological stress showed a significant depression of NK cell activity and of spleen weight. Compared to an equally stressed control group, administration of AGE (10 mL/kg) 24 h prior to and one hour before psychological stress caused a significant difference, with levels of NK cell activity and spleen weight nearly equal to those of unstressed controls (each $p < 0.01$) (Kyo, Uda, Ushijima et al., 1999).

Infectious Diseases

Fungal infections. Ajoene has been implicated as antifungal. Yoshida et al. (1987) tested various fractions isolated from an aqueous garlic extract in broth cultures of *Aspergillus niger* and *Candida albicans*. Ajoene proved to be more active than allicin as an antifungal; 95% inhibitory concentrations were < 20 mg/mL for both fungi; however, with the exception of *Staphylococcus aureus,* it was not active against the Gram-positive and Gram-negative bacteria tested.

Microbial infections. Garlic has broad-spectrum activity against many human pathogenic microorganisms (Harris et al., 2001). The primary active compound appears to be allicin (Adetumbi and Lau, 1983).

Garlic exhibits a broad spectrum antibiotic activity against Gram-positive and Gram-negative bacteria, including *Klebsiella, Corynebacterium, Mycobacterium,* and *Pasteurella* strains (Reuter, 1995). Aqueous garlic extract showed some degree of inhibition of growth of all the organisms tested except *Klebsiella;* however, none of the antibiotics tested showed any inhibitory effect on the resistant strains. Another in vitro study reported similar results for aqueous garlic extract, tracing the activity to allicin (Ahsan and Islam, 1996). Garlic extracts have shown promising in vitro activity against a variety of antibiotic-resistant bacteria, including clinical strains of *Staphylococcus, Escherichia coli, Proteus, Salmonella, Pseudomonas,* and *Klebsiella,* when tested in comparison with conventional antibiotics (Singh and Shukla, 1984).

Garlic has shown such potent activity against the so-called ulcer bug, *Helicobacter pylori,* that researchers have suggested its use in clinical trials in patients infected with the bug (Jonkers et al., 1999; O'Gara et al., 2000); however, the results of pilot studies in humans fail to support this use (Ernst, 1999; Graham et al., 1999). In one study, crushed garlic was more potent than several different commercial garlic tablets and showed a concentration-dependent, synergistic effect against *H. pylori* in combination with omeprazole in vitro (Jonkers et al., 1999). Undiluted garlic oil is a more potent inhibitor of *H. pylori* than garlic powder. The constituents responsible for in vitro anti-*H-pylori* activity were identified as diallyl sulfides, particularly allicin (MIC 4.0 µg/mL), which was far more potent than diallyl disulfide (MIC 100 to 200 µg/mL), although similar in potency to diallyl trisulfide (MIC 3 to 6 µg/mL) (O'Gara et al., 2000).

Viral infections. Therapeutic effects of garlic have been demonstrated against influenza virus A and B in mice when applied intranasally or by intramuscular injection. In addition, prophylactic application prolonged the survival time of infected mice (Reuter, 1995).

Tsai et al. (1985) reported that a commercial garlic extract showed activity against influenza and herpes simplex, but not Coxsackie viruses. The inhibitory effect was found from concentrations below those that caused damage to the cultured tissue cells.

Hughes et al. (1989) tested the effect of a commercial garlic product against a broad range of animal viruses. Incubation for 6 h in the presence of garlic extracts decreased the titer of poliovirus and parainfluenza-3. Bioassay-directed isolation of the active fraction yielded a compound identical to allicin.

Metabolic and Nutritional Functions

Antioxidant Activity

The cancer-preventive and liver-protective actions of many phytomedicines and their active phytochemicals are frequently attributable to antioxidant actions, and garlic falls into the same category. Several in vitro and in vivo studies have demonstrated that garlic extracts, as well as some of the sulfur-containing compounds, have potent effects in protecting the liver from damage due to exposure to carcinogens or other toxins. Of the constituents in garlic, the essential oil, alliin, S-allylmercaptocysteine (ASSC), and SAMC, have all shown antihepatotoxic activity in cultured liver cells exposed to carbon tetrachloride (CCl_4) or galactosamine. The mechanism of action was attributed to the inhibition of lipid peroxidation. In addition, alliin was more effective than vitamin E in preventing the formation of lipid peroxides in rat liver microsome preparations in vitro (Hikino et al., 1986).

In mice given acute hepatitis by exposure to hepatotoxins, oral administration of AGE, SAC, or ASAMC, were all effective in preventing the rise of serum enzymes considered markers for liver damage and in preventing liver necrosis (Nakagawa et al., 1988). SAMC (100 mg/kg p.o.) was by far the most potent, significantly reducing liver necrosis and lowering levels of marker enzymes. The researchers hypothesized that these compounds activate glutathione-related enzymes known to be involved in protecting liver tissues from oxidative damage. In addition, the same enzymes are known to function as potent scavengers of free radicals.

Heinle and Betz (1994) reported that rats fed a cholesterol-rich diet supplemented with garlic powder showed increased tissue levels of glutathione peroxidase and glutathione disulfide reductase (by 100% and 87%, respectively), compared to controls fed a cholesterol-rich diet without garlic powder. I'örök et al. (1994) demonstrated that garlic homogenates have significant in vitro radical-scavenging activity; the homogenates were particularly effective in quenching the radicals present in cigarette smoke. Ide and Lau (1999) showed that pretreatment with AGE could prevent the in vitro depletion of intracellular glutathione and the increase in lactate dehydrogenase-release induced by oxidized low density cholesterol (LDL) (significantly from ≥ 0.1 mg/mL). Similarly, in murine macrophages (J774 cells), pretreatment with AGE significantly dose-dependently suppressed oxidized LDL-induced peroxide production from ≥ 1 mg/mL. AGE also inhibited cytokine-induced NO production by macrophages (significantly from ≥ 2.5 mg/mL), and in a cell-free system exhibited dose-dependent hydrogen peroxide-scavenging activity (e.g., by 22.8% at 0.1 mg/mL). The researchers concluded that since AGE can ameliorate oxidative stress by scavenging peroxides in macrophages and endothelial cells and by modulating glutathione levels in endothelial cells, it may therefore be useful in preventing cardiovascular diseases and atherosclerosis (Ide and Lau, 1999).

Siegers, Röbke et al. (1999) examined the effect of garlic preparations on superoxide production in vitro in human granulocytes. An alliin-enriched garlic extract (8-10% alliin) with alliinase inactivated showed no inhibition of phorbol myristyl acetate (PMA)-induced superoxide production (1,000 μg/mL), whereas a garlic powder did (IC_{50} 390 μg/mL). When the two were combined as a 90% garlic powder plus 10% alliin-enriched garlic extract preparation, superoxide production was more potently inhibited (IC_{50} 295 μg/mL), although not as much as the ingredients in the reverse proportion could provide (IC_{50} 160 μg/mL). These results suggest that allicin, a metabolite of alliin, may be the active oxygen radical-scavenging elicitor (Siegers, Röbke et al., 1999).

Neurological, Psychological, and Behavioral Functions

Neurotoxicity/Neuroprotection

Numagami et al. (1996) tested garlic in a model of transient global ischemia in rats. Pretreatment of the rats with a high dose of an AGE (Wakunaga, 0.5 mL/kg i.p.) significantly inhibited the formation of edema of the ipsilateral hemisphere. A wide dosage range (0.08-0.5 mL/kg) significantly reduced the amount of brain water compared to the control group. S-allyl cysteine (SAC) also caused a significant reduction in the amount of water in the brain, and in neither treatment group were there any deaths. SAC caused a significant inhibition of free radical production in the brain and reduction in the size of brain infarct in animals treated with SAC compared to controls. The researchers found that the efficacy of SAC was comparable to that of the AGE in protecting against experimental brain ischemia in rats.

Moriguchi, Matsuura et al. (1997) reported that a phytoalexin in garlic known as "allixin" significantly promotes the survival of primary cultured neurons and increases the branching points of hippocampal neurons. Moriguchi, Saito et al. (1997) chronically administered an AGE (Wakunaga brand) as 2% of the diet of senescence accelerated mice with characteristic age-related brain atrophy. (The extract contained allicin < 0.01 mg/g and S-allyl cysteine 1.6-2.4 mg/g.) Compared to controls not fed the AGE, decreased brain weight was significantly prevented, as well as frontal cerebrum atrophy and the degree of senescence, as measured in skin coarseness and hair loss. In behavioral changes, the decrease of conditioned avoidance response was significantly and continuously ameliorated in the mice treated with the AGE, and the researchers also found evidence to suggest that the AGE elicited a preventive effect against learning impairment.

CLINICAL STUDIES

Studies indicate that garlic contains compounds which can inhibit platelet aggregation, increase fibrinolysis, lower blood pressure, and enhance antioxidant activity. However, Neil and Silagy (1994) note that there are difficulties in cross-comparison of studies due to the lack of standardization of many garlic preparations, and the methodological weaknesses of many of the earlier clinical trails.

Cardiovascular and Circulatory Disorders

Atherosclerosis

In a randomized, double-blind, placebo-controlled trail lasting 48 months in 152 patients (ages 40-80) diagnosed with advanced atherosclerotic plaques, Koscielny et al. (1999) reported a significant reduction in arteriosclerotic plaque formation in patients taking garlic powder tablets (900 mg/day, equivalent to Lichtwer Pharma AG, Berlin, LI 111) compared to placebo; however in a subsequent analysis of the trial it was determined that the effect was only significant in the female participants (Siegel and Klüssendorf, 2000). Compared to the placebo group, plaque volume in the garlic group showed a reduction of between 6% and 18%. In the ages of 50 to 80 years, the increase in plaque volume in the placebo group was 15.6% over the four-year treatment period, whereas those in the garlic group showed a reduction in plaque volume of 2.6%, indicating a regression in plaque volume. On the whole, those in the garlic group showed a constant plaque volume in the age span of 50 to 80 years, indicating a preventive effect. Results were measured in part using B-mode ultrasound and all the patients had a minimum of one major risk factor (e.g., high systolic BP, smoking, diabetes mellitus, or hypercholesterolemia). Excluded were pregnant patients and those taking omega-3 fatty acids, calcium antagonists, aspirin, and any other agents that might affect the primary outcome measurements of plaque volume changes in the femoral and common artery, as well as changes in the combined intimal-medial thickness of arterial vessel walls.

Byrne et al. (1999) employed samples obtained from a randomized, double-blind, placebo-controlled parallel trial on garlic (Kwai tablets, 900 mg/day) in moderately hypercholesterolemic volunteers conducted by Neil et al. (1996) to determine whether the lipids of patients taking the garlic preparation showed any difference in oxidative characteristics compared to the placebo group. Tests showed that there was no significant difference compared to placebo in lipoprotein(a) and other lipid/lipoprotein profiles (e.g., LDL, HDL, triglycerides, total cholesterol, Apo A, Apo B), nor in antibodies to oxidized LDL or the oxidative resistance of LDL (Byrne et al., 1999).

Cardiotonic; Cardioprotection

Legnani et al. (1993) tested the effect of a dried garlic preparation (Sapec, Lichtwer Pharma GmbH, Berlin, Germany) on platelet aggregation and fibrinolysis in ten healthy male volunteers, ages 20-26 years in a randomized, double-blind, placebo-controlled crossover study. The extract was standardized to contain 1.3% alliin and consisted of 300 mg tablets. For 14 days, subjects received 900 mg/day of the extract or placebo and after a 14-day washout period were crossed over to take the opposite preparation. Fibrinolytic measurements showed mean levels of tissue plasminogen activator levels were significantly higher after subjects received the garlic extract compared to the placebo. Platelet aggregation was significantly decreased after day 14 of the garlic treatment versus baseline and versus day seven of the garlic treatment or placebo. Collagen-stimulated β-thromboglobulin (β-TG) release in platelet-rich plasma of the volunteers after day 14 of the garlic treatment showed a significant decrease versus baseline and were significantly lower compared to placebo.

Breithaupt-Grögler et al. (1997) performed an observational study on a cross section of healthy, nonsmoking elderly Caucasian adults (ages 50-80) of both sexes not taking garlic regularly to determine differences in their cardiovascular health compared to a matched population of healthy elderly adults taking standardized garlic powder for at least two years. The average intake in the chronic garlic user group was 460 mg/day for 7.1 years and in neither group were subjects taking garlic under regular treatment with cholesterol-lowering agents, ACE inhibitors, or direct vasodilators. Subjects were also excluded who were endurance-trained athletes. Plasma lipid concentrations, heart rate, and blood pressure were not significantly different between the two groups ($n = 101$ each). The index measurement of elasticity of the aorta pulse wave velocity (PWV), however, did show a highly significant difference ($p < 0.0001$), with the chronic garlic users showing much better elasticity; a difference the researchers found was more pronounced in the older garlic users than the younger users. The elasticity of the aorta lessens with age, even without cardiovascular disease, and whether arterial function, left ventricular function, or myocardial perfusion, the whole cardiovascular system is affected by the health of the aorta. The researchers also found that with any increase in systolic blood pressure or age, the PWV index showed significantly less increase in the chronic garlic users compared to the comparison group ($p < 0.0001$). Statistical analyses revealed that the most crucial factors affecting PWV were systolic blood pressure and age. Confounding factors (casual sports activity, blood pressure, serum lipids and their subfractions, age, body mass index) were independent of the influence of garlic. No difference in PWV was detected between garlic users taking 300, 400, or 600 mg of standardized garlic/day, and age- or blood pressure-associated alterations in the stiffness of their aortas (Breithaupt-Grögler et al., 1997).

Cerebrovascular Dysfunctions

One hundred twenty volunteers, all with risk factors for cerebrovascular disease and an increased aggregation of platelets which was constant, were studied by Kiesewetter, Jung, Jung, Mroweitz, et al. (1993). The double-blind, placebo-controlled, parallel trial of coated garlic tablets (800 mg/day for four weeks) found that spontaneous platelet aggregation decreased by 56.3%, along with a decrease in circulating platelet aggregates of 10.3% (each $p < 0.01$). The parallel group component of the study revealed a significant difference in the ratio of circulating platelet aggregates ($p < 0.05$) compared to the placebo group, and there were no changes of any significance in the placebo group. Plasma viscosity showed a highly significant decrease in the garlic group after 28 days ($p < 0.0001$), at which time both diastolic and systolic blood pressures showed significant decreases in the garlic group. Platelet aggregation readings returned to baseline following a four-week washout phase.

Effects on Cholesterol and Lipid Metabolism

A large number of studies have shown beneficial effects of garlic preparations on cholesterol and lipid metabolism. Two meta-analyses, based on consolidations of data from controlled studies, concurred that daily ingestion of garlic cloves or dried garlic products, in doses as low as 600 mg/day to 10-20 g/day over periods of 4-12 weeks, can significantly lower serum cholesterol levels and serum triglycerides by an average of 9% to 12% (Silagy and Neil, 1994; Warshafsky et al., 1993). A more recent meta-analysis of garlic in the treatment of hypercholesterolemia was specific to changes in total cholesterol levels. Although the data suggest superior effects from garlic compared to placebo, the effect was modest enough to render the use of garlic for treating elevated cholesterol questionable. Out of 13 trials included in the meta-analysis, four reported no significant difference in total cholesterol levels compared to placebo (Stevinson et al., 2000), as did at least one trial since then (in moderately hypercholesterolemic patients) (Superko and Krauss, 2000). Large-scale, long-term trials of the effects of garlic on total cholesterol levels to obtain meaningful data are called for (Stevinson et al., 2000).

One of the possible reasons proposed for the high number of recent negative outcomes is lot to lot differences in allicin contents of Kwai enteric-coated tablets, one of the more studied garlic products (Lawson, 1998). Another possibility is that compared to Kwai tablets (Lichtwer Pharma GmbH, Berlin, Germany) manufactured during the positive trial outcomes, enteric-coated tablets used during the negative trials were significantly less resistant to acid-disintegration and released significantly less allicin. Dissolution tests of 24 brands of enteric-coated garlic tablets sold in the United States found that whereas nearly all contained the amounts of allicin they claimed to hold when they were powdered and placed in water, the release of allicin upon dissolution according to USP dissolution method 724A, which simulates gastrointestinal conditions to measure allicin-releasing potential, was dismal. Only one product (Garlicin, Nature's Way Products, Springville, UT) released a sufficiently high amount of allicin (94%) to meet the USP method dissolution requirement of a minimum 80% of its claimed allicin potential. Tablet allicin release varied 18-fold and for 83% of the brands tested, dissolution allicin release was <15% of the potential allicin found. The problem was shown to be largely the result of slow disintegration of the tablets and to excipients used in their manufacture which both contributed to impaired alliinase activity (Lawson and Wang, 2000). However, Stevinson et al. (2000) point out that negative results have also been found from other garlic preparations and that the relationship of allicin to the lipid-lowering effect of garlic remains to be established. At this, Stevinson et al. and Lawson and Wang admit that their meta-analysis of diverse garlic preparations was not ideal since these products may have held varying and different amounts of constituents.

Garlic was used in a trial of 35 hypercholesterolemic renal transplant patients who had been taught to use the Step I diet of the National Cholesterol Education Program and were then randomized to groups who would receive placebo or garlic tablets (Pure-Gar brand, 680 mg b.i.d. for 12 weeks; allicin content equivalent to 4.080 mg/day). Compared to placebo, the garlic treatment significantly lowered total serum cholesterol levels and LDL-c levels after the first six weeks, an effect which was sustained at 12 weeks. Although hyperlipidemia was still sufficiently severe in the garlic group to warrant consideration of standard therapy, these findings indicate that garlic may have a role combined with HMG-CoA reductase inhibitors in the treatment of hypercholesterolemic renal transplant patients, who typically have severe hyperlipidemia. In this combination, the dosage of HMG-CoA reductase inhibitor might be lowered, thereby lowering the chance of toxicity from these agents (Lash et al., 1998).

Thirty children ages 8-18 with familial hypercholesterolemia treated with a garlic extract (Kwai brand, 300 mg t.i.d. for eight weeks) in a randomized, double-blind, placebo-controlled clinical trial showed no significant difference compared to placebo in fasting total cholesterol, LDL-c, HDL-c, triglycerides, blood pressure, homocysteine, fibrinogen, lipoprotein(a), or apolipoprotein B-100 levels (McCrindle et al., 1998).

Prior to 1995, studies investigating the effects of garlic preparations on plasma lipids mostly showed an increase in HDL. In 49 patients with hyperlipoproteinemia treated with standardized garlic powder over 12 weeks, an increase of the HDL-2 fraction was found with a corresponding decrease of the HDL-3 fraction, suggesting an antiarteriosclerotic effect and indicating an increased transport of cholesterol from the peripheral vessels to the liver (Reuter, 1995).

Steiner et al. (1996) conducted a double-blind, placebo-controlled cross-over study of AGE in 41 moderately hypercholesterolemic men (ages 32-68; cholesterol levels of 220-290 mg/dL, or 5.7-7.5 mmol/L). Patients were advised to alter their diets in complete accordance with the Step I diet of the National Cholesterol Education Program for four weeks of the baseline period, after which they were given placebo or the AGE (Wakunaga brand, 7.2 g/day) for six months before being switched to either placebo or the garlic extract for a further four months. Total serum cholesterol compared to placebo decreased by 6.1%. LDL-c decreased by 4.6% compared to placebo, and systolic blood pressure decreased by an average of 5.5% compared to placebo. No significant change compared to placebo was found in HDL-c or triglyceride levels.

Neil et al. (1996) conducted a six-month double-blind, placebo-controlled, randomized parallel trial of standardized garlic powder (Kwai brand, 900 mg/day) in 115 moderately hypercholesterolemic subjects, of which 106 completed the trial. After a dietary advice intervention of six weeks, subjects had repeatedly shown total cholesterol levels of 6.0-8.5 mmol/L and LDL-c levels of 3.5 mmol/L or more (type IIa or type IIb hyperlipoproteinemia). Mean lipoprotein and lipid concentrations showed no significant difference compared to placebo.

Hypertension

In several randomized, controlled trials, researchers examined the effects of 600-900 mg daily doses of garlic powder on hypertensive men and women volunteers. Systolic blood pressure was lowered by about 11 mm Hg and diastolic pressure by about 6 mm Hg (Neil and Silagy, 1994).

In a study in 20 healthy volunteers, Barrie et al. (1987) reported that garlic oil and fresh garlic both significantly reduced platelet aggregation, serum cholesterol, and mean blood pressure. (Hypertension is one of the major risk factors of atherosclerosis.) McMahon and Vargas (1993) studied the effect of a high dose of standardized garlic extract (2,400 mg, 1.3% allicin) on patients with severe hypertension. They reported a significant reduction in sitting blood pressure from 5-14 h after receiving the dose, with no significant side effects. Another study in patients with mild hypertension found that supine diastolic blood pressure fell from 102 to 91 mm Hg after eight weeks of treatment, and to 89 mm Hg after 12 weeks of receiving 100 mg of standardized garlic powder t.i.d.. Serum cholesterol and serum triglycerides were also significantly reduced in the treatment group (Auer et al., 1990).

Peripheral Vascular Disorders

Microcirculatory disorders. Kiesewetter, Jung, Jung, Blume et al. (1993) reported that standardized garlic powder (800 mg/day for 12 weeks) was weakly effective in benefiting outpatient volunteers (80 patients ages 40-75, both sexes) with peripheral arterial occlusive disease stage II. Compared to the placebo group, the active treatment group showed a significant 46-meter increase in the distance they could walk (207.1m versus 161m), without pain ($p < 0.05$).

Endocrine and Hormonal Disorders

Diabetes

Allyl propyl sulfide administered orally (125 mg/kg) to normal volunteers resulted in an increase in blood insulin and a decrease in blood sugar concentration (Augusti, 1973). Others have reported that garlic supplementation displays hypoglycemic action in diabetics but not in controls (Ernst, 1987).

Immune Functions; Inflammation and Disease

Cancer

Cancer prevention. Several studies have pointed to SAC and diallyl sulfide as probable cancer-protective compounds in garlic (Welch et al., 1992; Takeyama et al., 1993; Wargovich, 1987; Nagabhushan et al., 1992). Garlic and its constituents are known to display cancer-preventive effects in a variety of in vitro and animal models. Epidemiological evidence for a cancer-preventive effect of garlic is found in eight epidemiological studies, seven that suggest a protective effect (Ernst, 1997). From meta-analyses of epidemiological studies on garlic and cancer, Fleischauer et al. (2000) concluded that high intakes of raw and cooked garlic combined (21 g or ≈ six cloves/ week), while not firmly associated with protection against colorectal and stomach cancers (because of confounding intakes of other vegetables, publication bias, varying estimations of dose, and other reasons), may be associated with a reduced incidence of these cancers. For garlic supplements, Fleischauer et al. (2001) concluded that any association with a reduced risk cancers will require further studies.

Through the use of genetic biomarkers, Hageman et al. (1997) studied the anticarcinogenic potential of garlic in nine healthy volunteers, all nonsmoking males. After eating a 50% cucumber:yogurt salad for a period of eight days followed by a washout period of seven days, the cucumber:yogurt salad was resumed with the addition of three grams of raw garlic for eight days. After eating the raw garlic-supplemented salad, in eight of the nine subjects, benzo[a]pyrene-DNA adduct levels were found to be reduced in ex vivo benzo[*a*]pyrene-treated peripheral blood lymphocytes compared to the cucumber salad without the addition of raw garlic. The difference was statistically significant ($p < 0.02$). At the same time, no effect on damage caused by oxidation in the DNA of white blood cells from the raw garlic-supplemented salad was found. Also significant was the increase in *N*-acetyltransferase activity ($p < 0.05$) in urinary metabolites of the volunteers after eating the garlic-supplemented salad for eight days. However, the most obvious beneficial effect was found after the period of consuming the cucumber/yogurt salad without the addition of garlic. Reductions in the benzo[*a*]pyrene-DNA adduct levels formed in peripheral blood lymphocytes showed a more significant reduction ($p < 0.01$), and there were significant reductions in oxidative damage to the DNA of white blood cells ($p < 0.01$). In conclusion, the consumption of garlic may afford protection against genetic damage from polycyclic aromatic hydrocarbons.

In the Netherlands, Dorant et al. (1996) conducted a large-scale prospective cohort study on the use of garlic supplements and the risk of rectum carcinoma among the same population. After the 3.3-year follow-up, no association between garlic supplement use and the risk for rectum and colon carcinoma in men and women combined was found. Also in the Netherlands, an epidemiological study on diet and cancer among 120,852 men and women (ages 55-69) by Dorant et al. (1994), which ran from 1986 to 1989, reported at 3.3 years of follow-up that subjects taking garlic supplements as their only dietary supplement showed a higher risk for lung carcinoma compared to those who did not take any dietary supplements. However, among those taking other dietary supplements, which included garlic supplements, there was a lower risk of lung carcinoma compared to subjects taking any other kind of dietary supplement. Dorant and colleagues concluded that a lowered risk of developing lung carcinoma did not seem to be associated with the use of garlic supplements.

In an open-label study, Gwilt et al. (1994) used acetaminophen to study the anticarcinogenic potential of garlic since its biodegradation shares metabolic pathways in common with carcinogens without being a carcinogen itself. Using this model, for three months, the researchers administered an AGE to 16 healthy volunteers (mean age 25.75 ± 3.96) with orange juice (10 mL/120 mL) between the hours of 6 p.m. and 10 p.m. Independent analysis of the garlic supplement (Wakunaga brand) reported the following contents: diallyl sulfide (6.91 µg/mL), diallyl disulfide (52.9 µg/mL), *S*-allyl-*L*-cysteine (1,890 µg/mL), methyl allyl disulfide (4.33 µg/mL), but not allicin (diallyl thiosulfinate). Each subject was administered 1 g acetaminophen (Tylenol caplets) immediately prior to taking the garlic supplement, four weeks after stopping the garlic supplement, and at the end of each month of the three-month treatment period. Five volunteers not included in the end results dropped out of the study due to various side effects (nosebleed, diarrhea, vomiting, and gas). The results showed that chronic use of the garlic extract had little effect, and it was concluded that the extract showed "limited potential" in the prevention of carcinogenesis (Gwilt et al., 1994).

In China, the cancer death rate of two provinces was compared, and the highest death rate from gastric cancer was found in the province with the lowest garlic intake (Dorant et al., 1993).

In a study of workers with heavy metal intoxication, garlic reduced the severity of symptoms, including the basophilic stippling of erythrocytes and excretion of porphyrins in the urine. Those workers who supplemented their diet with dried garlic showed a reduction of porphyrins in the urine (Reuter, 1995).

Immune Disorders

HIV/AIDS. Few human studies to date on the effect of garlic on the immune system have been done. In one pilot study, ten patients with documented HIV-positive antigens were given AGE starting with 5 g/day for the first six weeks, then increasing to 10 g/day for the following six weeks. Seven patients were able to complete the study, as three died during the study period. The study reported that six patients had NK cell activity restored to normal levels. In addition, helper:suppressor T cell ratios (T4:T8) reverted to normal in three patients and improved in two patients. Most patients reported improvement of symptoms associated with secondary infections. These symptoms included cryptosporidia, genital herpes, pansinusitis, and candidiasis of the oral cavity. The study concluded that further investigation of garlic as an immune enhancer, antimicrobial, and an antiviral in AIDS-related diseases is warranted (Abdullah et al., 1994).

Integumentary, Muscular, and Skeletal Disorders

Skin Disorders

An open trial of a 4% ajoene topical gel (Acugel) in the treatment of diagnostically confirmed tinea pedis infection (ringworm of the feet or athlete's foot) was conducted by Ledezma et al. (1996) in 34 soldiers of the Venezuelan Army. Ajoene-free gel applied in a previous trial was without efficacy. The active gel was applied twice daily for seven consecutive days and the results were evaluated by a dermatologist. In 65% of the soldiers, both feet were affected and in 88% interdigital lesions were found. Immediately following the last application of the gel, cultures taken showed no growth of the pathogenic fungi previously confirmed, and for 79% of the soldiers, there were no signs of the disease. For the remaining 21% who still showed desquamation and positive cultures, an additional seven days of treatment with the gel produced a complete cure. Cultures performed 90 days later showed negative in every case. The only side effect reported by the soldiers was a "slight burning sensation" only in the affected area which persisted for 3-5 min and became unnoticeable following three days of the treatment. The study group represented a difficult treatment population in that they shared communal bathrooms, wore tight-fitting boots, worked in a tropical environment, and were regularly training in the field. Moreover, the subjects wore the same boots they had on before the treatment began. Ledezma and colleagues also noted that since ajoene is readily extractable from an alcoholic extract of garlic cloves, it may be considered of expedient use in the developing world.

Ledezma et al. (1999) conducted a follow-up study with a randomized comparative analysis of a topical ajoene (0.6%) preparation in 60 Venezuelan soldiers infected with tinea corporis and tinea cruris. Results were compared to a topical preparation of terbinafine (1%). After 30 days, the healing rate was 77% in the ajoene group and 75% in the terbinafine group. At 60 days the rates of healing were 73% and 71% for the ajoene and terbinafine groups, respectively.

Metabolic and Nutritional Disorders

Antioxidant Activity

Many of the cancer chemoprotective, antiatherogenic, and liver-protective effects of garlic extracts are likely related to antioxidant constituents. Studies have shown, for instance, that dietary supplementation with garlic powder in healthy volunteers (600 mg/day) for two weeks reduced the susceptibility of lipoproteins to oxidation (–34%). These results were interpreted as evidence of the antiatherogenic activity of garlic constituents (Phelps and Harris, 1993).

DOSAGE

The German Commission E monograph recommends a dose of 4 g daily of fresh garlic, the equivalent, or 8 mg essential oil of garlic for supportive therapy to reduce blood lipids, and as a prophylactic against age-dependent vascular changes. The British Herbal Compendium and the British Herbal Pharmacopoeia recommend a dose of 2-4 g of the dried bulb t.i.d., or 2-4 mL of a 1:5 tincture in 45% alcohol t.i.d., or 0.03-0.12 mL of the oil t.i.d. The British Pharmaceutical Codex (1949) recommends a dose of 2-4 mL for the juice of fresh garlic, or 2-8 mL of garlic syrup.

According to work commissioned by the Center for Science in the Public Interest, 1/3 tsp of fresh garlic contains 5,660 mg of alliin, and about 590 mg of SAC (S-allyl cysteine). This amount is comparable to the most potent standardized garlic tablet (KAL Beyond Garlic), which contained 4,800 mg allicin, and 270 mg SAC per tablet. Competing products required the ingestion of 1-44 tablets to deliver comparable amounts of these active constituents. The least potent product tested was P. Leiner (private label). It required 44 tablets to deliver 5,020 mg of allicin and 2,020 mg of SAC (Schardt and Liebman, 1995). Because a variety of commercial extracts exist, as well as different standardization methods, specific recommendations for particular doses and standardization forms are difficult. Whether ingesting garlic powder, fresh garlic, or a standardized preparation, the daily dosage should contain about 5-6 mg of allicin, or 5-6 mg total thiosulfinates.

Impact of Cooking and Other Processing

Garlic has a wide spectrum of potentially beneficial therapeutic activities, and the sulfur-containing constituents of garlic are largely responsible for most of the therapeutic actions (e.g., allicin and the cysteine derivatives). The multiple sulfur-containing compounds in garlic are inherently unstable and readily react with other compounds. Cooking and other processing of garlic, such as steam distillation to obtain garlic oil, or drying and pulverizing to yield garlic powder, can have a significant impact on the composition and levels of sulfur-containing compounds in the garlic product. Ultimately, this will influence the therapeutic efficacy of the final product. For medicinal use, a standardized product would contain known amounts of the active compounds. Schardt and Liebman (1995) have listed levels of allicin and *S*-allyl cysteine (SAC) comparisons of some of the popular standardized, commercial garlic preparations. Stomach acid can inhibit formation of allicin and other thiosulfinates. Although enteric coating of the tablets could overcome this problem, following an in vitro drug release test (USP Method 724A), researchers have reported that most brands of enteric-coated garlic tablets released less than 10% of their stated content of allicin. The poor results were attributed to slow buffer disintegration and low alliinase activity (Lawson and Wang, 2000).

SAFETY PROFILE

Used extensively for culinary purposes, garlic shows no ill effects other than garlic odor on breath and skin. However, the safety of long-term use of concentrated extracts of garlic is unclear.

Contraindications

Therapeutic doses of garlic are not advised for individuals with prolonged blood clotting time (Newall et al., 1996) and, like aspirin, may be contraindicated prior to surgery due to decreased platelet aggregation leading to increased bleeding and subsequent postsurgical complications (German et al., 1995; Burnham, 1995). It has been estimated that abstinence from garlic for a minimum of seven days before surgery may be warranted, especially in cases where platelet-inhibiting agents are involved or postoperative bleeding is a concern (Ang-Lee et al., 2001).

Drug Interactions

Potential interactions of garlic with certain medications and therapies exist. In a recent literature review, no reports of garlic interacting with warfarin were found. In addition, data on the inhibition of platelet aggregation, at least in studies of healthy volunteers taking garlic, was conflicting (Vaes and Chyka, 2000). However, others have cautioned that therapeutic doses of garlic may interfere with existing hypoglycemic or anticoagulant therapies, such as warfarin, and may also potentiate the antithrombotic actions of antiinflammatory medications such as aspirin. Garlic may be synergistic with eicosapentenoic acid (EPA) from fish oil (Newall et al., 1996). The constituent ajoene, an inhibitor of platelet aggregation, was shown to synergistically potentiate the in vitro antiaggregatory effects of dypiridamole, forskolin, indomethicin, and prostacyclin in human platelets (Apitz-Castro et al., 1986). Whether similar synergistic potentiation of these agents could be obtained from the ingestion of garlic, even in large doses, is not known.

Dalvi (1992) reported that in rats, garlic oil significantly decreases hepatic CYP450 activity, indicating that the metabolism of a wide range of drugs may be inhibited by garlic products. Piscitelli et al. (2002) reported that plasma concentrations of the HIV-1 protease inhibiting drug saqinavir decreased by about 50% in adults taking a commercial garlic dietary supplement (GarliPure, Natrol) twice daily for 19 days. Based on analyses of the allicin and allin contents of the supplement, the dose was roughly equivalent to 8 grams of garlic cloves daily. Even after a ten-day washout period in which no garlic was taken, levels of the drug were still not up to baseline levels. The researchers note that because aged garlic, fresh garlic, and a commercial garlic product were all found to inhibit CYP3A4 metabolism in a model of human microsomes (Piscitelli et al., 2002, citing Foster et al., 2001), the bioavailability of other drugs besides saqinavir which are metabolized by the CYP3A4 enzyme may also be inhibited by garlic. Piscitelli et al. (2002) warn that the use of garlic supplements in patients taking saqinavir as the only protease inhibitor in their regimen should be avoided.

Pregnancy and Lactation

Use of garlic during pregnancy and lactation is widespread in some cultures, being that it is a daily foodstuff. As little as 1/3 tsp. of fresh garlic has an equivalent dose of important constituents as the strongest garlic tablet currently being sold (see Dosage). Thus, recommendations for use during pregnancy and lactation based on so described "reasonable" amounts or "amounts greatly exceeding amounts used in food" are subject to a wide range of interpretations depending on the culture.

Newall et al. (1996) report that garlic is abortifacient, affects the menstrual cycle, and is uteroactive, but they also note that there are no experimental or clinical reports on adverse reactions in pregnancy or lactation. The German Commission E monograph states no contraindication for pregnancy or lactation for doses of 4 gm/day or equivalent preparations (Blumenthal et al., 1998). Given the possible modulation of platelet aggregation and fibrinolysis, use of garlic in therapeutic doses during late pregnancy could conceivably increase blood loss during birth. However, no clinical reports have been found (see Special Precautions).

The *American Herbal Products Association's Botanical Safety Handbook* (McGuffin et al., 1997, p. 7) cites a statement by Watt and Breyer-Brandwijk (1962) that "oral administration [of fresh garlic] to children is said to be dangerous and even fatal." McGuffin et al. (1997) concluded from this statement that caution during lactation was warranted, even as they reiterated garlic's long history as a food. However, the dose of constituents received through breast milk is expected to be relatively small, even accounting for the volatility of the compounds, when compared to the dose received from direct feeding of garlic to an infant.

Hale (2000) notes that the transfer of garlic constituents into breast milk is likely but not reported. However, studies of breast-feeding infants showed that they nursed for longer periods and took in larger amounts of milk after their mothers ate garlic. The studies noted that the mothers' milk had a garlic odor that correlated with the heightened interest in nursing. In a follow-up study, the babies showed habituation to garlic when repeatedly exposed to garlicky milk and returned to their baseline nursing behavior (Mennella and Beauchamp, 1993). No adverse effects on these infants were noted during these studies. There is an ethnobotanical report of galactogogue use in India (Bingel and Farnsworth, 1994). No documented reports of adverse reactions are known from the literature (Hale, 2000), though gastric disturbances related to dietary garlic or onions have been noted in some sensitive babies.

Roberge et al. (1997) provided a well-documented case of burns to the breast resulting from the use of a fresh garlic poultice that a lactating mother applied to an undiagnosed skin condition on one breast. The baby continued to breast-feed without difficulty on the affected breast for the two days that the poultice was applied. It was speculated that the lactating breast may be especially susceptible to skin damage from fresh garlic applications (see Side Effects).

Side Effects

In a case report, an 87-year-old male received treatment for complete motor paralysis of the lower extremities which subsequently resolved after removal of a spinal hematoma. Because the patient showed a prolonged bleeding time, yet showed normal liver function, and no uremia and had no history of treatment with any agents known to cause such an effect, the spontaneous hematoma was associated with his habit of eating four cloves of garlic per day (2,000 mg/day) (Rose et al., 1990).

Garlic breath is caused by the release of allyl methyl sulfide from the gut and initially from the mouth after consuming garlic (Suarez et al., 1999). Garlic is generally considered nontoxic. In higher doses, and in raw form, however, garlic may be irritating to the digestive mucosa and cause nausea, diarrhea, vomiting, and burning of the mouth (Newall et al., 1996).

Contact dermatitis occasionally results from occupational exposure to garlic and garlic extracts (Añíbarro et al., 1997). Garlic is allergenic and the responsible allergens have been identified as diallyldisulphide, allylpropylsulphide, and allicin, though the latter may simply be an irritant (Newall et al., 1996). Contact dermatitis is common from exposure to garlic in allergic individuals (Kanerva et al., 1996), and urticaria, angioedema (Asero et al., 1998), rhinoconjunctivitis, asthma (Seuri et al., 1993), and anaphylaxis (Pérez-Pimiento et al., 1999) have been reported following exposure.

Special Precautions

See Side Effects.

Because of the potential of garlic to inhibit platelet function, its discontinuation for seven days prior to undergoing surgery may be prudent until the real risk is determined (Ang-Lee et al., 2001). Consumption of garlic extract tablets may interfere with occupational testing for exposure to allyl halides or allyl chloride and confound results (Rooij et al., 1996).

Toxicology

In Vitro Toxicity

No in vitro evidence of cytotoxicity has been reported in the Ree assay (Newall et al., 1996).

Mutagenicity

No evidence of genotoxicity has been reported in the Ames test (Newall et al., 1996). No evidence of genotoxicity in the micronucleus test was found in mice of either sex administered acute oral doses of garlic powder (2.5, 5.0 or 7.5 g/kg p.o.) (Abraham and Kesavan, 1984).

Toxicity in Animal Models

In an acute toxicity study, the LD_{50} of a garlic extract in male and female mice was > 30 mL/kg p.o., i.p. or s.c. In rats of either gender, the LD_{50} was > 30 mL/kg p.o. or s.c. In female rats, the i.p. LD_{50} was also > 30; however, at the same dose, 1 out of 10 females and 5 out of 10 male rats perished within 24 h. The cause was not found and no specific signs of toxicity attributable to garlic were observed in the rats that survived (Nakagawa et al., 1984). A chronic toxicity study in rats given garlic extract orally (2 g/kg 5 times per week for six months) found no toxic symptoms, nor were there any significant changes in urinary, hematological, histopathological, or serological parameters (Sumiyoshi et al., 1984).

REFERENCES

Abdullah, T.H., Kandil, O., Elkadi, A., and Carter, J. (1988). Garlic revisited: Therapeutic for the major diseases of our times. *Journal of the National Medical Association* 80: 439-445.

Abdullah, T.H., Kirkpatrick, D.V., and Carter, J. (1994). Enhancement of natural killer cell activity in AIDS with garlic. *Deutsche Zeitschrifte für Onkologie* 21: 52-53.

Abraham, S.K. and Kesavan, P.C. (1984). Genotoxicity of garlic, turmeric and asafoetida in mice. *Mutation Research* 136: 85-88.

Adetumbi, M.A. and Lau, B.H.S. (1983). *Allium sativum* (garlic), a natural antibiotic. *Medical Hypotheses* 12: 227-237.

Ahsan, M. and Islam, S.N. (1996). Garlic: A broad spectrum antibacterial agent effective against common pathogenic bacteria. *Fitoterapia* 67: 374-376.

Ali, M., Thomson, M., and Afzal, M. (2000). Garlic and onions: Their effect on eicosanoid metabolism and its clinical relevance. *Prostaglandins Leukotrienes and Essential Fatty Acids* 62: 55-73.

Ang-Lee, M.K., Moss, J., and Yuan, C.S. (2001). Herbal medicines and perioperative care. *Journal of the American Medical Association* 286: 208-216.

Añíbarro, B., Fontela, J.L., and De La Hoz, F. (1997). Occupational asthma induced by garlic dust. *Journal of Allergy and Clinical Immunology* 100: 734-738.

Apitz-Castro, R., Badimon, J.J., and Badimon, L. (1992). Effect of ajoene, the major antiplatelet compound from garlic, on platelet thrombus formation. *Thrombosis Research* 68: 145-155.

Apitz-Castro, R., Escalante, J., Vargas, R., and Jain, M.K. (1986). Ajoene, the antiplatelet principle of garlic, synergistically potentiates the antiaggregatory action of prostacyclin, forskolin, indomethacin and dypiridamole on human platelets. *Thrombosis Research* 42: 303-311.

Aqel, M.B., Gharaibah, M.N., and Salhab, A.S. (1991). Direct relaxant effects of garlic juice on smooth and cardiac muscles. *Journal of Ethnopharmacology* 33: 13-19.

Asero, R., Mistrello, G., Roncarolo, D., Antoniotti, P.L., and Falagiani, P. (1998). A case of garlic allergy. *Journal of Allergy and Clinical Immunology* 101: 427-428.

Auer, W., Eiber, A., Hertkorn, E., Hoehfeld, E., Koehrle, U., Lorenz, A., Mader, F., Merx, W., Otto, G., Schmid-Otto, B., et al. (1990). Hypertension and hyperlipidemia: Garlic helps in mild cases. *British Journal of Clinical Practice* 69(Suppl.): 3-6.

Augusti, K.T. (1973). Studies on the effects of a hypoglycemic principle from *Allium cepa* Linn. *Indian Journal of Medical Research* 61: 1066-1071.

Barrie, S.A., Wright, J.V., and Pizzorno, J.E. (1987). Effects of garlic oil on platelet aggregation, serum lipids, and blood pressure in humans. *Orthomolecular Medicine* 2: 15-21.

Berthold, H.K., Sudhop, T., and Bergmann, K. (1998). Effect of garlic oil preparation on serum lipoproteins and cholesterol metabolism: A randomized controlled trial. *Journal of the American Medical Association* 279: 1900-1902.

Bingel, A.S. and N.R. Farnsworth (1994). Higher plants as potential sources of galactogogues. In Wagner, H., Hikino, H., and Farnsworth, N.R. (Eds.). *Economic and Medicinal Plant Research,* 6 (pp. 1-54). New York: Academic Press, Inc.

Blumenthal, M., Busse, W.R., Goldberg, A., Gruenwald, J., Hall, T., Riggins, C.W., and Rister, R.S. (Eds.) (1998). *The Complete German Commission E Monographs.* Austin, TX: American Botanical Council.

Breithaupt-Grögler, K., Ling, M., Boudoulas, H., and Belz, G.G. (1997). Protective effect of chronic garlic intake on elastic properties of aorta in the elderly. *Circulation* 96: 2649-2655.

Burnham, B.E. (1995). Garlic as a possible risk for postoperative bleeding. *Plastic and Reconstructive Surgery* 95: 213 (letter).

Byrne, D.J., Neil, H.A.W., Vallance, D.T., and Winder, A.F. (1999). A pilot study of garlic consumption shows no significant effect on markers of oxidation or subfraction composition of low-density lipoprotein including lipoprotein(a) after allowance for noncompliance and the placebo effect. *Clinica Chimica Acta* 285: 21-33.

Choudhury, A.R., Das, T., and Sharma, A. (1997). Mustard oil and garlic as inhibitors of sodium arsenite-induced chromosomal breaks in vivo. *Cancer Letters* 121: 45-52.

Dalvi, R.R. (1992). Alterations in hepatic phase I and II biotransformation enzymes by garlic oil in rats. *Toxicology Letters* 60: 299-305.

Dirsch, V.M., Gerbes, A.L., and Vollmar, A.M. (1998). Aloene, a compound of garlic, induces apoptosis in human promyeloleukemic cells, accompanied by generation of reactive oxygen species and activation of nuclear factor κB. *Molecular Pharmacology* 53: 402-407.

Dorant, E., van den Brandt, P.A., and Goldbohm, R.A. (1994). A prospective cohort study on *Allium* vegetable consumption, garlic supplement use, and the risk of lung carcinoma in the Netherlands. *Cancer Research* 54: 6148-6153.

Dorant, E., van den Brandt, P.A., and Goldbohm, R.A. (1996). A prospective cohort study on the relationship between onion and leek consumption, garlic supplement use and the risk of colorectal carcinoma in the Netherlands. *Carcinogenesis* 17: 477-484.

Dorant, E., van den Brandt, P.A., Goldbohm, R.A., Hermus, R.J., and Sturmans, F. (1993). Garlic and its significance for the prevention of cancer in humans: A critical view. *British Journal of Cancer* 67: 424-429.

Efendy, J.L., Simmons, D.L., Campbell, G.R., and Campbell, J.H. (1997). The effect of the aged garlic extract, "Kyolic," on the development of experimental atherosclerosis. *Atherosclerosis* 132: 37-42.

Ensminger, E.H., Ensminger, M.E., Konlande, J.E., and Robson, J.R.K. (1994). *Foods and Nutrition Encyclopedia,* Second Edition. Boca Raton, FL: CRC Press.

Ernst, E. (1987). Cardiovascular effects of garlic *(Allium sativum):* A review. *Phytotherapy Research* 5: 83-89.

Ernst, E. (1997). Can Allium vegetables prevent cancer? *Phytomedicine* 4: 79-83.

Ernst, E. (1999). Is garlic an effective treatment for *Helicobacter pylori* infection? *Archives of Internal Medicine* 159: 2484-2485.

Fleischauer, A.T. and Arab, L. (2001). Garlic and cancer: A critical review of the epidemiologic literature. *Journal of Nutrition* 131(Suppl.): 1032S-1040S.

Fleischauer, A.T., Poole, C., and Arab, L. (2000). Garlic consumption and cancer prevention: Meta-analyses of colorectal and stomach cancer. *American Journal of Clinical Nutrition* 72: 1047-1052.

Foster, B.C., Foster, M.S., Vandenhoek, S., Krantis, A., Budzinski, J.W., Arnason, J.T., Gallicano, K.D., and Choudri, S. (2001). An in vitro evaluation of human cytochrome P450 3A4 and P-glycoprotein inhibition by garlic. *Journal of Pharmacy and Pharmaceutical Sciences* 4: 159-167.

German, K., Kumar, U., and Blackford, H.N. (1995). Garlic and the risk of TURP bleeding. *British Journal of Urology* 76: 518.

Graham, D.Y., Andersen, S.Y., and Lang, T. (1999). Garlic or jalapeño peppers for treatment of *Helicobacter pylori* infection. *American Journal of Gastroenterology* 94: 1200-1202.

Gwilt, P.R., Lear, C.L., Tempero, M.A., Birt, D.D., Grandjean, A.C., Ruddon, R.W., and Nagel, D.L. (1994). The effect of garlic extract on human metabolism of acetaminophen. *Cancer Epidemiology, Biomarkers and Prevention* 3: 155-160.

Hageman, G., Krul, C., van Herwijnen, M., Schilderman, P., and Kleinjans, J. (1997). Assessment of the anticarcinogenic potential of raw garlic in humans. *Cancer Letters* 114: 161-162.

Hahn, G. (1996). History, folk medicine, and legendary uses of garlic. In Koch, H.P. and Lawson, L.D. (Eds.), *Garlic: The Science and Therapeutic Application of Allium sativum L. and Related Species* (pp. 1-24). Baltimore, MD: Wilkins and Wilkins.

Hale, T. (2000). *Medications and Mother's Milk.* Amarillo, TX: Pharmasoft Medical Publications, pp. 298-299.

Harris, J.C., Cottrell, S.L., Plummer, S., and Lloyd, D. (2001). Antimicrobial properties of *Allium sativum* (garlic). *Applied Microbiology and Biotechnology* 57: 282-286.

Hayes, M.A., Rushmore, T.H., and Goldberg, M.T. (1987). Inhibition of hepatocarcinogenic responses to 1,2-dimethylhydrazine by diallyl sulfide, a component of garlic oil. *Carcinogenesis* 8: 1155-1157.

Heinle, H. and Betz, E. (1994). Effects of dietary garlic supplementation in a rat model of atherosclerosis. *Arzneimittel-Forschung/Drug Research* 44: 614-617.

Hikino, H., Tohkin, M., Kiso, Y., Namiki, T., Nishimura, S., and Takeyama, K. (1986). Antihepatotoxic actions of *Allium sativum* bulbs. *Planta Medica* 52: 163-168.

Hirao, Y., Sumioka, I., Nakagami, S., Yamamoto, M., Hatano, S., Yoshida, S., Fuwa, T., and Nakagawa, S. (1987). Activation of immunoresponder cells by the protein fraction from aged garlic extract. *Phytotherapy Research* 1: 161-164.

Hughes, B.G., Murray, B.K., North, J.A., and Lawson, L.D. (1989). Antiviral constituents from *Allium sativum. Planta Medica* 55: 114.

Ide, N. and Lau, B.H.S. (1999). Aged garlic extract attenuates intracellular oxidative stress. *Phytomedicine* 6: 125-131.

I'örök, R., Belagyi, J., Rietz, B., and Jacob, R. (1994). Effectiveness of garlic on the radical activity in radical generating systems. *Arzneimittel-Forschung/Drug Research* 44: 608-611.

Ip, C. and Lisk, D.J. (1995). Efficacy of cancer prevention by high-selenium garlic is primarily dependent on the action of selenium. *Carcinogenesis* 16: 2649-2652.

Ip, C., Lisk, D.J., and Thompson, H.J. (1996). Selenium-enriched garlic inhibits the early stage but not the late stage of mammary carcinogenesis. *Carcinogenesis* 17: 1979-1982.

Jain, M.K. and Apitz-Castro, R. (1994). Garlic: A matter for heart. In Chanalambous, G. (Ed.), *Spices, Herbs and Edible Fungi.* Amsterdam, New York: Elsevier.

Jonkers, D., van den Broek, E., van Dooren, I., Thijs, C., Dorant, E., Hageman, G., and Stobberingh, E. (1999). Antibacterial effect of garlic and omeprazole on *Helicobacter pylori. Journal of Antimicrobial Chemotherapy* 43: 837-839.

Kanerva, L., Estlander, T., and Jolanki, R. (1996). Occupational allergic contact dermatitis from spices. *Contact Dermatitis* 35: 157-162.

Kiesewetter, H., Jung, F., Jung, E.M., Blume, J., Mrowietz, C., Birk, A., Koscielny, J., and Wenzel, E. (1993). Effects of garlic coated tablets in peripheral arterial occlusive disease. *Clinical Investigator* 71: 383-386.

Kiesewetter, H., Jung, F., Jung, E.M., Mroweitz, C., Koscielny, J., and Wenzel, E. (1993). Effect of garlic on platelet aggregation in patients with increased risk of juvenile ischaemic attack. *European Journal of Clinical Pharmacology* 45: 333-336.

Koch, H.P., and Lawson, D. (Eds.) (1996). *Garlic: The Science and Therapeutic Application of Allium sativum L. and Related Species.* Baltimore, MD: Williams and Wilkins Publishing Co.

Koscielny, J., Klüßendorf, D., Latza, R., Schmitt, R., Radtke, H., and Siegel, G. (1999). The antiatherosclerotic effect of *Allium sativum. Atherosclerosis* 144: 237-249.

Krest, I. and Keusgen, M. (1999). Quality of herbal remedies from *Allium sativum:* Differences between alliinase from garlic powder and fresh garlic. *Planta Medica* 65: 139-143.

Kyo, E., Uda, N., Kasuga, S., Itakura, Y., and Sumiyoshi, H. (1999). Garlic as an immunomodulator. In Wagner, H. (Ed.), *Immunomodulatory Agents from Plants* (pp. 273-288). Basel, Switzerland: Birkhauser Verlag.

Kyo, E., Uda, N., Suzuki, M., Kakimoto, M., Ushijima, M., Kasuga, S., and Itakura, Y. (1998). Immunomodulation and antitumor activities of aged garlic extract. *Phytomedicine* 5: 259-267.

Kyo, E., Uda, N., Ushijima, M., Kasuga, S., and Itakura, Y. (1999). Prevention of psychological stress-induced immune suppression by aged garlic extract (AGE). *Phytomedicine* 6: 325-330.

Lamm, D.L. and Riggs, D.R. (2001). Enhanced immunocompetence by garlic: Role in bladder cancer and other malignancies. *Journal of Nutrition* 131(Suppl.): 1067S-1070S.

Larner, A.J. (1994). How does garlic exert its hypocholesterolemic action? The tellurium hypothesis. *Medical Hypotheses* 44: 295-297.

Lash, J.P., Cardoso, L.R., Mesler, P.M., Walczak, D.A., and Pollak, R. (1998). The effect of garlic on hypercholesterolemia in renal transplant patients. *Transplantation Proceedings* 30: 189-191.

Lau, B. (1989). Anticoagulant and lipid regulating effects of garlic *(Allium sativum).* In Spiller, G.A. and Seala, J. (Eds.), *New Protective Roles for Selected Nutrients* (pp. 295-325). New York: Liss.

Lawson, L.D. (1996). The composition and chemistry of garlic cloves and processed garlic. In Koch, H.P. and Lawson, L.D. (Eds.), *Garlic: The Science and Therapeutic Application of Allium sativum L. and Related Species* (pp. 37-107). Baltimore, MD: Wilkins and Wilkins.

Lawson, L. (1998). Garlic powder for hyperlipidemia—An analysis of recent negative results. *Quarterly Review of Natural Medicine* (Fall): 187-189.

Lawson, L.D. and Wang, Z.J. (2000). Low allicin release from garlic supplements: A major problem due to the sensitivities of alliinase activity. *Journal of Agricultural and Food Chemistry* 49: 2592-2599.

Ledezma, E., De Sousa, L., Jorquera, A., Sanchez, J., Lander, A., Rodriguez, E., Jain, M.K., and Apitz-Castro, R. (1996). Efficacy of ajoene, an organosulpher derived from garlic, in the short-term therapy of tinea pedis. *Mycoses* 39: 393-395.

Ledezma, E., Lopez, J.C., Marin, P., Romero, H., Ferrara, G., De Sousa, L., Jorquera, A., and Castro, A. (1999). Ajoene in the topical short-term treatment of tinea cruris and tinea corporis in humans: Randomized comparative study with terbinafine. *Arzneimittel-Forschung* 49: 544-547.

Legnani, C., Frascaro, M., Guazzaloca, G., Ludovici, S., Cesarano, G., and Coccheri, S. (1993). Effects of a dried garlic preparation on fibrinolysis and platelet aggregation in healthy subjects. *Arzneimittel-Forschung/Drug Research* 43: 119-122.

Leung, A.Y. and Foster, S. (1996). *Encyclopedia of Common Natural Ingredients Used in Food, Drugs, and Cosmetics*. New York: John Wiley and Son, Inc.

Liu, J.Z., Lin, R.I., and Milner, J.A. (1992). Inhibition of 7,12-dimethylbenz [a]anthracene-induced mammary tumors and DNA adducts by garlic powder. *Carcinogenesis* 13: 1847-1851.

Mabberley, D.J. (1990). *The Plant Book: A Portable Dictionary of the Higher Plants*. Cambridge, MA: Cambridge University Press.

Martin, N., Bardisa, L., Pantoja, C., Barra, E., Demetrio, C., Valenzuela, J., Barrios, M., and Sepulveda, M.J. (1997). Involvement of calcium in the cardiac depressant actions of a garlic dialysate. *Journal of Ethnopharmacology* 55: 113-118.

Martin, N., Bardisa, L., Pantoja, C., Vargas, M., Quezada, P., and Valenzuela, J. (1994). Antiarrhythmic profile of a garlic dialysate assayed in dogs and isolated atrial preparations. *Journal of Ethnopharmacology* 43: 1-8.

McCrindle, B.W., Helden, E., and Conner, W.T. (1998). Garlic extract therapy in children with hypercholesterolemia. *Archives of Pediatrics and Adolescent Medicine* 152: 1089-1094.

McGuffin, M., Hobbs, C., Upton, R., and Goldberg, A. (Eds.) (1997). *American Herbal Products Association's Botanical Safety Handbook*. Boca Raton, FL: CRC Press, pp. 6-7.

McMahon, F.G. and Vargas, R. (1993). Can garlic lower blood pressure? A pilot study. *Pharmacotherapy* 13: 406-407.

Mennella, J.A. and Beauchamp, G.K. (1993). The effects of repeated exposure to garlic-flavored milk on the nursling's behavior. *Pediatric Research* 34: 805-808.

Moriguchi, T., Matsuura, H., Itakura, Y., Katsuki, H., Saito, H., and Nishiyama, N. (1997). Allixin, a phytoalexin produced by garlic, and its analogues as novel exogenous substances with neurotrophic activity. *Life Sciences* 61: 1413-1420.

Moriguchi, T., Saito, H., and Nishiyama, N. (1997). Anti-aging effect of aged garlic extract in the inbred brain atrophy mouse model. *Clinical and Experimental Pharmacology and Physiology* 24: 235-242.

Nagabhushan, M., Line, D., Polverini, P., and Solt, D.B. (1992). Anticarcinogenic action of diallyl sulfide in hamster buccal pouch and forestomach. *Cancer Letters* 66: 207-216.

Nagourney, R.A. (1998). Garlic: Medicinal food or nutritious medicine? *Journal of Medicinal Food* 1: 13-28.

Nakagawa, S., Kasuga, S., and Matsuura, H. (1988). Prevention of liver damage by aged garlic extract and its components in mice. *Phytotherapy Research* 1: 1-4.

Nakagawa, S., Masamoto, K., Sumiyoshi, H., and Harada, H. (1984). [Acute toxicity test of garlic extract]. *Journal of Toxicological Sciences* 9: 57-60.

Neil, A. and Silagy, C. (1994). Garlic: Its cardioprotective properties. *Current Opinion in Lipidology* 5: 6-10.

Neil, H.A.W., Silagy, C.A., Lancaster, T., Hodgeman, J., Vos, K., Moore, J.W., Jones, L., Cahill, J., and Fowler, G.H. (1996). Garlic powder in the treatment of moderate hyperlipidaemia: A controlled trial and meta-analysis. *Journal of the Royal College of Physicians of London* 30: 329-334.

Newall, C.A., Anderson, L.A., and Phillipson, J.D. (1996). *Herbal Medicines: A Guide for Health Care Professionals.* London: The Pharmaceutical Press, pp. 129-133.

Numagami, Y., Sato, S., and Ohnishi, S.T. (1996). Attenuation of rat ischemic brain damage by aged garlic extracts: A possible protecting mechanism as antioxidants. *Neurochemistry International* 29: 135-143.

O'Gara, E.A., Hill, D.J., and Maslin, D.J. (2000). Activities of garlic oil, garlic powder, and their diallyl constituents against *Helicobacter pylori*. *Applied and Environmental Microbiology* 66: 2269-2273.

Orekhov, A., Tertov, V.V., Sobenin, I.A., and Pivovarova, E.M. (1995). Direct antiatherosclerosis-related effects of garlic. *Annals of Medicine* 27: 63-65.

Pedersen, M. (1994). *Nutritional Herbology: A Reference Guide to Herbs.* Warsaw, IN: Wendell W. Whitman Company.

Pedraza-Chaverri, J., Tapia, E., Medina-Campos, O.N., de los Angeles Granados, M., and Franco, M. (1998). Garlic prevents hypertension induced by chronic inhibition of nitric oxide synthesis. *Life Sciences* 62: 71-77.

Pérez-Pimiento, A.J., Moneo, I., Santaolla, M., de Paz, S., Fernandez-Parra, B., and Dominguez-Lazaro, A.R. (1999). Anaphylactic reaction to young garlic. *Allergy* 54: 626-629.

Phelps, S. and Harris, W.S. (1993). Garlic supplementation and lipoprotein oxidation susceptibility. *Lipids* 28: 475-477.

Pinto, J.T., Qiao, C., Xing, J., Rivlin, R.S., Protomastro, M.L., Weissler, M.L., Tao, Y., Thaler, H., and Heston, W.D. (1997). Effects of garlic thioallyl derivatives on growth, glutathione concentration, and polyamine formation of human prostate carcinoma cells in culture. *American Journal of Clinical Nutrition* 66: 398-405.

Piscitelli, S.C., Burstein, A.H., Welden, N., Gallicano, K.D., and Falloon, J. (2002). The effect of garlic supplements on the pharmacokinetics of saquinavir. *Clinical Infectious Diseases* 34: 234-238.

Polasa, K. and Krishnaswamy, K. (1997). Reduction of urinary mutagen excretion in rats fed garlic. *Cancer Letters* 114: 185-186.

Reuter, H.D. (1995). *Allium sativum* and *Allium ursinum*: Part 2. Pharmacology and medicinal application. *Phytomedicine* 2: 73-91.

Rivlin, R.S. (2001). Historical perspective on the use of garlic. *Journal of Nutrition* 131: 951S-954S.

Roberge, R.J., Leckey, R., Spence, R., and Krenzelok, E.J. (1997). Garlic burns of the breast. *American Journal of Emergency Medicine* 15: 548 (letter).

Rooij, B.M. de, Boogaard, P.J., Rijksen, D.A., Commandeur, J.N., and Vermeulen, N.P. (1996). Urinary excretion of *N*-acetyl-*S*-allyl-L-cysteine upon garlic consumption by human volunteers. *Archives of Toxicology* 70: 635-639.

Rose, K.D., Croissant, P.D., Parliament, C.F., and Levin, M.B. (1990). Spontaneous spinal epidural hematoma with associated platelet dysfunction from excessive garlic ingestion: A case report. *Neurosurgery* 26: 880-882.

Schaffer, E.M., Liu, J.Z., and Milner, J.A. (1997). Garlic powder and allyl sulfur compounds enhance the ability of dietary selenite to inhibit 7,12-dimethylbenz [a]anthracene-induced mammary DNA adducts. *Nutrition and Cancer* 27: 162-168.

Schardt, D. and Liebman, B. (1995). Powder wise . . . pill foolish. *Nutrition Action Newsletter* (July/August): 4-5.

Seuri, M., Taivanen, A., Ruoppi, P., and Tukiainen, H. (1993). Three cases of occupational asthma and rhinitis caused by garlic. *Clinical and Experimental Allergy* 23: 1011-1014.

Sheela, C.G. and Augusti, K.T. (1995). Effects of *S*-allyl-cysteine sulfoxide isolated from *Allium sativum* Linn and gugulipid on some enzymes and fecal excretions of bile acids and sterols in cholesterol fed rats. *Indian Journal of Experimental Biology* 33: 749-751.

Siegel, G. and Klüssendorf, D. (2000). The anti-atherosclerotic effect of *Allium sativum*: Statistics reevaluated. *Atherosclerosis* 150: 437-438 (letter).

Siegers, C.P., Röbke, A., and Pentz, R. (1999). Effects of garlic preparations on superoxide production by phorbol ester activated granulocytes. *Phytomedicine* 6: 13-16.

Siegers, C.P., Steffen, B., Röbke, A., and Pentz, R. (1999). The effects of garlic preparations against human tumor cell proliferation. *Phytomedicine* 6: 7-11.

Silagy, C. and Neil, A. (1994). Garlic as a lipid-lowering agent: Meta-analysis. *Journal of the Royal College of Physicians* 28: 2-8.

Singh, K.V. and Shukla, N.P. (1984). Activity on multiple resistant bacteria of garlic *(Allium sativum)* extract. *Fitoterapia* 55: 313-315.

Song, K. and Milner, J.A. (1999). Heating garlic inhibits its ability to suppress 7,12-dimethylbenz[*a*]anthracene-induced DNA adduct formation in rat mammary tissue. *Journal of Nutrition* 129: 657-661.

Steiner, M., Khan, A.H., Holbert, D., and Lin, R.I. (1996). A double-blind crossover study in moderately hypercholesterolemic men that compared the effect of aged garlic extract and placebo administration on blood lipids. *American Journal of Clinical Nutrition* 64: 866-870.

Stevinson, C., Pittler, M.H., and Ernst, E. (2000). Garlic for treating hypercholesterolemia: A meta-analysis of randomized clinical trials. *Annals of Internal Medicine* 133: 420-429.

Suarez, F., Springfield, J., Furne, J., and Levitt, M. (1999). Differentiation of mouth versus gut as site of origin of odiferous breath gases after garlic ingestion. *American Journal of Physiology* 276: G425-G430.

Sumiyoshi, H., Kanezawa, A., Masamoto, K., Harada, H., Nalagami, S., and Yokota, A. (1984). [Chronic toxicity test of garlic extracts in rats]. *Journal of Toxicological Sciences* 9: 61-75.

Superko, H.R. and Krauss, R.M. (2000). Garlic powder, effect on plasma lipids, postprandial lipemia, low-density lipoprotein particle size, high-density lipoprotein subclass distribution and lipoprotein(a). *Journal of the American College of Cardiology* 35: 321-326.

Takeyama, H., Hoon, D.S.B., Saxton, R.E., Morton, D.L., and Irie, R.F. (1993). Growth inhibition and modulation of cell markers for melanoma by *S*-allyl cysteine. *Oncology* 50: 63-69.

Tsai, Y., Cole, L.L., Davis, L.E., Lockwood, S.J., Simmons, V., and Wild, G.C. (1985). Antiviral properties of garlic: In vitro effects on influenza B, *Herpes simplex* and Coxsackie viruses. *Planta Medica* 51: 460-461.

Vaes, L.P.J. and Chyka, P.A. (2000). Interactions of warfarin with garlic, ginger, ginkgo, or ginseng: Nature of the evidence. *The Annals of Pharmacotherapy* 34: 1478-1482.

Wargovich, M.J. (1987). Diallyl sulfide, a flavor component of garlic *(Allium sativum)* inhibits dimethylhydrazine-induced colon cancer. *Carcinogenesis* 8: 487-489.

Warshafsky, S., Kamer, R.S., and Sivak, S.L. (1993). Effect of garlic on total serum cholesterol. *Annals of Internal Medicine* 119: 599-605.

Watt, J.M. and Breyer-Brandwijk, M.G. (1962). *The Medicinal and Poisonous Plants of Southern and Eastern Africa*. London: E. and S. Livingstone, Ltd.

Weber, N.D., Andersen, D.O., North, J.A., Murray, B.K., Lawson, L.D., and Hughes, B.G. (1992). In vitro virucidal effects of *Allium sativum* (garlic) extract and compounds. *Planta Medica* 58: 417-423.

Welch, C., Wuarin, L., and Sidell, N. (1992). Antiproliferative effect of the garlic compound *S*-allyl cysteine on human neuroblastoma cells in vitro. *Cancer Letters* 63: 211-219.

Yeh, Y.Y. and Yeh, S.M. (1994). Garlic reduces plasma lipids by inhibiting hepatic cholesterol and triaglycerol synthesis. *Lipids* 29: 189-193.

Yoshida, S., Kasuga, S., Hayashi, N., Ushiroguchi, T., Matsuura, H., and Nakagawa, S. (1987). Antifungal activity of ajoene derived from garlic. *Applied and Environmental Microbiology* 53: 615-617.

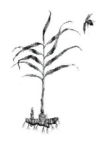

Ginger

BOTANICAL DATA

Classification and Nomenclature

Scientific name: *Zingiber officinale* Roscoe

Family name: Zingiberaceae

Common names: ginger, ingwer (Germany), gingembre (France), shen jiang (China), shokyo (Japan), adrak (India)

Description

Zingiber is believed to be native to the coastal regions of India. The name *Zingiber* is derived from a Sanskrit term used to describe a horn-shaped object. A perennial with a thick tuberous rootstock, *Zingiber* has an annual shoot with simple, alternate, lanceolate leaves, and a greenish-purple flower. The rhizome is aromatic and is the source of the dried powder spice. Ginger has been naturalized in Jamaica, China, Africa, and the West Indies and is cultivated in these and other tropical countries, including Indonesia and Australia (Schulick, 1994; Govindarajan, 1982).

HISTORY AND TRADITIONAL USES

Ginger has been cultivated in India since well before written history, and its use was documented by the Chinese as early as 400 B.C. Ginger is valued all over the world for its flavor and as a spice in food dishes. Traditionally, ginger has been used in folk medicine for indigestion, flatulence, diarrhea, malaria, fever, and a host of other health problems (Schulick, 1994). In traditional Arabian medicine, the rhizome is used in the treatment of sexual ailments and as an aphrodisiac (Qureshi et al., 1989). In China, ginger is used to detoxify meat, applied externally to relieve inflamed joints, and taken for gastrointestinal distress (Schulick, 1994). About 2000 years ago, Chinese doctors used dried ginger in the treatment of cough, "chest fullness," to arrest bleeding, promote perspiration, and to treat dysentery. Ginger was regarded as more efficacious if it was uncooked, and it was believed that prolonged use would give one the ability to "communicate with the spirit light" (Yang, 1997, p. 50). Today, processed ginger is used in an estimated 51% of Chinese herbal prescriptions (Sakai et al., 1988), and it is officially used in Chinese medicine in the treatment of diarrhea, abdominal pain, vomiting, abnormal uterine bleeding, cough, and dyspnea. The sun- or low temperature-dried rhizome *(gan jiang)* is processed by scalding until brown. The fresh rhizome *(shen jiang)* is used in treatments of the common cold, vomiting, cough, and to induce perspiration (Tu et al., 1992).

In traditional Indian medicine, ginger rhizome is used fresh and sundried (peeled and unpeeled). Apart from a host of culinary uses, dried ginger *(sonth)* is regarded as a memory-strengthener, aphrodisiac, digestive, and carminative. Uses include the treatment of nervous diseases, urinary incontinence, cough, colds, indigestion, colic, flatulence, vomiting, dyspepsia, chronic rheumatism, and stomach and bowel pains accompanied by fever (Nadkarni, 1976). Dried ginger is also one of the main ingredients of an herbal postpartum tonic used to recover from stress and weakness caused by pregnancy and childbirth (Puri et al., 2000). The juice of the fresh rhizome *(adrak)* is used as a diuretic and for the treatment of indigestion and biliousness. The juice is also used topically for the treatment of diarrhea by rubbing it around the navel area (Nadkarni, 1976), and in Assam, a paste made of the rhizome is applied topically for the relief of joint pains (Dutta and Nath, 1998). *Zingiber cassumunar* Roxb. is found from Sri Lanka to Tibet and is used for similar purposes as *Z. officinale* (Nadkarni, 1976).

Ginger was listed as an official herb in the *United States Pharmacopoeia* from 1820 to 1945 (Boyle, 1991).

CHEMISTRY

The most notable chemical constituents in ginger are the so-called "pungent principles," the gingerols, which give ginger its characteristic aroma. Also present are volatile oils, other oleoresin compounds, and starches, proteins, and lipids (Leung and Foster, 1996).

Lipid Compounds

Oils

The volatile oils in ginger vary according to the source of the plant material. The steam-distilled oil contains terpenoids, which usually include sesquiterpene hydrocarbons and monoterpene hydrocarbons. Other principal components include α-zingiberene, *ar*-curcumene, β-sesquiphellandrene, and β-bisaboene. When ginger is stored, the amount of *ar*-cumene increases and zingiberene and β-sesquiphellandrene decrease. Among other compounds identified in the oil are isovaleraldehyde, methyl allyl sulfide, camphene, sabinene, myrcene, limonene, and 1,8-cineole (Kami et al., 1972). From an acetone extract, Huang et al. (1991) isolated a diterpenoid identified as galanolactone.

Phenolic Compounds

The oleoresin contains the pungent principles as well as some nonpungent compounds. The pungent constituents comprise about 33% of the oleoresin and are called the gingerols, which are a series of homologous phenols with [6]-gingerol being the most common (Schulick, 1994).

Also pungent, but comprising a much smaller fraction of the oleoresin, are the shogaols. These anhydro-gingerols are formed during the drying of ginger. Other minor pungent compounds are paradols, gingediols, gingediacetates, gingerdiones, and gingerenones. Oleoresin is about 25% volatile oil (Schulick, 1994).

Other Constituents

Zingiber also contains starch, lecithins, and phosphatidic acid, saturated fatty acids (lauric, palmitic, and stearic), unsaturated acids (linoleic and oleic), and proteins (Schulick, 1994; Leung and Foster, 1996).

THERAPEUTIC APPLICATIONS

Research indicates that the rhizome of ginger possesses the following activities: antiemetic; promotes secretion of saliva and gastric juices; cholagogic; anti-inflammatory; carminative; spasmolytic; molluscicidal; antischistosomal; peripheral circulatory stimulant; increases peristalsis in the intestines; and enhances gastric motility (Mascolo et al., 1989; Adewunmi et al., 1990; Bradley, 1992; Schulick, 1994). Ginger is valued in traditional medicine for other gastrointestinal effects (Nadkarni, 1976), though studies are needed to confirm these actions.

PRECLINICAL STUDIES

Cardiovascular and Circulatory Functions

Atherosclerosis

Adult male albino rabbits fed an atherogenic diet for ten weeks and daily administration of a ginger extract (200 mg/kg p.o.) showed significantly less sever aortic atherosclerosis compared to the control group ($p < 0.001$). The effect was equally significant to another group administered gemfibrozil, although in this group the severity of atherosclerosis was a grade less than the ginger group (Bhandari et al., 1998).

Potential antiatherosclerotic effects of a standardized ethanolic extract of ginger were examined in atherosclerotic apolipoprotein E-deficient mice. The extract contained 14 mL/g essential oils, 40 mg/g pungent principles (including shogaols, gingerols, and zingerone), and 90 mg/g total polyphenols. Administered to their drinking water for ten weeks without any special diet, groups of these mice received daily doses of either 25 µg or 250 µg in 1.1% alcohol and water while controls received only the vehicle (1.1% alcohol and water). The ex vivo results showed remarkable effects in the ginger group compared to controls in reductions of LDL cholesterol oxidation. Measured in the TBARS assay, these results were 45% in the 25 µg/day group and 60% in those consuming 250 µg/day (each $p < 0.01$). In an in vitro examination of macrophages derived from the mice, those that received the ginger extract in either concentration showed significant reductions ($p < 0.01$) in their ability to incorporate oxidized LDL and to oxidize LDL (each $p < 0.01$). Basal levels of LDL-associated lipid peroxide showed a significant reduction (62%) only from the higher dose of the extract; however, a reduction in the ability of LDL to aggregate was significant from either dose (23% and 33%, respectively) compared to controls. Additional tests showed that the ginger extract was directly active against the oxidation of LDL. For example, copper ion-induced formation of lipid peroxides was dose-dependently inhibited by the extract (IC_{50} 5.0 mg/L) and by isolated constituents, shogaol and gingerol (IC_{50} 0.11 mg/ and 0.08 mg/L, respectively) (Fuhrman et al., 2000).

Cardiotonic; Cardioprotection

Following the observation of a potent, positive inotropic activity in isolated left atria of guinea pigs, Shoji et al. (1982) isolated and identified a number of cardiotonic principles of the dried rhizome which showed dose-dependent activity. In order of most to least potent, these were [8]-gingerol, [10]-gingerol, and [6]-gingerol. Since then, studies investigating the role of gingerol in heart function have shown that gingerols increase cardiac activity (Ohizumi et al., 1996). However, evidence that orally administered ginger extracts have such effects is lacking. No significant changes in heart rate or systolic blood pressure were found from a standardized ethanolic extract of ginger in rats at doses of 50 and 100 mg/kg p.o. (Weidner and Sigwart, 2000).

Cholesterol and Lipid Metabolism

A number of animal studies have shown significant cholesterol-lowering effects from ginger extracts (e.g., Bhandari et al., 1998; Sharma et al., 1996). The cholesterol-lowering effect appears to be due in part to the ability of ginger to stimulate the process in which cholesterol undergoes conversion to bile acids (Srivastava and Sambaiah, 1991). The constituents at least partly responsible appear to be [6]-gingerol, [10]-gingerol (Yamahara et al., 1985), and ZT or (E)-8β,17-epoxylabd-12-ene-15,16-dial (Tanabe et al., 1993).

Fuhrman et al. (2000) reported a significant decrease in plasma levels of LDL, VLDL, and triglycerides (58%, 36%, and 27%, respectively) in atherosclerotic apolipoprotein E-deficient mice fed an unpurified diet, along with a standardized ethanolic extract of ginger in their drinking water (250 µg/day in 1.1% alcohol for ten weeks) compared to controls. In addition, the plasma total cholesterol concentration dropped by 29% and the rate of cellular cholesterol synthesis in macrophages of the ginger-treated groups fell by 76% compared to controls. The standardized extract of ginger contained 14 mL/g essential oils, 40 mg/g pungent principles (including shogaols, gingerols, and zingerone), and 90 mg/g total polyphenols.

In rats fed a high-fat diet, a daily dose of an aqueous solution of ginger prepared from the dried and powdered rhizome (35 mg/kg p.o. for ten weeks) produced significant decreases (each $p < 0.01$) in total cholesterol, phospholipids, free fatty acids, and triglycerides compared to a high-fat diet control group. Decreases in these parameters were also significant compared to the control group ($p < 0.001$) from a daily dose of 70 mg/kg p.o. In rats fed a normal diet plus ginger, tissue free fatty acid levels also showed significant decreases compared to rats on the normal diet alone. In each organ measurement the effect was significant and greater from the higher dose, whether in aorta, intestine, liver (each $p < 0.001$), or kidney ($p < 0.01$). The decrease in free fatty acids was similarly significant in these organs when the high-fat diet plus ginger and the untreated high-fat diet groups were compared. Serum lipoproteins in the various study groups showed significant decreases from ginger with the same pattern of significance in LDL and VLDL cholesterol, and in the increased levels of HDL cholesterol in the ginger-treated rats compared to their respective controls. The atherogenic index (total cholesterol/HDL cholesterol) was also lower compared to control, except in those fed a normal diet compared to the control group administered ginger in the lower dose, whereas the higher dose caused a significant drop in the index regardless of the normal diet ($p < 0.001$). The lower dose used in this study was based upon a survey which calculated the average daily intake of ginger in the Indian population (Murugaiah et al., 1999).

Digestive, Hepatic, and Gastrointestinal Functions

Gastric Functions

The cancer chemotherapy agent cisplatin inhibits the gastric emptying rate and causes vomiting and nausea. Sharma and Gupta (1998) used ginger juice, an acetone extract of ginger, and a 50% ethanolic extract of ginger to test for antiemetic activity against cisplatin-induced gastric emptying rates in rats. The delay in gastric emptying induced by cisplatin (10 mg/kg i.p.) was significantly reversed by 30 min preadministration of the acetone extract (200 and 500 mg/kg p.o.), and at a rate similar to that of ondansetron (10 mg/kg p.o.), a 5-HT$_3$ receptor antagonist, compared to the control. However, the cisplatin-induced delay in gastric emptying was more significantly ameliorated by preadministration of ginger juice (4 mL/kg p.o., $p < 0.001$) than ondansetron (3 mg/kg p.o., $p < 0.01$), whereas the 50% ethanol extract was comparatively less effective at reversing the delay than either the acetone extract or the juice (significant only at 500 mg/kg p.o.). Based on studies proposing the involvement of free radical-induced release of serotonin and an antiserotonergic effect of ginger acetone extract, Sharma and Gupta (1998) surmised that either a free radical scavenging or an antiserotonergic mechanism may account for the reversal activities of ginger seen in their own study.

Sharma et al. (1997) tested the antiemetic activity of ginger extracts against cisplatin- and apomorphine-induced emesis in healthy mongrel dogs of either sex weighing 8-12 kg. Dogs administered either a 50% ethanolic or acetone extract (each at 200 mg/kg p.o.) of the rhizome 60 min prior to a 100% emetic dose of apomorphine (25 μg/kg i.v.) failed to show any difference in emetic episodes compared to controls. A further test using an aqueous extract of the rhizome also failed to prevent apomorphine-induced emesis and as a posttreatment against cisplatin-induced emesis. Dogs administered either of the solvent extracts of ginger (25 to 200 mg/kg p.o.) 30 min after a 100% emetic dose of cisplatin showed significant decreases ($p < 0.05$) in emetic episodes compared to controls, and an increase in emetic latency. The effect was dose-dependent. However, compared to a control group treated with granistron (0.5 mg/kg i.v.), the extracts (100 mg/kg) were less effective. The acetone extract provided complete protection from emesis in 20% of dogs, the ethanol extract in 0%, and granistron in 40%.

Kawai et al. (1994) identified the active antiemetic constituents of a methanolic extract of ginger used in copper sulfate pentahydrate-induced nausea in leopard and randid frogs as [6]-, [8]-, and [10]-gingerols and as [6]-, [8]-, and [10]-shogaols; the latter prolonging emetic latency more than any other (146.8% prolongation from 20 mg/kg p.o.).

Ginger was shown to enhance gastrointestinal motility in mice administered an acetone extract of the rhizome (75 mg/kg p.o.). The increase in motility was comparable to that of metoclopramide (10 mg/kg p.o.), a 5-HT$_3$ receptor antagonist. The orally active motility-enhancing constituents were identified as [6]-shogaol, [6]-, [8]-, and [10]-gingerol (Yamahara et al., 1990). After previous studies showed that pungent constituents of ginger and an extract of the rhizome exhibited antagonistic activity at serotonin receptors in isolated guinea pig ileum (Yamahara, Huang, Iwamoto, et al., 1989), an antiserotonergic effect was suspected when oral administration of [6]-gingerol (25 or 50 mg/kg p.o.) or an acetone extract of ginger (150 mg/kg p.o.) completely prevented cyclophosphamide-induced vomiting in male and female rodents—the same effect found from metoclopramide (25 mg/kg p.o.) (Yamahara, Huang, Naitoh et al., 1989).

[6]-gingerol inhibited serotonin-induced contractions in guinea pig ileum, which mostly contain 5-HT$_3$ receptors. The effect was considerably greater than in isolated rabbit aorta strips, which mainly contain 5-HT$_2$ receptors, or in rat fundus strips, which are richer in 5-HT$_1$ receptors (Yamahara, Huang, Iwamoto et al., 1989). From an acetone extract of ginger, Huang et al. (1991) isolated a diterpene, galanolactone, which showed 5-HT$_3$-receptor antagonist activity. However, as pointed out by Sharma et al. (1997), antioxidant activity of ginger may also be involved in the antiemetic effect since various antioxidants were shown to prevent cisplatin-induced emesis in dogs, and ginger has shown significant activity as a free radical scavenger (see Antioxidant Activity). They ruled out dopaminergic effects as a possible antiemetic activity of ginger when extracts of the rhizome failed to prevent apomorphine-induced emesis in dogs (Sharma et al., 1997).

Antiulcerogenic activity of ginger extracts in rats led to the isolation of various orally active constituents in both a water-soluble fraction and a lipophilic fraction of the rhizome. From the water-soluble fraction, 6-gingesulfonic acid was significantly active against the formation of hydrochloric acid/ethanol-induced gastric lesions in rats, and more potent than [6]-shogaol or [6]-gingerol isolated from the lipophilic fraction. Other less active constituents in the lipophilic fractions were identified as bisabolene-type sesquiterpenes, α-zingiberene, *ar*-curcumene, β-bisabolene, and α-sesquiphellandrene (Yoshikawa et al., 1994).

Fasted male rats administered powdered extracts of ginger rhizome (33.75 to 113.91 mg/kg p.o.) prior to pyloric ligature showed a dose-dependent inhibition of gastric acid production, which showed an increased pH and decreased hydrochloric acid concentration. At 62.01 mg/kg p.o., the ED_{50} of both extracts, the powdered extract made with acetone was more effective at reducing the gastric volume (–73.3%) than either cimetidine (32 mg/kg p.o.) or a powdered extract made with ethanol. Using the same doses against restraint stress-induced acute gastrointestinal lesions, administration of the extracts prior to the stress in fasted rats produced significant preventive effects: at 3 h, severity of the lesions was reduced 30.8% by the ethanol extract, 54.5% by the acetone extract, 53.8% by misoprostol (500 mg/kg p.o.), and 87.5% by cimetidine, compared to controls (Sertie et al., 1992).

Fasted male rabbits administered a methanolic extract and a water extract of ginger through an indwelling esophageal catheter showed different changes in gastric secretion according to the type of extract. After 3 h, either ginger extract at a dosage approximating that of the human dose used in traditional Chinese medicine caused significant decreases in gastric volume, acid output, and pepsin output compared to controls (each $p < 0.05$). Compared to cimetidine (50 mg/kg i.g.), the changes in gastric output from the water (169 mg/kg i.g.) or methanolic extract (114 mg/kg i.g.) were equally significant. However, by comparison, the methanolic extract was more potent at decreasing pepsin output than cimetidine or the water extract, which in turn was more effective at decreasing acid output and comparatively closer in potency to cimetidine than the methanolic extract (Sakai et al., 1989).

Hepatic Functions

Gingerols, shogaols, and diarylheptanoids and related analogues were screened for in vitro heptoprotective activity in the carbon tetrachloride-induced cytotoxicity assay using primary cultured rat hepatocytes. Gingerols were more active than shogaols with the most activity evident from [8]-gingerol and significant activity from [4]-gingerol to [14]-gingerol. The most potent shogaols were [7]- and [8]-shogaol. Among the diarylheptanoids, ten showed equally significant hepatoprotective activity (Hikino et al., 1985).

Endocrine and Hormonal Functions

Carbohydrate Metabolism; Antidiabetic Activity

The hypoglycemic activity of a hydro-ethanol extract of ginger was compared to tolbutamide. Two hours after rabbits were administered either substance at the same time as 1 g of glucose p.o., blood glucose levels showed significant decreases compared to a control group. At 4 h post administration, both the ginger extract and tolbutamide (each 100 and 300 mg/kg p.o.)

caused equally significant (each $p < 0.001$) and nearly equal decreases in blood glucose levels (37% and 43% versus 37% and 42%, respectively) compared to the control group (Mascolo et al., 1989). However, at doses of 25-100 mg/kg p.o., a standardized proprietary, ethanol extract of ginger containing a high amount of pungent principles (Institute of Drug Analysis, Copenhagen, Denmark, EV.EXT 33) was shown not to have a significant effect on blood glucose levels of rats compared to vehicle- (corn oil) or tolbutamide-treated controls (without oral glucose challenge) (Weidner and Sigwart, 2000).

Immune Functions; Inflammation and Disease

Cancer

Antiproliferative activity. Suzuki et al. (1997) found evidence of an antiproliferative effect from [6]-gingerol in mice with B16 melanoma as indicated by the inhibition of pulmonary metastasis, whereas [6]-shogaol was inactive. [6]-gingerol (0.07 mg/kg p.o.) exhibited a highly significant 75% inhibition of metastases ($p < 0.001$) and in a dose-dependent manner. When administered a water extract of ginger rhizome (7 mg/kg p.o.), the rate of inhibition was 89%. The mechanism of antiproliferative activity appears to be through activation of the immune system, particularly of CD8+ T cells.

Chemopreventive activity. Katiyar et al. (1996) studied the carcinogenesis-inhibiting (chemopreventive) activity of a methanol extract of ginger in a skin tumorigenesis model in mice. Topical application of the extract on the skin of mice subsequently exposed to the tumor inducer TPA (12-*O*-tetradecanoylphorbol-13-acetate) resulted in significant inhibition of tumor development and multiplication. TPA-induced tumorigenesis was significantly inhibited ($p < 0.0005$) by the ginger extract (2 mg/mouse; 56% inhibition). The same dose significantly inhibited TPA-induced cyclooxygenase ($p < 0.0005$) and lipoxygenase activity (38% to 72% inhibition). Epidermal ornithine decarboxylase activity induced by TPA was inhibited from pretreatment with the extract at 1-2 mg/mouse (46-55%, $p < 0.005$), and more significantly from 2-4 times the dose ($p < 0.0005$).

Park et al. (1998) examined the chemopreventive potential of topically applied [6]-gingerol using a two-stage skin carcinogenesis model in mice which used DMBA (7,12-dimethylbenz[*a*]anthracene) as the initiator of papillomagenesis following topical TPA. Compared to controls, [6]-gingerol (2.5 µmol) applied 30 min before each application of TPA caused a significant inhibition of papilloma formation ($p < 0.01$). In the same model, Surh et al. (1999) later showed that [6]-paradol was approximately equal to [6]-gingerol; however, [6]-paradol was far more potent at suppressing TPA-stimulated superoxide production in HL-60 cells. Lee and Surh (1998) proposed that the chemopreventive activity of ginger is likely due to the antiproliferative and apoptotic effects of [6]-gingerol and [6]-paradol. Both activities were shown in vitro in human promyelocytic leukemia cells (HL-60), suggesting that they may possess cytotoxic/cytostatic effects in vivo. Of the two, the minor constituent, [6]-paradol, was the more active (Lee and Surh, 1998). [6]-paradol occurs in greater quantities in other members of the ginger family (e.g., seeds of the African "grains of paradise," *Aframomum melegueta* K. Schum.) (Surh et al., 1999).

The environmental toxin benzo[*a*]pyrene (BaP) is carcinogenic, teratogenic, and embryotoxic in mice. A long-term study found that mice fed a diet containing the toxin developed a higher incidence of carcinoma/papillomas of the esophagus, tongue, and forestomach (Culp et al., 1998). BaP has shown the highest metabolism in cultured human cells of the bronchus, esophagus, and duodenum, followed by the transverse colon (Autrup et al., 1982). Using the Ames method, an in vitro assay of mutagenic activity, Sakai et al. (1988) found that a hot-water extract of ginger rhizome reduced the mutagenicity of BaP in two strains of *Salmonella typhimurium* (TA98 and TA 100). Whether this activity will translate to benefit humans is another matter; in part because the carcinogenicity of BaP varies from one species to the next and in the type and location of tumors that it causes to form (Weyand and Bevan, 1987).

Immune Functions

Immune modulation. Chang et al. (1995) examined the immunomodulating effect of ginger rhizome powder on the function of cytokines to see whether such effects might contribute to its medicinal uses in traditional Chinese medicine (TCM). The in vitro effects of a 50% ethanolic extract of the powdered rhizome was studied for effects on cytokine secretion in human peripheral blood mononuclear cells (PBMC). Incubated in PBMC at a concentration of 20 to 30 mg/mL for 18 or 24 h, the extract significantly augmented the secretion of interleukin-1β (IL-1β); however, higher concentration showed the opposite effect and the amounts that were secreted were small. The same dose-responsive result was found in the small amount of IL-6 secreted and the even smaller secreted amount of GM-CSF (granulocyte-macrophage-colony stimulating factor). The increase in secretion of tumor necrosis factor-α (TNF-α) by the extract was minor and insignificant. The researchers concluded that the effect of the extract on the secretion of cytokines by PBMC in vitro was a biphasic one; low concentrations had an augmenting effect, and higher concentrations had no effect or a suppressive effect of cytokine secretion. Incubation time was also important for cytokine secretion. After 18 to 24 h there was a significant augmentative effect from a low concentration of the extract, but not from an incubation time of 60 to 180 min. Based on the augmentative effect of the extract on cytokine secretion in vitro, a possible basis for clinical uses of ginger in TCM was offered, which would include a hematopoietic effect from IL-6 and GM-CSF and a pyrogenic effect from TNF-α and IL-1β.

Immunopotentiation. Puri et al. (2000) studied the immunopotentiating activity of a 50% ethanolic extract of ginger in BALB/c mice. They measured for effects on humoral immunity using plaque-forming cell counts (PFC) and the hemagglutinating-antibody (HA) titer assay to indicate antibody production and antibody levels, respectively, and the macrophage migration index (MMI) as an indication of cellular immunity and macrophage activation. After administration (25 mg/kg p.o. on seven consecutive days), the results showed a significant immunostimulatory effect, but only in the HA titer and PFC compared to the control ($p < 0.001$), suggesting that ginger primarily increases humoral immunity. According to the researchers, this observation may rationalize the traditional use of ginger for the treatment of chest and throat afflictions.

Infectious Diseases

Microbial infections. An 80% ethanolic extract residue of the rhizome moderately inhibited the growth of Gram-positive and Gram-negative bacteria *(Bacillus anthracis, B. subtilis, Escherichia coli 7075, E. coli Bp, Proteus mirabilis, Salmonella typhi H., Staphylococcus aureus, S. epidermis and S. haemolyticus),* yet failed to inhibit *Pseudomonas aeruginosa.* The minimum inhibitory concentrations (MICs) were 2.5-4.2 mg/mL (Mascolo et al., 1989). A 95% ethanolic extract residue inhibited the growth of *E. coli, Proteus vulgaris, Salmonella typhimurium, Staphylococcus aureus,* and *Streptococcus viridans,* but not that of *Pseudomonas aeruginosa* and *Streptococcus faecalis.* In this study, the MICs were much higher, at 25-50 mg/mL (Gugnani and Ezenwanze, 1985).

Parasitic infections. Goto et al. (1990) examined the effect of ginger constituents [6]-shogaol and [6]-gingerol on the pathogenic parasite *Anisakis,* the larvae of which are found in raw tuna, cuttlefish, halibut, mackerel, cod, and other fish. The popularity of Japanese cuisine in the West, in which raw fish is a main dish, could lead to a corresponding increased incidence of infection by the parasite. Therefore, garnishes such as ginger, which are traditionally eaten with raw fish in Japanese cuisine, need to be examined for potential anti-*Anisakis* activity.

Following their finding that an extract of ginger could kill the larvae of *Anisakis,* Goto et al. (1990) tested fractions of a methanolic extract of ginger to determine the most active constituents involved. Because the pungent fraction was most effective (100% lethality at 1% concentration), they tested the pungent principles [6]-shogaol and [6]-gingerol. With 100% lethality to *Anisakis* larvae, [6]-shogaol (62.5 µg/mL) showed 4 times the potency of [6]-gingerol. Although the amount of [6]-gingerol in the methanolic extract of ginger was not sufficient to be lethal to the larvae, 50 g/mL of [6]-gingerol with the addition of a small amount of [6]-shogaol (2.5 µg/mL) appeared to act synergistically: 23.8% of the larvae were killed and spontaneous movements were halted in 100% (Goto et al., 1990).

Datta and Sukul (1987) used residues from a 50% ethanol/water extract of the rhizome to treat dogs naturally infected with filariasis from *Dirofilaria immitis*. The microfilarial count was reduced by 98% after the last treatment phase and rose slowly after. At 55 days posttreatment (100 mg/kg s.c., daily for four days, in three cycles, with seven-day gaps), the microfilarial count was still reduced by 83%.

Inflammatory Response

An ethanolic extract of the rhizome (50 and 100 mg/kg p.o.) was tested against carrageenan-induced swelling of the hind-paw of the rat. Compared to untreated paws and rats treated with the same amounts of aspirin p.o., the extract at either dose produced a significant reduction in inflammation which was comparable to that of aspirin in degree of inhibition at either dose (22% and 23% inhibition and 38% and 39%, respectively). In a separate experiment, the ginger extract produced a significant and dose-dependent inhibition of prostaglandin release from rat peritoneal leukocytes in vitro (50-500 µg/mL) without affecting the process of phagocytosis; however, indomethacin (5 or 10 µg/mL) showed significantly greater potency (Mascolo et al., 1989). Potent in vitro inhibitors of prostaglandin biosynthesis in the rhizome were identified as [10]-dehydrogingerdione, [10]-gingerdione, [6]-gingerdione, [6]-dehydrogingerdione, and [6]-gingerol. With IC_{50}s of 1.0, 1.0, 1.6, 2.3, and 5.5 µM, respectively, most of them are more potent than one of the most potent prostaglandin biosynthesis inhibitors known, indomethacin (IC_{50} 4.9 µM) (Kiuchi et al., 1982).

In a rat model of severe paw and joint inflammation (chronic adjuvant arthritis), administration of ginger oil (33 mg/kg p.o.) 24 h before induction of arthritis and then daily for 25 days after, caused a significant anti-inflammatory effect. The ginger oil produced a significant suppression of joint swelling from days 2 to 22 ($p < 0.05$), which became highly significant on day 26 ($p < 0.001$). Paw swelling was significantly suppressed from days 18 to 26 ($p < 0.001$) (Sharma et al., 1994).

Park et al. (1998) reported a significant anti-inflammatory effect from the topical application of [6]-gingerol to the ears of mice (10 µmol/ear; 61% inhibition) against 12-*O*-teradecanoylphorbol-13-acetate (TPA)-induced by inflammation. At 20 µmol, topical [6]-gingerol also caused a significant inhibition of TPA-induced ornithine decarboxylase (ODC) activity in the skin of mice.

The effect of an ethanolic extract of ginger against fever—a marker of inflammation—was tested against yeast-induced fever in rats. Administered 15 h after yeast infection, the ginger extract (100 mg/kg p.o) caused a 38%

reduction in rectal temperature compared to controls, a potency comparable to the reference treatment, aspirin, at 50 mg/kg p.o. (Mascolo et al., 1989).

Using a standardized ethanolic extract of ginger (100 mg/kg p.o.) in rats, Weidner and Sigwart (2000) reported the absence of effects of blood coagulation, as evidenced by whole blood clotting, prothrombin, and activated partial thromboblastin times. Conversely, Bordia et al. (1997) found that an *n*-hexane extract of ginger powder (with *n*-hexane residues removed) exhibited a dose-dependent inhibition of adrenaline- and arachidonic acid (AA)-induced platelet aggregation in vitro, although it was comparatively more effective against the latter inducer. The extract also showed a dose-dependent inhibition of thromboxane formation (IC_{50} 16 ± 8 μg/mL). Guh et al. (1995) reported that [6]-gingerol exhibited a concentration-dependent (0.5-20 μM) in vitro inhibition of platelet aggregation in rabbit platelets against collagen- and AA-, but not against platelet-activating factor- or thrombin-induced aggregations. At the same concentrations, gingerol dose-dependently inhibited the release of prostaglandin D_2 and thromboxane B_2 formation elicited by AA. In platelet-rich human plasma, primary aggregation was not inhibited by gingerol (5 μM), but aggregation secondary to adrenaline and adenosine 5'-diphosphate was prevented, and the release of adenosine triphosphate (ATP) induced by the latter agents was blocked. [6]-gingerol (20 μM) also caused complete elimination of AA-induced phosphoinositide breakdown, though less potently than indomethacin (2 μM). The researchers concluded that the platelet aggregation-inhibitory activity of [6]-gingerol is the result of arachidonate metabolism-inhibition and secondary inhibition of thromboxane formation.

Cyclooxygenase-2 (COX-2) is an inducible enzyme involved in arachidonic acid metabolism which mediates inflammatory processes. When Tjendraputra et al. (2001) examined the effect of 17 different pungent principles of ginger on COX-2 in a model of intact cells using human airway epithelial cells, they found [8]-shogaol, [8]-paradol, and [10]-gingerol to be potent inhibitors of the enzyme (IC_{50}s 2.1, 3.4, and 3.7 μM, respectively). Inhibitors [8]-gingerol and [8]-gingerdiol were moderately strong in COX-2 activity (IC_{50}s 10 μM and 12.5 μM, respectively). The COX-2 inhibiting activity of these constituents was both structure- and concentration-dependent.

Metabolic and Nutritional Functions

Antioxidant Activity

[6]-gingerol has shown direct in vitro antioxidant activity as evidence by inhibition of xanthine oxidase (Chang et al., 1994) and phospholipid peroxidation (Aeschbach et al., 1994). In the DPPH (1,1-diphenyl-2-picrylhydrazyl) assay, direct scavenging of free radicals was shown from a standardized extract of ginger (Fuhrman et al., 2000) and from minor glucosides

isolated from fresh ginger rhizomes (6-gingerdiol and a related glucoside) (Sekiwa et al., 2000; Kikuzaki and Nakatani, 1993).

In albino rats, dietary ginger was shown to cause a significant decrease in subchronic pesticide-induced generation of oxygen free radicals and the resulting production of free radical-scavenging enzymes. Male albino rats were fed a standard diet containing powdered ginger (1% w/w) prepared from fresh rhizomes obtained in a local Indian market. Other groups received the standard diet with the addition of the pesticide malathion (20 ppm), the addition of both the ginger powder and malathion, and a fourth group received pesticide-free feed. After four weeks of the various dietary regimens, the results showed that compared to the rats with malathion in their feed, levels of lipid peroxidation in the ginger plus malathion group were significantly lower, as were and levels in the ginger-feed group without the pesticide (each $p < 0.001$). Levels of SOD (superoxide dismutase) activity in the malathion-treated rats increased threefold whereas in those receiving ginger in their feed the levels were unchanged and, by comparison, significantly different in the ginger plus malathion group ($p < 0.001$). Similar results were found in levels of erythrocyte catalase activity, blood glutathione content, erythrocyte glutathione peroxidase activity, serum glutathione reductase activity, and serum glutathione S-transferase activity (each $p < 0.001$) (Ahmed et al., 2000).

Receptor- and Neurotransmitter-Mediated Functions

The in vitro and in vivo antinociceptive activity of [6]- and [8]-gingerol, along with their metabolic precursor, zingerone, was compared to capsaicin—a known antinociceptive agent and activator of a VR1 receptor found in receptor neurons that mediate nociception to protons and heat. Evidence was found to suggest that both gingerols act as VR1 agonists since they increased the in vitro production of Ca^{2+} transients in capsaicin-sensitive dorsal root ganglia neurons and the transients were prevented by a VR1 receptor antagonist (capsazepine). The effectiveness of the ginger constituents as VR1 receptor activators was further evaluated following their topical application to the skin of rats. Capsaicin showed greater potency compared to [6]- and [8]-gingerol, which were equally effective, while zingerone was least effective. The authors concluded that as VR1 agonists, both [6]- and [8]-gingerol are prospective leads for the development of "a new class" of antinociceptive agents (Dedov et al., 2000).

Miscellaneous Pharmacological Activities

Male mice administered a 95% ethanol extract of the rhizomes in which the ethanol was removed (100 mg/kg p.o. for three months) developed a significant increase in sperm counts ($p < 0.05$) and highly significant increases in sperm motility and in the average weight of their seminal vesicles (each $p < 0.001$) (Qureshi et al., 1989).

CLINICAL STUDIES

Digestive, Hepatic, and Gastrointestinal Disorders

Gastric Disorders

Nausea. Micklefield et al. (1999) examined the effect of ginger on gastroduodenal motility (fasting and postprandial) in 12 male volunteers, ages 18 to 44 using gastroduodenal manometry. Subjects received either placebo or two 100 mg capsules of an extract of ginger rhizome (Dr. Willmar Schwabe GmbH and Co., Karlsruhe, Germany) corresponding to two grams of ginger rhizome. The prospective, randomized, placebo-controlled, double-blinded, two-period, crossover trial found that interdigestive motility was significantly increased by the ginger extract compared to placebo, and in the antrum ginger caused a significant decrease in contraction amplitudes. The researchers concluded that gastroduodenal motility was increased by oral ginger, both after a standard test meal and in the fasting state.

In a study of ginger on the gastric emptying rate, Phillips, Hutchinson, et al. (1993) conducted a placebo-controlled, double-blind, randomized, crossover trial of powdered ginger rhizome in 16 volunteers (aged 18 years plus), all in good health. The ginger powder was administered in 500 mg capsules and the placebo was indistinguishable in appearance, smell, and taste. Although no adverse effects were reported of any kind, one gram of ginger ingested at the same time as paracetamol had no effect on the gastric absorption rate compared to placebo.

Ernst and Pittler (2000) conducted a systematic review of double-blind, placebo-controlled, randomized clinical trials of ginger for the prevention of nausea and vomiting, finding six studies that met all of their inclusion criteria. The highest ranked trials were those of GrØntved et al. (1988) on seasickness in 80 subjects, and Arfeen et al. (1995) on postoperative nausea in 108 women. They concluded that, however promising, firm conclusions on the efficacy of ginger as an antiemetic are not possible until more sufficient clinical data is provided from rigorous studies. Examples of randomized, placebo-controlled clinical trials with ginger against nausea are provided as follows.

In a randomized, double-blind study, Riebenfeld and Borzone (1999) examined the comparative efficacy and tolerability of a standardized ginger root powder extract (Zintona, standardized to pungent phenolic compounds), and dimenhydrinate in identically marked capsules. Sixty matched subjects (ages 10-77) known to have a history of motion sickness sensitivity when traveling on rough seas, were randomly assigned to either the ginger group or the dimenhydrinate group: 500 mg 30 min prior to embarkation, followed by 500 mg/4 h over 48 h, and for the dimenhydrinate group, 100 mg 30 min prior to embarkation followed by 100 mg/4 h over 48 h. Subjects were monitored from September to March of the next year while passengers onboard a cruise ship. Every one of the subjects reported some motion sickness which was rated severe and of similar intensity in each of the treatment groups. The main symptoms reported were general malaise and nausea. Effectiveness of the ginger extract was rated very good ($n = 21$) or good ($n = 7$) in most cases. A similar result was shown in the dimenhydrinate group ($n = 15$ and $n = 12$, respectively). Tolerability was rated by the physicians as poor in zero cases for the ginger group and in ten cases for the dimenhydrinate group, while good tolerability was noted in 15 cases of the ginger group and only 3 in the dimenhydrinate group. Side effects amounted to 13.3% in the ginger groups and 40% in the dimenhydrinate group. These consisted of four cases in the ginger group (somnolence in three and headache in one), and 12 cases in the dimenhydrinate group (somnolence in eight, epigastric disturbances in two, cold sweating in one, and gastric acidity in one). The difference in tolerability was significant ($p < 0.001$) in favor of ginger. Total motion sickness mean scores revealed that dimenhydrinate was slightly more effective compared to the ginger group, although the difference was not statistically significant (Riebenfeld and Borzone, 1999).

Visalyaputra et al. (1998) conducted a randomized, double-blind, placebo-controlled trial of powdered ginger in the prevention of postoperative nausea and vomiting in 111 women (ages 20-40) undergoing elective gynecological diagnostic laparoscopy. The ginger powder and placebo was supplied in dark-colored, odorless capsules at a dosage of two 500 mg capsules 60 min prior to anesthesia (short-acting fentanyl followed by suxamethonium). Before induction of anesthesia, patients administered either placebo or ginger received i.v. injections of either saline or droperidol (1.25 mg), a neuroleptic anesthetic in the class of butyrophenones with antiemetic, antianxiety, and sedative effects. Thirty min before they were discharged, patients received two more capsules of either placebo or powdered ginger, resulting in a dosage of 2,000 mg of ginger in those who received ginger previous to laparascopy. The results showed that there was no significant difference in the incidence of postoperative nausea or vomiting in the groups that received placebo compared to those treated with ginger, or compared to ginger or placebo in combination with injections of either saline or droperidol.

Arfeen et al. (1995) conducted a randomized, double-blind, placebo-controlled trial of ginger powder (Blackmores Ltd., Sydney, Australia) in the prevention of postoperative nausea and vomiting in 108 women (ages 18-75) scheduled for gynecological laparascopic surgery. The encapsulated ginger powder was rendered indistinguishable in smell from that of the placebo (cellulose). One group received two capsules of ginger (one gram), another 500 mg ginger plus one capsule of placebo, and a third only placebo (two capsules). All patients received diazepam 60 min prior to anesthesia induced with vecuronium and thiopentone. During the 3 h postoperative assessment period, the incidence of moderate or severe nausea and vomiting in the group that received one gram of ginger powder was 36% and 31%, respectively, and 33% and 14% in the group that received 500 mg of ginger powder. The placebo group faired better with moderate or severe nausea in 22% and vomiting among 17%. Complaints of adverse effects reported in the three groups consisted of three in the 1 g ginger group (one each with severe heartburn, nausea, and burping), two in the 500 mg ginger group (one with a bloated feeling and flatulence, and the other burping), while in the placebo group one patient experienced the urge to burp and a sensation of feeling windy. In conclusion, the ginger powder was found to be ineffective in the prevention of postoperative nausea and vomiting.

Phillips, Ruggier, et al. (1993) studied the effect of the powdered root (1 g p.o.) as a potential antiemetic in a prospective, randomized, double-blind clinical trial in 120 women admitted for elective laproscopic surgery (gynecological). In a blinded fashion, placebo, ginger, or metoclopramide (10 mg) was administered in the form of two capsules per subject in each of three respective groups prior to anesthesia (atracurium following propofol and fentanyl). Although no assessment was made of nausea severity, the researchers found ginger significantly superior to placebo ($p < 0.006$) in reducing nausea, whereas the antinausea effect of metoclopramide compared to ginger was insignificant. The superior benefit of ginger was apparent in the number of patients who required antiemetics: placebo 38%; metoclopramide 32%; and ginger 15%, and in the incidence rates of nausea and vomiting: placebo 41%; metoclopramide 27%; and ginger 21%. Adverse effects were of very low incidence and showed no difference in occurrence between the study groups.

In a double-blind, randomized study on postoperative nausea, ginger was compared to metoclopramide and a placebo for antiemetic activity in 60 women who were about to undergo major gynecological surgery. Powdered ginger rhizome or placebo (1 g p.o.) was administered in colored capsules in addition to either a placebo injection or active injection (hyoscine and papaveretum). Both the placebo and the ginger capsules were flavored using a nonactive ginger flavoring and were indistinguishable when swallowed with water. The incidence of nausea in the two groups given either ginger or metoclopramide was similar (30% and 28%, respectively), although there were significantly fewer ($p < 0.05$) recorded instances of nausea in the groups that received ginger compared to the placebo group (51%). Incidence of nausea at any time during the study occurred in 45% of those administered ginger, in 50% of those administered metoclopramide, and in 70% of the placebo control group (Bone et al., 1990).

In another controlled double-blind study, Holtmann et al. (1989) reported that ginger root had no influence on artificially induced nystagmus in test subjects, suggesting a lack of action on the central nervous system.

In a double-blind, placebo-controlled study, GrØntved et al. (1988) recruited a group of 80 naval cadets, each of whom was given either 1 g of powdered ginger p.o. or a placebo while at sea. Symptoms of nausea were recorded once an hour during 4 h after treatment administration. Sweating and vomiting in the ginger group were 38% less than in the placebo group; however, there was no effect on vertigo or nausea compared to placebo and significant differences in reduced symptoms were only seen at the last (fourth) hour.

Inducing motion sickness using a rotating chair, Stewart et al. (1991) studied the motion sickness preventive effect of encapsulated fresh (1,000 mg, locally purchased) and powdered ginger (McCormick & Co., Hunt Valley, MD, 500 and 1,000 mg) in 28 volunteers (ages 18-44). Results were compared to placebo (lactose mixed with brown sugar), and to scopolamine (0.6 mg p.o.), and ginger at doses administered 15 or 60 min prior to inducing motion sickness. The study, which was not double-blinded or randomized, showed that ginger in either form or dosage was not significantly better than the placebo in preventing motion sickness, nor in altering gastric function in motion sickness compared to placebo, whereas scopolamine was significantly effective against motion sickness.

In contrast to the results of Stewart et al. (1991), Mowrey and Clayson (1982) reported good effects from ginger in a study of severe motion sickness. Each of 36 patients with histories of severe motion sickness received capsules containing either a placebo (powdered chickweed, *Stellaria media*), 100 mg of dimenhydrinate, or 940 mg of powdered ginger. Thirty minutes later they were blindfolded and spun in a mechanical chair until they asked to stop, or vomited. On average, the ginger group remained in the chair for 5.5 minutes, versus 3.5 minutes for those who received dimenhydrinate, and 1.5 minutes for the placebo group.

Immune Disorders; Inflammation and Disease

Inflammatory Response

Srivastava (1989) conducted an open study on thromboxane$_2$ (TBX$_2$) production in seven women volunteers (ages 25-65 years) who were instructed to ingest 5 g of fresh, raw ginger rhizome daily for seven days. Their diet was largely vegetarian. Venous blood collected before and after was reported to show a significant decrease in TXB$_2$ production in 6 of 7 volunteers (37%), thereby supporting previous in vitro results (see also, Preclinical Studies: Inflammatory Response). However, Lumb (1994) challenged this finding, pointing out that due to the diversity of readings the end result failed to reach statistical significance. Lumb then conducted a randomized, double-blind, placebo-controlled crossover study of ginger powder (2 g in capsules) in eight healthy male volunteers (ages not stated) and measured whole blood platelet aggregation, platelet count, and bleeding time before and at 3 h and 24 h postadministration. The results showed no significant differences compared to placebo in any of the measurements (Lumb, 1994).

Janssen et al. (1996) studied the effects of various ginger preparations on ex vivo platelet TBX_2 in a randomized, placebo-controlled, multiple crossover study. During three consecutive treatment periods of two weeks, healthy, nonsmoking volunteers of either sex ($n = 18$; ages 19-25 years) ingested either 40 g of cooked ginger stems, 15 g of raw, peeled ginger rhizome (Brazilian) or placebo (no ginger) in 125 g of vanilla custard ingested daily at the clinic and from supplied treatments over weekends. Blood work showed no abnormalities in any of the volunteers. Paracetamol was supplied in case of pain and they were instructed to abstain from dietary supplements for a period of four weeks preceding the trial. They were also told to abstain from products containing ginger or fatty fish while maintaining their normal dietary and drinking habits and level of exercise. Subjects also had to record any deviations from their normal habits of diet. The results showed no significant difference in TBX_2 production from either type of ginger compared to placebo. There were also no reports of adverse events and all subjects denied using aspirin during or four weeks prior to the study.

Bordia et al. (1997) conducted a placebo-controlled study to investigate the effects of Indian ginger on platelet aggregation in 60 subjects with coronary artery disease (CAD), half serving as the control group administered placebo. Before a two-week washout, all the CAD subjects were taking aspirin and nitrates and had healed from myocardial infarction over six months earlier. Ginger powder or placebo was administered in capsules at a dosage of 4 g/day for three months. Blood samples were taken every two weeks, and once a month the patients were evaluated for side effects and clinical symptoms. At 1.5 and 3 months, no affect was seen in the ginger group in either epinephrine- or adenosine diphosphate-induced platelet aggregation assays, and there was no change in their fibrinogen level and fibrinolytic activity. Despite this outcome, when ten patients from the ginger group were administered 10 g of the ginger powder in a single dose, both assays of platelet aggregation showed significant decreases (each $p < 0.05$) compared to ten patients from placebo control group after the same dose (Bordia et al., 1997).

The dissolution of fibrin (fibrinolysis) allows blood to thin. Fatty meals are known to increase the clotting of blood through the action of fibrin which is formed from fibrinogen during clotting. The effect of powdered ginger on fibrinolytic activity in healthy volunteers was investigated by Verma and Bordia (2001) in 30 adult males (ages 30-50). In a randomized, placebo-controlled study, blood samples were taken from the subjects after they had fasted and again four hours after they received slices of bread with 50 g of butter. The following week, they were given four capsules containing either placebo or ginger powder (625 mg/capsule) which were taken with the butter and bread. The fatty meal alone caused fibrinolytic activity to decrease by 18.8%, with or without placebo. With the ginger powder, fibrinolytic activity increased 6.7%, a highly significant difference compared to the effect of the fatty meal alone ($p < 0.001$). Compared to the effect of the fatty meal alone, this represented an increase in fibrinolytic activity of 31.5%. No side effects were found in any of the subjects. The researchers mention that an old custom in India is to add ginger to fatty meals.

Neurological, Psychological, and Behavioral Disorders

Receptor- and Neurotransmitter-Mediated Functions

Anecdotal reports of pain relief after the consumption of powdered ginger by individuals with osteoarthritis, rheumatoid arthritis, and muscle pain led Srivastava and Mustafa (1992) to conduct a questionnaire-based open trial of ginger in a group of 46 patients with osteoarthritis ($n = 18$), or rheumatoid arthritis ($n = 28$ including three with nonspecific arthritis) who had been taking powdered ginger for 3 months to 2.5 years. The self-reported dosage was calculated to be about 1-2 g per day which was considerably more than the amount the investigators suggested they take (0.5-1.0 g/day). Marked relief from pain was reported by 55% of the osteoarthritis patients and by 74% of the rheumatoid arthritis patients.

Bliddal et al. (2000) conducted a randomized, double-blind, placebo-controlled crossover design study on the pain-relieving effect of a ginger extract in 56 patients diagnosed with osteoarthritis (radiologically verified; 41 women and 15 men ages 24-87). Using three treatment periods lasting three weeks each, the pain-relieving effect of a standardized extract of Chinese ginger (Eurovita, Extract 33 in soft gelatin capsules; standardized to contain hydroxy-methoxy-phenyl compounds) was compared to ibuprofen and placebo. At the beginning of the study, the Lesquesne index of the patients ranged from 1 to 21.5 (mean 11.8) and the duration of their osteoarthritis ranged from 1 to 30 years (mean 7.7 years). Changes in their degree of pain were measured using the visual analogue scale (VAS). After a one-week washout period when the use of other pain-management substances was stopped, patients were randomly assigned to three-week treatment periods of ibuprofen (400 mg t.i.d), ginger extract (170 mg t.i.d.), and matching placebo (ibuprofen tablet- and ginger capsule-placebo t.i.d.). No washout periods were applied between the three treatment periods. No significant difference in the VAS was found from the ginger extract compared to placebo whereas the ibuprofen treatment produced a highly significant relief from pain compared to placebo or the ginger extract. No differences in range of motion were noted in any of the treatment periods and no significant difference in adverse effects were found between the three treatments. The researchers caution that because of carry over effects between the treatment periods which were without washouts, the results of their study may not accurately reflect the pain-relieving effects of ginger. For example, when they conducted an exploratory statistical analysis of the first period of treatment, the ginger extract and ibuprofen both showed significantly greater pain-relieving effects than placebo ($p < 0.05$ in the Chi-square test). They also mentioned that the three-week treatment period may have been inadequate to observe the effects of ginger extract in osteoarthritic pain and further suggested that future studies might employ more than one dose and even a more potent preparation of ginger.

Reproductive Disorders

Pregnancy and Labor Disorders

Vutyavanich et al. (2001) studied the effectiveness of ginger powder against nausea and vomiting in 67 pregnant women characterized as having less severe nausea and vomiting. The study was randomized, double-blinded, placebo-controlled, and parallel in design and the primary outcome was improvement in nausea which was measured using five-item Likert scales, a visual analogue scale, and an intention-to-treat analysis. The patients recruited were among new obstetric attendees of a prenatal clinic. Patients were administered identical appearing 250 mg capsules containing either placebo or ginger powder in a dosage of one gram per day in divided doses of 250 mg to be taken at bedtime and after each of three daily meals during four consecutive days. They were instructed to abstain from all other drugs and to eat frequent small meals low in fat and rich in carbohydrates and to report back for assessment after seven days. The results showed that a significant improvement had occurred in the nausea scores of the ginger group relative to their baseline scores and compared to the placebo group ($p = 0.014$), and that the significantly greater decrease in nausea was only evident on day four of the treatment period versus placebo. A day prior to treatment, 100% of the ginger group had vomiting episodes as did 94.3% of the placebo group. After day four of the treatment, 37.5% of the ginger group had vomiting episodes versus 65.7% of the placebo group. Subjective responses to treatment among the patients according to results of the Likert

scales found a significant difference, with 87.5% of the ginger group reporting improved symptoms versus 28.6% of the placebo group ($p < 0.001$)
(Vutyavanich et al., 2001).

None of the infants born to the participants subsequent to the trial showed
congenital anomalies and every infant was discharged "in good condition."
The patients had term deliveries in 96.9% of the placebo group and 91.4%
of the ginger-treated group. Headache was reported in 14.3% of the placebo
group and in 18.8% of the ginger group. The only other side effects reported
were in the ginger group with one patient each reporting heartburn, diarrhea
lasting one day, and abdominal discomfort; however, in no case was the side
effect more than minor, nor did it result in discontinuation of the trial prescription. The use of ginger during pregnancy has been cautioned against by
Backon (1991) who theorized that because ginger could affect receptor
binding of testosterone it could alter sex steroid-dependent differentiation at
the level of the fetal brain. Although this trial exposure to ginger lasted only
four days and the dosage was small, especially compared to amounts of ginger used in prepared foods (≥ 30 g), it is still possible that congenital anomalies or other "rare but significant adverse effects" may be undetected due to
the small number of patients thus far studied in trials of ginger (Vutyavanich
et al., 2001, p. 582).

Fischer-Rasmussen et al. (1990) conducted a double-blind, randomized,
crossover trial of powdered ginger rhizome in the treatment of hyperemesis
gravidarum in 27 women (ages 18-39). At the same dosage (250 mg q.i.d.
for four days), capsules of the ginger powder or placebo (lactose) were
taken in the second treatment phase (crossover) after a two-day washout period. No antiemetics were allowed and hyperemesis severity was scored before and after treatment according to degree of weight loss, nausea, and
vomiting. A symptom relief score was also applied to assess the treatment
and included patients' subjective assessments after each treatment period.
The results showed a significantly greater improvement in relief scores in
the ginger period compared to placebo ($p < 0.035$), and the most notable
change was in the reduced incidence of vomiting and the experience of nausea. Patient preference for treatment was also significantly higher for ginger
compared to placebo (70.4 versus 14.8% and 14.8% undecided) ($p < 0.003$).
No side-effects were reported and babies born to the women showed no de-
formities and were discharged in good condition. Apgar scores in all babies
were 9-10 (after 5 min). In the placebo group, one patient requested an abortion due to problems unrelated to treatment, and in the ginger group one patient spontaneously aborted (week 12 of gestation). It was noted that out of
27 pregnancies this one spontaneous abortion in early pregnancy was not
suspicious.

DOSAGE

Most clinical studies have used approximately one gram of powdered dried root per day. This seems to be an effective and safe dose. Other studies have used extracts of the fresh root, although the powdered root is considered more potent (Chang and But, 1986; Bradley, 1992; Fulder and Tenne, 1996). The German Commission E allows a daily dosage of 2-4 g of the rhizome or an equivalent preparation for use in the prevention of motion sickness or the treatment of dyspepsia (Blumenthal et al., 1998).

SAFETY PROFILE

Side Effects

The German Commission E states that side effects from ginger are unknown (Blumenthal et al., 1998). In a double-blind study of a standardized ginger extract (Zintona, 500 mg every 4 h for two days) in adults known to have sensitivity to motion sickness, side effects were reported by 13.3% of participants in the ginger group. These included somnolence in three and headache in one, both of which could have occurred from motion sickness rather than the ginger extract (Reibenfeld and Borzone, 1999). No side effects were reported in a double-blind study of motion sickness-sensitive children (ages four to eight) taking 250 mg of a standardized ginger extract every 4 h or as needed over two days (Careddu, 1999).

It has been theorized that overdosage could potentially appear in central nervous system problems or cardiac arrhythmias (Fulder and Tenne, 1996).

One case of inhibited platelet aggregation was reported in a patient who had consumed a presumably large amount of marmalade containing 15% raw ginger (Dorso et al., 1980); however, given that marmalades contain fruit products with antiaggregatory constituents (coumarins, flavonoids, etc.), in this case, ginger could hardly be singled out. See also Drug Interactions.

Contraindications

The German Commission E states that in cases of gallstones, ginger should only be used after consulting a physician (Blumenthal et al., 1998). See also, Pregnancy and Lactation.

Drug Interactions

At an oral dose of 100 mg/kg, a standardized ethanolic extract of ginger showed no significant effect on warfarin-prolonged blood coagulation in rats as measured by changes in activated partial thromboblastin, prothrombin, and whole blood clotting times (Weidner and Sigwart, 2000). Whether other ginger preparations would exhibit the same lack of drug interaction with warfarin is not known. A search of the literature for reported cases of drug interactions in patients taking ginger and warfarin found no instances in which the two were definitely linked (Vaes and Chyka, 2000). Subjects taking a dried ethanolic extract of ginger (4 g/day for three months) showed no significant change in platelet aggregation (Bordia et al., 1997), nor from powdered ginger at an acute dose of 2 g (Lumb, 1994). However, in a small, randomized, placebo-controlled trial in which healthy male volunteers (ages 30-50) were administered a fatty meal along with capsules containing ginger powder (2.5 g twice daily for seven days), platelet aggregation (adenosine diphosphate- and epinephrine-induced in vitro) was significantly inhibited compared to placebo.

Pregnancy and Lactation

As with garlic, ginger is a widely consumed foodstuff. In some cultures, daily ingestion of therapeutic doses (i.e., doses shown to have physiological activity) is common. In TCM, caution is advised in the use of ginger during pregnancy (Zhu, 1998). In TCM, however, medicinal doses of ginger may range up to 9 g/day. Newall et al. (1996) reports ginger as an abortifacient with uterotonic activity in related species. In Germany, ginger is contraindicated during pregnancy (Blumenthal et al., 1998) because of the hypothesis that ginger may inhibit testosterone binding. This is an untested hypothesis, and there is no evidence from any study to support it. No reports of miscarriage or birth defects from ginger have been reported (Fischer-Rasmussen et al., 1990; Vutyavanich et al., 2001). Small-scale studies involving pregnant women diagnosed with hyperemesis gravida showed no adverse effects on pregnancy or infant outcomes with doses of 1 g/day of dried ginger (see Reproductive Disorders: Pregnancy and Labor Disorders).

Ginger use during lactation is not associated with any reports of adverse effects, nor are any anticipated. Traditional use as an aid to recovery in the postpartum period is widespread in Asia, and infers common use during early lactation in these cultures (see History and Traditional Uses).

Special Precautions

Although studies thus far have shown ginger to be relatively safe, it is a strong in vitro thromboxane synthetase inhibitor and prostacyclin agonist; therefore, Backon (1986, 1987) cautioned that postoperative patients taking ginger as an antiemetic should be monitored closely. However, placebo-controlled clinical studies in healthy volunteers have shown that ginger exerts no significant effect on thromboxane levels (Lumb, 1994; Janssen et al., 1996).

Some individuals show contact allergic reactions to ginger. In one patch test study of common spices, reactions to ginger were more common than ten other common household spices (Futrell and Rietschel, 1993).

Toxicology

Mutagenicity

In reviewing the mutagenic studies of ginger and ginger constituents, Surh et al. (1998) noted that whereas in one study an ethanolic extract of the rhizome showed mutagenic activity (in *Salmonella typhimurium* TA 102 and TA 98) without metabolic activation, another found no mutagenic activity from ginger extract, and a third found that genotoxicity elicited by several carcinogens became suppressed by ginger extract, both in mammalian and bacterial cells.

With or without S9 mix, in *S. typhimurium* strains TA 1538 and TA 98, Nagabhushan et al. (1987) reported that an ethylether/ethanolic extract of ginger failed to induce revertants, yet it showed mutagenic activity in strains 1535 and TA 100 with S9 mix. Morimoto et al. (1982) reported that a water extract of fresh ginger *(Zingiber rhizoma)* was mutagenic in strain TA 100 (with or without rat liver S9 mix), whereas in either TA 98 or TA 100 a methanolic extract was not. Using a modified Ames test with *S. typhimurium* TA100 and TA98, Yamamoto et al. (1982) found no mutagenicity from a water and methanol extract of *Zingiber rhizoma,* but did find mutagenicity from an extract of *Zingiber siccatum rhizoma* (in *S. typhimurium* strains TA 100 with or without rat liver S9 mix, but not in strain TA 98). The former name refers to the fresh rhizome while the latter refers to the dried rhizome (Foster and Yue, 1992). The difference may be due to the presence of contaminants or to the balance of mutagenic and antimutagenic constituents of the two rhizome samples (Surh et al., 1998).

Shogaol and gingerol have shown mutagenic activity in the Ames test, whereas zingerone has been shown to dose-dependently suppress their mutagenic activity and showed no mutagenic activity with or without S9 mix in strains TA 98, TA 100, TA 1535, and TA 1538. Shogaol exhibited less mutagenic activity compared to gingerol in strains TA 100 and TA 1535 with S9 mix. No activity was found from either compound without S9 mix (Nagabhushan et al., 1987). Storage of ginger causes gingerol content to undergo conversion to shogaol and treatment of gingerol with alkali or heat converts it into zingerone (Nagabhushan et al., 1987, citing Bhagya and Govindrajan, 1979 and Connell and Sutherland, 1969).

Both [6]-gingerol and the freshly prepared juice of the rhizome accelerated chemically-induced mutagenesis in the Hs30 strain of *Escherichia coli* B/r. The observation was made after mixing the juice with either of two potently mutagenic furans. In a separate experiment, [6]-gingerol was found to be mutagenic by itself, so much so that it killed the bacteria; however, when the ginger juice was added, the mutagenic activity of [6]-gingerol was significantly suppressed. Subsequently, two [6]-gingerol-free fractions of the juice were isolated, which both caused a significant suppression of [6]-gingerol-induced mutagenesis whereas a fraction containing the gingerol was mutagenic (Nakamura and Yamamoto, 1982).

Toxicity in Animal Models

There is no reported LD_{50} because it has been impossible to feed lab rodents a sufficient amount of crude ginger to induce death. Doses of 3.0 g/kg and 3.5 g/kg of an ethanolic extract of ginger rhizome produced death by involuntary contractions of skeletal muscle in 10% to 30% of laboratory mice within 72 h of administration but doses of 2g or less were without toxic effects (Mascolo et al., 1989). Male mice administered a 95% ethanol extract of the rhizomes (with ethanol removed) at a dosage of 100 mg/kg p.o. for three months showed no significant change in abnormal sperm counts, total sperm counts, white blood cell counts, red blood cell counts, percentage of hemoglobin, mortality rate, average body weight, and average organ weights (heart, lung, liver, spleen, and kidneys). From an acute dose of 3 g/kg p.o., locomotor activity over 24 h was slightly reduced, but not after 1 g/kg p.o. (Qureshi et al., 1989). Groups of pregnant rats administered a standardized ginger extract from the sixth to fifteenth day of gestation at doses of 100, 333, and 1,000 mg/kg p.o. showed no signs of adverse effects, including reproductive performance, compared to untreated pregnant rats. Fetuses of the rats showed no teratogenic or embryotoxic effects (Weidner and Sigwart, 2001). The LD_{50}s of the main active constituents of ginger rhizome are 250-680 mg/kg for [6]-gingerol and [6]-shogaol, which is 3,500 to 9,000 times the normal adult human dose (Fulder and Tenne, 1996).

REFERENCES

Adewunmi, C.O., Oguntimein, B.O., and Furu, P. (1990). Molluscicidal and anti-schistosomal activities of *Zingiber officinale*. *Planta Medica* 56: 374-376.

Aeschbach, J., Loliger, J., Scott, B.C., Murcia, A., Butler, J., Haliwell, B., and Aruoma, O.I. (1994). Antioxidant actions of thymol, carbacol, 6-gingerol, zingerone and hydroxytyrolsol. *Food and Chemical Toxicology* 32: 31-36.

Ahmed, R.S., Seth, V., Pasha, S.T., and Banerjee, B.D. (2000). Influence of dietary ginger (*Zingiber officinale* Rosc) on oxidative stress induced by malathion in rats. *Food and Chemical Toxicology* 38: 443-450.

Arfeen, Z., Owen, H., Plummer, J.L., Ilsley, A.H., Sorby-Adams, R.A.C., and Doecke, C.J. (1995). A double-blind randomized controlled trial of ginger for the prevention of postoperative nausea and vomiting. *Anaesthesia in Intensive Care* 23: 449-452.

Autrup, H., Grafstrom, R.C., Brugh, M., Lechner, J.F., Haugen, A., Trump, B.F., and Harris, C.C. (1982). Comparison of benzo[*a*]pyrene metabolism in bronchus, esophagus, colon, and duodenum from the same individual. *Cancer Research* 42: 934-938.

Backon, J. (1986). Ginger inhibition of thromboxane synthetase and stimulation of prostacyclin: Relevance for medicine and psychiatry. *Medical Hypotheses* 20: 271-278.

Backon, J. (1987). Ginger and carbon dioxide as thromboxane synthetase inhibitors: Potential utility in treating peptide ulceration. *Gut* 28: 1323.

Backon, J. (1991). Ginger in preventing nausea and vomiting of pregnancy: A caveat due to its thromboxane synthetase activity and effect on testosterone binding. *European Journal of Obstetrics, Gynecology and Reproductive Biology* 42: 163 (letter).

Bhagya, G. and Govindrajan, V.S. (1979). Evaluation of spices and oleoresins. VIII. Improved separation of ginger and estimation of ginger by thin layer chromatography. *Journal of Food Quality* 2: 205-207.

Bhandari, U., Sharma, J.N., and Zafar, R. (1998). The protective action of ethanolic ginger *(Zingiber officinale)* extract in cholesterol-fed rabbits. *Journal of Ethnopharmacology* 61: 167-171.

Bliddal, H., Rosetzsky, A., Schlichting, P., Weidner, M.S., Andersen, L.A., Ibfelt, H.H., Christensen, K., Jensen, O.N., and Barslev, J. (2000). A randomized, placebo-controlled, cross-over study of ginger extracts and ibuprofen in osteoarthritis. *Osteoarthritis and Cartilage* 8: 9-12.

Blumenthal, M., Busse, W.R., Goldberg, A., Gruenwald, J., Hall, T., Riggins, C.W., and Rister, R.S. (Eds.) (1998). *The Complete German Commission E Monographs*. Austin, TX: American Botanical Council, pp. 135-136.

Bone, M.E., Wilkinson, D.J., Young, J.R., McNeil, J., and Charlton, S. (1990). Ginger root—A new antiemetic: The effect of ginger root on postoperative nausea and vomiting after major gynaecological surgery. *Anaesthesia* 45: 669-671.

Bordia, A., Verma, S.K., and Srivastava, K.C. (1997). Effect of ginger (*Zingiber officinale* Rosc.) and fenugreek (*Trigonella foenumgraecum* L.) on blood lipids, blood sugar and platelet aggregation in patients with coronary artery disease. *Prostaglandins, Leukotrienes and Essential Fatty Acids* 56: 379-384.

Boyle, W. (1991). *Official Herbs: Botanical Substances in the United States Pharmacopoeias 1820-1990*. East Palestine, OH: Buckeye Naturopathic Press, pp. 50-51.

Bradley, P. (Ed.) (1992). *British Herbal Compendium, 1*. Bournemouth, Dorset, England: British Herbal Medicine Association.

Careddu, P. (1999). Motion sickness in children: Results of a double-blind study with ginger (Zintona®) and dimenhydrinate. *Healthnotes Review of Complementary and Integrative Medicine* 6: 102-107.

Chang, C.P., Chang, J.Y., Wang, F.Y., and Chang, J.G. (1995). The effect of Chinese medicinal herb *Zingiberis rhizoma* extract on cytokine secretion by human peripheral blood mononuclear cells. *Journal of Ethnopharmacology* 48: 13-19.

Chang, H. and But, P. (Eds.) (1986). *Pharmacology and Applications of Chinese Materia Medica*, 1. Singapore: World Scientific.

Chang, W.S., Chang, Y.H., Lu, F.J., and Chiang, H.C. (1994). Inhibitory effects of phenolics on xanthine oxidase. *Anticancer Research* 14: 501-506.

Connell, O.W. and Sutherland, M.D. (1969). A re-examination of gingerol, shogaol and zingerone, the pungent principles of ginger (*Zingiber officinale* Roscoe). *Australian Journal of Chemistry* 22: 1033-1043.

Culp, S.J., Gaylor, D.W., Sheldon, W.G., Goldstein, L.S., and Beland, F.A. (1998). A comparison of the tumors induced by coal tar and benzo[*a*]pyrene in a 2-year bioassay. *Carcinogenesis* 19: 117-124.

Datta, A. and Sukul, N.C. (1987). Antifilarial effect of *Zingiber officinale* on *Dirofilaria immitis*. *Journal of Helminthology* 61: 268-270.

Dedov, V.N., Tran, V.H., Duke, C.C., and Roufogalis, B.D. (2000). Direct activation of the VR-1 receptor by natural gingerols: A new class of capsaicin VR-1 receptor agonists. *Phytomedicine* 7(Suppl. II): 52 (abstract SL-106).

Dorso, C.R., Levin, R.I., Eldor, A., Jaffe, E.A., and Weksler, B.B. (1980). Chinese food and platelets. *New England Journal of Medicine* 303: 756-757 (letter).

Dutta, M.L. and Nath, S.C. (1998). Ethno-medico botany of the Deories of Assam, India. *Fitoterapia* 69: 147-154.

Ernst, E. and Pittler, M.H. (2000). Efficacy of ginger for nausea and vomiting: A systematic review of randomized clinical trials. *British Journal of Anaesthesia* 84: 367-371.

Fischer-Rasmussen, W., Kjaer, S., Dahl, C., and Asping, U. (1990). Ginger treatment of hyperemesis gravidarum. *European Journal of Obstetrics and Gynecology, and Reproductive Biology* 38: 19-24.

Foster, S. and Yue, C. (1992). *Herbal Emissaries: Bringing Chinese Herbs to the West*. Rochester, VT: Healing Arts Press, p. 93.

Fuhrman, B., Rosenblat, M., Hayek, T., Coleman, R., and Aviram, M. (2000). Ginger extract consumption reduces plasma cholesterol, inhibits LDL oxidation and attenuates development of atherosclerosis in atherosclerotic, apolipoprotein E-deficient mice. *The Journal of Nutrition* 130: 1124-1131.

Fulder, S. and Tenne, M. (1996). Ginger as an anti-nausea remedy in pregnancy; the issue of safety. *HerbalGram* 38: 47-50.

Futrell, J.M. and Rietschel, R.L. (1993). Spice allergy evaluated by results of patch tests. *Cutis* 52: 288-290.

Goto, C., Kasuya, S., Koga, K., Ohtomo, H., and Kagei, N. (1990). Lethal efficacy of extract of *Zingiber officinale* (traditional Chinese medicine) or [6]-shogaol and [6]-gingerol in *Anisakis* larvae in vitro. *Parasitology Research* 76: 653-656.

Govindarajan, V.S. (1982). Ginger—Chemistry, technology, and quality evaluation. Part 1. *CRC Critical Reviews in Food Science and Nutrition* 17: 1-96.

GrØntved, A., Brask, T., Kambskard, J., and Hentzer, E. (1988). Ginger root against seasickness: A controlled trial on the open sea. *Acta Otolaryngologica* 105: 45-49.

Gugnani, H.C. and Ezenwanze, E.C. (1985). Antibacterial activity of extracts of ginger and African oil bean seed. *Journal of Communicable Diseases* 17: 233-236.

Guh, J.H., Ko, F.N., Jong, T.T., and Teng, C.M. (1995). Antiplatelet effect of gingerol isolated from *Zingiber officinale*. *Journal of Pharmacy and Pharmacology* 47: 329-332.

Hikino, H., Kiso, Y., Kato, N., Hamada, Y., Shioiri, T., Aiyama, R., Itokawa, H., Kiuchi, F., and Sanakawa, U. (1985). Antihepatotoxic actions of gingerols and diarylheptanoids. *Journal of Ethnopharmacology* 14: 31-39.

Holtmann, S., Clarke, A.H., Scherer, H., and Hohm, M. (1989). The anti-motion sickness mechanism of ginger: A comparative study with placebo and dimenhydrinate. *Acta Otolaryngologica* 108: 168-174.

Huang, Q., Iwamoto, M., Aoki, S., Tanaka, N., Tajima, K., Yamahara, J., Takaishi, Y., Yoshida, M., Tomimatsu, T., and Tamai, Y. (1991). Anti-5-hydroxytryptamine$_3$ effect of galanolactone, diterpenoid isolated from ginger. *Chemical and Pharmaceutical Bulletin* 39: 397-399.

Janssen, P.L., Meyboom, S., van Staveren, W.A., de Vegt, F., and Katan, M.B. (1996). Consumption of ginger (*Zingiber officinale* Roscoe) does not affect ex vivo platelet thromboxane production in humans. *European Journal of Clinical Nutrition* 50: 772-774.

Kami, T., Nakayama, M., and Hayashi, S. (1972). Volatile constituents of *Zingiber officinale*. *Phytochemistry* 11: 3377-3381.

Katiyar, S.K., Agarwal, R., and Mukhtar, H. (1996). Inhibition of tumor formation in SENCAR mouse skin by ethanol extract of *Zingiber officinale* rhizome. *Cancer Research* 56: 1023-1030.

Kawai, T., Kinoshita, K., Koyama, K., and Takahashi, K. (1994). Anti-emetic principles of *Magnolia obovata* bark and *Zingiber officinale* rhizome. *Planta Medica* 60: 17-20.

Kikuzaki, H. and Nakatani, N. (1993). Antioxidant effect of some ginger constituents. *Journal of Food Science* 58: 1407-1410.

Kiuchi, F., Shibuya, M., and Sankawa, U. (1982). Inhibitors of prostaglandin biosynthesis from ginger. *Chemical and Pharmaceutical Bulletin* 30: 754-757.

Lee, E. and Surh, Y.J. (1998). Induction of apoptosis in HL-60 cells by pungent vanilloids, [6]-gingerol and [6]-paradol. *Cancer Letters* 134: 163-168.

Leung, A.Y. and Foster, S. (1996). *Encyclopedia of Common Natural Ingredients*. Second Edition. New York: John Wiley and Sons, pp. 271-274.

Lumb, A.B. (1994). Effect of dried ginger on human platelet function. *Thrombosis and Haemostasis* 71: 110-111.

Mascolo, I., Jain, R., Jain, S.C., and Capasso, F. (1989). Ethnopharmacologic investigation of ginger (*Zingiber officinale*). *Journal of Ethnopharmacology* 27: 129-140.

Micklefield, G.H., Redeker, Y., Meister, V., Jung, O., Greving, I., and May, B. (1999). Effects of ginger on gastroduodenal motility. *International Journal of Clinical Pharmacology and Therapeutics* 37: 341-346.

Morimoto, I., Watanabe, F., Osawa, T., Okitsu, T., and Kada, T. (1982). Mutagenicity screening of crude drugs with *Bacillus subtilis* rec-assay and Salmonella/microsome reversion assay. *Mutation Research* 97: 81-102.

Mowrey, D.B. and Clayson, D.E. (1982). Motion sickness, ginger, and psychophysics. *Lancet* 1 (March 20): 655-657

Murugaiah, J.S., Namasivatam, N., and Menon, V.P. (1999). Effect of ginger (*Zingiber officinale* R.) on lipids in rats fed atherogenic diet. *Journal of Clinical Biochemistry and Nutrition* 27: 78-87.

Nadkarni, A.K. (1976). *Indian Materia Medica, 1.* Bombay, India: Popular Prakashan Pvt. Ltd., pp. 1308-1315.

Nagabhushan, M., Amonkar, A.J., and Bhide, S.V. (1987). Mutagenicity of gingerol and shogaol and antimutagenicity of zingerone in *Salmonella*/microsome assay. *Cancer Letters* 36: 221-233.

Nakamura, H. and Yamamoto, T. (1982). Mutagen and anti-mutagen in ginger, *Zingiber officinale*. *Mutation Research* 103: 119-126.

Newall, C.A., Anderson, L.A., and Phillipson, J.D. (1996). *Herbal Medicines: A Guide for Health Care Professionals.* London: The Pharmaceutical Press, pp. 135-137.

Ohizumi, Y., Sasaki, S., Shibusawa, K., Ishikawa, K., and Ikemoto, F. (1996). Stimulation of sarcoplasmic reticulum Ca^{2+}-ATPase by gingerol analogues. *Biological and Pharmaceutical Bulletin* 19: 1377-1379.

Park, K.K., Chun, K.S., Lee, J.M., Lee, S.S., and Surh, Y.J. (1998). Inhibitory effects of [6]-gingerol, a major pungent principle of ginger, on phorbol ester-induced inflammation, epidermal ornithine decarboxylase activity and skin tumor promotion in ICR mice. *Cancer Letters* 129: 139-144.

Phillips, S., Hutchinson, S.E., and Ruggier, R. (1993). *Zingiber officinale* does not affect gastric emptying rate: A randomized, placebo-controlled, crossover trial. *Anaethesia* 48: 393-395.

Phillips, S., Ruggier, R., and Hutchinson, S.E. (1993). *Zingiber officinale* (ginger)—An antiemetic for day case surgery. *Anaethesia* 48: 715-717.

Puri, A., Sahai, R., Singh, K.L., Saxena, R.P., Tandon, J.S., and Saxena, K.C. (2000). Immunostimulant activity of dry fruits and plant materials used in Indian traditional medical system for mothers after childbirth and invalids. *Journal of Ethnopharmacology* 71: 89-92.

Qureshi, S., Shah, A.H., Tariq, M., and Ageel, A.M. (1989). Studies on herbal aphrodisiacs used in Arab system of medicine. *American Journal of Chinese Medicine* 17: 57-63.

Riebenfeld, D. and Borzone, L. (1999). Randomized double-blind study comparing ginger (Zintona®) and dimenhydrinate in motion sickness. *Health Notes Review of Complementary and Integrative Medicine* 6: 98-101.

Sakai, K., Miyazaki, Y., Yamane, T., Saitph, Y., Ikawa, C., and Nishihata, T. (1989). Effect of extracts of Zingiberaceae herbs on gastric sections in rabbits. *Chemical and Pharmaceutical Bulletin* 37: 215-217.

Sakai, Y., Nagase, H., Ose, Y., Sato, T., Kawai, M., and Mizuno, M. (1988). Effects of medicinal plant extracts from Chinese herbal medicines on the mutagenic activity of benzo[*a*]pyrene. *Mutation Research* 206: 327-334.

Schulick, P. (1994). *Ginger: Common Spice and Wonder Drug,* Revised Edition. Brattleboro, VT: Herbal Free Press.

Sekiwa, Y., Kubots, K., and Kobayashi, A. (2000). Isolation of novel glucosides related to gingerdiol from ginger and their antioxidative activities. *Journal of Agricultural and Food Chemistry* 48: 373-377.

Sertie, J., Basile, A., Oshiro, T.T., Silva, F.D., and Mazella, A.A.G. (1992). Preventive anti-ulcer activity of the rhizome extract of *Zingiber officinale. Fitoterapia* 63: 155-159.

Sharma, I., Gusain, D., and Dixit, V.P. (1996). Hypolipidaemic and antiatherosclerotic effects of *Zingiber officinale* in cholesterol fed rabbits. *Phytotherapy Research* 10: 517-518.

Sharma, J.N., Srivastava, K.C., and Gan, E.K. (1994). Suppressive effects of eugenol and ginger oil on arthritic rats. *Pharmacology* 49: 314-418.

Sharma, S.S. and Gupta, Y.K. (1998). Reversal of cisplatin-induced delay in gastric emptying rate in rats by ginger *(Zingiber officinale). Journal of Ethnopharmacology* 62: 49-55.

Sharma, S.S., Kochupillai, V., Gupta, S.K., Seth, S.D., and Gupta, Y.K. (1997). Antiemetic efficacy of ginger *(Zingiber officinale)* against cisplatin-induced emesis in dogs. *Journal of Ethnopharmacology* 57: 93-96.

Shoji, N., Iwasa, A., Takemoto, T., Ishida, Y., and Ohizumi, Y. (1982). Cardiotonic principles of ginger (*Zingiber officinale* Roscoe). *Journal of Pharmaceutical Sciences* 71: 1174-1175.

Srivastava, K.C. (1989). Effect of onion and ginger consumption on platelet thromboxane production in humans. *Prostaglandins, Leukotrienes and Medicine* 35: 183-185.

Srivastava, K.C. and Mustafa, T. (1992). Ginger *(Zingiber officinale)* in rheumatism and musculoskeletal disorders. *Medical Hypotheses* 39: 342-348.

Srivastava, K. and Sambaiah, K. (1991). The effect of spices on cholesterol 7 alpha-hydroxylase activity and on serum and hepatic cholesterol levels in the rat. *International Journal for Vitamin and Nutrition Research* 61: 363-369.

Stewart, J.J., Wood, M.J., Wood, C.D., and Mims, M.E. (1991). Effects of ginger on motion sickness susceptibility and gastric function. *Pharmacology* 42: 111-120.

Surh, Y., Lee, E., and Lee, J.M. (1998). Chemoprotective properties of some pungent ingredients present in red pepper and ginger. *Mutation Research* 402: 259-267.

Surh, Y., Park, K.K., Chun, K.S., Lee, J.M., Lee, E., and Lee, S.S. (1999). Anti-tumor-promoting activities of selected pungent phenolic substances present in ginger. *Journal of Environmental Pathology, Toxicology and Oncology* 18: 131-139.

Suzuki, F., Kobayashi, M., Komatsu, Y., Kato, A., and Pollard, R.B. (1997). Keishi-ka-kei-to, a traditional Chinese herbal medicine, inhibits pulmonary metastasis of B16 melanoma. *Anticancer Research* 17: 873-878.

Tanabe, M., Chen, Y., Saito, K., and Kano, Y. (1993). Cholesterol biosynthesis inhibitory component from *Zingiber officinale*. *Chemical and Pharmaceutical Bulletin* 41: 710-713.

Tjendraputra, E., Tran, V.H., Liu-Brennan, D., Roufogalis, B.D., and Duke, C.C. (2001). Effect of ginger constituents and synthetic analogues on cyclooxygenase-2 enzyme in intact cells. *Bioorganic Chemistry* 29: 156-163.

Tu, G., Fang, Q., Guo, J., Yuan, S., Chen, C., Chen, J., Chen, Z., Cheng, S., Jin, R., Li, M., et al. (Eds.) (1992). *Pharmacopoeia of the People's Republic of China.* Guangzhou, China: Guangdong Science and Technology Press, pp. 215-216.

Vaes, L.P.J. and Chyka, P.A. (2000). Interactions of warfarin with garlic, ginger, Ginkgo, or ginseng: Nature of the evidence. *The Annals of Pharmacotherapy* 34: 1478-1482.

Verma, S.K. and Bordia, A. (2001). Ginger, fat and fibrinolysis. *Indian Journal of Medical Sciences* 55: 83-86.

Verma, S.K., Singh, J., Khamesra, R., and Bordia, A. (1993). Effect of ginger on platelet aggregation in man. *Indian Journal of Medical Research* 98: 240-242.

Visalyaputra, S., Petchpaisit, N., Sancharun, K., and Chouvaratana, R. (1998). The efficacy of ginger root on the prevention of postoperative nausea and vomiting after outpatient gynecological laparoscopy. *Anaesthesia* 53: 506-510.

Vutyavanich, T., Kraisarin, T., and Ruangsri, R.A. (2001). Ginger for nausea and vomiting in pregnancy: Randomized, double-masked, placebo-controlled trial. *Obstetrics and Gynecology* 97: 577-582.

Weidner, M.S. and Sigwart, K. (2000). The safety of a ginger extract in the rat. *Journal of Ethnopharmacology* 73: 513-520.

Weidner, M.S. and Sigwart, K. (2001). Investigation of the teratogenic potential of a *Zingiber officinale* extract in the rat. *Reproductive Toxicology* 15: 75-80.

Weyand, E.H. and Bevan, D.R. (1987). Species differences in disposition of benzo[*a*]pyrene. *Drug Metabolism and Disposition* 15: 442-448.

Yamahara, J., Huang, Q., Iwamoto, M., Kobayashi, G., Matsuda, H., and Fujimura, H. (1989). Active components of ginger exhibiting anti-serotonergic action. *Phytotherapy Research* 3: 70-71.

Yamahara, J., Huang, Q., Li, Y., Xu, L., and Fujimura, H. (1990). Gastrointestinal motility enhancing effect of ginger and its active constituents. *Chemical and Pharmaceutical Bulletin* 38: 430-431.

Yamahara, J., Huang, Q., Naitoh, Y., Kitani, T., and Fujimura, H. (1989). Inhibition of cytotoxic drug-induced vomiting suncus by a ginger constituent. *Journal of Ethnopharmacology* 27: 353-355.

Yamahara, J., Miki, K., Chisaka, T., Sawada, T., Fujimura, H., Tomimatsu, T., Nakano, K., and Nohara, T. (1985). Cholagogic effect of ginger and its active constituents. *Journal of Ethnopharmacology* 13: 217-225.

Yamamoto, H., Mizutani, T., and Nomura, H. (1982). Studies on the mutagenicity of crude drug extracts. I. *Yakugaku Zasshi* 102: 596-601.

Yang, S.Z. (1997). *The Divine Farmer's Materia Medica.* Boulder, CO: Blue Poppy Press, p. 50.

Yoshikawa, M., Yamaguchi, S., Kunimi, K., Matsuda, H., Okuno, Y., Yamahara, J., and Murakami, N. (1994). Stomachic principles in ginger. III. An anti-ulcer principle, 6-gingesulfonic acid, and three monoacyldigalactosylglycerols, gingerglycolipids A, B, and C, from *Zingiberis Rhizoma* originating in Taiwan. *Chemical and Pharmaceutical Bulletin* 42: 1226-1230.

Zhu, Y.P. (1998). *Chinese Materia Medica: Chemistry, Pharmacology and Applications.* Amsterdam, the Netherlands: Harwood Academic Publishers, p. 30.

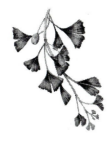

Ginkgo Biloba

BOTANICAL DATA

Classification and Nomenclature

Scientific name: *Ginkgo biloba* L. (formerly *Pterophyllus salisburiensis* Nelson and *Salisburia adiantifolia* Smith, and *S. macrophylla* Koch)

Family name: Ginkgoaceae

Common names: Ginkgo, maidenhair tree, forty-coin tree, arbre aux quarante ecus (French), Japanbaum (German), icho (Japanese), pai kuo yeh, white fruit (Chinese)

Some possibility for confusion of ginkgo *(G. biloba)* identity in the older literature exists. In 1797, an English botanist decided that the scientific name, *Ginkgo biloba,* given by Linnaeus, was "uncouth and barbarous," so he renamed it *Salisuburia adiantifolia* Sm., which never really became recognized. Because some features of ginkgo are similar to conifers, it was initially included in the family Taxaceae, but was later moved to its own family, the Ginkgoaceae (Huh and Staba, 1992).

Description

Ginkgo is a dioecious tree with male and female reproductive organs on different trees. At 20 years old, ginkgo trees are able to reproduce and ultimately develop naked seeds which have an outer fleshy layer. The female trees develop pendulous pairs of ovules at the tips of the short shoots which are mature at the time of pollination (Huh and Staba, 1992).

Ginkgo is among the oldest living species of trees on earth and for this reason some call it a "living fossil." Ginkgo flourished in large forests over 150 million years ago and almost became extinct during the last ice age. The wild stands that survived were in China and parts of Asia. Because of defor-

445

estation, ginkgo again became almost extinct, but is now being preserved by human cultivation. Ginkgo is grown for its ornamental value around the world and is a common street tree in urban areas due to its resistance to pollution, pests, and disease (Hobbs, 1991). Ginkgo grows well in temperate climes, including cold and Mediterranean temperate areas. Stands of ginkgo over 200 years old were recently catalogued in southern China. Fully mature, the tree can reach a height of 40 m; however, a specimen in Korea reached 65 meters with a girth of 14 meters (Del Tredici, 1991). In China and Japan, the oldest living specimens are found near Buddhist and Daoist temples (Del Tredici, 2000).

Young trees have a conical, coniferlike shape, and exhibit an interesting branching dimorphism. During the first year of shoot growth, elongated shoots are formed with leaves in a spiraling arrangement separated by nodes. As the long shoots mature, they develop "short shoots," also called lateral shoots or spur shoots. Light to deep-green leaves are borne in clusters at the end of both the long and short shoots each spring, which become golden-yellow in the fall during senescence. The leathery, fan-shaped leaves may appear with two lobes and resemble the maidenhair fern in shape and venation. The veins are dichotomous and parallel, arising from the two vascular strands within the petiole. In the fall the leaves turn a golden-yellow (Huh and Staba, 1992).

HISTORY AND TRADITIONAL USES

The name ginkgo is thought to come from the Chinese word *sankyo* or *yin-kuo,* meaning "hill apricot" or "silver fruit." This is in reference to the fully mature fruits produced by female trees which resemble apricots and have a smell like rotting flesh or rancid butter (Hobbs, 1991), a characteristic attributed to the content of butanoic and hexanoic acid in the sarcotesta, the fleshy layer of the outer part of the seeds. The same chemicals are responsible for the odor of romano cheese and rancid butter (Amato, 1993). The species name *biloba,* meaning two lobes, refers to the unique two-lobed leaves (Hobbs, 1991), which resemble a duck's foot, hence the old Chinese name *ya chio* (Huh and Staba, 1992).

Cultivation of ginkgo can be traced back nearly 1,000 years and the fruits of ginkgo have been used as both food and medicine for millennia. The fruits are prepared by fermentation and cooking and are considered a delicacy (Del Tredici, 1991). It is estimated that at least 63,000 kg of dried ginkgo seeds are produced in China each year (He et al., 1997). The elliptical seeds measure 1-1.5 cm in thickness and 1.5-2.5 cm in length. After removal of the white seed coat, the inner part is pale yellow to yellow-green (Yen, 1992). According to Hobbs (1991), in traditional Chinese medicine (TCM) the seeds are boiled and used as a tea to treat lung weakness and congestion (especially asthma), wheezing, coughing, vaginal candidiasis, frequent urination, cloudy urine, and excess mucus in the urinary tract (Hobbs, 1991). The unprocessed seed has been used to kill worms (Yen, 1992).

In Asian cuisine, the sarcotesta is removed before preparation of the seeds by boiling or roasting (Huh and Staba, 1992). In Malaya, the seeds are popularly used in making desserts and are recommended for nutritional gains believed to affect the brain, circulation, and eyes (Curtis-Prior et al., 1999). In Asia, it is also believed that eating the seeds will help digestion and lessen intoxication from wine (Huh and Staba, 1992). Other traditional uses of the seed kernel in Asia include cancer, kidney and bladder disorders, asthma, cough, intestinal worms, skin maladies, gonorrhea, and leukorrhea (Perry and Metzger, 1980). Usually boiled, the cooked seeds are said to have a flavor similar to that of sweet chestnuts (Del Tredici, 1991). The leaves are used much less and include the warming of chilblains (reddening, swelling and itching of the skin due to frostbite) using the juice of fresh leaves (Hori and Hori, 1997). Other herbs are frequently used in conjunction with ginkgo in TCM (Hobbs, 1991). A text from the fifteenth century in China mentions external application of the leaves in the treatment of head and skin sores and freckles (Del Tredici, 1991).

Medical use of ginkgo leaf extracts began in Germany in 1965 when the grandson of Dr. William Schwabe, Dr. Willmar Schwabe III, conducted experiments with a crude extract of the leaves in isolated guinea pig hearts. Noting potent effects, he went on to concentrate the flavonoid content and found even more potent effects which led to open label trials of the extract in humans. When the extract appeared to benefit patients with disorders of cerebral and peripheral blood flow, it was further developed into a commercial product which is currently known as EGb 761 (Drieu and Jaggy, 2000).

Today, ginkgo extract is enjoying worldwide popularity as a botanical medicine. In Germany, ginkgo leaf extract (standardized to contain 6% terpene glycosides and 24% ginkgo flavone glycosides; hereafter, ginkgo leaf extract or ginkgo extract) is one of the most popular single botanicals prescribed, with 5.24 million prescriptions written in 1988 alone (Chang and Chang, 1997). In the United States, ginkgo extract recently stepped into the "herbal spotlight," primarily due to heavy media coverage following an article in the *Journal of the American Medical Association* on the possible benefits of ginkgo extract in Alzheimer's patients (Le Bars et al., 1997).

CHEMISTRY

The constituents of primary interest in ginkgo leaf are ginkgolides and flavonoids (Huh and Staba, 1992) (see Figure 1).

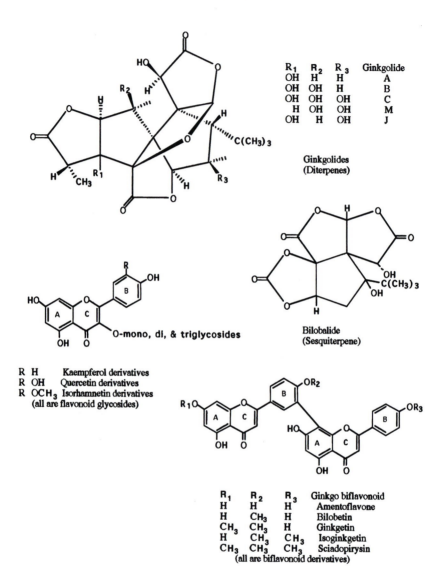

FIGURE 1. Major Active Constituents of *Ginkgo biloba*

Phenolic Compounds

Flavonoids

Flavonoids present in ginkgo leaf include flavones, biflavones, flavonols, tannins, and associated glycosides (Huh and Staba, 1992). In general, flavonoids are principally found in the leaves, although they are also present in many other parts of the plant. Including apigenin 7-O-glucoside, and luteolin 3(-O-glucoside, myricetin 3-O-glucoside (Sticher, 1993), there are about 20 flavonoid glycosides along with glucosides, quercetin, and kaempferol 3-rhamnosides and 3-rutinosides, p-coumaric esters of glucorhamnosides of quercetin and kaempferol (most with a 1''' → 2'' bond between sugars), and biflavones (all 3' → 8'' biflavones). The biflavones are amentoflavone, bilobetol, 5-methoxybilobetol, ginkgetin, isoginkgetin, and sciadopitysin. The plant part with the highest acylated flavonoid content is the bud, with a content three times greater in the fall than in the spring. The monomer content is also highest in the fall (Huh and Staba, 1992).

Ginkgo leaf extracts differ in flavonoid content. One of the main flavone marker chemicals used for standardization is the unique flavonoid, quercetin 3-O-(6'''-p-coumaroyl-glucosyl-1,4 rhamnoside) (Huh and Staba, 1992).

Terpenoid Compounds

Diterpenes

Ginkgolides (ginkgolides A, B, C, and J) in the leaves are diterpenes (terpene lactone ginkgolides): C (20) cage molecules that contain six rings of five carbons each, which involve a spirononane system, a tetrahydrofuran, three lactone groups, and a tert-butyl group (Huh and Staba, 1992).

Other Constituents

Ginkgo leaves contain flavan-3-ols, proanthocyanins and poly-isoprenoid-derived betulaprenols (similar to dolichol) in unusually high amounts (Huh and Staba, 1992). Other compounds of interest in the leaf include coumaroyl flavonol glycosides (Tang et al., 2001), ginnon, ginnol, 2-hexenal, and bilobalide (a terpenoid) (Huh and Staba, 1992), and in both the seeds and leaves, alkylphenols (cardols, cardanols), and ginkgolic (anacardic) acids (6-alkylsalicylic acids) (Irie et al., 1996). Kynurenic acid (Weber et al., 2001) and 6-hydroxykynurenic acid, which are related to quinoline-3-carboxylic acids, are also found in the leaves (Schennen and Hölzl, 1986; Matile, 1994) and in commercial *Ginkgo biloba* extracts (Grässel and Reuter, 1998). The essential oil of the heartwood is comprised of monoterpenes and sesquiterpenes; the seed contains bilobol, ginkgolic acid (phenolics), 4'-methoxypyridoxine (Huh and Staba, 1992), and ginkbilobin, an antifungal protein (Wang and Ng, 2000).

THERAPEUTIC APPLICATIONS

Ginkgo extract has many potential therapeutic applications and indications, including: failing memory, cognitive speed (loss of alertness), dementia, stroke, free radical damage in traumatic brain injury, Alzheimer's disease, and aging (Diamond et al., 2000).

PRECLINICAL STUDIES

Generally, the flavonoids in ginkgo leaf act as antioxidants by scavenging free radicals in the body, which result from oxidative processes, while the ginkgolides antagonize activities of inflammation and blood clotting associated with platelet-activating factor (PAF) (Chang and Chang, 1997). The majority of in vitro pharmacological studies on ginkgo leaf have been performed using a proprietary extract known as EGb 761 (Schwabe Gmbh, Germany) (DeFeudis, 1991).

Cardiovascular and Circulatory Functions

Ginkgo extract influences many components of the cardiovascular system, including arteries, veins, capillaries, blood components (e.g., erythrocytes, platelets), arterial blood flow, capillary perfusion, and venous return. Multiple actions are due to the heterogeneous nature of ginkgo extracts. Therefore, data interpretation is more difficult than in the case of a single chemical entity (DeFeudis, 1991).

Cardiotonic; Cardioprotection

Pietri et al. (1997) examined the potential antioxidant and cardioprotective effects of EGb 761 and the terpene constituent ginkgolide A on the hearts of male rats subjected to ischemia. Rats were pretreated on a daily basis with either substance or placebo for 15 days (EGb 761, 60 mg/kg p.o., and ginkgolide A, 4 mg/kg p.o.) at approximately equivalent dosages in humans of EGb 761 (240 mg/day). The human equivalent dose of ginkgolide A was based on the terpene content of EGb 761 of 6%. Anti-ischemic effects in either group of rats were significant compared to pretreatment. Significant functional improvements compared to placebo-treated rats were seen in postischemic functions of left ventricular end-diastolic pressure, left ventricular develop pressure, coronary flow, and the rate pressure product (each $p < 0.05$).

Peripheral Vascular Functions

In vitro studies by DeFeudis (1991) on isolated arterial preparations (rabbit aorta) indicated that ginkgo extract EGb 761 caused a reproducible concentration-dependent contraction of rabbit aortic strips involving catecholamine receptors. These studies further indicated that low concentrations of EGb 761 might influence catecholaminergic systems by an indirect mechanism; an action resembling that of tyramine more than norepinephrine. In addition, EGb 761 can relax rabbit aorta, probably via potentiation of the effects of endothelium-derived relaxing factor(s) (EDRF), which is spontaneously produced. Collectively, the experiments on the effect of EGb 761 on isolated veins, platelets, and arterial preparations support the theory of "trivasoregulation," and that cardiovascular diseases which have multifactorial origins are best treated with polyvalent agents. DeFeudis commented that with its actions of enzyme-inhibition and free radical scavenging (antioxidant), ginkgo extract may therefore be useful.

Kubota et al. (2001) demonstrated that in the aorta of rats, *Ginkgo biloba* extract causes vasodilation, and they identified quercetin as a major constituent responsible for the activity. Vaosodilation was mediated by an increase in intercellular calcium in endothelial cells of the aorta suggesting that the extract and quercetin activate calcium channels which have yet to be defined. The increase in calcium levels suggested that nitric oxide synthase (cNOS) may be activated which would enhance nitric oxide (NO) formation.

The overproduction of NO as a potential cause of damage to vascular walls led Cheung et al. (1999) to examine the effects of ginkgo on NO in human endothelial cells (ECV3C4, American Type Culture Collection) that express both calcium-independent and calcium-dependent forms of nitric oxide synthase (NOS) activities: inducible nitric oxide synthase (iNOS), and constitutive nitric oxide synthase (cNOS). A standardized ginkgo extract (Shanghai Luyuan Industry Company Ltd., 50 μg/mL) caused a significant reduction in the production of NO (30%), which was attended by a reduction in iNOS expression. Tests showed that the effect was not calcium-dependent, that calcium-dependent activity of NOS was essentially unchanged, and that the effect of the ginkgo extract on iNOS activity was not attributable to a direct action on NOS enzyme. The research also showed that the ginkgo extract did not affect endothelial cell DNA synthesis, although it did cause levels of iNOS protein to decrease by 27% at 50 μg/mL and by 43% at 100 μg/mL. The significance of these results is that NO (cNOS-derived) at normal levels in the body causes blood vessels to relax, inhibits the oxidation of lipoproteins, and decreases the aggregation of platelets and the adhesion of monocytes to vessel walls. Excess production of NO, and more so of iNOS, is believed to be toxic to vessel walls through oxidative mechanisms. Higher levels of NO have been found in atherosclerosis and in Alzheimer's disease. Researchers in the field of cardiovascular drug development have made numerous attempts to find iNOS inhibitors that will leave cNOS intact so as not to interfere with its vasodilating role in helping to maintain vessel tone.

Cheung et al. (2001) identified bilobalide and ginkgolides A and B as the constituents of EGb most likely responsible for selective inhibition of iNOS expression in human macrophages, but that had no effect on NO production by NO synthase in endothelial cells.

In vivo studies have generally mirrored or confirmed the results obtained from in vitro studies. Ginkgo extract EGb 761 exhibits in vitro antioxidant activities (which may be relevant to its relationship with EDRF), and ginkgolides have been shown to exhibit PAF-antagonist activity, potentially supporting the use of ginkgo extract in treating hypertensive states. EGb 761 has shown antiischemic activity in the CNS (central nervous system), and it is thought that ginkgolides, flavonoids, and bilobalide may all be involved. EGb 761 also exhibits effects on central neurotransmitter systems and behavior. Due to the possible involvement of several plant constituents, it is important for therapeutic purposes that the total extract is used (DeFeudis, 1991).

Thrombosis, Hemostasis, and Embolism

Ginkgolides A, B, and C were shown to be potent inhibitors of platelet-activating factor (PAF) by Braquet et al. (1985). PAF antagonism is the most notable single activity of ginkgo, attributed solely to the ginkgolides. In fact, ginkgolides, as natural PAF antagonists, have opened up a completely new area of understanding for the pharmacological basis of several other botanicals, including kadsurenone and futoxine from *Piper futokadsura,* swietemahonin A and E from *Swietenia mahogani,* and L-652,496 from *Tussilago farfara* (Braquet and Hosford, 1991).

Neurological, Psychological, and Behavioral Functions

Neurodegenerative Disorders

Alzheimer's disease. Because evidence strongly suggests that Alzheimer's disease may form or progress due to an accumulation of β-amyloid-derived peptides, Bastianetto, Ramassamy, et al. (2000) examined the effect of EGb 761 on the toxicity induced by β-amyloid (Aβ)-derived peptide on cultured hippocampal primary cells. In Alzheimer's disease, the hippocampus is the area most severely damaged. Cotreatment of the hippocampal cells with Aβ-derived peptides and EGb 761 revealed a concentration-dependent protective effect from EGb 761 on the neurons (10 μg/mL) and complete protection from a high concentration of the ginkgo extract (100 µg/mL). No such effect was found from the terpenoid fraction of EGb 761, but the flavonoid fraction provided protective effects, although of a less potent magnitude. Although less potent than EGb 761, the flavonoid fraction (10-50 µg/mL) also completely blocked the advent of cell death (apoptosis) and the accumulation of reactive oxygen species induced by Aβ in the hippocampal cells.

Yao et al. (2001) have shown that when added to Aβ protein, EGb 761 (30-300 µg/mL neuronal cells) dose-dependently inhibits apoptosis, cell death, an increase in glucose uptake, and Aβ-induced production of free radicals, with complete prevention at the highest dose. Vitamin E (100 µM/mL) was not effective in protecting neuronal cells from Aβ-induced cytotoxicity, whereas at all concentrations used, EGb 761 showed a significant effect ($p < 0.001$). Prevention of Aβ-induced apoptosis in PC12 cells (sympathetic nerve pheochromocytoma cell line) by EGb 761 was shown to be highly significant (by ANOVA analysis, $p < 0.0001$). However, pretreatment or posttreatment of the cells with EGb 761 did not protect against Aβ-induced cytotoxicity. The in vitro neuroprotective activity of EGb 761 when coincubated with neuronal cells exposed to Aβ raised the possibility that EGb 761 acts to inhibit the formation of neurotoxins derived from Aβ. Known as β-amyloid-derived diffusible neurotoxic soluble ligands (ADDLs), these neurotoxins are found in the brains of Alzheimer's disease patients in 12-fold greater levels than in normal brains. Further tests showed a dose-dependent inhibition of ADDL formation by EGb 761. As for what constituents are responsible, a flavonoid- and terpene-free preparation of EGb 761 also inhibited the formation of ADDLs, indicating that other constituents are involved.

Retinopathies. Studies by Baudouin et al. (1999) have shown that ginkgo can significantly ameliorate free radical-induced vitreoretinopathy (xanthine-xanthine oxidase-induced). In an experimental model of intraocular inflammation in rabbits, ginkgo significantly decreased the incidence of retinal detachment and the degree of vitreoretinal proliferation when administered seven days prior to vitreoretinopathy or 24 h after (100 mg/kg per day p.o.). The benefits of ginkgo were most evident in the complete absence of neovascularization versus an incidence in the control group of 38%, an incidence of retinal detachment/folding of 50% in the control group versus 12.5% to 25% in the ginkgo group, and of epiretinal membrane development in 12.5% to 25% of the ginkgo-treated rabbits versus 75% of the control group (Baudouin et al., 1999).

Grosche et al. (1995) studied the effect of ginkgo on the expression of the proto-oncogene Bcl-2 protein in Müller (glial) cells of male albino rats. This protein shows increased expression in hereditary rod photoreceptor cell degeneration, ganglion cell degeneration (experimentally induced), and in retinal neuronal damage. As the rats aged, the Müller cells showed a correspondingly greater expression of Bcl-2 protein, which also increased in light-damaged rat retinas. Two groups of retinal light-damaged rats aged 16 months (hereditary retinal dystropy-free) were assigned to a control group or a group administered ginkgo (EGb 761, 40 mg/kg in drinking water, 30 mL/day) for eight months. Approximately 50% of the photoreceptors of their eyes were absent due to light damage. At 24 months, when the treatment period ended, the number of photoreceptors lost, reduced glial-specific enzyme GS expression, and the transformed morphology of Müller cells were the same in both groups. However, ginkgo-treated rats showed no expression of the Bcl-2 protein in Müller cells whereas it was significantly expressed in Müller cells of 16- and 24-month-old rats, although barely at all in young control rats. Because the Bcl-2 protein is known to act in preventing apoptosis and necrosis mediated by free radicals, the researchers proposed that ginkgo, acting as a free radical scavenger and having shown protective effects against free radical damage to the retina, may act in such a way that it takes out the "trigger" that allows Bcl-2 expression.

De Kozak et al. (1994) examined the effect of ginkgo extract (EGb 761) and the platelet activating factor (PAF) antagonist ginkgolide BN 50730 (Institut Henri Beaufour, Courtaboeuf, France) in experimental autoimmune uveoretinitis in pigmented and albino rats as a model of severe acute inflammation largely affecting the choroid and retina. Daily administration of EGb 761 (100 mg/kg per day p.o.) or BN 50730 (50 mg/kg per day p.o.) one week prior to induced uveoretinitis and until death resulted in little inhibition of whole ocular inflammation. Yet, both EGb 761 and ginkgolide BN 50730 significantly reduced tissue damage to the outer layers of the retina by 50% ($p < 0.0004$ and $p < 0.001$, respectively); albeit, only in the albino rats.

Remé et al. (1992) suggested that PAF was involved in light- (400-450 lux white fluorescent light) and lithium-induced (2.6 g/kg rat chow) rod outer segment (ROS) lesion development of rats when administration of ginkgolide BN 50730 (25 mg/kg p.o.) beforehand caused significantly fewer ROS lesions. Doly et al. (1992) found results suggesting the involvement of PAF in vincristine-induced retinopathy when, compared to rats receiving vincristine alone, retinal damage was significantly reduced after pretreatment of the animals with ginkgolide BN 50730 (10 mg/kg p.o. daily × 10).

Droy-Lefaix et al. (1992) studied the ocular-protective effect of ginkgo extract (EGb 761) in rats with experimental chloroquine-induced retinopathy. Given that the retina is highly sensitive to peroxidation and that retinal function is greatly affected by PAF, it lends well to measuring effects of oxygenated free radicals and radical scavengers. Droy-Lafaix and colleagues used these factors to measure the effect of ginkgo in rats exposed to chloroquine, a widely used antimalarial drug with various impairing effects on the retina, which are probably due to localized, immunologically mediated inflammatory reactions. Electroretinogram (ERG) measurements showed deviations from normal in nerve connections and metabolism of the retina in all the chronic chloroquine-treatment rats (75 mg/kg p.o daily for 20 days). Rats pretreated with a high dosage of ginkgo extract (100 mg/kg p.o. daily) for ten days prior to chronic chloroquine treatment showed practically no deviation from normal ERG readings. Tests also showed that there was no alteration in ERG measurements in rats treated with the ginkgo extract alone compared to the controls. The researchers found it remarkable that the preventive use of EGb 761 could reduce retinal damage from chloroquine and concluded that it may be useful in preventing chloroquine-induced retinopathy and probably damage to the retina caused by other kinds of agents (Droy-Lefaix et al., 1992).

Baudouin et al. (1992) assessed the possible ocular-protective effect of ginkgo extract (EGb 761) in rabbits. A model of periretinal proliferation was used to simulate retinal detachment by means of an immunologically mediated inflammatory reaction, which in turn stimulated intraocular growth of vitreous stands. Their test followed observations of a possible immunologically mediated activation of cell proliferation that they observed in specimens from human cases of periretinal proliferative disorders, which are the main cause of retinal-origin blindness. Half the rabbits served as an untreated control group, and the other half received a high dosage of ginkgo extract (100 mg/kg p.o. t.i.d. for four to five weeks), at the same time as induced periretinal proliferation. Both groups showed intraocular cellular proliferation; however, in the ginkgo-treated group, development of cellular proliferation was delayed, less dense, and localized tractional retinal folding was found in only one eye versus all eyes in the untreated group. Furthermore, resolution of the proliferation was more rapid in the ginkgo group, and by the third week, vitreous membranes showed a progressive decrease. By the fourth and fifth weeks, the vitreous membranes had completely disappeared, accompanied by complete retinal reapplication, including the single incidence of tractional retinal detachment. These results contrasted sharply with those found in the control group, in which retinal detachment persisted along with preretinal membranes. The researchers also found evidence of intravitreal macrophages and lymphocytes in the rabbits, indicating an immune-mediated inflammatory response involved in the pathological state induced, which was hypothesized in the etiology of proliferative retinal diseases in humans (Baudouin et al., 1992).

Szabo et al. (1990) demonstrated that EGb 761 acts as a protective agent against free radicals in the retina. Bazan et al. (1987) suggested the involvement of PAF in the inflammatory activity found in an in vivo animal model of corneal injury induced by alkali burn. Drops of a PAF-antagonist ginkgolide (1% suspension of ginkgolide B, then codified BN 52021) administered to the injured eye specifically inhibited the production of hydroxyderivates and prostaglandins released during the inflammatory response.

Neurotoxicity/Neuroprotection

In vitro evidence supports the use of ginkgo extract in the treatment of neuronal diseases in which an excess of free radicals is involved. Cultured rat cerebellar granule cells subjected to oxidative stress were protected from apoptotic cell death following pretreatment with EGb 761. The pretreated cells also showed less oxidative damage, such as loss of cell membrane fluidity and altered membrane protein conformation (Wei et al., 2000). Cultured rat primary mixed hippocampal cells exposed to reactive oxygen species generated by nitric oxide (NO) inducers were completely protected from an accumulation of free radicals and decreased cell survival from cotreatment with either EGb 761 (10-100 μg/mL) or the flavonoid fraction of EGb 761 (25 μg/mL), but not from cotreatment with the terpenoid constituents. In hippocampal cells preexposed to an NO inducer (sodium nitroprusside or SNP), EGb 761 (50 μg/mL) or the flavonoid fraction (25 μg/mL) rescued the cells and blocked the production of protein kinase C induced by sodium nitroprusside (Bastianetto, Zheng et al., 2000).

Xin et al. (2000) showed that in vitro lipid peroxidation of rat cerebral granule cells is dose-dependently inhibited by EGb 761 (100 μg/mL). Through pretreatment with the ginkgo extract (20 μg/mL), apoptosis of the cells induced by hydroxyl radicals was shown to be significantly inhibited. Whereas the total flavonoid fraction and a mixture of the terpenes and flavonoids of the extract also protected the cells from apoptosis and oxidative damage induced by hydroxyl radicals, the terpene fraction was devoid of these actions and failed to show a synergistic effect when combined with the flavonoid fraction. In vitro studies of a standardized ginkgo leaf extract by Sloley et al. (2000) identified kaempferol as a potential neuroprotectant since it showed protective activity against NMDA-induced neuronal toxicity in rat cortical cultures; however, when administered to mice (100 mg/kg i.p.) it did not prevent chemically induced noradrenergic neurotoxicity.

Chandrasekaran et al. (2001) examined the neuroprotective effects of EGb 761 and bilobalide as pretreatments against ischemia-induced alterations of mitochrondrial gene expression and ischemia-induced neuronal death in male gerbils. EGb 761 was administered daily for seven days prior to ischemia at 50 mg/kg p.o., a human dose equivalent of 240 mg/day, and at 25 and 100 mg/kg p.o. in comparative dosage groups. Bilobalide was administered at daily doses of 3 and 6 mg/kg p.o. The results showed that damage to hippocampal areas from ischemia in the pretreated animals was significantly ameliorated by either substance. Bilobalide at 3 mg/kg provided a protective effect equal to EGb 761 at 50 mg/kg, and bilobalide at 6 mg/kg equal to or better than EGb 761 at 100 mg/kg. Compared to untreated controls, neurons in the hippocampal CA1 region of bilobalide-pretreated animals showed increased survival and higher levels of COX III mRNA. Therefore, bilobalide protected the animals from ischemia-induced damage to hippocampal neurons and ischemia-induced decrease in COX III mRNA. Similar results were found in the animals pretreated with EGb 761 and the results were dose-dependent. Chandrasekaran and colleagues (2001) noted that in cell-free studies bilobalide has shown negligible superoxide free radical scavenging activity and no in vitro or in vivo protection against oxidative stress-induced death of neurons. It would therefore appear that bilobalide affords neuronal protection by some mechanism other than antioxidation.

Amri et al. (1996) proposed that neuroprotective and antistress effects of EGb 761 are attributable to effects on the biosynthesis of glucocorticoids. Male rats administered EGb 761 at doses of 50 and 100 mg/kg p.o. for eight days showed a significant reduction in corticorsterone levels. EGb 761 also reduced expression of the peripheral-type benzodiazepine receptor, the result of which was a decrease in corticosteroid synthesis.

Psychological and Behavioral Functions

Anxiety and stress response. Porsolt et al. (1990) examined the effects of ginkgo extract in rats (EGb 761, 25 and 50 mg/kg p.o. twice daily × 5) using models of learned helplessness, behavioral despair (forced swimming test), shock-suppressed exploration, emotional hypophagia ("food consumption in a novel situation"), spontaneous exploration, the Vogel conflict test ("shock suppressed licking"), and memory using the passive-avoidance test. Ginkgo extract was effective as a preventive in the test for unavoidable shock as a model of learned helplessness, significantly reducing avoidance deficits compared to the untreated controls (50 mg/kg, $p < 0.05$), and was more effective than diazepam (4 mg/kg p.o. daily). Administered at the same time as the test, ginkgo-treated mice also showed reduced avoidance deficits, although not by a statistically significant amount compared to controls. Also, mice administered ginkgo (100 mg/kg p.o.) consumed significantly more food in the hypophagia test when the dosing was conducted prior to the test, but not after, in which diazepam produced an equally significant effect ($p < 0.01$). In all the other tests, ginkgo was not significantly effective given before or after the stress-inducing event. Porsolt and colleagues concluded that ginkgo extract appeared to ameliorate the effects of unavoidable stress in a way that could not be easily ascribed to either classical antidepressant or anxiolytic activity.

Cognitive functions. In a preliminary data-seeking study of *Ginkgo biloba* (form uncharacterized) for possible memory-enhancing effects, Gajewski and Hensch (1999) administered the leaves dissolved in water (12 mg/200 mL) in place of normal drinking water to two female and three male experimentally naive mice. Four phases using a different maze each time were employed in a total of 16 trials. Between each phase the mice received plain water for four days. Compared to plain water, the results showed that when the mice received ginkgo there was a decrease in wrong turns and a relative decrease in errors. In the first phase, the wrong-turn incidence decreased 8-60%. Among the 80% of mice showing improved performance scores, an improvement of 5-26% was evident when ginkgo was reintroduced as a water replacement, raising the possibility of an extended effect beyond the four-day plain-water period. The effect was seen again in phase four of the study. The results showed that when mice received ginkgo they made less errors, indicating a memory-enhancing effect.

Winter (1998) examined the cognitive behavioral and longevity effects of orally self-administered ginkgo extract (EGb 761, 50 mg/kg) in male rats, using a delayed, nonmatching-to-position task (DNMTP task) and continuous learning tasks. At this dose, their was a tendency towards fewer errors and fewer sessions before attaining criterion performance compared to the controls. A second set of experiments (DNMTP task) in male rats aged 20 months allowed varying doses of the extract immediately prior to one set of tests and 30 min before another, with control sessions before each dose. Errors were significantly reduced, indicating a dose-dependent effect of ginkgo (100 mg/kg, $p < 0.002$; 200 mg/kg, $p < 0.003$). At a specific dose of 200 mg/kg, rats aged 26 months showed a significant decrease ($p < 0.04$) in proactive (nonmnemonic) and retroactive (mnemonic) errors in the radial maze compared to controls. An unexpected finding was that the ginkgo-treated rats lived significantly longer ($p < 0.05$), yet weighed the same as control mice at death.

Receptor- and Neurotransmitter-Mediated Functions

Taylor (1988) reported that chronic oral administration of EGb 761 to aged rats caused an increase in hippocampal muscarinic receptors. However, no changes were found in binding capacity of radio-ligands with dopamine, μ-opiate, or α-adrenergic receptors. Huguet et al. (1994) investigated the effects of ginkgo extract (EGb 761, 50 mg/kg i.p. daily × 21) compared to placebo on the age-related decrease of serotonin receptor binding in the cerebral cortex of aged (24-month-old) and young male rats (four-month-old). No alteration in binding of 5-hydroxytryptamine ($5\text{-}HT_{1A}$) to $5\text{-}HT_{1A}$ receptors in the cerebral cortex membrane was found in the young rats from chronic ginkgo treatment, whereas in the aged rats, which had shown a significant 22% reduction in the number of maximal binding sites as a result of age, binding density increased 33%. Ginkgo may have a restorative effect on $5\text{-}HT_{1A}$ receptor binding in senescent rats in the cerebral cortex, which decreases as a result of aging. This age-related decrease has also been shown in the cerebral cortex of humans. The evidence suggests that the in-

crease in 5-HT$_{1A}$ receptors was not the result of modified synaptic serotonergic activity. A more likely explanation offered was that of a stimulation
receptor synthesis by ginkgo.

Ramassamy et al. (1992), using considerably higher doses of EGb 761
than Huguet et al. (1994), examined the neuromodulating effects of ginkgo
on cerebral cortex synaptosomes of mice. A significant increase in [^{3}H]5-
HT uptake (+25%, $p < 0.01$) was evident in cortex synaptosomes from mice
administered EGb 761 semichronically in a very high dosage (1000 mg/kg
p.o. twice daily × 4). In vitro studies with synaptosomes showed that in the
presence of clomipramine, a 5-HT uptake inhibitor, there was no increase in
[^{3}H]5-HT from EGb 761. In an attempt to identify the active fractions, the
researchers determined that whereas a quercetin- and a flavonoid-free form
of EGb 761 were inactive as [^{3}H]5-HT uptake-increasing constituents, a
terpene-free form of EGb 761 containing mostly flavonoids, was active.
[^{3}H]dopamine uptake in synaptosomes from striatum of mice showed no increase from EGb 761 in vitro. In ex vivo studies, Sloley et al. (2000) reported the absence of effects of a standardized ginkgo leaf extract (Acta
Pharmacal, Sunnyvale, CA; 150 mg/kg p.o.) on levels of 5-hydroxyindolacetic
acid, 5-hydroxytryptamine, noradrenaline, dopamine, and MAO in mouse
or rat brains. No ex vivo MAO inhibiting activity was shown from kaempferol,
(100 mg/kg p.o.) whereas it and isorhamnetin were active in vitro.

White et al. (1996) reported that ethanolic and aqueous extracts prepared
from fresh leaves and two commercial extract preparations of ginkgo (Nature's Way, Inc., Ginkgold, and General Nutrition Corp., Natural Brand)
caused in vitro inhibition of MAO-A and −B in rat brain mitochondria. Both
commercial extracts contained 50:1 leaf extracts standardized to contain
24% ginkgo flavone glycosides and one (Ginkgold) was identified as containing EGb 761. However, Fowler et al. (2000) reported that no significant
inhibition of brain MAO-A or −B in human volunteers administered a
ginkgo extract (EGb, 120 mg/day for one month) (see Psychological and
Behavioral Disorders: Receptor- and Neurotransmitter-Mediated Functions).

Immune Functions; Inflammation and Disease

Cancer

Antiproliferative activity. Ten phenolics from the sarcotestas (fleshy part
of the seeds) of ginkgo have shown inhibitory activity against phospho-
tidylinositol-specific phospholipase Cγ1 (PI-PLCγ1) in vitro (the most potent being phenolic acid C$_{17:1}$ or 6-[10' (Z)-heptadecenyl]salicylic acid with
an IC$_{50}$ value of 0.83 µg/mL) (Lee et al., 1998). PI-PLCγ1 is the critical enzyme acting in the signal transduction of hormones, growth factors, and
neurotransmitters. The enzyme became a target for new antitumor agents
due to the discovery of increased PI-PLCγ1 activity in human cancers (Noh

et al., 1994), including human glial tumors (Haas et al., 1991). This enzyme also aids in the progression and proliferation of human cancer (Noh et al., 1994; Hill et al., 1994).

All ten phenolic compounds also showed in vitro growth-inhibitory activity against human tumor cell lines, whether ovary or cancer cells (SKOV-3), or cancer cells of the lung (A-549), breast (MCF-7), bladder or (HT-1197), or colon (HCT-15). The activity of the most active phenolic acid against normal colon cells (CCD-18-Co) was less cytotoxic than in the colon cancer cell line (Lee et al., 1998).

Itokawa et al. (1987) reported remarkable antitumor activity from a methanolic extract of the sarcotestas of ginkgo against sarcoma 180 ascites in mice. Subsequent research identified cardenol and bilobol compounds as the most active constituents (each 40 mg/kg i.p.), inhibiting sarcoma 180 ascites by as much as 99.6% and 100%, respectively, following tumor cell implantation.

Metabolic and Nutritional Functions

Antioxidant Activity

Using a model of free radical production induced by UV irradiation of pheomelanin, Hibatallah et al. (1999) compared the antioxidant activity of a terpene-free ginkgo leaf extract containing 33% *Ginkgo* flavone glycosides to that of SOD (superoxide dismutase). The extract showed significant and dose-dependent inhibition of free radical production at concentrations of 8-320 μg/mL^{-1} with a maximum 22% inhibition from 160 μg/mL^{-1}. Increasing amounts resulted in diminished activity, with activity at half at the highest concentration. Two constituents of the extract were also tested. Kaempferol showed biphasic activity, inhibiting free radical generation by 14% up to a concentration of 80 μg/mL^{-1}, showing decreased activity at twice the concentration, and at the highest concentration (320 μg/mL^{-1}) pro-oxidant activity. Quercetin showed a dose-dependent inhibition of free radical production which became highly significant ($p < 0.001$) at 320 μg/mL^{-1}.

Tang et al. (2001) isolated eight coumaroyl flavonol glycosides from the dried leaves of mature ginkgo trees which showed potent antioxidant activity. Five of them were especially potent in the cyctochrome-*c* assay with IC$_{50}$s of 11.2 to 14.9 μg/mL. The most potent was quercetin 3-*O*-β-D-glucopyranoside.

Çeliköz et al. (1997) reported that the inhibition of necrosis of surgical skin flaps of rats by pretreatments with ginkgo extract (EGb 761, 100 mg/kg i.p.) or deferoxamine (150 mg/kg i.p.) were equally significant compared to the control group, and that each was superior to vitamin E (20 mg/kg i.m.) and vitamin C (340 mg/kg i.p.) as pretreatments compared to the control.

Rapin et al. (1998) demonstrated that male rats administered ginkgo extract (EGb 761, 50 mg/kg p.o. daily × 8) showed significantly increased cell viability and significantly decreased numbers of peroxyl radical-induced and spontaneously occurring apoptoses in hippocampal nerve cells ex vivo. They found similar results from the constituent ginkgolide B (2 mg/kg per day p.o. daily × 8) at a dosage/concentration/rat oral bioavailability representative of the percentage found in ginkgo extract. However, there was no activity from the constituent bilobalide in the same representative dosage. These results verified previous in vitro tests by Rapin et al. (1998); cell viability reached higher levels in cells treated with ginkgolide B at 0.4 µg/mL than untreated control cells.

Çeliköz et al. (1997) compared the antioxidant deferoxamine and *G. biloba* extract (EGb 761) in a rat groin island skin flap model to show rates of free radical scavenging activity and inhibition of skin flap necrosis. Rats were assigned to three groups: a ginkgo group (Tebokan, 5 mg/kg p.o. twice daily × 11); a deferoxamine group (Desferal, 20 mg/kg per day i.p. for 11 days); and a nontreatment control group. The rats began treatment one day before flap harvesting. At the tenth day the area of skin necrosis in the deferoxamine and the ginkgo groups was significantly less ($p < 0.001$) than that of the control group, while the ginkgo group showed significantly less skin necrosis than the deferoxamine group ($p < 0.05$). Antioxidant activity in the skin flap biopsies from the three groups, measured with estimates of superoxide dismutase (SOD), malondialdehyde (MDA), and glutathione peroxidase (GSH-Px), showed significantly higher levels in the two active treatment groups compared to the control group ($p < 0.001$), while the antioxidant activity of the ginkgo group was significantly less than that of the deferoxamine group ($p < 0.05$). Electron microscopic examination of the tissue structures of the three groups revealed a normal appearance in the two active treatment groups compared to the control group; however, ultrastructure of the dermis in the deferoxamine group was deteriorated, showing loss of the dermo-epidermal border, and preserved collagen showed a patchy distribution. The ginkgo group faired best, showing the dermo-epidermal junction, epidermis and dermis little different from normal, and with normal distribution of preserved collagen. The researchers noted that injury induced by ischemia-reperfusion causes skin flap failure and organ damage in a number of clinical interventions (e.g., stroke, organ transplantation, heart attack, hemorrhagic shock, and sepsis), and that reactive oxygen species are implicated in this tissue injury. Çeliköz and colleagues concluded that ginkgo extract is a preferable agent for administration post- and preoperatively for elective operations involving flap transfer operations.

Marcocci et al. (1994) examined the in vitro NO-scavenging effect of EGb 761 in an assay of nitrite formation (nitric oxide reacting with oxygen). Against the accumulation of sodium nitroprusside-generated nitric oxide,

EGb 761 dose-dependently inhibited nitrite accumulation by 40% of the control value (maximally at 300 μg/mL and half-maximally at 20 μg/mL). In an assay of nitric-oxide-induced oxidation of oxyhemoglobin, EGb 761 (IC_{50} 7.5 μg/mL) inhibited the rate of oxidation by 60% of the control value.

Barth et al. (1991) demonstrated that ginkgo extract (Schwabe, Tebonin = EGb 761) could inhibit the cyclosporine A-induced increase in malondialdehyde (MDA) in human liver cells in vitro. Total inhibition of CsA-induced lipid peroxidation occurred at a concentration of ginkgo extract of 50 μg/mL, while CsA-induced MDA was significantly and dose-dependently inhibited by ginkgo, starting at a lower concentration of 15 μg/mL. The addition of free iron ($FeCl_3$) to CsA resulted in a diminished ability of the ginkgo extract to inhibit the free radical production induced, though not completely.

CLINICAL STUDIES

Cardiovascular and Circulatory Disorders

Cerebrovascular Dysfunctions

Note that in Europe cerebral insufficiency is equal to early dementia (Itil et al., 1996). Kleijnen and Knipschild (1992a) examined 40 clinical studies on ginkgo in the treatment of cerebral insufficiency published from 1977-1991. Of these, only eight were judged to be well-performed, including four not cited by SØholm (1998): Wesnes et al., 1987; Haguenauer et al., 1986; Meyer, 1986; and Taillandier et al., 1986. These trials did not check for blindness of the placebo (inquiring of the patients as to whether they thought they had received the active or placebo medication) (Kleijnen and Knipschild, 1992a).

SØholm (1998) reviewed the clinical literature from 1975-1997 in which around 2,500 patients had participated in over 40 controlled trials of ginkgo. SØholm noted that from placebo-controlled studies in about 1,200 patients, cognitive symptoms were reduced by approximately 25% overall. Eleven of the clinical studies fulfilled the essential criteria for biometric parameter analysis used in testing clinical drugs: Le Bars et al., 1997; Kanowski et al., 1996; Vesper and Hänsgen, 1994; Grässel, 1992; Brüchert et al., 1991; Halama, 1991; Hofferberth, 1991; Maier-Hauff, 1991; Schmidt et al., 1991; Eckmann, 1990; and Vorberg et al., 1989. Hopfenmüller (1994) conducted a meta-analysis of clinical trials on ginkgo in the treatment of cerebral insufficiency and found seven that confirmed ginkgo extract was effective compared to placebo. Efficacy in treating both individual symptoms and the total complex of symptoms was calculated as significant compared to placebo ($p < 0.01$).

In reviewing the value of ginkgo as a substance to reduce declining mental function, Curtis-Prior et al. (1999) found the activities of ginkgo as a cerebral blood flow-enhancing, antioxidant, and free radical scavenging substance to be well-documented. Combined with the activity of antagonizing the pro-inflammatory platelet aggregating factor, as shown by Guinot et al. (1989) in healthy male volunteers, they assessed these activities as "compatible" with the benefits seen in clinical reports of ginkgo in treatments of dementia and cerebral insufficiency. At the same time, they lamented the over-reliance on self-assessment questionnaires in clinical trials of the extract to assess efficacy and suggested that for future, more objective assessments, the already tested and computerized Cambridge Neuropsychological Test Automated Battery (CANTAB) be employed.

Vesper and Hänsgen (1994) conducted a double-blind, placebo-controlled study in which they administered placebo or a ginkgo extract (LI 1370) for over 12 weeks to 90 outpatients (average age 62.7 years) diagnosed with cerebral insufficiency. A significant improvement in patient performance was noticed at the end of the treatment period, with the following parameters improved compared to placebo:

1. The quality of information processing stabilized in time-interval testing
2. Ability to attain consistent attentiveness over a long period of time while performing certain tasks, and ability to perform tasks which required the patient to quickly reorient and readapt
3. Improvement in visual memory with respect to parameters sensitive to cerebral insufficiency
4. Positive changes in subjective performance as tracked by the patient or by the people in the patient's environment

Peripheral Vascular Disorders

Intermittent claudication. The majority of trials of ginkgo extract in the treatment of peripheral vascular disturbances such as intermittent claudication have been performed on patients suffering from arterial occlusive diseases characterized as Stage IIb, according to the diagnostic criteria of Fontaine. Assessment of the overall value of ginkgo extract for this therapeutic category is difficult, as is usual in assessing drugs for chronic arteriopathies, because of the inherent interindividual variations in these diseases (DeFeudis, 1991). Pittler and Ernst (2000) conducted a meta-analysis of double-blind, placebo-controlled, randomized trials of ginkgo extracts in the treatment of intermittent claudication. Out of 12 trials, eight met their inclusion criteria. The researchers concluded that compared to placebo, ginkgo extract is an effective treatment for intermittent claudication. However, because exercise therapy is poorly complied with by patients with intermittent claudication, it was the opinion of the researchers that an overall 34 m increase in pain-free walking distance was modest and of "uncertain clinical relevance" (Pittler and Ernst, 2000, p. 276).

Schweizer and Hautmann (1999) compared the superiority of two dosages of EGb 761 (120 mg and 160 mg twice daily for 24 weeks) in 18 women and 56 men (ages 62-70) diagnosed with peripheral arterial occlusive disease (Fontaine's stage II). The randomized, double-blind, multicentric trial found no statistically significant difference between the dosages in pain intensity scores (obtained from walking distances), the time taken for ankle pressure afterwards to normalize, Doppler pressure arm-ankle difference and quotient thereof, or tolerance as determined from changes in heart rate, blood pressure, and other laboratory measurements. Compared to the lower dosage, the higher dosage showed statistically superior effects in pain-free walking distance after week 24 ($p = 0.0253$; a 5% superiority) and the maximum walking distance at weeks 18 and 24 ($p = 0.0133$ and $p = 0.0112$, respectively). Although the mean pain-free walking distance increased by over 50% in both dosage groups, patient and investigator assessments showed a slightly superior result from the higher dosage.

Peters et al. (1998) conducted a multicenter, randomized, placebo-controlled, double-blind trial of a ginkgo extract (EGb 761, 40 mg t.i.d. for 24 weeks) in 111 adult patients diagnosed with peripheral occlusive arterial disease (POAD) of the legs at stage IIb intermittent claudication (pain-free walking distance on a treadmill of less than 150 m). Treatment with the extract or placebo began after a two-week placebo run-in phase. The goal of the study was to detect a difference in the pain-free walking distance after treatment with the ginkgo extract, which was measured after weeks 8, 16, and 24 on a treadmill. Throughout the treatment period, the ginkgo group showed a more obvious and continuous increase in the mean pain-free walking distance until, at the end, the increase was 44.7 m compared to baseline after the two-week placebo run-in (108.5 m), versus a mean increase of 21.4 m in the placebo group. The difference was statistically significant at all three examination times in the ginkgo group ($p = 0.017$, $p = 0.007$, and $p = 0.016$ at week 24) compared to the placebo group. A clearer picture of the difference was evident in the mean maximum pain-free walking distances which were also significantly higher in the ginkgo group versus the placebo group at weeks 8, 16, and 24: +21.8 versus +10 m; +35.0 versus +19.3 m; and +61.1 compared to +25.0 m. Remarkably, the only side effects reported in any of the participants were gastric pain and heartburn in one patient in the placebo group. Peters and co-workers concluded that under the standardized measurements employed, ginkgo extract can significantly increase pain-free walking distances, and that the treatment was clinically relevant and well-tolerated and similar in efficacy to pentoxifylline in the treatment of POAD.

Mouren et al. (1994) conducted a randomized, placebo-controlled, double-blind, parallel study involving 20 patients diagnosed with claudicating atherosclerotic arterial occlusive disease of stage II. All patients were given placebo for 15 days under single-blind conditions, and then randomized into two groups receiving either placebo or ginkgo extract EGb 761 (320 mg/day). Transcutaneous oximetery (measuring the partial pressure of oxygen during exercise) was used to estimate local arterial perfusion and regional capillary perfusion. After four days of ginkgo extract, the areas of ischemia decreased by 38%, whereas in the placebo group they remained relatively unchanged. The difference was statistically significant.

Thomson et al. (1990) followed 37 patients with stage II peripheral vascular disease in a randomized, double-blind, placebo-controlled study. After an initial washout period, the patients received either placebo or a ginkgo extract (Tanakan) for six months. At 6, 12, and 24 weeks and before the beginning of treatment, effects were measured by claudication distance, A/B ratio, and Doppler ankle pressure response to exercise, together with recovery time and a 10 cm analogue scale (LAS) estimation of maximal pain severity. LAS scores were significantly improved in the ginkgo group after 24 weeks, and claudication distance was significantly increased compared to placebo. However, A/B ratio, Doppler ankle responses to exercise for any interval, and the postexercise recovery time all failed to show any significant change in either group. The researchers concluded that ginkgo extract was effective in improving claudication distance and pain associated with walking, although the Doppler studies failed to suggest gross improvement in perfusion of the leg in peripheral vascular disease.

Bauer (1984) followed 79 patients suffering from peripheral arteriopathy who were given placebo or ginkgo extract (Rökan, 40 mg/day) for six months in a double-blind, randomized clinical trial. Measurements of pain-free walking distance, maximum walking distance, and plesthymography recordings indicated ginkgo extract to be significantly superior to placebo. These results confirmed patient and physician overall assessments of the treatment.

Thrombosis, Hemostasis, and Embolism

Citing the presence of PAF in the mucosa of patients with active ulcerative colitis, Sandberg-Gertzén (1993) conducted a small open study using a standardized extract of ginkgo (Cedemin) in ten patients with the disease. The two men and eight women participants (ages 35-75) suffered from light to moderate symptoms yet showed light to severe pathological states upon sigmoidoscopic examination. Every evening for three weeks, the patients received the extract in the form of an enema in a dosage of 200 mg/100 mL of suspension. Two patients found some effect, five experienced no benefit, and in three the disease went into remission. Because these results were no better than placebo, Sandberg-Gertzén concluded that the ginkgo extract delivered as an enema appeared to be ineffective against distal ulcerative colitis (Sandberg-Gertzén, 1993).

Chung et al. (1987) examined the effect of a ginkgolide mixture (BN 52063) containing 40% ginkgolide A, 40% ginkgolide B, and 20% ginkgolide C on PAF in six nonatopic human subjects (ages 25-35) in a double-blind, placebo-controlled, crossover study. The researchers concluded that the ginkgolide mixture exhibited PAF inhibition in several measurements. Two hours after ingestion of 120 or 80 mg of the mixture, intradermal histamine- and PAF-induced weal and flare responses were inhibited in a dose-related manner. From a dose of 120 mg, the flare area was reduced by a mean of 62.4%, and the weal volume by a mean of 60%. Either dose inhibited PAF-induced platelet aggregation in platelet-rich plasma. The same mixture was also found to inhibit PAF-induced, but not ADP-induced, platelet aggregation. The researchers suggested that ginkgo may therefore be suitable for studies of diseases in which PAF is believed to play a significant role (e.g., asthma, bronchial hyperactivity).

Jung et al. (1990) examined the ability of a ginkgo extract (Lichtwer Pharma, GmbH, Kaveri) to influence peripheral circulation and blood fluidity of healthy volunteers ($n = 10$). The randomized, placebo-controlled, single-blind, crossover trial found that a single oral administration of the extract (45 ml) corresponding to a daily dose caused a significant increase in peripheral microcirculation of approximately 57% and a significant decrease in erythrocyte aggregation of 15.6%. No effect was found from either placebo or the extract on plasma viscosity, leukocyte counts, thrombocyte aggregation, numbers of circulating thrombocyte aggregates, thrombocyte counts, hematocrit, erythrocyte rigidity, heart rate, or blood pressure. However, in an open-label study in healthy volunteers ($n = 20$, ages 21-57) who ingested a *Ginkgo bilboa* extract for three months (Walgreens Co., Deerfield, Ill, 120 mg/day "at bedtime"), Kudolo (2000) reported a significant decrease in both diastolic ($p < 0.01$) and systolic blood pressure ($p < 0.05$). Bleeding times and fibrinogen levels after three months of the ginkgo extract showed no change.

Immune Disorders; Inflammation and Disease

Inflammatory Response

Hibatallah et al. (1999) conducted a simple-blind, placebo-controlled, randomized study of the anti-inflammatory activity of a topically applied terpene-free *Ginkgo* leaf extract compared to topical SOD and placebo. The ginkgo extract was applied in the form of an oil-in-water emulsion, the placebo in the form of the oil-in-water emulsion, and SOD was applied as a formulated carbomer gel (2000 units/mL^{-1}). These preparations were applied as a pretreatment twice daily for four days to six randomized areas (2 mg/cm^{-2}) on the inside of the forearms of ten healthy female volunteers (ages 23-28) who showed no signs of dermatological disease. The subjects were instructed to abstain from anti-inflammatory drugs for one week prior to the study, and from nicotine, coffee, or any other stimulants 3 h before commencing the study and until completion. In a model of exogenous free radical-induction, inflammation was induced by topical application of an aqueous solution of methyl nicotinate on the fifth day after occlusion of the sites for 3 h with a plastic film. The results showed that whereas there was no difference between the placebo and the control, compared to the placebo the ginkgo extract produced a significant reduction in methyl nicotinate-induced inflammation ($p < 0.01$). The best results were found from a 0.1% solution of the ginkgo extract which reduced inflammation by 37% and was equivalent in effect to the SOD gel (34% inhibition). Higher concentrations were less effective with 26% inhibition from a 0.2% solution ($p < 0.02$) and nonsignificant from a 0.3% solution.

Metabolic and Nutritional Disorders

Antioxidant Activity

In a prospective trial, Pietta et al. (1998) compared the total radical-trapping antioxidant potential (TRAP) of a ginkgo extract (100 mg ginkgolides and 400 mg ginkgo flavonoids) to that of an extract of green tea (400 mg total catechin tannins). The placebo-controlled study was conducted with 12 healthy subjects ages 20-25 years, none of whom were taking antioxidants and all of whom had a habitually low dietary flavonoid intake. Following a fast, the subjects ingested either a placebo (maltodextrin), ginkgo extract (~1.6 g), or green tea extract (600 mg). Tests of blood samples taken before ingestion of the substances and at each of 6 h following revealed a longer lasting and more rapid antioxidant potential of the ginkgo extract compared to the green tea extract. Yet in a separate assay of the total antioxidant potential of these extracts, green tea showed about twice the activity of the ginkgo extract (5.2 mM Trolox versus 2.4 mM Trolox value). Pietta et al. (1998) concluded, therefore, that in order to be useful, in vitro comparisons of the antioxidant activity of medicinal plants must be combined with in vivo comparisons.

Performance and Endurance Enhancement

Roncin et al. (1996) tested the prophylactic potential of ginkgo extract (EGb 761, 80 mg b.i.d. for 30 days, dispensed daily) in a placebo-controlled, randomized study on altitude sickness in 44 healthy, male mountain climbers (ages 28-31) undergoing an ascent in the Himalayas (1,800 to

5,200 m). Earlier investigations had found favorable results in related trials of the extract on preventing mountain sickness (a.k.a., high altitude sickness) (Ajasse, 1984), and on microcirculation of the extremities during exposure to cold (Clément et al., 1982). Inclusion criteria included a score of two or greater on the acute mountain sickness questionnaire in order to diagnose the illness; scores from which show a good correlation with the Environmental Symptom Questionnaire of Sampson et al. (1983), the main test used in the trial. Exclusion criteria included the long-term use of various prescription drugs that would interfere with the results (e.g., anticoagulants, calcium channel blockers, anti-ischemic agents), and rheological treatments. For pain, the subjects were asked to refrain from using aspirin. In addition to the questionnaires, peripheral vasomotor reactions were measured by plethysmography at room temperature, and functional disability was measured on a six-point scale for numbness, swelling of hands, pain, stiffness, and parasthesia. Despite the statistically significant difference in the active treatment group comprised of three ex-smokers and two smokers compared to the placebo group, which was unfavorable to the ginkgo group, the results still showed a highly significant protection from symptoms of altitude sickness in the ginkgo group and no patient dropped out of the trial. In the placebo group, 40.9% developed acute altitude sickness on the basis of cerebral factor versus no one in the ginkgo group. On the basis of respiratory factor, 13.6% in the ginkgo group developed acute altitude sickness versus 18.8% on placebo. The effect of cold showed a most noticeable difference with the placebo group deteriorating by 104% and the ginkgo group improving by 22.8% ($p < 10^{-6}$). Similar, highly significant results were found in favor of ginkgo over placebo by physician assessment, the acute mountain sickness questionnaire, and a vasomotor questionnaire. The decrease in vasomotor disorders affecting the extremities as measured by plethysmography was also highly significant ($p < 10^{-8}$) in the ginkgo group (Roncin et al., 1996).

Pharmacokinetics

Fourtillan et al. (1995) conducted a study on the bioavailability of bilobalide, and ginkgolides A and B. After a meal, an oral dose of a standardized ginkgo leaf extract (120 mg) was administered to 12 healthy volunteers of either sex. The results showed no change compared to the same dose under fasting conditions, except for slower absorption after the meal. Peak plasma concentrations of the compounds ranged from 11.5-21.1 ng/mL after a meal and from 16.5-33.3 ng/mL under fasting. The mean elimination half-lives for ginkgolide A were 4.5 h (fasting) and 3.95 h (after a meal). For ginkgolide B, they were 3.2 h (fasting) and 10.6 h (after a meal). The mean elimination half-life of bilobalide was 3.21 h (fasting) and 4.26 h (after a meal). Under fasting, urinary excretion of ginkgolide A was 72% of the oral dose, ginkgolide B was 41%, and bilobalide was 31% (Fourtillan et al., 1995).

The comparative bioavailability and pharmacokinetic parameters of flavonoid glycosides of standardized ginkgo leaf products (24% flavonoid glycosides) was examined in 18 healthy volunteers. In a randomized, cross-over design, the products were orally administered after an overnight fast in a single dose at intervals of at least five days in the form of drops, capsules (Agon Pharma GmbH, Wendlingen, Germany), and tablet formulations (Dr. W. Schwabe, Karlsruhe, Germany, Tebonin = EGb 761). Blood samples were taken before dosing and at 12 intervals afterward for serum assays of isorhamnetin, kaempferol, and quercetin. Each of the three flavonoid glycosides was rapidly absorbed and each showed similar elimination half-lives, total clearance and rate constants for elimination. Highest peak plasma concentrations were found from kaempferol which averaged 26.33 ng/mL from the capsules, 28.18 ng/mL from the drops, and 28.29 ng/mL from the tablets, and accorded with a relatively higher concentration of flavonoid glycoside in the ginkgo extract products (60.5%) compared to either the quercetin (23.7%) or isorhamnetin (15.8%). Isorhamnetin showed a higher mean value of AUC from the drops (up to 126.75%) compared to the results from the tablets. The researchers concluded that the three formulations were bio-equivalent (Wojcicki, et al., 1993).

Neurological, Psychological, and Behavioral Disorders

Neurodegenerative Disorders

Alzheimer's disease. Using data from placebo-controlled clinical trials of at least six month's duration, Wettstein (1999/2000) compared the efficacy of cholinesterase inhibitors (donepezil, metrifonate, rivastigmine, and tacrine) with those of EGb 761 in the treatment of Alzheimer's disease. When efficacy was compared based on delays in symptom progression, no large differences were evident except that in trials of tacrine, adverse reactions resulted in a high rate of drop outs. Based on these findings, Wettstein concluded that these agents "should be considered equally effective" (Wettstein, 1999/2000, p. 393). However, Oken et al. (1998), in a meta-analysis of clinical trials of ginkgo extract in the treatment of cognitive function in Alzheimer's disease, found only four out of 50 that met all six of the essential inclusion criteria used (Le Bars et al., 1997; Kanowski et al., 1996; Hofferberth, 1991; Wesnes et al., 1987). This amounted to 212 subjects in the placebo groups and the same number in the ginkgo groups. Quantitative analysis showed a significant ($p < 0.0001$) although modest effect size of the ginkgo treatment (at 120-240 mg/day for three to six months) when including the Alzheimer Disease Assessment Scale cognitive subtest (ADAS-cog). Oken and colleagues concluded that more research is needed to determine what functional improvements may result, the most effective dosage to use, and the active constituents of ginkgo extract in the treatment of cognitive impairment or dementia in Alzheimer's disease.

Maurer et al. (1998) used an extract of ginkgo (EGb 761, 240 mg/day for three months) in a double-blind, randomized, placebo-controlled parallel-group design trial in 20 patients diagnosed with mild to moderate dementia of the Alzheimer type (DAT). The placebo group showed deterioration while the ginkgo group showed a modest though significant improvement ($p < 0.013$). In the ADAS-cog, a psychometric test, the level of improvement was comparable to that of a cholinesterase inhibitor administered for the same length of time in another study. In addition, EEG and Clinical Global Impression tests showed indications of improvement in dynamic functional and psychopathological states in the ginkgo group. Maurer and colleagues noted that the improvements in attention and memory in mild to moderate DAT were evidenced in the topographic normalization of EEG recordings after the three-month treatment with ginkgo, but that this requires further confirmation. No adverse effects were reported and their data were in agreement with a meta-analysis on EGb 761 performed independently by Weiß and Kallischnigg (1991).

Le Bars et al. (1997) conducted a placebo-controlled, double-blind, randomized study of ginkgo extract EGb 761 (40 mg t.i.d. for 52 weeks) in 202 patients ages 45 and older to assess the efficacy and safety of the extract in patients with Alzheimer's disease or multi-infarct dementia, "without other significant medical conditions." The primary outcome measures were ADAS-cog, Geriatric Evaluation by Relative's Rating Instrument (GERRI), and Clinical Global Impression of Change (CGIC). In 27% of the patients taking EGb 761, an improvement of at least four points was seen for the ADAS-Cog compared to placebo ($o = 0.05$). For GERRI, 37% taking EGb 761 were considered improved compared to 23% taking placebo ($o = 0.003$), although no differences were seen for placebo in CGIC. In addition, no significant differences were seen compared to placebo regarding the safety profile of EGb 761.

An intent to treat analysis of the trial by Le Bars et al. (1997), based on a 26-week outcome in 244 patients who made the twenty-sixth week visit (73% of the EGb 761 group and 76% of the placebo group), arrived at the following conclusions: compared to baseline, a statistically significant worsening was evident in the placebo group in every area assessed; the EGb 761 group showed a slight improvement on the daily living and social behavior scores and cognitive assessment; 17% of those receiving EGb 761 showed worsened GERRI scores and 30% showed improved scores, whereas the placebo group showed 37% with worsened scores and 25% improved; 26% of those receiving EGb 761 showed a 4-point improvement or better on the ADAS-Cog versus 17% in the placebo group; and no significant difference was found in the safety profile of the two groups. These results compare favorably with those reported for tacrine at 160 mg/day or donepezil at 10 mg/day (Le Bars et al., 2000).

Cognitive disorders. van Dongen et al. (2000) conducted a 24-week, randomized, double-blind, placebo-controlled, parallel-group, multicenter trial of EGb 761 in 214 elderly patients (34 men and 180 women in their early eighties) in rest homes who were diagnosed with age-associated memory impairment or mild to moderate dementia (Alzheimer's or vascular). At random, after a three week run-in treatment period with placebo, patients received either the usual dosage of EGb 761 (160 mg/day), a high dose (240 mg/day; two tablets), or placebo. An intention to treat analysis found that compared to placebo there was no effect in the ginkgo groups on any of the outcome measures applied (clinical assessment for severity and presence of geriatric symptoms [SCAG], verbal learning [NAI-WL], digit memory span [NAI-ZN-G], trail-making speed [NAI-ZVT-G], depressive mood [GDS], and self-reported behavioral assessment based on instrumental daily life, and report marks of self-perceived memory and health status). Although no adverse effects were found to be associated with ginkgo, neither were there any benefits compared to placebo in either dosage group or in any subgroup. The researchers concluded that ginkgo was an ineffective treatment for "older patients with mild to moderate dementia or age-associated memory impairment" (van Dongen et al., 2000, p. 1192). The validity of this study has been criticized on the grounds that it was conducted in a population with too many types of memory loss to obtain meaningful results (Weber, 2000).

Winther et al. (1998) studied the effect of a ginkgo extract (GB-8) in elderly volunteers diagnosed with well-defined, mild to moderate age-related cognitive impairment in accordance with the Mini-Mental State Examination (MMSE). Volunteer selection was limited to those showing a score of 22-28 in the MMSE. Changes in blood pressure before and after the treatment period were also measured. The randomized double-blind, placebo-controlled study consisted of 54 patients (61-88 years old) who were assigned to either a placebo group, a low dosage group (40 mg t.i.d. for three months), or a high dosage group (80 mg t.i.d. for three months). After the first four weeks and at the end of the treatment period, results of the Wechsler Memory Scale test showed a significant improvement ($p < 0.016$) in the low dosage group, and tendency to improvement in the high dosage group compared to the placebo group, which showed no significant change. Results from the Memory Assessment Clinic Self-Rating Scale (MAC-S) at the start and after the end of the study revealed significant changes compared to baseline in the low and high dosage groups. Changes in the placebo group were less significant. In comparing the three groups using the cerebral insufficiency test, Winther and colleagues reported that compared to baseline, the low dosage group improved the most and that the improvement was highly significant ($p < 0.001$). As for blood pressure, a significant decrease ($p < 0.04$) was found only in diastolic pressure (73 to 68 mm Hg) and only in the low dosage group. The researchers concluded that the low dosage of ginkgo extract (GB-8) improved short-term verbal memory, attention, and concentration within the first four weeks of treatment in a homogenous group of elderly subjects with mild to moderate cognitive impairment (primarily due to the aging process), but showed no significance until the end of three months of treatment. They added that some patients in the high dosage group experienced side effects (sleep disturbances, dyspepsia, and dizziness). The change in diastolic BP might support the suggestion by others (Subhan and Hindmarch, 1984) that ginkgo improves cognitive function through a vasodilating activity. Winther et al. (1998) added that since the effect was clinically relevant it warranted further study in hypertensive patients.

Brautigam et al. (1998) studied the potential cognitive benefits of a water/alcohol extract (70% v/v) of ginkgo leaves (Geriaforce, Biohorma B.V., 1:4 extract; 0.34 mg/mL total ginkgolides and 0.20 mg/mL total flavone glycosides). The 24-week randomized, double-blind, placebo-controlled study involved 241 noninstitutionalized elderly patients (both sexes, ages 55-86) with self-reported concentration/memory complaints. Results were compared between a placebo group, a low-dose (40 drops or 1.9 mL 1:1 with placebo t.i.d.), and a high-dose ginkgo group (40 undiluted drops, or 1.9 mL t.i.d.). In the high-dose group, visual short-term memory (Benton test) improved significantly ($p = 0.0076$). The low-dose group showed an optimal increase in visual short-term memory of 26%, while respective increases of 18% and 11% were found in the high-dose and placebo groups. However, no improvements were found compared to placebo in the ginkgo groups in verbal short-term memory or verbal long-term memory. In a subgroup of patients who showed comparatively lower baseline scores at the start of the trial, a modest though significant improvement ($p < 0.02$) was evident in long-term memory/recognition improvement (Rey 2 test). The researchers concluded that while ginkgo extracts "might be promising" in cognitively-impaired elderly persons, further research with longer trials in patients with lower cognitive function using tests for sensomotoric and cognitive speed and accuracy are recommended.

Rai et al. (1991) conducted a six-month, double-blind, placebo-controlled study of ginkgo extract (Tanakan, 40 mg, t.i.d.) in 31 patients over the age of 50 who showed a mild to moderate degree of memory impairment. Digit copying subtests of the Kendrick battery performance improved at both 12 and 24 weeks, and the median speed of response on a computerized version of a classification task showed significant improvement over placebo after

24 weeks. The researchers concluded that ginkgo extract exhibited a beneficial effect on cognitive function in this group of patients.

Dementias. Kanowski et al. (1996) administered ginkgo extract (EGb 761, single dose 240 mg/day p.o. for six months) or placebo to 216 outpatients (ages > 55) diagnosed with mild (79%) or moderate (21%) multiinfarct dementia and primary dementia (senile or presenile primary degenerative, Alzheimer type), according to the DSM-III-R. Of the 156 subjects who completed the prospective randomized, double-blind, placebo-controlled trial, a significantly greater number showed improved responses in the ginkgo group (*p* < 0.05 in both the Clinical Global Impressions item two and Syndrom-Kurztest scores). An intent to treat analysis in 205 of the patients showed similar results. Also, the number of responders was significantly greater compared to the placebo group (*p* < 0.005). Among adverse events, 63 occurred in the ginkgo group with five serious events, versus 59 in the placebo group with two serious events. Although all serious adverse events could not be attributed to EGb 761, in five patients treated with the extract a number of possible reactions could not be ruled out: headache, allergic skin reactions, and gastrointestinal complaints in 4 cases; the latter being more intense in 9 patients in the placebo group (Kanowski et al., 1996).

In a double-blind, randomized trial, Weitbrecht and Jansen (1985) compared a three-month treatment with *Ginkgo biloba* extract versus placebo in a homogeneous population of 40 geriatric patients with primary degenerative dementia. The treatment was evaluated by patient self-evaluation, clinical geriatric scales, and psychomotor tests, which were carried out before the study and after 4, 8, and 12 weeks of treatment. By the eighth week, statistically significant improvements were found in the ginkgo group by psychometric tests and clinical scales.

Gebner et al. (1985) studied the effect of daily administration of ginkgo extract (3 × 40 mg) compared to placebo and 5 mg nicergoline in 60 patients with age-related mental deterioration. The subjects were assessed with a series of examinations and pharmaco-EEG before and at 4, 8, and 12 weeks. The EEG results revealed no advantage of ginkgo extract over the two reference drugs, but the vigilance of those who had a more unfavorable initial situation improved. The researchers concluded that ginkgo extract had a positive effect on geriatric subjects diagnosed with deterioration of mental performance and vigilance as reflected at the behavioral level. By contrast, very little improvement was noted in healthy subjects.

Retinopathies. In a randomized, prospective double-blind, crossover phase I clinical trial in 11 healthy volunteers (mean age 34), Chung et al. (1999) found that ocular blood flow velocity significantly increased with ginkgo extract (Ginkoba, 40 mg p.o. t.i.d. × 2). Ocular blood flow velocity was measured by color Doppler imaging and none of the patients had any history of either ocular or systemic disease or were taking systemic or topical medications concomitantly with the trial. The ophthalmic artery showed a significant increase in end diastolic velocity versus baseline compared to placebo, without altering arterial blood pressure, the heart rate, or intraocular pressure. No discomfort or side effects from the treatment were found. The researchers noted that despite increasing evidence that patients with glaucoma are burdened with poor ocular blood flow, current treatments neither document this fact nor offer treatments for the problem. Yet considerable research of late has focused upon optimum ocular circulation. Vascular abnormalities, such as deficits in ocular blood flow and altered vasodilation of choroidal circulation in glaucoma patients, may be some of the first signs of the disease.

Tinnitus. A systematic review of 19 clinical studies on the effects of EGb 761 on tinnitus (due to labyrinthine disorders or cerebrovascular insufficiency) found eight controlled trials that showed statistically significant results compared to reference drugs or placebo. Treatment periods lasted 4 to 12 weeks and best results were found in early onset tinnitus (Holstein, 2001).

Reisser and Weidauer (2001) conducted a comparative study of EGb 761 and the standard treatment for sudden deafness, pentoxifylline, in 71 patients presenting with sudden deafness (acute hearing loss). The randomized, reference-controlled, double-blind study was limited to patients without any previous treatment for the condition and who were not taking other rheological agents or had a history of kidney, heart, or liver diseases. After hospitalization, patients were randomly assigned to receive either daily (for ten days) infusions of either EGb 761 (200 mg dry extract, $n = 37$) plus the reference substance as a placebo, or pentoxifylline (300 mg, $n = 34$) plus the test substance (EGb 761) as a placebo. At the start of treatment, 39% of those being treated with EGb 761 had tinnitus compared to 41% of those in the pentoxyifylline group. Based on patient assessments, the results showed that there was no significant difference in tolerance or efficacy between pentoxifylline and EGb 761. However, the researchers could not exclude the possibility of a placebo effect. Among the EGb 761 group, one patient showed high blood pressure peaks which were presumed to be due to the carrier used in the infusion (Rheomacrodex), and another experienced drowsiness and tiredness. In the pentoxifylline group, one patient experienced itching of the feet and hands and another an allergic reaction to the carrier.

Drew and Davies (2001) conducted a double-blind, placebo-controlled trial of a ginkgo extract (LI 1370, 50 mg t.i.d. for 12 weeks) in 478 matched pairs of patients who had tinnitus for over one year and less than five years. Ranging in age from 18-70, the 956 otherwise healthy participants were given four questionnaires which rated changes in loudness and in how troublesome the symptoms of tinnitus were before, during, and after treatment.

The placebo was identical in appearance and supplied by the manufacturer of the ginkgo extract. The results showed no significant difference in outcome compared to placebo. Thirty-four participants in the ginkgo group reported improvement, and thirty-five in the placebo group reported the same.

Psychological and Behavioral Disorders

Cognitive functions-memory. Few studies have examined the cognitive effects of ginkgo extracts in healthy volunteers and in healthy, young volunteers, the results have been largely inconclusive (Moulton et al., 2001). In a randomized, double-blind, placebo-controlled trial in 50 healthy adults (ages 18-40 years) administered EGb (120 mg/day for 30 days), Stough et al. (2001) reported that, compared to placebo, subjects receiving the ginkgo extract showed significantly improved speed of information processing, executive processing, and working memory. Kennedy et al. (2000) conducted a placebo-controlled, double-blind, balanced, crossover design trial of a ginkgo leaf extract (Pharmaton SA, GK501) in three different acute doses (120 mg, 240 mg, 360 mg) or placebo in 20 healthy young volunteers (2 men and 18 women ages 19-24). Utilizing the Cognitive Drug Research computerized assessment battery, the researchers set out to determine whether acute doses of the extract had some consistent effect on changes in cognitive functions in quality of memory, accuracy of attention, and speeds of attention and memory. Apart from the use of birth control pills, none of the participants reported taking any medications and all claimed that they were in good health. For sufficient washout, the five study days were seven days apart. The results showed the clearest significant effects on the following factors of the assessment battery: enhanced speed on attention tasks at 2.5 and 6 h postdose from either 240 mg or 360 mg; quality of memory at 1 and 4 h postdose from either 120 mg or 240 mg; and speed of memory at 2.5 h postdose from 360 mg. Significant negative results were evident from the 240 mg dose on the accuracy of attention factor at 1 h postdose and speed of memory factor at 1, 2.5, 4, and 6 h postdose. In conclusion, although the 120 mg dose significantly enhanced performance at 1 and 4 h postdose in scores of quality of memory, the most significant effect was found in the performance speed of the subjects on tasks assessing attention which were time- and dose-dependent at 2.5, 4, and 6 h postdose from the 240 mg and 360 mg doses. The other significant outcomes, including the negative ones, were "not readily interpretable" (Kennedy et al., 2000, p. 421).

Rigney et al. (1999) conducted a more ambitious study on the psychomotor and memory performance effects of acute doses of a ginkgo extract (Lichtwer Pharma, Berlin, Germany, LI 1370). The goal of the study was to determine the optimum dose required for significant effects on memory and psychomotor performance using tests administered every hour for about 12 h. The five-way crossover study in 36 asymptomatic subjects made up of men and women ages 30-59 was randomized, double-blind, and placebo-controlled. The tests applied were the Stroop Task, the Digit Symbol Substitution Task, the Wrist Actigraphy, the Line Analogue Rating Scale for Sedation, the Leeds Sleep Evaluation Questionnaire, the short-term memory test, the Immediate and delayed recall of supraspan word lists, the Choice Reaction Time Task, and the Critical Flicker Fusion Task. Results were as follows: the most effective acute dose on cognitive enhancement was 120 mg in the morning (versus 50 or 100 mg t.i.d., a single 240 mg dose or placebo); enhancing effects on working memory were more pronounced than on selective attention or arousal; and the best results were seen in the subjects aged 50-59. However, no significant difference compared to placebo was seen from any dose of ginkgo extract in the Critical Flicker Fusion Task, the Stroop Task, the Digit Symbol Substitution Task, or in the Choice Reaction Time Task recognition component.

Subhan and Hindmarch (1984) tested the effect of a ginkgo extract (Tebonin in Germany and Tanakan in France) on information processing and cognitive ability in eight healthy female volunteers (ages 25-40). The subjects had to abstain from alcohol and caffeine on the test days and their diet was standardized. Other than birth control pills, patients were excluded if they were taking any medications, had a history of psychiatric disease, or were even possibly pregnant. The study was double-blinded, placebo-controlled, and used a crossover design with tests administered an hour after subjects were given the ginkgo extract in different doses (120, 240, 600 mg), or placebo. The tests were Choice Reaction Time, Critical Flicker Fusion, Sternberg memory scanning, and a subjective rating of drug effects. A one-week washout period was used between each of the four randomized drug administrations with tests. The results showed no significant placebo-drug differences, and no significant improvements in any of the tests at any of the dosages except for the Sternberg test at 600 mg of the ginkgo extract, a result that was highly significant ($p < 0.0001$) compared to placebo.

Depression. Schubert and Halama (1993) investigated the effect of EGb 761 (80 mg × t.i.d. for eight weeks) in 40 patients (ages 51-78) suffering from episodes of depression combined with mild to moderate cerebral dysfunction. For a minimum of three months, the patients showed a lack of response to treatment with tetracyclic and tricyclic antidepressants (e.g., amitriptyline, doxepin, maprotiline, trimipramine). While maintaining their antidepressant medications, half of the patients received the ginkgo extract while the other half received placebo. The randomized, placebo-controlled, double-blind study found highly significant results at four weeks into the study, with the Hamilton Depression Scale (HAMD) decreasing from 14 to 7 in the active treatment group. Results were still significant after eight weeks ($p < 0.01$) and cognitive functions also showed significant improvement in the ginkgo group.

Psychoses. Zhang et al. (2001) conducted a clinical study on the effect of EGb (Honghui Pharmaceutical Company, Guangxi, China) on changes in clinical rating scores when added to haloperidol in treatment-resistant chronic schizophrenia inpatients. Ranging in age from 44 to 52, the patients (35 women and 47 men) all met the criteria for schizophrenia according to the ICD-10 and had an average history of the disease of 21 to 29 years. Pregnant or breast-feeding patients, alcohol abusers, and those with severe physical disease or other mental disorders were excluded. After a seven-day psychotropic-drug withdrawal period, the patients were divided into two groups: one received haloperidol (10-24 mg/day) plus EGb (tablets, 360 mg/day) and the other received the same dosage of haloperidol plus a placebo of identical appearance. The treatment lasted 12 weeks and 30 healthy volunteers (ages 22-61) served as the control group. Among the three groups, there was no significant difference in the number who smoked and the amount of cigarettes each smoked in a day. The patients who were treated with both halperidol and the ginkgo extract showed significant improvement in scores on the SANS (Scale for the Assessment of Negative Symptoms) and the SAPS (Scale for the Assessment of Positive Symptoms), which was also significant compared to before treatment ($p < 0.05$). Those treated with halperidol plus placebo showed a significant improvement only in the SANS compared to before treatment. In conclusion, while showing no evidence of causing side effects, EGb appeared to both increase the effect of haloperidol and alleviate its side effects. Similar results were reported by Zhang, Zhou, Zhang et al. (2001) in a double-blind, placebo-controlled, parallel-group trial of EGb in 109 patients with treatment-resistant schizophrenia. Because reports have suggested that schizophrenic patients show high levels of free radical production, Zhang, Zhou, Su, and colleagues (2001) made a further test of SOD levels. Before treatment, the patients showed higher levels of SOD compared to the healthy controls. After treatment these levels showed a significant decrease in the haloperidol plus ginkgo group ($o = 0.021$), but not in the halperidol alone group. The higher production of free radicals may be associated with medical conditions in which there is an increase in catecholamine metabolism and the increased levels of SOD in these patients might have been the result of hyperdopaminergic activity in schizophrenia. Through antioxidant mechanisms, EGb might have improved the efficacy of haloperidol and/or improved scores by alleviating the increased production of free radicals associated with increased catecholamine metabolism in schizophrenia (Zhang et al., 2000).

Seasonal affective disorder (SAD). In 17 patients (ages 26-68 years) diagnosed with seasonal affective disorder (SAD), Lingaerde et al. (1999) conducted a randomized, double-blind, placebo-controlled, parallel group study of ginkgo extract PN246 (Bio-Biloba, Pharma Nord, Vejle, Denmark,

120-160 mg/day) as a possible means of preventing winter depression. The extract used was standardized to contain 7 mg terpene lactones and 24 mg flavone glycosides per coated tablet. After the ten-week trial (extended to a period of two years), Lingaerde and colleagues reported no significant difference compared to placebo.

Receptor- and Neurotransmitter-Mediated Functions

In a study by Fowler et al. (2000), pretreatment with EGb 761 (60 mg b.i.d. for one month) in ten normal subjects (ages 38-76; 8 women and 2 men) was examined for effects on MAO inhibition by means of PET scans and radiolabelled L-deprenyl and clorgyline, which respectively inactivate MAO A and B. Fowler et al. (2000) found that although their tests did not rule out MAO inhibition in other organs of the body, compared to baseline PET scans with the radiolabelled agents, the one-month treatment with EGb 761 had no effect on any of the brain regions they measured ($n = 9$), either for MAO A or B. In addition, there was no change in arterial plasma time activity curves for MAO A or B. As a caveat, patients with dementia and elderly subjects may differ in the reactivity of their cerebral vasculature compared to normal subjects. Contrary to a commonly reported adverse effect of ginkgo as a substance that antagonizes platelet activating factor, upon the removal of arterial catheters the researchers observed increased clotting time in their subjects.

Reproductive Disorders

Infertility (Male)

Sikora et al. (1998) studied the effect of ginkgo (EGb 761, 240 mg/day, p.o.) in 32 men diagnosed with erectile dysfunction which was suspected to be of vasculogenic origin. The 24-week, placebo-controlled, double-blind, randomized trial used diagnostic measurements that included nocturnal penile tumescence and rigidity recording (NPTR), duplex-sonography, dynamic cavernosometry, and examinations of drug-induced tumescence, before and after the treatment period. The drop-out rate (reasons not stated) was relatively high, leaving just 23 patients for follow-up examination. Overall, the results showed no significant benefit from the ginkgo extract, which was in contrast to earlier results from an uncontrolled preliminary study.

An elderly patient taking selective serotonin reuptake inhibitor (SSRI) medication for major depression reported improved libido and erections after taking ginkgo to enhance his memory. When he went off the ginkgo, his sexual difficulties returned, and when he began taking ginkgo again they went into remission (Cohen and Bartlik, 1998). Based on these observations, and the fact that no consistently effective pharmacological agent has been found that reliably treats SSRI-induced sexual dysfunction, Cohen and Bartlik conducted an open trial of ginkgo (form not stated) in depressive men and women suffering from the same side effect. The patients were being treated with various kinds of antidepressants (bupropion, venlafaxine, nefazodone, fluoxetine, phenelzine, sertaline, Vivactil, and paroxetine), the majority receiving SSRIs. Decreased libido was experienced by 76%, inhibited or delayed orgasm by 54%, and for 19% there were difficulties with erections. Various pharmacological means were attempted without satisfactory results, including yohimbine, buspirone, lower dosages of the antidepressants, and amantadine. While maintaining their antidepressant medications, 63 patients received ginkgo extract at an average dosage of 207 mg/day for 28 days (60 mg q.i.d. to 120 mg t.i.d.). Cohen and Bartlik reported that 84% of the patients found relief from their antidepressant-induced sexual dysfunction, with more female patients (30/33) finding relief than males (23/30). No side effects or drug interactions from the ginkgo treatment were reported. A more recent, open-label study of ginkgo (uncharacterized; 300 mg t.i.d. for one month) in 22 patients (9 men and 13 women) with SSRI-induced sexual dysfunction also reported an absence of side effects, but little if any effect on sexual function (Ashton et al., 2000).

Menopause

Tamborini and Taurelle (1993) conducted a double-blind, placebo-controlled, multicenter trial of ginkgo (EGb 761, 80 mg twice daily) in 165 women between the ages of 18 and 45 who experienced congestive symptoms of PMS. These symptoms were present in all the patients during seven days of the cycle and consisted of edema of the extremities, pain in the breast, and abdomino-pelvic distention accompanied by neuropsychological problems. Treatment with the ginkgo extract or placebo was received by the patients for two menstrual cycles after an observational cycle, and initiated from day 16 of the first cycle until day five of the second cycle. Patient self-evaluations during the treatment phase and evaluations by practitioners before and after treatment were used to judge the efficacy of the ginkgo extract. Of the 143 patients who completed the trial, a significant difference was found in the ginkgo group versus the placebo group in the amelioration of congestive symptoms ($p < 0.07$), which was especially noticeable in those affecting the breast ($p < 0.03$), as well as edema of the extremities ($p < 0.05$). Significant improvements were also seen in neuropsychological symptoms (irritability-aggression) compared to placebo ($p < 0.001$), and the tolerability of the treatment was judged to be good or very good by 86% of the patients. Patient evaluation scores were significantly higher in favor of the ginkgo extract versus placebo ($p < 0.07$) and in the evaluation of the practitioners ($p < 0.01$).

Respiratory and Pulmonary Disorders

Allergies and Asthma

Ten patients with exercise-induced asthma were studied (Wilkens et al., 1990) for the effect of single-dose and short-term treatment with the PAF-antagonist BN 52063, which is a mixture of ginkgolides A, B, and C (molar ratio 2:2:1). Inhalation of BN 52063 was not found to have beneficial effects on pulmonary function, but short-term treatment by mouth appeared to provide partial protection against exercise-induced bronchoconstriction and antagonized platelet secretion of Beta-TG and PF4. The researchers noted that further studies were warranted to more decisively evaluate the role of this mixture in asthma therapy.

DOSAGE

In Europe, ginkgo extract is administered clinically at the total daily dosage of 120-240 mg of a standardized extract containing at least 24% ginkgo flavone glycosides and 6% terpene lactones (ginkgolides and bilobalides) for a period of at least eight weeks (Chang and Chang, 1997; Blumenthal et al., 1998). The German Commission E recommends administration for a period of not less than eight weeks in the treatment of chronic conditions, and a review of benefits before exceeding three months (Blumenthal et al., 1998).

SAFETY PROFILE

There is general agreement of a low risk associated with ginkgo extract products (Woerdenbag and van Beek, 1997). Possible serious side effects have rarely been noted in any of the numerous clinical trials on ginkgo extract, and those that were noted were not significantly different from those experienced with placebo (e.g., Kanowski et al., 1996).

The following case reports are summarized as examples of the difficulty inherent in evaluating the safety of ginkgo in the absence of large-scale case-controlled studies.

Commercial ginkgo leaf extract products available in the United States (Ganzera et al., 2001) and from other countries have shown considerable variability, both in their total contents of terpenes (1.24 to 2.64 mg/tablet in European products and 0 to 5.18 mg/tablet in Chinese domestic products), and individual terpenes (i.e., ginkgolides A, B, and C, and bilobalide). Several European ginkgo products have shown highly consistent amounts of total and individual terpenes from batch to batch (e.g., Ginaton, Tanakan, EGb 761). For example, among individual terpenes, the bilobalide content of seven out of ten different Chinese domestic brands of ginkgo tablets was zero and the highest amount detected was 0.48 mg/tablet. In eight different Chinese domestic ginkgo extracts, the bilobalide content was 0 to 1.98%. In samples of Ginaton ($n = 3$) and Tanakan tablets ($n = 4$) from Europe, bilobalide content was more consistent, with 1.03-1.30 mg/tablet and 1.10-1.28 mg/tablet, respectively (Peishan et al., 2001). Among nine different ginkgo (tablets and capsules) products sold in the United States (California and Mississippi) claiming to contain a standardized extract of ginkgo leaf, contents of individual terpenelactones (ginkgolides A, B, C, and J, and bilobalide) showed remarkable variation, ranging from a total of 7.2 mg/g to 32.6 mg/g (Ganzera et al., 2001). Of more immediate concern is that among 14 samples of *Ginkgo biloba* leaf products manufactured in China, 13 were found to contain the neurotoxins ginkgolic acids at levels that were 16 to 733 times that of an acceptable standardized extract (Chiu et al., 2002), or 5 ppm. A survey of ginkgo products sold in the United States for ginkgolic acid content has, to our knowledge, not been conducted. The fact that the majority of imported ginkgo extracts are from China (Drieu and Jaggy, 2000) is sufficient cause for such a survey. In any case, bioequivalence of ginkgo extracts to EGb 761, which includes safety, has yet to be shown (Robbers and Tyler, 1999; Drieu and Jaggy, 2000).

Vale (1998a) reported a possible association of ginkgo extract with subarachnoid hemorrhage in an elderly man taking 120-160 mg/day who already had shown a slightly increased bleeding time. Gilbert (1997) reported a case of left frontal subdural hematoma in a 72-year-old woman whose use of ginkgo (50 mg times t.i.d. for five to six months) coincided with the duration of her complaints of dizziness and memory impairment. Rowin and Lewis (1996) reported the case of a patient who developed spontaneous bilateral subdermal hematomas following ingestion of 120 mg *Ginkgo biloba* extract daily. Whether the hematomas were caused by the ginkgo extract remains unknown, but the prolonged bleeding time of 15 min and 9.5 min (normal range = 3.0-9.0 min) during self-administration of the extract improved to within normal ranges (to 6.5 min and 6.5 min) 35 days after discontinuation. Due to the demonstrated PAF-inhibiting ability of ginkgo extract, further investigation of possibly clinically relevant antiplatelet effects of ginkgo extract is suggested, especially for longer duration treatments beyond normal clinical trial times (Rowin and Lewis, 1996). Skogh (1998) expressed doubts about this association, noting that no inhibition of platelet aggregation is found from the "usual dose" of *Ginkgo biloba* extract. In reply, Vale (1998b) summarily dismissed these doubts, partly by citing the manufacturer of the extract (Schwabe Laboratories, Germany). According to the product literature, the patient clearly regarded the product as a "platelet aggregation factor antagonist." Vale admitted that while the case did not prove a causal association with ginkgo, he warned to carefully monitor herbal extracts to "prevent rare but potential disastrous results" (Vale, 1998b, p. 1146).

Benjamin et al. (2001) provided a case report of a male taxi driver who developed a spontaneous intracerebral hemorrhage after taking a ginkgo leaf extract for 18 months at a dosage of 40 mg t.i.d. During that period, the patient had not regularly taken any proprietary drugs nor any other dietary supplement. The patient was a nonsmoker without a history of vascular problems, diabetes, or hypertension and evidence showed no recent ingestion of alcohol (Benjamin et al., 2001). Intracerebral hemorrhage appears to be more commonly found in association with diabetes mellitus, hypertension, quantity of alcohol ingested within the past week, and anticoagulant drug therapy, while subarachnoid hemorrhage appears to be more frequently associated with cigarette smoking (Juvela, 1996). Nothing abnormal was apparent in blood tests, and he showed no sign of vascular abnormality. Initially, he was in a confused state with severe pain in his right temple and behind his right eye and was unable to stand. He was diagnosed with left-sided neglect, left hemiparesis, left hemianopia, midline shift, edema, and a right hematoma. A week later the left-sided neglect became severe and while the left hemianopia persisted he developed profound topographical disturbance. The patient remained with a left inferior quadranopia. Although the researchers admitted that the connection of ginkgo to hemorrhage was anecdotal, they advise physicians who encounter spontaneous hemorrhage to be aware of the herbal remedies that their patients are taking and to record them.

Contraindications

Ginkgo biloba products are contraindicated for individuals with hypersensitivity to the plant or its products (Blumenthal, 1998).

Granger (2001) reported two cases of recurrent seizures in elderly epileptic patients "with well-controlled epilepsy" (Gregory, 2001, p. 523) who had done nothing to alter their medications except for the addition of ginkgo products (120 mg daily). One patient had been seizure-free for the preceding two years and the other for seven years. In both cases, seizures stopped after discontinuation of the ginkgo and no other cause for the seizures was found. Granger found that mice pretreated with ginkgo (50 mg/kg i.p.) showed more picxrotoxin-provoked seizures and less protection from carbamazepine and sodium valproate (valproic acid) (Granger citing Manocha et al., 1996 and Manocha et al., 1997), drugs used in the treatment of generalized tonic-clonic seizures and cortical myoclonus, respectively, as evidence in support of the possible contraindication for ginkgo in epileptic patients. However, evidence to support the contraindication in epileptics is still lacking.

Gregory (2001) noted six reports of seizure temporally associated with the use of ginkgo products adding that several other cases occurred in which ginkgo was an ingredient of the associated products. He acknowledged that how seizures might be caused by ginkgo remains unclear, but offered the contamination of leaf products with the seeds as a possible explanation.

Mossabeb et al. (2001) reported that in skin prick tests in polysensitized plant-allergic patients ($n = 95$) and serological tests in rabbits, no evidence of type I allergenic activity was found from the parenteral *Ginkgo biloba* extracts Tebonin (= EGb 761) and Tebofortan. Had these subjects been allergic to the Anacardiaceae family and the extract contained more than the limited amount of ginkgolic acids, the outcome might have been different.

Based on provocation tests in animals and humans, allergic reactions to crude ginkgo leaf extracts have been attributed to a number of alkylphenols, including ginkgolic acids (Koch et al., 2000). These are potent contact allergens found more abundantly in the seeds (Woerdenbag and van Beek, 1997). The German Commission E prohibits the sale of ginkgo extracts containing more than 5 ppm of these acids (Blumenthal et al., 1998). Levels above that present a hazard to persons who are allergic to plants of the cashew family (Anacardiaceae) because they contain alkylphenols (urushiols) which have been shown to cross-react with alkyphenols in ginkgo. This is of particular importance to North Americans because 50-85% of them have become sensitized to the cashew family (e.g., poison ivy, poison sumac, poison oak, mango, cashew) (Koch et al., 2000). The widely used EGb 761 is manufactured to remove alkylphenols and is reported to contain 2 ppm (Siegers, 1999). However, evidence suggests that other allergenic substances may still be present in ginkgo leaf extracts which remain to be elucidated (Koch et al., 2000) (see Special Precautions).

Drug Interactions

The potential of a standardized extract of ginkgo leaf (Tanakan, Ipsen, France) to effect the hepatic microsomal drug oxidation system was investigated in a randomized, double-blind, placebo-controlled trial in 24 healthy volunteers (ages 19-35). Activity was compared to phenytoin. At a daily oral dose of 400 mg for 13 days, the ginkgo extract caused no significant change in the elimination half-life of antipyrine compared to baseline or placebo, whereas it decreased when subjects were treated with phenytoin. The difference compared to placebo or the ginkgo extact was significant ($p < 0.05$). The demonstrated lack of effect on the hepatic microsomal drug metabolism system led the researchers to conclude that the ginkgo extract "would not alter the metabolism of concomitant medications which are metabolized by this system" (Duche et al., 1989, p. 168).

Whether ginkgo extract may potentiate or have additive effects when combined with sedative medications is not known with certainty. In a double-blind, placebo-controlled, randomized crossover trial in 12 women, Schultz et al., 1998 reported that a single dose of ginkgo extract (LI 1370, 150 mg) produced an increase in subjective tiredness (measured with a visual analogue scale). However, Marcilhac et al. (1998) found no effect on plasma levels of corticosterone and ACTH in stressed rats chronically administered EGb 761 at a dosage of 50 mg/kg p.o. for 14 days.

Galluzzi et al. (2000) reported the case of an 80-year-old woman with Alzheimer's disease who, after being switched from vitamin E (600 mg/day) and donepezil (5 mg/day at bedtime) to replace an unsatisfactory treatment with bromazepam (3.5 mg/day) alone for mild anxiety, restlessness, and irritability, entered a coma after a further switch in treatment to a ginkgo product (EGb 761, 80 mg twice daily) in addition to the sedative trazodone (20 mg twice daily). In total, she had received 320 mg EGb 761 plus 100 mg trazodone within a period of 50 h. The patient then became drowsy and showed an unstable gait and an hour later fell asleep and could not be awoken, even by a slap to the face. Her Glasgow coma scale read 6/15 and her blood pressure measured 120/55 mmHg. She awoke following treatment with intravenous flumazenil (1 mg). The researchers hypothesized that as ligands for the benzodiazepine receptor, flavonoids in the ginkgo extract may have increased GABAergic activity which was further increased by trazodone, even though ginkgo is not a sedative and trazodone is not a benzodiazepine receptor ligand (Galluzzi et al., 2000). According to a ten-point scoring system designed to estimate the probability of herb-drug interactions, this interaction was scored as "possible" (Fugh-Berman and Ernst, 2001).

Matthews (1998) reported the possible association of intracerebral hemorrhage with the use of ginkgo in a 78-year-old woman who was also taking warfarin due to coronary artery bypass surgery five years earlier. In addition, she was suffering from sick sinus syndrome, and had a pacemaker and hypertension. She had taken ginkgo for two months when she suddenly developed severe apraxia. A CT scan revealed a left parietal hemorrhage. After hospitalization and some recovery, a follow-up one month later found that she still had some apraxia. Fugh-Berman and Ernst (2001) rate both this case and the following one as "possible" herb-drug interactions.

Rosenblatt and Mindel (1997) reported the case of a 70-year-old man who developed bleeding from the margin of the iris of his right eye one week after beginning daily ingestion of a ginkgo extract (two 40 mg tablets of 50:1 extract/day). He was also taking aspirin (325 mg/day) since a coronary bypass three years earlier. Examination revealed no evidence of trauma to the eye or of vascular occlusion or ischemia. A three-month follow-up indicated that the patient had no recurrence of the bleeding after he stopped taking the ginkgo product, and he maintained his daily dose of aspirin. Vaes and Chyka (2000) reviewed four cases of spontaneous bleeding temporally associated with ginkgo extracts including the latter case report. They concluded that ginkgo "may affect bleeding time through interference with platelet function" (Vaes and Chyka, 2000, p. 1481).

German authorities have reported no interactions with other drugs (Blumenthal et al., 1998). It is important to note that no definite drug interactions have been reported, even though those taking ginkgo extract are often taking many other drugs simultaneously (Chang and Chang, 1997; Kleijnen and Knipschild, 1992b).

Pregnancy and Lactation

German authorities report no precautions for the use of ginkgo extract in pregnant or lactating women (Chang and Chang, 1997; Blumenthal et al., 1998); however, human data on the safety of using ginkgo extracts on fertility, lactation, or pregnancy are lacking (Woerdenbag and van Beek, 1997; Woerdenbag and DeSmet, 2000).

No adverse reports of excessive blood loss during delivery associated with ginkgo use have been made, though it may be a risk factor (see Special Precautions).

Gingko is one of the few herbs for which any pharmacokinetic data are available, which are preferred data for assessing risk from medicine during lactation. Pharmacokinetic studies of ginkgo constituents indicate that only small amounts of terpene lactones or flavone glycosides accumulate in the serum (in the range of nanograms/mL). Serum levels set the limit on the amount of constituents available to enter into breast secretory cells and on through these cell membranes into the milk compartment. Serum half-life of the terpene lactones is also relatively short (in the range of 3-4 hrs), thus reducing the possibility of accumulation in the infant (see Pharmacokinetics). Anecdotal self-observations of a moderate increase in milk flow with ginkgo use have been made by lactation specialists (personal communication Humphrey, 2001). Increased blood flow to breast tissue is known to increase milk flow. The potential usefulness of gingko extracts as an alternative medication for treating Reynaud's disease of the nipple is currently unexplored.

Side Effects

In rare cases, mild gastrointestinal complaints, headache, and allergic skin reactions have been reported (Blumenthal et al. 1998; Kleijnen and Knipschild, 1992a). In a recent clinical study on ginkgo in 241 institutionalized elderly men and women (ages 55-86), among 197 patients who completed the trial, 25 dropped out due to side effects, of which there were nine from the placebo group and eight each in the high-dose and low-dose ginkgo groups (80 or 40 mg t.i.d. for three months, respectively). These side effects were mostly dizziness and gastrointestinal complaints. However, no differences in the number of placebo group patients compared to ginkgo group patients with gastrointestinal complaints was found. One patient in the high-dose group dropped out due to facial nerve pain, and two in the high-dose group dropped out because of "mild gastric bleeding" (Brautigam et al., 1998). In a review of clinical trials on EGb 761, the profile of adverse events showed no difference compared to placebo (Le Bars and Kastelan, 2000).

Special Precautions

To avoid the chance of bleeding, patients about to undergo surgery should stop taking ginkgo 36 h beforehand (Ang-Lee et al., 2001). To date (2002), at least four cases have been reported of spontaneous bleeding in patients taking ginkgo extracts (Matthews, 1998; Gilbert, 1997; Rosenblatt and Mindel, 1997; Rowin and Lewis, 1996) (see Drug Interactions), and one case of postoperative bleeding (Fessenden et al., 2001). In an open-label study, healthy volunteers administered a single oral dose of a standardized ginkgo extract (Tanakan, 15 mL) showed only transient ex vivo inhibition of platelet aggregating factor (PAF)-induced aggregation of platelets (maximally at 2-4 h post-administration), without any change in coagulation parameters concomitant to the extract, no significant changes in bleeding times, and no adverse effects (Guinot et al., 1989). Yet in other clinical studies, in order to achieve antagonist effects on PAF with even the most potent of the platelet aggregation inhibiting ginkgolides (ginkgolide B) doses of 80 to 120 mg and more were required (Chung et al., 1987; Duchier et al., 1989). The matter of bleeding episodes and ginkgo use remains unresolved and may be related to discrepancies in the composition of the extracts used (Peishan et al., 2001).

Jung et al. (1990) examined the ability of a ginkgo extract (Lichtwer Pharma, GmbH, Kaveri) to influence peripheral circulation and blood fluidity of healthy volunteers ($n = 10$). The randomized, placebo-controlled, single-blind, crossover trial found that a single oral administration of the extract (45 ml) corresponding to a daily dose caused a significant increase in peripheral microcirculation of approximately 57% and a significant decrease in erythrocyte aggregation of 15.6%. No effect was found from either placebo or the extract on plasma viscosity, leukocyte counts, thrombocyte aggregation, numbers of circulating thrombocyte aggregates, thrombocyte counts, hematocrit, erythrocyte rigidity, heart rate, or blood pressure. However, in an open-label study in healthy volunteers ($n = 20$ ages 21-57) who ingested a *Ginkgo biloba* extract for three months (EGb 761, 120 mg/day "at bedtime"), Kudolo (2000) reported a significant decrease in both diastolic ($p < 0.01$) and systolic blood pressure ($p < 0.05$). Bleeding times and fibrinogen levels after three months of the ginkgo extract showed no change. Even so, further studies using double-blinded protocols are needed to resolve the matter.

In the same study, Kudolo (2000) observed that after the three-month treatment period, there were increases in plasma fasting levels of pancreatic β-cell C-peptide and insulin levels which showed significant increases during oral glucose tolerance tests (OGTT) ($p < 0.001$). Because hyperinsulinemia precedes the onset of insulin resistance syndrome, atherosclerotic cardiovascular disease, and non-insulin-dependent diabetes mellitus (NIDDM), Kudolo (2000) called for long-term studies to establish the safety of ginkgo extracts in relation to pancreatic β-cells. Side effects were reported by 12 of the subjects (60%) who complained of hunger. Among them, two subjects reported experiencing the shakes and occasional and "momentary dizzy spells" when they missed meals. Kudolo (2000) concluded that because the two subjects who experienced "the shakes" showed increased C-peptide and insulin levels, the complaints may have been caused by hypoglycemia. Such an effect appears to be in contrast to effects in male rats administered EGb 761 (50 or 150 mg/kg p.o. for 15 days) in which no changes were found in mean arterial blood pressure or the concentration of glucose in blood. The only significant decrease in glucose utilization was found from the lower dose and only in the frontoparietal somatosensory cortex (Duverger et al., 1995).

In a subsequent open-label study of EGb 761 (same lot number) Kudolo administered the extract to NIDDM patients ($n = 20$) at the same daily dosage as the healthy, normoglycemic volunteers. Two groups were studied: one with hyperinsulinemia ($n = 12$) and one with pancreatic exhaustion ($n = 8$) taking oral hypoglycemic agents. Among the hyperinsulinemic patients, half were taking oral hypoglycemics and half were diet controlled. Kudolo (2001) found that after three months of taking the extract, those with pancreatic exhaustion showed twice the pancreatic β-cell response, as evidenced in C-peptide and insulin level increases in response to glucose loading. Among the NIDDM patients with hyperinsulinemia taking oral hypoglycemic agents, plasma insulin levels in response to glucose loading showed a lower area under the curve (AUC) compared to pre-ginkgo tests. However, no significant changes in the pancreatic β-cell insulin secretory response were seen in the diet-controlled hyperinsulinemic NIDDM group. Whether patients were taking oral hypoglycemics or not, the extract failed to improve glucose metabolism during the OGTT. When those taking medication were compared to those with pancreatic exhaustion, ginkgo extract appeared to produce a significant increase in the pancreatic β-cell response to OGTT, with the insulin AUC showing an increase of over 92% in parallel with an increase in the C-peptide AUC of 90%. Adverse reactions were not found; however, Kudolo cautioned that concomitant use of ginkgo extracts with sulfonylureas (e.g., glipizide, glyburide) may be of concern because of a risk of hypoglycemic episodes owing to the finding that both agents stimulate an increase in pancreatic β-cell activity. Although further studies are needed to determine the dangers of ginkgo in patients taking oral hypoglycemics or the lack thereof, Kudolo (2001) raised the possibility of ginkgo interfering with the potency of these agents, possibly by increasing their rate of clearance and probably by increasing clearance of insulin by the liver. However, contrary to Kudolo's findings, Appleton (2000) points out that in ten trials of EGb 761 in diabetics and nondiabetics spanning the years 1980 to 1998, no adverse effects of any significance were found on blood glucose levels and laboratory results of glucose control.

The raw fruits of ginkgo have been reported to be toxic (especially to children) and have caused at least one fatality (Hobbs, 1991). An aqueous extract of the seed administered to guinea pigs (11 mg/kg p.o.) produced auditory hyperalgesia, leg paralysis, and opisthontonus, clonic convulsions (Woerdenbag and van Beek, 1997). In China, Del Tredici (1991) was warned that consumption of any more than seven of the nuts at a time would cause "toxic side effects." If eaten in sufficient quantity, it is believed that the raw seeds can cause unconsciousness, convulsions, and death ("gin-nan food poisoning") (Benjamin et al., 2001). In most cases of food poisoning attributed to the seeds, subjects had ingested 20-50 seeds and a minimum of six seeds. Over a period of 30 years, poisoning from the seeds produced a lethality of approximately 27% (Arenz et al., 1996). Children under age six are more vulnerable than adults and comprise about 74% of all cases. It is presently advised in Japan that children consume no more than five seeds per day and that they not eat the seeds every day (Wada, 2000).

The toxin responsible for ginkgo poisoning is believed to be ginkgotoxin (4'-O-methylpyridoxine), a neurotoxin with antivitamin B_6 and potent convulsant activity. Ginkgotoxin occurs in both the leaves and boiled seeds of *G. biloba*. Due to its ability to inhibit GABA (4-aminobutyric acid) formation from glutamate in the brain, ginkgotoxin has the potential to cause seizures. One method of treating ginkgo seed food poisoning is the administration of vitamin B_6 in the form of pyridoxal phosphate. Mice treated with one of the constituents of the leaves (bilobalide, 10-30 mg/kg per day p.o.) showed a decrease in symptoms from ginkgotoxin-induced poisoning (Wada, 2000).

The highest amounts of ginkgotoxin have been detected in the outer seed coat (Arenz et al., 1996), which is reported to be toxic regardless of roasting (Sowers et al., 1965). However, amounts detected in the boiled seeds or leaf-based medications were found to be so low as to not present a problem of toxicity from their ingestion (Arenz et al., 1996). Medicinal preparations of ginkgo are usually only prepared from the leaves or the cooked or processed fruits (Hobbs, 1991).

Ginkgolic acids (alkylphenols), such as bilobol, cardanols, cardols, and ginkgol, are potential toxic principles in the leaves which must be removed to avoid gastrointestinal and allergenic reactions (Baron-Ruppert and Luepke, 2001; Westendorf and Regan, 2000; Siegers, 1999).

Reactions reported in patients after taking ginkgo preparations containing ginkgolic acids and ginkgols consisted of gastroenteritis, proctitis, stomatitis, and effects on the mouth mucosa (Woerdenbag and De Smet, 2000). The German Federal Health Agency requires manufacturers of ginkgo products to limit the amount of ginkgolic acids to $\leq$ 5 ppm (Blumenthal et al., 1998). In the preparation of EGb 761, most of the alkylphenols are eliminated so that the content is about 2 ppm (Siegers, 1999).

Cytotoxicity of ginkgo extracts containing ginkgolic acids was demonstrated in human small intestine cells (407 cells), human hepatoma cells (HepG2 cells), pig and rhesus monkey kidney cells (LLC-PK1 and LLc-MK2 cells), kerotinocytes (HaCaT cells), and in the neutral red cytotoxicity assay. Among these, kidney cells from pigs (renal tubulus cells) showed by far the greatest sensitivity to ginkgolic acids (Siegers, 1999).

In the popliteal lymph node assay in mice, an aqueous/alcoholic extract of the leaves produced immunotoxicity. Ginkgolic acids were almost entirely responsible (Jaggy and Koch, 1997). Dose-dependent neurotoxic effects were found in cultured chick embryonic neurons exposed to a mixture of ginkgolic acids at a concentration of 50 μM or more. Ahlemeyer et al. (2001) concluded that such toxic effects are not expected to occur in humans because the content of ginkgolic acids in standardized extracts is required to be less than 5 ppm. However, the researchers could not discount the possibility of ginkgolic acids accumulating in the body and concluded, therefore, that these lipophilic chemicals should be removed from ginkgo extracts as much as possible.

In the hen's egg test (HET), a fraction of the leaf extract containing 16% ginkgolic acids and 6.7% biflavones at a dose of 33 ppm caused half the chick embryos to die. A fraction containing 58% ginkgolic acids and a far smaller concentration of biflavones (0.02%) produced an LD_{50} of 64 ppm, suggesting that the biflavones and perhaps other constituents in ginkgo leaf extracts may be capable of amplifying the toxic effects of ginkgolic acids (Baron-Ruppert and Luepke, 2001). Ideally, ginkgo extracts should contain zero ginkgolic acids.

In traditional Chinese medicine, use of ginkgo is contraindicated in "excess" conditions in which there is acute infection with fever (Hobbs, 1991).

Toxicology

Mutagenicity

In the Ames test (with or without metabolic activation in rat liver S9-mix and using five different TA strains of *Salmonella typhymurium*), extracts of a ginkgo leaf extract showed no in vitro mutagenicity. In vivo tests of the extract in mice ($\geq$ 20 g/kg p.o. using the micronucleus test and the Ames test with *S. typhymurium* strain TA 1537) found no mutagenicity. Using the chromosome aberration test in human lymphocytes, concentrations of the extract $\geq$ 100 mg/mL were devoid mutagenic effects. Administered to rats for 104 weeks, the leaf extract was devoid of carcinogenic effects at oral doses of 4, 20, and 100 mg/kg (Woerdenbag and van Beek, 1997, p. 57).

Toxicity in Animal Models

The acute oral LD_{50} of ginkgo leaf extract (standardized to contain 6% terpene glycosides and 24% ginkgo flavone glycosides) in mice was found at 7.725 g/kg, and $\geq$ 10 g/kg in rats was without lethality. Chronic oral dosing of ginkgo leaf extract (500 mg/kg per day for six months) in rats found no histological, biochemical, or hematological damage, and kidney and liver function was unaltered. The same findings were made in dogs (400 mg/kg per day for six months) from oral dosing except that at 100 mg/kg "light and transient vasodilatory effects" were noticed in the head which were pronounced at 400 mg/kg after 35 days (Woerdenbag and van Beek, 1997, p. 57).

Oral doses of ginkgo leaf extract in rats ($\leq$ 1600 mg/kg per day) and rabbits ($\leq$ 900 mg/kg per day) did not affect reproduction and caused no teratogenic effects. Other toxicity studies in animals found no indications of mutagenicity, teratogenicity, or embryotoxicity (Woerdenbag and van Beek, 1997).

REFERENCES

Ahlemeyer, B., Selke, D., Schaper, C., Klumpp, S., and Krieglstein, J. (2001). Ginkgolic acids induce neuronal death and activate protein phosphatese type-2C. *European Journal of Pharmacology* 430: 1-7.

Ajasse, D. (1984). Le mal des montagnes. Un essai thérapeutique à double insu à 7700 mètres. [The illness of the mountains. A double-blind therapeutic trial at 7700 meters]. *La Vie Médicale* 19: 749-750.

Amato, I. (1993). Sniffing out the origins of ginkgo-stink. *Science* 261: 1389.

Amri, H., Ogwuegbu, S.O., Boujrad, N., Drieu, K., and Papadopoulos, V. (1996). In vivo regulation of peripheral-type benzodiazepine receptor and glucocorticoid synthesis by *Ginkgo biloba* extract 761 and isolated ginkgolides. *Endocrinology* 137: 5707-5718.

Ang-Lee, M.K., Moss, J., and Yuan, C.S. (2001). Herbal medicines and perioperative care. *Journal of the American Medicine Association* 286: 208-216.

Appleton, G. (2000). Does Ginkgo supplementation cause insulin resistance? *Health Notes Review of Complementary and Integrative Medicine* 7: 298-300.

Arenz, A., Klein, M., Fiehe, K., Gross, J., Drewke, C., Hemscheidt, T., and Leistner, E. (1996). Occurrence of neurotoxic 4'-*O*-methylpyridoxine in *Ginkgo biloba* leaves, *Ginkgo* medications and Japanese *Ginkgo* food. *Planta Medica* 62: 548-551.

Ashton, A.K., Ahrens, K., Gupta, S., and Masano, P.S. (2000). Antidepressant-induced sexual dysfunction and *Ginkgo biloba*. *American Journal of Psychiatry* 157: 836-837 (letter).

Baron-Ruppert, G. and Luepke, N.P. (2001). Evidence for toxic effects of alkylphenols from *Ginkgo biloba* in the hen's egg test (HET). *Phytomedicine* 8: 133-138.

Barth, S.A., Inselmann, G., Engemann, R., and Heidemann, H.T. (1991). Influences of *Ginkgo biloba* on cyclosporin A induced lipid peroxidation in human liver microsomes in comparison to vitamin E, glutathione and *N*-acetylcysteine. *Biochemical Pharmacology* 41: 1521-1526.

Bastianetto, S., Ramassamy, C., Dore, S., Christen, Y., Poirier, J., and Quirion, R. (2000). The *Ginkgo biloba* extract (EGb 761) protects hippocampal neurons against cell death induced by β-amyloid. *European Journal of Neuroscience* 12: 1882-1890.

Bastianetto, S., Zheng, W.H., and Quirion, R. (2000). The *Ginkgo biloba* extract (EGb 761) protects and rescues hippocampal cells against nitric oxide-induced toxicity. *Journal of Neurochemistry* 74: 2268-2277.

Baudouin, C., Ettaiche, M., Fredj-Reygrobellet, D., Droy-Lefaix, M.T., Gastaud, P., and Lapalus, P. (1992). Effects of *Ginkgo biloba* extracts in a model of tractional retinal detachment. *Lens and Eye Toxicity Research* 9: 513-519.

Baudouin, C., Pisella, P.J., Ettaiche, M., Goldschild, M., Becquet, F., Gastaud, P., and Droy-Lafaix, M.T. (1999). Effects of EGb 761 and superoxide dismutase in an experimental model of retinopathy generated by intravitreal production of superoxide anion radical. *Graefe's Archives for Clinical and Experimental Ophthalmology* 237: 58-66.

Bauer, U. (1984). 6-Month double-blind randomized clinical trial of *Ginkgo biloba* extract versus placebo in two parallel groups in patients suffering from peripheral arterial insufficiency. *Drug Research* 34: 716-720.

Bazan, H.E.P., Braquet, P., Reddy, S.T.K., and Bazan, N.G. (1987). Inhibition of the alkali burn-induced lipoxygenation of arachidonic acid in the rabbit cornea in vivo by a platelet activating factor antagonist. *Journal of Ocular Pharmacology* 3: 357-365.

Benjamin, J., Muir, T., Briggs, K., and Pentland, B. (2001). A case of cerebral haemorrhage—Can *Ginkgo biloba* be implicated? *Postgraduate Medical Journal* 77: 112-113.

Blumenthal, M., Busse, W.R., Goldberg, A., Gruenwald, J., Hall, T., Riggins, C.W., and Rister, R.S. (Eds.) (1998). *The Complete German Commission E Monographs*. Austin, TX: American Botanical Council, pp. 136-138.

Braquet, P. and Hosford, D. (1991). Ethnopharmacology and the development of natural PAF antagonists as therapeutic agents. *Journal of Ethnopharmacology* 32: 135-139.

Braquet, P.G., Spinnewyn, B., Braquet, M., Bourgain, R.H., Taylor, J.E., Etienne, A., and Drieu, K. (1985). BN 52021 and related compounds: A new series of highly specific PAF-acether receptor antagonists isolated from *Ginkgo biloba* L. *Blood Vessels* 16: 558-572.

Brautigam, M.R.H., Blommaert, F.A., Verleye, G., Castermans, J., Jansen Steur, E.N.H., and Kleijnen, J. (1998). Treatment of age-related complaints with *Ginkgo biloba* extract: A randomized double blind placebo-controlled study. *Phytomedicine* 5: 425-434.

Brüchert, E., Heinrich, S.E., and Ruf-Kohler, P. (1991). Wirksamkeit von LI 1370 bei älteren patienten mit hirnleistungsschwäche. Multizentrische doppelblindstudie des fachverbandes Deutsche allgemeinärzte. *Münchener Medizinische Wochenschrift* 133(Suppl. 1): S9-S14.

Çeliköz, B., Aydin, A., Kubar, A., Kisa, U., and Selmanpakoglu, N. (1997). The effects of *Ginkgo biloba* extract and deferoxamine on flap viability. *European Journal of Plastic Surgery* 20: 197-201.

Chandrasekaran, K., Mehrabian, Z., Spinnewyn, B., Drieu, K., and Fiskum, G. (2001). Neuroprotective effects of bilobalide, a component of the *Ginkgo biloba* extract (EGb 761), in gerbil global brain ischemia. *Brain Research* 922: 282-292.

Chang, J.Y. and Chang, M.N. (1997). Medicinal uses of *Ginkgo biloba. Today's Therapeutic Trends* 15: 63-74.

Cheung, F., Siow, Y.L., Chen, W.Z., and Karmin, O. (1999). Inhibitory effect of *Ginkgo biloba* extract on the expression of inducible nitric oxide synthase in endothelial cells. *Biochemical Pharmacology* 58: 1665-1673.

Cheung, F., Siow, Y.L., and O, K. (2001). Inhibition by ginkgolides and bilobalide of the production of nitric oxide in macrophages (THP-1) but not in endothelial cells (HUVEC). *Biochemical Pharmacology* 61: 503-510.

Chiu, A.E., Lane, A.T., and Kimball, A.B. (2002). Diffuse morbilliform eruption after consumption of *Ginkgo biloba* supplement. *Journal of the American Academy of Dermatology* 46: 145-146.

Chung, H.S., Harris, A., Kristinsson, J.K., Ciulla, T.A., Kagemann, C., and Ritch, R. (1999). *Ginkgo biloba* extract increases ocular blood flow velocity. *Journal of Ocular Pharmacology and Therapeutics* 15: 233-240.

Chung, K.F., McCusker, M., Page, C.P., Dent, G., Guinot, P., and Barnes, P.J. (1987). Effect of a ginkgolide mixture (BN 52063) in antagonizing skin and platelet responses to platelet activating factor in man. *Lancet* 1 (January 31): 248-251.

Clement, J.L., Livescchi, G., Jimenez, C., Morino, S., Drevard, R., and Eclache, J.P. (1982). Modifications vasomotrices des extrémités de l'exposition à des conditions thermiques défavorables. Méthodologie et résultat de l'étude de l'extrait de *Ginkgo biloba. Actualité d'Angéiologie* 7: 3-8.

Cohen, A.J. and Bartlik, B. (1998). *Ginkgo biloba* for antidepressant-induced sexual dysfunction. *Journal of Sex and Marital Therapy* 24: 139-143.

Curtis-Prior, P., Vere, D., and Fray, P. (1999). Therapeutic value of *Ginkgo biloba* in reducing symptoms of decline in mental function. *Journal of Pharmacy and Pharmacology* 51: 535-541.

DeFeudis, F.V. (1991). *Ginkgo biloba Extract (EGb 761): Pharmacological Activities and Clinical Applications.* Paris: Elsevier.

De Kozak, Y., Faure, J.P., Thillaye, B., Ruchoux, M.M., Doly, M., Droy-Lefaix, M.T., and Braquet, P. (1994). *Ginkgo biloba* extract (EGb 761) and platelet-activating factor antagonist protect the retina in experimental autoimmune uveoretinitis. *Ocular Immunology and Inflammation* 2: 231-237.

Del Tredici, P. (1991). Ginkgos and people: A thousand years of interaction. *Arnoldia* 51: 2-15.

Del Tredici, P. (2000). The evolution, ecology, and cultivation of *Ginkgo biloba*. In van Beek, T.A. (Ed.), *Ginkgo Biloba* (pp. 7-23). Amsterdam, the Netherlands: Harwood Academic.

Diamond, B.J., Shiflett, S.C., and Schoenberger, N.E. (2000). *Ginkgo biloba* extract: Mechanisms and clinical indications. *Archives of Physical Medicine and Rehabilitation* 81: 668-678.

Doly, M., Millerin, M., Bonhomme, B., Droy-Lefaix, M.T., and Braquet, P. (1992). Inhibition of vincristine-induced retinal impairments by a specific PAF antagonist. *Lens and Eye Toxicity Research* 9: 529-535.

Drew, S. and Davies, E. (2001). Effectiveness of *Ginkgo biloba* in treating tinnitus: Double blind, placebo controlled trial. *British Medical Journal* 322 (January 13): 1-6.

Drieu, K. and Jaggy, H. (2000). History, development and constituents of EGb 761. In van Beek, T.A. (Ed.), *Ginkgo biloba* (pp. 267-277). Amsterdam, The Netherlands: Harwood Academic.

Droy-Lefaix, M.T., Vennat, J.C., Besse, G., and Doly, M. (1992). Effect of *Ginkgo biloba* extract (EGb 761) on chloroquine induced retinal alterations. *Lens and Eye Toxicity Research* 9: 521-528.

Duche, J.C., Barre, J., Guinot, P., Duchier, J., Cournot, A., and Tillement, J.P. (1989). Effect of *Ginkgo biloba* extract on microsomal enzyme induction. *International Journal of Pharmacology Research* 9: 165-168.

Duchier, J., Cournot, A., Hosford, D., et al. (1989). Clinical studies on the tolerance and effects of BN 52021 on PAF-induced platelet aggregation and skin reactivity in healthy volunteers. In Braquet, P. (Ed.), *Ginkgolides: Chemistry, Biology, Pharmacology and Clinical Perspectives*, vol. 2 (pp. 987-994). Barcelona: J.R. Prous.

Duverger, D., Defeundis, F.V., and Drieu, K. (1995). Effects of repeated treatments with an extract of *Ginkgo biloba* (EGb 761) on cerebral glucose utilization in the rat: An autoradiographic study. *General Pharmacology* 26: 1375-1383.

Eckmann, F. (1990). Hirnleistungsstörungen—Behandlung mit Ginkgo-biloba-extrakt [Cerebral insufficiency—Treatment with *Ginkgo biloba* extract. Time of onset of effect in a double-blind study with 60 inpatients]. *Fortschritte der Medizin* 108: 557-560.

Fessenden, J.M., Wittenborn, W., and Clarke, L. (2001). *Ginkgo biloba:* A case report of herbal medicine and bleeding postoperatively from a laparoscopic cholecystectomy. *The American Surgeon* 67: 33-35.

Fourtillan, J.B., Brisson, A.M., Girault, J., Ingrand, I., Decourt, J.P., Drieu, K., Jouenne, P., and Biber, A. (1995). Propriétés pharmacocinétiques du bilobalide et des ginkgolides A et B chez le sujet sain après administrations intraveineuses et orals d'extrait de *Ginkgo biloba* (EGb 761) [Pharmacokinetics of biobalide, ginkgolide A and ginkgolide B in healthy volunteers following oral and intravenous administrations of *Ginkgo biloba* (EGb 761)]. *Thérapie* 50: 137-144.

Fowler, J.S., Wang, G.J., Volkow, N.D., Logan, D., Franceschi, D., Franceschi, M., MacGregor, R., Shea, C., Garza, V., Liu, N., et al. (2000). Evidence that *Ginkgo biloba* does not inhibit MAO A and B in living human brain. *Pharmacology Letters* 66: 141-146.

Fugh-Berman, A. and Ernst, E. (2001). Herb-drug interactions: Review and assessment of report quality. *British Journal of Clinical Pharmacology* 52: 587-595.

Gajewski, A. and Hensch, S.A. (1999). *Ginkgo biloba* and memory for a maze. *Psychological Reports* 84: 481-484.

Galluzi, S., Zanetti, O., Binetti, G., and Frisoni, G.B. (2000). Coma in a patient with Alzheimer's disease taking low dose trazodone and *Ginkgo biloba*. *Journal of Neurology, Neurosurgery and Psychiatry* 68: 679-680 (letter).

Ganzera, M., Zhao, J., and Khan, I.A. (2001). Analysis of terpenelactones in *Ginkgo biloba* by high performance liquid chromatography and evaporative light scattering detection. *Chemical and Pharmaceutical Bulletin* 49(9): 1170-1173.

Gebner, B., Voelp, A., and Klasser, M. (1985). Study of the long-term action of a *Ginkgo biloba* extract on vigilance and mental performance as determined by means of quantitative pharmaco-EEG and psychometric measurements. *Arzneimittel-Forschung/Drug Research* 35: 1459-1465.

Gilbert, G.J. (1997). *Ginkgo biloba. Neurology* 48: 1137 (letter).

Granger, A.S. (2001). *Ginkgo biloba* precipitating epileptic seizures. *Age and Aging* 30: 523-525.

Grässel, E. (1992). Einfluss von Rökan auf die geistige leistungsfähigkeit. Placebokontrollierte doppelblindstudie unter computerisierten messbedingungen bei patienten mit zerebraler insuffizienz. In Diehm, C. and Müller, D. (Eds.), *Rökan, Ginkgo biloba EGb 761*. Berlin, Germany: Springer-Verlag.

Grässel, I. and Reuter, G. (1998). Analysis of 6-hydroxykynurenic acid in *Ginkgo biloba* and *Ginkgo* preparations. *Planta Medica* 64: 566-570.

Gregory, P.J. (2001). Seizure associated with *Ginkgo biloba?* *Annals of Internal Medicine* 134: 344 (letter).

Grosche, J., Härtig, W., and Reichenbach, A. (1995). Expression of glial fibrillary acidic protein (GFAP), glutamine synthetrase (GS), and Bcl-2 protooncogene protein by Müller (glial) cells in retinal light damage of rats. *Neuroscience Letters* 185: 119-122.

Guinot, P., Caffrey, E., Lambe, R., and Darragh, A. (1989). Tanakan inhibits platelet-activating-factor-induced platelet aggregation in healthy male volunteers. *Haemostasis* 19: 219-223.

Haas, N., McDanel, H., Godwin, A., Humphrey, P., Bigner, S., and Wong, A. (1991). Specific expression of phospholipase Cγ2 in human glial tumors. *Proceedings of the American Association of Cancer Research* 32: 17 (abstract).

Haguenauer, J.P., Cantenot, F., Koskas, H., and Pierart, H. (1986). Traitement des troubles de l'équilibre par l'extrait de *Ginkgo biloba*. Étdue multicentrique à double insu face au placebo [Treatment of disturbed equilibrium with *Ginkgo biloba* extract. A multicenter double-blind, placebo-controlled study]. *Presse Medical* (Paris) 15: 1569-1572.

Halama, P. (1991). *Ginkgo biloba*. Wirksamkeit eines spezialekstrakts bei patienten mit zerebraler insuffizienz [Effectiveness of special extracts in patients with cerebral insufficiency]. *Münchner Medizinische Wochenschrift* 133: 190-194.

He, S.A., Yin, G., and Pang, Z.J. (1997). Resources and prospects of *Ginkgo biloba* in China. In Hori, T., Ridge, R.W., Tulecke, W., Del Redicini, P., Tremouillaux-Guiller, J., and Tobe, H. (Eds.), *Ginkgo biloba—A Global Treasure* (pp. 373-383). Tokyo, Japan: Springer-Verlag.

Hibatallah, J., Carduner, C., and Poelman, M.C. (1999). In-vivo and in-vitro assessment of the free radical-scavenger activity of *Ginkgo* flavone glycosides at high concentration. *Journal of Pharmacy and Pharmacology* 51: 1435-1440.

Hill, S.R., Bonjouklian, R., Powis, G., Abraham, R.T., Ashendel, C.L., and Zalkow, L.H. (1994). A multisample assay for inhibitors of phosphatidylinositol phospholipase C: Identification of naturally occurring peptide inhibitors with antiproliferative activity. *Anti-Cancer Drug Design* 9: 353-361.

Hobbs, C. (1991). *Ginkgo: Elixir of Youth*. Capitola, CA: Botanica Press.

Hofferberth, B. (1991). Ginkgo-biloba-spezialekstrakt bei patienten mit hirnorganischem psychosyndrom. Prufung der wirksamkeit mit neurophysiologischen und psychometrischen methoden [*Ginkgo biloba* special extract in patients with organic brain syndrome]. *Münchner Medizinische Wochenschrift* 133(Suppl. 1): 30-33.

Holstein, N. (2001). Ginkgo-spezialextrakt EGb 761 in der tinnitus-therapie. Ein ubersicht uber die ergebnisse der durchgefuhrten klinischen prufungen [Ginkgo special extract EGb 761 in tinnitus therapy. An overview of results of completed clinical trials]. *MMW Fortschritte der Medizin* 118: 157-164 (English abstract).

Hopfenmüller, W. (1994). Nachweis der therapeutischen wirksamkeit eines *Ginkgo biloba*-spezialekstraktes. Meta-analyse von 11 klinischen studien bei patienten mit himleistungsstörungun im alter [Evidence for a therapeutic effect of *Ginkgo biloba* special extract. Meta-analysis of 11 clinical studies in patients with cerebrovascular insufficiency in old age]. *Arzneimittel-Forschung/Drug Research* 44: 1005-1013 (English abstract).

Hori, S. and Hori, T. (1997). A cultural history of *Ginkgo biloba* in Japan and the generic name *Ginkgo*. In Hori, T., Ridge, R.W., Tulecke, W., Del Tredici, P., Tremouillaux-Guiller, J., and Tobe, H. (Eds.), *Ginkgo biloba: A Global Treasure. From Biology to Medicine* (pp. 385-411). Tokyo: Springer-Verlag.

Huguet, F., Drieu, K., and Pirpiou, A. (1994). Decreased cerebral 5-HT$_{1A}$ receptors during aging: Reversal by *Ginkgo biloba* extract (EGb 761). *Journal of Pharmacy and Pharmacology* 46: 316-318.

Huh, H. and Staba, E.J. (1992). The botany and chemistry of *Ginkgo biloba* L. *Journal of Herbs, Spices and Medicinal Plants* 1: 92-124.

Humphrey, S. (2001). Sheila Humphrey, RN, BSc, ICBLC, personal communication with INPR, September.

Irie, J., Murata, M., and Homma, S. (1996). Glycero-3-phosphate dehydrogenase inhibitors, anacardic acids, from *Ginkgo biloba*. *Bioscience, Biotechnology and Biochemistry* 60: 240-243.

Itil, T.M., Erlap, E., Tsambis, E., Itil, K.Z., and Stein, U. (1996). Central nervous system effects of *Ginkgo biloba,* a plant extract. *American Journal of Therapeutics* 3: 63-73.

Itokawa, H., Totsuka, N., Nakahara, K., Takeya, K., Lepoittevin, J.P., and Asakawa, Y. (1987). Antitumor principles from *Ginkgo biloba* L. *Chemical and Pharmaceutical Bulletin* 35: 3016-3020.

Jaggy, J. and Koch, E. (1997). Chemistry and biology of alkylphenols from *Ginkgo biloba* leaves. *Pharmazie* 52: 735-738.

Jung, C., Mrowietz, H., Kiesewetter, H., and Wenzel, E. (1990). Effect of *Ginkgo biloba* on fluidity of blood and peripheral microcirculation in volunteers. *Arzneimittel Forschung/Drug Research* 40: 589-593.

Juvela, P. (1996). Prevalence of risk factors in spontaneous intracerebral hemorrhage and aneurysmal subarachnoid hemorrhage. *Archives of Neurology* 53: 734-740.

Kanowski, S., Herrmann, W.M., Stephan, K., Wierich, W., and Horr, R. (1996). Proof of efficacy of the *Ginkgo biloba* special extract EGb 761 in outpatients suffering from mild to moderate primary degenerative dementia of the Alzheimer's type or multi-farct dementia. *Pharmacopsychiatry* 29: 47-56.

Kennedy, D.O., Scholey, A.B., and Wesnes, K.A. (2000). The dose-dependent cognitive effects of acute administration of *Ginkgo biloba* to healthy young volunteers. *Psychopharmacology* 151: 416-423.

Kleijnen, J. and Knipschild, P. (1992a). *Ginkgo biloba* for cerebral insufficiency. *British Journal of Clinical Pharmacology* 34: 352-358.

Kleijnen, J. and Knipschild, P. (1992b). *Ginkgo biloba. Lancet* 340: 1136-1139.

Koch, E., Jaggy, H., and Chatterjee, S.S. (2000). Evidence for immunotoxic effects of crude *Ginkgo biloba* L. leaf extracts using the popliteal lymph node assay in the mouse. *International Journal of Immunopharmacology* 22: 229-236.

Kubota, Y., Tanaka, N., Umegaki, K., Takenaka, H., Mizuno, H., Nakamura, K., Shinozuka, K., and Kunitomo, M. (2001). *Ginkgo biloba* extract-induced relaxation of rat aorta is associated with increase in endothelial intracellular calcium level. *Life Sciences* 69: 2327-2336.

Kudolo, G.B. (2000). The effect of 3-month ingestion of *Ginkgo biloba* extract on pancreatic β-cell function in response to glucose-loading in normal glucose tolerant individuals. *Journal of Clinical Pharmacology* 40: 647-654.

Kudolo, G.B. (2001). The effect of 3-month ingestion of *Ginkgo biloba* extract (EGb 761) on pancreatic β-cell function in response to glucose loading in individuals with non-insulin-dependent diabetes mellitus. *Journal of Clinical Pharmacology* 41: 600-611.

Le Bars, P.L. and Kastelan, J. (2000). Efficacy and safety of a *Ginkgo biloba* extract. *Public Health Nutrition* 3: 495-499.

Le Bars, P.L., Katz, M.M., Berman, N., Itil, T.M., Freedman, A.M., and Schatzberg, A.F. (1997). A placebo-controlled, double-blind, randomized trial of an extract of *Ginkgo biloba* for dementia. *Journal of the American Medical Association* 278: 1327-1332.

Le Bars, P.L., Kieser, M., and Itil, K.Z. (2000). A 26-week analysis of a double-blind, placebo-controlled trial of the *Ginkgo biloba* extract EGb 761 in dementia. *Dementia and Geriatric Cognitive Disorders* 11: 230-237.

Lee, J.S., Cho, Y.S., Park, E.J., Kim, J., Oh, W.K., Lee, H.S., and Ahn, J.S. (1998). Phospholipase Cg1 inhibitory principles from the sarcotestas of *Ginkgo biloba*. *Journal of Natural Products* 61: 867-871.

Lingaerde, O., Foreland, A.R., and Magnusson, A. (1999). Can winter depression be prevented by *Ginkgo biloba* extract? A placebo-controlled trial. *Acta Psychiatrica Scandinavica* 100: 62-66.

Maier-Hauff, K. (1991). LI 1370 nach cerebraler aneurysma-operation. Wirksamkeit bei ambulanten patienten mit störungen der hirnleistungsfähigkeit. *Münchner Medizinische Wochenschrift* 133(Suppl. 1): 34-37.

Manocha, A., Pillai, K.K., and Husain, S.Z. (1996). Influence of *Ginkgo biloba* on the effect of anticonvulsants. *Indian Journal of Pharmacology* 28: 84-87.

Manocha, A., Pillai, K.K., and Husain, S.Z. (1997). Effect of *Ginkgo biloba* on chemshock in mice. *Indian Journal of Pharmacology* 29: 198-200.

Marcilhac, A., Dakine, N., Bourhim, N., Guillaume, V., Grino, M., Drieu, K., and Oliver, C. (1998). Effect of chronic administration of *Ginkgo biloba* extract or ginkgolide on the hypothalamic-pituitary-adrenal axis of the rat. *Life Sciences* 62: 2329-2340.

Marcocci, L., Maquire, J.J., Droy-Lefair, M.T., and Packer, L. (1994). The nitric oxide-scavenging properties of *Ginkgo biloba* extract EGb 761. *Biochemical and Biophysical Research Communications* 201: 748-755.

Matile, P. (1994). Fluorescent ideoblasts in autumn leaves of *Ginkgo biloba*. *Botanica Helvetica* 104: 87-92.

Matthews, M.K. (1998). Association of *Ginkgo biloba* with intracerebral haemorrhage. *Neurology* 50: 1933-1934 (letter).

Maurer, K., Ihl, R., Dierks, T., and Frolich, L. (1998). Clinical efficacy of *Ginkgo biloba* special extract EGb 761 in dementia of the Alzheimer type. *Phytomedicine* 5: 417-424.

Meyer, B. (1986). Étude multicentrique randomisée à double insu face au placebo du traitement des acouphènes par l'extrait de *Ginkgo biloba* [A multicenter randomized double-blind study of *Ginkgo biloba* extract versus placebo in the treatment of tinnitus]. *Presse Medicale* (Paris) 15: 1562-1564.

Mossabeb, R., Kraft, D., and Valenta, R. (2001). Evaluation of the allergenic potential of *Ginkgo biloba* extracts. *Wiener Klinische Wochenschrift* 113: 580-587.

Moulton, P.L., Boyko, L.N., Fitzpatrick, J.L., and Petros, T.V. (2001). The effect of *Ginkgo biloba* on memory in healthy male volunteers. *Physiology and Behavior* 73: 659-665.

Mouren, X., Caillard, P., and Schwartz, F. (1994). Study of the anti-ischemic action of EGb 761 in the treatment of peripheral arterial occlusive disease by TcPo2 determination. *Angiology* 45: 413-417.

Noh, D.Y., Lee, Y.H., Kim, S.S., Kim, Y.I., Ryu, S.H., Suh, P.G., and Park, J.G. (1994). Elevated content of phospholipase C-γ1 in colorectal cancer tissues. *Cancer* 73: 36-41.

Oken, B.S., Storzbach, D.M., and Kaye, J.A. (1998). The efficacy of *Ginkgo biloba* on cognitive function in Alzheimer's disease. *Archives of Neurology* 55: 1409-1415.

Peishan, X., Yuzhen, Y., Haoquan, Q., and Qiaoling, L. (2001). Fluorophotometric thin-layer chromatography of *Ginkgo* terpenes by postchromatographic thermochemical derivatization and quality survey of commercial *Ginkgo* products. *Journal of the Association of Official Analytical Chemists International* 84: 1232-1241.

Perry, L.M. and Metzger, J. (1980). *Medicinal Plants of East and Southeast Asia: Attributed Properties and Uses.* Cambridge, MA: The MIT Press, p. 160.

Peters, H., Kieser, M., and Hölscher, U. (1998). Demonstration of the efficacy of *Ginkgo biloba* special extract EGb 761® on intermittent claudication—A placebo- controlled, double-blind multicenter trial. *VASA* 27: 106-110.

Pietri, S., Maurelli, E., Drieu, K., and Calcasi, M. (1997). Cardioprotective and antioxidant effects of the terpenoid constituents of *Ginkgo biloba* extract (EGb 761). *Journal of Molecular and Cellular Cardiology* 29: 733-742.

Pietta, P., Simonetti, P., and Mauri, P. (1998). Antioxidant activity of selected medicinal plants. *Journal of Agricultural and Food Chemistry* 46: 4487-4490.

Pittler, M.H. and Ernst, E. (2000). *Ginkgo biloba* extract for the treatment of intermittent claudication: A meta-analysis of randomized trials. *The American Journal of Medicine* 108: 276-281.

Porsolt, R.D., Martin, P., Lenegre, A., Fromage, S., and Drieu, K. (1990). Effects of an extract of *Ginkgo biloba* (EGB 761) on "learned helplessness" and other models of stress in rodents. *Pharmacology, Biochemistry and Behavior* 36: 963-971.

Rai, G.S., Shovlin, C., and Wesnes, K.A. (1991). A double-blind, placebo-controlled study of *Ginkgo biloba* extract (Tanakan®) in elderly outpatients with mild to moderate memory impairment. *Current Medical Research and Opinion* 12: 350-355.

Ramassamy, C., Christen, Y., Clostre, F. and Costentin, J. (1992). The *Ginkgo biloba* extract, EGb 761, increases synaptosomal uptake of 5-hydroxytryptamine: In vitro and ex-vivo studies. *Journal of Pharmacy and Pharmacology* 44: 943-945.

Rapin, J.R., Zaibi, M., and Drieu, K. (1998). In vitro and in vivo effects of an extract of *Ginkgo biloba* (EGb 761), ginkolide B, and bilobalide on apoptosis in primary cultures of rat hippocampal neurons. *Drug Development Research* 45: 23-29.

Reisser, C.H. and Weidauer, H. (2001). *Ginkgo biloba* extract EGb 761 or pentoxifyline for the treatment of sudden deafness: A randomized, reference-controlled, double-blind study. *Acta Oto-laryngologica* 121: 579-584.

Remé, C., Wei, Q., Munz, K., Jung, H., Doly, M., and Droy-Lefaix, M.T. (1992). Light and lithium effects in the rat retina: Modification by the PAF antagonist BN 52021. *Graefe's Archive for Clinical and Experimental Ophthalmology* 230: 580-588.

Rigney, U., Kimber, S., and Hindmarch, I. (1999). The effects of acute doses of standardized *Ginkgo biloba* extract on memory and psychomotor performance in volunteers. *Phytotherapy Research* 13: 408-415.

Robbers, J.E. and Tyler, V.E. (1999). *Tyler's Herb of Choice. The Therapeutic Use of Phytomedicinals*. Binghamton, NY: The Haworth Press, p. 145.

Roncin, J.P., Schwartz, F., and D'Arbigny, P. (1996). EGb 761 in control of acute mountain sickness and vascular reactivity to cold exposure. *Aviation, Space, and Environmental Medicine* 67: 445-452.

Rosenblatt, M. and Mindel, J. (1997). Spontaneous hyphema associated with ingestion of *Ginkgo biloba* extract. *New England Journal of Medicine* 336 (April 10): 1108 (letter).

Rowin, J. and Lewis, S.L. (1996). Spontaneous bilateral subdural hematomas associated with chronic *Ginkgo biloba* ingestion. *Neurology* 46: 1775-1776.

Sampson, J.B., Cymerman, A., Burse, R., Maher, J.T., and Rock, P.B. (1983). Procedures for the measurement of Acute Mountain Sickness. *Aviation, Space and Environmental Medicine* 54: 1063-1073.

Sandberg-Gertzén, H. (1993). An open trial of cedemin, a *Ginkgo biloba* extract with PAF-antagonistic effects for ulcerative colitis. *American Journal of Gastroenterology* 88: 615-616 (letter).

Schennen, A. and Hölzl, J. (1986). 6-Hydroxykynurensäure, die erste *N*-haltige verbindung aus den blättern von *Ginkgo biloba* [6-Hydroxykynurenic acid, the first *N*-containing compound from the *Ginkgo biloba* leaf]. *Planta Medica* 52: 235-236.

Schmidt, U., Rabinovici, K., and Lande, S. (1991). Einfuß eines Ginkgo-biloba-spezialextraktes auf die befindlichkeit bei cerebraler insuffizienz. *Münchener Medizinische Wochenschrift* 133(Suppl. 1): S15-S18.

Schubert, H. and Halama, P. (1993). Primär therapieresistente depressive verstimmung älterer patienten mit hirnleistungsstörungen: Wirksamkeit der kombination von *Ginkgo-biloba*-extrakt EGb 761 antidepressiva [Depressive episode primarily unresponsive to therapy in elderly patients: Efficacy of *Ginkgo biloba* extract EGb 761 in combination with antidepressants]. *Geriatrie Forschung* 3: 45-53.

Schulz, H., Jobert, M., and Hübner, W.D. (1998). The quantitative EEG as a screening instrument to identify sedative effects of single doses of plant extracts in comparison with diazepam. *Phytomedicine* 5: 449-458.

Schweizer, J. and Hautmann, C. (1999). Comparison of two dosages of *Ginkgo biloba* extract EGb 761 in patients with peripheral occlusive disease Fontaine's stage IIb: A randomized, double-blind, multicentric clinical trial. *Arzneimittel-Forschung* 49: 900-904.

Siegers, C.P. (1999). Cytotoxicity of alkylphenols from *Ginkgo biloba*. *Phytomedicine* 6: 281-283 (letter).

Sikora, R., Sohn, M.H., Engelke, B., and Jakse, G. (1998). Randomized, placebo-controlled study on the effects of oral treatment with *Ginkgo biloba* extract in patients with erectile dysfunction. *The Journal of Urology* 159(Suppl. 5): 240 (abstract).

Skogh, M. (1998). Extracts of *Ginkgo biloba* and bleeding or haemorrhage. *Lancet* 352: 1145-1146 (letter).

Sloley, B.D., Urichuk, L.J., and Coutts, R.T. (2000). Identification of kaempferol as a monoamine oxidase inhibitor and potential neuroprotectant in extracts of *Ginkgo biloba* leaves. *Journal of Pharmacy and Pharmacology* 52: 451-459.

SØholm, B. (1998). Clinical improvement of memory and other cognitive functions by *Ginkgo biloba*: Review of relevant literature. *Advances in Therapy* 15: 54-65.

Sowers, W.F., Weary, P.E., Collins, O.D., and Cawley, E.P. (1965). Ginkgo-tree dermatitis. *Archives of Dermatology* 91: 452-456.

Sticher, O. (1993). Quality of *Ginkgo* preparations. *Planta Medica* 59: 2-11.

Stough, C., Clarke, J., Lloyd, J., and Nathan, P.J. (2001). Neuropsychological changes after 30-day *Ginkgo biloba* administration in healthy participants. *International Journal of Neuropsychopharmacology* 4: 131-134.

Subhan, Z. and Hindmarch, I. (1984). The psychopharmacological effects of *Ginkgo biloba* extract in normal healthy volunteers. *International Journal of Clinical and Pharmacological Research* 4: 89-93.

Szabo, M.E., Droy-Lefaix, M.T., Doly, M., Carre, C., and Braquet, P. (1990). Ischemia and reperfusion-induced histologic changes in the rat retina: Demonstration of a free radical-mediated mechanism. *Investigative Ophthalmology and Visual Science* 31: 1471-1478.

Taillandier, J., Ammar, A., Rabourdin, J.P., Ribeyre, J.P., Pichon, J., Niddam, S., and Pierart, H. (1986). Traitement des troubles du vieillissement cérébral par l'extrait de *Ginkgo biloba* [Treatment of cerebral aging disorders with *Ginkgo biloba* extract. A longitudinal multicenter double-blind drug vs. placebo study]. *Presse Medicale* (Paris) 15: 1583-1587.

Tamborini, A. and Taurelle, R. (1993). Intérêt de l'extrait standardisé de *Ginkgo biloba* (EGb 761) dans la prise en charge des symptômes congestifs du syndrome prémenstruel [Value of standardized *Ginkgo biloba* extract (EGb 761) in the management of congestive symptoms of premenstrual syndrome]. *Revue Francaise de Gynecologie et D'Obstetrique* 88: 447-457.

Tang, Y., Lou, F., Wang, J., Li, Y., and Zhuang, S. (2001). Coumaroyl flavonol glycosides from the leaves of *Ginkgo biloba*. *Phytochemistry* 58: 1251-1256.

Taylor, J.E. (1988). Binding of neuromediators to their receptors in rat brain: Effect of chronic administration of *Ginkgo biloba* extract. In Fünfgeld, E.W. (Ed.), *Rökan (Ginkgo biloba). Recent Results in Pharmacology and Clinic* (pp. 103-108). New York: Springer-Verlag.

Thomson, G.J.L., Vohra, R.K., Carr, M.H., and Walker, M.G. (1990). A clinical trial of *Ginkgo biloba* extract in patients with intermittent claudication. *International Angiology* 9: 75-78.

Vaes, L.P.J. and Chyka, P.A. (2000). Interactions of warfarin with garlic, ginger, ginkgo, or ginseng: Nature of the evidence. *The Annals of Pharmacotherapy* 34: 1478-1482.

Vale, S. (1998a). Subarachnoid hemorrhage associated with *Ginkgo biloba*. *Lancet* 352: 36 (letter).

Vale, S. (1998b). Letter to the editor. *Lancet* 352: 1146.

van Dongen, M.C., van Rossum, E., Kessels, A.G., Seilhorst, H.J., and Knipschild, P.G. (2000). The efficacy of ginkgo for elderly people with dementia and age-associated memory impairment: New results of a randomized trial. *Journal of the American Geriatrics Society* 48: 1183-1194.

Vesper, J. and Hänsgen, K.D. (1994). Efficacy of *Ginkgo biloba* in 90 outpatients with cerebral insufficiency caused by old age: Results of a placebo-controlled, double-blind trial. *Phytomedicine* 1: 9-16.

Vorberg, G., Schenk, N., and Jansen, W. (1989). Wirksamkeit eines neuen Ginkgo-biloba-extraktes bei 100 patienten mit zerebraler insuffizienz [Effectiveness of a new *Ginkgo biloba* extract tested on 100 patients with cerebral insufficiency]. *Herz and Gefäße* 9: 936-941.

Wada, K. (2000). Food poisoning by Ginkgo seeds: The role of 4-*O*-methylpyridoxine. In van Beek, T.A. (Ed.), *Ginkgo Biloba* (pp. 453-465). Amsterdam, The Netherlands: Harwood Academic.

Wang, H. and Ng, T.B. (2000). Ginkobilobin, a novel antifungal protein from *Ginkgo biloba* seeds with sequence similarity to embryo-abundant protein. *Biochemical and Biophysical Research Communications* 279: 407-411.

Weber, M., Dietrich, D., Grässel, I., Reuter, G., Seifert, G., and Steinhäuser, C. (2001). 6-Hydroxykynurenic acid and kynurenic acid differently antagonize AMPA and NMDA receptors in hippocampal neurons. *Journal of Neurochemistry* 77: 1108-1115.

Weber, W. (2000). Ginkgo not effective for memory loss in elderly. *Lancet* 344 (October 14): 1333.

Wei, T., Ni, Y., Hou, J., Chen, C., Zhao, B., and Xin, W. (2000). Hydrogen perox-ide-induced oxidative damage and apoptosis in cerebellar granule cells: Protec-tion by *Ginkgo biloba* extract. *Pharmacological Research* 41: 427-433.

Weiß, H. and Kallischnigg, G. (1991). *Ginkgo biloba*-extrakt (EGb 761. Meta-analyse von studien zum nachweis der therapeutischen wirksamit bei hirn-leistungsstörungen bzw. periperer arterieller verschlußkrankheit [*Ginkgo biloba* extract (EGb 761). Meta-analysis of studies, in order to prove the therapeutic ef-fectiveness on brain output disturbances with respect to peripheral arterial occlu-sive disease]. *Münchner Medizinische Wochenschrift* 133: 138-142.

Weitbrecht, W.V. and Jansen, W. (1985). Double-blind and comparative (*Ginkgo biloba* versus placebo) therapeutic study in geriatric patients with primary de-generative dementia—A preliminary evaluation. In Agnoli, A., Rapin, J.F., Scapagnini, V., and Weitbrecht, W.V. (Eds.), *Effects of Ginkgo biloba Extract on Organic Cerebral Impairment*. London: John Libbey Eurotext Ltd.

Wesnes, K., Simmons, D., Rook, M., and Simpson, P. (1987). A double-blind pla-cebo-controlled trial of Tanakan in the treatment of idiopathic cognitive impair-ment in the elderly. *Human Psychopharmacology* 2: 159-169.

Westendorf, J. and Regan, J. (2000). Genotoxic and tumor promoting activity of ginkgolic acids in primary rat hepatocytes. *Phytomedicine* 7(Suppl. 2): 104 (ab-stract P-105).

Wettstein, A. (1999/2000). Cholinesterase inhibitors and Ginkgo extracts – Are they comparable in the treatment of dementia? *Phytomedicine* 6: 393-401.

White, H.L., Scates, P.W., and Cooper, B.R. (1996). Extracts of *Ginkgo biloba* leaves inhibit monoamine oxidase. *Life Sciences* 58: 1315-1321.

Wilkens, J.H., Wilkens, H., Uffmann, J., Bovers, J., Fabel, H., and Frolich, J.C. (1990). Effects of a PAF-antagonist (BN 52063) on broncho-constriction and platelet activation during exercise-induced asthma. *British Journal of Clinical Pharmacology* 29: 85-91.

Winter, J.C. (1998). The effects of an extract of *Ginkgo biloba*, EGb 761, on cogni-tive behavior and longevity in the rat. *Physiology and Behavior* 63: 425-433.

Winther, K., Randlov, C., Rein, E., and Eydbjorg, M. (1998). Effects of *Ginkgo biloba* extract on cognitive function and blood pressure in elderly subjects. *Cur-rent Therapeutic Research* 59: 881-888.

Woerdenbag, H.J. and De Smet, P.A.G.M. (2000). Adverse effects and toxicity of *Ginkgo* extracts. In van Beek, T.A. (Ed.), *Ginkgo biloba* (pp. 443-451). Amster-dam: Harwood Academic Publishers.

Woerdenbag, H.J. and van Beek, T.A. (1997). *Ginkgo biloba*. In De Smet, P.A.G.M., Keller, K., Hänsel, R., and Chandler, R.F. (Eds.), *Adverse Effects of Herbal Drugs* (pp. 51-66). Volume 3. New York: Springer-Verlag.

Wojcicki, J., Gawrinska-Szklarz, B., Bieganowski, W., Patalan, M., Smulki, H., Samochowiec, L., and Zakrzewski, J. (1993). Comparative pharmacokinetics and bioavailability of flavonoid glycosides of *Ginkgo biloba* after a single oral administration of three formulations to healthy volunteers. *Materia Medica Polona* 27: 141-146.

Xin, W., Wei, T., Chen, C., Ni, Y., Zhao, B., and Hou, J. (2000). Mechanisms of apoptosis in rat cerebellar granule cells induced by hydroxyl radicals and the effects of EGb 761 and its constituents. *Toxicology* 148(2-3): 103-110.

Yao, Z.X., Drieu, K., and Papadopoulos, V. (2001). The *Ginkgo biloba* extract EGb 761 rescues the PC12 neuronal cells from β-amyloid-induced cell death by inhibiting the formation of β-amyloid-derived diffusible neurotoxic ligands. *Brain Research* 889: 181-190.

Yen, K.Y. (1992). *The Illustrated Chinese Materia Medica. Crude and Prepared.* Taipei, Taiwan: SMC Publishing, Inc., p. 171.

Zhang, X.Y., Zhou, D.F., Su, J.M., and Zhang, P.Y. (2001). The effect of extract of *Ginkgo biloba* added to haloperidol on superoxide dismutase in inpatients with chronic schizophrenia. *Journal of Clinical Psychopharmacology* 21: 85-88.

Zhang, X.Y., Zhou, D.F., Zhang, P.Y., Wu, G.Y., Su, J.M., and Cao, L.Y. (2001). A double-blind, placebo-controlled trial of *Ginkgo biloba* added to haloperidol in treatment-resistant patients with schizophrenia. *International Journal of Clinical Psychiatry* 62: 878-883.

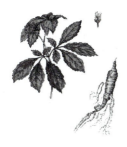

Ginseng

BOTANICAL DATA

Classification and Nomenclature

Scientific name: *Panax ginseng* C.A. Meyer; synonyms:
P. quinquefolius L. var. *ginseng* (C.A. Meyer) Regel & Maack;
P. quinquefolius L. a. *coreensis* Siebold; *P. schinseng* Nees.

Family name: Araliaceae

Common names: ginseng (English and German), Korean ginseng, Chinese ginseng, Asiatic ginseng, Oriental ginseng, Panax de Chine (French) (De Smet, 1993), ren shen (China) (Foster and Yue, 1992)

Description

Panax ginseng is an herbaceous, perennial plant, native to the damp woodlands of Northern China and Korea. When mature (after four to six years), it has a taproot, reaches 61 cm in height with a single stalk, and displays five-lobed palmate leaves with greenish-white flowers in an umbel. The fruits are red, berrylike, and contain two hard seeds. Although extremely rare in the wild, ginseng is cultivated in Korea, northeastern China, Russia, and Japan. After the plant is harvested, the root is prepared in one of two ways, which results in either white or red ginseng (Foster and Yue, 1992).

White ginseng refers to *Panax ginseng* which has been peeled and then dried. It has a yellowish-brown appearance, a hard structure, and brown speckles appear on the inside of the woody core. Red *P. ginseng* is the same root, but is steamed before being peeled and then dried. The color is a deep reddish-brown. Due to the steaming process, diagonal slices of the root reveal a translucent surface, which is also reddish-brown (Yen, 1992). In the Orient, red ginseng has been preferred over white ginseng, whereas in the European community white ginseng is the most common type used in ginseng products (Sticher, 1998).

There are presently 11 species and one variety of *Panax* (Wen, 2001). Some congeners of *Panax ginseng* are also valued for their medicinal properties, including *P. quinquefolius* L. (North American ginseng), *P. notoginseng* (Burk) F.H. Chen (sanqi ginseng, China), *P. pseudoginseng* (Himalayan ginseng), and *P. japonicum* C.A. Meyer (Japanese ginseng) (Okrent, 1994; Foster and Yue, 1992). Siberian ginseng, *Eleutherococcus senticosus* (Rupr. & Maxim.) Maximowicz, is not a true ginseng, though it is a member of the same plant family, Araliaceae.

HISTORY AND TRADITIONAL USES

Ginseng (Panax ginseng) is mentioned in the oldest Chinese pharmacopoeia, *Shen-Nung Pen T'sao Ching* (Yang, 1998), and references to ginseng in other Chinese texts date back to ancient times. Because these written records are preceded by centuries-old oral tradition, ginseng may have been known in Chinese ethnopharmacology for as many as 5,000 years.

The Chinese do not take ginseng to cure a disease, but rather as a tonic for increasing energy and a sense of well-being. In *Shen Nung's Materia Medica* (196 A.D.), ginseng was described as a nontoxic ("Superior") herb that "brightens the eyes, opens the heart, and sharpens the wits." It was also purported to check palpitations from fright, eliminate evil "qi," quiet the "essence spirit," and prolong life (Yang, 1998). The leaves have been used in the treatment of fevers (Foster and Yue, 1992). In the *Pharmacopoeia of the People's Republic of China,* ginseng is indicated for reinforcing the "vital" energy, restoring the "normal pulse," calming the nerves, remedying collapse, and promoting the production of body fluid (Tu et al., 1992). Western scientific study of *P. ginseng* began approximately 48 years ago. Interest in ginseng has grown steadily since, and today ginseng is one of the most extensively researched botanicals (Okrent, 1994).

CHEMISTRY

The primary constituents of *Panax ginseng* roots are saponins which occur in concentrations of approximately 1% to 3% (Shibata et al., 1985).

Ginsenosides

Ginsenosides are considered the pharmacologically active components of ginseng. There are at least 13 different ginsenosides in *P. ginseng;* all are triterpene glycosides in the form of saponins. They have a tetracyclic structure based on one of three aglycones (sapogenins): 20(S)-protopanaxadiol (ginsenosides Rb_1, Rb_2, Rc, and Rd); 20(S)-protopanaxatriol (ginsenosides Re, Rf, Rg, Rg_1, Rg_2, and Rh_1); and oleanolic acid (ginsenoside R_o) (Shibata et al., 1985). More recently isolated ginsenosides include Rg_5 (Lee, Lee, Kim et al., 1997) and Rs_3 (Baek et al., 1997). After traditional heat-processing (steaming at 98-100°C for 2-3 h) of the raw root to produce "red ginseng," it is assumed that the malonylginsenosides, mRb_1, mRb_2, and mRc, are converted to Rb_1, Rb_2, and Rc, respectively (Yamaguchi et al., 1988). Upon steaming the root at 100°C for 2 h, ginsenosides Rg_3, Rg_5, and F_4 were produced, after their absence in the raw root (Kim et al., 2000). The most abundant ginsenosides in *P. ginseng* are Rb_1 and Rg_1 (Shibata et al., 1985; Chuang et al., 1995), which generally occur in a ratio of from 1 to 3 (Awang, 2000; Ma et al., 1996). The other main ginsenosides in *P. ginseng* are Rb_2, Rc, Re, and Rd. Together with Rb_1 and Rg_1, they account for about 90% of the total ginsenoside content of the root (Court, 2000).

Ginsenoside concentrations are twice as high in the lateral roots than in the main root, and concentrations in the root hairs may be twice that of the lateral roots (Shibata et al., 1985). Among 44 ginseng products analyzed for ginsenoside content, concentrations ranged from 1.9% to 9.0% (Cui et al., 1994), and in another study, the content in powdered preparations sold in the United States varied from 0.28% to 4.2% (Harkey et al., 2001).

Acetylenic Compounds

P. ginseng contains panaxynol, panaxtriol, panaxdiol, β-elemene, and other acetylene compounds (Shibata et al., 1985), such as panaxytriol (Lu et al., 1998).

Peptidoglycans

Panaxans A, B, C, D, and E are peptidoglycans of *P. ginseng* (Shibata et al., 1985). Others include panaxans A to F (Hikino et al., 1985), I to L (Oshima et al., 1985), M to P (Konno and Hikino, 1987), Q to U (Konno et al., 1985), and the protein-bound acid polysaccharides ginsenan PA (Tomoda et al., 1994), ginsenan PB (Tomoda et al., 1993), ginsenan S-IA, ginsenan S-IIA (Sonoda et al., 1998), and ginsan (Kim et al., 1998).

Volatile Oil

Concentrations of approximately 0.05% of the volatile oil panacene have been reported in *P. ginseng* (Shibata et al., 1985).

Other Constituents

Other compounds reported include free- and glucoside-bound sterols, 8-32% starch, low molecular weight polysaccharides, pectin, vitamins,

0.1-0.2% choline, minerals, simple sugars, some ginseng flavonoids (Shibata et al., 1985), and *Panax ginseng* NFG (*P. ginseng* nerve growth factor) (Murase et al., 1994).

THERAPEUTIC APPLICATIONS

The actions most commonly ascribed to *P. ginseng* are adaptogenic and tonic. An adaptogen was defined by Brekhman and Dardymov (1969) as a substance which acts to enhance nonspecific resistance to various external and internal stresses. However, the usefulness of the term adaptogen is questionable (Davydov and Krikorian, 2000). Early research in animals showed that ginseng has fatigue-inhibiting and radioprotective actions, and that it stimulated the immune system (Brekhman and Dardymov, 1969). Research in China has focused on the possibility of antiaging, anticancer, and antiarrhythmic effects of ginsenosides, and nootropic effects of ginseng (Chen and Dou, 1998).

Although ginseng was initially tested in humans by Brekhman, animal experimentation has been used to support his results in humans. Tests in mice were used to assess the limits of physical exhaustion after ginseng use, and it was concluded that ginseng had a fatigue-inhibiting action (Shibata et al., 1985).

Some of the properties ascribed to ginseng appear contradictory and are probably due to the large variation of extract preparations. These include slight CNS-stimulant action, CNS-depressant action, tranquilizing action, cholinergic action, histamine-like action, hypotensive, hypertensive, papaverine-like action, serotonin-like action, ganglion stimulant action, analgesic, antipyretic, anti-inflammatory, no antihistamine-like action, and antihistamine-like action (Shibata et al., 1985).

Attempts were made to resolve these conflicting results by studying the activities at each step of fractionation. In general, the aqueous extracts showed a stimulative action, whereas the methanolic extracts revealed mainly sedative action. The actions of the individual ginseng saponins were investigated as follows: ginsenoside Rb_1 exhibited CNS-sedative, analgesic, anticonvulsant, antipyretic, tranquilizing, and hypotensive actions, whereas ginsenoside Rg_1 showed weak CNS-stimulating, hypertensive, and fatigue-inhibiting actions. Ginsenoside Rg_1 showed a slight CNS-stimulating activity in lower doses, and at higher doses a sedative activity which was ascribed to toxic effects (Shibata et al., 1985).

Ginseng is not usually regarded as having specific disease-fighting properties, but rather has been proposed to act with the body to help adjust and adapt to stressful conditions. This has been suggested as one of the reasons for seemingly contradictory results obtained in studies. Ginseng's non-specific ability to balance a variety of metabolic functions is thought to be responsible for the spectrum of results that have been reported (Shibata et al., 1985; Fulder, 1993).

PRECLINICAL STUDIES

Cardiovascular and Circulatory Functions

Thrombosis, Hemostasis, and Embolism

Park et al. (1996) found indications of an antithrombotic effect of ginseng. They compared the effect of ginseng in rats fed a basal diet supplemented with corn oil (15% w/w), and rats fed the same basal diet supplemented with corn oil plus a lipophilic fraction (0.0025% of the total diet) of ginseng powder from fresh six-year-old roots of *P. ginseng*. Comparisons of blood platelet activity between the two dietary groups yielded significant findings. Platelet aggregation was affected by the addition of the lipophilic fraction (LF) to the diet, significantly inhibiting both thrombin-induced platelet aggregation and intrinsic blood coagulation ($p < 0.01$). In collagen-stimulated platelets from rats on the LF plus corn oil feed, the LF had significantly increased the level of platelet cGMP in vitro and in vivo, and produced a fourfold increase in levels of cAMP. The latter effect appeared to be synergistic with an increase in cGMP levels and the ratio of cAMP to cGMP showed no significant change despite the increase. Without a possible explanation, Park et al. (1996) also reported a significant increase in kidney weight in the rats fed the corn oil plus LF feed compared to the corn oil feed group.

Effects on Cholesterol and Lipid Metabolism

Studies in animals have shown that biosynthesis of high density lipoproteins (HDL) increases with ginseng administration, while total cholesterol and the low density lipoproteins (LDL), which are thought to contribute to heart disease, decrease (Dixit et al., 1991; Park et al., 1996). In contrast, Ismail et al. (1999) reported no significant hypolipidemic activity in a feeding study with rabbits fed a 2% cholesterol-enriched diet of which 2% consisted of ginseng (uncharacterized). The aortic walls of the ginseng-diet group showed massive intimal plaques and endothelial damage, comparable to those of hypercholesterolemic rabbits. Inoue et al. (1999), using a cyclophosphamide-induced model of hyperlipidemia in rabbits, found a significant decrease in serum total cholesterol and triglyceride levels in the animals administered the isolated total saponin fraction of ginseng (10 mg p.o./day for four weeks), but found no significant change in HDL levels.

Kwon et al. (1999) attributed the cholesterol-lowering activity of ginseng to a mild in vitro inhibiting activity of sapogenins on acyl-CoA:cholesterol acyltransferase (ACAT). The sapogenins strongly inhibited rat liver microsomal ACAT. Protopanaxadiols and protopanaxatriols derived from ginseng were shown to be active inhibitors of the enzyme, especially (20R)-proto-panaxatriol (IC_{50} 6 µM), (20R)-protopanaxadiol (IC_{50} 10 µM), and (20R)-panaxtriol (IC_{50} 12 µM).

Digestive, Hepatic, and Gastrointestinal Functions

Hepatic Functions

The liver regenerating effects of ginseng were studied by Cui (1997) in 66% hepatectomized male rats using the mitotic index (MI) to measure liver regeneration. Thirty rats were administered a ginseng root extract (un-characterized, 125 mg/kg per day p.o.) starting three days prior to hepa-tectomy, with half receiving twice the dose in two divided doses daily. In addition, two groups of six rats each received either ginsenoside Rg_1 or ginsenoside Rb_1 (2.5 mg/kg per day p.o.). With the exception of the six-day, 125 mg/kg per day dose, all treatments were administered for three days and longer. After hepatectomy in the 125 mg/kg per day group, a significant increase in the MI was evident on days two ($p < 0.05$) and three ($p < 0.01$), which normalized after a further three days. The same dose administered twice daily produced a dose-dependent increase in the MI. At two days posthepatectomy, ginsenoside Rg_1, at a dose nearly equal to the estimated amount found in the root extract (2-5%), produced a significant increase in the MI ($p < 0.01$), whereas ginsenoside Rb_1 did not. Cui speculated that the latter result may have been due to inactivation of Rb_1 by the oral route (see Pharmacokinetics). He also noted that food intake is known to affect liver regeneration in hepatectomy results, but in this study, the extract had no effect on the amount of food consumed by the rats. Water intake did increase, but is not known to affect liver regeneration. Insulin is another factor affecting liver regeneration, but no increase in insulin secretion was found. In blood analyses, no differences in levels of total protein, albumin, glutamic pyruvic transaminase (GPT), alkaline phosphatase, total bilirubin, blood urea nitrogenase (BUN), or plasma glucose were found. Total cholesterol and triglyceride levels showed significant decreases ($p < 0.05$ and $p < 0.01$, respectively), and body fat retroperitoneal white adipose tissue (RPWT) weight showed a significant decrease ($p < 0.01$) three days after hepatectomy, an effect that tended toward dose-dependency from the ginseng extract, as evidenced by the greater drop in value from the higher dose. However, the Lee Index was unchanged.

Endocrine and Hormonal Functions

Carbohydrate Metabolism; Antidiabetic Activity

Ginseng has long been used in traditional Chinese medicine (TCM) to ameliorate the effects of diabetes, and recent studies in animals suggest that ginseng has hypoglycemic actions. The chemical constituents thought to be responsible for the hypoglycemic effects are five glycans (polysaccharides, panaxans A to E), adenosine, a carboxylic acid, a peptide, and a fraction designated DPG-3-2. In addition, other glycans from ginseng have shown hypoglycemic activity in animals (i.e., panaxans M, N, O, and P) (Konno and Hikino, 1987). The ginsenosides appear to have no direct role in the blood sugar-modulating activity of ginseng (Konno et al., 1984; Ng and Yeung, 1985).

Hypothalamic and Pituitary Functions

In another study, ginseng saponins produced an increase in adrenal cyclic adenosine monophosphate (cAMP) in rats. However, this did not occur in hypophysectomized rats. Therefore, the ginseng saponins were thought to act directly on the hypothalamus or the pituitary to secrete adrenocorticotropic hormone (ACTH), which stimulates the adrenal cortex and promotes corticosteroid synthesis (Hiai et al., 1979; Avakian and Evonuk, 1979; Fulder, 1981, 1993). In accordance, some of the pharmacological and biochemical actions of ginseng have been attributed to interactions with the hypothalamic-pituitary-adrenal axis and enhanced corticosteroid synthesis (Hiai et al., 1979; Fulder, 1981, 1993).

A mixture of ginsenosides administered to rats (Rb_1, Rb_2, Rc, Rd and Re; 70 mg/kg i.p.) produced a significant increase in plasma ACTH and corticosterone levels which lasted up to one hour and then fell rapidly over the next 90-120 min after an initial drop 20 min postadministration. Plasma corticosterone remained at high levels 90 min after administration, whereas ACTH had dropped to 50% of the maximum increase. Smaller doses (5-40 mg/kg i.p.) were also active and caused a dose-dependent increase in corticosterone. Ginsenosides Rb_2 and Rd (35 mg/kg i.p.) were shown to be especially active and the researchers concluded that the increase in plasma levels resulted from stimulation of corticosterone secretion by the adrenals (Hiai et al., 1979). However, Pearce et al. (1982) pointed out that intraperitoneal injection itself is able to change plasma corticosterone and ACTH levels.

Even if this hypothalamic-pituitary-adrenal theory can be proved, just how physiologically important the increased secretion of glucocorticoids is during stress has recently been called into question (Marcilhac et al., 1998). A study in monkeys indicated that basal amounts of glucocorticoid secretion may be all an organism requires for adapting to stressful events (Udelsman et al., 1986). Agents that inhibit hypersecretion of glucocorticoids in stressful events may be more desirable. Organisms subjected to high amounts of glucocorticoids over long periods may develop adverse effects, including metabolic dysfunctions, hypertension, immunosuppression, and neurotoxicity. Marcilhac et al. (1998) suggested that in some individuals such effects could render an underlying disease state worse and even bring on disease states, if the individual is so predisposed.

Lee, Chung, Lee, Lee, et al. (1997) demonstrated that ginsenoside Rg_1, although found only in trace amounts in ginseng, is a functional ligand of glucocorticoid receptor at a half-maximal concentration of 1-10 μM in vitro, and that it activates a glucocorticoid-responsive reporter gene. Pearce et al. (1982) demonstrated that ginseng extract (3.96% ginsenosides by reference to Rg_1) has a modest binding activity for mineralcorticoid and progesterone receptors, no estrogen receptor binding activity, and a fairly high receptor binding activity for glucocorticoid in vitro. They noted that given a near complete absorption of ginseng from oral administration, the concentrations needed to affect steroid receptor binding were readily achievable, although modest. Given that the level of absorption of ginsenosides by the oral route is only 20%, Hobbs (1996), citing an unpublished study by Büchi and Jenny (1984), remarked that unless rather high dosages are used, there is some doubt as to whether enhanced glucocorticoid synthesis would occur.

Reproductive Hormone Interactions

Liu et al. (2001) examined the in vitro estrogenic activity of a methanolic extract of ginseng roots in a number of assays. In estrogen receptor-positive endometrial adenocarcinoma (Ishikawa) cells, the extract failed to induce expression of the progesterone receptor gene *(PR)*, exhibited no binding activity in estrogen receptors (both alpha and beta human recombinant types), and showed no evidence of inducing an estrogenic response in the cells according alkaline phosphate activity. However, in an estradiol-responsive breast cancer cell line (S30 cells), the extract induced up-regulation of the estrogen-inducible gene presenelin-2 *(pS2)*, as did a methanolic extract of North American ginseng *(Panax quinquefolius)* roots. These results suggest that, rather than a direct effect on the estrogen receptor, ginseng may modulate elements of estrogen receptor function (Liu et al., 2001).

Immune Functions; Inflammation and Disease

Cancer

Antiproliferative activity. Research with mice suggests that ginseng may have potent antitumor effects. Lu et al. (1998) describe panaxytriol as a potent antitumor compound isolated from the root, which is currently of interest as a potential new antitumor agent. They also synthesized the compound in an optically pure form.

Various mechanisms appear to be involved in the tumor-inhibiting activity of ginseng. Kim et al. (1999) found evidence to suggest that ginsenoside Rs_3 induces apoptosis in human hepatoma cells (SK-HEP-1 cells) by a selective increase in levels of $p21^{WAF1}$ and p53. Ginsenoside Rs_3 is a diol-type saponin recently derived from the root of *P. ginseng*. Previously, Kim and colleagues had shown that Rh_2 also induced apoptosis in the same human hepatoma cells.

Lee, Chung, Lee, Kim, et al. (1997) reported a tumor inhibition rate of 56.3% against B16 melanoma in mice treated with ginsan (200 mg/kg i.p.), a purified acidic polysaccharide (MW 150,000) derived from an ethanol insoluble fraction of the root. Against benzo[*a*]pyrene-induced tumors in mice (autochthonous lung tumors), the polysaccharide (1 mg/mL drinking water ad libitum) inhibited tumor incidence by 70%. In both tumor models, the results were significant compared to untreated mice ($p < 0.05$). In both studies, ginsan was administered weeks after tumor induction.

Administered to tumor cell (B16-F10)-colonized mice in combination with recombinant interleukin-2 (rIL-2), ginsan caused a more significant inhibition of melanoma metastasis than either rIL-2 or ginsan alone (Kim et al., 1998). Both Lee, Chung, Lee, Kim, et al. (1997) and Kim et al. (1998) suggest that ginsan could serve as an immunostimulating agent in the treatment of cancerous diseases.

Byun et al. (1997) showed that ginsenoside Rh_1 and Rh_2 inhibit cellular proliferation of a human ascites cell line (HRA), noting that Rh_2 has also shown tumor growth inhibition against mouse melanoma. Intracellular activity of protein kinase C was also inhibited by Rh_1 and Rh_2, and the researchers raised the possibility of using ginsenosides as anticancer agents.

Shinkai et al. (1996) found that Rg_3 could potently and dose-dependently inhibit the invasion of human pancreatic adenocarcinoma (PSN-1), rat ascites hepatoma MM1 (by 98.8% from 32 μm), human small cell lung carcinoma (OC10), and B16FE7 melanoma cells in vitro, but not tumor cell proliferation. In the same model, they found no tumor cell-inhibitory activity from ginsenoside Rh_1 or Rh_2, the 20(R)-ginsenosides Re, Rh_1, Rc, and Rb_1, and little from 20(S)-ginsenoside Rg_3, 29(R)-ginsenoside Rg_2, or ginsenoside Rb_2.

In an experimental in vivo model of pulmonary metastasis in mice using a highly metastatic melanoma cell line (mouse melanoma B16FE7), Shinkai et al. (1996) found significant antimetastatic activity from injections of Rg_3 (4.3-29.0 μM into the lateral tail vein).

Sato et al. (1994) reported that Rb_2 (10-500 μg/mouse i.v.) produced a dose-dependent inhibition of tumor-induced (B16-B6 melanoma) angiogenesis in mice. When Rb_2 was administered in a higher dosage by the oral route (2 mg/mouse), the formation of new capillaries which feed tumor growth was significantly inhibited ($p < 0.001$). Lung metastases were dose-dependently inhibited by Rb_2 (100 μg/mouse i.v.).

Park et al. (1997) reported apoptosis-inducing activity by ginsenoside Rh_2 in human hepatoma SK-HEP-1 cells. Liu et al. (2000) demonstrated that ginsenoside Rg_3 exhibits antiproliferative activity in the human prostate carcinoma cell line LNCaP (IC_{50} 650 mM), whereas six other ginsenosides were inactive (i.e., Rd_2, Re, Rf, Rg_1, Rg_2, and Ro). Incubation with 250 μM of Rg_3 for 48 h resulted in the cells losing their adherent property. Rg_3 suppressed prostate specific antigen (PSA) expression, expression of proliferating cell nuclear antigen (PCNA), and the expression of both 5α-reductase and androgen receptor. Rg_3 also showed apoptotic-inducing activity in the prostate cancer cells in which it interfered with caspase-3 and Bcl-2, apoptosis-related genes. Lee et al. (2000) reported that IH-901 or 20-O-β-D-glucopyranosyl-20(S)-protopanaxdiol (one of the bacteria metabolites of ginseng protopanaxadiol saponins found in rats and humans after oral administration of ginseng extract), induces apoptosis in the human myeloid leukemia cell line, HL-60. Treatment of the cells caused mitochondrial cytochrome c to be released into the cytosol but had no effect on expression of antiapoptotic protein Bcl-2. The researchers described the suppression of HL-60 cell growth as dramatic, with an IC_{50} of 24.3 μM at 96 h. Ginsenoside Rb_1 had no effect on the proliferation of the leukemia cells (Lee et al., 2000).

In multidrug-resistant P388 leukemia cells in vitro, dammarane-type triterpenoids, 20(S)-protopanaxdiol, ginsenoside Rh_2, compound K, and especially potent, quasipanaxtriol, were shown to enhance the cytotoxicity of daunomycin and vinblastine (Hasegawa et al., 1995).

Chemopreventive activity. Oral administration of ginseng powder extract (1 mg/mL ad libitum) reduced the incidence of tumors and also retarded the growth of chemically-induced tumors (Yun et al., 1983; Yun and Kim, 1988), including aflatoxin B_1- and urethane-induced tumors (Yun et al., 1983). In an animal model of colon cancer (DMH, 1,2-dimethylhydrazine-induced aberrant crypt foci as preneoplastic lesions), diets containing 1% red (steamed and dried root) or white ginseng (peeled and then dried root) powders were fed to 125 DMH-treated Fischer 344 male rats. Compared to DMH-treated control rats that did not receive red ginseng in their diet, development of aberrant crypt foci (ACF) in the colon of ginseng-fed rats was significantly inhibited, and more effectively than in rats receiving white ginseng. White ginseng caused a decrease in the number of total aberrant crypt foci in the rat colon, but the decrease in the frequency of large ACF was not significant.

Keum et al. (2000) studied the chemopreventive effects of a methanol extract of ginseng prepared after heat-processing the root using a higher temperature (steamed at 120ºC for 3 h and then dried) than is normally used to produce red ginseng. This resulted in a product with higher concentrations of the ginsenosides Rg_3, Rg_5, Rg_6, Rh_2, Rh_3, Rh_4, and Rs_3, referred to as heat-processed neo-ginseng (NGMe). Female mice topically treated with tumor-promoting agents (DMBA followed by topical TPA a week later) received topical treatment with NGMe prior to TPA. A 0.5% solution of NGMe inhibited the development of papilloma by approximately 90% and treatment with a 0.1% solution resulted in complete inhibition of papilloma formation. TPA-stimulated production of TNF-α was significantly inhibited by the NGMe pretreatments, however basal levels of TNF-α were not affected.

Lee, Lee, Hui, et al. (1998) reported that three major metabolites of ginseng saponins, produced by bacteria in the intestines of humans, showed antigenotoxic activity in vitro. Significant activity was shown by these metabolites against benzo[*a*]pyrene-induced clastogenicity in the chromosome aberration assay and mutagenicity in the *Salmonella typhimurium* bacterial mutation assay. In rats and humans administered ginseng extracts orally, Hasegawa et al. (1996) identified these ginsenoside metabolites as 20(*S*)-protopanaxadiols. Hasegawa et al. (1995) also reported that 20(*S*)-protopanaxadiol enhanced the in vitro antitumor activity of the anticancer agents daunomycin and vinblastine against multidrug-resistant leukemia P388 cells.

Immune Functions

The ability of ginseng to modify the reactions to various stresses and to boost the immune system is suggested by its effects on cellular and metabolic function (Scaglione et al., 1990). Ginseng also appears to stimulate protein biosynthesis, an action with numerous implications for immune system function; however, this remains to be confirmed in clinical studies (Fulder, 1981).

Immunopotentiation. Kim et al. (1998) studied the activity of ginsan, a purified acidic polysaccharide (MW 150,000) derived from an ethanol insoluble fraction of the root. In activating spleen cells to cytotoxicity toward a range of tumor cells in vitro, the activity of ginsan was 12 times that of lentinan, a potent immunopotentiating polysaccharide used clinically in Japan which is derived from the shiitake mushroom *(Lentinula edodes)*. Spleen cell proliferation was also significantly greater from ginsan compared to lentinan ($p < 0.01$). Compared to untreated cells, ginsan increased proliferation 160-fold.

Four acid polysaccharides derived from a hot water extract of ginseng root significantly increased the production of interleukin-8 in human monocytes and monocytic leukemia cells (THP-1 cells) in vitro. Among them, ginsan-S-IIA was most potent, concentration-dependently enhancing interleukin-8 (IL-8) production in THP-1 cells tenfold. Ginsan-S-IIA was also the most potent at increasing production of IL-8 in normal human monocytes, and, just as in THP-1 cells, increased expression of IL-8 mRNA. Tests also indicated that the acid polysaccharides of ginseng have an effect mainly on monocytic cells and none on T cells or the production of IL-2. The researchers caution that because IL-8 is a proinflammatory cytokine, an increase in its production might adversely affect areas of the body already affected by inflammation (Sonoda et al., 1998).

In mice administered ginsan (200 mg/kg i.p.), Lee, Chung, Lee, Kim, et al. (1997) found significant immunomodulating activity and no toxic effects at a dosage of 1 g/kg i.p. or p.o. Among the many in vitro activities found, ginsan activated B and T cell proliferation and the cytotoxic capacity of macrophages by 39.5%, which then became cytotoxic to leukemic cells (L929); significantly increased macrophage production of reactive nitrogen ($p < 0.01$); activated spleen cells which then showed cytotoxicity against P815 mastocytoma cells; and generated activated killer cells with demonstrable cytotoxicity against tumor cells, a function evidently involving various cytokines (γ-interferon, interleukin-2, interleukin-1, and tumor necrosis factor-α) (Lee, Chung, Lee, Kim et al., 1997).

Kim et al. (1997) studied the effects of long-term (52 days) oral administration of a ginseng extract (50% ethanol extract of four-year-old "white ginseng" root) on immunoglobulin and serum proteins in female mice, starting from the ages of 4-11 weeks. They examined the effects of 30 and 150 mg/kg, which corresponded to dosages for a 60 kg person of 8 g/day and 40 g/day, an amount obtainable from 2-10 g/day of a 4:1 ginseng extract, and stated to be a "usual" dosage in traditional Oriental medicine (Kim et al., 1997). However, this dosage is higher than that cited by authorities on the traditional dosage (1-9 g/day) (Hobbs, 1996; Tu et al., 1992). Kim et al. (1997) reported that serum levels of γ-globulin significantly decreased by 18% from the low dosage and by 44% from the high dosage. Although there was a significant increase in the level of α_1-globulin of 24% from either dosage, they found no increases in levels of albumin, the ratio of albumin to globulin, β- and α_2- globulin, and total protein. From the high dosage, various immunoglobulin isotypes (IgA, IgM, IgG_1, IgG_{2a}, IgG_{2b}, IgG_3) significantly decreased (by 31%, $p < 0.05$). No other immunoglobulin isotypes showed a significant change. Given that the same action could increase cytotoxicity to allograft cells, this would probably make the higher dosage prohibitive in organ transplant patients. Further studies are needed to determine any different effects in male mice, and to determine which proteins in the α_1-globulin fraction (significantly increased by either dosage) might also be increased, among them, prothrombin, thyroid-binding globulin, α_1-glycoprotein, α_1-lipoprotein, and α_1-antitrypsin (Kim et al., 1997).

Liu et al. (1995) demonstrated that Rg_1 increased the in vitro proliferative response of lymphocytes derived from aged (65-78 years old) and young people (25-30 years old). Membrane fluidity of lymphocytes, whether those of the young or aged, was significantly stimulated by Rg_1 ($p < 0.05$, in the presence of phytohemmagglutin). Proliferative responses, surface antigen presentation, and the percentage of interleukin-2 receptor positive cells, all lower in the lymphocytes of the elderly subjects, were restored to normal by Rg_1.

Inflammatory Response

Platelet activating factor receptor binding antagonistic activity was shown from ginsenosides (20-ginsenoside Rg_3 and 20(S)-ginsenoside Rg_3 in vitro (IC_{50} 9.2×10^{-5} M and 4.9×10^{-5} M, respectively), yet 17 other ginsenosides showed no activity (Jung et al., 1998).

Metabolic and Nutritional Functions

Antioxidant Activity

Working with the *SOD1* gene from the rat, which is nearly identical to that of humans and a major antioxidant enzyme, Kim et al. (1996) found transcription of the gene induced by saponins of ginseng. Rb_1 showed much weaker activity compared to Rb_2, which happens to occur in more abundant amounts in ginseng. *SOD1* (Cu,Zn-superoxide dismutase) is a major catalyzer of oxygen free radicals that renders superoxide radicals into hydrogen peroxide and oxygen. It has been reported to decrease cardiotoxic and cytotoxic effects of anticancer agents and to prevent both tumor promotion and initiation. *SOD1* has also shown a protective effect against damage of ischemic tissue caused by reperfusion, and the over-expression of this gene in flies was associated with an increase in their average life span. Although Rb_2 proved the most potent activator, a threefold increase in *SOD1* was found from a mixture of ginseng saponins Rb_1, Rb_2, and minor fractions. The transcription factor through which Rb_2 activates the *SOD1* gene was identified as AP2, and showed increased protein levels after treatment with Rb_2. These results suggest that Rb_2 can increase cellular levels of the antioxidant enzyme *SOD1* by accelerating AP2 autoregulation, which in turn raises the amount of *SOD1* in cells. Kim et al. (1996) suggest that their findings may offer a molecular basis for the life span-increasing activity of ginseng saponins.

Pharmacokinetics

From recent in vitro, in vivo, and human studies, it is evident that ginsenosides undergo hydrolysis by intestinal bacteria which transform them into more absorbable forms and that these are the main active principles of ginseng (Hasegawa et al., 1996, 1997). Five metabolites were identified in the blood and urine of humans administered ginseng extract (150 mg/kg p.o.) as 20(S)-protopanaxdiols (Hasegawa et al., 1996). Ginsenoside Rb_1 is poorly absorbed by the oral route. Bacteria in the lower intestine of humans that hydrolyze Rb_1, such as *Eubacterium* sp. A-44, transform the ginsenoside into compound K, which is absorbed and appears in plasma (Akao et al., 1998). Rats orally administered the diol group saponin Rb_1 showed little of the compound in their digestive tract (Odani et al., 1983), and mice failed to show either the ginsenoside or its middle metabolites in their plasma; however, 20-*O*-β-D-glucopyranosyl-20(S)-protopanaxdiol was detected as a final metabolite which was also produced when Rb_1 was hydrolyzed by a bacteria *(Prevotella oris)* isolated from human intestines (Hasegawa et al., 1997). The same intestinal bacteria metabolite is formed from hydrolysis of ginsenosides Rb_2 and Rc (Hasegawa et al., 1996). Among the human intestinal bacteria with the ability to hydrolyze ginsenosides to respective ginsenoside metabolites, *P. oris* appears to be a major species (Hasegawa et al., 1997). It would follow that individuals lacking the intestinal bacteria required for ginsenoside metabolites to appear in blood plasma, whether due to dietary or other factors, may not receive the same benefits from ginseng. It is anticipated that pharmacological activities of these intestinal bacteria metabolites will increasingly be the focus of future activity studies on *P. ginseng*.

Neurological, Psychological, and Behavioral Functions

Neurotoxicity/Neuroprotection

Takahashi and Tokuyama (1998) have shown that when given daily as a pretreatment to mice, ginseng (100 mg/kg p.o.) could completely abolish the inhibitory effect on tolerance development to morphine from foot-shock stress. They suggested, therefore, that this effect may result from antistress activities of ginseng and that ginseng may be clinically useful in the prevention and treatment of opioid dependence. However, ginseng had no effect on the impact of psychological stress on the development of tolerance. Higher dosages (200 mg/kg i.p.) produced results that might suggest a potential for the use of ginseng in the prevention and treatment of methamphetamine and cocaine dependence.

Oh et al. (1997) reported that mice pretreated with the total saponin fraction of ginseng (50 or 100 mg/kg i.p.), twice before a high dose of methamphetamine (10 mg/kg s.c.), then showed a significantly smaller ($p < 0.01$) decrease in striatal dopamine after methamphetamine (MAP), compared to a saline-pretreated control. They also found a significantly higher level of the dopamine metabolite 3,4-dihydroxyphenylacetic acid (DOPAC) compared to controls treated with saline.

Psychological and Behavioral Functions

Cognitive functions. It has long been suggested that ginseng may influence monoamines in the brain (Petkov, 1978). Recent research has clarified this suggestion. In an investigation of the possible mechanisms of nervous system effects of ginseng, Tachikawa et al. (1999) found in vitro evidence that certain ginsenosides exert potent effects on various key receptors. Notable among their findings was that at 1-100 μM, ginsenoside Rg_3 strongly inhibited a wide range of receptors: neurotensin, γ-aminobutyric acid, nicotine, muscarine, and histamine, and Rg_2 strongly inhibited nicotine and γ-aminobutyric acid receptors.

Murase et al. (1994) isolated a nerve-growth factorlike component from the root powder of ginseng (686 ng/kg) which was indistinguishable from mouse NGF, immunologically, physiochemically, and biologically. Remarkably enough, the factor derived (molecular mass 25 kDa) showed near-equivalent activity to mouse NGF in stimulating neurite outgrowth in vitro, and showed no antigenic difference. NGF—a nerve growth factor required for growth, development, and survival of sensory and sympathetic neurons—plays the same vital role in cholinergic neurons in the basal forebrain. Although any physiological role for the factor had yet to be determined, *P. ginseng* NGF (3.9 ng/mL) stimulated neurite outgrowth in both the dorsal root ganglia assay and the sympathetic ganglion assay.

Watanabe et al. (1991) compared the dopaminergic and spontaneous motor activity of young and old rats administered a water extract of ginseng orally for four weeks (1.8% concentration, corresponding to 7 g of dried root/kg per day). During the dark period, the old rats displayed a significant increase in spontaneous motor activity which reached the level of young rats in a control group during the same period. Conversely, the young rats treated with ginseng extract showed a significantly decreased spontaneous motor activity in the dark period. Curiously, neither group showed any change in motor activity during the light period. As for dopaminergic activity, levels of striatal dopamine in the old rats before receiving ginseng showed no significant difference compared to the young rats. In rats that ingested the ginseng water extract for 5 weeks, levels remained the same. However, dopamine utilization after ginseng ingestion was affected differently in the old rats compared to the young rats. Although dopamine receptor mechanisms showed no change in either group, during the day, the old rats showed inhibited striatial dopamine utilization while the young rats showed increased utilization. The reason for these opposite effects was unclear. To clarify the action of ginseng on dopamine, the researchers have called for further studies using clinically relevant dosages of ginseng (2-3 g/day) instead of the considerably higher dosage which yielded their perplexing observations (7 g/kg per day).

In a study of ginseng's effects on memory, learning, and locomotor ability in rats, Petkov and Mosharrof (1987) used a commercial, standardized (4% ginsenosides), freeze-dried aqueous extract of ginseng (G115). Prior to beginning the tests, groups of rats were administered different dosages of the extract (3 to 300 mg/kg p.o.) for ten days. Tests began on day ten, 1 h after the last dose. Against the memory-impairing effect of scopolamine (2 mg/kg i.p.), ginseng (30 mg/kg p.o.) prevented memory impairment. In the step-down passive avoidance test alone, only a pretreatment dosage of 30 mg/kg p.o. caused any significant increase in memory retention. In a test of learning and retention (shuttle-box test) conducted 14 days after the last pretreatment dose, they found a significant increase ($p < 0.01$) in these capabilities from 10 and 30 mg/kg p.o. On learning (staircase maze training and positive reinforcement), the best results were found in animals pretreated with ginseng at 10 mg/kg p.o. In a test of locomotor activity effects (treadmill training), male animals pretreated with the ginseng extract at 30 mg/kg p.o. showed a pronounced increase in locomotor activity compared to controls, whereas female animals showed no change. At a pretreatment dosage of 100 mg/kg p.o, however, both sexes showed an even greater increase in locomotor activity of 2.5 times in the females and 3 times in the males. The researchers suggested that the latter result could be attributed to an anti-fatigue effect of ginseng.

An earlier study using the same extract in rats showed that after several days of pretreatment at 20 mg/kg p.o., the animals performed better in memory and learning tests than from pretreatment with 100 mg/kg p.o. In some indices, the higher dosage appeared to have impaired memory and learning. Petkov and Mosharrof (1987) concluded that their findings served to confirm data from similar, previous research, which demonstrated that under certain conditions, higher dosages of ginseng show indications of impairing conditioned-reflex activity. However, Lewis et al. (1983), in a blinded study in mice on stamina in cold water-swimming trials, found no differences of any significance compared to distilled water in tests of a simple *Panax ginseng* root infusion (corresponding to 303.63 mg of dried root/day), whether the animals consumed the infusion for 38, 46, or 96 days.

Petkov (1978) reported that at a low dosage (20 mg/kg p.o. for three days), an alcoholic-aqueous extract of ginseng (1:5 ginseng extract) caused a highly significant improvement in memory retention and learning indices in male rats ($p < 0.001$). The extract also caused a significant increase in the transport of ^{14}C-DL-phenylalanine across the blood-brain barrier (30 mg/kg p.o. for five days in male rats). Less significant results were obtained from 100 mg/kg p.o, an effect the authors ascribed to either a possible deterioration of the memory and learning indices or even to unreliable differences in the memory and learning indices. In either event, they suggested that correct dosage might be a deciding factor in obtaining favorable results.

Receptor- and Neurotransmitter-Mediated Functions

Eight ginseng saponin fractions and a total *n*-butanol extract of the dried roots were tested in whole rat brain synaptosomes for neurotransmitter reuptake effects. Tsang et al. (1985) found only two active fractions: fraction three containing 80% ginsenoside Rd and unidentified ginsenosides, and fraction five containing 2% Rd, 40% Rc, and 45% Rb_1 and Rb_2. At a low concentration (50 μg/mL), the total *n*-butanol extract also caused a significant and dose-dependent inhibition of neurotransmitter uptake, showing a potency somewhere between that of fractions three and five, and with the order of neurotransmitter uptake inhibited (least to greatest) in comparatively greater contrast: leucine (Leu) < 2-deoxyglucose (2-DG) < serotonin (5-HT) = norepinephrine (NE) = dopamine (DA) < gamma-aminobutyrate (GABA) < glutamic acid (Glu). From least to most inhibited, the following order of neurotransmitters were inhibited by fraction three at the low concentration: leucine (Leu) < 2-DG < DA < 5-HT < Glu < GABA < NE. At 50% of the overall activity of fraction three, fraction five (at the same low concentration) was found to contain 2% ginsenoside Rd compared to 80% in fraction three. The difference in composition may have been responsible for the difference in potency, but at the same time, still other ginsenosides may have been active. The order of neurotransmitters inhibited by fraction five at the lowest concentration was similar to that of fraction three: Leu < GABA < 2-DG < Glu < 5-HT < Da < NE. Also notable was the finding that neurotransmitters were more affected by the subfractions and the total *n*-butanol extract itself than the metabolic substrates 2-FG and Leu, which implied that the activity of the effective extracts was a specific action rather than a surface action. The reuptake of GABA was inhibited more than any other neurotransmitter tested; however, this was only the case at much higher concentrations of the *n*-butanol extract (500 μg/mL, 34% reuptake inhibition) or fractions three and five (100 μg/mL, 40% and 25%, respectively), either of which are less likely to be physiological from oral doses of ginseng extracts. At the lower concentration, the greatest inhibition produced by these respective ginseng preparations was found in glutamic acid (13%) and NE (27% and 12%) (Tsang et al., 1985).

Reproductive Disorders

Sexual Dysfunctions (Male)

The sexual stimulant or aphrodisiac nature of ginseng, which has been long-alluded to in Oriental folk medicine, appears to have some basis in fact, at least in the laboratory. Yamamoto et al. (1977) found in vitro evidence suggesting that saponins of ginseng may be responsible for increasing protein and DNA synthesis in rat testes. Chen and Lee (1995) and later Choi et al. (1998) reported that ginseng extract dose-dependently relaxed the corpus cavernosal tissue of rabbits in vitro starting from a concentration of 1 mg/mL, and that the action was mediated by an increase in the sequestration of intracellular calcium and from corporal sinusoids by an increase in the release of nitric oxide (NO) (Choi et al., 1998), the main mediator of penile erection, and/or cyclic GMP, which mediates the vascular smooth muscle relaxing activity of NO (Gillis, 1997). However, the results of Choi et al. (1998) also suggested that an α-adrenergic blocking activity by ginseng extract may be involved in the relaxing effect on the smooth muscle of the corpus cavernosum. Furthermore, a potassium channel opening-induced hyperpolarizing effect was found which the researchers suspect may also be involved in the relaxing effect of the extract. Therefore, multiple actions could be at work in the smooth muscle relaxing activity observed.

Choi et al. (1999) found further evidence of the erectile-enhancing effect of ginseng in normal male rats and male rabbits administered red Korean ginseng extract for three months (Korean Ginseng and Tobacco Research Institute, Taejon, Korea; 50% ethanol extract, 50 mg/kg p.o. daily in physiological saline). Intracavernosal pressure, but not systemic blood pressure, was significantly higher ($p < 0.01$) in the ginseng-treated rabbits and rats compared to the placebo-treated controls (physiological saline only p.o.), an effect that may have been due to improved local penile peripheral circulation. In vitro tests of corpus cavernosum tissue from the rabbits showed that the action was due to an endothelium-derived relaxing factor and enhancement of the peripheral neurophysiology. Rabbit cavernosal muscle showed significantly increased relaxation after the three-month treatment period compared to controls. The same results were found in the ginseng extract-treated rats compared to the control group ($p < 0.01$).

Yoshimura et al. (1998) studied the effect of ginseng saponin in male mice displaying no copulatory behavior following housing over a prolonged time, which provided the researchers with a model of psychogenic impotence. The crude saponins and some individual saponins of ginseng (Rb_1, Rb_2, Rg_1, Ro) were administered right after the male mice were housed individually and stopped a day prior to tests of sexual behavior with virgin female mice. Dose-dependently, mice administered the crude saponins (50 and 100 mg/kg i.p. daily) showed a significant increase in mounting from either dosage, and an increase in intromission incidence (100 mg/kg) compared to saline-treated control mice. Mounting frequency was also significantly higher in the crude saponin-treated mice (100 mg/kg) compared to the control ($p < 0.01$), but not in the frequency of intromission. Among the ginsenosides tested, only Rg_1 (10 mg/kg i.p. daily) showed significant activity, increasing both the incidences and frequency of mounting and intromission. The researchers concluded that Rg_1 potently exerts preventive effects on copulatory disorder caused by social stress in male mice.

In another study, Kim et al. (1976) reported that male rats administered ginseng showed high levels of nucleic acids in their testicles, and gonad weight increased in both male and female rats administered an alcoholic extract of ginseng. They also reported a significant increase in various mating behaviors of male rats administered ginseng extract subcutaneously.

CLINICAL STUDIES

The scientific literature on *Panax ginseng* is prolific and often displays inconsistent results (Shibata et al., 1985; Vogler et al., 1999; Bahrke and Morgan, 2000). There are several reasons for this, among which is the fact that different procedures are used in the preparation of extracts. For instance, while some studies employ pure ginsenosides, others use fractions of root extracts. Another factor influencing clinical results is that in traditional Chinese medicine *Panax ginseng* is usually prescribed at a low dosage for a long period of time, a situation that is difficult to replicate in a clinical study (Shibata et al., 1985).

Cardiovascular and Circulatory Disorders

Vascular Insufficiency

Cerebrovascular dysfunctions. Quiroga (1982) conducted a double-blind study on 45 patients suffering from cerebrovascular deficits. Subjects received either G115 standardized ginseng extract (100 mg b.i.d.), Hydergina (a vasoactive preparation containing 1.5 mg of actives), or placebo. Using the outcome measurement of cerebral flow, the use of Hydergina was very favorable with an improvement quotient of 58.43%. The outcome with G115 was rated favorable with an improvement quotient of 34.36%. Placebo treatment groups showed improvement quotients of 0.72% and 0.31% or no response.

Quiroga and Imbriano (1979) studied G115 in 134 patients who received a dosage of two capsules per day (200 mg/day) for the first month and one capsule per day for the next two consecutive months. Clinical, hematological, radiological, and rheographic examinations were conducted at the end of three months with the following results: in 36% the effects were very favorable, for 54% the effects were favorable, and 10% showed no response. These ratings were based on the following respective criteria:

1. recovery of cerebral flow with subsequent increase of flow in both cerebral carotid systems;
2. small modifications in the elasticity of the arteries or in the first lead of the rheoencephalogram; and
3. no cardiohemodynamic changes, interpreted as an absence of "inotropic myocardial changes."

Endocrine and Hormonal Disorders

Diabetes

Sotaniemi et al. (1995) reported benefits from a ginseng tablet product (Dansk Droge, Copenhagen, Denmark) in newly diagnosed diabetic patients who participated in a small, double-blind, placebo-controlled, multicenter trial. Sixteen men and 20 women (ages 52-66) were randomly assigned to receive either placebo or ginseng tablets at 100 mg or 200 mg daily for eight weeks after a run-in period of eight weeks. The patients were counseled to maintain a diet made up of 30% fat, 20% protein, and 50% carbohydrate, to self-monitor their blood glucose levels, and to set a goal of reducing the body weight by a minimum of 2 kg. Among the patient parameters monitored in the trial were physical activity, serum lipids, body weight, fasting blood glucose, glycosalted hemoglobin A_{1c} (HbA_{1c} or "glycated hemoglobin"), serum aminoterminalpropeptide (PIINP), mood, memory, vigor, well-being, and psychophysical performance. The researchers reported that the results showed benefits from either dosage of the ginseng tablets versus placebo. In most measurements, greater significance and number of improved parameters were found in the higher dosage group. Although memory, lipid values, and body weight showed no significant change in either ginseng group compared to placebo, well-being, physical activity, and glucose response (oral glucose tolerance test and reduced HbA_{1c} levels) were significantly improved in the 200-mg group compared to the 100-mg and placebo groups. Vigor was significantly improved in both ginseng dosage groups though more so in the 200-mg group. Mood and psychophysical performance were significantly improved in both ginseng dosage groups, fasting blood glucose reached normal levels in 8/24 patients in both of the ginseng groups (versus two subjects in the placebo group), and the higher ginseng dosage group showed a significant reduction in serum PIINP. No side effects were found in any of the treatment groups. The researchers concluded that the benefits of ginseng on fasting blood glucose levels in NIDDM patients may be due to a number of factors, including changes in physical activity, diet, improved self-management (psychophysical activation), improved insulin sensitivity, increased glycogen storage, and reduced collagen synthesis. In summary, Sotaniemi and co-workers declared that their study showed that by activating psychophysical performance and mood, ginseng may facilitate improvements in glucose balance, and as an adjunctive therapy may be useful in managing NIDDM (Sotaniemi et al., 1995). This study has been criticized as ambiguous on the grounds of significant differences in the baseline characteristics of the treatment groups, which includes HbA_{1c} levels, and the poorly characterized nature of the ginseng product used (Vuksan et al., 2000).

Immune Disorders; Inflammation and Disease

Cancer

Cancer prevention. Chemopreventive effects of ginseng were reported by Lee, Lee, and Kim (1998) in a double-blind, randomized study of 15 male smokers and five nonsmokers (ages 19-31) given 1.8 g of red ginseng or placebo daily for four weeks. Antioxidant levels in the plasma of smokers increased while carbonyl contents and 8-OHdG (8-hydroxydeoxyguanosine) levels showed a significant ($p < 0.05$) time-dependent decrease in comparison to smokers on placebo. The nonsmokers were described as having never smoked a cigarette and the smokers were described as having used at least 20 cigarettes a day for the past two years. Both groups were also described as "healthy." At baseline, carbonyl contents, a measure of protein oxidation, showed a significantly higher level in smokers compared to nonsmokers. After taking ginseng for four weeks, the carbonyl content in the smokers showed a time-dependent decrease of 21.3%, whereas the placebo-smoker group showed no decrease. The 8-OHdG levels, used to measure oxidative DNA damage, were also significantly higher in the smokers compared to the non-smokers at baseline. After four weeks of ginseng, the mean level of 8-OHdG had time-dependently decreased by 31.7%. In addition, there was a linear increase in the level of ginsenoside Rb_1 in the smokers on ginseng. Although this was a preliminary study, the researchers found a significant correlation between red ginseng and decreased oxidative damage.

Yun and Choi (1990) studied 905 pairs of case studies which were matched by age, sex, and date of admission to the Korea Cancer Center Hospital in Seoul, Korea. Of the 905 pairs of cases, 562 (62%) reported a history of ginseng intake, as opposed to 674 (75%) controls. The odds ratio of cancer to ginseng intake was 0.56 (95% confidence interval). Statistical trends showed a highly significant decrease ($p < 0.001$) in the proportion of cancer cases with increasing frequency of ginseng intake (over 1-3 times/year, 4-11 times/year, and at least once monthly) for males as well as female users of ginseng, including the use of fresh ginseng extract, fresh ginseng extract combined with fresh sliced ginseng, white ginseng extract, and white ginseng powder. A significant reduction in cancer incidence was not found from intake of fresh ginseng juice, fresh ginseng slices, or white ginseng tea. Although the most effective forms in this study were found to be ginseng powder and extract, data for red ginseng use was insufficient to make a statistical analysis with sufficient weight to be reliable. For reasons as yet unknown, the cancer preventive effect of ginseng was much more significant in males ($p < 0.00001$) than females ($p < 0.05$).

In a later study of 1,987 pairs, Yun and Choi (1995) found a correlation between ginseng intake and a decreased risk of developing certain cancers. A dose-response relationship was indicated from the increase in frequency and duration of ginseng usage in association with decreasing risk of cancer frequency. Regardless of whether subjects had started to take ginseng between the ages of 30 and 39 or after the age of 60, a cancer-preventive effect was evident after one year of ginseng use which thereafter increased with the duration of consumption. The odds ratios were 0.47 for cancer of the lip, oral cavity, and pharynx; 0.36 for stomach cancer; 0.42 for colorectal cancer; 0.48 for liver cancer; 0.22 for pancreatic cancer; 0.18 for laryngeal cancer; 0.55 for lung cancer; and 0.15 for ovarian cancer. No positive association of decreased risk and ginseng intake was established with the following cancers: female breast, uterine cervix, urinary bladder, and thyroid gland. The odds ratio for ginseng users was 0.50 compared to nonusers. In the types of ginseng used, the best odds ratio was found in users of red ginseng (OR = 0.20), white ginseng extract (OR = 0.30), and fresh ginseng extract (OR = 0.37). No decreased risk of cancer was evident from the use of white ginseng tea, fresh ginseng juice, or slices of fresh ginseng. Comparing smokers who used ginseng to nonsmoking ginseng users, the smokers showed decreased risks for developing cancers of the lung, lip, pharynx, oral cavity, and liver, but not of the colorectum, stomach, or esophagus.

In reviewing the evidence from both of his studies' experimental and epidemiological data for the cancer-preventive activity of ginseng, Yun (1996) concluded that all the data supported the effect. He emphasized that ginseng "should be recognized as a functional food for cancer prevention" and encouraged continued research of its chemopreventive effect internationally (Yun, 1996, p. S80).

Immunomodulation

In a controlled, single-blind study, Scaglione et al. (1994) investigated the immunomodulatory effect of ginseng extract (G115) in 40 smokers diagnosed with chronic bronchitis. After an eight-week treatment period, the phagocytosis index (PHI, rate or index of phagocytosis) and the phagocytosis fraction (PHF, phagocytic alveolar macrophages) of the ginseng group showed significant increases ($p < 0.001$) compared to the placebo group, as measured by in vitro phagocytic activity against *Candida albicans*. The percentage of *C. albicans* killed by alveolar macrophages (intracellular killing) from the ginseng group was also highly significant compared to the placebo group. By increasing the activity of alveolar macrophages, such an immunomodulating effect may be capable of preventing or treating respiratory disorders of an infective or immunological nature (Scaglione et al., 1994).

The immunomodulatory effect of ginseng was tested by Scaglione et al. (1990) in a double-blind study involving 60 healthy volunteers (ages 18-50). Group A was treated with an aqueous extract of ginseng (Pharmaton, Switzerland, 100 mg), while group B, which served as the control group, received lactose. Group C received 100 mg capsules of standardized ginseng extract (G115), one capsule every 12 h for eight weeks. Blood samples were drawn before the treatment, at the fourth week, and at the eighth week. Parameters studied included chemotaxis of PMNs, phagocytosis index (PHI), phagocytosis fraction (PHF), intracellular killing (IK), total lymphocytes (T3), T helper (T4) subset, T suppressor (T8) subset, blastogenesis of circulating lymphocytes, and natural killer (NK) cell activity. Groups A and C showed increased chemotaxis by the fourth week and at the eighth week group C showed even more increased chemotaxis. PHI and PHF were enhanced by the eighth week in group A (aqueous extract) with the enhancement much higher in group C starting at the fourth week. IK began to show a significant increase by the fourth week for both groups A and C. Total lymphocytes were enhanced at the fourth week for both groups A and C and by the eighth week the increases became highly significant ($p < 0.001$). The T4 subset showed an increase in both groups A and C, while group C showed a faster and more significant rise. The T8 subset appeared not to be significantly affected. The T4:T8 ratio showed a significant enhancement only in group C starting at the fourth week. Blastogenesis showed significant increases for both groups A and C, with faster increases evident in group C. Overall, the researchers concluded that the standardized ginseng extract showed stronger and broader immunostimulating activities than the aqueous extract, and that both extracts showed significant activity compared to the control group (Scaglione et al., 1990).

The immunomodulatory effects of ginseng were studied in a preliminary randomized, placebo-controlled, double-blind study of a ginseng extract standardized to contain ginsenosides in a predetermined composition (Pharmagin, New Century Pharma, Seoul, Korea). Twenty healthy young adult males (ages 21-22) taking no medications and without any serious past illness received either placebo or the standardized extract, 300 mg/day p.o. for eight weeks. Peripheral blood was collected for analysis of lymphocyte populations and T cell subsets. Compared to placebo, the ginseng group showed significant decreases in the number of total white cells (leukocytes), monocytes, and neutrophils at week eight and at week four a significant decrease in neutrophils. However, no other significant differences compared to placebo were found, whether in body weight, numbers of basophils, differential and total leukocyte counts, ratio of CD4/CD8 cells (compared to initial values in both groups), nor in the percentage of CD3, CD8, CD19, and

CD25 cells. Apart from the absence of significant changes in lymphocyte subsets and peripheral blood leukocytes, the researchers noted that the extract may have contained "slightly stronger foreign substances" compared to the placebo (undefined). They also point out that other studies in animals and humans have shown that the ginseng saponin Rg_1 exerted significantly greater effects on immunological functions of aged subjects than in the young (Srisurapanon et al., 1997).

Metabolic and Nutritional Disorders

Performance and Endurance Enhancement

Bahrke and Morgan (1994), in a critical review of the clinical studies of ginseng on physical performance to date, concluded that they offered "little evidence" of efficacy, the absence of which may have been due to poor study designs, including the lack of controls/control groups and relevant variables. More recent, well-designed studies have also shown a lack of benefit from ginseng on physical performance. In a critical review of studies on performance enhancement from ginseng published since their earlier review, Bahrke and Morgan (2000) arrived at much the same conclusion, stating that their analysis had "not resolved the equivocal nature of research evidence involving animals or humans" (p. 114). Poor study designs prevailed, leaving the question of "whether or not ginseng possesses efficacy" as a performance-enhancing and fatigue-modifying agent unanswered.

An eight-week double-blind, placebo-controlled, randomized trial in 19 healthy women (ages 21-35) found no significant benefits from ginseng (G115, 200 mg/day, equivalent to 1 g of *P. ginseng* root) compared to placebo in work capacity, energy metabolic responses, acute recovery (VO_2, VE, heart rate, and RER), or blood levels of lactic acid (Engels et al., 1996). In a similar way, an eight-week, randomized, double-blind, placebo-controlled trial in 36 healthy men (ages 21-28) given ginseng in two dosages (G115, 200 mg and 400 mg/day) found no effect on graded maximal exercise, changes in oxygen utilization, or improvements in capacity for aerobic work from either dosage level compared to placebo (Engels and Wirth, 1997).

In China, a 12-week, controlled trial of red ginseng (900 mg, t.i.d.) in 64 volunteers was conducted to test for changes in exercise capacity and information processing in old-aged (65-74 years) and middle-aged people (55-64 years). The middle-aged group on ginseng was reported to show benefits in information processing performance, spatial ability (trail-making test), speed of processing information (choice and finger simple reaction times), and in exercise performance in these tasks. For the elderly group on ginseng, however, there was no change in exercise capacity to perform these tasks, nor in any tests of information processing speed. Choi (1998) concluded that whereas their results indicate that ginseng provides no benefit to the elderly in speed of information processing, it may benefit middle-aged people for the same kind of tasks.

McNaughton et al. (1989) compared the ergogenic effects of *Panax ginseng* to eleuthero *(Eleutherococcus senticosus)* and placebo in 15 male and 15 female athletes. The group taking *Panax ginseng* (uncharacterized, 1 g/ day each morning for six weeks) showed significant improvements compared to placebo in maximal oxygen uptake (VO$_2$max) ($p < 0.01$), recovery time ($p < 0.05$), quadriceps strength (av. 18%; $p < 0.05$), and pectoral strength (av. 22%; $p < 0.01$). The group taking eleuthero only showed significant improvements in pectoral strength (av. 13%; $p < 0.05$), and quadriceps strength (av. 15%; $p < 0.05$), versus placebo.

Forgo et al. (1981) investigated the influence of ginsenosides on physical and mental capability and its effects on gonadal hormones in a 12-week, double-blind study in 60 male and 60 female participants. The researchers administered 100 mg of standardized *P. ginseng* root extract (G115) twice a day and compared the results to a placebo (gelatin capsules containing glycerin oil). Capsules were taken in the morning and at midday with meals. Four tests were administered before, during, and after the study to evaluate reaction times, pulmonary function, sex hormones in the blood, and subjective self-assessment of condition. In the reaction test, there was a significant difference between those given G115 and those given placebo, but only in subjects ages 40-60. In the pulmonary test, those given G115 performed better, with the most notable improvement in men ages 40-60. No changes were found in sex hormone production for either group. Self-assessed results indicated benefits in the G115 group, with males and females ages 40-60 reporting the most significant improvement.

In a three-month, double-blind study involving 60 elderly men and women, the effect of a standardized ginseng extract (G115, 1 g/day) on general physical subjective condition, physical fitness, mental alertness, attitude to life/mood, concentration/memory, and sleep behavior was analyzed. Beneficial results were noted after several weeks of treatment with G115, especially on reaction time, two-hand coordination, recovery period, subjective complaints, and recovery quotient. Ginseng also appeared to exert a beneficial influence on the lungs, oxygen intake, and sleep (Dorling et al., 1980).

Neurological, Psychological, and Behavioral Disorders

D'Angelo et al. (1986) conducted a double-blind clinical study on the effect of G115 on the mental and psychomotor performance of healthy volunteers. Sixteen male participants were given 100 mg of the extract twice a day for a duration of 12 weeks. The researchers reported that the ginseng extract tended to improve results in the cancellation, mental arithmetic, logical de-duction, choice reaction time, and auditory reaction time tests. However, the only statistically significant improvement was in mental arithmetic. No side effects were reported. SØrensen and Sonne (1996) reported similar results in a double-blind, randomized, test-retest study in 112 volunteers ages 40-70. After receiving ginseng tablets (Gerimax, Dansk Droge A/S, 400 mg/day for eight to nine weeks), mental performance results showed no significant differences in either group in abstract thinking.

Psychological and Behavioral Disorders

Rosenfeld (1989) conducted a study to evaluate the effects of G115 on asthenia (i.e., fatigue attributed to psychophysical stress). Fifty patients were each given 2,100 mg capsules of G115 daily for 56 days. At the end of the trial period, the researchers found that treatment with G115 appreciably improved scores in the Tolouse, Weschler-Bellevue, and Sandoz Clinical Assessment-Geriatric (SCAG) tests. No adverse effects were reported.

The effect of ginseng on performance and feeling of well-being was investigated in a double-blind, crossover study of 12 nurses on night duty. Results were compared to placebo and daytime work. Ginseng improved the self-rating scores for competence, mood, and performance in one of the psychophysiological tests, but in some other variables it rated negatively in "bodily feelings" (i.e., sweating, palpitations, difficulty breathing, tension, tiredness, and agitation) (Hallstrom et al., 1982).

Depression. In a study on the effects of ginseng (powdered six-year-old roots, 1,500 mg/day in tablet form) on functional deterioration in the form of depression or fatigue, Fulder et al. (1984) conducted a ten-day, double-blind, randomized, crossover trial in 49 geriatric patients (~60 years of age) of both sexes. The ginseng group showed slightly better results in the Object Learning, digit span, and concentration tests compared to the placebo group. However, the results were not significant. In the psychophysical reactivity tests, the ginseng group showed a highly significant difference ($p < 0.001$) in the number-copying-in-3-min component, and significant results in the digit span and paired association components (both $p < 0.05$) compared to placebo. No significant difference between placebo and ginseng was found in the objects learned or the concentration components. Subjective reports of significant improvement in symptomology, well-being, and depressive feelings occurred more frequently during the ginseng-treatment periods than during the placebo-treatment periods. The dosage used was in conformance with commercial supplier-recommended levels in the West, which were less than those used in traditional Chinese medicine. No changes in blood pressure were found and there were no side effects except for a mild case of diarrhea in one patient who continued in the trial. From the results of these and still other tests, Fulder and colleagues summarized their results as follows: ginseng caused a slight reduction in memory tests, yet improved performance in speed tests (general responses in letter copying); although performance showed significant changes, the results were obfuscated by the factor of trial participation, which was especially the case in test results of cognitive, function, general well-being, and mood, which showed only little improvement from ginseng. Using analogue scales, the researchers noted the while patients showed a slight increase in energy and alertness during the trial, their sleep was slightly poorer and they were less happy. Fulder et al. (1984) noted that because psychopharmacological agents for geriatric patients usually show benefits after a few weeks, it would have been advisable to administer ginseng at a higher dosage (ideally 2-3 g/day) for a much longer period.

Reproductive Disorders

Menopause

Wiklund et al. (1999) conducted a randomized, placebo-controlled, multicenter parallel group study of ginseng extract (G115) on quality of life in postmenopausal women complaining of climacteric symptoms. Changes in quality of life were assessed using various self-administered questionnaires (Psychological General Well-Being Index, Women's Health Questionnaire, and Visual Analogue Scales for assessing changes in climacteric symptoms). Prior to inclusion in the study, subjects received a physical exam consisting of vaginal ultrasound to measure endometrial thickness, vaginal pH, pap smear, heart rate, blood pressure, weight, and height. Further tests were taken at random, including urine analysis, estradiol and follicle-stimulating hormone (FSH) levels, and plasma FSH and estradiol levels, which were measured a second time at the final visit. At baseline, the placebo ($n = 193$) and ginseng groups ($n = 191$) were well-matched for age (mean age 53 years), weight, height, blood pressure, heart rate, and a normal rating upon gynecological examination. After a two-week run-in period, patients received either placebo or ginseng (100 mg, "two capsules in the morning after breakfast") for a period of 16 weeks. The results showed no significant differences between the treatment groups in the following outcome measurements: tolerability and safety parameters (levels of FSH and estradiol, vaginal pH, vaginal cytology, endometrial thickness), Women's Health Questionnaire (vasomotor symptoms, sleep problems, menstrual problems), and Visual Analogue Scales (climacteric complaints). No significant difference was found in the number of subjects who reported adverse events in the placebo ($n = 77$) and ginseng groups ($n = 80$). The most commonly reported adverse events consisted of cold (11.7%), diarrhea and gastrointestinal complaints (10.4%), and migraine and headache (4.7%). In the Psychological General Well-Being Index, the ginseng group showed statistically significant improvements compared to placebo in scores of well-being ($p = 0.09$), depression ($p = 0.04$), and general health ($p = 0.09$). However, the total score of the Psychological General Well-Being Index in the ginseng group "showed only a tendency for slightly better overall symptomatic relief ($p < 0.1$)" (Wiklund et al., 1999, p. 89).

Sexual Dysfunctions (Male)

In a placebo-controlled study, Choi et al. (1995) found no change in premature ejaculation, intercourse frequency, and duration and frequency of morning erections in 90 erectile dysfunction patients treated with either red ginseng extract (1,800 mg/day), placebo, or trazadone (25 mg at bedtime) for three months. In no case were symptoms aggravated by the treatments, and although serum testosterone showed a slight increase in the ginseng group, testosterone and prolactin levels showed no significant change, nor in the other groups. Eighty-one of the men were diagnosed with psychogenic erectile dysfunction and the remaining nine with a mild vasculogenic type. The only changes of any statistical significance by comparison to the other treatment groups were found in the ginseng group with increases in libido in 50%, sexual satisfaction in 43.3%, penile tumescence during erection in 53.5%, penile rigidity during erection in 50%, and decreased early detumescence in 23.3% (all $p < 0.05$). Overall, the researchers gave the ginseng group a therapeutic efficacy rating of 60% and the other groups 30% each. They noted that although the ginseng group showed clearly superior results, when tested for changes in erection induced by audiovisual stimulation there was no change compared to baseline. The researchers proposed that an explanation of the erectile activity of ginseng would be found in a combination of anxiolytic, antidepressive, vasodilating activities, and the effect of improved microvascular flow.

Miscellaneous Pharmacological Activities

Following positive results in mice and rats (Choi et al., 1984; Huh et al., 1985; Lee et al., 1987), a pilot study on the alcohol-clearing effect of ginseng was conducted in humans. Each serving as their own control, 14 healthy male volunteers between the ages of 25 and 35 drank 25% ethanol at a dosage of 72 g/kg over 45 min. Blood samples were taken 40 min after the last drink. One week after the control test, the volunteers drank the same dosage of alcohol again, only this time it was mixed with an extract of ginseng providing a dose of 3 g. The extract was prepared using dried roots heated three times in water ($100ºC$) at ten times the volume of the roots for 8 h and then freeze-dried. Blood alcohol levels of the volunteers were 35.2% lower when ginseng was combined with the alcohol compared to straight alcohol. Individual results 40 min after the ginseng-alcohol test showed that for 70% of the subjects, blood alcohol levels were 32% to 51% lower compared to levels after drinking straight alcohol, and that for 20% they were lower by 14% to 18%. For one volunteer there was no change (Lee et al., 1987).

DOSAGE

Many recent clinical trails have used the extract G115, commercially known as Ginsana, which has a standardized ginsenoside content. Generally, 100 mg of ginseng extract, standardized to $\geq 5\%$ ginsenoside, and Rb_1 $\geq 0.75\%$, with an optimal ratio of $Rg_1:Rb_1$ of ≥ 0.5, is taken twice daily. According to the *British Herbal Compendium*, the dosage of ginseng is generally 0.6-2 g of the dried root taken in decoction in the morning. Equivalent extracts are not recommended for continuous use beyond three months without discontinuing for one month (Bradley, 1992). The daily dose of the dried root is traditionally 1-9 g (Hobbs, 1996).

SAFETY PROFILE

Cases of ill effects from ginseng in humans have been reported. In one study reported by Siegel (1979), 22 out of 133 participants in a study experienced adverse effects after long-term doses of up to 15 g/day (mean dosage 3 g/day). These effects included sleeplessness, skin problems, anxiety, and diarrhea. Siegel (1979) termed these adverse effects Ginseng Abuse Syndrome (GAS); however, due to the lack of controls, lack of data about the participants, lack of intake control, concomitant use of caffeine in high amounts, and administration of a wide variety of ginseng products with no information about product ingredients, Siegel himself later retracted some of his conclusions regarding this and another study he conducted (Hobbs, 1996).

One reported case of Stevens Johnson syndrome (SJS) associated with ginseng use has been reported. A 27-year-old male ginseng-user took two "pills" of ginseng (concentration not stated) during three days while on a course of prescribed antibiotics and aspirin for a sore throat. He developed SJS and toxic epidermal necrosis. Because SJS can be associated with corticosteroids (among other drugs), it is plausible that ginseng contributed in this case, although the researchers gave no information on the type of supplement taken (Dega et al., 1996). SJS is characterized as a skin disease often resulting from an immunological reaction to circulating immune complexes. Painful blisters form in the mouth and eyes, the palms often develop a dark purple area or blisters circled with erythema, and the patient feels and appears afflicted with fever. In half of all cases, no cause has been found; however, infections (herpes simplex, *Mycoplasma pneumoniae,* and *Strep-*

tococcus), penicillin, NSAIDS, corticosteroids, sulfonamides, barbiturates, and other drugs may be suspected (Parker, 1996; Dega et al., 1996).

Palmer et al. (1978) reported a case of what appeared to be hormonal side effects from ginseng in an elderly woman, age 70. She had been regularly taking a powdered ginseng product ("Gin Seng") and experiencing a feeling of general "well-being"; however, after three weeks on the powder she developed tender and swollen breasts with diffuse nodules. When she went off the product, her symptoms "settled," and on two further occasions they returned after she resumed the powder. Serum prolactin measurements showed nothing abnormal whether she was taking the powder or not. The researchers noted that the product was composed of the roots of several *Panax* species and speculated that it may have had "mild hormonal activity." Obviously, contamination of the product cannot be ruled out.

Excessive intake of ginseng is reported to cause side effects of sleeplessness and hypertension (Bradley, 1992).

Contraindications

Ginseng is contraindicated in acute infections, especially those involving fever. It also may be contraindicated in hypertension, and in use with stimulants; for example, with large amounts of caffeine (Bradley, 1992). Due to immunopotentiating activity (Scaglione et al., 1990, 1994), ginseng may also be contraindicated in organ transplant patients and patients being treated with immunosuppressive agents.

Drug Interactions

A suggested possible interaction with warfarin in a patient taking 300 mg/day of a standardized *P. ginseng* extract was reported when the production of clotting factor was apparently antagonized (Janetzky and Morreale, 1997). However, such an interaction was not shown in rats concomitantly administered a high dosage of ginseng root decoction (20 g/kg p.o. for five days) and a single dose of warfarin (20 mg/kg p.o.). From further tests, no significant effect on the pharmacodynamics and/or pharmacokinetics of warfarin was found from ginseng (Zhu et al., 1999).

Some researchers have suggested that ginseng could possibly potentiate monoamine oxidase inhibitors (Blumenthal, 1997). Two cases are reported of putative drug interactions with the MAO inhibitor phenelzine. In one case, a woman, age 64, experienced headache, tremulousness, and insomnia when she drank ginseng tea while on the drug (60 mg/day) (Shader and Greenblatt, 1985); and in the other case, a woman, age 42, taking ginseng and bee pollen concurrent with phenelzine (45 mg/day), lorazepam (1 mg q.i.d.) and triazolam (0.5 mg at bedtime) experienced maniclike symptoms (Jones and Runikis, 1987). According to a 10-point scoring system for the probability of herb-drug interactions developed by Fugh-Berman and Ernst (2001), the first case does not provide enough data to be evaluated, and in the second case an herb-drug interaction is "possible."

Pregnancy and Lactation

The *British Herbal Compendium* to the *British Herbal Pharmacopoeia* states that ginseng is contraindicated in pregnancy and lactation (Bradley, 1992). Caution should always be used during pregnancy. However, the German Commission E monograph states no contraindications for pregnancy or lactation for doses of 1-2 g/day (Blumenthal et al., 1998).

A very popular and old traditional use of ginseng among Asians is to take the root during pregnancy in the belief that it will give the mother and her baby added "energy" (Chin, 1991, citing Fok et al., 1985). Chin (1991) conducted a survey on the use of ginseng among 1,000 delivering women presenting at a hospital in Hong Kong in 1990. After eliminating those who were uncertain of its use in their pregnancy and those with multiple births, 88 out of 913 delivering patients confirmed that they had used ginseng during pregnancy. A matching control group of 88 patients (parity- and age-matched) who claimed not to have used ginseng during their pregnancy and delivered during the time of the ginseng users was used to compare outcomes. No stillbirths or neonatal deaths occurred in either group and no significant differences were found between the groups in birth weights, Apgar scores, delivery modes, incidences of preterm births, antepartum hemorrhage (ginseng $n = 1$ versus control group $n = 3$), primary postpartum hemorrhage (ginseng $n = 1$ versus control group $n = 3$), or gestational diabetes mellitus/impaired glucose tolerance (WHO criteria defined) (ginseng $n = 6$ versus control group $n = 2$). However, the incidence of preeclampsia was significantly higher in the control group ($n = 8$ versus ginseng $n = 1$). Based on the results of his survey, Chin (1991) advised that research be conducted on the use of ginseng in the prevention and possible treatment of preeclampsia. At the same time, he cautioned against the use of ginseng in pregnancy without a randomized clinical trial to show what benefits it may have in this application.

Newall et al. (1996) describe rat and rabbit studies showing no fetal abnormalities and a long-term rat study in which ginseng was fed to two successive generations of animals with no teratogenicity observed. The report (Koren et al. 1990) of an apparently androgenized infant born to a mother who used "ginseng" during her pregnancy and during early breastfeeding has been refuted (Awang, 1991). Subsequent examination of the product found that it contained "siberian ginseng." Analysis of the product clearly showed that it contained neither *Panax* nor *Eleulotherococcus* ginseng but another plant, *Periploca sepium,* known to contain potentially toxic constituents.

Ginseng has been studied as a treatment for mastitis in dairy cows (Hu et al., 1995). An anecdote describing the successful treatment of mastitis with ginseng and homeopathic pokeweed in one mother was recently commented upon (Lawrence, 2001). No reports of adverse effects with the use of *Panax* ginseng during lactation are known.

Side Effects

There are no reported side effects other than those noted.

Special Precautions

A case of overdosage was reported (Ryu and Chien, 1995) in which two female patients (age 28) developed severe headaches, cerebral arteritis, chest tightness, nausea, and vomiting following ingestion of a large quantity of a 22% alcohol extract of ginseng: 200 mL derived from about 25 g of dry root in a single dose.

Radish is reported to be a folk remedy for ginseng intoxication (Chang and But, 1986).

Due to a lack of information on the pharmacokinetics of ginseng, precautions concerning the length of its discontinuation prior to surgical operations are difficult to determine. Ang-Lee et al. (2001) suggest a "probably prudent" time of seven days or more.

Toxicology

Toxicity in Animal Models

A freeze-dried, water-soluble extract of ginseng administered to mice produced an oral LD_{50} of 10 g/kg. By i.p. injection, the LD_{50} was (2 g/kg (Shoji and Kisara, 1975).

Toxicological investigations with laboratory animals indicate that only extremely high doses of ginseng cause significant side effects. Added to the diet of beagle dogs for 13 weeks, G115 (1.5-15 mg/kg per day) produced no toxic effects (Owen, 1981). Another study in rats found no detrimental or toxicological effects of G115 in F0, F1, and F2 generations from doses up to 15 mg/kg per day. A study in mice and rats found the oral LD_{50} of G115 exceeded 1,000 mg/kg. Additional in vivo data on G115 over time confirmed the relative safety of oral ingestion in laboratory animals (Owen, 1981; Hess et al., 1983). A recent study supports the need to repeat these experiments and for the publication of unpublished toxicological studies to replace the arguably dated safety information cited (Sharma et al., 1999).

When administered to male rabbits and rats as part of their feed (100 mg/kg per day for 30-60 days), G115 was reported to have caused a reduction in testicular germ cell counts, size and number of Leydig cells, decreased levels of endoplasmic reticulum, contents of protein, glycogen and sialic acid, a decrease in motile sperm production of 77%, increased testicular cholesterol, and delayed spermiation with sperm heads only found in tubule basal regions in further stages of spermatogenesis. At 60 days, most tubules displayed only preleptotene spermatocytes, Sertoli cells, and spermatogonia. Collectively, the results suggested complete cessation of spermatogenesis in association with changes in luteinizing hormone and follicle-stimulating hormone (Sharma et al., 1999).

REFERENCES

Akao, T., Kida, H., Kanaoka, M., Hattori, M., and Kobashi, K. (1998). Intestinal bacterial hydrolysis is required for the appearance of compound K in rat plasma after oral administration of ginsenoside Rb₁ from *Panax ginseng*. *Journal of Pharmacy and Pharmacology* 50: 1155-1160.

Ang-Lee, M.K., Moss, J., and Yuan, C.S. (2001). Herbal medicines and perioperative care. *Journal of the American Medical Association* 286: 208-216.

Avakian, E.V. and Evonuk, E. (1979). Effect of *Panax ginseng* extract on tissue glycogen and adrenal cholesterol depletion during prolonged exercise. *Planta Medica* 36: 43-48.

Awang, D.V.C. (1991). Maternal use of ginseng and neonatal androgenization. *Journal of the American Medical Association* 265: 1828 (letter).

Awang, D.V.C. (2000). The neglected ginsenosides of North American ginseng (*Panax quinquefolius* L). *Journal of Herbs, Species and Medicinal Plants* 7(2): 103-109.

Baek, N.I., Kim, J.M., Park, J.H., Ryu, J.H., Kim, D.S., Lee, Y.H., Park, J.D., and Kim, S.I. (1997). Ginsenoside Rs₃, a genuine dammarane glycoside from Korean red ginseng. *Archives of Pharmaceutical Research* 20: 280-282.

Bahrke, M.S. and Morgan, W.P. (1994). Evaluation of the ergogenic properties of ginseng. *Sports Medicine* 18: 229-248.

Bahrke, M.S. and Morgan, W.P. (2000). Evaluation of the ergogenic properties of ginseng: An update. *Sports Medicine* 29: 113-133.

Blumenthal, M. (1997). *Popular Herbs in the U.S. Market: Therapeutic Monographs*. Austin, TX: American Botanical Council, pp. 37-38.

Blumenthal, M., Busse, W.R., Goldberg, A., Gruenwald, J., Hall, T., Riggins, C.W., and Rister, R.S. (Eds.) (1998). *The Complete German Commission E Monographs*. Austin, TX: American Botanical Council, p. 90.

Bradley, P.R. (Ed.) (1992). *British Herbal Compendium*, 1. Bournemouth, Dorset, England: British Herbal Medicine Association, pp. 115-118.

Brekhman, I.I. and Dardymov, I.V. (1969). New substances of plant origin which increase nonspecific resistance. *Annual Review of Pharmacology* 9: 419-430.

Büchi, K. and Jenny, E. (1984). On the interference of the standardized ginseng extract G115 and pure ginsenosides with agonists of the progesterone receptor of human myometrium. Report dated January 18. Delray Beach, FL: Ginsana USA Corporation (unpublished).

Byun, B.H., Shin, I., Yoon, Y.S., Kim, S.I., and Joe, C.O. (1997). Modulation of protein kinase C activity in NIH 3T3 cells by plant glycosides from *Panax ginseng. Planta Medica* 63: 389-392.

Chang, H.M. and But, P.P.H. (Eds.) (1986). *Pharmacology and Applications of Chinese Materia Medica*, 2. Hong Kong: World Scientific.

Chen, X. and Lee, T.J.F. (1995). Ginsenosides-induced nitric oxide-mediated relaxation of the rabbit corpus cavernosum. *British Journal of Pharmacology* 115: 15-18.

Chen, Y.J. and Dou, D.Q. (1998). Recent advances in studies on *Panax ginseng* in China. In *The 7th International Symposium on Ginseng, Seoul, Korea, September 22-25, 1998, Program and Abstracts*. Seoul, Korea: The Korean Society of Ginseng, p. 83 (poster).

Chin, R.K.H. (1991). Ginseng and common pregnancy disorders. *Asia-Oceania Journal of Obstetrics and Gynaecology* 17: 379-380.

Choi, C.W., Lee, S.I., and Huh, K. (1984). [Effects of ginseng on the hepatic alcohol metabolizing enzyme system activity in chronic alcohol-treated mice]. *Korean Journal of Pharmacology* 20: 13-21.

Choi, H.K., Seong, D.H., and Rha, K.H. (1995). Clinical efficacy of Korean red ginseng for erectile dysfunction. *International Journal of Impotence Research* 7: 181-186.

Choi, J. (1998). The effects of red ginseng intake and exercise on information processing performance in the middle-aged and elderly. In *The 7th International Symposium on Ginseng, Seoul, Korea, September 22-25, 1998, Program and Abstracts*. Seoul, Korea: The Korean Society of Ginseng, p. 101 (poster).

Choi, Y.D., Rha, K.H., and Choi, H.K. (1999). In vitro and in vivo experimental effect of Korean red ginseng on erection. *The Journal of Urology* 162: 1508-1511.

Choi, Y.D., Xin, Z.C., and Choi, H.K. (1998). Effect of Korean red ginseng on the rabbit corpus cavernosal smooth muscle. *International Journal of Impotence Research* 10: 37-43.

Chuang, W.C., Wu, H.K., Sheu, S.J., Chiou, S.H., Chang, H.C., and Chen, Y.P. (1995). A comparative study on commercial samples of Ginseng Radix. *Planta Medica* 61: 459-465.

Court, W.E. (2000). *Ginseng: The Genus Panax*. Amsterdam, the Netherlands: Harwood Academic.

Cui, J., Garle, M., Eneroth, P., and Bjorkhem, I. (1994). What do commercial ginseng preparations contain? *Lancet* 344: 134 (letter).

Cui, X. (1997). Orally administered ginseng extract stimulates liver regeneration in partially hepectomized rats. *Acta Medica et Biologica* 45: 161-166.

D'Angelo, L., Grimaldi, R., Caravaggi, M., Marcoli, M., Perucca, E., Lecchini, S., Frigo, G.M., and Crema, A. (1986). A double-blind, placebo controlled clinical study on the effect of a standardized ginseng extract on psychomotor performance in healthy volunteers. *Journal of Ethnopharmacology* 16: 15-22.

Davydov, M. and Krikorian, A.D. (2000). *Eleutherococcus senticosus* (Rupr. & Maxim.) Maxim. (Araliaceae) as an adaptogen: A closer look. *Journal of Ethnopharmacology* 72: 345-393.

Dega, H., Laporte, J., Frances, C., Herson, S., and Chosidow, O. (1996). Ginseng as a cause for Stevens-Johnson syndrome? *Lancet* 347: 1344.

De Smet, P.A.G.M. (Ed.) (1993). *Adverse Effects of Herbal Drugs,* 1. Berlin, Germany: Springer-Verlag.

Dixit, V.P., Jain, P., Bhandari, K., and Purohit, A.K. (1991). Effects of ginseng (G-115) on serum lipids of hyperlipidaemic rhesus monkeys (*Macaca mulatta*). *Indian Journal of Pharmaceutical Sciences* 52: 88-91.

Dorling, E., Kirchdorfer, A.M., and Rücker, K.H. (1980). Haben ginsenoside einfluss auf das leistungsvermögen? Ergebnisse einer doppelblindstudie [Do ginsenosides influence the performance?]. *Notabene Medici* 10: 241-246, translation.

Engels, H.J., Said, J.M., and Wirth, J.C. (1996). Failure of chronic ginseng supplementation to affect work performance and energy metabolism in healthy adult females. *Nutrition Research* 16: 1295-1305.

Engels, H.J. and Wirth, J.C. (1997). No ergogenic effects of ginseng (*Panax ginseng* C.A Meyer) during graded aerobic exercise. *Journal of the American Dietetic Association* 97: 1110-1115.

Fok, T.F., Lau, S.P., and Hui, C.W. (1985). Chinese herbs in pregnancy and neonatal jaundice. *Hong Kong Journal of Pediatrics* 2: 138-144.

Forgo, I., Kayasseh, L., and Staub, J.J. (1981). Effect of a standardized ginseng extract on general well-being, reaction capacity, pulmonary function, and gonadal hormones. *Medizinische Welt* 32: 751-756.

Foster, S. and Yue, C. (1992). *Herbal Emissaries.* Rochester, VT: Healing Arts Press, pp. 102-112.

Fugh-Berman, A. and Ernst, E. (2001). Herb-drug interactions: Review and assessment of report reliability. *British Journal of Clinical Pharmacology* 52: 587-595.

Fulder, S.J. (1981). Ginseng and the hypothalamic-pituitary control of stress. *American Journal of Chinese Medicine* 9: 112-118.

Fulder, S.J. (1993). *The Book of Ginseng.* Rochester, VT: Healing Arts Press.

Fulder, S.J., Kataria, M., and Gethyn-Smith, B. (1984). A double-blind clinical trial of *Panax ginseng* in aged subjects. In *Proceedings of the 4th International Ginseng Symposium.* Daejeon, Korea: Korea Ginseng and Tobacco Research Institute, pp. 215-223.

Gillis, C.N. (1997). *Panax ginseng* pharmacology: A nitric oxide link? *Biochemical Pharmacology* 54: 1-8.

Hallstrom, C., Fulder, S., and Carruthers, M. (1982). Effect of ginseng on the performance of nurses on night duty. *Comparative Medicine East and West* 6: 277-282.

Harkey, M.R., Henderson, G.L., Gershwin, M.E., Stern, J.S., and Hackman, R.M. (2001). Variability in commercial ginseng products: An analysis of 25 preparations. *American Journal of Clinical Nutrition* 73: 1101-1106.

Hasegawa, H., Sung, J.H., and Benno, Y. (1997). Role of human intestinal *Prevotella oris* in hydrolyzing ginseng saponins. *Planta Medica* 63: 436-440.

Hasegawa, H., Sung, J.H., Matsumiya, S., and Uchiyama, M. (1996). Main ginseng saponin metabolites formed by intestinal bacteria. *Planta Medica* 62: 453-457.

Hasegawa, H., Sung, J.H., Matsumiya, S., Uchiyama, M., Inouye, Y., Kasai, R., and Yamasaki, K. (1995). Reversal of daunomycin and vinblastine resistance in multidrug-resistant P388 leukemia in vitro through enhanced cytotoxicity by terpenoids. *Planta Medica* 61: 409-413.

Hess, F.G. Jr., Parent, R.A., Cox, G.E., Cox, G.E., and Becci, P.J. (1983). Effects of subchronic feeding of ginseng extract G115 in beagle dogs. *Food and Chemical Toxicology* 21: 95-97.

Hiai, S., Yokoyama, H., Oura, H., and Yano, S. (1979). Stimulation of pituitary-adrenocortical system by ginseng saponin. *Endocrinologica Japonica* 26: 661-665.

Hikino, H., Oshima, Y., Suzuki, Y., and Konno, C. (1985). Isolation and hypoglycemic activity of panaxans F, G and H, glycans of *Panax ginseng* roots. *Shoyakugaku Zasshi* 39: 331-333.

Hobbs, C. (1996). *The Ginsengs: A User's Guide*. Santa Cruz, CA: Botanica Press.

Hu, S., Concha, C., Cooray, R., and Holmberg, O. (1995). Ginseng-enhanced oxidative and phagocytic activities of polymorphonuclear leucocytes from bovine peripheral blood and stripping milk. *Veterinary Research* 26: 155-61.

Huh, K., Park, C.M., Lee, S.I., and Choi, C.W. (1985). [The effect of ginseng (butanol fraction) on the acetaldehyde metabolism in mice]. *Yakhak Hoeji* 29: 18-26.

Inoue, M., Wu, C.Z., Dou, D.Q., Chen, Y.J., and Ogihara, Y. (1999). Lipoprotein lipase activation by red ginseng saponins in hyperlipidemia model animals. *Phytomedicine* 6: 257-265.

Ismail, M.F., Gad, M.Z., and Hamdy, M.A. (1999). Study of the hypolipidemic properties of pectin, garlic and ginseng in hypercholesterolemic rabbits. *Pharmacological Research* 39: 157-166.

Janetzky, K. and Morreale, A.P. (1997). Probable interaction between warfarin and ginseng. *American Journal of Health-System Pharmacy* 54: 692-693.

Jones, B.D. and Runikis, A.M. (1987). Interaction of ginseng with phenelzine. *Journal of Clinical Psychopharmacology* 7: 201-202 (letter).

Jung, K.Y., Kim, D.S., Oh, S.R., Lee, I.S., Lee, J.J., Park, J.D., Kim, S.I., and Lee, H.K. (1998). Platelet activating factor antagonistic activity of ginsenosides. *Biological and Pharmaceutical Bulletin* 21: 79-80.

Keum, Y.S., Park, K.K., and Surh, Y.J. (2000). Antioxidant and anti-tumor promoting activities of the methanol extract of heat-processed ginseng. *Cancer Letters* 150: 41-48.

Kim, C., Choi, H., Kim, C.C., Kim, J.K., and Kim, M.S. (1976). Influence of ginseng on mating behavior of male rats. *American Journal of Chinese Medicine* 4: 163-168.

Kim, K.H., Lee, Y.S., Jung, I.S., Park, S.Y., Chung, H.Y., Lee, I.R., and Yun, Y.S. (1998). Acidic polysaccharide from *Panax ginseng,* ginsan, induces Th1 and macrophage cytokines and generates LAK cells in synergy with rIL-2. *Planta Medica* 64: 110-115.

Kim, S.E., Lee, Y.H., Park, J.H., and Lee, S.K. (1999). Ginsenoside-Rs3, a new diol-type ginseng saponin, selectively elevates protein levels of p53 and p21^{WAF1} leading to induction of apoptosis in SK-HEP-1 cells. *Anticancer Research* 19: 487-492.

Kim, W.Y., Kim, J.M., Han, S.B., Lee, S.K., Kim, N.D., Park, M.K., Kim, C.K., and Park, J.H. (2000). Steaming of ginseng at high temperature enhances biological activity. *Journal of Natural Products* 63: 1702-1704.

Kim, Y.H., Park, K.H., and Rho, H.M. (1996). Transcriptional activation of the Cu,Zn-superoxide dismutase gene through the AP2 site by ginsenoside Rb$_2$ extracted from a medicinal plant, *Panax ginseng. Journal of Biological Chemistry* 271: 24539-24543.

Kim, Y.W., Song, D.K., Kim, W.H., Lee, K.M., Wie, M.B., Kim, Y.H., Kee, S.H., and Cho, M.K. (1997). Long-term oral administration of ginseng extract decreases serum Gamma-globulin and IgG$_1$ subtype in mice. *Journal of Ethnopharmacology* 58: 55-58.

Konno, C. and Hikino, H. (1987). Isolation and hypoglycemic activity of panaxans M, N, O, and P, glycans of *Panax ginseng* roots. *International Journal of Crude Drug Research* 25: 53-56.

Konno, C., Murakami, M., Oshima, Y., and Hikino, H. (1985). Isolation and hypoglycemic activity of panaxans Q, R, S, T and U, glycans of *Panax ginseng* roots. *Journal of Ethnopharmacology* 14: 69-74.

Konno, C., Sugiyama, K., Kano, M., Takahashi, M., and Hikino, H. (1984). Isolation and hypoglycemic activity of panaxans A, B, C, D, and E, glycans of *Panax ginseng* roots. *Planta Medica* 50: 434-438.

Koren, G., Randor, S., Martin, S., and Danneman, D. (1990). Maternal ginseng use associated with neonatal androgenization. *Journal of the American Medical Association* 264: 2866 (letter).

Kwon, B.M., Kim, M.K., Baek, N.I., Kim, D.S., Park, J.D., Kim, Y.K., Lee, H.K., and Kim, S.I. (1999). Acyl-CoA: Cholesterol acyltransferase inhibitory activity of ginseng sapogenins, produced from the ginseng saponins. *Bioorganic and Medicinal Chemistry Letters* 9: 1375-1378.

Lawrence, R.A. (2001). A thirty-five-year-old woman experiencing difficulty with breastfeeding. *Journal of the American Medical Association* 285: 73-80.

Lee, B.H., Lee, S.J., Hui, J.H., Lee, S., Sung, J.H., Huh, J.D., and Moon, C.K. (1998). In vitro antigenotoxic activity of novel ginseng saponin metabolites formed by intestinal bacteria. *Planta Medica* 64: 500-503.

Lee, B.M., Lee, S.K., and Kim, H.S. (1998). Inhibition of oxidative DNA damage, 8-OHdG, and carbonyl contents in smokers treated with antioxidants (vitamin E, vitamin C, β-carotene and red ginseng). *Cancer Letters* 132: 219-227.

Lee, F.C., Ko, J.H., Park, J.K., and Lee, J.S. (1987). Effects of *Panax ginseng* on blood alcohol clearance in man. *Clinical and Experimental Pharmacology and Physiology* 14: 543-546.

Lee, K.Y., Lee, S.K., Kim, S.I., Park, J.H., and Lee, S.K. (1997). Ginsenoside-Rg$_5$ suppresses cyclin E-dependent protein kinase activity via up-regulation of p21^{WAF1} with concomitant down-regulation of cdc25A in SK HEP-1 cells. *Anticancer Research* 17: 1067-1072.

Lee, S.J., Ko, W.G., and Lee, B.H. (2000). Induction of apoptosis by a novel intestinal metabolite of ginseng saponin via cytochrome *c*-mediated activation of caspase-3 protease. *Biochemical Pharmacology* 60: 677-685.

Lee, Y., Chung, E., Lee, K.Y., Lee, Y.H., Huh, B., and Lee, S.K. (1997). Ginsenoside-Rg$_1$, one of the major active molecules from *Panax ginseng,* is a functional ligand of glucocorticoid receptor. *Molecular and Cellular Endocrinology* 133: 135-140.

Lee, Y.S., Chung, I.S., Lee, I.R., Kim, K.H., Hong, W.S., and Yun, Y.S. (1997). Activation of multiple effector pathways of immune system by the antineoplastic immunostimulator acidic polysaccharide ginsan isolated from *Panax ginseng*. *Anticancer Research* 17: 323-332.

Lewis, W.H., Zenger, V.E., and Lynch, R.G. (1983). No adaptogenic response of mice to ginseng and *Eleutherococcus* infusions. *Journal of Ethnopharmacology* 8: 209-214.

Liu, J., Burdette, J.E., Xu, H., Gu, C., van Breemen, R.B., Bhat, K.P., Booth, N., Constantinou, A.I., Pezzuto, J.M., Fong, H.H., et al. (2001). Evaluation of estrogenic activity of plant extracts for the potential treatment of menopausal symptoms. *Journal of Agricultural and Food Chemistry* 49: 2472-2479.

Liu, J., Wang, S., Liu, H., Yang, L., and Nan, G. (1995). Stimulatory effect of saponin from *Panax ginseng* on immune function of lymphocytes in the elderly. *Mechanisms of Aging and Development* 83: 43-53.

Liu, W.K., Xu, S.X., and Che, C.T. (2000). Antiproliferative effect of ginseng saponins on human prostate cancer cell line. *Life Sciences* 67: 1297-1306.

Lu, W., Zheng, G., and Cai, J. (1998). First total synthesis of panaxytriol, a potent antitumor agent isolated from *Panax ginseng*. *Synlett* (July) (7): 737-738.

Ma, Y., Mai, L., Malley, L., and Doucet, M. (1996). Distribution and proportion of major ginsenosides and quality control of ginseng products. *Chinese Journal of Medicinal Chemistry* 6: 11-21.

Marcilhac, A., Dakine, N., Bourhim, N., Guillaume, V., Grino, M., Drieu, K., and Oliver, C. (1998). Effect of chronic administration of *Ginkgo biloba* extract or ginkgolide on the hypothalamic-pituitary-adrenal axis in the rat. *Life Sciences* 62: 2329-2340.

McNaughton, L., Egan, G., and Caelli, G. (1989). A comparison of Chinese and Russian ginseng as ergogenic aids to improve various facets of physical fitness. *International Clinical Nutrition Review* 9: 32-35.

Murase, K., Yamamoto, T., and Hayashi, K. (1994). Nerve growth factor-like immunoreactive substance in *Panax ginseng* extract. *Bioscience, Biotechnology, and Biochemistry* 58: 1638-1641.

Newall, C.A., Anderson, L.A., and Phillipson, J.D. (1996). *Herbal Medicines: A Guide for Health Care Professionals.* London: The Pharmaceutical Press, pp. 145-150.

Ng, T.B. and Yeung, H.W. (1985). Hypoglycemic constituents of *Panax ginseng*. *General Pharmacology* 6: 549-552.

Odani, T., Tanizawa, H., and Takino, Y. (1983). Studies on the absorption, distribution, excretion and metabolism of ginseng saponins. III. The absorption, distribution and excretion of ginsenoside Rb_1 in the rat. *Chemical and Pharmaceutical Bulletin* 31: 1059-1066.

Oh, K.W., Kim, H.S., and Wagner, G.C. (1997). Ginseng total saponin inhibits the dopaminergic depletions induced by methamphetamine. *Planta Medica* 63: 80-81.

Okrent, N. (1994). Ginseng. *Townsend Letter for Doctors* (February/March) (127): 162-168, 304-309.

Oshima, Y., Konno, C., and Hikino, H. (1985). Isolation and hypoglycemic activity of panaxans I, J, K and L, glycans of *Panax ginseng* roots. *Journal of Ethnopharmacology* 14: 255-259.

Owen, R.T. (1981). Ginseng—A pharmacological profile. *Drugs of Today* 17: 343-351.

Palmer, B.V., Montgomery, A.C.V., and Monteiro, J.C.M.P. (1978). Ginseng [sic] and mastalgia. *British Medical Journal* 1 (May 13): 1284.

Park, H.J., Lee, J.H., Song, Y.B., and Park, K.H. (1996). Effects of dietary supplementation of lipophilic fraction from *Panax ginseng* on cGMP and cAMP in rat platelets and on blood coagulation. *Biological and Pharmaceutical Bulletin* 19: 1434-1439.

Park, J.A., Lee, K.Y., Oh, Y.J., Kim, K.W., and Lee, S.K. (1997). Activation of caspase 3 protease via a Bcl-2-insensitive pathway during the process of ginsenoside Rh_2-induced apoptosis. *Cancer Letters* 121: 73-81.

Parker, F. (1996). Skin diseases of general importance. In Bennett, J.C. and Plum, F. (Eds.), *Cecil Textbook of Medicine,* Twentieth Edition (p. 2206). Philadelphia, PA: W.B. Saunders Company.

Pearce, P.Y., Zois, I., Wynne, K.N., and Funder, J.W. (1982). *Panax ginseng* and *Eleutherococcus senticosus* extracts—In vitro studies on binding to steroid receptors. *Endocrinologica Japonica* 29: 567-573.

Petkov, V. (1978). Effect of ginseng on the brain biogenic monoamines and 3,5-AMP system. *Arzneimittel-Forschung/Drug Research* 28: 388-393

Petkov, V.D. and Mosharrof, A.H. (1987). Effects of standardized ginseng extract on learning, memory, and physical capabilities. *American Journal of Chinese Medicine* 15: 19-29.

Quiroga, H.A. (1982). [Comparative double-blind study of the action of Ginsana G115® and Hydergin® on cerebrovascular deficits]. *Orientación Médica* 31: 201-202, translation.

Quiroga, H.A. and Imbriano, A.E. (1979). [The effect of *Panax ginseng* extract on cerebrovascular deficits]. *Orientación Médica* 28: 86-87, translation.

Rosenfeld, M. (1989). Evaluation of the efficacy of standardized ginseng extract in patients with psychophysical asthenia and neurological disorders. *La Semana Medica* 173: 148-154.

Ryu, S.J. and Chien, Y.Y. (1995). Ginseng-associated cerebral arteritis. *Neurology* 45: 829-830.

Sato, K., Mochizuki, M., Saiki, I., Yoo, Y.C., Samukawa, K., and Azuma, I. (1994). Inhibition of tumor angiogenesis and metastasis by a saponin of *Panax ginseng*, ginsenoside-Rb$_2$. *Biological and Pharmaceutical Bulletin* 17: 635-639.

Scaglione, F., Cogo, R., Cocuzza, C., Arcidiacono, M., and Beretta, A. (1994). Immunomodulatory effects of *Panax ginseng* C.A. Meyer (G115) on alveolar macrophages from patients suffering with chronic bronchitis. *International Journal of Immunotherapy* 10: 21-24.

Scaglione, F., Ferrara, F., Dugnani, S., Falchi, M., Santoro, G., and Fraschini, E. (1990). Immunomodulatory effects of two extracts of *Panax ginseng* C.A. Meyer. *Drugs Under Experimental and Clinical Research* 16: 537-542.

Shader, R.I. and Greenblatt, D.J. (1985). Phenelzine and the dream machine— Ramblings and reflections. *Journal of Clinical Psychopharmacology* 5: 65 (editorial).

Sharma, K.K., Sharma, A., Chaturvedi, M., Verma, P.K., Joshi, S.C., and Dixit, V.P. (1999). Testicular dysfunction in rat/rabbit following *Panax ginseng* (G-115 Fr.I) feeding. *International Ginseng Conference '99 Programme and Abstracts,* July 8-11, 1999, Hong Kong. Hong Kong, China: BDG Communications Management Ltd.

Shibata, S., Tanaka, O., Shoji, J., and Saito, H. (1985). Chemistry and pharmacology of *Panax*. In Wagner, H., Hikimo, H., and Farnsworth, N.R. (Eds.), *Economic and Medicinal Plant Research,* 1. (pp. 217-284). New York: Academic Press.

Shinkai, K., Akedo, H., Mukai, M., Imamura, F., Isoai, A., Kobayashi, M., and Kitagawa, I. (1996). Inhibition of in vitro tumor cell invasion by ginsenoside Rg$_3$. *Japanese Journal of Cancer Research* 87: 357-362.

Shoji, T. and Kisara, K. (1975). [Pharmacological studies of crude drugs showing antitussive and expectorant activity (Report 1)—The combined effects of some crude drugs in antitussive activity and acute toxicity. *Oyo Yakuri [Pharmacokinetics]* 10: 407-415.

Siegal, R.K. (1979). Ginseng abuse syndrome—Problems with the panacea. *Journal of the American Medical Association* 241: 1614-1615.

Sonoda, Y., Kasahara, T., Mukaida, N., Shimizu, N., Tomoda, M., and Takeda, T. (1998). Stimulation of interleukin-8 production by acidic polysaccharides from the root of *Panax ginseng. Immunopharmacology* 38: 287-294.

SØrensen, H. and Sonne, J.A. (1996). Double-masked study of the effects of ginseng on cognitive functions. *Current Therapeutic Research* 57: 959-968.

Sotaniemi, E.A., Haapakoski, E., and Rautio, A. (1995). Ginseng therapy in non-insulin-dependent diabetic patients. *Diabetes Care* 18: 1373-1375.

Srisurapanon, S., Apibal, S., Siripol, R., Rungroeng, K., Cherdrugsi, P., Vanich-Angkul, V., and Timvipark, C. (1997). The effect of standardized ginseng extract on peripheral blood leukocytes and lymphocyte subsets: A preliminary study in young healthy adults. *Journal of the Medical Association of Thailand* 80(Suppl. 1): S82-S85.

Sticher, O. (1998). Getting to the root of ginseng. *Chemtech* 28: 26-32.

Tachikawa, E., Kudo, K., Harada, K., Kashimoto, T., Miyate, Y., Kakizaki, A., and Takahashi, E. (1999). Effects of ginseng saponins on responses induced by various receptor stimuli. *European Journal of Pharmacology* 369: 23-32.

Takahashi, M. and Tokuyama, S. (1998). Pharmacological and physiological effects of ginseng on actions induced by opioids and psychostimulants. *Methods and Findings in Experimental and Clinical Pharmacology* 20: 77-84.

Tomoda, M., Hirabayashhi, K., Shimizu, N., Gonda, R., and Ohara, N (1994). The core structure of ginsenan PA, a phagocytosis-activating polysaccharide from the root of *Panax ginseng. Biological and Pharmaceutical Bulletin* 17: 1287-1291.

Tomoda, M., Takeda, K., Shimizu, N., Gonda, R., Ohara, N., Takada, K., and Hirabayashi, K. (1993). Characterization of two acidic polysaccharides having immunological activities from the root of *Panax ginseng. Biological and Pharmaceutical Bulletin* 16: 22-25.

Tsang, D., Yeung, H.W., Tso, W.W., and Peck, H. (1985). Ginseng saponins: Influence on neurotransmitter uptake in rat brain synaptosomes. *Planta Medica* 51: 221-224.

Tu, G., Fang, Q., Guo, J., Yuan, S., Chen, C., Chen, J., Chen, Z., Cheng, S., Jin, R., Li, M., et al. (Eds.) (1992). *Pharmacopoeia of the People's Republic of China.* Guangzhou, China: Guangdong Science and Technology Press, pp. 163-164.

Udelsman, R., Ramp, J., Galluci, W.T., Gordon, A., Lipford, E., Norton, J.A., and Loriaux, D.L. (1986). Adaptation during surgical stress. A re-evaluation of the role of glucocorticoids. *Journal of Clinical Investigation* 77: 1377-1381.

Vogler, B.K., Pittler, M.H., and Ernst, E. (1999). The efficacy of ginseng: A systematic review of randomized clinical trials. *European Journal of Clinical Pharmacology* 55: 567-575.

Vuksan, V., Stevenpiper, J.L., Koo, V.Y.Y., Francis, T., Beljan-Zdravkovic, U., Xu, Z., and Vidgen, E. (2000). American ginseng (*Panax quinquefolius* L.) reduces postprandial glycemia in nondiabetic subjects and subjects with type 2 diabetes mellitus. *Archives of Internal Medicine* 160: 1009-1013.

Watanabe, H., Ohta, H., Imamura, L., Asakura, W., Matoba, Y., and Matsumoto, K. (1991). Effect of *Panax ginseng* on age-related changes in the spontaneous motor activity and dopaminergic nervous system in the rat. *Japanese Journal of Pharmacology* 55: 51-56.

Wen, J. (2001). Species diversity, nomenclature, phylogeny, biogeography, and classification of ginseng genus (*Panax* L., Araliaceae). In Punja, Z.K. (Ed.), *Utilization of Biotechnological, Genetic and Cultural Approaches for North American and Asian Ginseng Improvement*. Proceedings of the International Ginseng Workshop. Vancouver, B.C., Canada: Simon Fraser University Press.

Wiklund, I.K., Mattsson, L.A., Lindgren, R., and Limoni, C. (1999). Effects of a standardized ginseng extract on quality of life and physiological parameters in symptomatic postmenopausal women: A double-blind, placebo-controlled trial. *International Journal of Clinical Pharmacology Research* 19: 89-99.

Yamaguchi, H., Kasai, R., Matsura, H., Tanaka, O., and Fuwa, T. (1988). High-performance liquid chromatographic analysis of acidic saponins of ginseng and related plants. *Chemical and Pharmaceutical Bulletin* 36: 3468-3473.

Yamamoto, M., Kumagai, A., and Yamamura, Y. (1977). Stimulatory effect of *Panax ginseng* principles on DNA and protein synthesis in rat testes. *Arzneimittel-Forschung/Drug Research* 27: 1404-1405.

Yang, S.Z. (1998). *The Divine Farmer's Materia Medica: A Translation of the Shen Nong Ben Cao Jing*. Boulder, CO: Blue Poppy Press, Inc., pp. 24-25.

Yen, K.Y. (1992). *The Illustrated Chinese Materia Medica, Crude and Prepared*. Taipei, Taiwan: SMC Publishing Inc., pp. 40-41.

Yoshimura, H., Kimura, N., and Sugiura, K. (1998). Preventive effects of various ginseng saponins on the development of copulatory disorder induced by prolonged individual housing in male mice. *Methods and Findings in Experimental and Clinical Pharmacology* 20: 59-64.

Yun, T.K. (1996). Experimental and epidemiological evidence of the cancer-preventive effects of *Panax ginseng* C.A. Meyer. *Nutrition Reviews* 54(Suppl.): S71-S81.

Yun, T.K. and Choi, S.Y. (1990). A case-control study of ginseng intake and cancer. *International Journal of Epidemiology* 19: 871-876.

Yun, T.K. and Choi, S.Y. (1995). Preventive effect of ginseng intake against various human cancers: A case-control study on 1,987 pairs. *Cancer Epidemiology, Biomarkers and Prevention* 4: 401-408.

Yun, T.K., Yun, Y.S., and Han, I.W. (1983). Anticarcinogenic effect of long-term oral administration of red ginseng on newborn mice exposed to various chemical carcinogens. *Cancer Detection and Prevention* 6: 515-525.

Yun, Y.S. and Kim, S.H. (1988). Inhibition of development of benzo[*a*]pyrene-induced mouse pulmonary adenoma by several natural products in medium-term bioassay system. *Journal of the Korean Cancer Association* 20: 133-142.

Zhu, M., Chan, K.W., Ng, L.S., Chang, Q., Chang, S., and Li, R.C. (1999). Possible influences of ginseng on the pharmacokinetics and pharmacodynamics of warfarin in rats. *Journal of Pharmacy and Pharmacology* 51: 175-180.

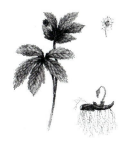

Goldenseal

BOTANICAL DATA

Classification and Nomenclature

Scientific name: *Hydrastis canadensis* L.

Family name: Ranunculaceae

Common names: goldenseal, yellow root, jaundice root, turmeric root, eye root, Indian dye, yellow puccoon, ground raspberry

Description

Hydrastis canadensis is a perennial herbaceous plant found in rich shady woods and moist meadows in eastern North America, especially in Ohio, northern Kentucky, Indiana, and Virginia, whereas in Canada it is restricted to southwestern Ontario (Sinclair and Catling, 2000). Populations of goldenseal in the wild have nevertheless been greatly diminished in recent years due to overcollection and habitat loss, which has placed this plant on the endangered-species list. Due to concerns about overharvesting and increasing market demand, it is now commercially cultivated across the country, and especially in the Blue Ridge Mountains (Foster, 1991; Snow, 1996).

Goldenseal grows to about 30 cm in height with a simple, hairy stem, usually bearing a single-lobed basal leaf and two-lobed cauline leaves near the top. The flower is terminal, solitary, and erect, with small greenish-white sepals and no petals; it blooms in May and June. The fruit is an oblong, compound, orange-red berry containing two black seeds in each carpel. The medicinal rhizome is horizontal and irregularly knotted, bears numerous long slender roots, and is bright yellow with an acrid scent (Foster, 1991; Duke, 1985).

The name *goldenseal* comes from the yellow scars left on the rhizome by the stem that bursts forth every spring; these scars resemble the imprint of an old-fashioned wax letter seal. *Hydrastis* is a Greek word meaning "to accomplish with water" (Duke, 1985; Snow, 1996).

Recently, other species of plants purported to be *H. canadensis* have been sold in place of the bulk dried herb on the U.S. wholesale market. This substitution is due to the high market price goldenseal now commands and the shortage of cultivated supply. Care must be taken in ascertaining accurate identification of dried material (Snow, 1996; Govindan and Govindan, 2000).

HISTORY AND TRADITIONAL USES

Native Americans used goldenseal both as a dye and as a medicinal plant. Medicinal use in treating inflammatory conditions induced by allergy or infection appears to have been based on goldenseal's ability to soothe the mucous membranes that line the respiratory, digestive, and genitourinary tracts. Native Americans taught the first European settlers to use goldenseal root to treat skin diseases, ulcers, gonorrhea, and arrow wounds. Both the Iroquois and the Cherokee used goldenseal extensively. Folk use included treatments of sore eyes, hepatitis, menstrual difficulty, dyspepsia, and fever. Goldenseal became known as one of the most powerful North American medicinal plants and was included in the *U.S. Pharmacopoeia* from 1831-1936, and then in the *National Formulary* until 1960 (Foster, 1991; Duke, 1985). Goldenseal is used as a treatment for canker sores and sore mouth (Govindan and Govindan, 2000); many herbal practitioners advise that gargling with a solution of goldenseal can arrest a sore throat much more effectively than ingesting the same amount of the root in capsule form (Bergner, 1996).

The root of goldenseal supplied Native Americans with a brilliant yellow dye for coloring their clothing and weapons, as well as for painting their skin (Duke, 1985).

In Chinese medicine, three species of *Coptis,* a related genus, are used for many of the same functions as goldenseal, such as problems affecting the heart, liver, gallbladder, stomach, and large intestine (Chang and But, 1986). Other medicinal plants containing berberine include Oregon grape root (*Mahonia aquifolium* [Pursh] Nutt.) and Amur corktree (*Phellodendron amurense* Rupr.) (Leung and Foster, 1996).

CHEMISTRY

Nitrogenous Compounds

Alkaloids

The primary active constituents of goldenseal are the isoquinoline alkaloids hydrastine (1.5% to 4%) and berberine (0.5% to 6%) (Leung and

Foster, 1996). Goldenseal contains lesser amounts of the alkaloids berberastine, canadine (tetrahydroberberine), canadaline, 1-α-hydrastine, isohydrastindine, (s)-corypalmine, and (s)-isocorypalmine (Genest and Hughes, 1969; Gleye and Stanislas, 1972; Leone et al., 1996; Messana et al., 1980).

Other Constituents

Other constituents include meconin, chlorogenic acid, lipids, resin, starch, sugars, and a small amount of volatile oil (Leung and Foster, 1996).

THERAPEUTIC APPLICATIONS

Many herbal practitioners consider goldenseal to be indispensable for its many documented activities: digestive, antibiotic, immunostimulatory, uterotonic, choleretic, carminative, antidiarrheal, antifungal, and antimicrobial (Murray, 1995; Mills and Bone, 2000).

Goldenseal's medicinal effects are mostly attributed to the isoquinoline alkaloid berberine, on which exists the most clinical data (Leung and Foster, 1996). Some studies have begun investigating the other abundant alkaloid, hydrastine (Snow, 1996). Hydrastine is a central nervous system (CNS) stimulant and has direct myocardial and intestinal smooth-muscle-depressant effects (Brinker, 1998). The *British Herbal Compendium* by Bradley (1992) states that the activity of goldenseal is mainly due to hydrastine, which is vasoconstrictive and active on the nervous, reproductive, respiratory, and cardiac systems. Both berberine and hydrastine are choleretic, spasmolytic, sedative, and antibacterial; canadine is a stimulant to uterine muscle (Bradley, 1992).

PRECLINICAL STUDIES

Cardiovascular and Circulatory Functions

Arrythmia

Berberine was shown by Huang et al. (1992) to inhibit experimental ventricular arrhythmias induced by aconitine, ouabain, and barium chloride in rats by 62%. In the same study, 8/18 dogs with induced ischemic left ventricular heart failure administered berberine showed dramatic alleviation of left ventricular failure. The underlying mechanism of the positive inotropic effect of berberine is thought to be due to stimulation of the β-receptor of the myocardial cell membrane and to direct action on the myocardium. The reduction of systemic vascular resistance shown was reported as being due to significant vasodilating and α-adrenergic blocking activity.

Cardiotonic; Cardioprotection

Protective effects of berberine were shown against anoxia and re-oxygenation damage in the rat heart. Berberine significantly reduced creatine phosphokinase released during the reoxygenation period, and ultra-structural damage was reduced (Zhou et al., 1993). At a low concentration (1×10^{-6} M, approximating an amount found in the therapeutic use of berberine-containing herbs used in Chinese medicine), berberine caused significant in vitro relaxation of norepinephrine-tensed isolated rat aorta, but only in the presence of endothelium. Lower concentrations of berberine were ineffective (Wong, 1998). In isolated mesenteric arteries of rats, berberine exhibited vasorelaxant activity, which was partly ameliorated upon the removal of endothelium. Berberine also inhibited the proliferation of isolated rat aortic smooth muscle cells in vitro (IC_{50} 2.3×10^{-5} M) (Ko et al., 2000).

Digestive, Hepatic, and Gastrointestinal Functions

Diarrhea

Extracts of berberine-containing plants (*Berberis aristata* and others) have been used as antidiarrheal medications in Ayurvedic medicine in India and in the traditional medicine of China for the past 3,000 years (Chang and But, 1986). An antisecretory effect of berberine is noted to be limited to certain kinds of diarrhea (Rabbani et al., 1987). Berberine sulfate was shown to inhibit the intestinal secretory response induced by *Vibrio cholerae* and *Escherichia coli* by 70% in vivo. However, the drug was effective when given either before or after enterotoxin binding (Sack and Froelich, 1982). In the human colon (in vitro), berberine was shown to inhibit ion transport. Based on studies using a human model of intestinal ion transport, the antisecretory activity of berberine appears to be due to a direct action on epithelial cells, possibly through the blockade of potassium channels (Taylor et al., 1999).

Hepatic Functions

Rats pretreated with berberine (4 mg/kg p.o. twice daily) showed significantly reduced levels of alkaline phosphatase (ALP) and serum transaminases (ALT and AST) following a single toxic dose of acetaminophen (640 mg/kg p.o.) compared to controls. Carbon tetrachloride (CCl_4)-induced (1.5 mL/kg p.o.) hepatotoxicity was also significantly ameliorated by pretreatment with berberine in rats, although not as much as the protection afforded against acetaminophen. In posttreatment tests, berberine (4 mg/kg p.o.) administered 6 h after treating rats with acetaminophen (640 mg/kg p.o.) caused serum levels of ALP, AST, and ALT to decrease significantly compared to controls not posttreated with berberine; however, the hepatotoxic effects of CCl_4 were not ameliorated by berberine as a posttreatment (Janbaz and Gilani, 2000).

Endocrine and Hormonal Functions

Adrenal Functions

Berberine has shown α-adrenergic antagonistic activities in isolated animal organs. In rabbit aorta, berberine antagonized the actions of phenylephrine and norepinephrine (Ölmez and Ilhan, 1992). In studies with male rat anococcygeus muscle, Yao et al. (1987) found that berberine acted like yohimbine and prazosin in showing competitive blocking activity against α_1- and α_2-adrenoreceptors. In a similar study, Yao et al. (1989) reported that berberine could relax 5-hydroxytryptamine-induced muscle contractions. Palmery et al. (1996) have shown that an extract of goldenseal exhibits an inhibitory action on adrenaline-induced contractions in rat thoracic aorta in vitro (IC_{50} 8.79×10^{-7} M). The constituents responsible were identified as the alkaloids canadaline (IC_{50} 2.60×10^{-6} M), berberine (IC_{50} 3.25×10^{-6} M), and canadine (IC_{50} 5.18×10^{-6} M). Including the inactive alkaloid β-hydrastine, the alkaloid mixture showed an IC_{50} of 2.86×10^{-7} M. Therefore, Palmery and colleagues concluded that the mixture of active alkaloids, producing a greater adrenolytic action than any one alone, acted synergistically. Moreover, acting in a dose-dependent manner, the total extract of the roots and rhizomes was able to inhibit contractions induced by higher doses of adrenaline, whereas the individual alkaloids did not. Palmery and colleagues concluded that these alkaloids appear to account for the vasoconstrictive activity of goldenseal, which led to its popular use.

Immune Functions; Inflammation and Disease

Cancer

Antiproliferative activity. In vitro antiproliferation of six types of esophageal cancer lines was found from coculturing the cells with berberine (ID_{50} 0.11 to 0.90 µg/mL) (Wu et al., 1998). The in vitro proliferation of human myeloma cells was inhibited by berberine (IC_{50} 5 M) by a mechanism that appeared to be due partly to a direct blockade of potassium channels (Iizuka et al., 2000).

Antitumor activity of berberine was demonstrated in Swiss albino mice with Dalton's lymphoma ascites tumors. From consecutive daily intraperitoneal administration of the alkaloid at a nontoxic dose (100 mg/kg i.p.

for ten days), ascites-bearing mice showed a significant 32% increase in life span ($p < 0.001$) compared to untreated controls. Oral administration of berberine resulted in a 5% increase in life span and then only from a dose of 250 mg/kg. However, against solid tumors induced by Dalton's lymphoma ascites cells, the same dosage of berberine administered orally produced a significant decrease in tumor volume compared to controls (1.5 cm^3 versus 5.06 cm^3, $p < 0.001$). The result against solid tumors was also significant from berberine administered intraperitoneally compared to untreated controls (0.86 cm^3 versus 5.5 cm^3, $p < 0.01$) (Anis et al., 1999).

Chemopreventive activity. Berberine has shown dose-dependent in vitro inhibitory activity against the tumor-inducing chemical arylamine and the activity of its major metabolizing enzyme, N-acetyltransferase (NAT), in human bladder tumor cells (Chung, Wu, Chu, et al., 1999), human colon tumor cells (Lin, Chung, et al., 1999), and human leukemia cells (Chung et al., 2000).

Animal studies indicate that berberine suppresses the promoting effect of teleocidin on skin-tumor formation. Based on folk use of goldenseal as an anti-inflammatory, investigations by Nishino et al. (1986) found that berberine sulfate could inhibit the activity of inflammatory tumor promoters 12-O-tetradecanoylphorbol-13-acetate (TPA) and teleocidin in vitro. In addition, the compound appeared to inhibit the stimulation of $^{32}P_i$ incorporation into phospholipids of cell membranes and hexose transport activity, and was shown to have antitumor-promoting activity in two-stage carcinogenesis experiments on mouse skin. In mice treated with the tumor-inducing substance teleocidin, those that received an application of berberine sulfate prior to weekly teleocidin treatments developed far fewer tumors than untreated control mice.

Chemotherapy adjunct treatments. Swiss albino mice implanted with Dalton's lymphoma ascites tumor cells were treated seven days later with whole body hyperthermia (43°C for 30 min) with and without concomitant berberine (250 mg/kg p.o. for ten days). In the combined treatment group, berberine produced a synergistic effect, with the volume of the resulting solid tumors that formed showing significant reduction of 78% (1.74 cm^3 versus 3.43 cm^3 in the hyperthermia-only-treated mice and 4.3 cm^3 in the untreated control group). Synergistic reductions in tumor volume were also found with orally administered berberine in combination with radiation treatment and with cyclophosphamide, resulting in 76% and 82% reductions in tumor volume, respectively (Anis et al., 1999).

Cytotoxicity. In vitro cytotoxic activity of berberine has been demonstrated in a wide variety of tumor cells (Iwasa et al., 2001). At a concentration of 10 ppm or less, berberine has shown cytotoxic activity against human uterus carcinoma (Hela), human ovary carcinoma (SVKO$_3$), and human larynx carcinoma (Hep-2) cells (Orfila et al., 2000). Selective and dose-dependent cytotoxicity was shown from berberine against C6 glioma cells at concentrations of 10-100 mg/mL without considerable toxicity against NIH 3T3 fibroblast cells (Korkmaz et al., 2000). Berberine induced apoptotic cell death through the induction of morphological changes and internucleosomal DNA fragmentation in leukemia cells (Kumazawa et al., 1984). In human leukemia cells (HL-60), berberine-induced apoptosis was shown to be associated with telomerase activity and down-regulation of nucleophosmin/B23 (Wu et al., 1999). Time- and dose-dependent inhibition of activator protein-1 activity of human hepatoma cells (KIM-1) was shown from berberine at concentrations of 0.3 μM (IC$_{50}$ approximately 1 μM). Nearly complete inhibition was found from berberine at 10 μM (Fukuda et al., 1999).

Immune Functions

Immunopotentiation. Rehman et al. (1999) examined the effects of continuous treatment with a goldenseal-root extract (Eclectic Institute, Sandy, Oregon) on antigen-specific immunity in male rats over a six-week treatment period (6.6 g in glycerin solvent/L drinking water) compared to glycerin-only-treated rats. Drinking water was provided in addition to the goldenseal-extract drinking water. No significant difference was found in the consumption levels of treated and nontreated controls. Limited to recording changes in immunoglobulins G and M, Rehman and colleagues found no significant difference in IgG levels during the first three weeks and a trend toward lower levels in the last three weeks of treatment, compared to the controls which reached significance on day 42 only. IgM levels became significantly higher in the goldenseal group on day 4 and were still significantly higher on days 11 and 15, after which they showed no significant difference compared to levels in the control group. The authors commented that IgM levels peaked at days 7 through 10 and then declined after animals received a booster injection of a keyhole limpet hemocyanin (KLH) antigen, which was used to elicit anti-KHL IgG and IgM antibodies for measurement (days 0, 14, and 28). The goldenseal-treated rats showed an augmented IgM response for the first two weeks and no augmentation in the IgG response. The effect amounted to an accelerated antibody response, which permitted a more rapid increase in levels of IgM or an enhancement of "the acute primary IgM response." Rehman and colleagues also commented that further studies of immunomodulatory medicinal plants should take the matter of time dependence into consideration to pinpoint times of maximal effects.

Berberine alkaloids have shown potent macrophage-activating activity, which in turn induces cytostatic activity against tumor cells. In mice, and in vitro against human brain tumors, berberine produced an average of 91% tumor inhibition against six malignant brain-tumor cell lines (Werbach and Murray, 1994).

Infectious Diseases

Fungal infections. The overgrowth of *Candida* on mucous membranes responds well to the use of goldenseal extract. Berberine sulfate has demonstrated antifungal activity against *Candida albicans, C. tropicalis, Trichophyton mentagrophytes, Microsporum gypseum, Cryptococcus neoformans,* and *Sporotrichum schenkii* (Amin et al., 1969) (see also the following section, Microbial Infections).

Microbial infections. Although studies on the antimicrobial activity of berberine are numerous, those on goldenseal are lacking, despite the fact that the herb is more commonly used. A recent in vitro study of antimicrobial activity was conducted using two goldenseal products sold commercially in the United States. The ground-up powder of an encapsulated product (Nature's Way Goldenseal Herb) dissolved in 70% ethanol was referred to as "pure goldenseal." A goldenseal extract (Extract of Goldenseal, Herbs Etc.) providing a goldenseal concentration of 336 mg/mL was referred to as "tincture." The control was 70% ethanol. Pure goldenseal failed to inhibit totally the growth of *Pseudomonas aeruginosa,* even at a concentration of 10,000 μg/mL, leaving the minimum inhibitory concentration (MIC) unknown. By comparison, penicillin was active at 8,000 μg/mL. Against the growth of *Staphylococcus aureus,* the MIC was 300-2,000 μg/mL, and against *Streptococcus pyogenes* 4,000 μg/mL (penicillin MIC = 0.98 μg/mL in both). The tincture showed significantly more activity against *S. pyogenes* and *S. aureus* than the ethanol control, but against *P. aeruginosa* the effective concentrations were not significantly different from that of the control and were so high (8,000-10,000 μg/mL) that a MIC was not established. Knight (1999) notes that the pure goldenseal showed significantly more activity than the tincture against *S. pyogenes,* whereas against *S. aureus* the reverse was true. Also noted was the fact that ethanol is known to be synergistic with antibacterial agents and that, in the case of the goldenseal products tested, this action seemed to be at work for *S. aureus* but was not apparent in the case of *S. pyogenes.* The evidence also suggested that the activity found could be attributed to the presence of berberine, and that at the 3-4% concentration known for goldenseal the activity against *S. aureus* and *S. pyogenes* of the products tested appeared proportional (Knight, 1999).

Berberine has a broad spectrum of antibiotic activity which shows up against various bacteria, including *Vibrio cholerae, Shigella, Pseudomonas, Escherichia coli, Proteus,* protozoa such as *Entamoeba histolytica, Trichomonas, Giardia, Leishmania,* and various fungi (Amin et al., 1969; Ghosh et al., 1985; Kaneda et al., 1991). Berberine sulfate and berberine hydrochloride have shown activity against *Entamoeba histolytica* and have been used in the chemotherapy of indolent ulcers and diarrheas (Amin et al., 1969). Berberine sulfate has shown antimicrobial activity against a more rapid antibacterial activity in vitro than tetracycline and chloramphenicol on

Vibrio cholerae, against which it acted as a bacteriocide. On *Staphylococcus aureus,* at concentrations of 35 and 50 mg/mL, berberine was bacteriostatic. In both of these organisms, the same concentrations inhibited RNA and protein synthesis almost immediately; otherwise, little effect on DNA synthesis occurred at these concentrations. The decrease in content of RNA by more than 50% suggested at least a partial enzymatic degradation (Amin et al., 1969).

Certain microbial agents can block the adherence of microorganisms to host cells at doses much lower than those needed to kill cells or to inhibit cell growth. Strategies that interrupt the adhesive functions of bacteria before host-tissue invasion occurs may be an effective prophylactic approach against bacterial infectious diseases. Berberine sulfate has shown direct interference with the adherence of group A *Streptococci* to host cells by way of two distinct mechanisms: (1) by releasing the adhesin lipoteichoic acid (LTA) from the *Streptococcal* cell surface, and (2) by directly preventing or dissolving lipoteichoic acid-fibronectin complexes. Berberine caused an eightfold increase in the release of lipoteichoic acid, the major ligand responsible for adherence of *Streptococci* to epithelial cells, fibronectin, and hexadecane (Sun et al., 1988).

A "total" standardized extract of goldenseal tested for relative killing time of various microorganisms in a low-density inoculum showed the most activity at 1 mL undiluted, and dose dependently at two dilutions, accordingly weaker activity. Scazzocchio et al. (1998) found least activity from the standardized extract and four derivative alkaloids against *Escherichia coli* and *Candida albicans.* Compared to the alkaloids tested, however, the undiluted standardized extract showed the most potent activity, killing the fungus at 15 s versus 1-2 h for the alkaloids (canadaline, canadine, berberine, and β-hydrastine). Undiluted, berberine was the most potent alkaloid against *C. albicans* (killing time, 1 h at 3.0 mg/mL), equivalent to the standardized extract at 50% dilution. Against the various microorganisms tested, canadaline showed the most potent activity, although against *Streptococcus sanguis, Pseudomonas aeruginosa,* and *Staphylococcus aureus* it was equivalent to berberine at the same dose (3 mg/mL). Canadaline killed *C. albicans* at over 2 h. The results suggested that benzylisoquinoline alkaloids with an open C ring, such as canadaline, appear to show greater antimicrobial activity. In most of the microorganisms tested, canadine also showed more potency than berberine (Scazzocchio et al., 1998). The minimum inhibitory concentration of canadaline against *S. aureus* and *S. sanguis* was 0.25 mg/mL (Scazzocchio et al., 2001).

A concentration-dependent inhibitory activity was shown from berberine (0.08-160 μM) against 21 strains of *Helicobacter pylori* obtained from human peptic-ulcer patients. However, even at the highest concentration tested, the maximum inhibition in any strain was 88% (Chung, Wu, Chang, et al., 1999).

Parasitic infections. The protozoan parasite *Leishmania donovani* and its treatment with berberine chloride was studied by Ghosh et al. (1985) using hamsters. Berberine was effective in reducing by 90% the number of parasitic amastigotes in the liver and spleen in long-term infections, and was much better tolerated at levels of 50 and 100 mg/kg per day than the medication pentamidine. Both drugs interfere with macromolecular biosynthesis in prokaryotic and eukaryotic cells. Ghosh and colleagues note that berberine interacts with various naturally occurring DNAs.

In vitro studies and strong anecdotal evidence indicate that goldenseal is effective at inhibiting the growth of protozoan parasites such as *Entamoeba histolytica, Giardia lamblia, Trichomonas vaginalis,* and *Leishmania donovani.* Berberine induces morphological changes in the parasites, often changing the form and size of the vacuole. It does not have the mutagenic side effects of metraonidazole, the current agent of choice for treating these conditions, yet it has in some cases appeared equally effective (Kaneda et al., 1991).

Based on the ability of D-hydrastine to dissolve *Echinococcus granulosus* cysts in mice, Ye et al. (1989) showed that it may be a promising agent for treating hydatidosis (cysts resulting from infection by a larval stage of the tapeworm *E. granulosus*). The alkaloid disturbs organelles, microtubules, mitochondria, and Golgi complexes, and causes pits in the cyst cell membrane. The researchers reported a "profound intracellular effect" from D-hydrastine at dosages of 3.75 mg/kg per day for 20 days (Ye et al., 1989).

Integumentary, Muscular, and Skeletal Functions

Connective Tissue Functions

Berberine-type alkaloids inhibit the activity of elastase, a serine proteinase that degrades elastin, an important structural component of blood vessels, lung, skin, and other tissues. Tanaka et al. (1992) suggest that berberine-type alkaloids might therefore be effective in certain inflammatory diseases, such as pulmonary emphysema, chronic bronchitis, arthritis, and rheumatoid arthritis. The enzyme elastase also degrades collagen, proteoglycan, and fibronectin.

Osteoporosis

In a rat model of postmenopausal osteoporosis, berberine was administered to ovariectomized rats at doses of 30 and 50 mg/kg per day p.o. Compared to controls, the lumbar bone-mass density of the berberine-treated rats showed significantly less loss. The effect was dose dependent and without causing an increase in plasma levels of estradiol (Li et al., 1999).

Neurological, Psychological, and Behavioral Functions

Receptor- and Neurotransmitter-Mediated Functions

Berberine *has shown* concentration-dependent noncompetitive MAO inhibitory activity in vitro in mouse brain mitochondria (IC_{50} 98.2 μM; 39.1% inhibition at 50 μM) (Lee et al., 1999). At a concentration of 20 μM for 24 h, berberine inhibited the biosynthesis of dopamine in PC12 cells by 53.7% (IC_{50} 18.6 μM). Evidence indicated that inhibition of MAO was not through modulation of tyrosine hydroxylase (TH) gene expression but through inhibition of TH activity (Shin et al., 2000).

Respiratory and Pulmonary Functions

A relaxing effect was shown from an ethanolic extract of goldenseal roots in carbachol-precontracted guinea pig trachea (Cometa et al., 1998). Complete relaxation of carbachol-precontracted isolated guinea pig trachea was obtained from a total extract of the roots in a cumulative dose of 5 μg/mL. Further studies have shown that the constituents responsible are the alkaloids canadaline, canadine, berberine, and β-hydrastine (EC_{50} 2.4, 11.9, 34.2, 72.8 μg/mL, respectively). Although as yet unclear, the activity appears to involve interactions of the alkaloids with adenosine and adrenergic receptors (Abdel-Haq et al., 2000).

CLINICAL STUDIES

Cardiovascular and Circulatory Disorders

Arrhythmia

In a study of 200 patients with ventricular tachyarrhythmias, berberine treatment (dose not specified in summary) resulted in significant reductions in the number of beats/hour. No side effects were noted except for mild gastroenterologic symptoms in some patients (Werbach and Murray, 1994). In China, berberine is a class III antiarrhythmic agent; oral berberine (tablets, 1.2 g/day) is reportedly of value in the treatment of ventricular premature beats in patients with congestive heart failure. However, the safety and pharmacokinetics of oral berberine in such patients is only now beginning to be determined (Zeng and Zeng, 1999).

Digestive, Hepatic, and Gastrointestinal Disorders

Diarrhea

In a randomized controlled study, the efficacy of berberine sulfate in the treatment of diarrhea due to enterotoxigenic *E. coli* (ETEC) and *Vibrio cholerae* was evaluated in 165 patients. After 24 h, a significant percentage of patients who received 400 mg berberine sulfate in a single oral dose no longer had diarrhea, or 42% versus 20% prior to treatment. The berberine sulfate group showed significantly reduced stool volumes for three consecutive 8-h periods following treatment. In patients with cholera given 400 mg berberine sulfate, the mean 8-h stool volume was significantly lower in the second 8-h period (mean of 2.22 L) versus controls (mean of 2.79 L). However, patients who received 1,200 mg berberine sulfate in conjunction with tetracycline (1,000 mg) did not show a significant reduction in stool volume compared to those who received tetracycline alone. No side effects were noted in any treatment group receiving berberine sulfate. The results suggest that berberine can be an effective and safe antisecretory drug for ETEC diarrhea but that it has only slight activity against cholera and is not additive with tetracycline (Rabbani et al., 1987).

To reduce the need for treatment using oral and intravenous fluid in patients with severe diarrhea due to cholera and similar bacterial enteric infections, agents that reverse the stimulation of secretion of water and electrolytes by cholera toxin and the related toxins of enterotoxigenic *E. coli* are actively being sought. In a study by Khin-Maung-U et al. (1985), 400 adults presenting with acute watery diarrhea were entered into a randomized placebo-controlled, double-blind clinical trial of berberine, tetracycline, and a tetracycline-plus-berberine combination to study the antisecretory and vibriostatic effects of berberine. Of 185 patients with cholera, those given tetracycline or tetracycline plus berberine showed considerably reduced volume and frequency of diarrheal stools, duration of diarrhea, and volume of required intravenous and oral rehydration fluid. Berberine did not produce an antisecretory effect but did reduce the volume of excretion. When administered with tetracycline, a conflict appeared to exist in antibiotic activity, as those patients remained sick for a longer period. It was hypothesized that the vibriostatic action of tetracycline may have been antagonized by berberine. The authors concluded that the dosages of berberine, when administered alone, may have to be larger than the 100 mg q.i.d. used in their study.

In a study of 65 children under five years of age affected with acute diarrhea, a superior response was observed in those receiving berberine tannate (25 mg every 6 h) compared to those receiving standard antibiotic therapy. Berberine tannate was effective against diarrhea caused by *Escherichia coli, Shigella, Salmonella,* and *Klebsiella* (Sack and Froelich, 1982).

In 200 adult patients with acute diarrhea, standard antibiotic treatment in conjunction with berberine hydrochloride (150 mg p.o./day) resulted in a faster recovery than in patients given antibiotic therapy alone. In an additional 30 patients treated with berberine hydrochloride alone, diarrhea was arrested in all with no side effects or toxicity (Kamat, 1967).

Gastric Disorders

Parasitic diseases. Pediatric patients five months to 14 years of age infected with giardiasis were divided into two groups, one test group administered berberine (10 mg/kg per day) and one control group receiving a standard antigiardial drug (metronidazole). After ten days, 90% of the berberine group showed negative stools, versus 95% in the metronidazole group; at one month, 83% of the berberine group remained negative, compared to 90% of the metronidazole group (Gupte, 1975). In another study, berberine (5 mg/kg p.o. per day for six days) was superior to placebo (vitamin B complex syrup) in the treatment of 40 patients (ages one to 10 years) diagnosed with giardiasis. Sixty-eight percent of the patients in the berberine group showed no signs of *Giardia* in their stools. Three of these patients complained of side effects (giddiness, abdominal distention, and headache, respectively). Remarkably, 25% of the placebo-treated patients also showed no signs of *Giardia* in their stools after six days of treatment (Choudhry et al., 1972).

Hepatic Diseases

Cirrhosis. Berberine (600-800 mg p.o. per day) is reported to have corrected hypertyraminemia in patients with alcohol-related liver cirrhosis. Berberine prevented the elevation of serum tyramine following oral tyrosine load by inhibiting bacterial tyrosine decarboxylase in the large intestine. The accumulation of tyramine causes lowering of peripheral resistance, resulting in high cardiac output, reduction in renal function, and cerebral dysfunction (Watanabe et al., 1982).

DOSAGE

The dose of goldenseal is based on berberine or hydrastine content. As goldenseal preparations vary widely in quality, standardized extracts are preferred. For best results, an extract standardized to contain 5% total alkaloids, calculated as hydrastine or berberine, is recommended. For a standardized extract, the recommended dose is 250-500 mg, t.i.d. (Werbach and Murray, 1994).

Practitioners have recommended the following doses be taken t.i.d.:
Dried root as decoction: 0.5-1.0 g
Tincture (1:10, 60% ethanol): 2-4 mL

Fluid extract (1:1, 60% ethanol): 0.3-1.0 mL (Bradley, 1992; Newall et al., 1996)

Standardized extract (5% hydrastine): 250-500 mg/day (Werbach and Murray, 1994)

SAFETY PROFILE

Contraindications

Goldenseal is contraindicated in individuals with high blood pressure (Newall et al., 1996, citing the *British Herbal Pharmacopoeia, 1983*).

One study concluded that berberine sulfate is inappropriate for the treatment of newborn infants with prenatal jaundice. According to Bergner (1996), some practitioners recommend that goldenseal not be administered to children under two years of age. Brinker (1998) cautions against the local use of goldenseal to treat purulent ear discharge because of a possible underlying rupture in the eardrum. He also lists goldenseal as a bitter herb that could ostensibly aggravate gastrointestinal irritations.

Berberine is contraindicated for infants with a deficiency of glucose-6-phosphate-dehydrogenase. This follows the observation that shortly after these infants were administered berberine-containing herbs, they developed hemolytic anemia and jaundice. After a subsequent ban of berberine-containing herbs by the government of Singapore in 1979, incidences of jaundice dropped, whereas they remained at a high level among infants in southern China and Hong Kong. Using serum from neonates, in vitro tests of herbal teas rich in berberine showed bilirubin protein binding was decreased and that the effect was at least partly due to berberine (De Smet, 1997).

Drug Interactions

In herbal medicine, goldenseal is widely believed to enhance the activity of other botanicals; however, no studies are available to support this contention. In one study, a combination of berberine and tetracycline was no more effective than tetracycline alone in relieving diarrheal symptoms in cholera patients (Rabbani et al., 1987).

Yao et al. (1987) found berberine acted like yohimbine and prazosin in showing competitive blocking activity against α_1- and α_2-adrenoreceptors. Therefore, goldenseal may have an additive effect with those agents.

In vitro studies using various colon, gastric, and oral-cancer cell lines pretreated with berberine (32 μM) 24 h before their treatment with the anticancer drug Taxol (paclitaxel) found the anticancer activity of the agent was compromised (Lin, Liu, Wu, et al., 1999). Others have made similar observations in murine and human hepatoma cell lines in which berberine compromised the retention of chemotherapy agents (tamoxifen and verapamil) in tumor cells (Lin, Liu, Lui, et al., 1999). In vivo studies are required to clarify these potential drug interactions with berberine.

Mice pretreated with berberine (4 mg/kg p.o.) in a single dose showed significantly prolonged phenobarbital-induced (60 mg/kg i.p.) sleeping time and increased toxicity, resulting in 100% death from a sublethal dose of strychnine (0.3 mg/kg i.p.). These results strongly suggest inhibition of the drug-metabolizing enzymes hepatic cytochrome P450s (Janbaz and Gilani, 2000). Among 21 commercial ethanolic herbal extract products sold in Canada, in vitro inhibitory activity on cytochrome P450 3A4 (CYP3A4) was found in about 66% of the products. Significant inhibition of CYP3A4 was shown at concentrations of less than 10% of their full-strength source preparations. An extract of goldenseal (*Hydrastis canadensis,* 0.03% full strength) was the most potent inhibitor (Budzinski et al., 2000).

Pregnancy and Lactation

Herbs that contain berberine are not recommended for use during pregnancy. Berberine has been shown to cause uterine contractions in experimental animals (De Smet, 1992; Murray, 1995; Bradley, 1992) and to cause displacement of bilirubin in vitro and in rats (Chan, 1993) (see Special Precautions). No information is available regarding the safety of goldenseal for breast-feeding women or their infants. *The American Herbal Product Association's Botanical Safety Handbook* (McGuffin et al., 1997) does not provide cautionary information about the use of goldenseal during lactation. Goldenseal and berberine-containing plants are usually considered nontoxic (Newall et al., 1996), and few side effects are known at the recommended dosages. Tyler (1999) stated that berberine and hydrastine are not orally available, which would infer no milk entry. This lack of oral bioavailability of berberine is refuted by recent animal (Janbaz and Gilani, 2000; Anis et al., 1999; Li et al., 1999) and human studies (Zeng and Zeng, 1999). There are no pharmacokinetic studies of goldenseal to confirm to what extent this may be true. Use by breast-feeding mothers of babies with jaundice or a deficiency of glucose-6-phosphate-dehydrogenase should be carefully scrutinized (see Contraindications). In vitro tests of serum from neonates fed berberine-containing herbal teas showed bilirubin protein binding was decreased and that the effect was at least partly due to berberine (De Smet, 1997). The applicability of this and other similar findings to lactation should be viewed in perspective, however, as the dose of plant constituents received in direct feeding with herbal teas is many times larger than the dose possible to receive through breast milk. Quantification of oral availability, serum levels, and degree, if any, of milk entry are sorely needed.

Side Effects

Little data on the side effects of goldenseal are available. *The American Herbal Product Association's Botanical Safety Handbook* (McGuffin et al., 1997) lists goldenseal as a class 2b herb, i.e., an herb that should not be used during pregnancy. This source notes that the use of goldenseal as an ingredient in nonmedicinal oral-use products is prohibited under Canadian government regulations.

Berberine is well tolerated up to a dose of 500 mg. Above that, side effects have been reported: eye and skin irritation, nephritis and kidney irritation, nosebleed, lethargy, and dyspnea (Blumenthal et al., 1998).

Special Precautions

Goldenseal and berberine-containing plants are usually considered nontoxic (Newall et al., 1996), and are generally nontoxic at the recommended dosages; however, higher dosages may interfere with metabolism of vitamin B (Duke, 1985). Tinctures may cause irritation of the mucous membranes (Brinker, 1998).

Chan (1993) reported that berberine caused in vitro displacement of bilirubin showing tenfold the potency of a known bilirubin displacer (phenylbutazone) and 100-fold the potency of a related berberine-type alkaloid (papaverine). Administered to rats, berberine (1 and 2 mg/kg i.p. per day for one week), berberine caused bilirubin serum protein binding to significantly decrease. The effect was a displacement and persistent elevation in serum levels of total and unbound bilirubin. Therefore, Chan cautioned against the use of medicinal plants containing high amounts of berberine in cases of jaundice, in neonates, and in pregnancy.

Bergner (1996) reports that large doses over a long duration can overstimulate and eventually exhaust the mucous membranes. At this, he cites the traditional Chinese medical point of view that bitter herbs taken inappropriately can injure the spleen.

Duke (1985) warns that topical overdose can cause skin or membrane ulceration; for that reason, Duke warns against its traditional use as a douche. Foster (1991) counters that this fear stems from Millspaugh's 1887 homeopathic text, *American Medical Plants,* and that modern studies have not been able to confirm this.

Toxicology

Toxicity in Animal Models

The oral LD_{50} in mice of berberine is variously reported at 3.29 mg/10 g to 1,000 mg/kg body weight, suggesting that toxicity is extremely low

(Snow, 1996). The German Commission E gives the LD_{50} of berberine in mice as 24.3 mg/kg i.p. (Blumenthal et al., 1998). Others report that in Swiss albino mice the acute i.p. LD_{50} of berberine is 500 mg/kg and the chronic LD_{50} is 150 mg/kg for ten days (Anis et al., 1999).

REFERENCES

Abdel-Haq, H., Cometa, M.F., Palmery, M., Leone, M.G., Silvestrini, B., and Saso, L. (2000). Relaxant effects of *Hydrastis canadensis* L. and its major alkaloids on guinea pig isolated trachea. *Pharmacology and Toxicology* 87: 218-222.

Amin, A.H., Subbaiah, T.V., and Abbasi, K.M. (1969). Berberine sulfate: Antimicrobial activity, bioassay and mode of action. *Canadian Journal of Microbiology* 15: 1067-1076.

Anis, K.V., Kuttan, G., and Kuttan, R. (1999). Role of berberine as an adjuvant response modifier during tumour therapy in mice. *Pharmacy and Pharmacology Communications* 5: 697-700.

Bergner, P. (1996). Goldenseal and the common cold: The antibiotic myth. *Medical Herbalism* 8: 1-10.

Blumenthal, M., Busse, W.R., Goldberg, A., Gruenwald, J., Hall, T., Riggins, C.W., and Rister, R.S. (Eds.) (1998). *The Complete German Commission E Monographs* (pp. 309-310). Austin, TX: American Botanical Council.

Bradley, P.R. (1992). *British Herbal Compendium* (pp. 119-120). Bournemouth, Dorset, England: British Herbal Medicine Association.

Brinker, F. (1998). *Herb Contraindications and Drug Interactions,* Second Edition. Sandy, OR: Eclectic Medical Publications.

Budzinski, J.W., Foster, B.C., Vandenhoek, S., and Arnason, J.T. (2000). An in vitro evaluation of human cytochrome P450 3A4 inhibition by selected commercial herbal extracts and tinctures. *Phytomedicine* 7: 273-282.

Chan, E. (1993). Displacement of bilirubin from albumin by berberine. *Biology of the Neonate* 63(4): 201-208.

Chang, H.M. and But, P.P.H. (Eds.) (1986). *Pharmacology and Applications of Chinese Materia Medica.* Singapore: World Scientific.

Choudhry, V.P., Sabir, M., and Bhide, V.N. (1972). Berberine in giardiasis. *Indian Pediatrics* 9: 143-146.

Chung, J.G., Chen, G.W., Hung, C.F., Lee, J.H., Ho, C.C., Chang, H.L., Lin, W.C., and Lin, J.G. (2000). Effects of berberine on arylamine *N*-acetyltransferase activity and 2-aminofluorene-DNA adduct formation in human leukemia cells. *American Journal of Chinese Medicine* 28: 227-238.

Chung, J.G., Wu, L.T., Chang, S.H., Lo, H.H., Hsieh, S.E., Li, Y.C., and Hung, C.F. (1999). Inhibitory actions of berberine on growth and arylamine *N*-acetyltransferase activity in strains of *Helicobacter pylori* from peptic ulcer patients. *International Journal of Toxicology* 18: 35-40.

Chung, J.G., Wu, L.T., Chu, C.B., Jan, J.Y., Ho, C.C., Tsou, M.F., Lu, H.F., Chen, G.W., Lin, J.G., and Wang, T.F. (1999). Effects of berberine on arylamine *N*-acetyltransferase activity in human bladder tumour cells. *Food and Chemical Toxicology* 37: 319-326.

Cometa, M.F., Abdel-Haq, H., and Palmery, M. (1998). Spasmolytic activities of *Hydrastis canadensis* L. on rat uterus and guinea pig trachea. *Phytotherapy Research* 12(Suppl.): S83-S85.

De Smet, P.A.G.M. (Ed.) (1992). *Adverse Effects of Herbal Drugs,* Vol. 1. New York: Springer-Verlag.

De Smet, P.A.G.M. (1997). Notes added in proof. In De Smet, P.A.G.M., Keller, K., Hänsel, R., and Chandler, R.F. (Eds.), *Adverse Effects of Herbal Drugs,* Vol. 3 (pp. 229-240). New York: Springer-Verlag.

Duke, J.A. (1985). *Handbook of Medicinal Herbs.* Boca Raton, FL: CRC Press.

Foster, S. (1991). *Goldenseal.* Botanical Series Leaflet No. 309. Austin, TX: American Botanical Council.

Fukuda, K., Hibiya, Y., Mutoh, M., Koshiji, M., Akao, S., and Fujiwara, H. (1999). Inhibition of activator protein 1 activity by berberine in human hepatoma cells. *Planta Medica* 65: 381-383.

Genest, K. and Hughes, D.W. (1969). Natural products in Canadian pharmaceuticals. IV. *Hydrastis canadensis. Canadian Journal of Pharmaceutical Sciences* 4: 41-45.

Ghosh, A.K., Bhattacharyya, F.K., and Ghosh, D.K. (1985). *Leishmania donovani:* Amastigote inhibition and mode of action of berberine. *Experimental Parasitology* 60: 404-413.

Gleye, J. and Stanislas, E. (1972). Alkaloids in underground parts of *Hydrastis canadensis.* Presence of 1-α-hydrastine. *Plantes Medicinales et Phytotherapie* 6: 306-310.

Govindan, M. and Govindan, G. (2000). A convenient method for the determination of the quality of goldenseal. *Fitoterapia* 71: 232-235.

Gupte, S. (1975). Use of berberine in the treatment of giardiasis. *American Journal of Diseases of Children* 129: 866.

Huang, W.M., Yan, H., Jin, J.M., Yu, C., and Zhang, H. (1992). Beneficial effects of berberine on hemodynamics during acute ischemic left ventricular failure in dogs. *Chinese Medical Journal* 105: 1014-1019.

Iizuka, N., Miyamoto, K., Okita, K., Tangoku, A., Hayashi, H., Yosino, S., Abe, T., Morioka, T., Hazama, S., and Oka, M. (2000). Inhibitory effect of Coptidis Rhizoma and berberine on the proliferation of human esophageal cancer cell lines. *Cancer Letters* 148: 19-25.

Iwasa, K., Moriyasu, M., Yamori, T., Turuo, T., Lee, D.U., and Wiegrebe, W. (2001). In vitro cytotoxicity of the protoberberine-type alkaloids. *Journal of Natural Products* 64: 896-898.

Janbaz, K.H. and Gilani, A.H. (2000). Studies on preventive and curative effects of berberine on chemical-induced hepatotoxicity in rodents. *Fitoterapia* 71: 25-33.

Kamat, S.A. (1967). Clinical trial with berberine hydrochloride for the control of diarrhea in acute gastroenteritis. *Journal of Associated Physicians of India* 15: 525-529.

Kaneda, Y., Torii, M., Tanaka, T., and Aikawa, M. (1991). In vitro effects of berberine sulphate on the growth and structure of *Entamoeba histolytica, Giardia lamblia* and *Trichomonas vaginalis. Annals of Tropical Medicine and Parasitology* 85: 417-425.

Khin-Maung-U, Myo-Khin, Nyunt-Nyunt-Wai, Aye-Kyaw, and Tin-U (1985). Clinical trial of berberine in acute watery diarrhoea. *British Medical Journal* 291: 1601-1605.

Knight, S.E. (1999). Goldenseal *(Hydrastis canadensis)* versus penicillin: A comparison of effects on *Staphylococcus aureus, Streptococcus pyogenes,* and *Pseudomonas aeruginosa. Bios* 70: 3-10.

Ko, W.H., Yao, X.Q., Lau, C.W., Law, W.I., Chen, Z.Y., Kwok, W., Ho, K., and Huang, Y. (2000). Vasorelaxant and antiproliferative effects of berberine. *European Journal of Pharmacology* 399: 187-196.

Korkmaz, S., Kosar, M., Baser, K.H.C., and Ozturk, Y. (2000). Effects of berberine on C6 glioma and NIH 3T3 fibroblast cell lines. In 3rd International Congress on Phytomedicine, October 11-13, 2000, Munich, Germany, Abstracts. *Phytomedicine* 7(Suppl. 2): 123 (abstract P-150).

Kumazawa, Y., Itagaki, A., Fukumoto, M., Fujisawa, H., Nishimura, C., and Nomoto, K. (1984). Activation of peritoneal macrophages by berberine-type alkaloids in terms of induction of cytostatic activity. *Journal of Immunopharmacology* 6: 587-592.

Lee, S.S., Kai, M., and Lee, M.K. (1999). Effects of natural isoquinoline alkaloids on monoamine oxidase activity in mouse brain: Inhibition by berberine and palmatine. *Medical Science Research* 27: 749-751.

Leone, M.G., Cometa, M.F., Palmery, M., and Saso, L. (1996). HPLC determination of the major alkaloids extracted from *Hydrastis canadensis* L. *Phytotherapy Research* 10: S45-S46.

Leung, A.Y. and Foster, S. (1996). *Encyclopedia of Common Natural Ingredients Used in Food, Drugs, and Cosmetics.* New York: John Wiley and Sons, Inc.

Li, H., Miyahara, T., Tezuka, Y., Namba, T., Suzuki, T., Dowaki, R., Watanabe, M., Nemoto, N., Tonami, S., Seto, H., et al. (1999). The effect of Kampo formulae on bone resorption in vitro and in vivo. II. Detailed study of berberine. *Biological and Pharmaceutical Bulletin* 22: 391-396.

Lin, H.L., Liu, T.Y., Lui, W.Y., and Chi, C.W. (1999). Up-regulation of multidrug resistance transporter expression by berberine in human and murine hepatoma cells. *Cancer* 85: 1937-1942.

Lin, H.L., Liu, T.Y., Wu, C.W., and Chi, C.W. (1999). Berberine modulates expression of *mdr1* gene product and the responses of digestive track cancer cells to paclitaxel. *British Journal of Cancer* 81: 416-422.

Lin, J.G., Chung, J.G., Wu, L.T., Chen, G.W., Chang, H.L., and Wang, T.F. (1999). Effects of berberine on arylamine *N*-acetyltransferase activity in human colon tumor cells. *American Journal of Chinese Medicine* 27: 265-275.

McGuffin, M., Hobbs, C., Upton, R., and Goldberg, A. (1997). *American Herbal Product Association's Botanical Safety Handbook*. Boca Raton, FL: CRC Press.

Messana, I., La Bua, R., and Galeffi, C. (1980). The alkaloids of *Hydrastis canadensis* L. (Ranunculaceae). Two new alkaloids: Hydrastidine and isohydrastindine. *Gazzetta Chimica Italiana* 110: 539-543.

Mills, S. and Bone, K. (2000). *Principles and Practice of Phytotherapy* (pp. 286-296). New York, NY: Churchill Livingstone.

Murray, M.T. (1995). *The Healing Power of Herbs* (pp. 162-172). Rocklin, CA: Prima Publishing.

Newall, C.A., Anderson, L.A., and Phillipson, J.D. (1996). *Herbal Medicine: A Guide for Health-Care Professionals* (pp. 151-152). London: The Pharmaceutical Press.

Nishino, H., Kitagawa, K., Fujiki, H., and Iwashima, A. (1986). Berberine sulfate inhibits tumor-promoting activity of teleocidin in two-stage carcinogenesis on mouse skin. *Oncology* 43: 131-134.

Ölmez, E. and Ilhan, M. (1992). Evaluation of the α-adrenoreceptor antagonistic action of berberine in isolated organs. *Arzneimittel-Forschung/Drug Research* 42: 1095-1097.

Orfila, L., Rodriguez, M., Colman, T., Hasegawa, M., Merentes, E., and Arvelo, F. (2000). Structural modification of berberine alkaloids in relation to cytotoxic activity in vitro. *Journal of Ethnopharmacology* 71: 449-456.

Palmery, M., Cometa, M.F., and Leone, M.G. (1996). Further studies of the adrenolytic activity of the major alkaloids from *Hydrastis canadensis* L. on isolated rabbit aorta. *Phytotherapy Research* 10(Suppl.): S47-S49.

Rabbani, G.H., Butler, T., Knight, J., Sanyal, S.C., and Alam, K. (1987). Randomized controlled clinical trial of berberine sulfate therapy for diarrhea due to enterotoxigenic *Escherichia coli* and *Vibrio cholerae*. *The Journal of Infectious Diseases* 155: 979-984.

Rehman, J., Dillow, J.M., Carter, S.M., Chou, J., Le, B., and Maisel, A.S. (1999). Increased production of antigen-specific immunoglobulins G and M following in vivo treatment with medicinal plants *Echinacea angustifolia* and *Hydrastis canadensis*. *Immunology Letters* 68: 391-395.

Sack, R.B. and Froelich, J.L. (1982). Berberine inhibits intestinal secretory response of *Vibrio cholerae* and *Escherichia coli* enterotoxins. *Infection and Immunity* 35: 471-475.

Scazzocchio, F., Cometa, M.F., and Palmery, M. (1998). Antimicrobial activity of *Hydrastis canadensis* extract and its major isolated alkaloids. *Fitoterapia* 69(Suppl): 58-59.

Scazzocchio, F., Cometa, M.F., Tomassini, L., and Palmery, M. (2001). Antibacterial activity of *Hydrastis canadensis* extract and its major alkaloids. *Planta Medica* 67: 561-564 (letter).

Shin, J.S., Kim, E.I., Kai, M., and Lee, M.K. (2000). Inhibition of dopamine biosynthesis by protoberberine alkaloids in PC12 cells. *Neurochemical Research* 25: 363-368.

Sinclair, A. and Catling, P.M. (2000). Status of goldenseal, *Hydrastis canadensis* (Ranunculaceae), in Canada. *Canadian Field-Naturalist* 114: 111-120.

Snow, J.M. (1996). *Hydrastis canadensis* L. (Ranunculaceae). *Protocol Journal of Botanical Medicine* 2: 25-28.

Sun, D., Courtney, H.S., and Beachey, E.H. (1988). Berberine sulfate blocks adherence of *Streptococcus pyogenes* to epithelial cells, fibronectin, and hexadecane. *Antimicrobial Agents and Chemotherapy* 32: 1370-1374.

Tanaka, T., Metori, K., Mineo, S., Hirotani, M., Furuya, T., and Kobayashi, S. (1992). Inhibitory effects of berberine-type alkaloids on elastase. *Planta Medica* 59: 200-202.

Taylor, C.T., Winter, D.C., Skelly, M.M., O'Donoghue, D.P., O'Sullivan, G.C., Harvey, B.J., and Baird, A.W. (1999). Berberine inhibits ion transport in human colonic epithelia. *European Journal of Pharmacology* 368: 111-118.

Tyler, V.E. (1999). Phytomedicines: Back to the future. *Journal of Natural Products* 62: 1589-1592.

Watanabe, A., Obata, T., and Nagashima, H. (1982). Berberine therapy of hypertyraminemia in patients with liver cirrhosis. *Acta Medica Okayama* 36: 277-281.

Werbach, M.R. and Murray, M.T. (1994). *Botanical Influences on Illness: A Sourcebook of Clinical Research* (pp. 114-115). Tarzana, CA: Third Line Press.

Wong, K.K. (1998). Mechanism of the aortic relaxation induced by low concentrations of berberine. *Planta Medica* 64: 756-757.

Wu, H.L., Hsu, C.Y., Liu, W.H., and Yung, B.Y.M (1999). Berberine-induced apoptosis of human leukemia HL-60 cells is associated with down-regulation of nucleophosmin/B23 and telomerase activity. *International Journal of Cancer* 81: 923-929.

Wu, S.N., Yu, H.S., Jan, C.R., Li, H.F., and Yu, C.L. (1998). Inhibitory effects of berberine on voltage- and calcium-activated potassium currents in human myeloma cells. *Life Sciences* 62: 2283-2294.

Yao, W.X., Fang, D.C., Cheng, B., and Jiang, M.X. (1987). Blocking action of berberine on α_2- and α_1-adrenoreceptors in rat vas deferens and anococcygeus muscle. *Journal of Tongji Medical University* 7: 233-238.

Yao, W.X., Fang, D.C., Xia, G.J., and Jiang, M.X. (1989). Blocking action of berberine on various receptors in rat anococcygeis muscle. *Journal of Tongji Medicinal University* 9: 86-90.

Ye, Y.C., Chen, Q.M., Hai, P., Chai, F.L., and Zhou, S.X. (1989). Effect of d-hydrastine on the ultrastructure of several experimental *Echinococcus granulosus* cyst in mice. *Chung Kuo Yao Li Hseuh Pao* 10: 185-187.

Zeng, X. and Zeng, X. (1999). Relationship between the clinical effects of berberine on severe congestive heart failure and its concentration in plasma studied by HPLC. *Biomedical Chromatography* 13: 422-444.

Zhou, J., Xuan, B., and Li, D.X. (1993). Effect of tetrahydroberberine on ischemic and reperfused myocardium in rats. *Chang Kuo Yao Li Hsueh Pao* 14: 130-133.

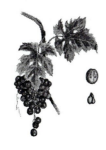

Grape Seed

BOTANICAL DATA

Classification and Nomenclature

Scientific name: *Vitis vinifera* L. and *V. coignetiae*

Family name: Vitaceae

Common names: grape seed, grape seed extract, muskat

Description

Vitis vinifera is native to Asia Minor, south of the Black and Caspian Seas. However, with cultivation, *V. vinifera* has spread eastward through Turkey, Iran, Pakistan, India, and China, and westward into the Americas. *Vitis vinifera* can also be found in the moderate regions of South Africa, Australia, and New Zealand (Cormier and Do, 1993; Bombardelli and Morazzoni, 1995).

HISTORY AND TRADITIONAL USES

The use of *Vitis vinifera* for medicinal purposes can be traced to ancient times (Bombardelli and Morazzoni, 1995). References to the medicinal properties of grapes have been found among the following: Hippocrates, Theophrastus, Dioscorides, Pliny, Galen, and the ancient Egyptians. Sap obtained from young branches has been used for treating skin diseases and eye inflammation. The leaves have been used for the treatment of diarrhea, hemorrhage, varicose veins, and hemorrhoids, while the juice of unripe fruits has been employed in the treatment of throat infections. On the other hand, the fruit of *V. vinifera* has been employed in folk medicine for treating various conditions, including cachexia, cancer, cholera, smallpox, diarrhea,

569

hoarseness, scurvy, ophthalmia, and skin, kidney, and liver diseases. Grape seed oil is reported to have laxative, antacid, and cholagogic properties and to be useful in treating burns and slow-healing ulcers (Bombardelli and Morazzoni, 1995).

CHEMISTRY

Grape seeds are generally obtained as a by-product of wine production. They account for 20% to 26% of the pomace produced from pressing grapes.

Phenolic Compounds

Tannins

The major phenolic constituents of grape seed are proanthocyanidins (also called procyanidin oligomers, PCOs, procyanidins, or condensed tannins) (Peng et al., 2001). PCOs are composed of two basic structural units: the catechins and the leucocyanidins. Upon heating in an acid medium, PCOs yield cyanidin (Bombardelli and Morazzoni, 1995; Ricardo Da Silva et al., 1991).

A standardized PCO extract used in France for treating microcirculatory disorders contains a mixture of procyanidin dimers, trimers, tetramers, and oligomers of up to seven units. Dimers represent approximately 15% of the total oligomeric fraction. In addition, small amounts of catechin and epicatechin are present (Bombardelli and Morazzoni, 1995).

Other Constituents

Grape seeds contain 16% crude protein, 23% fat, 48% fiber, a number of pigments, and several essential amino acids (Kamel et al., 1985). Inorganic nutrients in grape seeds include iron, calcium, zinc, copper, phosphorus, magnesium, and potassium.

THERAPEUTIC APPLICATIONS

Grape seed extracts (and specific wine fractions) display a wide range of pharmacological activities, including cardioprotective, antioxidant, free radical-scavenging, vasorelaxant, antimutagenic, collagen-protecting, anti-inflammatory, and capillary-reinforcing activity.

PRELIMINAL STUDIES

Cardiovascular and Circulatory Functions

Arrhythmia

A procyanidolic oligomer fraction of a grape seed extract (Endotelon), containing dimers, monomers, and a small amount of trimers, was shown to inhibit angiotensin I-converting enzyme in vitro. Administered to rabbits prior to angiotensin I and II (i.v.), the procyanidolic oligomer fraction (5 mg/kg i.v.) caused a significant inhibition of hypertensive responses (Meunier et al., 1987).

Atherosclerosis

The potential antiatherosclerotic effects of procyanidin-rich (73.4% procyanidins) extracts of grape seed at 0.1% and 1% in the diets (w/w) of cholesterol-fed rabbits for eight weeks were examined against peroxyl radical-mediated lipid peroxidation. Plasma taken from the extract-fed rabbits at four weeks showed a significant decrease ($p < 0.05$) in cholesteryl ester hydroperoxides compared to the controls fed the cholesterol-enriched diet alone. Total cholesterol and malondialdehyde (MDA) contents in the aortic arch of rabbits fed either concentration of the extract showed a significant decrease compared to the control group, and the MDA content of the thoracic aorta was also significantly decreased. Rabbits on either dosage of the extract also showed significantly fewer atherosclerotic plaques in their aortic arch but not in their thoracic arch. The higher dosage of extract produced a more significant decrease than the lower dosage ($p < 0.01$ versus $p < 0.05$) compared to the control group. In the atherosclerotic lesions, a decrease in the number of foam cells in oxidized low-density lipoprotein (LDL)-positive cells was evident in the extract-fed rabbits. Using human plasma, the researchers found that in LDL the extract could inhibit oxidation of cholesteryl linoleate, but not in LDL from plasma in which the extract and plasma were preincubated, suggesting that the procyanidin-rich extract could enhance resistance of plasma to lipid peroxidation, although accumulation of the procyanidins in LDL did not occur. In conclusion, Yamakoshi and colleagues suggested that the antiatherosclerotic activity of the grape seed procyanidins is likely related to the inhibition of LDL peroxidation located in the arterial wall (Yamakoshi et al., 1999).

Cardiotonic; Cardioprotection

Ischemic conditions are known to precipitate the production of superoxide anions and other toxic oxygen free radicals. These reactive molecular species induce alteration of cellular membranes and inhibition of membrane-associated enzymes by lipid peroxidation.

In the rabbit heart, procyanidins did not show any intrinsic contractile activity. However, they caused a dose-dependent reduction in ventricular contracture during ischemia (Maffei Facinó et al., 1996)—specifically, administration of procyanidins: decreased coronary perfusion pressure; improved cardiac mechanical performance following reperfusion; substantially increased release of prostaglandins in both preischemic and reperfusion periods; and suppressed irregularity in heart rhythm.

In a series of experiments, Maffei Facinó et al. (1996) showed that the cardioprotective effects of procyanidins are mediated by the following: (1) scavenging of oxygen-centered radicals (hydroxyl and peroxyl) and (2) sequestration of the cations Fe^{+2} and Cu^{+2} that catalyze formation of harmful hydroxyl radicals in the presence of superoxide/hydrogen peroxide. By reducing the concentrations of oxyradicals, procyanidins also suppress the nonenzymatic metabolism of arachidonic acid and thus promote the production of prostaglandins.

Sato et al. (1999) reported ex vivo cardioprotective effects from a grape seed extract (GSE) administered to rats in a high dosage (ActiVin, batch # 609016, 100 mg/kg p.o. daily for three weeks). Compared to controls, the hearts of rats administered the GSE showed significantly faster recovery from postischemic mycocardial infarction, significantly smaller infarct mass and size, and significantly higher aortic flow, but no difference in coronary flow.

Cholesterol and Lipid Metabolism

A laboratory-made extract of grape seed (73.4% procyanidins) at 0.1% and 1% (= 270 mg/kg p.o.) of the diets (w/w) of male New Zealand rabbits fed a 1% cholesterol diet produced a significant decrease in low-density lipoprotein cholesterol (LDL-c) at six weeks, but at eight weeks there was no significant change compared to untreated controls on the same diet (Yamakoshi et al., 1999). In male New Zealand rabbits fed normal and 1% cholesterol diets, a ten-week administration of a procyanidin-rich grape seed extract (Endotelon, 50 mg/kg p.o. per day) failed to change blood cholesterol levels in either group. However, the grape seed extract caused a significant reduction in the amount of cholesterol bound to aortic elastin relative to the untreated and cholesterol-fed rabbits (Wegrowski et al., 1984).

Peripheral Vascular Functions

Procyanidins are potent inhibitors of proteases, such as collagenase, elastase, hyaluronidase, and β-glucuronidase. This protease-inhibitory activity thus provides the basis for the vasoprotective properties of these compounds (Maffei Facinó et al., 1994).

Procyanidins are perhaps best known for their effects on capillary permeability and fragility. Intravenous injection of collagenase increases capillary permeability in such tissues as brain, aorta, and myocardium and thus provides a useful animal model for assessing the effects of increased capillary permeability. In this model, overall protection from the effects of collagenase was obtained by pretreatment with procyanidins (50 mg/kg p.o. per day for 21 days) (Bombardelli and Morazzoni, 1995).

The proteolytic enzyme elastase contributes to the destruction of elastic fibers and conjunctive tissue. Jonadet et al. (1983) compared the in vitro elastase-inhibiting activities (I_{50}) of anthocyanosides derived from three sources and found the following order of greatest to least inhibiting activity: grape seed (0.13 mg/mL), bilberry *(Vaccinium myrtillus)* (0.20 mg/mL), and pine bark *(Pinus maritimus)* (0.31 mg/mL). Animal experiments with the same anthocyanosides administered intraperitoneally in rodents showed the same order of potency.

The following grape products relaxed precontracted smooth muscle of intact aortic rings and in vascular tissue increased the levels of the secondary messenger guanosine 3',5'-cyclic monophosphate (cyclic GMP or cGMP): grape skin extracts from red and white grapes, grape juice, red wine, and the grape skin components quercitin and tannic acid (Fitzpatrick et al., 1993). These products were ineffective when the endothelium was removed, suggesting that the effect was dependent on specific mediators found within the endothelium. Both the vasorelaxant effect and the increase in cGMP levels were reversed by *N*-nitro-*L*-arginine and *N*-monomethyl-*L*-arginine, two competitive inhibitors of nitric oxide synthetase, suggesting that the endothelium-dependent vasorelaxant activity of these grape products are mediated by the nitric oxide-cGMP pathway. Such vasorelaxant effects, if they occur in vivo, may be expected to contribute to a reduced incidence of coronary heart disease.

Digestive, Hepatic, and Gastrointestinal Functions

Gastric Functions

Saito et al. (1998) compared the ulcer-inhibiting activity of a low flavanol content GSE (LFCE = 40.9%) to that of a high flavanol content GSE (HFCE = 81.3%) and pine bark extract (PBE = 53.9%) in rats. LFCE inhibited acidified ethanol-induced acute gastric mucosal injury by 82% from a dosage of 200 mg/kg p.o. At the same dosage, HFCE showed approximately 98% inhibition and PBE about 50% inhibition. Among the procyanidins tested, (+)-catechin showed no inhibitory activity (200 mg/kg p.o.), nor did dimeric or trimeric procyanidins or procyanidin B-3. However, at the same dosage, tetramers, pentamers, and hexamers showed very significant activity (all $p < 0.001$). From further tests, the authors concluded that the gastroprotective activity appears to be due to the longer molecular procyanidin oligomers in GSE (i.e., hexamers and pentamers) and that the demonstrably weaker activity of pine bark extract may owe to the lower concentration of longer procyanidin oligomers.

Bagchi et al. (1999) studied the gastroprotective effects of a procyanidin-rich, standardized water-ethanol extract powder of red grape seeds (Inter-Health Nutraceuticals, Benicia, CA, IH636, batch # AV 609016) (Bagchi et al., 2000). They demonstrated that, as a pretreatment, the GSE ameliorated damage to the gastric mucosa and intestinal mucosa of female rats exposed to daily (for 15 days) chronic stress or acute stress in the water-immersion restraint stress test. The preventive effect of the pretreatment (100 mg/kg per day p.o.) was evident in the complete absence of gastro-intestinal lesions versus their occurrence in the controls not treated with the extract. Also, rates of mucosal lipid peroxidation (measured by changes in thiobarbituric acid-reactive substances, or TBARS) significantly decreased by 22.8% in the chronic stress model and by 15.3% in the acute stress model compared to the control groups. Superoxide anion production in the gastric mucosa, but not the intestinal mucosa, increased in unstressed rats treated with the GSE by about 20% compared to untreated controls; however, in stressed rats, production of the free radical showed a significant decrease in the GSE-pretreated rats compared to controls as well as in both the intestinal and gastric mucosa (by about 26.3% and 18.7% in the chronic stress study and by 24.4% and 17.2%, respectively). Likewise, pretreatment with the GSE produced significant decreases of stress-induced DNA fragmentation in both the intestinal and gastric mucosa in chronic (by 21% and 26%, respectively) and acute stress models (by 12% and 14%, respectively) compared to the controls. Yet in unstressed rats, the GSE (100 mg/kg per day p.o. for 15 days) actually increased DNA fragmentation in the intestinal and gastric mucosa (by 70% and 30%, respectively) compared to unstressed, untreated controls. Similarly, membrane microviscosity of the intestinal mucosa and gastric mucosa showed significant increases in unstressed rats treated with the same dosage of the GSE and in stressed rats pretreated with the extract significant decreases occurred in both chronic and acute stress tests.

Hepatic Functions

Ray et al. (1999) examined the protective effects of a procyanidin-rich extract of grape seed (InterHealth Nutraceuticals, Concord, CA) against the liver-damaging effects of high doses of acetaminophen (Tylenol) on mouse livers. The GSE contained an admixture of a small amount of high molecular and monomeric proanthocyanosides plus 6.8% tetrameric, 13% trimeric, and > 54% dimeric forms—a profile common to red grape seeds. Mice administered the GSE for seven days (100 mg/kg p.o.) then received a hepatotoxic dose of acetaminophen (400 mg/kg i.p.) on the same day after the last dose of GSE were found to resemble the untreated controls. Mice treated with acetaminophen alone showed significant weight loss, little active movement, and greater leakage of alanine aminotransferase (ALT) ($29,813 \pm 463$ U/L versus 2792 ± 78 U/L), an indicator of cellular liver damage. Even a three-day pretreatment with the GSE resulted in a far healthier group of mice compared to those treated only with acetaminophen, but no appreciable difference in ALT occurred. At a dose of 500 mg/kg i.p., 44% of those mice treated only with acetaminophen died, whereas no mice perished from the same dose of acetaminophen in the group treated with the GSE for seven days beforehand. In mice pretreated for three days with the GSE, only 28% died. Microscopic examination of liver cells showed close to complete protection, including an absence of apoptotic cells, from the seven-day pretreatment versus the state of liver cells from mice treated only with acetaminophen. The increase in DNA fragmentation from acetaminophen (500 mg/kg i.p.) compared to controls was also significantly reduced by pretreatment with the GSE for seven days compared to acetaminophen alone (157% versus 478%).

Immune Functions; Inflammation and Disease

Cancer

Chemopreventive activity. Procyanidins reduce the spontaneous mutation rate of yeast cells without affecting the rate or yield of cell division (Liviero et al., 1994). At a concentration of 25 mg/mL, procyanidins decreased the spontaneous mutation rate of yeast mitochondria by 65%, while the rate of spontaneous mutation in yeast cell nuclei was reduced by 92%. The antimutagenic effects of procyanidins provide a rationale for the use of these compounds as chemopreventive agents.

Joshi et al. (1999) studied the in vitro chemopreventive effects of a GSE powder (ActiVin, batch # 609016) in cultured Chang cells, a nonmalignant human epithelial cell line, against the growth-inhibitory effects of the chemotherapy agents idarubicin (30 nM) and 4HC (4-hydroxyperoxycyclophosphamide) (1 μg/mL). The oligomeric procyanidin content of the extract was 54% dimeric, 13% trimeric, and 7% tetrameric. Monomers and flavonoids made up 6% of the extract. In the presence of the GSE (25 μg/mL), the growth-inhibitory effect of 4HC was significantly ameliorated ($p < 0.05$); in the case of idarubicin, growth inhibition was completely prevented by the GSE. In contrast, when the same concentration of the GSE was added to the culture of epithelial cells without the presence of a chemotherapy agent, growth of the cells was significantly stimulated ($p < 0.05$). Evidence of the chemopreventive effect of the GSE was also found in the rates of apoptosis of the epithelial cells in the presence of the chemotherapeutic agents. Without the extract, the rate of cells undergoing apoptosis from treatment with 4HC was 18%, and 8% when cotreated with the GSE. For idarubicin-treated cells, the rate of apoptosis was 35%, and 11% in the presence of GSE. Further, Joshi and colleagues showed that whereas antiapoptotic protein (Bcl-2) expression was decreased in the epithelial cells by idarubicin, treatment with the GSE prevented the down-regulation.

Bomser et al. (1999) investigated the preventive effects of a grape seed polyphenolic fraction (GSPF) (Traconol, Traco Labs, Inc., Champaign, IL) against chemically induced tumors on mouse skin. Before topical application of the tumor promoter, TPA (12-O-tetradecanoylphorbol-13-acetate), the same area of the skin of female CD-1 mice was topically treated with the GSPF (0 to 30 mg). As measured by myeloperoxidase (MPO), a marker of inflammation, and ornithine decarboxylase (ODC), a marker of tumor promotion, their activities showed significant and dose-dependent decreases in mice pretreated with the GSPF at doses of 5 to 30 mg. Accordingly, MPO activity was inhibited by 43% to 73% and ODC activity was inhibited by 27% to 70% compared to controls. After 15 weeks, pretreatment with the GSPF at doses of 5, 10, and 20 mg reduced tumor incidence by 63%, 51% and 94%, respectively, compared to controls.

In the mouse skin two-stage carcinogenesis protocol, using DMBA (7,12-dimethylbenz[a]anthracene) as the initiator of tumors followed with TPA as the promoter, Zhao et al. (1999) studied the chemopreventive effects of a GSPF (95% w/w polyphenols with procyanidin B5 at 19% and B5-3'-gallate at 15% the major constituents). After 20 weeks, the skin of female SENCAR mice topically treated with the GSPF in doses of 0.5 mg and 1.5 mg after the chemical initiation of tumors showed a highly significant ($p < 0.001$) inhibition of tumors per mouse (65% and 80%, respectively), incidence of tumors per mouse (35% and 65%, respectively), and volume of tumors per mouse (50% to 87%) compared to controls. However, per tumor volume and tumor growth was not significantly different compared to the controls. Zhao and colleagues associated the inhibition of tumor promotion by the GSPF with in vitro antioxidant activity using the epidermal lipid peroxidation assay employing SENCAR mouse epidermal microsomes. With this, they identified the most active antioxidant constituent as procyanidin B5-3'-gallate, which exhibited a concentration-dependent inhibition of epidermal lipid peroxidation and at a concentration of 0.04 mM, produced 100% inhibition—a rate attained only by vitamin E and catechin at concentrations of 1.0 mM. In order of greatest to least activity in the assay, the IC_{50}s of other procyanidin constituents and reference antioxidants was as follows: procyanidin B5-3'-gallate, procyanidin C1, procyanidin B5, procyanidin B2, catechin, vitamin E , and vitamin C (Zhao et al., 1999).

Cytotoxicity. Four solvent extracts of the seeds and peels of a Japanese variety of grape vine (*V. vinifera* "Koshu") were compared for in vitro cytotoxicity against human oral salivary gland tumor cells (HSG) and human squamous cell carcinoma cells (HSC-2), as well as nonmalignant human oral gingival fibroblasts (HGF). Radical scavenging against superoxide anion generated in the hypoxanthine/xanthine oxidase reaction was also measured. All four extracts of the peel were only weakly active in any of the cell lines. Two of the seed extracts (70% methanol extracts) displayed greater cytotoxicity against HSC-2 (CC_{50} 146 and 154 µg/mL, respectively) than either HSG (CC_{50} 221 and 243 µg/mL, respectively) or the nonmalignant HGF cells, against which all the extracts showed only weak activity ($CC_{50} > 500$ µg/mL). All the seed extracts scavenged superoxide, yet the same two with greatest scavenging activity were also the most cytotoxic to the tumor cell lines (Shirataki et al., 2000).

Agarwal, Sharma, and Agarwal (2000) studied the in vitro activity of a grape seed polyphenolic fraction (GSPF) (Traco Labs Inc., Champaign, IL) against the growth of androgen-independent human prostate carcinoma (DU145) cells. Cell cycle and apoptotic death assays were performed after incubating the DU145 cells with the GSPF. No inhibition of cell growth was evident from concentrations of 10 or 25 µg/mL; however, higher concentrations significantly inhibited growth of the DU145 cells compared to controls ($p < 0.001$), showing inhibition rates of 27%, 39%, and 76% from respective concentrations of 50, 75, and 100 µg/mL. Besides the concentration-dependent activity, cell death was also time dependent with significantly greater rates of cell death after longer periods of treatment (up to six days). Evidence was found that the inhibiting activity of the GSPF on DU145 cells may be attributed to a significant inhibition of the autocrine growth factor receptor feedback loop of constitutively active MAPK/ERK1 (mitogen-activated protein kinase/extracellular signal-regulated protein kinase-1), which allows these cells to grow autonomously. Compared to controls, a dose of 50 µg/mL of the GSPF decreased phosphorylated ERK1 by 93% after 72 h and by 88% after only 24 h (each $p < 0.001$). ERK2 was also significantly decreased, although to a lesser degree (70% after 72 h at doses of 25, 50, or 75 µg/mL). Since a number of cell-cycle regulators are suspected factors of uncontrolled growth of cells in the growth factor receptor-autocrine loop, Agarwal, Sharma, and Agarwal (2000) investigated the effects of the GSPF on several of these regulators. On cyclin-dependent kinases (CDKs) in prostate carcinoma cells, significant decreases were evident in levels of CDK4 after 24 h exposure (25, 50, or 75 µg/mL resulting in decreases of 30%, 40%, and 90%, respectively; each $p < 0.001$). Evidence was also found of increased arrest of cell-cycle progression (G1 phase) and of apoptotic cell death by the GSPF. After 48 h incubation, the three concentrations of the GSPF caused DNA fragmentation in the DU145 cells, which was only stronger after 72 h. The pattern of fragmentation was similar to that of the positive control, paclitaxel. To obtain some confirmation of this effect, the researchers used the same conditions and three doses of the GSPF in an androgen-dependent human prostate carcinoma cell line (LNCaP). After two days, no significant inhibition of growth was evident from 10-100 µg/mL, but after four or six days concentrations of 25-100 µg/mL produced inhibition rates of 10% to 96% and $\geq$ 53% cell death (Agarwal, Sharma, and Agarwal, 2000). Similar growth-inhibitory effects in DU145 cells were reported by Bhatia and Agarwal (2001) from the catechin EGCg from green tea leaves, silymarin from milk thistle, and genistein from soybeans. After days of incubation with these substances at concentrations of 50 µM, in vitro growth of DU145 cells was significantly inhibited by EGCg (76%), genistein (80%), and silymarin (50%).

Turning their attention to breast cancer, Agarwal, Sharma, Zhao, et al. (2000) tested a polyphenolic fraction of grape seeds (GSPF) against a line of estrogen-independent human breast carcinoma (MDA-MB468) cells. The same fraction was previously described by Zhao et al. (1999) in a study in mice against chemically induced skin tumors as containing 95% w/w polyphenols with procyanidin B5 at 19% and B5-3'-gallate at 15% as the major constituents. Agarwal, Sharma, Zhao, and colleagues examined the effects of the GSPF (25, 50, or 75 µg/mL) on cultures of the MDA-MB468 cells with much the same parameters used in the study on prostate carcinoma cells, reviewed above (Agarwal, Sharma, and Agarwal, 2000). Again, the results were highly encouraging. Briefly, after 24 to 72 h in MDA-MB468 cells at the three concentrations tested, the GSPF produced highly significant rates of inhibition of cell-cycle regulators (G1 phase regulators cyclin D1 and CDK4) and activation of MAPKs (mitogen-activated protein kinases, ERK1/2, and p38). It also caused a significant induction of Cip1/p21 levels which showed a 2.7-fold increase at the highest dose and resulted in G_1 arrest. Although without induction of apoptosis, terminal differentiation of the MDA-MB468 cells preceded their demise. Compared to controls, treatment of the cells with the GSPF at a dose of 50 µg/mL resulted in growth inhibition rates at 24, 48, and 72 h of 44%, 46%, and 52% ($p < 0.001$), respectively, and from a dose of 75 µg/mL, higher rates were obtained (77%, 86%, and 88%, respectively). When the cell growth pattern was followed for 72 h after washing out the grape seed fraction, evidence was found of an irreversible inhibitory effect of the GSPF, as opposed to a wholly cytostatic effect on the breast cancer cells. The researchers suggested that, based on their results, the GSPF requires further investigation as a potential interventive and/or preventive agent in the battle against breast cancer and that these studies would need to include bioavailability and toxicity.

Ye et al. (1999) assessed the in vitro cytotoxicity of a commercially available proanthocyanidin-rich powder extract of grape seed (InterHealth Nutraceuticals, IH636, batch # AV 609016) in normal human gastric mucosal cells and normal J774A.1 murine macrophage cells, and compared the effects with those obtained in human cancer cell lines (MCF-7 breast cancer, CRL-1739 gastric adenocarcinoma, A-427 lung cancer, and K562 chronic myelogenous leukemic cells). Cultured with these cells at 25 and 50 mg/mL, time- and concentration-dependent growth inhibition was found in all the cancer cell lines except K562 cells, which showed no significant change. Greatest growth inhibition from the grape seed extract (50 mg/mL after 72 h) was found in human lung cancer (48%) and breast cancer cell lines (47%). In both the normal human gastric mucosal cells and normal J774A.1 murine macrophage cells, however, cell growth increased, both time and concentration dependently. The greatest increase in growth was found in the gastric mucosal cells (18%) from 50 mg/mL after 72 h.

Inflammatory Response

Degranulation of mast cells releases other mediators of inflammation, including leukotrienes and platelet activating factor (PAF). Leukotrienes and PAF are implicated in asthma, arthritis, allergies, skin inflammation, and increased vascular permeability (leakage). Free radicals also activate the release of histamine and other mediators of inflammation. In turn, these mediators of inflammation produce more free radicals and thus perpetuate the inflammatory process. By effectively scavenging free radicals, procyanidins inhibit activation of inflammatory mediators (Schwitters and Masquelier, 1993).

The inflammatory process involves several mediators, including indoleamine histamine. Release of histamine into the circulation results in increased capillary permeability. Histamine is made available in microcirculation by two pathways: (1) a direct pathway involving decarboxylation of the amino acid histidine, and (2) an indirect pathway involving the release of histamine from vesicles of degranulating mast cells (Schwitters and Masquelier, 1993). Procyanidins appear to inhibit both pathways.

Procyanidins administered orally for six days at a dose of 6 mg/kg per day inhibited carrageenan-induced paw edema in the rat (Bombardelli and Morazzoni, 1995). Procyanidins inhibit the release of histamine from mast cells by blocking the activation of the enzyme hyaluronidase during degranulation of mast cells. The dual action of procyanidins suggests that these compounds should be effective anti-inflammatory agents. In fact, procyanidins have shown twice the anti-inflammatory activity of phenylbutazone (Blaszo and Gabor, 1980). Procyanidins, as well as epi-(+)-catechin, also inhibit the enzyme histidine decarboxylase, thereby preventing the production of histamine by this pathway (Kakegawa et al., 1985).

Procyanidins have also been shown to inhibit platelet aggregation (Chang and Hsu, 1989) with the potency of some procyanidin oligomers comparable to that of aspirin.

Sen and Bagchi (2001) reported that a grape seed procyanidin extract (GSPE) (ActiVin, batch # AV 609016) exhibits in vitro activity in human endothelial cells indicative of anti-inflammatory activity at the level of inducible adhesion molecule expression. Sen and Bagchi studied the in vitro regulatory effects of the GSPE on two types of adhesion molecules: vascular cell adhesion molecule-1 (VCAM-1) and intracellular adhesion molecule-1 (ICAM-1); these inducible glycoproteins play a role in processes of cell adhesion and show considerable modification in conditions of atherosclerosis, ischemia-reperfusion injury, chronic inflammation, cancer, and diabetes. The researchers add that cell adhesion molecules are known to be activated by oxidants, proinflammatory cytokines (e.g., TNF-α), HIV-1-tat-protein, and phorbol 12-myristate 13-acetate (PMA). In primary human umbilical vein endothelial cells (HUVEC) pretreated with the GSPE at doses of 1-5 µg/mL, VCAM-1 protein expression induced by tumor necrosis factor-α (TNF-α) was significantly down-regulated. The researchers ruled out cytotoxic activity as being responsible for the effect and showed that, at the doses used, gene expression of VCAM-1 was also inhibited by the GSPE. However, ICAM-1 protein expression showed a slight up-regulation at these doses. At the same pretreatment doses, the GSPE significantly decreased TNF-α-induced adherence of Jurkat T-lymphocytes to the endothelial cells, an effect presumed to have been mediated by an NF-κB-dependent pathway. However, an NF-κB reporter assay ruled that out. Given the low concentrations of the GSPE required to inhibit agonist-induced VCAM-1 expression, the researchers suggest that it may have potential use in the treatment of conditions involving altered expression of the adhesion molecule, including inflammatory conditions (Sen and Bagchi, 2001).

Integumentary, Muscular, and Skeletal Functions

Connective Tissue Functions

Collagen is the most abundant protein in the human body. This protein is a key component upholding the integrity of tendons, ligaments, cartilage, blood vessels, bone, skin, and the dermis. Procyanidins and other flavonoids are particularly effective at stabilizing collagen and preventing its destruction (Harmand and Blanquet, 1978; Masquelier et al., 1981; Tixier et al., 1984).

Procyanidins are presumed to affect collagen metabolism by

1. cross-linking with collagen fibers, thereby reinforcing the natural cross-linking of collagen that forms the so-called collagen matrix of connective tissues (Tixier et al., 1984);
2. preventing free-radical damage through their antioxidant and free-radical-scavenging action (Meunier et al., 1989);
3. inhibiting enzymatic cleavage of collagen by the enzymes collagenase, elastase, and hyaluronidase secreted by white blood cells during inflammation and microbes during infection (Maffei Facinó et al., 1994); and
4. preventing the synthesis and release of compounds that promote inflammation, such as histamine, serine proteases, prostaglandins, and leukotrienes (Schwitters and Masquelier, 1993).

Follicular Activity

Grape seed procyanidins (3 μM) stimulated the growth of C3H mouse hair follicle cells in vitro by 230% compared to controls, a degree of activity considerably higher than that of minoxidil (160% from 400 μM). Hair-cycle-converting activity (telogen to anagen phase) was shown in the dorsal hair of C3H mice from a 3% grape seed procyanidin solution at a topical dosage of 200 μL/day per mouse for 19 days. At day 19, 80-90% of the shaven area was covered in hair, compared to no hair growth from topical application of epicatechin, 90-100% from 1% minoxidil, and approximately 30-40% in the untreated control group. No side effects or inflammatory responses were seen in any group (Takahashi et al., 1998).

Skin Diseases

Khanna et al. (2001) examined the effect of a GSPE (ActiVin, batch # 005004) which contains a small amount of resveratrol (5,000 ppm) on in vitro vascular endothelial growth factor (VEGF) expression in a line of human keratinocyte cells (HaCaT). VEGF is thought to play the dominant role in stimulating the development of new cells (angiogenesis) in wounds, and its expression is induced by oxidants and cytokines produced by the actions of neutrophils and macrophages at wound sites as part of the inflammation process which attends wounds. Khanna and colleagues demonstrated that in keratinocytes pretreated with the GSPE (2.5-10 μg/mL), oxidant-induced gene expression of VEGF becomes up-regulated. The gene expression of VEGF and the release of VEGF protein induced by the cytokine tumor necrosis factor-α (TNF-α) was also increased by pretreating the keratinocytes with the GSPE (2.5-15 μg/mL). The researchers concluded their results confirmed an old belief that condensed tannins or procyanidins promote the healing of wounds and that GSPE may be of benefit in the management of "wound healing and other related skin disorders" (Khanna et al., 2001, p. 42).

Metabolic and Nutritional Functions

Antioxidant Activity

The antioxidant property of procyanidins appears to derive from both direct and indirect actions. Direct actions are those that scavenge oxygen free radicals, while indirect actions are those that inactivate promoters of oxygen free-radical formation.

Direct actions. Free radicals interact with a wide range of molecules, such as proteins, membrane lipids, and nucleic acids, to initiate a cascade of events that culminate in pathologic conditions, including ischemia/reperfusion damage, heart disease, arthritis, cancer, and chronic neurodegenerative processes. Free-radical damage has also been implicated in aging. Procyanidins are particularly effective scavengers of superoxide anion, hydroxyl radical anion, and lipid peroxyl radicals (Maffei Facinó et al., 1996; Meunier et al., 1989). By trapping these activated oxygen species, procyanidins inhibit lipid peroxidation.

Indirect actions. Phenolic extracts from red wine markedly inhibit oxidation of low-density lipoprotein (LDL) catalyzed by Cu^{+2} (Frankel et al., 1993). At a 1,000-fold dilution, these extracts were 1.5 times more effective than α-tocopherol (vitamin E). Similarly, grape juice dose dependently inhibits Cu^{+2}-catalyzed oxidation of LDL in vitro (Lanningham-Foster et al., 1995). A 1,000-fold dilution of grape juice (total content of phenolic substances equivalent to 0.018 mmol gallic acid equivalents/mL) delayed the onset of lipid peroxidation by as much as 11 h relative to the control. The antioxidant activity of procyanidins is attributed to their ability to form stable complexes with Cu^{+2} (or Fe^{+2}), cations known to catalyze the formation of oxyradicals (Maffei Facinó et al., 1996). The antioxidant activity of procyanidins is approximately 50 times greater than that of vitamin C and vitamin E (Bombardelli and Morazzoni, 1995).

Leukocyte activation during inflammation results in (1) degranulation and subsequent release of lysosomal proteases and (2) an increase in oxyradicals. The abnormally high levels of both proteases and active oxygenated species combine to damage elastic fibers and endothelial membranes (Schwitters and Masquelier, 1993).

Bagchi et al. (1997) compared the concentration-dependent in vitro oxygen free-radical-scavenging potentials of a commercial GSE (InterHealth Nutraceuticals, Concord, CA) to those of vitamin E succinate, vitamin C, and catalase plus superoxide dismutase (SOD) (Sigma Chemical Co., St. Louis, MO). Differences in antioxidant potential in xanthine oxidase-generated systems were measured using a chemoluminescence assay for hydroxyl radical production and a cytochrome *c* reduction assay for superoxide anion production. The researchers demonstrated that although all the antioxidants showed a dose-dependent inhibition of oxygen free radicals, the scavenging activity of the GSE was superior to that of either vitamin C or vitamin E succinate. In the cytochrome *c* reduction assay, the GSE at concentrations of 5, 25, 50, 100, and 200 mg/L inhibited superoxide anion production by 17%, 59%, 72%, 81%, and 89%, respectively, and at the same concentrations in the chemoluminescence assay inhibited hydroxyl radical production by 18%, 60%, 70%, 78%, and 90%, respectively.

Yamaguchi et al. (1999) examined the in vitro superoxide anion, hydroxyl radical, and methyl radical suppressing activities of a grape seed extract (Kikkoman Corp., Tokyo; ethanol extract of grape seeds containing 38.7% procyanidins and 2.40% monomeric flavanols) in the $H_2O_2/NaOH/DMSO$ system measured by a spin trapping electron spin resonance (ESR) method. Comparisons were made to the activity of the GSE using ascorbic acid, β-carotene, and *dl*-α-tocopherol. The GSE exhibited little suppressant activity on the methyl radical, a slight inhibitory effect on the hydroxy radical, and superior suppression of the superoxide anion; compared to *dl*-α-tocopherol, the IC_{50} of the GSE (nearly 0.00005%) was ten times smaller, and compared to ascorbic acid, 30 times smaller. The activity of β-carotene against superoxide anion production was even lower. Indeed, the activities of the various antioxidants showed variable results depending on the radical being scavenged. For example, while β-carotene showed specificity for the hydroxyl radical, *dl*-α-tocopherol showed specificity for the methyl radical. It showed less activity than ascorbic acid against the hydroxyl radical and exhibited nearly the same activity as ascorbic acid against the superoxide anion. Using different preparations of the GSE, superoxide anion scavenging activity was shown to be mainly dependent upon procyanidin content. As they showed using synthetic oligomers, greater superoxide scavenging activity was evident with the greatest degree of polymerization, pentamers showing the greatest activity and catechin the least.

Castillo et al. (2000) compared the in vitro antioxidant activity of a GSE prepared from the seeds of two varieties each of red and white grape vines grown in Murcia, Spain, to those of ascorbic acid, diosmin (a flavone found in lemons), rutin (flavonol), and (+)-catechin (monomer favan-3-ol). Antioxidant activity was measured by their ability to scavenge the ABTS·+ radical cation (prepared from 2,2'-azinobis(3-ethylbenzothiazoline-6-sulphonic acid diammonium salt through manganese dioxide). According to their Trolox equivalent antioxidant capacities (TEAC values), the GSE extract showed the greatest scavenging activity (TEAC 8.21 mM), followed in potency by rutin (2.75), catechin (1.37), diosmin (1.14), and ascorbic acid (1.12).

Castillo et al. (2000) tested the radioprotective effects of the mutivarietal GSE they prepared in male mice exposed to whole-body X-irradiation (48 cGy) and compared its potency to those of five substances which had previously shown radioprotective effects in rodents: ascorbic acid, DMSO, diosmin, PTU (6-n-propyl-2-thiouracil-6c), and rutin. DMSO (dissolved in water), diosmin, and rutin (also dissolved in DMSO) were each administered by injection (0.6 mL into the lumen gastric) 6 h prior to X-irradiation, whereas ascorbic acid, the GSE extract, and PTU were administered orally as 0.2% of the drinking water five days prior to X-irradiation. According to the frequencies of micronucleated polychromatic erythrocytes (MnPCEs) as a measure of DNA damage in the bone marrow of the irradiated mice, the most active preventive treatment was the GSE, which was followed in potency by rutin, DMSO, ascorbic acid, PTU, and diosmin.

Procyanidins are potent noncompetitive inhibitors of xanthine oxidase (Meunier et al., 1987), an enzyme that promotes the formation of superoxide anion. Bouhamidi et al. (1998) reported that a natural mixture of grape seed procyanidins completely inhibited ultraviolet-C (UV-C)-induced peroxidation of polyunsaturated fatty acids (PUFAs) at low concentrations (2 mg/mL) in vitro. At the same concentration, PUFA contents of mouse brain and mouse liver microsomes irradiated with UV-C were totally protected by the grape seed procyanidin mixture ($p < 0.001$). However, using epigallocatechin gallate and epigallocatechin monomers (equivalent to epicatechin 1.45 mg/L), no protection against UV-C-induced lipid peroxidation of mouse liver microsomes was found.

Sato et al. (1999) showed that after administration to rats for three weeks (100 mg/kg p.o.), a GSE (ActiVin, batch # 60916) caused coronary perfusates to show a significant decrease in malondialdehyde, indicating less oxidative stress and lipid peroxidation compared to the controls. The in vitro tests showed peroxyl radical scavenging activity from the extract at 10 µg/mL, comparable to that of Trolox at 25 µg/mL. In vitro scavenging of γ-irradiation-induced hydroxyl radicals by the extract (10 µg/mL) was comparable to that of DMSO (1 mM).

Koga et al. (1999) measured the antioxidant ability of blood plasma in rats an hour after the administration of a GSE (250 mg/kg p.o.). Measured according to copper ion-mediated oxidation, the difference in antioxidant potential of blood plasma from GSE-treated rats compared to rats administered water only was significant ($p < 0.01$), peaked at 15 min postadministration, and still showed a significant difference for another 105 minutes before falling after 2 h. Even at 8 h postadministration, the plasma obtained from the GSE group continued to show a higher resistance to oxidation compared to that of control rat plasma, even though the difference was not statistically significant. Plasma metabolites of the active treatment group were identified as gallic acid (9.2 μM), (–)-epicatechin (1.9 μM), and (+)-catechin (1.6 μM).

Pharmacokinetics

Following oral administration, gastrointestinal absorption of procyanidins is rapid, and maximum blood levels are observed within 45 min. The half-life is estimated to be 5 h. After a single oral dose of 50 mg/kg, 70% is eliminated within the first 24 h, with 6% as carbon dioxide, 19% in the urine, and 45% in the feces. The major fecal metabolite is ethylcatechol, while the major urinary metabolites are hippuric acid, ethylcatechol, and μ-hydroxyphenylpropionic acid. A commercially available procyanidin-phosphatidylcholine complex was shown to display higher absorption (Bombardelli and Morazzoni, 1995).

CLINICAL STUDIES

Procyanidins (as the active constituent of GSE) have been employed for the treatment of a variety of conditions. These include inflammation, edema, allergies, wound healing, diabetic retinopathy, atherosclerosis, microcirculatory disorders, varicose veins, capillary fragility, macular degeneration, poor night vision, ocular photosensitivity, and increased platelet aggregation. Because of their collagen-protecting activity, procyanidins have been used in dermatology for the treatment of skin conditions secondary to venous insufficiency, or excessive exposure to the sun. Due to their free radical-scavenging properties, procyanidins are used as the active ingredient in cosmetics designed to protect the skin from free-radical-induced damage. Their antimutagenic effects suggest potential chemopreventive properties.

Cardiovascular and Circulatory Disorders

Peripheral Vascular Disorders

Microcirculatory disorders. A randomized, placebo-controlled double-blind study by Lesbre and Tigaud (1983) in 20 patients diagnosed with capillary hyperpermeability and hepatic cirrhosis found significant improvements in the capillary fragility index compared to placebo ($p < 0.05$) in patients receiving a GSE (150 mg procyanidins b.i.d. for eight weeks). Three patients in each group complained of mild gastrointestinal disturbances.

In a double-blind placebo-controlled study of 92 patients with peripheral venous insufficiency, procyanidins (300 mg/day for 28 days) improved functional measures used to assess the treatment (i.e., pain, paresthesias, nocturnal cramps, and edema) by more than 50%. The medication was effective in 75% of patients, resulting in a 41% increase in venous function over the placebo group (Bombardelli and Morazzoni, 1995). In another study, a single oral dose of 150 mg of procyanidins was shown, by objective measurements, to increase venous tone in patients with widespread varicose veins (Royer and Schmidt, 1981).

A placebo-controlled study of GSE by Sarrat (1981) was conducted in 30 patients ages 26-55 without varicose veins. They received 150 mg of grape seed oligomeric procyanidins, a semisynthetic flavonoid product known as diosmin, or placebo daily for 30 days. Those who received the GSE showed significantly fewer indications of functional problems that could develop from impaired backflow of venous blood compared to either of the other two other groups: heaviness of the legs, cramps, itching, abnormal sensations such as burning and prickling, and the sensation of swelling. Sarrat therefore suggested that the extract might be effective in treating the functional problems that could later develop into varicose veins.

In a double-blind study, Delacroix (1981) investigated the effect of a standardized GSE (Endotelon, 150 mg/day for 30 days) in 50 female patients (ages 20-60), most with pregnancy-related chronic venous insufficiency. A comparative treatment group received diosmin (450 mg/day for 30 days). Active treatment began following a 30-day placebo period when the patients were randomly assigned to either treatment group. Although both treatments were effective in reducing symptoms of peripheral venous insufficiency, the GSE was superior in terms of rapidity of action and duration of activity. In the diosmin group, 45% became symptom free versus 65% in the GSE group, and a significant decrease in varicose veins occurred compared to baseline in the GSE group, but not in the diosmin group. Significant toxicity was absent from either agent and side effects were minor. Specifically, some patients reported transient epigastric discomfort in both treatment groups, while vertigo and nausea were reported by some in the GSE group, although in no case was either treatment discontinued due to side effects. Among the 20 pregnant patients (+2 months), no contraindications were found (Delacroix, 1981).

Thébaut et al. (1985) performed a double-blind placebo-controlled study of a standardized GSE (Endotelon, 100 mg t.i.d. for 28 days) in 71 patients diagnosed with peripheral venous insufficiency (ages 24-62), the majority of whom were female (92% on placebo and 97% on extract) and had suffered from venous disease for over seven years. Compared to the placebo group, those receiving the GSE showed a significant improvement ($p < 0.01$) in symptoms (nocturnal cramps, leg heaviness, edema, and tingling). In all, 75% of those in the active treatment group improved compared to 41% on placebo. Four patients dropped out of the trial due to side effects: three on the extract owing to gastrointestinal complaints, itchy scalp, or headache, and one on placebo due to gastrointestinal complaints. Other side effects reported were from six patients in the placebo group (malaise, gastrointestinal complaints, asthenia, constipation, and itchy scalp), and three in the extract group (gastrointestinal complaints, allergic reactions, and headaches) (Thébaut et al., 1985).

Lymphedema. Pecking et al. (1989) conducted a double-blind placebo-controlled study of a GSE (Endotelon) in the treatment of postsurgical edema in 63 women (ages 33-64) who had undergone surgery for breast cancer. Patients received 150 mg of the extract twice daily for six months. Symptoms of edema affecting the arms included tension of the skin, pain, and difficulty moving the arms and shoulders. During the first six weeks, no difference compared to placebo was evident; however, after this period and at six months, a significant difference occurred, with the extract-treated patients showing amelioration of all three symptoms. The researchers attributed the effect to improved intralymphatic transport.

Vascular permeability. In a double-blind study of 25 diabetic and hypertensive patients, the effects of procyanidins (150 mg/day) were compared to placebo. In the procyanidin group, capillary resistance increased by 23% while no change was observed in the placebo group (Lagrue et al., 1981). Using a similar dose of procyanidins in an open trial on 28 diabetic and hypertensive patients, capillary resistance was found to increase by 18% (Lagrue et al., 1981).

A double-blind study of a standardized GSE (Endotelon, 50 mg procyanidins/dose) was conducted by Dartenuc et al. (1980) in 37 hospitalized patients (average age 74.7). Diagnosed with capillary fragility in various pathological contexts, the patients received the extract (50 mg procyanidins b.i.d.) or placebo over a period of 15 days. Capillary resistance improved in ten out of 21 patients on the active treatment and in three out of 12 on placebo.

Metabolic and Nutritional Disorders

Antioxidant Activity

Nuttall et al. (1998) conducted a single-blinded, randomized, placebo-controlled crossover study to examine the antioxidant activity of a GSE (Indena, Leucoselect-phytosome) in 20 healthy nonsmoking volunteers, ages 19-31. The subjects all maintained a standardized dietary pattern and none took vitamin supplements. Subjects received the encapsulated extract (standardized to contain 150 mg of grape procyanidins/capsule) in a dosage of 300 mg/day for five days, or placebo, and again after two weeks of washout during the second treatment period in which the subjects taking placebo were crossed over to active treatment. The results showed that, as measured using an enhanced chemoluminescence assay (citing Whitehead et al., 1992), the mean total antioxidant capacity of serum from those taking the grape procyanidin extract significantly increased compared to baseline but showed no significant change in the placebo group. The increases on day 1 and day 5 of supplementation were comparable and significant compared to baseline at 30 and 60 minutes postadministration ($p < 0.05$ and $p < 0.01$, respectively) and continued to show a significant difference ($p < 0.01$) at 180 min postadministration on day 1 and until 120 min on day 5. Nuttall and colleagues made note of the fact that the results were comparable to those found in a study using the same method of measuring antioxidant capacity in which the active treatment was red wine (5.7 mL/kg).

Neurological, Psychological, and Behavioral Disorders

Retinopathies

Procyanidins were investigated in a double-blind placebo-controlled study of 75 patients suffering from ocular stress caused by a visual display unit. Patients receiving procyanidins at a dose of 300 mg/day for 60 days showed significant improvement in contrast sensitivity relative to the control group. A global improvement of subjective symptoms was also reported (Bombardelli and Morazzoni, 1995). In another study of 91 myopic patients, retinal function (adaptometric curve) was reported to have improved following a dose of 300 mg/day administered over 28 days (Bombardelli and Morazzoni, 1995).

Twenty-six patients with diabetic retinopathy were treated with a daily dose of 100 mg procyanidins for an average of 51 days. The researchers concluded that the treatment had an undisputedly favorable effect on the disease, especially with respect to microaneurisms and exudates (Schwitters and Masquelier, 1993).

In a study of 30 retinopathy patients suffering from microaneurism, hemorrhage, and neovascularization after capillary hypoxia, researchers reported that it was possible to stabilize these retinopathic lesions when procyanidins were administered at 50 mg t.i.d. (Schwitters and Masquelier, 1993).

In a comparative study, Corbe et al. (1988) investigated the possible ocular-strengthening and -protective effects of a GSE (Endotelon) in 100 subjects without ophthalmological pathology. Half the subjects received 200 mg/day for five weeks while the other half went untreated. Compared to the untreated control group, visual adaptation to low-intensity light (night morphoscopic vision) and visual performance following glare as measured with a nyctometer both improved in the extract-treated group. The results were supported in ergovision tests, which showed a stabilization of ocular performances under conditions of change in the light from normal to glare.

Vérin et al. (1978) reported that in a double-blind placebo-controlled study among patients diagnosed with atherosclerotic retinopathy, those who received an extract containing grape seed procyanidins (100 mg/day for one year) showed improved visual acuity or remained stable in 29 out of 30 cases.

DOSAGE

For preventive purposes, a daily dose of 50 mg is recommended. This dose compares with the average daily intake of flavonoids in the diet, which is estimated to be 25 mg. When bound forms are used, such as PCO-phosphatidylcholine, the dose should be maintained at 150 mg. For therapeutic purposes, a daily dose of between 100 and 300 mg is indicated. This dosage is comparable to those utilized in most therapeutic clinical studies (Bombardelli and Morazzoni, 1995). These recommendations are based on a standardized extract containing 80%-85% procyanidin oligomers.

SAFETY PROFILE

Contraindications

Due to the platelet antiaggregatory activity of some procyanidin oligomers being comparable to aspirin (Chang and Hsu, 1989), GSE may be contraindicated in persons taking anticoagulant/blood thinning medications and if taken prior to surgery.

Drug Interactions

One important indirect effect of procyanidins appears to be their ability to act synergistically with vitamin C. Guinea pigs on a diet either suboptimal in vitamin C or devoid of vitamin C developed scurvy and died within a few weeks. When the suboptimal dose of dietary vitamin C (5 mg/kg p.o.) was supplemented with a 20 mg/kg p.o. daily dose of oligomeric procyanidins, the animals fared almost as well as those receiving a full complement of vitamin C (Schwitters and Masquelier, 1993).

Pregnancy and Lactation

No teratogenic effects have been found from procyanidins in pregnant chicks, mice, or rabbits at doses ten times higher than the mean therapeutic dose of 150 mg/day and therefore should be safe during pregnancy (Masquelier, 1990). Among 20 pregnant patients (+2 months), no contraindications were found from a standardized GSE (Endotelon, 150 mg p.o. per day for 30 days) compared to placebo (Delacroix, 1981).

There is no specific information on the safety of procyanidins during lactation, though no adverse effects are known or anticipated. Grape seed extracts may pose a risk of increased bleeding during birth (see Contraindications).

Toxicology

Mutagenicity

The genomic DNA of adult male ICR (CD-1) mice treated with a procyanidin-rich GSE (IH636 Grape Seed Proanthocyanidin Extract or ActiVin, 100 mg/kg p.o.) daily for three or seven days showed no alterations in integrity (Ray et al., 1999).

Toxicity in Animal Models

In acute toxicity studies of procyanidins, the LD_{50} values for rats and mice were greater than 4,000 mg/kg following oral dosing. At a daily oral dose of 60 mg/kg, procyanidins were well tolerated for six months in rats and for 12 months in dogs. No evidence of toxicity was obtained (Bombardelli and Morazzoni, 1995). The acute oral LD_{50} of a procyanidin-rich GSE (IH636 or ActiVin) in fasted mice of either sex is reported to be > 5 g/kg (by gastric tube). Necropsy revealed no gross findings. In rats of either sex, the systemic toxicity NOEL (no-observed-effect-level) for a single dermal application of this GSE to the clipped, intact skin for 24 h was 2 g/kg. From the same route, the dermal LD_{50} of the GSE was determined be > 2 g/kg. Erythema induced by this dose in the 24-h exposure period was very slight in all ten animals, and apart from a very slight desquamation in three, dermal effects had completely resolved by day 12 or sooner. The clipped, intact skin of rabbits to which a single 500 mg dose of the GSE was applied showed a moderate irritation (primary irritation index = 2.7) (Bagchi et al., 2000).

Grape seed oil and its isolated constituents are generally considered safe. At the time of this writing, at least one proprietary grape seed extract (ActiVin, Dry Creek Nutrition, Inc., Modesto, CA) was approved by the Flavor and Extract Manufacturers Association (FEMA) as GRAS (generally recognized as safe) (Dry Creek, 2001). However, some minor constituents of the Oriental subspecies *Vitis coignetiae* have shown hepatoxicity in mice. Interestingly, this biological activity is counterbalanced by the striking hepatoprotective activity of ε-viniferin, a more abundant constituent of the extract (Oshima et al., 1995).

REFERENCES

Agarwal, C., Sharma, Y., and Agarwal, R. (2000). Anticarcinogenic effect of a polyphenolic fraction isolated from grape seeds in human prostate carcinoma DU145 cells: Modulation of mitogenic signaling and cell-cycle regulators and induction of G_1 arrest and apoptosis. *Molecular Carcinogenesis* 28: 129-138.

Agarwal, C., Sharma, Y., Zhao, J., and Agarwal, R. (2000). A polyphenolic fraction from grape seeds causes irreversible growth inhibition of breast carcinoma MDA-MB468 cells by inhibiting mitogen-activated protein kinases activation and inducing G_1 arrest and differentiation. *Clinical Cancer Research* 6: 2921-2930.

Bagchi, D., Bagchi, M., Stohs, S.J., Das, D.K., Ray, S.D., Kuszynski, C.A., Joshi, S.S., and Preuss, H.G. (2000). Free radicals and grape seed proanthocyanidin extract: Importance in human health and disease prevention. *Toxicology* 148: 187-197.

Bagchi, D., Garg, A., Krohn, R.L., Bagchi, M., Tran, M.X., and Stohs, S.J. (1997). Oxygen free radical scavenging abilities of vitamins C and E, and a grape seed proanthocyanidin extract in vitro. *Research Communications in Molecular Pathology and Pharmacology* 95: 179-189.

Bagchi, M., Milnes, M., Williams, C., Balmoori, J., Ye, X., Stohs, S., and Bagchi, D. (1999). Acute and chronic stress-induced oxidative gastrointestinal injury in rats, and the protective ability of a novel grape seed proanthocyanidin extract. *Nutrition Research* 19: 1189-1199.

Bhatia, N. and Agarwal, R. (2001). Detrimental effect of cancer preventive phytochemicals silymarin, genistein and epigallocatechin 3-gallate on epigenetic events in human prostate carcinoma DU145 cells. *The Prostate* 46: 98-107.

Blaszo, G. and Gabor, M. (1980). Oedema-inhibiting effect of procyanidin. *Acta Physiologica Academiae Hungaricae* 65: 235-240.

Bombardelli, E. and Morazzoni, P. (1995). *Vitis vinifera* L. *Fitoterapia* 66: 291-317.

Bomser, J.A., Singletary, K.W., Wallig, M.A., and Smith, M.A.L. (1999). Inhibition of TPA-induced tumor promotion in CD-1 mouse epidermis by a polyphenolic fraction from grape seeds. *Cancer Letters* 135: 151-157.

Bouhamidi, R., Prevost, V., and Nouvelot, A. (1998). High protection by grape seed proanthocyanidins (GSP) of polyunsaturated fatty acids against UV-C-induced peroxidation. *Plant Biology and Pathology* 321: 31-38.

Castillo, J., Benavente-Garcia, O., Lorente, J., Alcaraz, M., Redondo, A., Ortuno, A., and Del Rio, J.A. (2000). Antioxidant activity and radioprotective effects against chromosomal damage induced in vivo by X-rays of flavan-3-ols (procyanidins) from grape seeds (*Vitis vinifera*): Comparative study versus other phenolic and organic compounds. *Journal of Agricultural and Food Chemistry* 48: 1738-1745.

Chang, W.C. and Hsu, F.L. (1989). Inhibition of platelet aggregation and arachidonate metabolism in platelets by procyanidins. *Prostaglandins Leukotrienes and Essential Fatty Acids* 38: 181-188.

Corbe, C., Boissin, J.P., and Siou, A. (1988). Sens lumineux et circulation choriorétinenne. Etude de l'effet des O.P.C. (Endotelon) [Chromatic sense and chorioretinal circulation. Study of the effect of O.P.C. (Endotelon)]. *Journal Francais D'Ophtalmologie* 11: 453-460.

Cormier, F. and Do, C.B. (1993). *Vitis vinifera* L. (grapevine): In vitro production of anthocyanins. *Biotechnology, Agriculture and Forestry* 24: 373-386.

Dartenuc, J.Y., Marache, P., and Choussat, H. (1980). Résistance capillaire en gériatrie: Etude d'un microangioprotecteur = Endotélon [Capillary resistance in geriatrics: A study of a microangioprotector = Endotelon]. *Bordeaux Médical* 13: 903-907.

Delacroix, P. (1981). Étude en double aveugle de l'endotelon dans l'insuffisance veineuse chronique [Double-blind trial of Endotelon® in chronic venous insufficiency]. *La Revue de Médecine* (27-28): 1793-1802.

Dry Creek (2001). Press release: ActiVin grape seed extract earns GRAS approval. Modesto, CA: Dry Creek Nutrition, Inc., June 7. Accessed June 22 at <http://www.activin.com/Press%20Trade.htm>.

Fitzpatrick, D.F., Hirschfield, S.L., and Coffe, R.G. (1993). Endothelium-dependent vasorelaxing activity of red wine and other grape products. *American Journal of Physiology* 265: H774-H778.

Frankel, E.N., Kanner, J., German, J.B., Parks, E., and Kinsella, J.E. (1993). Inhibition of oxidation of human low-density lipoprotein by phenolic substances in red wine. *Lancet* 341: 454-457.

Harmand, M.F. and Blanquet, P. (1978). The fate of total flavonolic oligomers (OGFT) extracted from *Vitis vinifera* L. in the rat. *European Journal of Drug Metabolism and Pharmacokinetics* 1: 15-30.

Jonadet, M., Meunier, M.T., and Bastide, P. (1983). Anthocyanosides extraits de *Vitis vinifera,* de *Vaccinium myrtillus* et de *Pinus maritimus*. I. Activités inhibitrices vis-à-vis de l'élastase in vitro. II. Activités angioprotectrices comparées in vivo [Anthocyanosides extracted from *Vitis vinifera, Vaccinium myrtillus* and *Pinus maritimus*. I. Elastase-inhibiting activities in vitro. II. Compared angioprotective activities in vivo]. *Journal de Pharmacie de Belgique* 38: 41-46.

Joshi, S.S., Kuszynski, C.A., Benner, E.J., Bagchi, M., and Bagchi, D. (1999). Amelioration of the cytotoxic effects of chemotherapeutic agents by grape seed proanthocyanidin extract. *Antioxidants and Redox Signaling* 1: 563-570.

Kakegawa, H., Matsumoto, H., Endo, K., Satoh, T., Nonaka, G., and Nishioka, I. (1985). Inhibitory effects of tannins on hyaluronidase activation and on the degranulation from rat mesentery mast cells. *Chemical Pharmaceutical Bulletin* 33: 5079-5082.

Kamel, B.S., Dawson, H., and Kakuda, Y. (1985). Characteristics and composition of melon and grape seed oils and cakes. *Journal of the American Oil Chemists' Society* 62: 881-883.

Khanna, S., Roy, S., Bagchi, D., Bagchi, M., and Sen, C.K. (2001). Upregulation of oxidant-induced VEGF expression in cultured keratinocytes by a grape seed proanthocyanidin extract. *Free Radical Biology and Medicine* 31: 38-42.

Koga, T., Moro, K., Nakamori, K., Yamakoshi, J., Hosoyama, H., Kataoka, S., and Ariga, T. (1999). Increase of antioxidative potential of rat plasma by oral administration of proanthocyanidin-rich extract from grape seeds. *Journal of Agricultural and Food Chemistry* 47: 1892-1897.

Lagrue, G., Olivier-Martin, F., and Grillot, A. (1981). [A study of the effects of procyanidol oligomers on capillary resistance in hypertension and in certain nephropathies]. *La Semaine des Hopitaux de Paris* 57: 1399-1401.

Lanningham-Foster, L., Chen, C., Chance, D.S., and Loo, G. (1995). Grape extract inhibits lipid peroxidation of human low density lipoprotein. *Biological and Pharmaceutical Bulletin* 18: 1347-1351.

Lesbre, F.X. and Tigaud, J.D. (1983). [The effect of Endotelon on the capillary fragility index of a specified controlled group: Cirrhosis patients]. *Gazette Medicale* 90: 24-28.

Liviero, L., Puglisi, P.P., Morazzoni, P., and Bombardelli, E. (1994). Antimutagenic activity of procyanidins from *Vitis vinifera*. *Fitoterapia* 65: 203-209.

Maffei Facinó, R., Carini, M., Aldini, G., Berti, F., Rossoni, G., Bombardelli, E., and Morazzoni, P. (1996). Procyanidines from *Vitis vinifera* seeds protect rabbit heart from ischemia/reperfusion injury: Antioxidant intervention and/or iron and copper sequestering ability. *Planta Medica* 62: 495-502.

Maffei Facinó, R., Carini, M., Aldini, G., Bombardelli, E., Morazzoni, P., and Morelli, R. (1994). Free radical scavenging action and anti-enzyme activities of procyanidines from *Vitis vinifera*. A mechanism for their capillary protection. *Arzneimittel-Forschung/Drug Research* 44: 592-601.

Masquelier, J. (1990). [Procyanidolic oligomers]. *Parfumes Cosmetiques, Arômes* 95: 89-95.

Masquelier, J., Dumon, J., and Dumas, J. (1981). [Stabilization of collagen with procyanidolic oligomers]. *Acta Therapeutica* 7: 101-105.

Meunier, M.T., Duroux, E., and Bastide, P. (1989). [Free-radical scavenging activity of procyanidolic oligomers and anthocyanosides with respect to superoxide anion and lipid peroxidation]. *Plantes Medicinales et Phytotherapie* 23: 267-274.

Meunier, M.T., Villie, F., Jonadet, M., Bastide, J., and Bastide, P. (1987). Inhibition of angiotensin I converting enzyme by flavonolic compounds: In vitro and in vivo studies. *Planta Medica* 53: 12-15.

Nuttall, S.L., Kendall, M.J., Bombardelli, E., and Morazzoni, P. (1998). An evaluation of the antioxidant activity of a standardized grape seed extract, Leucoselect®. *Journal of Clinical Pharmacy and Therapeutics* 23: 385-389.

Oshima, Y., Namao, K., Kamijou, A., Matsuoka, S., Nakano, M., Terao, K., and Ohizumi, Y. (1995). Powerful hepatoprotective and hepatotoxic plant oligostilbenes isolated from the Oriental medicinal plant *Vitis coignetiae* (Vitaceae). *Experientia* 51: 63-66.

Pecking, A., Desprez-Curely, J.P., and Megret, G. (1989). Oligomères pro-cyanidoliques (Endotelon) dans le traitement des lymphoedèmes post-thérapeutiques des membres supérieurs [Oligomeric procyanidins (Endotelon) in the post-therapeutic treatment of the upper limbs]. *Congrès International d'Angiologie,* Toulouse, France, October 4-7, 1989, pp. 69-72.

Peng, Z., Hayasaka, Y., Iland, P.G., Sefton, M., Hoj, P., and Waters, E.J. (2001). Quantitative analysis of polymeric procyanidins (tannins) from grape (*Vitis vinifera*) seeds by reverse phase high-performance liquid chromatography. *Journal of Agricultural and Food Chemistry* 49: 26-31.

Preuss, H.G., Montamarry, S., Echard, B., Scheckenbach, R., and Bagchi, D. (2001). Long-term effects of chromium, grape seed extract, and zinc on various metabolic parameters of rats. *Molecular and Cellular Biochemistry* 223: 95-102.

Ray, S.D., Kumar, M.A., and Bagchi, D. (1999). A novel proanthocyanidin IH636 grape seed extract increases in vivo Bcl-XL expression and prevents ace-tominophen-induced programmed and unprogrammed cell death in mouse liver. *Archives of Biochemistry and Biophysics* 369: 42-58.

Ricardo Da Silva, J.M., Rigaud, J., Cheynier, V., Cheminat, A., and Moutounet, M. (1991). Procyanidin dimers and trimers from grape seeds. *Phytochemistry* 30: 1259-1264.

Royer, R.J. and Schmidt, C.L. (1981). [Evaluation of venotropic drugs by venous gas plethysmography: A study of procyanidolic oligomers]. *La Semaine des Hôpitaux de Paris* 57: 2009-2013.

Saito, M., Hosoyama, H., Ariga, T., Kataoka, S., and Yamaji, N. (1998). Anti-ulcer activity of grape seed extract and procyanidins. *Journal of Agricultural and Food Chemistry* 46: 1460-1464.

Sarrat, L. (1981). Abord thérapeutique des troubles fonctionnela des membres inférieurs par un microangioprotecteur l'Endotelon [Therapeutic approach to the disordered function of the lower limbs by means of the microangioprotector, Endotelon]. *Bordeaux Médical* 11: 685-688.

Sato, M., Maulik, G., Ray, P.S., Bagchi, D., and Das, D.K. (1999). Cardioprotective effects of grape seed proanthocyanidin against ischemic reperfusion injury. *Journal of Molecular and Cellular Cardiology* 31: 1289-1297.

Schwitters, B. and Masquelier, J. (1993). *OPC in Practice. Bioflavonols and Their Application.* Rome, Italy: Alfa Omega.

Sen, C.K. and Bagchi, D. (2001). Regulation of inducible adhesion molecule ex-pression in human endothelial cells by grape seed proanthocyanidin extract. *Molecular and Cellular Biochemistry* 216: 1-7.

Shirataki, Y., Kawase, M., Saito, S., Kurihara, T., Tanaka, W., Satoh, K., Sakagami, H., and Motohashi, N. (2000). Selective cytotoxic activity of grape peel and seed extracts against oral tumor cell lines. *Anticancer Research* 20: 423-426.

Takahashi, T., Kamiya, T., and Yokoo, Y. (1998). Proanthocyanidins from grape seeds promote proliferation of mouse hair follicle cells in vitro and convert hair cycle in vivo. *Acta Dermato-Venereologica* 78: 428-432.

Thébaut, J.F., Thébaut, P., and Vin, F. (1985). Étude de l'Endotelon® dans les manifestations fonctionelles de l'insuffisance veineuse périphérique. Résultats d'une en double aveugle portant sur 92 patients [Study of Endotelon® in functional manifestations of peripheral venous insufficiency. Results of one double-blind carried out on 92 patients]. *Gazette Médicale* 92: 96-100.

Tixier, J.M., Godeau, G., Robert, A.M., and Hornbeck, W. (1984). Evidence by in vivo and in vitro studies that binding of pycnogenols to elastin affects its rate of degradation by elastases. *Biochemical Pharmacology* 33: 3933-3939.

Vérin, M.M.P., Vildy, A., and Maurin, J.F. (1978). Rétinopathies et O.P.C. [Retinopathies and O.P.C.]. *Bordeaux Médical* 11: 1467-1474.

Wegrowski, J., Robert, A.M., and Moczar, M. (1984). The effect of procyanidolic oligomers on the composition of normal and hypercholesterolemic rabbit. *Biochemical Pharmacology* 33: 3491-3497.

Whitehead, T.P., Thorpe, G.H.G., and Maxwell, S.R.J. (1992). Enhanced chemoluminescence assay for antioxidant capacity in biological fluids. *Analytica Chemica Acta* 266: 265-277.

Yamaguchi, F., Yoshimura, Y., Nakazawa, H., and Ariga, T. (1999). Free radical scavenging activity of grape seed extract and antioxidants by electron spin resonance spectrometry in an H_2O_2/NaOH/DMSO system. *Journal of Agricultural and Food Chemistry* 47: 2544-2548.

Yamakoshi, J., Kataoka, S., Koga, T., and Ariga, T. (1999). Proanthocyanidin-rich extract from grape seeds attenuates the development of aortic atherosclerosis in cholesterol-fed rabbits. *Atherosclerosis* 142: 139-149.

Ye, X., Krohn, R.L., Liu, W., Joshi, S.S., Kuszynski, C.A., McGinn, T.R., Bagchi, M., Preuss, H.G., and Stohs, S.J. (1999). The cytotoxic effects of a novel IH636 grape seed proanthocyanidin extract on cultured human cancer cells. *Molecular and Cellular Biochemistry* 196: 99-108.

Zhao, J., Wang, J., Chen, Y., and Agarwal, R. (1999). Antitumor promoting activity of a polyphenolic fraction isolated from grape seeds in mouse skin two-stage initiation-promotion protocol, and identification of procyanidin B5-3'-gallate as the most effective antioxidant constituent. *Carcinogenesis* 20: 1737-1745.

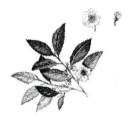

Green Tea

BOTANICAL DATA

Classification and Nomenclature

Scientific name: *Camellia sinensis* (L.) Kuntze

Family name: Theaceae

Common names: The English word *tea* is thought to be derived from the Malay word *teh* or the Chinese (Amoy dialect) word *t'e*. The word was originally pronounced *tay* when the Dutch introduced both the word and the beverage to England around 1655. It is still pronounced this way in certain British dialects, but the customary pronunciation, *tee*, although originating in the 1600s, gained predominance only in the eighteenth century (Gutman and Ryu, 1996).

The Mandarin Chinese term *ch'a* is the origin of other tea terms in other languages. Together, these two terms, *t'e* and *ch'a*, are the basis of all other common names for tea. The Dutch and Portuguese, the first major tea importers, probably introduced these terms into European languages and the Middle East, along with the commodity itself (Gutman and Ryu, 1996).

Cultivated tea was originally classified as two species, *Thea sinensis* and *Thea bohea* by Linnaeus in 1752; later, this classification was revised and *Thea sinensis* became the designation for the small-leaved Chinese variety and *Thea assamica* designated the large-leaved Assam plant. Both cultivated tea and nontea plants are today classified in a single genus, *Camellia,* in the family Theaceae (Gutman and Ryu, 1996).

Description

Camellia sinensis occurs variably as an evergreen shrub (growing to one meter) or as a tree (up to 15.24 meters in height). Trimming keeps the plant at a height suitable for picking the leaves for tea. The leaves are elliptic, dark green, glossy, alternate, and toothed, 5-14 cm in length, and 1.9-5 cm wide. The white flowers, which have five to six sepals and seven to eight petals, measure 2.5 cm across with stamens half as long united below. The fruit appears as a cap and contains one to several seeds that yield an oil (Bailey and Bailey, 1976).

HISTORY AND TRADITIONAL USES

Archaeological evidence (Jelinek, 1978) indicates that tea leaves steeped in boiling water were consumed by *Homo erectus pekinensis* more than 500,000 years ago. Chinese legend, described in the *Cha Ching* (Tea book) around C.E. 780, attributes tea drinking to one of the earliest Chinese herbalists, King Shen Nong, circa 2700 B.C.E.. Indian legend claims that tea was brought to China by Siddhartha Guatama Buddha during his travels in that country (Gutman and Ryu, 1996).

Today, botanic evidence suggests that both India and China, as well as Burma and Thailand, can lay claim to the origin of cultivated tea. Wild-type plants have been found in the forests of these countries which appear to be the ancestors of the present-day cultivars. Although genuine wild-type plants may no longer exist, previous explorations have determined that wild tea once grew from Nepal north and eastward to Formosa, the Liu-Kiu Islands, and southern Japan (Gutman and Ryu, 1996).

Tea was introduced to the West by Turkish traders in the sixth century. It was introduced as a commercial commodity into Tibet by the Song dynasty between 960-1127. The Dutch, followed by the British, established the tea trade between Europe and the Far East around 1600. The British pioneered the plantation-style cultivation of tea in India and Ceylon, and the Dutch developed tea cultivation in Java and Sumatra. China lost its dominance of the tea industry in 1850 when its exports were exceeded by those of India and Ceylon (Weatherstone, 1992).

In the traditional medicine of India, green tea is recorded as a mild excitant, stimulant, diuretic, and astringent, and the leaf-infusion of tea was formerly used to remedy fungal infections caused by insects (Nadkarni, 1976). In traditional Chinese medicine (TCM), green tea has been used as an astringent, cardiotonic, central nervous system stimulant, and diuretic (Keys, 1991). Other uses in TCM include the treatment of flatulence, regulation of body temperature, promotion of digestion, and improvement of mental processes (Snow, 1995).

CHEMISTRY

Nitrogenous Compounds

Alkaloids

Tea is a popular beverage because it contains methylxanthines, primarily caffeine with trace amounts of theophylline and theobromine. Tea commonly contains about half as much caffeine as a comparable volume of coffee (50-100 mg/cup versus 100-200 mg/cup), and the amounts of other methylxanthines present are pharmacologically insignificant. Caffeine is a competitive adenosine antagonist and potent central nervous system (CNS) stimulant which stimulates the cortical and medullary regions of the brain and, at high doses, the spinal cord. Caffeine is a CNS, respiratory, cardiac, and skeletal-muscle stimulant; it causes coronary dilation, smooth-muscle relaxation, and diuresis (Rall, 1980). Acute activity studies suggest that caffeine is harmful to the cardiovascular system and aggravates hypertension; however, the results of long-term administration of caffeine do not support this contention (Robertson et al., 1981).

Phenolic Compounds

Polyphenolics

Most of the therapeutic benefits of green tea are due to the catechins, which are polyphenols with a flavonoid structure (see Figure 1). Four major green tea catechins exist, namely (–)-epicatechin (EC), (–)-epigallocatechin (EGC), (–)-epicatechin gallate (ECg), and (–)-epigallocatechin gallate (EGCg), with lesser amounts of catechin derivatives also present. The *epi* designation refers to the stereochemistry at position 3, where the hydrogen is attached in the β position. In the catechins, the C ring of the flavonoid skeleton, like that of catechol, contains two ortho aromatic hydroxyls, while in the gallocatechins the C ring contains an ortho-trihydroxyl substitution similar to pyrogallol. The C3 hydroxyl can be esterfied with gallic acid to yield gallocatechin gallate (GCg) or epigallocatechin gallate (EGCg), which can easily be oxidized to quinone structures by oxygen or enzymes. It is this property that makes these catechins potent antioxidants and free-radical scavengers. Epigallocatechin gallate (EGCg) is the most potent antioxidant of the series, and this compound is considered the most physiologically active (Harbowy and Ballentine, 1997; Mitscher et al., 1997).

The catechins comprise approximately 30% to 42% of the total green tea solids, and a typical cup of green tea contains between 300 and 400 mg polyphenols, of which 10-30 mg is EGCg. Some commercial green tea extracts contain up to 97% polyphenols (Harbowy and Ballentine, 1997; Mitscher et al., 1997).

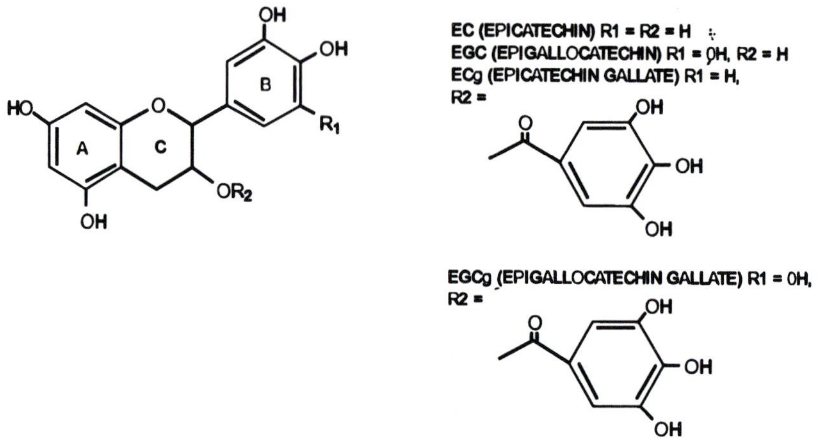

FIGURE 1. Catechins from Green Tea

Other Constituents

In addition to catechins and methylxanthines, other constituents present in green tea beverage include: flavonols, which are closely related to catechins but have a higher level of oxidation in ring C; theogallin, a condensation product of gallic acid and quinic acids; theanine, an *N*-methyl derivative of glutamine whose presence is said to correlate with green tea quality; trigalloylglucose, different than pentagalloylglucose (tannic acid), which is not present; minerals, including relatively high levels of aluminum and manganese; trace levels of carotenoids and volatile oils which are negligible nutritionally but essential for the aroma and other sensory qualities of tea (Harbowy and Ballentine, 1997; Mitscher et al., 1997; Gutman and Ryu, 1996); and the chlorophyll-related compounds, pheophytins a and b (Higashi-Okai et al., 2000).

Tea Processing

The best quality teas are derived from the young shoots, or flushes, comprising the first two or three leaves, plus the growing bud. Poor quality teas, used in the manufacture of instant teas and brick tea, are made from leaves further down the stem (Gutman and Ryu, 1996). Three main varieties of tea are recognized. *Black tea,* the most prevalent commercial variety, is prepared by allowing enzymatic oxidation to take place shortly after picking; during the drying and curing process, the action of enzymes present in the tea leaves (*O*-diphenol oxidases, also known as polyphenol oxidases) lead to an oxidative polymerization termed fermentation. Catechin and other phenolics present in the leaves polymerize to form brown or reddish compounds known as theaflavins and thearubigins, compounds responsible for the characteristic color of black tea infusions. *Oolong teas,* which are characteristically reddish or yellow in color, result from a partial fermentation. *Green tea* is unfermented; postharvest processing, in the form of thermal treatments consisting of either roasting or sweating, are applied as soon as possible after harvesting to arrest the enzymatic oxidation process of the catechins, to which most of the health benefits of tea are ascribed. The composition of green tea, therefore, is similar to that of the fresh, unprocessed leaves (Harbowy and Ballentine, 1997; Graham, 1992).

PRECLINICAL STUDIES

The pharmacological activities of green tea polyphenols have been investigated in preclinical studies, using both in vitro and animal test systems, with many of these investigations focusing on antioxidant activities. It is interesting to note that the freshly picked leaves of *Camellia sinensis* contain a peroxidase (TcAPX II) with the highest specific activity for ascorbate as a reducing substrate ever recorded. This discovery is of great interest to plant physiologists owing to the potential function of the enzyme as an antioxidant formed in plants in response to aerobic stress (Kvaratskhella et al., 1999).

Metabolic and Nutritional Disorders

Antioxidant Activity

The total antioxidant activity (TAA) of green tea, standardized to contain 70% catechin polyphenols (Greenselect), was measured by Pietta et al. (1998) according to the Trolox equivalent antioxidant capacity method of Miller and Rice-Evans (1996). By comparison, the mean TAA of green tea extract (5.12 mM Trolox) was far higher than those of many popular herbal extracts. In order of most to least activity, they included dry standardized extracts of bilberry (Indena, Milan, Italy, 25% anthocyanins), grape seed OPC (Leucoselect), grape skin (Specchiasol, Verona, Italy), *Ginkgo biloba* (Ginkgoselect, 24% flavone glycosides, at 2.57 mM Trolox), pine bark (Dèrivès Rèsiniques et Terpèniques, Dax, France, Oligopin, 22% total flavanols), *Ginkgo biloba* (Ginkgoselect, 15% flavone glycosides), witch hazel (Indena, 16.7% tannins, as hamamelitannin), *Ginkgo biloba* (Ginkgoselect, 11% flavone glycosides), propolis EPID (Specchiasol, Verona, Italy, 3.1% flavonoids), hawthorn (Indena, 1.8% vitexin 2"-*O*-rhamnoside), artichoke (14% caffeoyl derivatives), *Panax ginseng* (15% ginsenosides), passionflower (4% isovitexin), and *Echinacea* sp. (4.5%

echinacoside); the latter three (Indena) at < 0.32 mM Trolox (Pietta et al., 1998).

Lin et al. (1998) found that rats fed a basal diet mixed with powdered green tea leaves (2.5%) for 63 weeks showed significantly higher activity levels of superoxide dismutase in blood serum ($p < 0.0005$), as well as significantly increased hepatic activity levels of GST (glutathione S-transferase) and catalase (both $p < 0.05$).

Paquay et al. (2000) reported that green tea potently scavenges nitric oxide (NO) in vitro and, although less potent than red wine, its potency was about five times that of black tea. The most active constituent was EGCg, which also inhibited the induction of inducible NO synthetase (iNOS), as did green tea, and with about twice the potency of black tea. At the inhibition of peroxynitrate, green tea exhibited greater than twice the activity of black tea. In this aspect, it was calculated (prepared at 3 g/L) to be similar to red wine and 25 times higher than that of white wine.

In the suppression of auto-oxidation of linoleic acid, Higashi-Okai et al. (2000) reported higher in vitro antioxidant activity from pheophytins a and b (chlorophyll-related substances found in the nonpolyphenolic fraction) than in either vitamin E or EGCg. Pheophytins a and b were also more potent than EGCg in the scavenging of superoxide anion generated in mouse macrophages. In both assays the effects of pheophytins a and b were dose dependent.

Incubated with human aortic endothelial cells, LDL oxidation mediated by these cells was significantly and dose-dependently inhibited by catechin and epicatechin derived from green tea, as measured by the inhibition of conjugated dienes. Inhibition ranged from 3.9% to 98% from two commercial green tea powder extracts at concentrations of 0.08-5 ppm. The catechin derivatives and the extracts of green tea also showed dose-dependent inhibitory activity against end-stage lipid peroxide decomposition product formation and early lipid peroxidation product formation (Pearson et al., 1998). Others have shown that human LDL copper-catalyzed peroxidation is significantly inhibited by green tea and green tea polyphenols in vitro, beginning to show significant activity at 0.5 µg/mL ($p < 0.05$) and 0.1 µg/mL ($p < 0.01$), respectively. At the same concentration as green tea, theanine also showed a significant inhibitory activity at twice the incubation time ($p < 0.05$), whereas caffeine required three times the incubation time to reach the same level of inhibitory significance (Yokozawa and Dong, 1997).

Cardiovascular and Circulatory Functions

Effects on Cholesterol and Lipid Metabolism

Lin et al. (1998) noted a significant decrease in the weight of rats after 63 weeks on a basal diet to which powdered green tea leaves were admixed

(2.5%), without any effect on amounts of feed or water consumed compared to controls on the basal diet alone. At week 15, the green tea group weighed 12% less ($p < 0.05$), and between week 15 and the end of the study at week 63, they showed an average weight loss compared to the controls of 10-18% ($p < 0.0005$) and 100% survived. A significant hypolipemic effect was found in the green tea group in total serum cholesterol, triglyceride, and LDL-cholesterol levels at week 27 ($p < 0.05$), but by week 63 serum LDL-c was not significantly different from the control group. HDL-c showed no significant change relative to the controls at any time.

Watanabe et al. (1998) reported that an aqueous methanol extract of green tea potently inhibited acetyl-CoA carboxylase activity in vitro. The main active constituent was identified as (–)-epigallocatechin gallate (IC_{50} 3.1×10^{-4} M), while almost the same potency was shown for (–)-epicatechin gallate and (–)-epigallocatechin gallate. The inhibition of acetyl-CoA carboxylase activity by green tea was found to be greater than that of black tea, pooal tea, enokitake mushrooms, *Panax ginseng*, Welsh onion, and other foodstuffs.

Long-term feeding of green tea polyphenols to rats produced significant reductions in lipids and lipid peroxides in plasma, liver, and kidney. In older animals (3-19 months), lipid peroxides, triglycerides, total cholesterol, and phospholipids were significantly decreased in the serum of the group fed green tea polyphenols as 1% of their diet. Weight gain was reduced only in young rats, and the livers and kidneys of rats in this group had normal weights compared to the controls. These results suggest a hypocholesterolemic effect of long-term feeding of green tea polyphenols (Sano et al., 1995).

In experimental hyperlipidemic rats, a six-week supplementation with green tea polyphenols resulted in significant reductions of serum cholesterol and triglycerides and significant elevations of serum high-density lipoprotein (HDL) compared to controls (Shen et al., 1993). In another study, mice fed an atherogenic diet supplemented with green tea constituents did not show elevated cholesterol levels in their blood, but their serum triglyceride and HDL levels were unaffected (Yamaguchi et al., 1991).

Peripheral Vascular Functions

Huang et al. (1999) have shown that (–)-epicatechin exhibits a concentration-dependent vasorelaxing effect on the endothelium-intact rat mesenteric artery and significantly increases the tissue content of cyclic GMP of these arteries ex vivo. Tests showed that the endothelial mechanisms responsible appear to involve an increase in the release of nitric oxide and an increase in intracellular calcium.

Thrombosis, Hemostasis, and Embolism

Hot water extracts of green tea and green tea catechins dose-dependently inhibited platelet aggregation in washed rabbit platelets, while EGCg suppressed platelet aggregation induced by collagen, thrombin, and platelet aggregating factor (Sagesaka-Mitane et al., 1990). The ability of green tea constituents catechin and epicatechin to inhibit platelet aggregation in human platelets was tested in vitro using platelets obtained from healthy human volunteers ($n = 15$). The catechins were each (20-200 µg/mL) incubated with the platelets for 5 min prior to inducing aggregation with arachidonic acid, epinephrine, or adenosine diphosphate. At their highest concentrations, epicatechin inhibited aggregation by 94% and catechin by 68%, yet tests showed no significant alteration of blood coagulation enzymes by either tannin, whether in thrombin, prothrombin, or thromboplastin levels (Neiva et al., 1999).

Kang et al. (1999) studied the antithrombotic activity of EGCg and green tea catechins (GTC) in rats in a model of murine pulmonary thrombosis. In addition, they examined the ex vivo effects of GTC and EGCg on platelet aggregation in rats and mice and in vitro using human platelets. Rats administered GTC (10 to 100 mg/kg p.o.) 90 min prior to the induction of thrombosis (collagen- and epinephrine-induced) showed significant protection from death or paralysis owing to pulmonary thrombosis. Protection afforded by GTC was dose-dependent and significant at all doses. Protection ranged from 40.0% from 10 mg/kg to 85.0% from 100 mg/kg. EGCg produced similar results, and 10 mg/kg afforded protection (45.5%) comparable to that of aspirin at 50 mg/kg (47.4%). In a separate experiment, Kang and co-workers examined the ex vivo effects of GTC and EGCg on mouse tail bleeding times. At doses of 4 and 10 mg/kg i.p. 60 min prior to testing, both substances caused a significant prolongation of bleeding times, which were comparable to aspirin (10 mg/kg i.p.). Significant inhibition of adenosine diphosphate- and collagen-induced ex vivo platelet aggregation (53.3% and 39.3%, respectively) was also shown from rats administered GTC (100 mg/kg p.o.). Dose-dependent in vitro antiaggregatory effects of GTC and EGCg on platelet-rich human plasma were shown against epinephrine-, collagen-, calcium ionophore-, and ADP-induced platelet aggregation, whereas aspirin failed to inhibit ADP-induced aggregation. The in vitro effects of GTC and EGCg on blood coagulation enzymes in platelet-rich human plasma were examined in doses of 0.1, 0.5, and 1 mg/mL. No significant changes were found in either the thrombin time, the activated partial thromboplastin time, or the prothrombin time, suggesting to Kang and colleagues that the antithrombotic effect of GTC and EGCg may be facilitated by the inhibition of platelet aggregation rather than by any direct effect on thrombin/thromboplastin formation.

As mentioned in the previous section, the amino acid theanine (2-amino-5-(*N*-ethylcarboxylamido)pentanoic acid) is a potent inhibitor of thrombin-stimulated thromboxane formation in whole blood. Ali et al. (1990) also measured significantly reduced levels of thromboxane in adult and juvenile rats fed unprocessed tea leaves for eight weeks. However, feeding of processed leaves failed to produce this result. In vitro experiments also provided evidence for cardioprotective effects of green tea constituents and suggested a possible role in preventing atherosclerosis. The amino acid theanine, which is unique to tea, inhibited thromboxane formation in rabbit whole blood stimulated by thrombin. When the amino acid was fed to rats for eight weeks, significant decreases in plasma thromboxane were measured as was a decrease in cholesterol (Ali et al., 1990).

Digestive, Hepatic, and Gastrointestinal Functions

Hepatic Functions

Animal studies indicate a hepatoprotective action for green tea and its components. Lin et al. (1998) noticed a significant increase in liver catalase and glutathione *S*-transferase activity in rats fed a powdered green tea-supplemented (2.5%) basal diet for 63 weeks. Male rats fed a diet consisting of 0.5% instant green tea powder (Thomas J. Lipton, New Jersey) in their drinking water showed 20%-30% less hepatic nuclear aflatoxin B_1-DNA binding compared to rats without green tea in their drinking water. When the rats were pretreated with the instant green tea powder (two or four weeks at 0.5% of their drinking water), glutathione *S*-transferase placental form-positive hepatocytes induced by aflatoxin B_1 were inhibited by 60%-70%. The researchers concluded that green tea appears to modulate aflatoxin B_1 metabolism in rats (Qin et al., 1997).

Hasegawa et al. (1995) administered green tea to mice in drinking water for two weeks prior to a single i.p. injection of the carcinogen 2-nitropropene. Liver nuclear 8-hydroxydeoxyguanosine levels and hepatoxicity parameters were determined 8 and 16 h after treatment. Green tea suppressed the increase in 8-hydroxydeoxyguanosine in liver nuclear DNA by 50% at both time points; similarly, time-dependent elevations of 2-nitropropene-induced liver enzymes were prevented by the green tea treatment. Although green tea had no obvious effect on decreases in serum lipid peroxide or triglyceride levels associated with carcinogen exposure, histopathological examination showed effective protection against hepatic degenerative changes at 15 h. Green tea extract was more effective than EGCg alone at the same concentration, indicating that other hepatoprotective constituents were present in the crude extract.

D-galactosamine has been used as a model for viral hepatitis; injection into rats causes fulminant hepatitis within 48 h, as shown by marked increases in levels of serum aspartate aminotransferase (AST), alanine amino transferase (GPT), alkaline phosphatase (ALP), and decreases in serum protein and cholesterol levels. Animals administered a water extract of green tea in doses from 50-200 mg/kg were protected from these responses (Hayashi et al., 1992).

Endocrine and Hormonal Functions

Carbohydrate Metabolism; Antidiabetic Activity

The crude catechin tannin fraction (90% catechin tannins) administered to rats (either 60 or 80 mg p.o.) before orally administered soluble starch caused a significant suppression of increases in serum glucose and insulin concentrations, whereas from 40 mg p.o. little suppression occurred compared to controls. In the same method of administration using sucrose instead of starch, the catechin fraction suppressed the increases in plasma insulin and glucose at oral doses of 10 and 80 mg, but not at 5 mg p.o. Sucrase activity in the groups treated with the catechin tannin fraction (5, 10, and 80 mg) was significantly lower compared to controls for 2 h after they received the starch. Similarly, intestinal α-amylase activity showed little increase in the catechin-treated group (40, 60, and 80 mg) compared to their respective controls (Matsumoto et al., 1993).

Genitourinary and Renal Functions

Renal Functions

In a model of renal failure in male rats, Yokozawa et al. (1997) studied the kidney-protective activity of individual green tea polyphenols and a green tea polyphenol mixture (Sunphenon, Taiyo Kagaku Co., Yokkaichi, Japan) as a water extract of green tea. Administered in the drinking water, the water extract (10-20 mg/kg per day for 25 days) caused a significant decrease ($p < 0.05$) in blood levels of the uremic toxin methylguanidine, which otherwise accumulates as kidney failure progresses. Among the individual tannins showing methylguanidine-inhibiting activity, (−)-epigallocatechin 3-*O*-gallate (EGCg) and (−)-epicatechin 3-*O*-gallate (ECg) were the most effective, and dose dependently so beginning at 2.5 mg/kg per day. These individual tannins showed more potent activity than the total polyphenol mixture.

Immune Functions; Inflammation and Disease

Cancer

Antiproliferative activity. In vitro studies have shown that EGCg can inhibit the growth of both human and mouse leukemic cells (Otsuka et al., 1998), and human stomach cancer cells (KATO III cells) (Hibasami et al., 1998; Okabe et al., 1999). It is postulated that the inhibition of carcinogenesis caused by green tea polyphenols might be orchestrated through the modulation of phase II enzymes in the liver, which may metabolize carcinogens toward inactivation (Bu-Abbas et al., 1998). After rats were fed an infusion of green tea as 2.5% (w/v) of their drinking water for four weeks, only one phase II liver enzyme (glucuronosyl transferase) showed any significant increase ($p < 0.05$). However, the green tea infusion at 5% (w/v) of the drinking water caused two liver enzymes to increase significantly: glucuronosyl transferase ($p < 0.001$) and glutathione *S*-transferase ($p < 0.01$). Activity of the antioxidant enzyme catalase in the liver was significantly inhibited ($p < 0.001$) at this dosage, and cytosolic protein showed a slight decrease ($p < 0.05$). At 2.5% (w/v) of the drinking water, which approximates the concentration consumed by humans, the infusion caused no significant decrease in catalase activity or cytosolic protein content. However, at this concentration, black tea, which contains far fewer flavanols than green tea, showed the most activity in stimulating hepatic phase-II activities. Glutathione *S*-transferase activity (GST) ($p < 0.01$) and glucuronidation of 2-aminophenol were both enhanced by black tea at 2.5% (w/v), whereas neither green tea or decaffeinated black tea caused any significant increase in GST and only a modest enhancement of 2-aminophenol glucuronidation. The researchers concluded, therefore, that neither caffeine nor flavanols—two of the most abundant compounds found in tea—were responsible for the increase in phase-II liver enzyme activity and that the constituents involved had yet to be determined (Bu-Abbas et al., 1998).

Significant increases in certain phase-II enzyme activities were reported by Lin et al. (1998) in a long-term feeding study of green tea as part (2.5%) of a basal diet in rats. Based on serum marker-enzyme levels, glutathione *S*-transferase activity and catalase activity showed a significant increase after 63 weeks of the tea-supplemented diet. However, the activity of superoxide dismutase (SOD) and liver GSH (glutathione) content (both antioxidative principles in the body) showed no significant change.

Bridge, Sun, Peter, et al. (1998) identified EGCg and infusions of green tea as inhibitors of an NADH oxidase known as quinol (NADH) oxidase, or NOX. The activity of NOX is needed by normal cells for growth. Cancer cells can express NOX all the time, whereas normal cells do so only when dividing. An overactive form of NOX, known as tumor-associated NOX (tNOX), plays a significant role in the ability of tumor cells to grow (Bridge,

Sun, Peter, et al., 1998). Moreover, tNOX is found in the blood serum of cancer patients but not of healthy individuals (Chueh et al., 1998).

Bridge, Sun, Peter, et al. (1998) explained that while infusions of black tea inhibited tNOX activity at a dilution of 1:10, green tea infusions were active at dilutions from 1:100 to as low as 1:1,000. Significantly, EGCg inhibited tNOX activity without inhibiting healthy cell NOX activity; e.g., whereas EGCg showed tumor-inhibiting and cytocidal activity against human mammary cancer cells (8T-20) in vitro, it had no cytotoxic effect on normal human mammary cells (MCF-10A cells). Cancer cells in the presence of EGCg were found to undergo apoptosis following a complete inhibition of growth (Bridge, Sun, Peter, et al., 1998). Furthermore, EGCg was a more potent inhibitor of a breast cancer cell line (4T1) affecting mice than sulfonylurea (LY181984)—a potent antitumor compound and inhibitor of tNOX—or capsaicin from cayenne pepper *(Capsisum annuum)* (Bridge, Sun, Wu, et al., 1998).

Other in vitro studies (Mitscher et al., 1997) have shown that green tea extracts and polyphenolics positively influence metabolic processes associated with cancer initiation and tumor growth. Green tea polyphenols have been shown to inhibit DNA synthesis in cultured mouse erythroleukemia cells and in rat hepatoma cells. Water extracts of green tea as well as EGCg inhibited activation of protein kinase C by teleocidin, a tumor promoter, and also inhibited the growth of lung and mammary tumor cells in culture.

Jankun et al. (1997) have postulated that the antitumor activity of green tea derives from inhibition of urokinase-type plasminogen activation (uPA), an enzyme that human cancers use for cellular invasion of healthy cells and to metastasize. Agents that inhibit uPA have caused complete remissions of tumors in mice and can otherwise decrease the size of tumors. Jankun and colleagues, aware of the fact that, to date, such agents are either too toxic for use in humans or too weak to be effective, scanned for new inhibitors of uPA examining 190,000 compounds in chemical databases. Among them, EGCg showed up, which bound to uPA in such a way that it would interfere with the enzyme and inhibit its activity. They confirmed this in an amidolytic assay of the enzyme and compared the activity to a known uPA inhibitor (amiloride) used in the treatment of cancer. EGCg was weaker and required higher concentrations than amiloride; however, as Jankun and colleagues point out, the maximum allowable dose of amiloride is 20 mg, whereas a single cup of green tea contains over seven times that amount in EGCg. They surmise that so much uPA inhibitor could reduce cancer incidence in humans and/or reduce the size of existing tumors.

The induction of apoptosis of cancer cells by EGCg is the focus of an increasing number of studies on green tea. Working with human epidermoid carcinoma (A431) cells, Ahmad et al. (2000) have shown that the apoptotic activity of EGCg involves the arrest of the cell cycle in phases G_0-G_1, which results in an irreversible process whereby the cancer cells cannot repair the damage done and subsequently perish through apoptosis. Their research of protein kinase complexes involved in the apoptotic activity of EGCg led them to investigate a cell-cycle regulating complex of *cki-cyclin-cdk;* cyclin-dependent kinase (cdk) and their inhibitors, proteins known as cyclin-dependent kinase inhibitor (cki), which together (cki-cyclin-cdk) constitute one of the main regulators of the cell cycle. Cancer cells are known to be defective at points that the cki-cyclin-cdk machinery regulates and so have become enticing targets for the development of agents that will intervene against their growth. Synthetic agents that act as cell-cycle inhibitors of tumor cells are currently undergoing clinical study in cancer patients as a new generation of anticancer drugs, and Ahmad and colleagues believe that EGCg and other green tea polyphenols could also become agents used in the management of neoplastic disease. While their research of EGCg is ongoing, Ahmad and co-workers have shown that its ability to facilitate cell-cycle dysregulation of cancer cells appears to be mediated through an up-regulation of all the major cyclin-dependent kinase inhibitors involved in the cell-cycle phase G_0/G_1 (Ahmad et al., 2000). A growing body of evidence indicates that the ability of EGCg to deregulate the cell-cycle phase G_0/G_1 in cancer cells is due to inhibition of the transcription factor nuclear factor-kappaB (NF-κB) (Lin and Lin, 1997; Yang, De Villiers, et al., 1998; Nomura et al., 2000), an effect seen only in normal cells from high concentrations of EGCg (Ahmad et al., 2001).

Paschka et al. (1998) identified EGCg as the active component in green tea that induced in vitro apoptosis in several types of human prostate cancer cells (DU145, LNCaP, and PC-3). Growth of the androgen-dependent human prostate cancer cell line LNCaP was inhibited by 90% from 1 μM of EGCg. Bhatia and Agarwal (2001) compared the in vitro growth-inhibiting activity of EGCg to those of genistein and silymarin in DU145 cells at the same concentration (50 μM). After five days of treatment the respective rates of inhibition were 76%, 80%, and about 50%. Gupta et al. (2000) investigated the apoptosis-inducing, cell-cycle-deregulating, and cell-growth-inhibiting activities of EGCg on both androgen-insensitive (DU145 cells) and androgen-sensitive human prostate carcinoma (LNCaP) cells in vitro. EGCg was added to cultures of the cells and incubated for 48 h. The results showed that the growth of both types of prostate carcinoma cells was inhibited (dose dependently and time dependently at concentrations of 10-80 μg/mL) and that EGCg had induced apoptosis and DNA fragmentation (40 and 80 μg/mL). After 48 h of treatment with four concentrations of EGCg (10, 20, 40, and 80 μg/mL), dose-dependent apoptosis was evident in both types of cells with slightly greater activity in the androgen-insensitive DU145 cell line (i.e., 13.9%, 19.1%, 42.2%, and 58.8% apoptosis, respectively). From DNA cell-cycle analyses of the cells, it was found that EGCg treatment resulted in a significant induction of the cyclin kinase inhibitor

WAF1/p21, which in turn appeared to mediate arrest of the G_0/G_1 cell cycle in both types of prostate cancer cells.

In a preliminary study, Li et al. (2000) measured the apoptotic activity and antiproliferative effect of green tea polyphenols (GTPs) and EGCg by adding them to cultures of peripheral blood T lymphocytes (PBLs) derived from adult T-cell leukemia patients ($n = 3$) and healthy volunteers (controls). After three days of incubation, growth of the PBLs derived from healthy controls was minimally inhibited by either GTPs or EGCg at 3-9 µg/mL and showed definite inhibition at 27 mg/mL, whereas the growth of PBLs from the leukemia patients was inhibited by 3-27 µg/mL of GTPs or EGCg. Evidence of apoptotic activity and significant DNA fragmentation was found in the PBLs from the leukemia patients from either EGCg of GTPs at 27 µg/mL, while little apoptotic activity and no DNA fragmentation was evident in PBLs of the healthy controls. Based on previous studies determining the absorption and concentration of GTPs and EGCg in human plasma, the authors estimated that from drinking ten cups of green tea it would be possible for one to achieve a plasma concentration of 5-9 µg/mL, which would allow a 50% growth inhibition of the adult T-cell leukemia cells.

Research shows that green tea prevents tumor growth partly by inhibiting angiogenesis, i.e., through the suppression of blood supply to tumors by suppression of new blood vessel formation. In vitro tests by Cao and Cao (1999) found that EGCg may inhibit the growth of blood vessels by inhibition of endothelial cell growth, since nonendothelial cells, such as smooth-muscle cells of rats or T241 fibrosarcoma cells, showed no inhibitory response. In a bovine endothelial cell proliferation assay designed to measure capillary endothelial cell proliferation, EGCg showed significant proliferation-inhibitory activity ($p < 0.005$) at a concentration of 10 µg/mL^{-1}. In the chick chorioallantoic membrane assay, EGCg significantly and dose-dependently (1-100 µg/disc) inhibited the growth of new blood vessels. Finally, when a water extract of green tea was tested in mice as 1.25% of the drinking water, it caused a highly significant ($p < 0.0001$) inhibition of vascular endothelial growth factor-induced corneal neovascularization, compared to a water-only control group. Blood vessel length was inhibited by 55% and corneal neovascularization area by 70%. Since vascular endothelial growth factor (VEGF) is one of the most potent endothelial factors known, this is a significant result in itself. As the researchers point out, this finding has implications for the treatment and possible prevention of other diseases critically affected by angiogenesis, such as blindness resulting from diabetes (Cao and Cao, 1999).

In mice with a type of tumor known to be highly insensitive to doxorubicin (M5076 ovarian sarcoma), administration of green tea powder (100 mg/kg p.o. daily for four days) enhanced the antitumor activity of the agent

(2 mg/kg i.p. daily for four days) 2.5-fold, whereas no tumor inhibition was seen from doxorubicin alone. The combination resulted in 45% inhibition of tumor growth. Tissue examination revealed that significantly more doxorubicin was concentrated in the tumors in the group of mice treated with green tea powder plus doxorubicin than in mice treated with the anticancer agent alone. Researchers found no increase in doxorubicin in normal cells as a result of green tea, nor in tests with green tea components caffeine and theanine. Rather, they reported that both theanine and green tea caused doxorubicin concentrations in the heart to decrease. Given that doxorubicin causes cardiac toxicity, this finding may have clinical relevance. Green tea powder or theanine, a component of green tea, plus doxorubicin resulted in even lower concentrations of the anticancer agent in the heart (Sadzuka et al., 1998).

Others have reported in vitro apoptotic activity from green tea constituents (polyphenols and epigallocatechin-3-gallate) against various human cancer cell lines: human prostate carcinoma cells (DU145), human carcinoma keratinocytes cells (HaCaT), human epidermoid carcinoma cells (A431), mouse lymphoma cells (L5178Y) (Ahmad et al., 1997), human colorectal adenocarcinoma cells (Caco-2), human breast ductal cancer cells (Hs578T) (Chen et al., 1998), and human lung cancer cells (PC-9) (Suganuma et al., 1999).

The root of the tea plant (*Camellia sinensis* var. *assamica*) has also shown antiproliferative activity. After soaking the roots in 50% aqueous methanol, the resulting solid residue dissolved in water was administered to two dosage groups (5 mg/kg and 10 mg/kg i.p. daily for nine days, respectively) of male mice, a day after tumor initiation (Ehrlich ascites carcinoma). These groups were compared to a control group treated with saline and another group treated with the anticancer agent 5-fluorouracil (5-FU) (10 mg/kg i.p. per day for nine days). The median survival time of the lower dosage tea root extract (TRE) group was greater than the saline control group (32 days versus 19 days, respectively), and 3/11 mice were cured. The higher dosage TRE group showed a median survival time of 60 days and 4/9 mice were cured. No cures were found in the 5-FU treatment group. All the mice found cured were still alive five months later and showed no signs of adverse effects. No signs of toxicity were found in either TRE treatment group, whether in the pathology of vital organs, or body weight and appearance. Blood cells counts, including white and red blood cells, lymphocytes, and neutrophils, were abnormal in the untreated tumor-bearing mice compared to normal mice. In the higher dosage TRE group, the treatment restored these cell counts to normal and in the cured mice they remained normal 60 days later. The authors also showed evidence suggesting that the effect of TRE is partly immunological, since peritoneal macrophage levels were increased in the higher dosage TRE group (Sur and Ganguly, 1994).

Chemopreventive activity. In vitro studies have shown that EGCg can inhibit the growth of chemically induced lung tumors (Yang, Yang, et al., 1998). In addition, the nonpolyphenolic fraction contains chlorophyll-related substances (pheophytin a and b) which, when topically applied, potently suppressed the formation of skin tumors in mice in a two-stage tumor promotion model (Higashi-Okai, Oyani, et al., 1998). Topical applications or oral feeding of green tea polyphenols inhibited mouse skin tumor formation induced by combinations of mutagens, tumor promoters, and ultraviolet light (Mukhtar et al., 1994; Wang, Huang, et al., 1992). Another study demonstrated the inhibition by green tea and EGCg of lung tumorigenesis in mice induced by *N*-nitrosodiethylamine (NDMA) and the tobacco carcinogen 4-(methylnitrosoamino)-1-(3-pyridyl)-1-butanone (Xu et al., 1992). Similar results have been reported in animal studies with green tea on the development of cancers of the esophagus (Han and Xu, 1990), forestomach (Wang, Agarwal, et al., 1992; Oguni et al., 1992), duodenum and small intestine (Fujita et al., 1989), colon (Yamane et al., 1991; Narisawa and Fukaura, 1993), liver (Qin, 1991; Chung and Liu, 1991), pancreas (Hiura et al., 1997), mammary gland (Hirose et al., 1994), and prostate (Liao et al., 1995).

Green tea inhibits the formation of nitrosamine in vitro (Nakamura and Kawabata, 1981) and in vivo (Wu et al., 1993) and the formation of nitrate-induced tumors in animals (Xu and Han, 1990; Oguni et al., 1992). Green tea catechins, especially EGCg, inhibit in vitro damage to DNA induced by acidic nitrate and inhibit acid nitrate-induced tyrosine nitration (Rice-Evans, 1999). In a study of seven types of tea drunk in China, out of 145 samples tested green tea was the most effective at blocking the in vitro formation of *N*-nitrosmorpholine (NMOR) under simulated gastric fluid condition (by 89.04%), an effect correlated with polyphenol contents, notably catechins. Furthermore, low concentrations of green, black, or oolong tea increased the in vitro formation of NMOR whereas higher amounts inhibited its formation (Wu et al., 1993).

In many of these studies, EGCg has been implicated as the most active of the green tea catechins. However, female rats on a regular diet containing 0.5% of an extract of green tea standardized to contain 58.4% EGCg showed no significant difference in DMBA-induced mammary tumor incidence and size compared to untreated controls, although a tendency toward inhibited mammary tumor development at the stage of tumor promotion was evident. Curiously, a diet containing a green tea extract with a higher concentration of EGCg (81%) was less effective (Hirose et al., 1997).

Kostyuk et al. (2000) examined the in vitro protective effects of green tea extract (41.2% total polyphenols) and the polyphenols ECG and EGCg against asbestos-induced cellular injury to macrophages. Whereas exposure to chrysotile or crocidolite asbestos caused rat peritoneal macrophages to undergo cell lysis and to release LDH (lactose dehydrogenase), these effects were dose-dependently inhibited by the addition of increasing amounts of green tea extract or the polyphenol constituents. Chrysotile asbestos- and crocidolite asbestos-induced hemolysis of red blood cells was also dose-dependently inhibited by green tea extract and the polyphenols in vitro. Test results indicated that asbestos toxicity appears to be closely related to cell injury caused by overproduction of radical oxygen species.

Schut and Yao (2000) investigated the chemopreventive activity of green and black teas in female F-344 rats exposed to a carcinogen that forms in the process of cooking proteinaceous meats such as chicken, fish, and red meats. Known as PhIP or 2-amino-1-methyl-6-phenylimidazo[4,5-b]pyridine, this chemical is the most abundant carcinogen in a class of highly mutagenic heterocyclic amines. Previous studies had shown that certain tea polyphenols and both green and black tea inhibit the mutagenicity of PhIP in bacteria. In the Fischer 344 rat, PhIP is known to induce prostate and colon tumors in males and lymphomas and mammary tumors in females. Since both types of tea were previously shown to inhibit PhIP adduct formation in the colon of male F-344 rats, chemoprevention was measured in terms of DNA adduct formation in the females rats. For six weeks, groups of the rats received a standard diet with antioxidant ingredients removed and either drinking water or water containing infusions of green tea or black tea (each 2% wt/vol). During the last three weeks they were treated with the carcinogen daily by gavage. Compared to controls on plain drinking water, adduct formation on days 1 and 8 after cessation of the PhIP treatment was significantly lower in the colons of rats receiving green tea (40.0% and 75.0%, respectively) but only on day 1 in the black tea group (by 40.0%). Adduct levels in the small intestine were also significantly lower in the green and black tea groups, but only on day 8 (54.4% and 81.8%, respectively). Adduct levels in mammary epithelial cells were significantly lower in the green tea group on both days (33.3% and 80.0%, respectively), but not in the black tea group. However, liver adducts were significantly lower in both tea groups on both days. Changes in adduct levels in other organs (lungs, heart, spleen, pancreas, kidneys, stomach, cecum, and white blood cells) were not significantly different compared to controls.

A chemopreventive activity against prostate cancer was shown by Gupta et al. (1999) using a polyphenolic fraction of green tea. Significant in vitro activity was found from the fraction against ornithine decarboxylase (ODC), an enzyme known to be overexpressed in the prostatic fluid of patients with prostate cancer. Stimulated by androgens, ODC functions as a growth and development rate regulator of normal prostate cells and those affected by tumors. Human prostate cancer cells (LNCaP cells) treated with testosterone induced the activity of ODC, whereas pretreatment with the polyphenol fraction (20-60 µg/mL) of green tea significantly inhibited the induction; at 40 µg/mL the polyphenol fraction almost completely inhibited the testosterone-induced mRNA expression of ODC. Further in vitro tests revealed that pretreatment with the polyphenol fraction dose-dependently inhibited the testosterone-induced increase in growth of LNCaP cells (e.g., by 71% from 80 μg/mL, the highest dose tested). Carrying their studies to rats, Gupta and colleagues reported that as 0.2% of the rats' drinking water for seven days, the polyphenolic fraction caused a 54% decrease in ODC activity induced by testosterone. Similar results were found in the prostate glands of mice. Testosterone treatment caused a twofold increase in ODC activity, whereas mice that drank the polyphenolic fraction in their drinking water showed a 40% inhibition of the testosterone-induced increase in ODC activity. However, in both animal experiments, feeding the polyphenolic fraction alone had no effect on ODC activity.

Another group (Nakamura et al., 1992) investigated the effects of four kinds of tea extracts on neoplastic transformation of Balb/C mouse epidermal cells induced by 12-O-tetradecanoylphorbol-13-acetate (TPA). Hot water extracts of green, black, pu-erh, and oolong tea decreased the TPA-induced transformation by 70%, 67%, 32%, and 46%, respectively. The green tea ethylacetate fraction, containing the highest concentration of catechins, exhibited the highest activity (68.8% of total activity). Other fractions of green tea ($CHCl_3$, n-BuOH, aqueous) had much lower levels of activity. In black tea, however, the aqueous fraction was the most active with 43.2% of the total activity. Therefore, both green tea and black tea appear to inhibit tumor promotion and the green tea catechins and other high molecular weight substances contribute to this activity.

Osawa et al. (1992) showed that tea polyphenols inhibited mutagenicity induced during lipid peroxidation in the red blood cell membrane, and that the polyphenols acted as oxygen radical scavengers during the microsomal activation of carcinogens, such as 2-hydroxy-napthylamine. The researchers investigated the structure/activity relationships related to the antioxidant activity of tea polyphenols. Against lipid peroxidation in an adriamycin-induced microsome preparation and a t-butylhydroperoxide-induced erythrocyte ghost test system, presence of the gallic acid moiety was found to be an important structural feature contributing to the antioxidant activity.

The mutagen/carcinogen benzo[a]pyrene, when metabolically activated to an epoxydiol, can bind to DNA. Green tea polyphenolics not only inhibit this epoxidation reaction but also bind to the epoxy derivative in place of DNA, thus acting as an intercepting agent preventing the compound from binding with DNA, thereby circumventing subsequent mutagenic events (Wood et al., 1982).

The antimutagenic properties of green tea extracts and individual catechins have been examined by several groups of investigators using various in vitro test systems. For instance, Wang et al. (1989) tested the antimutagenic activity of a water extract of green tea with a concentrate of green tea polyphenols and EGC using *Salmonella typhimurium* tester strains TA100 and TA98, and various promutagens: including benzo[*a*]pyrene, aflatoxin B_1, and metabolically activated polycyclic aromatic hydrocarbons. All concentrates were highly antimutagenic yet not toxic to the test system. When ranked as inhibitors of aryl carbon hydroxylase activity using benzo[*a*]pyrene as the substrate in cultured hepatic and epidermal cells, the inhibition was dose dependent with the following order of activity: epigallocatechin gallate > green tea phenolics > epicatechin gallate > epigallocatechin > epicatechin > catechin. Horikawa et al. (1994), utilizing *S. typhimurium* tester strain T98 challenged with S9-activated benzo[*a*]pyrene, found a similar rank order: epigallocatechin gallate > epigallocatechin > catechin > epicatechin.

Various studies suggest that the antimutagenic properties of green tea extracts and green tea phenolics result primarily from antioxidant actions which interfere with the metabolic formation of mutagens (Mitscher et al., 1997). However, Bu-Abbas et al. (1997), in a study of fully characterized green tea flavanol fractions, concluded that their role in the antimutagenic activity of green tea is limited. They found no association between antimutagenic activity and any individual flavanol in the Ames test against the mutagens benzo[*a*]pyrene, Glu-P-1, nitrosopyrrolidine, or 2-aminoanthracene. Yet marked inhibition of mutagenic activity was demonstrated by the fractions containing various flavanols. The authors concluded, therefore, that the major constituents responsible for the potent antimutagenic activity of green tea would appear to be something else contained in the flavanol fraction (Bu-Abbas et al., 1997). In addition, the chlorophyll-related constituents of green tea leaves, pheophytin a and b, have shown antigenotoxic activity and are derived from the nonpolyphenolic fraction (Higashi-Okai, Taniguchi, et al., 1998).

Aqueous extracts of green tea in concentrations customarily consumed by humans caused a very marked dose-dependent inhibition of Aroclor 1254-hepatic S9-mediated mutagenicity caused by heterocyclic amines and polycyclic aromatic hydrocarbons, as well as isoniazid-induced S9-mediated mutagenicity of nitrosamines. Direct acting mutagens (e.g., 9-amino acridine and *N*'-methyl-*N*'-nitronitrosoguanidine) were also inhibited, but less than those requiring metabolic activation. When the aqueous green tea extract was added after metabolic activation, some inhibition of mutagenicity was measured with the effect being significantly less than that obtained when the extract was added prior to oxidative activation (Bu-Abbas et al., 1994).

Immunopotentiation. Hu et al. (1992) reported that EGCg, ECg, and theaflavin digallate (TF3) show strong enhancing effects on B-cells, which significantly increased their production in vitro. Tannic acid and gallic acid were only somewhat active. Tests showed that the immunoenhancing activity was not macrophage mediated. The effect of EGCg was very much dose dependent, whereby the opposite reaction was evident beyond a certain dose. For example, in the direct plaque-forming cell response to sheep red blood cells, EGCg (0.01 to 0.5 μg/mL) enhanced the response by 39% to 309%. But above those amounts, it caused the response to be suppressed. B-cell proliferation, spontaneous and LPS-induced, showed a similar pattern, with large doses suppressing and smaller doses enhancing B-cell proliferation. Compared to LPS, the effect of EGCg was almost the same at the same doses, indicating a potent immunoenhancing effect.

Immunoprotection. Katiyar, Matsui, et al. (1999) studied the effect of topical EGCg on human skin irradiated with ultraviolet B (UVB) in an effort to determine protective effects against immunological functions besides protection against erythema. Studies in mice had shown sunscreen provided no protection against UVB-induced local cutaneous or systemic immunological functions, despite protecting against sunburn. UVB was applied at an equivalent dose of 4 MED (minimal erythema dose) to the buttocks of healthy adults who volunteered for the study. Prior to the irradiation, skin areas (2.5 cm^2) received topically applied EGCg (3 mg/100 μL acetone), no treatment, and a vehicle only (acetone). The area of skin treated with EGCg 30 min prior showed significantly less erythema at 48 h postirradiation compared to the other treatments. As for immunological effects of UVB exposure, the skin left untreated showed increased infiltration of monocytes/macrophages and neutrophils, which are primarily responsible for generating radical oxygen species that can lead to skin damage. By comparison, the skin pretreated with EGCg showed fewer dead cells and an inhibition of macrophage/neutrophil infiltration, as measured by tissue levels of myeloperoxidase. Katiyar, Matsui, and colleagues (1999) noted that cyclooxygenase activity was induced in mouse skin by the application of tumor promoter and in human skin following UVB irradiation. Topical pretreatment with EGCg also significantly inhibited UVB-induced cyclooxygenase activity in the skin of the volunteers, as shown by significantly less prostaglandin (PG) metabolite formation. EGCg pretreatment inhibited PGE$_2$ formation by 64% ($p < 0.0005$), while PGD$_2$ and PGF$_{2\alpha}$ formation were inhibited by 55% and 47%, respectively. Katiyar, Challa, et al., (1999) found evidence in mice to suggest that in addition to reducing the quantities of neutrophils and CD11b+ monocytes/macrophages that infiltrate inflammatory lesions of the skin (held to be a causative factor in immunosuppression induced by UV light), the protection afforded by topically applied EGCg (3 mg/mouse) against UVB-induced immunosuppression may additionally result from a greatly decreased production of IL-10 in the draining lymph nodes and skin and a marked increase in the production of IL-12 in the draining lymph nodes (Katiyar, Challa, et al., 1999). A subsequent study on human skin exposed to UV radiation confirmed that pretreatment with

EGCg caused a significant reduction in the number of infiltrating neutrophils and CD11b+ monocytes/macrophages (Katiyar et al., 2001).

Infectious Diseases

Microbial infections. Yam et al. (1998) explain that antimicrobial activity was recognized from a water extract of *Camellia sinensis* (tea) as long as 90 years ago. They attribute the activity to an indirect action through inhibition of bacterial enzymes, and a direct action in the form of bactericidal and bacteriostatic effects. In their own research, they found extracts of green tea reversed the methicillin resistance of methicillin-resistant *Staphylococcus aureus*. Working with Japanese sencha green tea, they prepared an extract by freeze-drying the filtered liquid produced from 2 g of dry, powdered sencha tea leaves, to which 100 mL of boiling water was added. A synergistic activity was evident against methicillin-resistant *S. aureus* when the extract was combined with either methicillin or benzylpenicillin. In these tests, the amount of green tea extract required was far less than that showing direct inhibition of the bacteria. Either the extract at a 100-fold dilution or 8 mg/L of methicillin showed little growth-inhibitory activity alone against strains of methicillin-resistant *S. aureus*. But when combined, the inhibition of growth was greater than 200 mg/L of methicillin alone and lasted 24 h or more. The authors reported significant synergistic activity in all 40 of the methicillin-resistant *S. aureus* strains tested. At 40- to 200-fold dilutions, the extract converted the resistant strains to show sensitivity to methicillin. Yam and colleagues also reported that a 250-fold dilution of the extract inhibited the synthesis of a resistance-conferring substance (PBP2') produced by a strain of *S. aureus* by greater than 90%, and inhibited synthesis of PBP1. The authors note that the ability of the extract to inhibit PBP2' production by methicillin-resistant *S. aureus* could represent an important means of countering the resistance of pathogenic bacteria to antimicrobial agents, and also because green tea has a history of thousands of years of use by literally billions of people without adverse effects, this resource becomes all the more enticing (Yam et al., 1998).

Ikigai et al. (1993) found green tea extracts inhibited the growth in cultures of a variety of bacterial pathogens, including resistant strains of *Staphylococcus aureus*. The extract proved more active than the individual phenolics (i.e., EC and EGCg) (Ikigai et al., 1993).

In vitro studies have shown that green tea polyphenolics can inhibit the growth of *Streptococcus mutans,* the bacteria that causes dental caries, by reducing their adhesion to the tooth surface and possibly by interfering with the action of glucosyltransferase (Mitscher et al., 1997; Sakanaka et al., 1992), an enzyme produced by the bacteria that initiates the decay process. Among the main catechins, greater inhibition of *S. mutans* was found from gallocatechin (GC) than EGCg or EGC (Sakanaka et al., 1989). However, against the in vitro growth of a plaque bacteria most often found in adults with advanced periodontitis *(Porphyromonas gingivalis),* EGCg was by far the most active green tea polyphenol (Sakanaka et al., 1996).

In vitro studies also indicate an inhibitory action of oolong tea polyphenols on glucosyltransferase of *Streptococcus mutans,* and an inhibition of adhesion of *S. mutans* to saliva-coated hydroxyapatite discs (Mitscher et al., 1997). In another study, green tea polyphenols were given to rats at various percentages of their drinking water (0.1% to 0.5%) for 40 days along with a cariogenic diet. The 0.1% polyphenol supplementation significantly reduced total fissure caries lesions by about 40% without toxicity (Sakanaka et al., 1992).

Green tea extracts inhibited the growth of cariogenic streptococci, including *S. mutans,* an effect possibly mediated by inhibition of the synthesis of insoluble glucans. ECG and EGCg also interfered with the sucrose-dependent adherence of these bacterial cells, and at low concentrations (Mitscher et al., 1997). Along the same line of inquiry, Horiba and colleagues (1991) tested extracts of four varieties of green tea against 24 bacterial pathogens isolated from infected root canals. The extracts inhibited the growth or were bactericidal against 18 of the 24 strains tested.

Viral infections. In studies on the infectivity of influenza type A and B viruses in cultured canine kidney cells, Nakayama et al. (1993) reported that concentrations of EGCg as low as 1 µmol effectively inhibited the absorption of the virus to the cell membranes, along with the plaque formation that develops subsequent to infection. This concentration was about 100 times lower than the concentration of amantadine, an anti-influenza drug, required to produce a comparable effect. When the polyphenol was added to the cell cultures after they were exposed to the virus, however, plaque formation was not inhibited, suggesting that the polyphenol exhibits a preventive action, inhibiting the virus from entering the cells.

EGCg and EC were reported to be relatively potent inhibitors in vitro of reverse transcriptase and RNA polymerase in cell-free systems (10 and 20 ng/mL, respectively). However, the concentrations required to inhibit reverse transcriptase in cell cultures were cytotoxic (Nakane and Ono, 1990).

Inflammatory Response

With in vitro methods, Higashi-Okai, Taniguchi, et al. (1998) recently identified nonpolyphenolic constituents in green tea leaves, pheophytin a and b, as inhibitors of human polymorphonuclear neutrophil (PMN) activation. Chemotaxis and oxygen free-radical generation by functional PMNs was also inhibited by these chlorophyll-related compounds, as well as the release of the inflammatory cytokine interleukin-1β by PMNs.

CLINICAL STUDIES

Clinical investigations of the potential health benefits of green tea and its extracts are relatively few; however, epidemiological studies in various human populations and cohorts provide evidence suggesting that the regular ingestion of green tea can have important health benefits.

Cardiovascular and Circulatory Disorders

Cardiotonic; Cardioprotection

In a randomized short-term study in 60 smokers ($\geq$ 10 cigarettes/day; all volunteer subjects judged to be healthy), de Maat et al. (2000) investigated the effects of black tea and green tea in combination with green tea polyphenols (GTPs) on various indicators of cardiovascular risk compared to a control group administered mineral water. The treatment period lasted four weeks during which time two groups of the volunteers were administered freeze-dried extracts of either black tea or green tea (500 mg) in tea bags with the instruction to consume six cups of the tea per day (150 mL), which would result in a dosage of 3 g of tea solids/day. Another group was instructed to ingest 24 capsules of GTPs/day (150 mg GTPs/capsule), which was equivalent to consuming 9 g of green tea solids or 18 cups of green tea/day. The flavonoid compositions of the teas and the catechin tannin composition of the GTPs were determined using reverse phase HPLC. The subjects were further instructed to abstain from red wine and any other tea and not to consume more than two 100 mL glasses of fruit juice or two oranges/day. From analyses of blood samples taken during the run-in phase and at day 29 of the treatment phase, no significant effects on cardiovascular risk factors were found in either of the tea groups or the GTP group compared to the controls, whether in plasma levels of inflammatory system markers of risk (C-reactive protein, IL-1β, IL6, and TNF-α) or hemostatic factors of vWF (von Willebrand factor), uPA (urokinase-type plasminogen activator), FVIIa (activated factor VII), and plasminogen activator inhibitor-1 (PAI-1) (de Maat et al., 2000).

Starting in 1960, a large investigation of 12,763 middle-aged men from seven countries examined the relationship between dietary intake of flavonoids and heart disease (Hertog et al., 1995). A strong positive correlation between flavonoid content of the diet and a lower risk of heart disease was found in these men. Mortality rates from heart disease varied greatly between different countries and flavonoid intake resulted in 1/4 of the differences. Following up on the Netherlands arm of the study, Hertog and co-workers (1993) compared the flavonoid intake of 805 elderly men with their risk for cardiovascular disease over a five-year period. The primary source of flavonoids in their diet was apples (10%), tea (61%), and onions (13%). Hertog and colleagues found that the volume of flavonoids in the diet inversely correlated to the risk of death from heart disease and that the risk of nonfatal heart attack was similarly inversely correlated. Men with the highest intake of flavonoids had half the risk of those with the lowest intake.

In a study of black tea in 20,000 middle-aged Norwegian men and women, those who drank five or more cups/day had lower levels of cholesterol than those who did not drink tea; for men the figure was 9.3 mg/dL lower, and for women 5.8 mg/dL lower. Black tea drinkers were less likely to die from a heart attack, and systolic blood pressure in these groups was inversely related to tea consumption (Stensvold et al., 1992).

Cerebrovascular Dysfunctions

Loss of mental acuity and cognitive functions with age has been associated with free-radical damage to brain tissues and to the circulatory system which brings oxygen and nutrients to the brain. Therefore, the antioxidant nature of green tea polyphenols might have a protective or restorative effect on cerebrovascular impairment. A Chinese study reported on 46 patients with dementia or other age-related cerebrovascular deficits who were given green tea polyphenol supplements for one month. Ninety-one percent of the dementia patients and 60% of those with verbal disorders showed significant improvement. The treatments appeared to be most effective when initiated in the early stages of the disease (Mitscher and Dolby, 1998).

Effects on Cholesterol and Lipid Metabolism

Tsubono and Tsugane (1997) randomly selected 207 men (mean age 44.4) and 164 of their wives (mean age 41.4 years) from five regions in Japan for inclusion in an analysis of cholesterol levels after drawing their blood two weeks earlier. Extensive controls were employed for dietary and other factors affecting health, including smoking/nonsmoking, nutrient intake, alcohol intake, education, physical activity, district of origin, intake of animal fats, fatty acids, coffee, and oolong tea, and other factors. Among the women, green tea was consumed at the rate of at least one cup/day by 68% and on average they drank 3.1 cups/day. Among the men, 69% drank at least one cup/day and on average consumed 3.5 cups/day. Following adjustments for both dietary and nondietary factors, the researchers found no significant effect of green tea consumption on lipid profiles, whether of triglycerides, total cholesterol, or HDL cholesterol.

In contrast, a Japanese study of 1,371 men aged 40 and older, Imai and Nakachi (1995) found that green tea consumption was strongly correlated with lower cholesterol levels, even after correcting for age, smoking, alcohol use, and body weight; men who drank ten or more cups/day had significantly lower cholesterol levels, with LDL cholesterol decreased and HDL cholesterol elevated. The tea drinkers also had a decreased atherogenic index. Consumers of more than ten cups/day also had decreased levels of hepatological markers in serum, including aspartate aminotransferase, alanine transferase, and ferritin. The subjects in the study who smoked had greatly elevated levels of lipid peroxides in their blood, but of those smokers who were also among the heaviest consumers of green tea, lipid peroxide profiles were similar to those of nonsmokers (Imai and Nakachi, 1995). The contrasting results above may be attributable to the length of green tea use and other dietary differences between the Japanese study group of Imai and Nakashi (1995) and the relatively small Dutch group ($n = 64$) in the study by Princen et al. (1998).

Digestive, Hepatic, and Gastrointestinal Disorders

Buccal Health

Krahwinkel and Willershausen (2000) conducted a randomized, double-blind, placebo-controlled clinical study on the effects of green tea catechins and polyphenols on gingival inflammation in 47 volunteer dental students (24 females and 23 males, mean age 25.76 years). Among those excluded from the trial were chain smokers (> 15 cigarettes/day), those with fewer than 20 teeth, pregnant individuals, permanently medicated individuals, and anyone with rheumatic complaints, profound periodontal disease, and metabolic or systemic diseases. Outcomes were primarily measured after seven days and another 21 days of the treatment period according to bacterial plaque accumulation and degree of inflammation of the gingiva. All subjects received a dental cleaning before the treatment period and were instructed to maintain their regular dental hygiene without changing from their usual toothbrush and toothpaste. At random, the subjects received chew candies containing either placebo or green tea extract (1.55%) with instruction to chew eight candies per day, chewing each of them for 5 min (= 40 min of chewing/day) with an interval of one hour between candies. The results showed that after four weeks of chewing the candies the placebo group developed a slight increase in the approximal plaque index (API) and sulcus bleeding index (SBI) versus a slight decrease in gingival inflammation and of both indices in the green tea group; however, the difference was not significant.

Genitourinary and Renal Disorders

Renal Disorders

Researchers in China examined the influence of green tea polyphenol supplements in 25 patients with chronic renal failure due to diabetes, hypertensive renal disease, or infections. Half received the standard treatment (low salt, high protein diet) while the other half received the standard treatment plus green tea polyphenols. The latter group showed significant improvements in renal function, as measured by improved blood and urine profiles, edema, lumbago, and dizziness. Similar results were reported in a study at Long Sai Hospital in China in 60 patients with chronic renal failure. Kidney functions in the green tea-supplemented group were significantly improved after one to two months, versus those receiving standard care alone (Mitscher and Dolby, 1998). Serum methylguanidine and the methylguanidine/creatinine ratio were measured in 50 chronic kidney hemodialysis patients administered a mixture of green tea polyphenols (Sunphenon, 200 mg b.i.d.) in the form of a jelly for six months. After this time, the mean serum concentration of methylguanidine showed a significant decrease of 30% compared to baseline, as did the methylguanidine/creatinine ratio at the second month (from 4.12×10^{-3} to 3.86×10^{-3}), which continued throughout the period of green tea polyphenol administration (Ninomiya et al., 1997).

Immune Disorders; Inflammation and Disease

Cancer

Cancer prevention. Tsubono et al. (2001) conducted a population-based, prospective-cohort study on green tea and gastric cancer in northern rural Japan (Miyagi Prefecture), an area with a high incidence of gastric cancer. The study was performed over a period of eight years in 26,311 residents age 40 and older (14,409 women and 11,902 men). After adjusting for peptic ulcer, alcohol, smoking, health insurance type, age, sex, and dietary elements, the authors found no association between the risk of gastric cancer and consumption of green tea at amounts of less than one to five or more cups (100 mL) per day. Intervention trials and large cohort studies are ongoing in Japan to better determine associations between gastric cancer incidence and the consumption of green tea (Tsubono et al., 2001).

Quantities of tea consumed, when reported in cohort and case-control studies, vary widely. At least ten cups/day was associated with a decreased risk of gastric cancer in Northern Kyushu, Japan (Kono et al., 1988); a decreased incidence of all cancers in Saitama Prefecture, Japan, was found from at least three cups/day (about 100-125 mg EGCg) (Imai et al., 1997); a decrease in cancer incidence in Shanghai, China, was associated with at least one cup of freshly brewed green tea/week for a minimum of six months during the past five years (Yu et al., 1995); one cup/week for six months or longer was associated with lower risks of developing pancreatic or colorectal cancers in Shanghai (Ji et al., 1997); five or more cups/day was associated with a decreased recurrence of breast cancer at stages I and II ($p < 0.05$) but not stage III in Japanese women. In the latter study, no association was found between tamoxifen use, radiotherapy, or chemotherapy and use of green tea in the decreased risk of breast cancer recurrence. Suggesting further studies, the authors noted that the significance of consuming green tea before breast cancer was clinically diagnosed or when taken after surgical intervention could not be determined with their data (Nakachi et al., 1998).

A prospective study of gastric cancer incidence among Japanese people (5,610 men and 6,297 women) residing in Hawaii found green tea consumption positively associated with gastric cancer (Galanis et al., 1998), a finding also reported in a hospital-based case-control study of 210 Taiwanese men and women recently diagnosed with stomach cancer. However, the positive association was of only slight statistical significance ($p < 0.10$) (Lee et al., 1990).

Kohlmeier et al. (1997) reviewed the epidemiologic literature suggesting an association (either positive or negative) between tea consumption and cancer prevention in stomach, colon, and lung cancers and concluded that unequivocal evidence of protective effects of tea drinking on cancers could not be derived from the existing data. With respect to stomach cancer, Kohlmeier and colleagues asserted that no convincing claims could be made for a protective effect of tea because of the shortcomings of the studies. They concluded that if a beneficial association exists between tea drinking and stomach cancer, the effect is likely to be significant only in high-risk populations having a high intake of tea. In the case of colon cancer, the evidence seemed to suggest that green tea consumption had a protective effect against the development of colon cancer; however, many of these studies suffered from the same kinds of methodological weaknesses that influenced the stomach cancer studies. They suggested that a meta-analysis of the data might considerably strengthen the conclusions. Only four epidemiologic studies on the influence of tea drinking on lung cancer were reviewed, emphasizing again the problems of a limited number of studies and serious methodological flaws, in particular the failure to account for the confounding effects of smoking. In two of the lung cancer studies, the incidence of cancer was actually higher in the tea-consuming populations, but the researchers state that no conclusions can be justified due to the inadequate study design and failure to control for confounding variables.

Yang and Wang (1993) reviewed the epidemiological studies on associations between tea and various types of cancers. They cited ten studies which found no correlation between pancreatic cancer and tea consumption, while one case-control study had found a positive correlation and two studies showed a negative correlation. In addition, the authors recounted that two studies indicated a negative association between tea consumption and uterine cancer.

A positive correlation has been postulated between tea consumption and the development of esophageal cancer, based on findings that higher incidences occur in geographical regions where tea consumption is high relative to water consumption. Yang and Wang (1993) point out that other studies did not support this, although evidence did seem to suggest that consumption of very hot tea, rather than tea per se, was a significant risk factor for esophageal cancer. With respect to stomach cancer, significant negative correlations have been reported between the incidence and green tea consumption, and case-control studies in Japan indicated that individuals consuming green tea frequently or in larger quantities had a lower risk of developing gastric cancer. The authors note that in other case control studies, however, including Buffalo, New York, Kansas City, Missouri, Nagoya, Japan, Piraeus, Greece, Milan, Italy, and Spain and Turkey, no statistical association between tea consumption and stomach cancer was found; nor were statistical associations found between tea consumption and bladder, urinary tract, or breast cancer. Contradictory findings were found for colon and rectal cancer; three studies indicated a positive association with tea drinking and three indicated a negative association. Similarly, with respect to liver, kidney, and lung cancers, studies have found both positive and negative correlations. No correlations have been found between tea consumption and nasopharyngeal cancers.

Yang and Wang (1993) pointed to the difficulties inherent in interpreting the data derived from cohort and case-control studies of this kind, emphasizing that often a lack of information existed on the type, quantity, and temperature of the tea consumed, and problems occurred in adjusting for confounding factors, such as smoking and alcohol. The fact that black tea is predominantly consumed in the West while green tea is the usual beverage of choice in Japan, and that both green and black teas are consumed in China, was given as a further variable adding to the complexity of such studies and contributing to their lack of consistency and often contradictory conclusions. More recently, Chow et al. (1999) of the National Cancer Institute, Division of Cancer Epidemiology and Genetics, cited these and other inconsistencies in the epidemiological data available and called for further research on the influence of tea on cancer risk in humans. They advise that until that time, the influence of tea on cancer incidence remains inconclusive (Chow et al., 1999). Shim et al. (1995) compared the chemopreventive effect of coffee and green tea among 52 male smokers (ages 20-52) judged clinically healthy. The subjects were selected from 357 males who completed a questionnaire designed to eliminate confounding subjects, such as those who had been exposed to alcohol, radiation, or toxic chemicals or who had a preexisting disease. The subjects selected were male smokers who were regular coffee drinkers or regular green tea drinkers (two to three cups/day for six months) and male smokers and nonsmokers who drank neither beverage.

All the smokers smoked more than ten cigarettes/day. Noting that frequencies of sister chromatid exchange (FSCE) in the peripheral lymphocytes (mitogen-stimulated) affords a far more sensitive marker of mutagenic activity than measuring chromosomal aberrations, Shim and colleagues compared the FSCE of the three groups of smokers to a group of nonsmokers. At the outset, the FSCE of smokers was significantly higher (35%) compared to nonsmokers. Measured after six months, the FSCE of coffee-drinking smokers showed no statistically significant difference compared to smokers. The FSCE was significantly higher among the smokers who did not drink coffee or green tea regularly compared to smokers who were regular green tea drinkers, and, most notably, the FSCE of the green tea-drinking smokers was not significantly different from that of the nonsmokers.

Hamajima et al. (1999) conducted a phase-II study of the effect of green tea extract (polyphenon capsules, Mitsui Norin Co., Ltd., Tokyo) on serum pepsinogen levels in outpatients of both sexes (ages 40-69) who previously underwent gastroscopy at a cancer hospital and were found without stomach disease. Pepsinogen levels were measured as an indicator of gastric atrophy, since atrophic gastritis is recognized as a risk factor for developing stomach cancer. The patients measured for pepsinogen levels were divided into two groups: 77 (mean age 57.8) who would take two capsules of the nondecaffeinated green tea extract (100 mg/capsule, standardized to contain 50% epigallocatechin gallate) after each of three daily mealtimes for one year, and 86 patients (mean age 58.9) who would take one capsule/day after breakfast for one year. The majority of these subjects drank at least three cups of tea/day and six capsules/day was equivalent to ten cups/day. Measured by radioimmunoassay, pepsinogen levels in the one capsule/day group increased by an average of 3.5 ng/mL, which was not significantly different from levels of the six capsules/day group at 3.1 ng/mL. Alcohol, tea, and smoking were found to have no effect on pepsinogen levels. Hamajima and colleagues concluded that average pepsinogen levels are not affected by green tea polyphenol capsules.

Wu et al. (1993) conducted a preliminary study on endogenous *N-nitrosation using method A of the N*-nitrosoproline (NPRO) test (citing Ohshima and Bartsch, 1981, 1988) in 14 healthy male volunteers (nonsmokers) recruited to drink green tea either before or after breakfast while following a controlled diet. After two days on the diet, one group ingested sodium nitrate (300 mg) 60 min before breakfast while the other group took the same dose after breakfast. After another 30 min, they ingested 300 mg proline. On day five, they drank green tea (5 g boiled in 500 mL water) at the same time as the sodium nitrate was ingested and 30 min later, the 300 mg proline.

In a second study, black tea was used under the same experimental conditions. The results showed that either green or black tea potently inhibited *N*-nitrosation and that drinking the tea after meals worked better than taking it before meals. Remarkably, compared to controls on the control diet alone, the levels of NPRO excreted by tea drinkers were not significantly different. In yet a further study in 12 men and women, they used the same experimental design except that a low-nitrate control diet was employed (only vegetables low in nitrates or < 200 mg/kg). The results of this study suggested that a daily dosage of 1,000 mg of green tea blocks only partially the endogenous formation of nitrate-induced NPRO, whereas three to five times that amount blocks its formation completely. This effect was also shown in a separate study in ten healthy male volunteers on the original control diet for 23 days who ingested green tea polyphenols at a dosage of 480 mg/day (equivalent to 3 g green tea). In those taking the green tea polyphenols, NPRO excretion was decreased to a rate (0.21) comparable to that of the green tea at 3 g/day (0.23), which was an even lower rate than that of the controls on the diet alone who were not treated with proline or sodium nitrate (0.30).

Vermeer et al. (1999) investigated the effects of green tea and vitamin C on the formation and 24-h urinary excretion of two N-nitroso carcinogens, N-nitrosopiperdine (NPIP) and N-nitrosodimethylamine (NDMA). Both compounds undergo endogenous formation in humans following environmental nitrates. The authors note that the endogenous formation of N-nitroso compounds (NOC) in humans by nitrosation has been linked to an increased risk of developing cancers (bladder, gastric, nasopharyngeal, and esophageal) (citing Mirvish, 1995) and that their formation largely occurs in the stomach. Healthy, nonsmoking female volunteers ($n = 25$, ages 18-46 years) taking no vitamin supplements or medications during or prior to the study were entered in the control week during which time they were instructed to refrain from foods rich in nitrates while their background urinary NDMA levels were established. To increase NDMA levels, each day during the seven-day treatment period the subjects received a meal containing low levels of nitrates which contained fish to supply nitrosatable precursors, plus 220 mg of nitrate in water, a dose based on the mean weight of the participants to arrive at an acceptable daily intake amount. At the same time as the meal and nitrate, subjects received a 250-mg tablet of vitamin C and freeze-dried green tea powder (Thomas J. Lipton, "lyophilized tea solids") dissolved in boiling water (500 mg/100 mL) for ingestion during the day with four cups/day (2 g) in one test week and eight cups/day (4 g) in a second test week at the following intervals: morning (one or two cups), during the fish meal at the clinic, and afternoon and evening. In the second test week, the amount of vitamin C taken with the fish meal was increased to 1 g. Nitrate levels were determined according to a kit method (Boehringer Mannheim Kit no. 905658) and NPIP and NDMA in the urinary excretions were analyzed using a previously reported GC-MS method (Vermeer et al., 1999).

After five test weeks, each alternated with a control week, the results showed that although the levels of nitrate excretion in the test weeks were significantly increased versus the control weeks (Wilcox, $p = 0.0001$), the average level of NDMA excreted in urine was far less when vitamin C was added to the protocol, although the 250 mg dose of the vitamin produced about the same decrease as the 1 g dose. During the last three days of either dose, levels of urinary NDMA decreased to levels found in the control weeks. These levels were also significantly decreased compared to the first test week in which the subjects received only nitrate and the fish meal ($p = 0.0001$). Similar results were found from the 2 g dose of green tea with a significant decrease in urinary NDMA ($p = 0.0035$) during the last three days, compared to test week one. However, unlike all the other interventions, the 4 g dose of green tea produced a significant *increase* ($p = 0.0001$) in urinary excretion of NDMA in the last three days when compared to levels in test week one, yet no NDMA (or NPIP) was detected in the green tea itself. As for NPIP levels, urinary excretion showed no relationship to intakes of vitamin C, green tea, or the composition of the diet, as also observed in a previous study. Even so, the mean level of NPIP excreted during the 4 g green tea test appeared higher in comparison to all other test weeks (Vermeer et al., 1999).

In discussing these differences, Vermeer and co-workers (1999) point out that in low concentration in vitro, some phenolics are known to form nitroso derivatives and that these can act to catalyse nitrosation of *N*-nitroso compounds (citing Pignatelli et al., 1982; others). Nakamura and Kawabata (1981) reported that green tea showed the strongest catalytic effect for NDMA, versus NPIP, NDEA (*N*-nitrosodiethylamine), and NPYR (*N*-nitrosopyrrolodine). Vermeer et al. (1999) were at a loss to explain how the higher dose of green tea resulted in an increased urinary extraction of NDMA, since previous studies reported that contrary to the catalyzing effect of low doses, higher amounts of phenolic compounds had the opposite effect, inhibiting the formation of *N*-nitrosamine. Nitrosation was catalyzed by phenolic compounds only when the molar ratio was phenolic:nitrite of < 1 and was inhibited at a ratio of > 1 (citing Wu et al., 1993). Indeed, in their study they had calculated that the ratio was polyphenols:nitrite > 1. Therefore, their conclusion for the present was that either in vitro nitrosation mechanisms are different from in vivo ones or the increase in NDMA formation they found from the higher dose of green tea is the result of some unknown mechanism. In the meantime, they suggest that a dose of eight cups of green tea/day carries the risk of an increased formation of carcinogenic NDMA (Vermeer et al., 1999)—albeit in subjects consuming a daily meal rich in amines (nitrosatable precursors) and nitrate and without the use of antioxidants such as vitamins C or E (Vermeer et al., 1999).

Immunomodulation

Immunoprotection. The chemopreventive effect of the polyphenolic fraction of green tea (GTP) was investigated against UV-light-induced DNA damage to human skin, a well-known factor in the development of skin cancer. Damage was primarily measured according to the formation of cyclobutane pyrimidine dimers (CPDs) in the buttock skin of six Caucasian subjects of either sex (ages 25-35) in good health. The authors of the study note that CPDs represent the main form of UV-light-induced damage to the chromosomal DNA of the skin, which is an important factor in the induction of skin cancer and immune suppression. GTP was topically applied (3 mg/ skin site per 50 µL of acetone = approximately 1 mg/cm² skin area) 20 min before exposure to UVB light. In a dose-response study on UVB-induced CPD formation, GTP was applied in doses of 1-4 mg/skin site per 50 µL acetone. The results showed that pretreatment with GTP inhibited the UVB-induced erythema response and CPD formation. At the highest minimal erythema dose of UVB exposure (4.0), CPD formation was inhibited by 60% and by 81% at the lowest minimal dose (0.5). Against the highest dose of UVB exposure, topical pretreatment of the buttocks skin with the polyphenolic fraction caused a dose-dependent decrease in the formation of CPDs in the dermis and the epidermis (Katiyar et al., 2000).

Researchers in China conducted a study of green tea polyphenols in 60 patients undergoing radiation or chemotherapy for various types of cancers. Patients receiving supplementation with green tea polyphenols for one month, starting on the first day of the therapy, maintained stable white blood cell counts throughout their treatment. Those receiving a standard medication for maintaining blood quality experienced decreasing numbers of white blood cells over the treatment period; those given no supplemental medications showed very dramatic drops in white blood cell counts, suggesting that the tea polyphenolics were beneficial in maintaining the blood profile in patients undergoing radiation or chemotherapy (Mitscher and Dolby, 1998).

Another unpublished study from China reported on 60 patients who had low white blood cell counts from a variety of diseases, 31 of whom had various cancers and were undergoing radiation and chemotherapy. After taking green tea supplements for 30 days, 60% of the patients showed an increase in white blood cell counts of more than 50%, and 31% showed their counts had increased by 30% to 50%. Also important, patients with low white cell counts resulting from radiation therapy showed a 100% response to green tea polyphenols; patients receiving chemotherapy had a good but less dramatic response. Blood counts in most patients remained normal for at least two months after supplementation was suspended; no serious side effects were noted (Mitscher and Dolby, 1998).

Infectious Diseases

Microbial infections. In a clinical study, Ooshima et al. (1994) administered thorough dental examinations and assessed the levels of bacteria in the mouths of 35 volunteers (ages 18-29). The volunteers followed different regimens for two periods, each four days long. In the first period, they ate a normal diet but refrained from brushing or performing other oral hygiene procedures, except for rinsing their mouths with a solution of tea polyphenols after each meal and before bedtime. In the second regimen, the same procedure was followed except the rinse did not contain any active ingredients. Bacterial counts and follow-up dental exams were performed at the end of each period. In 34 volunteers, bacterial counts were reduced and plaque deposition was significantly decreased by the polyphenol treatment, even though none of the patients had been brushing or flossing. The results suggested that the tea polyphenols inhibit plaque deposition.

Metabolic and Nutritional Disorders

Aging and Senescence; Longevity Enhancement

One study examined the effects of regular green tea ingestion on longevity in 3,380 Japanese women over a nine-year period. All of the women were teachers of the Japanese tea ceremony and were at least 50 years old at the start of the study. As green tea is a major component of the tea ceremony, it was assumed that these women ingested more than an average amount. The researchers recorded all deaths that occurred in this group over nine years and compared the incidence of mortality to that of other Japanese women throughout Japan during the same period. They found a smaller percentage of the green tea drinkers died (280 versus 512 in the general population) and concluded that green tea was indicated as a possible protective factor against several diseases of high mortality, such as heart disease, cancer, and cerebrovascular diseases (Sadakata et al., 1992).

Epidemiological studies of green tea have focused mainly on two areas: cancer and, fewer in number, cardiovascular diseases. In the absence of well-designed, multicenter clinical trials involving large numbers of subjects, epidemiological studies on the influence of green tea consumption on disease incidences in large population samples can provide evidence for or against the potential preventive and therapeutic benefits of regular green tea ingestion. Such studies are often complicated, however, by the existence of confounding behavioral or dietary factors (e.g., smoking, alcohol consumption) and the lack of quantitative information on the amount, frequency, and consistency of tea ingestion by subjects in the study cohort or case-control population. Therefore, these studies are usually indicative rather than definitive of probable effects. For those reasons, epidemiological studies on the

long-term use of green tea have turned up both positive and negative correlations with disease incidences.

Antioxidant Activity

Laboratory studies indicate that the flavonoids of green tea (polyphenols
or catechins) are responsible for the antioxidant properties of tea and, by extension, most of the health benefits may be traceable to this antioxidant activity. In a study at the University of Nebraska, ten volunteers were fed a
controlled diet over a 14-day period including the following beverages at
each meal: green tea, black tea, decaffeinated black tea, or a nontea beverage. Urine, blood, and feces were collected and analyzed for polyphenolics;
those given green tea had the highest levels of polyphenolics, followed by
black tea, decaffeinated black tea, and no tea. These results established that
green tea polyphenolics are bioavailable (He and Kies, 1994).

Elmets et al. (2001) treated the skin of six volunteers with various concentrations of green tea polyphenols (GTPs) in a study of protection from
damage caused by UVA. Pretreatment of the skin with topical solutions containing 2.5% to 10% GTPs produced dose-dependent protection from UV-
induced erythema in all six volunteers. A 10% GTP solution provided almost
complete protection against erythema up to three days after UV exposure,
although protection afforded by a 2.5% solution was still judged to be excellent. Biopsy specimens from the volunteers showed that pretreatment with a
2.5% solution of GTPs reduced the number of sunburned cells by 66% and
reconstituted Langerhans cells by 58%. Greater protection was afforded
from higher concentrations. In vitro studies showed that damage to DNA
after UV irradiation was significantly reduced by pretreatment of skin with
a 5% GTP solution.

Hodgson et al. (2000) noted that to date four studies on the antioxidant
effect of tea failed to show that the oxidation of LDL cholesterol is inhibited
ex vivo. Suspecting that the negative results of previous studies may have
owed to methods whereby the antioxidant polyphenols present in the water-
soluble fraction of the serum were isolated from LDL particles, they examined ex vivo cupric ion (Cu^{2+})-induced lipoprotein oxidation following
acute ingestion of green and black teas by healthy volunteers, but without
first isolating lipoproteins from serum. Twenty healthy male volunteers
(ages 35-73 years), all nonsmokers, were recruited under various exclusion
criteria, including a history of major diseases, use of dietary supplements or
medications, regular coffee or tea consumption averaging less than one cup
per day, and a body mass index of more than 33. Subjects were instructed to
maintain their usual diet for the duration of the four-week study and before
each visit went without caffeine-containing beverages for at least the prior
12 h. Treatment consisted of four hot beverages (black tea, green tea, water
matched to the caffeine content of the teas, and water) taken randomly at the

clinic at four intervals of at least one week apart and as close as possible to the same day and same time as the first acute dose. The tea infusions were prepared using 7.9 g of leaves/400 mL boiled water. The total polyphenolic and gallic acid contents of the black and green tea infusions were 19% and 18% and 103 mg and 102 mg, respectively. Blood samples were taken before and one hour after the beverage was consumed; urine samples were taken before and 1.5 h after consumption. Antioxidant activity in serum was calculated by assaying total peroxyl-radical trapping potential. The results showed that compared to water, the difference in lipoprotein oxidation from black tea was of borderline significance ($p < 0.05$) and that green tea produced an insignificant trend toward increased total antioxidant activity of serum ($p < 0.09$). Total antioxidant activity one hour after ingestion of black or green tea was meager (about 3% and 4%, respectively). The researchers concluded that longer studies are required to settle the issue of whether green or black tea attenuates the oxidation of lipoproteins and that these studies will require more suitable markers of oxidative stress.

Miura et al. (2000) investigated the effect of green tea polyphenols (GTPs) on low-density lipoprotein (LDL) oxidation ex vivo measured according to Cu^{2+}-mediated oxidation. A polyphenol-rich extract of green tea (Polyphenon E) containing 58.4% EGCg and 78.8% total catechins was administered to 22 healthy males (ages 22-32 years), 12 of whom were smokers. The dosage of 300 mg b.i.d., immediately before breakfast and dinner for seven days (after a seven-day baseline period), was roughly equivalent to consuming seven to eight cups of green tea/day (100 mL/cup). The control group was not administered the green tea extract. All the volunteers were normolipidemic and were not taking dietary supplements, vitamins, or medications. During the study, they followed an undisclosed dietary regimen which restricted their beverage intake to vegetable or fruit juice and black or green tea. The results showed no significant differences between the groups in plasma levels of TBARS (thiobarbituric acid-reactive substances), vitamin C, and lipids (cholesterol and triglycerides) either before or after the treatment period and between smokers and nonsmokers. However, after the treatment period, the GTP group showed a significant increase in β-carotene levels ($p < 0.01$) and vitamin E levels showed a tendency to increase compared to the controls. Plasma concentrations of EGCg showed a highly significant increase in the GTP group in both free and conjugated forms ($p < 0.001$) whereas they showed no change in the controls. Finally, the change in Cu^{2+}-mediated LDL oxidation ex vivo between the groups was significantly different with an increase in lag time in the GTP group of 13.7 min for both smokers and nonsmokers compared to baseline ($p < 0.05$) versus no change of any significance in the controls. By extrapolation, a similar study with vitamin E found the lag time of LDL oxidation increased by 15 min after 200 to 400 mg/day. The researchers estimate that nearly the same result was achieved in the present study from about 480 mg/day of the GTP preparation. In discussing their results and the failure of other studies to find any significant prolongation in the Cu^{2+}-mediated LDL oxidation lag time, Miura and colleagues (2000) note that in one other study in which the LDL oxidation lag time was significantly prolonged ($p < 0.01$) (by 8 min after black tea, 750 mL/day for four weeks) (Ishikawa et al., 1997), the subjects ($n = 14$) were also healthy males of about the same age (21 to 25 years) who adhered to a dietary regimen. These parameters are in contrast to those of the negative studies wherein the ages of subjects were more diverse, both males and females were enrolled, and their diets were unaltered. Besides these differences, the researchers contend that they also failed to analyze the data using the paired Student's t-test, which would have allowed the elimination of factors related to age, sex, and genetic and environmental factors (Miura et al., 2000).

Nakagawa et al. (1999) tested the antioxidant effects of a standardized green tea extract (Sunphenon DCF-1) on the plasma of 18 healthy male volunteers (nonsmokers, ages 23-41), all employees of a laboratory involved in the study. The dosage was one tablet containing 254 mg of catechin tannins (equivalent to drinking two cups of green tea) after a 12 h fast. One hour later, their plasma showed 267 pmol EGCg/mL plasma. Levels of phosphatidylcholine hydroperoxide (PCOOH) as a marker of oxidized lipoproteins were significantly and rapidly decreased in the green tea group: 44.6 pmol/mL in the green tea group versus 73.7 pmol/mL in the control, a change inversely correlated with the increased levels of EGCg and concentrations of PCOOH. In vitro tests also demonstrated that plasma containing catechin exhibits a high resistance to copper-dependent lipid peroxidation. The researchers concluded that their results indicate that by increasing the antioxidant capacity of human plasma the ingestion of green tea catechins lowers the risk of cardiovascular disease. Their study also showed that after 6 h levels of EGCg in the volunteers reached zero or close to it after peaking at 1 to 2 h. Nakagawa and co-workers noted that in a study by van het Hof et al. (1997) in which subjects ingested 900 mL of green tea/day for one month, the reported absence of antioxidant activity 12 h after the last dose would be expected, owing to the relatively short half-life of tea catechins in human plasma.

In the Netherlands, Princen et al. (1998) performed a randomized, single-blind, placebo-controlled parallel study of 64 healthy smokers (males and females, ages 22-46, ten or more cigarettes/day) to examine the effect of black tea, green tea, green tea polyphenols (GTP), or water on plasma antioxidants and plasma LDL oxidation ex vivo. Subjects were forbidden to add milk to their tea, told to adhere to their regular diet, had to refrain from consuming red wine or tea (apart from the prescribed tea), and were asked either to drink more than 100 mL of fruit juice or to eat more than two oranges/day. The treatment period lasted four weeks and no adverse effects were found. No changes were found in plasma levels or LDL levels of vitamin E in either the black tea (150 mL or 6 cups/day) or green tea group (150 mL or 6 cups/day) compared to the control group (mineral water, 150 mL/day). However, the GTP group (6 capsules q.i.d. = 900 mg GTP q.i.d.) showed a significant *decrease* in plasma levels of vitamin E and LDL vitamin E content compared to the control group ($p = 0.102$). Yet neither the black tea, green tea, nor GTP group showed any significant difference in ex vivo LDL oxidation, despite an estimated 3.5-fold greater amount of catechins in green tea compared to black tea. The plasma from one subject in each treatment group showed significantly increased lag times in vitro from the addition of GTP directly into the copper ion and AAPH oxidation assays, as expected from earlier research results. Thus, Princen and colleagues concluded that GTP remains unproven as an in vivo antioxidant of LDL, and that neither GTP, green tea, nor black tea have any ex vivo antioxidant effect on LDL (Princen et al., 1998).

A similar study by van het Hof et al. (1997) in nonsmokers ($n = 45$) also found no significant change in LDL resistance to oxidation ex vivo after four weeks of consuming either green or black tea compared to mineral water (six cups/day) when they measured the antioxidant activity of plasma after the subjects had fasted for up to 12 h. However, as noted by Nakagawa et al. (1999), because of a relatively short half-life of EGCg by the time they measured antioxidant activity plasma levels of green tea, catechin levels would have been zero or close to it. Serafini et al. (1996) indicated as much in a study on the total radical trapping ability of plasma (TRAP assay) by black and green teas in vitro. Ten healthy adults were randomly divided into two groups; after an overnight fast, five drank about two cups of green tea (Birko Chinese green tea, KI, 300 mL) while the second group of five adults drank the same amount of black tea (Twinnings Earl Grey). The teas were prepared by allowing the leaves (2.0 g) to steep in boiling tap water (100 mL) for 90 s before filtering and no sweetener was added. Blood samples were collected prior to drinking and at 30, 50, and 80 min after. Both green and black tea increased plasma TRAP values compared to those of five controls who drank the same amount of plain tap water. In the green tea group, TRAP values peaked at 30 min and showed an average increase of 40% over basal levels. At 80 min after consuming the tea, TRAP values had returned almost to basal levels. In the black tea group, TRAP values increased 48%, peaked at 50 min, and were close to baseline values at 80 min. Serafini and colleagues speculated that the rapidity of the change in antioxidant capacity suggested that the polyphenols were absorbed in the upper part of the gastrointestinal tract. The overall antioxidant effect measured according to AUC (area under the curve) values from individual responses during the course of the observation period showed that the values for green tea (21.3 ± 4.3) and black tea (14.3 ± 5.8) were greater than those of the control group. These results differed significantly in a second experiment in which whole pasteurized milk (100 mL) was added to the teas: the AUC values in both tea groups became nearly zero, an effect, the authors surmised, resulting from the binding of the tannins to the protein in the milk to form a complex that would be more difficult to absorb in the upper gastrointestinal tract. However, when tested in vitro the TRAP values with milk added to the teas showed no decrease from their original antioxidant capacities against chemically induced peroxidation of human plasma. Plain green tea was about five times more efficient than plain black tea: 17,850 µM versus 3,542 µM, respectively (Serafini et al., 1996). It has been suggested that results from TRAP assay may be attended with a higher than desirable degree of variability (Miller and Rice-Evans, 1996).

In an acute dosage study, Leenen et al. (2000) investigated the plasma antioxidant effects of black and green teas with and without milk in a crossover design study in ten males and 11 females (ages 18-70 years), all nonsmokers in good health and on no particular diet. Controls received water with or without milk. None of the participants were taking medications, dietary supplements, or mineral or vitamin supplements. At baseline and at time points up to 2 h after the drinking of the teas and water, antioxidant activity was measured from fasting blood samples using the FRAP assay which measures the ferric reducing ability of plasma. The beverages were administered at least two days apart at dosages of 300 mL and at 240 mL plus 60 mL pasteurized whole milk. The teas were prepared using freeze-dried solids (Lipton, Englewood Cliffs, NJ, Lipton Research Blend) dissolved in boiled mineral water (noncarbonated) with 2 g of solids per 300 mL (equivalent to about three cups of tea). Total catechins in the black and green teas were shown to be 0.07 g/g and 0.32 g/g, respectively, and the content of EGCg was close (41% and 37%, respectively). The results showed that plasma FRAP activity compared to baseline was significantly enhanced (about 2%) by black tea compared to water ($p < 0.001$) at each time point tested (30, 60, 90, and 120 min). The same result was found with green tea except that the increase in plasma FRAP was about 3% and was significantly larger at the 30-min interval. No significant differences were evident in the responses of men compared to women, and the addition of milk had no significant effect on FRAP activity. However, a significant difference was evident in the women who showed 27% lower FRAP values compared to the men ($p < 0.001$) at all time points. Over the two-hour observation period, the antioxidant potential of plasma showed a greater increase from green tea compared to black tea ($p < 0.05$), which was about a 1.5 times greater increase. At the same time, plasma catechins rose about five times more compared to the rise after black tea which reflected the higher content of catechins in the green tea. Peak levels of plasma antioxidant activity and catechins were found at 90 min with black tea and 60 min with green tea. After 90 min, plasma FRAP activity showed a significant decline in all the treatment groups ($p < 0.001$). Similar results were found by Benzie et al. (1999) who used the FRAP assay to assess renal excretion, systemic distribution, and absorption of antioxidant polyphenols of green tea in healthy adults ($n = 12$), in addition to changes in the antioxidant potential of plasma. Excretion of the polyphenols peaked at 60-90 min and the peak increase in plasma FRAP after ingestion of green tea (400 mL) was found at 20-40 min. The mean 40-min increase in FRAP was 4%, and although a correlation between the dose taken and the peak increase in FRAP (40 min) was not evident, the absorption of the polyphenols resulted in a significant increase in the antioxidant potential of plasma ($p < 0.001$).

Freese et al. (1999) conducted a double-blind, placebo-controlled study in 20 healthy women (nonsmoking, ages 23-50) to determine whether green tea affects antioxidant status during a controlled high linoleic acid (9%) diet consisting of a mixture of natural foods. None of the subjects were taking medications except for one receiving percutaneous estrogen replacement therapy. For four weeks, green tea or placebo was taken during meals in 300-mg capsules (Itoen Co., Tokyo, 27% polyphenols w/w): three with breakfast, four with lunch, and three with dinner, along with a special diet. The daily dose of green tea extract was equivalent to ten cups of green tea per day. A two-week period preceding the intake of green tea or placebo was devoted to decreasing the oxidative stress of the subjects by replacing dietary unsaturated fats with dietary saturated fats. The results showed that the short-term intake of green tea extract had no effect on serum lipid levels, nitric oxide synthesis, oxidative stress, blood coagulation, or thromboxane formation in the healthy females on a cholesterol-lowering diet. Scarcely any effect on blood coagulation factors occurred and no side effects were found in any of the subjects. Although some indication of a decrease in thrombin production occurred, tests indicated that the anticoagulant effects of green tea are not mediated by way of thrombin inhibition. The only noticeable indication of a significant ($p < 0.05$) decrease in oxidative stress was found in decreased plasma levels of malondialdehyde in the green tea group, a nonspecific marker of lipid peroxidation.

In 12 healthy volunteers (ages 20-25), Pietta et al. (1998) examined the total antioxidant activity of green tea extract (600 mg, equivalent to 400 mg total green tea catechins) compared to a ginkgo extract (1.6 g equivalent to 100 mg ginkgolides and 400 mg ginkgo flavonoids) and placebo (maltodextrin). None of the volunteers were taking antioxidant supplements and all had a habitually low intake of flavonoids. Following an overnight fast and subsequent ingestion of the test substances, venous blood was tested for total radical-trapping ability (TRAP) once each hour after they ingested the test substances for 6 h, and compared to TRAP from blood taken before ingestion. Using the Trolox equivalent antioxidant capacity method of Miller and Rice-Evans (1996), Pietta and co-workers found a longer-lasting and more rapid TAA from the ginkgo extract compared to the green tea extract, despite the fact that in vitro tests using the same methods showed the green tea extract to have a higher TAA (5.2 mM Trolox) than the ginkgo extract (2.4 mM Trolox) (Pietta et al., 1998). This result serves to emphasize the need for in vivo tests to confirm more immediate in vitro data.

Obesity and Weight Loss

Dulloo et al. (1999) conducted a double-blind, placebo-controlled randomized study of the thermogenic effects of a green tea extract (Arkopharma Laboratories, Nice, France, Exolise, standardize to contain 25% catechins) in ten healthy, nonsmoking male volunteers (ages 24-26 years). The study also sought to determine the effects of the extract on 24-h energy expenditure (EE) and whether a thermogenic effect of green tea could be found apart from its caffeine content, a known thermogenic. The study was based on in vitro results in which the extract was shown to be effective in stimulating thermogenesis in peripheral tissue and more so than could be accounted for by its caffeine content (citing Dulloo et al., 1996). The subjects ranged from lean to mildly obese and all had eaten a typical Western diet for many years with a daily intake of methylxanthines of 100 to 200 mg. Throughout the study period (five to six weeks) the subjects received a weight-maintenance diet made up of ≈ 47% carbohydrates, ≈ 40% fat, and ≈ 13% protein which was fed at a rate of 1.4 times their estimated basal energy requirement. On three occasions, at intervals of five to ten days, each of the subjects spent 24 h in a respiratory chamber in which the same conditions of sleeping period, patterns of physical activity, sedentary lifestyle, and meals were applied. After abstaining from methylxanthine-containing beverages and foods for 24 h prior to the three trials, they each received capsules containing either the green-tea extract (containing 90 mg EGCg and 50 mg caffeine), 50 mg caffeine, or placebo (cellulose). The dosage was two capsules with each of three daily meals. With EGCg providing ≈ 72% of the catechin intake, total catechin intake from each two-capsule dose was 125 mg (Dulloo et al., 1999).

Dulloo et al. (1999) reported a significantly higher total 24-h EE in the green tea phase compared to caffeine or placebo (by 2.8 and 3.5% respectively; each $p < 0.05$), which was significantly higher across treatments ($p < 0.01$). Diurnal EE was also significantly higher in the green tea phase compared to placebo or caffeine ($p < 0.01$). Despite the magnitude of increase in the thermogenic response, no correlation was evident relative to the body mass index (BMI or percentage of fat) of the subjects. Respiratory quotients (RQs) showed a significant decrease in the green tea phase compared to placebo or caffeine at total 24 hr, nocturnal, and diurnal periods. In

80% of the subjects the difference in RQ compared to placebo was substantial ($p < 0.01$). Yet the magnitude of decrease in the RQ showed no correlation to the BMI. The oxidation of fat was also significantly increased after the green tea phase compared to placebo and caffeine ($p < 0.001$), and the placebo and caffeine phases showed no significant difference. Fat oxidation accounted for 41.5% of the 24-h EE during the green tea phase and 31.6% during the placebo phase. This difference was also highly significant ($p < 0.001$). Urinary catecholamine excretion showed no significant difference except in the green tea phase in the total 24-h period when norepinephrine excretion was higher ($p < 0.05$) compared to the caffeine or placebo phases. Heart rate measured during the first 8 h in the respiratory chamber showed no significant difference in any of the treatment phases and no subject reported side effects of any kind. The researchers calculated that the increase in metabolic rate produced by the green tea extract represented an increase of $\approx 4\%$ in the 24-h EE and, by extrapolation, an increase in the thermogenesis of the daily EE of 35% to 43% or 328 kJ/day. In conclusion, they propose that the green tea extract holds the potential of being able to modulate body composition and weight through changes in substrate utilization and energy expenditure (Dulloo et al., 1999).

Green tea polyphenolics have been shown to inhibit the activity of amylase, a carbohydrate-digesting enzyme present in saliva. By inhibiting this enzyme, researchers theorized that green tea polyphenolics may favor the slow digestion of carbohydrates, which prevents sharp spikes of insulin in the blood and favors fat burning over fat storage. In a small, double-blind placebo-controlled study of 60 middle-aged obese women (30-45 years old), subjects were placed on a diet of 1,800 calories/day and randomly assigned either to a green tea supplement (Arkopharma Laboratories, Carros, France, Phytotrim) group or to a placebo supplement group. Capsules were taken at each meal for 30 days (250 mg × 8/day in three divided doses starting with 500 mg at breakfast). After two weeks, the green tea group had lost twice as much weight as those given a placebo on the same diet. After the full four-week treatment period, the women in the green tea group had lost three times as much weight as the placebo group (2.9 kg versus 0.935 kg, respectively). Compared to the placebo group, the green tea group also showed a significantly greater reduction in waist size (-0.48 ± 0.97 cm versus -2.1 ± 1.37 cm). In addition, blood triglyceride levels in the green tea group showed a significant decrease compared to the placebo group (-0.207 ± 0.195 g/L versus -0.033 ± 0.14 g/L). No side effects, including sleep loss, were reported (Lecomte, 1985).

Pharmacokinetics; Pharmacodynamics

A bioavailability study of decaffeinated (> 0.1%) green tea (Lipton, Englewood Cliffs, NJ) was conducted in 18 healthy adult volunteers at Memorial Sloan-Kettering Cancer Center in New York City (Yang, Chen, et al., 1998). Using green tea solids dissolved in 500 mL hot water, they found no significant increase in maximum plasma concentrations of green tea catechins from an oral dose of 4.5 g, suggesting a saturation level is achieved at a dose of 3 to 4.5 g. Following ingestion of the green tea (4.5 g), plasma levels of (–)-epigallocatechin, (–)-epicatechin, and EGCg peaked at from 1.5 to 2.5 h and were undetectable after 24 h. The time to reach maximum plasma concentrations of EC and EGC (1.3-1.8 h) was shorter than that of EGCg (1.6-2.7 h). Although dosage increases of these polyphenols had no affect on these times, the urinary elimination half-life of EGCg (5.0-5.5 h) was longer than EC and/or EGC (2.5-3.4 h). Total urinary (–)-epicatechin (EC) and (–)-epigallocatechin (EGC) showed greater than 90% excretion within 8 h, but EGCg was not excreted and a dose-response relationship between increased dosages of green tea and urinary excretion of urinary EC and EGC was not found (Yang, Chen, et al., 1998).

Dalluge et al. (1997) devised a simple and efficient microscale method for the separation and detection of EGCg and six of the biologically active catechin tannins of green tea in human plasma.

The most abundant polyphenol in green tea, EGCg is widely distributed in the organs of male and female mice 24 h after oral administration. The highest amounts of radiolabeled EGCg were found in the order of stomach > colon > small intestine in females, and colon > stomach > small intestine in males. In other organs the levels of radiolabeled EGCg incorporated were highest in the order of liver > brain > kidney > lung in female mice, and in the order of liver > kidney > brain > lung in males. Blood levels were practically equal in both sexes after 24 h. A second single dose administered orally to female mice 6 h later resulted in as high as 5.9 times the amount of EGCg already distributed following the first dose. Levels were enhanced fourfold in the bone, bladder, brain, liver, lung, and pancreas, and 1.3- to 2.0-fold in the digestive tract. At 24 h, levels of EGCg were enhanced in the same organs greater than threefold compared to the single administration. As the researchers note, their data suggest that the Japanese tradition of drinking green tea throughout the day may result in a higher concentration of green tea polyphenols being maintained than from infrequent dosing (Suganuma et al., 1998).

By the topical route, EGCg (10% w/w) in the form of a hydrophilic ointment at a dose of 17 mg EGCg showed an uptake of 1% to 20% on mouse or human skin. Systemic levels of EGCg were negligible, however, and EGCg showed transdermal penetration only in mouse skin (Dvorakova et al., 1999).

DOSAGE

In traditional Chinese medicine, loose green tea is used in a dose of 4-7 g as required (Keys, 1991). Standardized extracts of green tea polyphenols are currently offered on the supplement market which contain, typically, 60% to 80% and as high as 97% polyphenols. In France, green tea powder extract is combined with a calorie-restricted diet (1,800 calories/day) as a means of weight management in obese, middle-aged women in a dosage of 8 g/day in three divided doses with meals (2 g/breakfast, 3 g/lunch, 3 g/evening meal) (Lecomte, 1985).

One cup of green tea contains over 250 mg of polyphenols (Yang and Wang, 1993), making the ingestion of ten cups/day equivalent to more than 2,500 mg of total polyphenols. Others have estimated that the average Japanese green tea aficionado will ingest up to 1,000 mg of EGCg/day (Yoshizawa et al., 1987).

SAFETY PROFILE

Toxicology

Vermeer et al. (1999) found evidence in human female volunteers to suggest that drinking eight or more cups of green tea per day (800 mL providing 4 g of freeze-dried tea solids/day) combined with a dietary intake of nitrates of 220 mg and a daily meal of amine-rich foods that provide nitrosatable precursors (e.g., fish)—without the use of antioxidant supplements such as vitamins C or E—could pose a risk of increased formation of carcinogenic NDMA (*N*-nitrosodimethylamine); however, half that dose decreased NDMA levels.

Indications from epidemiological studies suggest that regular tea ingestion is correlated with an increase in esophageal cancers in some regions where tea consumption is high relative to water consumption, although other evidence indicates that this is related more to the consumption of very hot beverages (> 130°F), rather than to tea consumption per se (Yang and Wang, 1993; Dhar et al., 1993).

Evidence derived from epidemiological data indicates that long-term consumption of ten or more cups of green tea/day is without adverse effects and may be associated with significant health benefits (Mitscher et al., 1997). In a year-long phase-II observatory study (without a placebo control) (Hamajima et al., 1999), 101 Japanese men and women (ages 40-69 years) ingested one capsule/day of a decaffeinated green tea extract standardized to contain 50% EGCg (Polyphenon capsules, Mitsui Norin Co., Ltd., Tokyo). From a daily dosage of 100 mg after breakfast, the subjects showed no serious adverse effects. Abdominal discomfort was reported by 13 subjects (12.9%). In the same study, no serious adverse effects were reported among a group of 83 Japanese men and women taking two capsules t.i.d. after meals for one year. However, a significantly higher ($p < 0.05$) incidence of diarrhea occurred compared to the one capsule/day group. One patient complained of resumed menstruation accompanied with abdominal pain; another of sleeplessness; one of constipation; five of diarrhea; and five of abdominal discomfort. In total, 14.4% reported adverse events.

In an earlier phase-I study in ten volunteers (five women and five men), a dosage of six capsules of the extract taken daily for three months was without serious adverse effects. Blood pressure was not affected by the high dosage of the extract, nor were any abnormalities detected in blood tests of saturation percent of iron, platelet counts, red and white blood cell counts, hematocrit, iron, total iron binding capacity, hemoglobin, uric acid, urea nitrogen, glucose, creatinine, triglycerides, total cholesterol, HDL cholesterol, LDH, GOT, GPT, or γ-GTP. Among these subjects, one woman complained of sleeplessness despite the extract having been decaffeinated (Hamajima et al., 1999).

Neither EGCg or the polyphenolic fraction of green tea (GTP) showed any cytotoxicity in the MTT (colorimetric) assay in human washed platelets at a final concentration of 20 mg/mL at various times from 0 to 120 min (Kang et al., 1999). In a confluent culture of normal human lung fibroblast cells (WI38), EGCg (50 and 200 μM) induced apoptosis in less than 5% of the cells after 24 hr (Chen et al., 1998).

Toxicity in Animal Models

Little evidence of long- or short-term toxicity of green tea or green tea extracts exists. Mice given 1.25% green tea extract as the sole source of water for 30 weeks failed to develop liver tumors or any signs of liver toxicity (NCI, 1996).

After 63 weeks, Lin et al. (1998) reported that serum creatinine levels as a measure of kidney disease or injury showed no significant change in rats fed a basal diet to which powdered green tea leaves were added as 2.5% of the total diet. Similarly, liver enzyme levels were normal at 27 weeks and at week 63 of the green tea-supplemented diet; neither kidney nor livers showed any microscopic lesions; and 100% of the rats survived. Water and food intake showed no significant difference compared to controls, yet the average body weight of the green tea group significantly decreased by 12% at week 15 ($p < 0.05$), and from week 15 to the end of the experiment at week 63 by 10-18% ($p < 0.0005$).

Animal studies indicate that green tea (Gomes et al., 1995) and (–)-epicatechin have potentially beneficial effects in models of diabetes (Ahmad et al., 1989; Chakravarthy et al., 1982). However, one study has suggested that the regular consumption of tea by children increases their risk for developing insulin-dependent (type I) diabetes (Vertanen et al., 1994).

Side Effects

A randomized crossover study on the effect of 400 mL of green tea containing 180 mg caffeine was performed to determine its effect on blood pressure in healthy, nonsmoking adults (ages 25-72). The subjects had either mild systolic hypertension or high-normal systolic blood pressure (SBP > 130 mm Hg and < 150 mm Hg) and diastolic blood pressure (DBP) of < 100 mm Hg. The study found that at 30 min and 1 h after drinking the tea, a nonsignificant increase occurred in either DBP or SBP compared to changes from drinking 400 mL of water or black tea containing the same amount of caffeine (180 mg/400 mL). No changes in heart rate were found from drinking green tea at these times. However, black tea caused BP to increase significantly at 30 min postingestion compared to caffeine in water at 30 min postingestion. The 24-h ambulatory measurement also showed no significant changes in blood pressure compared to black tea or caffeine in water, and neither black nor green tea showed any significant influence on the ambulatory heart rate. Although the researchers advised that other changes may be seen from a longer period of study than their seven-day investigation showed, they concluded that green tea had no effect of any significance on ambulatory or acute BP and the regular ingestion of tea by individuals with moderately elevated BP does not result in significantly changed BP over a period of seven days (Hodgson et al., 1999).

Excessive consumption of caffeine, present in green tea and some green tea extracts, is known to cause typical caffeine effects, such as nervousness, insomnia, and restlessness, in some individuals. These symptoms can be avoided by the use of a decaffeinated green-tea extract or by reducing the dosage (Mitscher and Dolby, 1998). In a study of premenopausal Japanese women (ages 21-42), "high intakes" of nondecaffeinated green tea or coffee were reported to show a significant association with sex-hormone binding globulin (SHBG) on days 11 and 22 of the menstrual cycle. The association of increased levels of SHBG with the risk of breast cancer (Nagata et al., 1998) would suggest that for premenopausal women, decaffeinated green tea products are preferable to nondecaffeinated products.

Drug Interactions

From in vitro studies, the antimicrobial activity of methicillin or benzylpenicillin against methicillin-resistant *Staphylococcus aureus* was found to be increased by a dilute water extract of green tea (Yam et al., 1998). Others have shown that green tea polyphenols act synergistically to enhance the growth inhibition and apoptosis of human lung cancer cells (PC-9) treated with tamoxifen or with suldinac. Inactive amounts of EGCg and tamoxifen or suldinac in cotreatments of PC-9 cells showed significant apoptotic activity. An eightfold increase in apoptosis was observed when inactive amounts of EGCg and suldinac were combined. The same effect was reported in cotreatments with suldinac and EGCg against mouse colon adenocarcinoma cells (Colon 26 cell line) using inactive amounts of suldinac, and with tamoxifen against human breast cancer cells (MCF-7 cell line) (Suganuma et al., 1999). In addition, animal studies indicate that the anticancer agent doxorubicin may be modulated by green tea (p.o.), resulting in an increase in antineoplastic activity (Sadzuka et al., 1998).

Because one cup of green tea contains up to 142 mg of EGCg (Yang and Wang, 1993), individuals taking aspirin or other anticoagulant substances on a daily basis should be aware of potential additive effects and consult with their physicians before regular consumption of green tea or green tea supplements. EGCg has been shown to completely inhibit collagen-induced platelet aggregation at a concentration of 0.2 mg/mL in vitro, an effect found to be comparable to aspirin (Sagesaka-Mitane et al., 1990). In a case report seemingly contradicting this potential, a 44-year-old man who consumed 1.13-3.78 L of green tea/day for approximately one week, while maintaining his intake of warfarin as a thromboembolic prophylaxis, showed a significantly decreased international normalization ratio (INR). After discontinuing the tea, his INR increased toward previous levels. The researchers reporting the case suggested that the content of vitamin K in green tea may have been responsible for the antagonizing effect on warfarin (Taylor and Wilt, 1999).

Contraindications

Green tea and green tea polyphenols should not be ingested by infants, as evidence suggests that doses of more than 250 mL/day may interfere with iron metabolism and result in microcytic anemia (Merhav et al., 1985). No other specific contraindications have been identified.

Pregnancy and Lactation

Although no specific contraindications exist for the consumption of green tea or green tea extracts in pregnancy or during lactation, women who are pregnant or lactating are advised to seek the advice of a health care professional regarding high doses of concentrated products.

In Japan, it is generally believed that green tea should be avoided before and after the intake of iron preparations. However, a recent study conducted with anemic pregnant patients using sodium ferrous citrate found no differences between a tea-drinking group and a non-tea-drinking group in terms of hemoglobin content, serum iron, and total iron binding capacity; all were markedly improved after administration of the iron supplement and no differences were found between the treatment groups (Mitamura et al., 1989).

No studies on the bioavailability of green tea polyphenols in breast milk have been conducted. As a rule of thumb, only about 1 percent of compounds ingested by the mother enters the milk, so large doses of polyphenols would not be expected to enter milk, although they are rapidly and widely distributed to the brain and other body compartments (see Pharmacokinetics; Pharmacodynamics). There is evidence that green tea may interfere with iron metabolism in infants (Merhav et al., 1985). Such direct feeding of tea to infants would deliver a dose of polyphenols many times larger than that possible to receive through breast milk. A recent study in southern China (He et al., 2001) documented adverse effects for infants given teas directly, compared to their fully breast-fed cohorts not given teas. Unfortunately, no details about the teas were included in this study. Drinking green tea is widespread in China and other Asian countries as well as in the United States and has not been associated with any adverse effects during lactation, excepting those infants especially sensitive to caffeine.

Special Precautions

Tea has a low sodium content but a high potassium content. Patients with end-stage renal disease must restrict their potassium intake; therefore, tea consumption could be deleterious to this group (Mitscher et al., 1997).

In a study of seven patients diagnosed with green tea-induced asthma, Shirai et al. (1997) found one patient who showed no histamine response (bronchial and skin) and five (71%) who showed a dose-dependent release of histamine in response to EGCg. In four healthy controls and four asthmatics, no reaction to EGCg was found at any concentration tested. Evidence that the allergic reaction is mediated by IgE was established by a washed whole blood method (Shirai et al., 1997). Conversely, in animal experiments EGCg and gallocatechin gallate have shown dose-dependent antiallergic activity (Ohmori et al., 1995). Other studies have been inconclusive and the results may be related to methods of aging, agent preparation, and the condition of the patients tested (Shirai et al., 1994).

EGCg was found to be the major constituent in green tea powder that provoked asthma and immediate skin reactions in three asthmatic patients who worked in a tea factory. Similar results were found for black and oolong tea (Shirai et al., 1994).

Samman et al. (2001) reported a significant decrease in the absorption of nonheme iron in young women (ages 19-39; $n = 10$) after they consumed meals containing a polyphenol-rich green tea extract (Nestec, Luassanne, Switzerland, Licosa-P/The Chinois), 9.32% by weight polyphenols. Compared to results from meals without the addition of the extract, the decrease was 28%. The green tea extract polyphenol content in each meal was 37.3 mg.

REFERENCES

Ahmad, F., Khalid, P., Khan, M.M., Rastogi, A.K., and Kidwai, J.R. (1989). Insulin like activity in (–)-epicatechin. *Acta Diabetologica Latina* 26: 291-300.

Ahmad, N., Chen, P., and Mukhtar, H. (2000). Cell cycle dysregulation by green tea polyphenol epigallocatechin-3-gallate. *Biochemical and Biophysical Research Communications* 275: 328-334.

Ahmad, N., Feyes, D.K., Nieminen, A.L., Agarwal, R., and Mukhtar, H. (1997). Green tea constituent epigallocatechin-3-gallate and induction of apoptosis and cell cycle arrest in human carcinoma cells. *Journal of the National Cancer Institute* 89: 1881-1886.

Ahmad, N., Gupta, S., and Mukhtar, H. (2001). Green tea polyphenol epigallocatechin-3-gallate differentially modulates nuclear factor κB in cancer cells versus normal cells. *Archives of Biochemistry and Biophysics* 376: 338-346.

Ali, M., Afzal, M., Gubler, C.J., and Burka, J.F. (1990). A potent thromboxane formation inhibitor in green tea leaves. *Prostaglandins, Leukotrienes and Essential Fatty Acids* 40: 281-283.

Bailey, L.H. and Bailey, E.Z. (1976). *Hortus Third* (pp. 208-210). New York: Macmillan General Reference.

Benzie, I.F.F., Szeto, Y.T., Strain, J.J., and Tomlinson, B. (1999). Consumption of green tea causes rapid increase in plasma antioxidant power in humans. *Nutrition and Cancer* 34: 83-87.

Bhatia, N. and Agarwal, R. (2001). Detrimental effect of cancer preventive phytochemicals silymarin, genistein and epigallocatechin 3-gallate on epigenetic events in human prostate carcinoma DU145 cells. *The Prostate* 46: 98-107.

Bridge, A., Sun, P., Peter, A.D., Morré, D.M., and Morré, D.J. (1998). How green tea prevents cancer. In K. Wilson (Ed.), *1998 ASCB Annual Meeting, Selected Biomedical Abstracts* (pp. 9-10). American Society for Cell Biology 38th Annual Meeting, December 12-16, San Francisco, CA. Bethesda, MD: American Society of Cell Biology.

Bridge, A., Sun, P., Wu, L.Y., Morré, D.M., and Morré, D.J. (1998). Cancer-specific NADH oxidase (tNOX) a molecular target for the active principle of green tea? *Molecular Biology of the Cell* 9: 184A (abstract).

Bu-Abbas, A., Clifford, M.N., Walker, R., and Ioannides, C. (1994). Marked antimutagenic potential of aqueous green tea extracts: Mechanism of action. *Mutagenesis* 9: 325-331.

Bu-Abbas, A., Clifford, M.N., Walker, R., and Ioannides, C. (1998). Contribution of caffeine and flavanols in the induction of hepatic phase II activities by green tea. *Food and Chemical Toxicology* 36: 617-621.

Bu-Abbas, A., Copeland, E., Clifford, M.N., Walker, R., and Ioannides, C. (1997). Fractionation of green tea extracts: Correlation of antimutagenic effect with flavanol content. *Journal of the Science of Food and Agriculture* 75: 453-462.

Cao, Y. and Cao, R. (1999). Angiogenesis inhibited by drinking tea. *Nature* 398 (April 1): 381.

Chakravarthy, B.K., Gupta, S., and Gode, K.D. (1982). Functional Beta cell regeneration in the islets of pancreas in alloxan diabetic rats by (–)-epicatechin. *Life Sciences* 31: 2693-2697.

Chen, Z.P., Schell, J.B., Ho, C.T., and Chen, K.Y. (1998). Green tea epigallocatechin gallate shows a pronounced growth inhibitory effect on cancerous cells but not on their normal counterparts. *Cancer Letters* 129: 173-179.

Chueh, P.J., Kim, C., Morré, D.M., and Morré, D.J. (1998). Isolation and expression cloning of a tumor-associated NADH oxidase (tNOX) that is a potential pancancer marker. *Molecular Biology of the Cell* 9: 184A (abstract).

Chung, C.H. and Liu, T.C. (1991). Comparative study of the inhibitory effect of green tea, coffee, and levamisole on the hepatocarcinogenic action of diethylnitrosoamine. *Chinese Journal of Oncology* 13: 193-195.

Chow, W.H., Blot, W.J., and McLaughlin, J.K. (1999). Tea drinking and cancer risk: Epidemiological evidence. *Proceedings of the Society for Experimental Biology and Medicine* 220: 197 (abstract).

Dalluge, J.J., Nelson, B.C., Thomas, J.B., Welch, M.J., and Sander, L.C. (1997). Capillary liquid chromatography/electrospray mass spectrometry for the separation and detection of catechins in green tea and human plasma. *Rapid Communications in Mass Spectrometry* 11: 1753-1756.

de Maat, M.P., Pijl, H., Kluft, C., and Princen, H.M. (2000). Consumption of black and green tea had no effect on inflammation, haemostasis and endothelial markers in smoking healthy individuals. *European Journal of Clinical Nutrition* 54: 757-763.

Dhar, G.M., Shah, G.N., and Naheed, B.H., et al. (1993). Epidemiological trend in the distribution of cancer in Kashmir Valley. *Journal of Epidemiology and Community Health* 47: 290-292.

Dulloo, A.G., Duret, C., Rohrer, L., Girardier, L., Mensi, N., Fathi, M., Chantre, P., and Vandermander, J. (1999). Efficacy of green tea extract rich in catechin polyphenols and caffeine in increasing 24-h energy expenditure and fat oxidation in humans. *American Journal of Clinical Nutrition* 70: 1040-1045.

Dulloo, A.G., Seydoux, J., and Girardier, L. (1996). Tealine and thermogenesis: Interactions between polyphenols, caffeine and sympathetic activity. *International Journal of Obesity and Related Metabolic Disorders* 20(Suppl. 7): 71 (abstract).

Dvorakova, K., Dorr, R.T., Valcic, S., Timmermann B., and Alberts D. (1999). Pharmacokinetics of the green tea derivative, EGCG, by the topical route of administration in mouse and human skin. *Cancer Chemotherapy and Pharmacology* 43: 331-335.

Elmets, C.A., Singh, D., Tubesing, K., Matsui, M., Katiyar, S., and Mukhtar, H. (2001). Cutaneous photoprotection from ultraviolet injury by green tea polyphenols. *Journal of the American Academy of Dermatology* 44: 425-432.

Freese, R., Basu, S., Hietanen, E., Nair, J., Nakachi, K., Bartsch, H., and Mutanen, M. (1999). Green tea decreases plasma malondialdehyde concentration but does not affect other indicators of oxidative stress, nitric oxide production, or hemostatic factors during a high-linoleic acid diet in healthy females. *European Journal of Nutrition* 38: 149-157.

Fujita, Y., Yamane, T., Tanaka, M., Kuwata, K., Okuzumi, J., Takahashi, T., Fujiki, H., and Okuda, T. (1989). Inhibitory effect of (–)-epigallocatechin gallate on carcinogenesis with *N*-ethyl-*N'*-nitrosoguanidine in mouse duodenum. *Japanese Journal of Cancer Research* 80: 503-505.

Galanis, D.J., Kolonel, L.N., Lee, J., and Nomura, A. (1998). Intakes of selected foods and beverages and the incidence of gastric cancer among the Japanese residents of Hawaii: A prospective study. *International Journal of Epidemiology* 27: 173-180.

Gomes, A., Vedasiromoni, J.R., Das, M., Sharma, R.M., and Ganguly, D.K. (1995). Antihyperglycemic effect of black tea *(Camellia sinensis)* in rat. *Journal of Ethnopharmacology* 45: 223-226.

Graham, H.N. (1992). Green tea composition, consumption, and polyphenol chemistry. *Preventive Medicine* 21: 334-350.

Gupta, S., Ahmad, N., Mohan, R.R., Husain, M.M., and Mukhtar, H. (1999). Prostate cancer chemoprevention by green tea: In vitro and an in vivo inhibition of testosterone-mediated induction of ornithine decarboxylase. *Cancer Research* 59: 2115-2120.

Gupta, S., Ahmad, N., Nieminen, A.L., and Mukhtar, H. (2000). Growth inhibition, cell-cycle dysregulation, and induction of apoptosis by green tea constituent (–)epigallocatechin-3-gallate in androgen-sensitive and androgen-insensitive human prostate carcinoma cells. *Toxicology and Applied Pharmacology* 164: 82-90.

Gutman, R.L. and Ryu, B.H. (1996). Rediscovering tea. *HerbalGram* 37: 34-48.

Hamajima, N., Tajima, K., Tominaga, S., Matsuura A., Kuwabara, M., and Okuma, K. (1999). Tea polyphenol intake and changes in serum pepsinogen levels. *Japanese Journal of Cancer Research* 90: 136-143.

Han, C. and Xu, Y. (1990). The effect of Chinese tea on occurrence of esophageal tumor induced by *N*-nitroso-methylbenzylamine in rats. *Biomedical and Environmental Science* 3: 35-42.

Harbowy, M.E. and Ballentine, D.A. (1997). Tea chemistry. *CRC Critical Reviews in Plant Sciences* 16: 415-480.

Hasegawa, R., Chujo, T., Sai-Kato, K., Umemura, T., Tanimura, A., and Kurokawa, Y. (1995). Preventive effects of green tea against liver oxidative DNA damage and hepatotoxicity in rats treated with 2-nitropropane. *Food Chemistry and Toxicology* 33: 961-970.

Hayashi, M., Yamazoe, H., Yamaguchi, Y., and Kunitomo, M. (1992). [Effects of green tea extract on galactosamine-induced hepatic injury in rats]. *Nippon Yakurigaku Zasshi* 100: 391-399.

He, Y.H. and Kies, C. (1994). Green and black tea consumption by humans: Impact on polyphenol concentration in feces, blood, and urine. *Plant Foods for Human Nutrition* 46: 221-229.

Hertog, M.G., Feskens, E.J., Holloman, P.C., Katan, M.B., and Kromhout, D. (1993). Dietary antioxidant flavonoids and risk of coronary heart disease. The Zutphen elderly study. *Lancet* 342: 1007-1011.

Hertog, M.G., Kromhout, D., Aravanis, C., Blackburn, H., Buzina, R., Fidanza, F., Giampaoli, S., Jansen, A., Menotti, A., Nedeljkovic, S., et al. (1995). Flavonoid intake and long-term risk of coronary heart disease and cancer in the Seven Countries Study. *Archives of Internal Medicine* 155: 381-386.

Hibasami, H., Komiya, T., Achiwa, Y., Ohnishi, K., Kojima, T., Nakanishi, K., Akashi, K., and Hara, Y. (1998). Induction of apoptosis in human stomach cancer cells by green tea catechins. *Oncology Reports* 5: 527-529.

Higashi-Okai, K., Oyani, S., and Okai, Y. (1998). Potent suppressive activity of pheophytin a and b from the non-polyphenolic fraction of green tea *(Camellia sinensis)* against tumor promotion in mouse skin. *Cancer Letters* 129: 223-228.

Higashi-Okai, K., Taniguchi, M., and Okai, Y. (1998). Potent suppressive activity of pheophytin a and b from non-polyphenolic fraction of green tea *(Camellia sinensis)* against the activation of oxygen radical generation, cytokine release and chemotaxis of human polymorphonuclear neutrophils (PMNs). *Journal of Fermentation and Bioengineering* 85: 555-558.

Higashi-Okai, K., Taniguchi, M., and Okai, Y. (2000). Potent antioxidative activity of non-polyphenolic fraction of green tea *(Camellia sinensis)*—Association with pheophytins a and b. *Journal of the Science of Food and Agriculture* 80: 117-120.

Hirose, M., Hoshiya, T., Akagi, K., Futakuchi, M., and Ito, N. (1994). Inhibition of mammary gland carcinogenesis by green tea catechin and other naturally occurring antioxidants in female Sprague-Dawley rats pretreated with 7,12 dimethylbenz[*a*]-anthracene. *Cancer Letters* 83: 149-156.

Hirose, M., Mizoguchi, Y., Yaono, M., Tanaka, H., Yamaguchi, T., and Shirai, T. (1997). Effects of green tea catechins on the progression or late promotion stage of mammary gland carcinogenesis in female Sprague-Dawley rats pretreated with 7,12-dimethylbenz[*a*]anthracene. *Cancer Letters* 112: 141-147.

Hiura, A., Tsutsumi, M., and Satake, K. (1997). Inhibitory effect of green tea extract on the process of pancreatic carcinogenesis induced by *N*-nitro-sobis-(2-oxypropyl)amine (BOP) and on tumor promotion after transplantation of *N*-nitro-sobis-(2-hydroxypropyl)amine (BHP)-induced pancreatic cancer in Syrian hamsters. *Pancreas* 15: 272-277.

Hodgson, J.M., Puddey, I.B., Burke, V., Beilin, L.J., and Jordan, N. (1999). Effects on blood pressure of drinking green and black tea. *Journal of Hypertension* 17: 457-463.

Hodgson, J.M., Puddey, I.B., Croft, K.D., Burke, V., Mori, T.A., Caccetta, R.A., and Beilin, L.J. (2000). Acute effects of ingestion of black and green tea on lipoprotein oxidation. *American Journal of Clinical Nutrition* 71: 1103-1107.

Horiba, N., Maekawa, Y., Ito, M., Matsumoto, T., and Nakamura, H. (1991). A pilot study of Japanese green tea as a medicament: Antibacterial and bactericidal effects. *Journal of Endodontics* 17: 122-124.

Horikawa, K., Mohri, T., Tanaka, Y., and Tokiwa, H. (1994). Moderate inhibition of mutagenicity and carcinogenicity of benzo[*a*]pyrene, 1,6-dinitropyrene and 3,9-dinitrofluoranthene by Chinese medicinal herbs. *Mutagenesis* 9: 523-526.

Hu, Z.Q., Toda, M., Okubo, S., Hara, Y., and Shimamura, T. (1992). Mitogenic activity of (–)epigallocatechin gallate on B-cells and investigation of its structure-function relationship. *International Journal of Immunopharmacology* 14: 1399-1407.

Huang, Y., Chan, N.W.K., Lau, C.W., Yao, X.Q., Chan, L.F., and Chen, Z.Y. (1999). Involvement of endothelium/nitric oxide in vasorelaxation induced by purified green tea (–)-epicatechin. *Biochemica et Biophysica Acta. General Subjects* 1427: 322-328.

Ikigai, H., Nakae, T., Hara, Y., and Shimamura, T. (1993). Bactericidal catechins damage the lipid bilayer. *Biochimica et Biophysica Acta* 1147: 132-136.

Imai, K. and Nakachi, K. (1995). Cross sectional study of effects of drinking green tea on cardiovascular and liver diseases. *British Medical Journal* 18: 693-696.

Imai, K., Suga, K., and Nakachi, K. (1997). Cancer-preventive effects of drinking green tea among a Japanese population. *Preventive Medicine* 26: 769-775.

Ishikawa, T., Suzukawa, M., Ito, T., Yoshida, H., Ayaori, M., Nishikawa, M., Yonemura, A., and Hara, Y. (1997). Effect of tea flavonoid supplementation on the susceptibility of low-density lipoprotein to oxidative modification. *American Journal of Clinical Nutrition* 66: 261-266.

Jankun, J., Selman, S.H., and Swiercz, R. (1997). Why drinking green tea could prevent cancer. *Nature* 387 (June 5): 561.

Jelinek, J. (Ed.) (1978). *Illustrated Encyclopedia of Prehistoric Man*. Paris: Grund.

Ji, B.T., Chow, W.H., Hsing, A.W., McLaughlin, J.K., Dai, Q., and Gao, Y.T. (1997). Green tea consumption and the risk of pancreatic and colorectal cancers. *International Journal of Cancer* 70: 255-258.

Kang, W.S., Lim, I.H., Yuk, D.Y., Chung, K.H., Park, J.B., Yoo, H.S., and Yun, Y.P. (1999). Antithrombotic activities of green tea catechins and (–)-epigallocatechin gallate. *Thrombosis Research* 96: 229-237.

Katiyar, S.K., Afaq, F., Perez, A., and Mukhtar, H. (2001). Green tea polyphenol (–)-epigallocatechin-3-gallate treatment of human skin inhibits ultraviolet radiation-induced oxidative stress. *Carcinogenesis* 22: 287-294.

Katiyar, S.K., Challa, A., McKormick, T.S., Cooper, K.D., and Mukhtar, H. (1999). Prevention of UVB-induced immunosuppression in mice by the green tea polyphenol (–)-epigallocatechin-3-gallate may be associated with alterations in IL-10 and IL-12 production. *Carcinogenesis* 20: 2117-2124.

Katiyar, S.K., Matsui, M.S., Elmets, C.A., and Mukhtar, H. (1999). Polyphenolic antioxidant (–)-epigallocatechin-3-gallate from green tea reduces UVB-induced inflammatory responses and infiltration of leukocytes in human skin. *Photochemistry and Photobiology* 69: 148-153.

Katiyar, S.K., Perez, A., and Mukhtar, H. (2000). Green tea polyphenol treatment of human skin prevents formation of ultraviolet light B-induced pyrimidine dimers in DNA. *Clinical Cancer Research* 10: 3864-3869.

Keys, J.D. (1991). *Chinese Herbs: Their Botany, Chemistry, and Pharmacodynamics* (pp. 189-190). Rutland, VT: Charles E. Tuttle Company.

Kohlmeier, L., Weterlings, K.G.C., Steck, S., and Kok, F.J. (1997). Tea and cancer: An evaluation of the epidemiologic literature. *Nutrition and Cancer* 27: 1-13.

Kono, S., Ikeda, M., Tokudome, S., and Kuratsune, M. (1988). A case-control study of gastric cancer and diet in northern Kyushu, Japan. *Japanese Journal of Cancer* 79: 1067-1074.

Kostyuk, V.A., Potapovich, A.I., Vladykovskaya, E.N., and Hiramatsu, M. (2000). Protective effects of green tea catechins against asbestos-induced cell injury. *Planta Medica* 66: 762-764.

Krahwinkel, T. and Willershausen, B. (2000). The effect of sugar-free green tea chew candies on the degree of inflammation of the gingiva. *European Journal of Medical Research* 54: 463-467.

Kvaratskhella, M., Winkel, C., Naldrett, M.T., and Thorneley, R.N.F. (1999). A novel high activity cationic ascorbate peroxidase from tea *(Camellia sinensis)*— A class III peroxidase with unusual substrate specificity. *Journal of Plant Physiology* 154: 273-282.

Lecomte, A. (1985). [Clinical study of weight loss using Arkogelules green tea] (in French) [Green tea 'Arkocaps'/Phytotrim® double-blind trial clinical results; extract in English]. *Revue de l'Association Mondiale de Phytotherapie* (1): 36-40, June. Cited in M.R. Werbach and M.T. Murray. (1994), *Botanical Influences on Illness* (p. 249). Tarzana, CA: Third Line Press.

Lee, H.H., Wu, H.Y., Chuang, Y.C., Chang, A.S., Chao, H.H., Chen, K.Y., Chen, H.K., Lai, G.M., Huang, H.H., and Chen, C.J. (1990). Epidemiologic characteristics and multiple risk factors of stomach cancer in Taiwan. *Anticancer Research* 10: 875-882.

Leenen, R., Roodenburg, A.J.C., Tijburg, L.M.B., and Wiseman, S.A. (2000). A single dose of tea with or without milk increases plasma antioxidant activity in humans. *European Journal of Clinical Nutrition* 54: 87-92.

Li, H.C., Yashiki, S., Sonoda, J., Lou, H., Ghosh, S.K., Byrnes, J.J., Lema, C., Fujiyoshi, T., Karasuyama, M., and Sonoda, S. (2000). Green tea polyphenols induce apoptosis in vitro in peripheral blood T lymphocytes of adult T-cell leukemia patients. *Japanese Journal of Cancer Research* 91: 34-40.

Liao, S., Umekita, Y., Guo, J., Kokontis, J.M., and Hiipakka, R.A. (1995). Growth inhibition and regression of human prostate and breast tumors in athymic mice by tea epigallocatechin gallate. *Cancer Letters* 96: 239-243.

Lin, Y.L., Cheng, C.Y., Lin, Y.P., Lau, Y.W., Juan, I.M., and Lin, J.K. (1998). Hypolipidemic effect of green tea leaves through induction of antioxidant and phase II enzymes including superoxide dismutase, catalase, and glutathione *S*-transferase in rats. *Journal of Agricultural and Food Chemistry* 46: 1893-1899.

Lin, Y.L. and Lin, J.K. (1997). (–)-Epigallocatechin-3gallate blocks the induction of nitric oxide synthase by down-regulating lipopolysaccharide-induced activity of transcription factor nuclear factor-κB. *Molecular Pharmacology* 52: 465-472.

Matsumoto, N., Ishigaki, F., Ishigaki, A., Iwashina, H., and Hara, Y. (1993). Reduction of blood glucose levels by tea catechin. *Bioscience, Biotechnology and Biochemistry* 57: 525-527.

Merhav, H., Amitai, Y., Palti, H., and Godfrey, S. (1985). Tea drinking and microcytic anemia in infants. *American Journal of Clinical Nutrition* 41: 1210-1213.

Miller, N.J. and Rice-Evans, C. (1996). Spectrophotometric determination of antioxidant activity. *Redox Reports* 2: 161-171.

Mirvish, S.S. (1995). Role of *N*-nitroso compounds (NOC) and *N*-nitrosation in etiology of gastric, esophageal, nasopharyngeal and bladder cancer and contribution to cancer of known exposures to NOC. *Cancer Letters* 93: 17-48.

Mitamura, T., Kitazono, M., Yoshimura, O., and Yakushiji, M. (1989). [The influence of green tea upon the improvement of iron deficiency anemia with pregnancy treated by sodium ferrous citrate]. *Acta Obstetrica et Gynaecologica Japonica* 41: 688-694.

Mitscher, L.A. and Dolby, V. (1998). *The Green Tea Book: China's Fountain of Youth.* Garden City, NY: Avery Publishing Group.

Mitscher, L.A., Jung, M., Shankel, D., Dou, J.K., Steele, L., and Pillai, S.P. (1997). Chemoprotection: A review of the potential therapeutic anti-oxidant properties of green tea *(Camellia sinensis)* and certain of its constituents. *Medicinal Research Reviews* 17: 327-365.

Miura, Y., Chiba, T., Miura, S., Tomita, I., Umegaki, K., Ikeda, M., and Tomita, T. (2000). Green tea polyphenols (flavan 3-ols) prevent oxidative modification of low density lipoproteins: An ex vivo study in humans. *Journal of Nutritional Biochemistry* 11: 216-222.

Mukhtar, H., Katiyar, S.K., and Agarwal, R. (1994). Green tea and skin—Anticarcinogenic effects. *Journal of Investigative Dermatology* 102: 3-7.

Nadkarni, K.M. (1976). *Indian Materia Medica*, Vol. 1. (pp. 247-249). Bombay, India: Popular Prakashan Pvt. Ltd.

Nagata, C., Kabuto, M., and Shimizu, H. (1998). Association of coffee, green tea, and caffeine intakes with serum concentrations of estradiol and sex hormone-binding globulin in premenopausal Japanese women. *Nutrition and Cancer* 30: 21-24.

Nakachi, K., Suemasu, K., Suga, K., Takeo, T., Imai, K., and Higashi, Y. (1998). Influence of green tea on breast cancer malignancy among Japanese patients. *Japanese Journal of Cancer Research* 89: 254-261.

Nakagawa, K., Ninomiya, M., Okubo, T., Aoi, N., Juneja, L.R., Kim, M., Yamanaka, K., and Miyazawa, T. (1999). Tea catechin supplementation increases antioxidant capacity and prevents phospholipid hydroperoxidation in plasma of humans. *Journal of Agricultural and Food Chemistry* 47: 3967-3973.

Nakamura, M. and Kawabata, T. (1981). Effect of Japanese green tea on nitrosamine formation in vitro. *Journal of Food Science* 46: 306-307.

Nakamura, Y., Harada, S., Kawase, I., Matsuda, M., and Tomita, I. (1992). Inhibition of in vitro neoplastic transformation by tea ingredients. In abstracts of papers presented at the First International Symposium on the Physiological and Pharmacological Effects of *Camellia sinensis* (Tea), New York City, March 4-5, 1991. *Preventive Medicine* 21: 331-333 (abstract).

Nakane, H. and Ono, K. (1990). Differential inhibitory effects of some catechin derivatives on the activities of human immunodeficiency virus reverse transcriptase and cellular deoxyribonucleic acid polymerases. *Biochemistry* 20: 2841-2845.

Nakayama, M., Suzuki, K., Toda, M., Okubo, S., Hara, Y., and Shimamura, T. (1993). Inhibition of the infectivity of influenza virus by tea polyphenols. *Antiviral Research* 21: 289-299.

Narisawa, T. and Fukaura, Y. (1993). A very low dose of green tea polyphenols in drinking water prevents *N*-methyl-*N*-nitrosourea-induced colon carcinogenesis in F334 rats. *Japanese Journal of Cancer Research* 84: 1007-1009.

NCI, DCPC, Chemoprevention Branch and Agent Development Committee (1996). Clinical development plan: Tea extracts, green tea polyphenols, epigallocatechin gallate. *Journal of Cellular Biochemistry* 26S: 236-257.

Neiva, T.J.C., Morais, L., Polack, M., Simoes, C.M., and D'Amico, E.A. (1999). Effects of catechins on human blood platelet aggregation and lipid peroxidation. *Phytotherapy Research* 13: 597-600.

Ninomiya, M., Sakanaka, S., Juneja, L.R., Kim, M., Yamazaki, N., Ito, Y., and Yokozawa, T. (1997). Suppressive effect of uremic toxin formation by green tea polyphenols. *Abstracts of Papers (American Chemical Society)* 213: AGFD 171.

Nomura, M., Ma, W., Chen, N., Bode, A.M., and Dong, Z. (2000). Inhibition of 12-O-tetradecanoylphorbol-13-acetate-induced NF-κB activation by tea polyphenols, (–)-epigallocatechin gallate and theaflavins. *Carcinogenesis* 21: 1885-1890.

Oguni, I., Cheng, S.J., Lin, P.Z., and Hara, Y. (1992). Protection against cancer risk by Japanese green tea. In abstracts of papers presented at the First International Symposium on the Physiological and Pharmacological Effects of *Camellia sinensis* (Tea), New York City, March 4-5, 1991. *Preventive Medicine* 21: 331-333 (abstract).

Ohmori, Y., Ito, M., Kishi, M., Mizutani, H., Katada, T., and Konishi, H. (1995). Antiallergic constituents from oolong tea stem. *Biochemical and Pharmaceutical Bulletin* 18: 683-686.

Ohshima, H. and Bartsch, H. (1981). Quantitative estimation of endogenous nitrosation in humans by monitoring of *N*-nitrosoproline excreted in urine. *Cancer Research* 41: 3658-3662.

Ohshima, H. and Bartsch, H. (1988). Urinary *N*-nitrosamino acids as an indices of exposure to *N*-nitroso compounds. In H. Barrtsch, K. Hemminki, and I.K. O'Neill (Eds.), *Methods for Detecting DNA Damaging Agents in Humans: Applications in Cancer Epidemiology and Prevention*. IARC Publication No. 89. Lyon, France: International Agency for Research on Cancer.

Okabe, S., Ochiai, Y., Aida, M., Park, K., Kim, S.J., Nomura, T., Suganuma, M., and Fujiki, H. (1999). Mechanistic aspects of green tea as a cancer preventive: Effect of components on human stomach cancer cell lines. *Japanese Journal of Cancer Research* 90: 733-739.

Ooshima, T., Minami, T., Aono, W., Yamura, Y., and Hamada, S. (1994). Reduction of dental plaque deposition in humans by oolong tea extract. *Caries Research* 28: 146-149.

Osawa, T., Kumon, H., Nakayama, T., Kawakishi, S., and Hara, Y. (1992). Tea polyphenols as antioxidants. In abstracts of papers presented at the First International Symposium on the Physiological and Pharmacological Effects of *Camellia sinensis* (Tea), New York City, March 4-5, 1991. *Preventive Medicine* 21: 331-333 (abstract).

Otsuka, T., Ogo, T., Eto, T., Asano, Y., Suganuma, M., and Niho, Y. (1998). Growth inhibition of leukemic cells by (−)-epigallocatechin gallate, the main constituent of green tea. *Life Sciences* 63: 1397-1403.

Paquay, J.B.G., Haenen, G.R.M.M., Stender, G., Wiseman, S.A., Tijburg, L.B.M., and Bast, A. (2000). Protection against nitric oxide toxicity by tea. *Journal of Agricultural and Food Chemistry* 48: 5768-5772.

Paschka, A.G., Butler, R., and Young, C.Y.F. (1998). Induction of apoptosis in prostate cancer cell lines by the green tea component, (−)-epigallocatechin-3-gallate. *Cancer Letters* 130: 1-7.

Pearson, D.A., Frankel, E.N., Aeschbach, R., and German, J.B. (1998). Inhibition of endothelial cell mediated low-density lipoprotein oxidation by green tea extracts. *Journal of Agricultural and Food Chemistry* 46: 1445-1449.

Pietta, P., Simonetti, P., and Mauri, P. (1998). Antioxidant activity of selected medicinal plants. *Journal of Agriculture and Food Chemistry* 46: 4487-4490.

Pignatelli, B., Bereziat, J.C., Descotes, G., and Bartsch, H. (1982). Catalysis of nitrosation in vitro and in vivo in rats by catechin and resorcinol and inhibition by chlorogenic acid. *Carcinogenesis* 3: 1045-1049.

Princen, H.M.G., van Duyvenvoorde, W., Buytenhek, R., Blonk, C., Tijburg, L.B., Langius, J.A., Meinders, A.E., and Pijl, H. (1998). No effect of consumption of green and black tea on plasma lipid and antioxidant levels and on LDL oxidation in smokers. *Arteriosclerosis, Thrombosis and Vascular Biology* 18: 833-841.

Qin, G.Z. (1991). Effects of green tea extract on the development of aflatoxin B_1-induced precancerous enzyme altered hepatocellular foci in rats. *Chinese Journal of Preventive Medicine* 25: 332-334.

Qin, G., Gopalan-Kriczky, P., Su, J., Ning, Y., and Lotlikar, P.D. (1997). Inhibition of aflatoxin B_1-induced initiation of hepatocarcinogenesis in the rat by green tea. *Cancer Letters* 112: 149-154.

Rall, T.W. (1980). The xanthines. In A.G. Gilman, L.S. Goodman, and A. Gilman (Eds.), *The Pharmacological Basis of Therapeutics* (pp. 592-607). New York: Mac Millan.

Rice-Evans, C. (1999). Implications of the mechanisms of action of tea polyphenols as antioxidants in vitro for chemoprevention in humans. *Proceedings of the Society for Experimental Biology and Medicine* 220: 262-266.

Robertson, D., Wade, D., and Workman, R. (1981). Tolerance to the humoral and hemodynamic effects of caffeine in man. *Journal of Clinical Investigations* 67: 1111-1117.

Sadakata, S., Fukao, A., and Hisamichi, S. (1992). Mortality among female practitioners of Chanoya (Japanese "Tea-ceremony"). *Tohoku Journal of Experimental Medicine* 166: 475-477.

Sadzuka, Y., Sugiyama, T., and Hirota, S. (1998). Modulation of cancer chemotherapy by green tea. *Clinical Cancer Research* 4: 153-156.

Sagesaka-Mitane, Y., Miwa, M., and Okada, S. (1990). Platelet aggregation inhibitors in hot water extract of green tea. *Chemical and Pharmaceutical Bulletin* 38: 790-793.

Sakanaka, S., Aizawa, M., Kim, M., and Yamamoto, T. (1996). Inhibitory effects of green tea polyphenols on growth and cellular adherence of an oral bacterium, *Porphyromonas gingivalis*. *Bioscience, Biotechnology and Biochemistry* 60: 745-749.

Sakanaka, S., Kim, M., Taniguchi, M., and Yamamoto, T. (1989). Antibacterial substances in Japanese green tea extract against *Streptococcus mutans,* a cariogenic bacterium. *Agricultural and Biological Chemistry* 53: 2307-2311.

Sakanaka, S., Shimura, N., Aizawa, M., Kim, M., and Yamamoto, T. (1992). Preventive effect of green tea polyphenols against dental caries in conventional rats. *Bioscience, Biotechnology, and Biochemistry* 56: 592-594.

Samman, S., Sandstrom, B., Toft, M.B., Bukhave, K., Jensen, M., Sorensen, S., and Hansen, M. (2001). Green tea or rosemary extract added to foods reduces nonheme-iron absorption. *American Journal of Clinical Nutrition* 73: 607-612.

Sano, M., Takahashi, Y., Yoshino, K., Shimoi, K., Nakamura, Y., Tomita, I., Oguni, I., and Konomoto, H. (1995). Effect of tea (*Camellia sinensis* L.) on lipid peroxidation in rat liver and kidney: A comparison of green and black tea feeding. *Biological and Pharmaceutical Bulletin* 18: 1006-1008.

Schut, H.A.J. and Yao, R. (2000). Tea as a potential chemopreventive agent in PhIP carcinogenesis: Effects of green tea and black tea on PhIP-DNA adduct formation in female F-34 rats. *Nutrition and Cancer* 36: 52-58.

Serafini, M., Ghiselli, A., and Ferro-Luzzi, A. (1996). In vivo antioxidant effect of green and black tea in man. *European Journal of Clinical Nutrition* 50: 28-32.

Shen, X., Lu, R., Tang, J., and Chen, R. (1993). A study on the hypolipidemic and anticoagulant effects of tea polyphenols in rats. *Acta Nutrimenta Sinica* 15: 147-151.

Shim, J.S., Kang, M.H., Kim, Y.H., Roh, J.K., Roberts, C., and Lee, I.P. (1995). Chemopreventive effect of green tea (*Camellia sinensis*) among cigarette smokers. *Cancer Epidemiology, Biomarkers and Prevention* 4: 387-391.

Shirai, T., Sato, A., Chida, K., Hayakawa, H., Akiyama, J., Iwata, M., Taniguchi, M., Reshad, K., and Hara, Y. (1997). Epigallocatechin gallate-induced histamine release in patients with green tea-induced asthma. *Annals of Allergy, Asthma, and Immunology* 79: 65-69.

Shirai, T., Sato, A., and Hara, Y. (1994). Epigallocatechin gallate. The major causative agent of green tea-induced asthma. *Chest* 106: 1801-1805.

Snow, J.M. (1995). *Camellia sinensis* (L.) Kuntze (Theaceae). *The Protocol Journal of Botanical Medicine* (Autumn): 47-51.

Stensvold, I., Tverdal, A., Solvoll, K., and Foss, O.P. (1992). Tea consumption: Relationship to cholesterol, blood pressure, and coronary and total mortality. *Preventive Medicine* 21: 546-553.

Suganuma, M., Okabe, S., Kai, Y., Sueoka, N., Sueoka, E., and Fujiki, H. (1999). Synergistic effects of (–)-epigallocatechin gallate with (–)-epicatechin, suldinac, or tamoxifen on cancer-preventive activity in the human lung cancer cell line PC-9. *Cancer Research* 59: 44-47.

Suganuma, M., Okabe, S., Oniyama, M., Tada, Y., Ito, H., and Fujiki, H. (1998). Wide distribution of [^{3}H](–)-epigallocatechin gallate, a cancer preventive tea polyphenol, in mouse tissue. *Carcinogenesis* 19: 1771-1776.

Sur, P. and Ganguly, D.K. (1994). Tea plant root extract (TRE) as an antineoplastic agent. *Planta Medica* 60: 106-109.

Taylor, J.R. and Wilt, V.M. (1999). Possible antagonism of warfarin by green tea. *Annals of Pharmacotherapy* 33: 426-428.

Tsubono, Y., Nishino, Y., Komatsu, S., Hsieh, C.C., Kanemura, S., Tsuji, I., Nakatsuka, H., Fukao, A., Satoh, H., and Hisamichi, S. (2001). Green tea and the risk of gastric cancer in Japan. *New England Journal of Medicine* 344: 632-636.

Tsubono, Y. and Tsugane, S. (1997). Green tea intake in relation to serum lipid levels in middle-aged Japanese men and women. *Annals of Epidemiology* 7: 280-284.

van het Hof, K.H., de Boer, S.M., Wiseman, S.A., Lien, N., Weststrate, J.A., and Tijburg, L.B.M. (1997). Consumption of green or black tea does not increase resistance of low-density lipoprotein to oxidation in humans. *American Journal of Clinical Nutrition* 66: 1125-1132.

Vermeer, I.T.M., Moonen, E.J.C., Dallinga, J.W., Kleinjans, J.C.S., and van Maanen, J.M.S. (1999). Effect of ascorbic acid and green tea on endogenous formation of *N*-nitrosodimethylamine and *N*-nitrosopiperidine in humans. *Mutation Research* 428: 353-361.

Virtanen, S.M., Rasanen, L., Aro, A., Ylonen, K., Lounamaa, R., Akerblom, H.K., Tuomilehto, J., Vertanen, S.M., Rasanen, L., Aro, A., et al. (1994). Is children's or parents' coffee or tea consumption associated with the risk for type I diabetes mellitus in children? *European Journal of Clinical Nutrition* 48: 279-285.

Wang, Z.Y., Agarwal, R., Kahn, W.A., and Mukhtar, H. (1992). Protection against benz[*a*]pyrene- and *N*-nitrosodiethylamine-induced lung and forestomach tumorigenesis in A/J mice by water extracts of green tea and licorice. *Carcinogenesis* 13: 1491-1494.

Wang, Z.Y., Cheng, S.J., Zhou, Z.C., Athar, M., Khan, W.A., Bickers, D.R., and Mukhtar, H. (1989). Antimutagenic activity of green tea polyphenols. *Mutation Research* 223: 273-285.

Wang, Z.Y., Huang, M.T., Ferraro, T., Wong, C.Q., Lou, Y.R., Reuhl, K., Iatropoulos, M., Yang, C.S., and Conney, A.H. (1992). Inhibitory effect of green tea in the drinking water on tumorigenesis by ultraviolet light and 12-*O*-tetradecanoylphorbol-13-acetate in the skin of SKH-1 mice. *Cancer Research* 52: 1162-1170.

Watanabe, J., Kawabata, J., and Niki, R. (1998). Isolation and identification of acetyl-CoA carboxylase inhibitors from green tea *(Camellia sinensis)*. *Bioscience, Biotechnology, and Biochemistry* 62: 532-534.

Weatherstone, J. (1992). Historical introduction. In K.C. Willson and M.N. Clifford (Eds.), *Tea: Cultivation to Consumption* (pp. 1-23). New York: Chapman and Hall.

Wood, A.W., Huang, M.T., Chang, R.L., Newmark, H.L., Lehr, R.E., Sayer, J.M., Jerina, D.M., and Conney, A.H. (1982). Inhibition of the mutagenicity of bayregion diol epoxides of polycyclic aromatic hydrocarbons by naturally occurring plant phenols: Exceptional activity of ellagic acid. *Proceedings of the National Academy of Sciences, USA* 79 (Part 1: Biological Sciences): 5513-5517.

Wu, Y.N., Wang, H.Z., Li, J.S., and Han, C. (1993). The inhibitory effect of Chinese tea and its polyphenols on in vitro and in vivo *N*-nitrosation. *Biomedical and Environmental Sciences* 6: 237-258.

Xu, Y. and Han, C. (1990). The effects of Chinese tea on the occurrence of esophageal tumor induced by *N*-nitrosomethylbenzylamine formed in vivo. *Biomedical and Environmental Sciences* 3: 406-412.

Xu, Y., Ho, C.T., Amin, S.G., Han, C., and Chung, F.L. (1992). Inhibition of tobacco-specific nitrosamine-induced lung tumorigenesis in A/J mice by green tea and its major polyphenol as anti-oxidants. *Cancer Research* 52: 3875-3879.

Yam, T.S., Hamilton-Miller, J.M.Y., and Shah, S. (1998). The effect of a component of tea *(Camellia sinensis)* on methicillin resistance, PBP2' synthesis, and Beta-lactamase production in *Staphylococcus aureus*. *Journal of Antimicrobial Chemotherapy* 42: 211-216.

Yamaguchi, Y., Hayashi, M., Yamazoe, H., and Kumitomo, M. (1991). [Preventive effects of green tea extract on lipid abnormalities in serum, liver and aorta of mice fed an atherogenic diet]. *Nippon Yakazigaku Zasshi* 97: 329-337.

Yamane, T., Hagiwara, N., Tatteishi, M., Akachi, S., Kim, M., Okuzumi, J., Kitao, Y., Inagake, M., Kuwata, K., and Takahashi, T. (1991). Inhibition of azoxymethane-induced colon carcinogenesis in rat by green tea polyphenol fraction. *Japanese Journal of Cancer Research* 82: 336-339.

Yang, C.S., Chen, L., Lee, M.J., Balentine, D., Kuo, M.C., and Schantz, S.P. (1998). Blood and urine levels of tea catechins after ingestion of different amounts of green tea by human volunteers. *Cancer Epidemiology, Biomarkers and Prevention* 7: 351-354.

Yang, C.S. and Wang, Z.Y. (1993). Tea and cancer. *Journal of the National Cancer Institute* 85: 1038-1049.

Yang, C.S., Yang, G.Y., Landau, J.M., Kim, S., and Liao, J. (1998). Tea and tea polyphenols inhibit cell hyperproliferation, lung tumorigenesis, and tumor progression. *Experimental Lung Research* 24: 629-639.

Yang, F., De Villiers, W.J.S., McClain, C.J., and Varilek, G.W. (1998). Green tea polyphenols block endotoxin-induced tumor necrosis factor-production and lethality in a murine model. *Journal of Nutrition* 128: 2334-2340.

Yokozawa, T. and Dong, E. (1997). Influence of green tea and its three major components upon low-density lipoprotein oxidation. *Experimental and Toxicologic Pathology* 49: 329-335.

Yokozawa, T., Dong, E., and Oura, H. (1997). Proof that green tea tannin suppresses the increase in the blood methylguanidine level associated with renal failure. *Experimental and Toxicologic Pathology* 49: 117-122.

Yoshizawa, S., Horiuchi, T., Fujiki, H., Yoshida, T., Okuda, T., and Sugimura, T. (1987). Antitumor promoting activity of (–)-epigallocatechin gallate, the main constituent of "tannin" in green tea. *Phytotherapy Research* 1: 44-47.

Yu, G.P., Hiseh, C.C., Wang, L.Y., Yu, S.Z., Li, X.L., and Jin, T.H. (1995). Green tea consumption and risk of stomach cancer: A population-based case-control study in Shanghai, China. *Cancer Causes and Control* 6: 532-538.

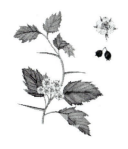

Hawthorn

BOTANICAL DATA

Classification and Nomenclature

Scientific name: *Crataegus laevigata* (Poiret) DC., also known as *C. oxyacantha* L.

Family name: Rosaceae

Common names: hawthorn, English hawthorn, haw, whitethorn, may flower, may, quickthorn, maybush, aubepine, shan-zha (Mandarin) (Wicke, 1994; Djumlija, 1994; Hobbs and Foster, 1990)

Description

Nearly 1,000 species of *Crataegus* have been described in the literature, although today approximately only 280 species are thought to exist. *Crataegus* are native to the northern temperate climate zones in eastern Asia, Europe, and eastern North America. Many of these species are valued for their nutritional, medicinal, and ornamental uses. *Crataegus* species grow as shrubs or small, widely spreading trees. The branches have long, slender thorns, and the leaves are trilobed, pinnate, and oval. The five-petaled flowers are small, usually white or pink, and grow in corymbs on long stalks. The fruits are red with white meat and a large stone, and have the appearance of tiny apples (Hoffmann, 1995; Weiss, 1988).

Crataegus oxyacantha has three- to five-lobed leaves with uneven indentations, especially near the tip of the leaf. The individual lobes of the leaf are more rounded in form. The leaves, twigs, and flower stems are all hairless. Compared to those of *C. monogyna,* the leaves are more pointed at the tips and the lobes are deeper and more pronounced. *Crataegus monogyna* has only one pistil (as the scientific name implies) whereas *C. oxyacantha* may have two or three (Weiss, 1988).

HISTORY AND TRADITIONAL USES

Hawthorn fruits have been popular since ancient Greek and Roman times, when their use was associated with the ritual of marriage. However, it was not until the Renaissance in Europe that hawthorn became valued for its medicinal properties when it was administered for digestive ailments. In the late 1800s, European doctors began to use the plant for heart disease. Hawthorn has also been used in traditional Chinese medicine (TCM) for much longer than in Europe (Djumlija, 1994). The fruit of hawthorn (*C. pinnatifida* Bge. var. major N.E. Br.) is mentioned in the oldest-written pharmacopoeia in China in which it is listed as being used to improve digestion and for improving other maladies. Currently in China, the specially prepared dried ripe fruit is used to stimulate digestion and promote stomach function, and is administered in treatments of epigastric distention, abdominal pain, diarrhea, hyperlipemia, and amenorrhea due to "blood stasis" (Tu et al., 1992; Yao et al., 1996). The fruits of various species of *Crataegus* were used by the Indians of Canada and the United States as a food, and the roots, bark, sapwood, sap, small branches (without leaves), and spines (thorns) served medicinal purposes (Moerman, 1998).

Crataegus monogyna and *C. pentagyna* have similar pharmacological activities to those of *C. laevigata* and are sometimes used as alternatives (Hobbs and Foster, 1990).

CHEMISTRY

Hawthorn contains a number of biologically active constituents including flavonoids, amines, triterpenoids, purine derivatives, and others (Hobbs and Foster, 1990; Ammon and Handel, 1981).

Nitrogenous Compounds

Amino Acids

Crataegus contains several amino acids, such as free glutamine, methionine sulfoxide, aspartic acid, asparagine, glutamic acid, sarcosine, citrulline, proline, glycine, alanine, and valine (Hobbs and Foster, 1990).

Miscellaneous Nitrogenous Compounds

Amines isolated from hawthorn include *O*-methoxyphene-thylamine, tyramine, phenethylamine, and isobutylamine. Hawthorn contains β-phenylethylamine, ethylamine, dimethylamine, trimethylamine, isoamylamine, ethanolamine, choline, acetylcholine, and polyamines, such as spermindine (Hobbs and Foster, 1990).

Phenolic Compounds

Flavonoids

The major flavonoid glycosides in hawthorn are vitexin-4'-rhamnoside, rutin, quercetin, and hyperoside. The flowers and leaves contain the highest concentration of flavonoids in this plant and the fruits contain the lowest. Other important flavonoids in hawthorn are proanthocyanidins, including oligomeric proanthocyanidins with varying degrees of polymerization, catechin-1-epicatechin, cyanidin, and anthocyanidin. Hawthorn also contains anthocyanins, leucocyanidin, and some macromolecular polyphenolic compounds, including oligomeric leucocyanidin, polymeric (–)-epicatechin, polymeric leucocyanidin, and a copolymer of leucocyanidin with (–)-epicatechin. Cyanidin chloride was also isolated from hawthorn (Ficarra et al., 1990; Hobbs and Foster, 1990).

Terpenoid Compounds

Triterpenes

Hawthorn contains the following triterpenic acids: crataegus acid, cinnamic acid, oleanolic acid, ursolic acid, acantolic acid, neoteogolic acid, 2-α-hydroxy-oleanic acid (syn., crataegolic acid). The total content of terpenoids in the leaves is 0.5%-1.4%; fruit, 0.3%-1.4%; and blossoms, 0.7%-1.2% (Hobbs and Foster, 1990; Djumlija, 1994). The fruits of *C. pinnatifida* Bunge. var. *pilosa* Schneider contain ursolic acid, euscapic acid, and corosolic acid (2α-hydroxyursolic acid) (Ahn et al., 1998).

Other Constituents

Hawthorn contains the phenylpropanoid derivatives chlorogenic acid and caffeic acid, steric acid, pectin, citric acid, saccharides, sorbitol, saponins, proteins, and fats. The following nutrient analysis was obtained from the fruits: vitamin B_1 (1.2 ppm), vitamin B_2 (0.6 ppm), vitamin C (805 ppm), vitamin E (19 ppm), potassium (43.15-170.55 mg/100 g), calcium (10-61.4 mg/100 g), magnesium (4.8-18 mg/100 g), iron (0.8-2.6 mg/100 g), zinc (0.4-1.4 mg/100 g), and 1.1% protein, as well as sugars and pectin (Hobbs and Foster, 1990; Djumlija, 1994).

THERAPEUTIC APPLICATIONS

Recent therapeutic uses of hawthorn concern cardiovascular effects, especially in regard to atherosclerosis, hypertension, and congestive heart failure. It is also indicated in dyspepsia, fluid retention, and for helping digestion. Hawthorn has collagen-stabilizing properties that are believed to render it useful for treating rheumatoid arthritis and other inflammatory conditions. The various flavonoids in hawthorn are believed to work synergistically to potentiate the action of the extract; although flavonoids are identified as the principle pharmacologically active constituent, no specific flavonoid is used singly to assess the biological activity of hawthorn (Hobbs and Foster, 1990; Djumlija, 1994).

Hawthorn has shown a number of beneficial actions on the heart and cardiovascular system. Hawthorn dilates the coronary arteries, improves blood supply to the heart, and may also improve the tone of heart muscle walls in patients with low blood pressure. Hawthorn stabilizes heart contractions and improves the metabolic functioning of the heart, thus increasing the pumping force (a positive inotropic effect). The main actions of hawthorn are as follows: cardiotonic and trophorestorative; coronary and peripheral vasodilator; cardiac antispasmodic; amphoteric to blood pressure; sedative; antiarrhythmic; diuretic; astringent; antiscorbutic; antidiarrheal; and collagen stabilizing (Djumlija, 1994).

PRECLINICAL STUDIES

Cardiovascular and Circulatory Functions

Atherosclerosis

Proanthocyanidins in hawthorn are regarded as being active in preventing the buildup of arterial plaque. This activity is based upon a strengthening effect exhibited by flavonoids of hawthorn on collagen matrices in arterial walls. Hawthorn also acts to dilate the coronary vessels, which improves blood flow to the heart (Djumlija, 1994).

An alcoholic tincture of the berries of *C. oxycantha* was administered to male rats (5 mL/kg per day p.o. for six weeks) during which time they were fed a high-cholesterol diet. Compared with rats fed the same diet without the hawthorn tincture, the hawthorn-treated rats showed significantly lower levels of plasma total cholesterol ($p < 0.01$), VLDL, LDL, and a significantly lower atherogenic index (each $p < 0.001$). Comparing changes in lipid profiles of their livers, the hawthorn group showed significantly lower liver total cholesterol and liver cholesterol biosynthesis (each $p < 0.001$), while fecal bile acid levels and liver bile acids (cholic and deoxycholic acids) were significantly higher (each $p < 0.001$). Binding of ^{125}I-LDL to liver plasma membranes was only slightly increased in the rats fed the high-cholesterol diet, whereas in the group treated with hawthorn binding of ^{125}I-LDL was clearly enhanced. When maximum binding capacity was examined, the increase was also slight in the untreated group (+ 25%) and, by comparison, significantly higher in the hawthorn group (+ 45%, $p < 0.01$), suggesting that the extract caused liver plasma membrane LDL binding sites to increase significantly in number. However, differences in binding affinity showed no significant alteration in either group. The researchers note that in rats, guggulsterone, derived from *Commiphora mukul,* was also reported to enhance LDL catabolism by way of hepatic receptors (Rajendran et al., 1996).

Cardiotonic; Cardioprotection

In an ex vivo animal model of cardiac ischemia, a water-soluble extract of the leaves and flowers containing 3.31% oligomeric procyanidins (Dr. Willmar Schwabe GmbH and Co., Karlsruhe, Germany) showed a significant cardioprotective effect, without affecting aortic pressure and heart rate. The extract significantly accelerated reperfusion-induced recovery of the energy metabolism and inhibited ischemia-induced accumulation of lactate. The research indicated that although the extract protected the myocardium from reperfusion- and ischemia-induced damage of the heart, the effect was weak when compared with calcium channel blockers and β-adrenoreceptor antagonists (Nasa et al., 1993).

Flavonoids in hawthorn are thought to inhibit cellular phosphodiesterase and increase cellular concentrations of cAMP, which may account for some of the cardiotonic properties of the botanical (Schüssler et al., 1991). The inhibition of thromboxane A_2 (TXA_2) may also play a significant role in the cardiological effects of hawthorn. In an in vitro study, a hydroalcoholic extract of the dried flower heads *(C. oxycantha)* inhibited the biosynthesis of TXA_2 (ID_{30} 0.88 mg/mL^{-1}). The most active constituents of the hawthorn extract in the assay were (–)-epicatechin, (+)-catechin, and quercetin dihydrate (each 0.05 mg/mL^{-1}), while at higher concentrations (0.1 and 0.2 mg/mL^{-1}) hyperoside, vitexin-2"-O-rhamnoside, and vitexin were also active (Vibes et al., 1994).

In an in vitro study, a hawthorn extract containing greater than 2% hyperoside and 5.1% procyanidins (Emil Flaschman AG, Germany, batch no. 30364.01) and a procyanidin-rich fraction (flavonoid free) derived from the extract caused a significant endothelium-dependent relaxing effect on isolated rat aortic rings contracted with phenylephrine. In each case the effect was concentration dependent; the procyanidin fraction produced 18-fold greater activity, and no effect was found in the aorta without endothelium. Flavonoid constituents of hawthorn (i.e., vitexin, rutin, and hyperoside) were inactive. The maximally effective doses of the extract and the procyanidins (10^{-4} and 10^{-5} g/mL, respectively) also caused a significant 3.2- and 4.2-fold increase in the contents of cGMP, respectively; again, only in endothelium-intact aorta. The results of further tests suggested that nitric oxide (NO) production in the vascular endothelium was increased by the procyanidin fraction, an effect that appears to involve activation of tetra-ethylammonium-sensitive K+ channels (Kim et al., 2000). However, others have shown that a proprietary extract of the leaves with flowers (WS 1442, standardized to contain 18.7% oligomeric procyanidins and containing the flavonoids hyperoside, rhamnoside, rutin, vitexin, and others) has no effect on cAMP; yet it was shown to produce an effect on the Na+/K+-ATPase of human cardiac muscle tissue similar to that of digitalis (Schwinger et al., 2000).

The inotropic action of hawthorn extracts was investigated on isolated human myocardium (right auricular trabeculae) taken from patients with coronary heart disease who did not experience heart failure (nonfailing controls), from patients with congestive heart failure (left ventricular myocardium, New York Heart Association [NYHA] stage IV), and on left ventricular papillary muscle strips from terminal heart failure (heart transplant) patients. The hawthorn extracts tested were a special dry extract of the leaves with flowers (WS 1442, an active substance derived from Crataegutt 450, Dr. Willmar Schwabe, Karlsruhe, Germany) and three fractions derived from it, named fraction A, a flavone-enriched fraction, and B and C, which the researchers leave uncharacterized. In membranes of failing myocardium, no evidence of interaction with the adenylate cyclase system was found from the three fractions; however, fractions A and B and WS 1442 showed evidence of a significant concentration-dependent influence on sacrolemmal Na+/K+-ATPase. Fraction A (EC_{50} 51 µg/mL) was about twice as potent as either fraction B or WS 1442. In left ventricular papillary muscle strips from terminal heart failure patients, significant increases in force of contraction were found from fraction A and WS 1442 (+0.6 and +0.4 mN, respectively) at concentrations of 100 µg/mL, yet no inotropic effects were found from fractions B or C. The increases appeared to involve transient Ca^{2+} since in electrically driven right auricular trabeculae from coronary heart disease patients *without* heart failure, either WS 1442 or fraction A (each 50 µg/mL) produced a significant increase in force of contraction while they significantly increased the intracellular Ca^{2+} transient. The same effect was found from ouabain, a cardiac glycoside; however, fraction B was inactive. An unexpected finding was that like fraction A and WS 1442 (+0.7 and +0.9 mN, respectively), fraction B also increased force-frequency in left ventricular myocardium from patients with congestive heart failure (+ 0.5 mN), although at the same concentration (100 µg/mL) fraction C was inactive. The researchers concluded that the actions of WS 1442 appear to be similar to those of cardiac glycosides with a cAMP-independent positive inotropic action (Schwinger et al., 2000).

A standardized hawthorn extract (Crataegutt) orally administered to nonanesthetized dogs on a regular basis (1.5-9 g/day) resulted in a significant, dose-dependent increase in local left ventricular blood flow (Mavers and Hensel, 1974). Ventricular muscle fiber preparations from rabbits fed a diet containing a standardized hawthorn extract (Crataegutt, 5 mg/100 g feed for six weeks) showed a significantly smaller decrease in membrane potential and amplitude of action potential resulting from hypoxic conditions compared to control tissue from rabbits fed unsupplemented feed (Kanno et al., 1976).

Clinical studies have supported the activity of hawthorn in this regard, and researchers suggest that hawthorn possesses a mechanism distinct from that of other cardiac remedies. For example, unlike digitalis, which affects contractile fibers, hawthorn improves the utilization of oxygen and energy by the heart, resulting in improved heart function. These actions may help to explain the purported ability of hawthorn to stem age-induced changes in the myocardium (Hoffman, 1995; Murray, 1995).

Cholesterol and Lipid Metabolism

An aqueous-alcoholic tincture prepared from the pulp of ripe hawthorn berries *(C. oxycantha)* administered to rats (5 mL/kg p.o. for six weeks) along with a hyperlipidemic diet was reported to cause a significant decrease in aortic and hepatic deposits of fats and significantly lower levels of VLDL, LDL, phospholipids, and triglycerides while improving atherogenic ratio (Shanthi et al., 1994).

Hypertension

Hawthorn lowers blood pressure by effecting a number of changes in cardiovascular function. It dilates coronary vessels, increases the ability of the heart to function, and inhibits angiotensin-converting enzyme (ACE). Studies have established a direct relationship between the amount of procyanidins in extracts of hawthorn and the hypotensive (and beta-blocking) effects of the extract. In vivo studies have also shown that hawthorn acts dose dependently in decreasing systolic, diastolic, and mean blood pressure (Djumlija, 1994).

In an in vitro assay of angiotensin-converting enzyme (ACE)-inhibiting activity, a methanolic extract of the leaves and flowers of *C. monogyna/ C.oxycantha* (Lichtwer, Berlin, Germany, batch 461457) showed significant though moderate activity, inhibiting ACE by about 33% at a concentration of 0.33 mg/mL. About 11% of the extract consisted of a mixture of oligomeric procyanidins. Individual procyanidins (procyanidins B_2 and C_1) as well as flavonoids derived from hawthorn, vitexin, isovitexin, and (–)-epicatechin also exhibited significant ACE-inhibitory activity in the ranges of 21% to 46%. The most active were isovitexin and procyanidin C_1, which inhibited ACE by 46% and 45%, respectively (Lacaille-Duboise et al., 2001).

Digestive, Hepatic, and Gastrointestinal Functions

Gastric Functions

Hawthorn's gastrointestinal activities are as yet scarcely understood. Studies thus far have shown that the fruit contains lipase, which promotes lipolysis, along with crataegolic acid, a substance thought to improve the activity of proteolytic enzymes, thereby improving digestion (Wicke, 1994; Hobbs and Foster, 1990).

Immune Functions; Inflammation and Disease

Cancer

Cytotoxicity. Corosolic acid was identified in the fruits of *Crataegus pinnatifida* var. pilosa as a potent inhibitor of protein kinase C (PKC). This activity may be related to its cytotoxic action against the in vitro growth of various human tumor cell lines (A549, HeLa S$_3$, K-562, and SNU-C$_4$) (ED$_{50}$ 0.4-5.0 µg/mL). Ursolic acid derived from the fruits also showed activity against the tumor cell lines (ED$_{50}$ 1.4-12.5 µg/mL) but was much less potent as a PKC inhibitor than corosolic acid, which decreased PKC activity by 95% at a concentration of 0.1 µg/mL (versus a decrease of 43% from ursolic acid at 50 µg/mL) (Ahn et al., 1998). Corosolic acid (2α-hydroxyursolic acid) has also shown potent glucose transport-inhibitory activity in Ehrlich ascites tumor cells (Murakami et al., 1993).

Inflammatory Response

In a screening study of plants to detect inhibitory activity against adenosine 5'-diphosphate-induced platelet aggregation, Rogers et al. (2000) reported that a methanolic extract of *C. monogyna* fruit showed significant activity ($p < 0.01$), inhibiting ACE by about 25%. The resulting release of 5-HT in this assay was also inhibited by the hawthorn berry extract, by about 75% ($p < 0.01$). The researchers' use of this assay, which was previously used to test feverfew, was to screen plants for potential antimigraine activity, a traditional use for hawthorn berries in Australia. When they removed protein-precipitating polyphenolic tannins from the extract by adding PVP (polyvinyl pyrrolidone), the resulting extract still showed activity, inhibiting the release of [14C]5-HT by about 85%—an effect apparently not due to tannins.

Ahumada et al. (1997) reported a weak in vitro inhibitory activity of the triterpene fraction of the freshly collected leaves, stems, and twigs *(C. monogyna)* against phospholipase A$_2$. This fraction contained a high content of cycloartenol (80% to 87%). A significant 34.12% inhibition ($p < 0.05$) of snake *(Naja naja)* venom phospholipase A$_2$ was found only from a relatively high concentration of the triterpene fraction (10.65 μg) compared to mepacrine (1.8 μg). The triterpene fraction was also tested in rats with carrageenan-induced hind-paw edema. At 3 h after the induced inflammation, relatively high concentrations of the triterpene fraction (100, 200, and 400 mg/kg p.o.) caused a significant anti-inflammatory effect (ED_{50} 244.5 mg/kg; $p < 0.05$). However, at 5 h only 400 mg/kg p.o. produced a significant degree of anti-inflammatory activity (ED_{50} 351 mg/kg p.o.; $p < 0.01$). On the ability of the triterpene fraction to inhibit the aggregation of leukocytes during carrageenan-induced inflammation in mice, the authors compared the activity to that of indomethicin and prednisolone (each at 100 mg/kg p.o.). The triterpene fraction caused a significant and dose-dependent inhibition of leukocyte infiltration (ED_{50} 146.1 ± 32 mg/kg p.o.). The lowest dose (100 mg/kg p.o.) was significantly more effective than indomethicin ($p < 0.01$). From twice the dose, the result was highly significant (64.70%, $p < 0.001$) and comparable to that of prednisolone (Ahumada et al., 1997).

Metabolic and Nutritional Functions

Antioxidant Activity

A comparative study of antioxidant activities of flavonoid fractions from medicinal plants on lecithin liposomes showed hawthorn fruits were the least active among them. Concentrations required to inhibit oxidation by 50% (IC_{50}) were 60 μM for *Crataegus oxyacantha,* compared to 55 μM for grape seeds, 38 μM for Japanese quince, and 32 μM for rose hips (Gabrielska et al., 1997). Another group tested the total phenolic content of hawthorn flowers *(C. monogyna)* for antioxidant activity against reactive oxygen species hydrogen peroxide and hypochlorous acid. For the solvent extract of the flowers, the IC_{50} concentrations against hydrogen peroxide and hypochlorous acid were 12.88 ± 0.47 and 35.18 ± 0.34 mg/mL, respectively. The most active antioxidant constituents of the flower extract were shown from the flavonoid fraction and from proanthocyanidin B_2 (Rakotoarison et al., 1997).

In tests of a standardized extract of hawthorn (WS 1442), the flavone-free, oligomeric procyanidin-rich (OPC) fraction (21.3% of WS 1442) exhibited potent in vitro radical scavenging activity (lipid peroxidation inhibiting IC_{50} 0.3 μg/mL) and human neutrophil elastase inhibitory activity (IC_{50} 0.84 μg/mL). The extract itself was also active, whereas the flavone-rich fraction (14.9% of WS 1442) showed half the activity. Rats orally administered the OPC fraction (20 mg/kg per day) showed a similar degree of protection from ischemia-reperfusion-induced pathologies as those administered WS 1442 (100 mg/kg p.o. per day) (Chatterjee et al., 1997).

In a lipid peroxidation assay, freeze-dried methanolic extracts of hawthorn *(C. monogyna)* flowers, leaves, and fruits were compared for antioxidant activity when collected at different stages of maturity. Total phenolic content and antioxidant activity showed obvious correlation, with plant parts highest in phenols showing the greatest activity. The content of (–)-epicatechin and proanthocyanidins in the plant parts correlated with the highest rates of antioxidant activity, whereas little activity was found from aqueous extracts containing mostly chlorogenic acid, vitexin 2"-*O*-rhamnoside, or polymeric proanthocyanidins. Accordingly, malondialdehyde formation was most inhibited by the flower buds and leaves collected in May (91%) and less so by the young leaves with young flower buds, the mature leaves, or the green fruits (79%, 76%, and 75%, respectively). Coincidentally, both the same organs and that stage of maturity were those recommended for harvesting hawthorn in pharmacopoeial texts (Bahorun et al., 1994).

Mice fed a water extract of *C. pinnatifida* berries for 90 days at a concentration of 5 mg/mL showed significantly increased ($p < 0.01$) levels of SOD (superoxide dismutase) activity in their livers. The increase in SOD was 137% in females and 109% in the males. In addition, lipid peroxidation (according to changes in thiobarbituric acid reactive substance formation in livers) showed a significant decrease ($p < 0.05$) (Dai et al., 1987).

CLINICAL STUDIES

Clinical studies have focused primarily on the cardiotonic activities of hawthorn. In Europe, hawthorn extract (of the flowers and leaves) is widely regarded for its ability to potentiate the action of cardiac glycosides and is often used in combination with digitalis. Studies indicate that hawthorn is an effective cardioprotectant in the treatment of congestive heart failure and early stages of mild arrhythmias.

Cardiovascular and Circulatory Disorders

Cardiotonic; Cardioprotection

A 5:1 powder extract of the leaves and flowers standardized to contain 18.75% oligomeric procyanidins (Crataegus extract WS 1442, Willmar Schwabe Pharmaceuticals, Karlsruhe, Germany) was clinically tested to further confirm efficacy and safety in patients diagnosed with mild congestive heart failure corresponding to New York Heart Association class II (NYHA II). The computer-randomized, placebo-controlled double-blind study was conducted in 40 outpatients of either sex (29 women and 11 men ages 40-80) administered the extract in capsules or matching placebo (80 mg t.i.d.) for 12 weeks. Efficacy was measured according to impaired exercise tolerance using bicycle exercise (primary outcome variable) and the pressure-rated product (heart rate multiplied by systolic blood pressure multiplied by 10^{-2}) was employed as a secondary outcome variable. Concomitant medications were allowed if maintained at a constant dosage, except for other hawthorn preparations, angiotensin-converting enzyme (ACE) inhibitors, calcium antagonists, cardiac glycosides, or diuretics, which required a seven-day washout period before commencing treatment with placebo or the trial medication (WS 1442). Except for one patient in the placebo group who withdrew because of an allergic skin reaction, the rest of the patients completed the trial and gave no reports of adverse events. The results showed that exercise tolerance decreased in the placebo-treated group by more than 15%, whereas it increased in the hawthorn group by over 10%, a difference of borderline significance ($p = 0.06$). In the secondary outcome measure of the pressure-rated product, the difference failed to reach significance ($p = 0.11$). Laboratory tests revealed good tolerance to the extract with no significant changes during therapy compared to normal values in the following: ESR (erythrocyte sedimentation rate), serum glutamate pyruvate transaminase (= alanine transaminae) (SGPT), serum glutamic oxaloacetic transaminase (SGOT), gamma-glutamyltransferase (γ-GT), cholesterol, glucose, creatine, uric acid, urea, bilirubin, calcium chloride, potassium, sodium, thrombocytes, erythrocytes, hemoglobin, hematocrit, and leukocytes (Zapfe jun, 2001).

Holubarsch et al. (2000) reported on the progress made in the SPICE trial (Survival and Prognosis: Investigation of *Crataegus* Extract WS 1442 in CHF trial), a randomized, multicenter, double-blind, placebo-controlled international trial of WS 1442 underway in Europe in about 120 centers. The primary outcome variable is the time to first cardiac event in adult patients of either sex diagnosed with heart failure NYHA-II-III. Nine secondary outcome variables are being used to evaluate efficacy: safety is being evaluated according to laboratory values and adverse events. Eligible patients, all with reduced ventricular ejection fraction, are being treated with WS 1442 or placebo in addition to their regular treatments with conventional therapies for chronic heart failure (i.e., only ACE inhibitors, β-adrenoreceptor blockers, digitoxin or digoxin, and diuretics). The placebo is identical in appearance to the hawthorn extract, which is being taken in a high dosage: two film-coated tablets daily; each 450-mg tablet of WS 1442 containing a dry extract of *Crataegus* leaves with flowers (4 to 6.6:1 solvent; ethanol 45%) standardized to contain 84.3 mg oligomeric procyanidins. After a 28-day placebo run-in phase, male and female patients meeting eligibility for entry are being followed for up to two years. Presently, over 1,600 patients are participating in the trial. Results are expected sometime in the year 2002.

Prior to the SPICE trial, Tauchert et al. (1999) conducted a multicenter utilization observational study in which they monitored 1,011 cardiac patients (cardiac insufficiency stage NYHA II) who were treated with WS 1442 (Crataegutt novo 450, one 450-mg tablet b.i.d.) for 24 weeks. In short, after the 24 weeks, nearly 66% of patients reported that they felt better or much improved; nocturia and ankle edema were reduced by 83% in half of the patients; cardiac performance was improved, as shown in reduced BP, the difference in pressure/heart rate product, and increased maximal exercise tolerance. Fewer patients showed arrhythmias, ST depressions, and, at their maximum exercise levels, ventricular extrasystoles, indicating an improvement in myocardial perfusion. Other beneficial changes were noted in improved ejection fraction, slower rest pulse, and greater numbers of days and nights in which patients were normorhythmic. Over 75% of physicians rated the efficacy of the treatment as good or very good and over 98% rated the tolerance to treatment in the patients as good or very good.

Tauchert et al. (1994) conducted a multicenter, double-blind comparative study of a hawthorn extract (LI 132, Faros 300, Lichtwer Pharma GmbH, Germany; 300 mg p.o. t.i.d.) in 132 patients diagnosed NYHA stage II stable heart failure. Captopril (12.5 mg p.o. t.i.d.) served as the compared drug and both treatments were administered for eight weeks with a run-in period of seven days. The main confirmatory measure was exercise tolerance on a stationary bicycle on days 7, 28, and 56. Secondary criteria consisted of patient scores for five symptoms typical of NYHA II stable heart failure, as well as the pressure-rated product (heart rate multiplied by systolic blood pressure multiplied by 10^{-2}). The patients consisted of 53 men and 79 women ages 56-68. Over the course of the treatment period, the hawthorn group showed a significant increase in exercise tolerance (from 83 to 97 watts), a decrease in the pressure rated product, and a decrease in the severity and frequency of symptoms (of about 50%). The same results were found in the Captopril group, with exercise tolerance increasing significantly from 83 to 99 watts. No side effects of a serious nature were found in the hawthorn group, and only one patient in the Captopril group discontinued therapy owing to adverse effects. The authors also reported not a single significant difference when they compared the treatment groups for the target parameters.

Schmidt et al. (1994) studied the effect of a hawthorn extract (LI 132) in patients diagnosed with chronic heart failure of the NYHA functional class II. Seventy-eight patients received either a hawthorn extract (600 mg/day) or placebo. Treatment occurred over eight weeks with a washout phase of one week. The parameters used to assess the efficacy of the hawthorn extract were derived from changes in patient working capacity on an ergometer bicycle. Between days 0 and 56, the working capacity of those taking LI 132 increased by 28 watt (median), whereas for the placebo group the median increase was only 5 watt. Therefore, those taking the hawthorn extract exhibited a statistically significant ($p < 0.001$) increase in working capacity.

There were also significant decreases in systolic blood pressure, heart rate, and pressure rate product in the hawthorn group.

Förster et al. (1994) conducted a randomized, placebo-controlled, double-blind clinical trial of a hawthorn extract (LI 132, Faros 300, Lichtwer Pharma GmbH, Germany; 300 mg p.o. t.i.d.) in 69 patients (39 women and 30 men ages 40-62) diagnosed with moderately reduced left ventricular ejection fraction. The patients were monitored for changes in ergospirometric values using oxygen uptake, tolerance period to reach the anaerobic threshold, and the time to reach discontinuation of exercise to confirm the changes. After a treatment period of eight weeks, the group administered the hawthorn extract showed an extended mean time to reach their anaerobic threshold of 30 s compared to a mean prolongation time of 2 s in the placebo group ($p < 0.05$). No side effects were attributed to the active treatment and Förster and colleagues found significant ($p < 0.01$) improvements in the subjective state of the patients taking the hawthorn extract.

In a randomized double-blind study, Leuchtgens (1993) administered an extract of hawthorn standardized to contain 15 mg procyanidin oligomers per 80 mg capsule (WS 1442, or Crataegutt forte). Thirty patients diagnosed with NYHA functional class II cardiac insufficiency were given capsules of the extract b.i.d. for eight weeks. The main parameters were alteration in the pressure-times-rate product on a bicycle ergometer and a subjective assessment of improvement through a questionnaire. The secondary parameters were exercise tolerance, change in heart rate, and arterial blood pressure. Compared to placebo, the group receiving the hawthorn extract exhibited a statistically significant increase in performance in primary and secondary parameters with no adverse reactions.

In a small, randomized placebo-controlled study, 18 volunteers (mean age 35) received either sugar-coated pills of a hawthorn extract (CRAT, Kneipp Planzen-Dragees Weissdorn, t.i.d. for four weeks) or placebo. Although no differences were found in resting cardiovascular rates, the sum of the exercise (upright cycle ergometry) rate-pressure indices were significantly decreased in the group administered the hawthorn extract (Hellenbrecht et al., 1990).

A standardized extract of hawthorn (Crataegutt, 3 mg procyanidin oligomers per 60 mg capsule; t.i.d. for six weeks) was administered to 36 elderly multimorbid patients (ages 62-84) suffering from decreased cardiac performance (NYHA stages I and II) in a placebo-controlled, double-blind crossover study. Exercise tolerance, pressure heart rate product, physician ratings, and psychological parameters were used to measure the results. The extract caused a highly significant improvement in cardiac function. The early termination of exercise sessions decreased in the hawthorn group, and the heart rate during and after exercise showed a significant improvement versus the placebo group. In addition, the patients all reported an increased sense of well-being (O'Conolly et al., 1986).

In a double-blind study, 46 patients with angina pectoris were treated with either *Crataegus pinnatifida* leaves or placebo. The antianginal effective rates were 84.8% for those administered hawthorn, and 37% for those given placebo ($p < 0.01$). Overall, the researchers assessed hawthorn as beneficial to the patients with angina pectoris (Weng et al., 1984).

A placebo-controlled double-blind study in 80 patients with heart disease of ischemic and/or hypertensive origin in NYHA functional classes II and III was conducted to evaluate the efficacy of Crataegutt versus placebo. The group that received the hawthorn extract showed highly significant improvements in subjective symptoms, cardiac function, dyspnea, palpitations, and cardiac edemas. However, no difference was found in ECGs (Iwamoto et al., 1981).

Peripheral Vascular Disorders

Intermittent claudication. A hawthorn extract standardized to procyanidins appeared to exhibit similar benefits to those of procyanidolic oligomers derived from grape seed when tested in 20 patients with intermittent claudication. Injection of the extract improved blood flow and walking distance in all of the patients (Werbach and Murray, 1994).

DOSAGE

Clinical studies have varied in the source of the hawthorn (leaf with flower) powder extract used but have been roughly equivalent in dosage to a flower and leaf extract standardized to 1.8% vitexin-4'-rhamnoside, or 20% procyanidins (Murray, 1995). According to the German Commission E, the recommended dosage for a water-ethanol extract of the leaf with flower is 160-900 mg/day, provided that the extract contains 30-168.7 mg procyanidins or 3.5-19.8 mg flavonoids (Blumenthal et al., 1998). Since the Commission E recommended dosage range was written in 1994, however, Schulz et al. (2001) point out that clinically effective dosages have been in the range of 600-900 mg/day. According to the *British Herbal Pharmacopoeia,* the dosage of the dried fruit is 0.3-1.0 g t.i.d. which may be supplied by an infusion. For a 1:5 tincture in 45% alcohol of the fruit, the dosage given is 1-2 mL t.i.d., and for a 1:1 liquid extract in 25% alcohol the dosage given is 0.5-1.0 mL t.i.d. (Newall et al., 1996).

SAFETY PROFILE

Clinical trials have reported no adverse reactions from long-term use of hawthorn (Weiss, 1988); adverse events have occurred only rarely in clinical trials.

Contraindications

See Pregnancy and Lactation.

Drug Interactions

Animal studies suggest that hawthorn may potentiate the action of digitalis, other cardiotonic drugs (e.g., digitoxin, digoxin), and medicinal plants containing cardiac glycosides (e.g., *Digitalis lantana, D. purpurea, Adonis vernalis*) (Semm, 1952; Hahn et al., 1960; Trunzler and Schuler, 1962; Brinker, 1998).

Pregnancy and Lactation

The German Commission E monograph indicates no known contraindication during pregnancy or lactation (Blumenthal et al., 1998). The *American Herbal Products Association's Botanical Safety Handbook* lists no cautions specific to pregnancy or lactation (McGuffin et al., 1997). No cases of adverse effects during pregnancy or lactation are documented. Due to the fact that most women who would use hawthorn are well past the childbearing years, there has been little concern of the safety of hawthorn in pregnant or lactating patients (Hobbs and Foster, 1990). Whether the German Commission E's lack of safety concerns reflects this thinking is unknown. However, in reality, women of reproductive age do develop cardiac problems requiring medical intervention (American Academy of Pediatrics, 2001).

Side Effects

In a study of 3,664 NYHA stage I or II heart failure patients administered a standardized extract of hawthorn (Faros 300, 300 mg t.i.d.) by private practice physicians, a total of 72 adverse reactions were reported by 1.3% of the patients ($n = 48$). Among these were 24 complaints of gastrointestinal effects, which the physicians associated with the extract in seven cases. Other side effects reported by the patients were associated by the physicians in 3/10 reports of palpitations, 2/7 reports of headaches, and 2/7 reports of vertigo. In addition, physicians associated use of the extract in single reports of sleeplessness, apprehension, and circulatory problems (Schulz et al., 2001).

Special Precautions

Individuals taking beta-blockers to lower blood pressure are cautioned that hawthorn may cause a slight rise in blood pressure (Weiss, 1988). See previous section on Drug Interactions.

Toxicology

In Vitro Toxicity

In an in vitro cytogenetic test system using cultured human lymphocytes, a hydroalcoholic extract of hawthorn blossoms and leaves (WS 1442, Dr. Willmar Schwabe, Karlsruhe, Germany), standardized to contain 18.75% oligomeric procyanidins, showed no evidence of clastogenic activity (with or without S9 mix) (Schlegelmilch and Heywood, 1994).

Mutagenicity

In the mouse micronucleus assay, a hydroalcoholic extract of hawthorn blossoms and leaves (WS 1442, Dr. Willmar Schwabe, Karlsruhe, Germany), standardized to contain 18.75% oligomeric procyanidins, showed no evidence of mutagenicity or toxicity in the bone marrow of male or female mice (CD-1) that were administered the extract orally (5 g/kg). The same extract showed no mutagenicity in the Ames test. In a gene mutation assay (the mouse lymphoma test), the extract failed to show any mutagenic potential (Schlegelmilch and Heywood, 1994).

Toxicity in Animal Models

The oral LD_{50} of hawthorn was found to be 18.5 mL/kg in mice administered a standardized liquid extract (Ammon and Handel, 1981). A commercial hydroalcoholic extract of hawthorn blossoms and leaves (WS 1442, Dr. Willmar Schwabe, Karlsruhe, Germany), standardized to contain 18.75% oligomeric procyanidins, failed to cause any deaths in male and female mice (NMRI) or rats (Sprague-Dawley, CD strain) at an acute dosage of 3 g/kg p.o., or about 1,000 times the human oral dose (2.7 mg/kg per day). By the intraperitoneal route, the extract produced dyspnea, sedation, tremor, and piloerection in both types of animals, and an LD_{50} of 750 mg/kg i.p. in the rat and of 1,170 mg/kg i.p. in the mouse (Schlegelmilch and Heywood, 1994).

Oral administration of the extract in rats at dosages of 30, 90, and 300 mg/kg (100 times the human dose) for 26 weeks caused only a slight decrease in body weight in the males at the higher dosages; no other organ system was affected. At the same dosage in beagle dogs administered the extract in capsules, no specific organ toxicity was found. From the highest dose (300 mg/kg per day p.o.), at week 26 the males showed a slight increase in blood glucose and a significant decrease in absolute spleen weights ($p < 0.10$) compared to control; however, no morphological change was evident in their spleens and no explanation could be found for the difference. In the females, creatine levels showed a slight though insignificant elevation at week 13, also from the highest dose (Schlegelmilch and Heywood, 1994).

REFERENCES

Ahn, K.S., Hahm, M.S., Park, E.J., Lee, H.K., and Kim, I.H. (1998). Corosolic acid isolated from the fruit of *Crataegus pinnatifida* var. *pilosa* is a protein kinase C inhibitor as well as a cytotoxic agent. *Planta Medica* 64: 468-470.

Ahumada, C., Sáenz, T., Garcia, D., De La Puerta, R., Fernandez, A., and Martinez, E. (1997). The effects of a triterpene fraction isolated from *Crataegus monogyna* Jacq. on different acute inflammation models in rats and mice. Leucocyte migration and phospholipase A_2 inhibition. *Journal of Pharmacy and Pharmacology* 49: 329-331.

American Academy of Pediatrics Committee on Drugs (2001). The transfer of drugs and other chemicals into human milk. *Pediatrics* 108:776-789.

Ammon, H.P.T. and Handel, M. (1981). *Crataegus,* toxicology and pharmacology. *Planta Medica* 43: Part I, 105-120; Part II, 209-239; Part III, 313-322.

Bahorun, T., Trotin, F., Pommery, J., Vasseur, J., and Pinkas, M. (1994). Antioxidant activities of *Crataegus monogyna* extracts. *Planta Medica* 60: 490-498.

Blumenthal, M., Busse, W.R., Goldberg, A., Gruenwald, J., Hall, T., Riggins, C.W., and Rister, R.S. (Eds.) (1998). *The Complete German Commission E Monographs* (pp. 142-144). Austin, TX: American Botanical Council.

Brinker, F. (1998). *Herb Contraindications and Drug Interactions,* Second Edition (pp. 82-83). Sandy, OR: Eclectic Medical Publications.

Chatterjee, S.S., Koch, E., Jaggy, H., and Krzeminski, T. (1997). [In vitro and in vivo investigations on the cardioprotective effects of oligomeric procyanidins in a *Crataegus* extract from leaves with flowers]. *Arzneimittel-Forschung/Drug Research* 79: 821-825.

Dai, Y.R., Gao, C.M., Tian, Q.L., and Yin, Y. (1987). Effect of extracts of some medicinal plants on superoxide dismutase activity in mice. *Planta Medica* 53: 309-310.

Djumlija, L.C. (1994). Medicinal plant review: *Crataegus oxyacantha. Australian Journal of Medical Herbalism* 6: 37-42.

Ficarra, P., Ficarra, R., de Pasquale, A., Monforte, M.T., and Calabro, M.L. (1990). High performance liquid chromatography of flavonoids in *Crataegus oxyacantha* L. IV. Reversed-phase high-pressure liquid chromatography in flower, leaf and bud extractives of *Crataegus oxyacantha* L. *Il Farmaco* 45: 247-255.

Förster, A., Förster, K., Bühring, M., and Wolfstadter, H.D. (1994). *Crataegus* bei maßig reduzierter linksventrikulärer auswurffraktion—Ergospirometrische verlaufsuntersuchung bei 72 patienten in doppelblinden vergleich mit plazebo [*Crataegus* for moderately reduced left ventricular ejection fraction—Ergospirometric monitoring study with 72 patients in a double-blind comparison with placebo]. *Munchener Medizinische Wochenschrift* 136 (Suppl. 1): S21-S26.

Gabrielska, J., Oszmianski, J., and Lamer-Zarawska, E. (1997). Protective effect of plant flavonoids on the oxidation of lecithin liposomes. *Pharmazie* 52: 170-171.

Hahn, F., Klinkhammer, F., and Oberdorf, A. (1960). [Preparation and pharmacological investigation of a new therapeutic agent obtained from *Crataegus oxycantha*]. *Arzneimittel Forschung/Drug Research* 10: 825-829.

Hellenbrecht, D., Saller, R., Ruckbeil, C., and Buhrinhg, M. (1990). Randomized placebo-controlled study with *Crataegus* on exercise tests and challenge by catecholamines in healthy subjects. *European Journal of Pharmacology* 183: 525-526 (poster).

Hobbs, C. and Foster, S. (1990). Hawthorn: A literature review. *HerbalGram* 22: 19-33.

Hoffmann, D. (1995). Hawthorn: The heart helper. *Alternative and Complementary Therapies* (April/May): 191-192.

Holubarsch, C.J., Colucci, W.S., Meinertz, T., Gaus, W., and Tendera, M. (2000). Survival and prognosis: Investigation of *Crataegus* extract WS 1442 in congestive heart failure (SPICE)—Rationale, study design and study protocol. *European Journal of Heart Failure* 2: 431-437.

Iwamoto, M., Ishizaki, T., and Sato, T. (1981). Klinische wirkung von Crataegutt® bei herzerkrankungen ischamischer und/oder hypertensiver genese: Ein multizentrische doppelblindstudie [The clinical effect of Crataegutt® in heart disease of ischemic or hypertensive origin: A multicenter double-blind study]. *Planta Medica* 42: 1-16.

Kanno, T., Suga, T., and Yamamoto, M. (1976). Reduction of the hypoxia-induced depression in the intracellular electrical activity of the ventricular muscle fibers of the rabbit fed on food containing Crataegutt®. *Japanese Heart Journal* 17: 512-520.

Kim, S.H., Kang, K.W., Kim, K.W., and Kim, N.D. (2000). Procyanidins in *Crataegus* extract evoke endothelium-dependent vasorelaxation in rat aorta. *Life Sciences* 67: 121-131.

Lacaille-Dubopis, M.A., Franck, U., and Wagner, H. (2001). Search for potential angiotensin converting enzyme (ACE)-inhibitors from plants. *Phytomedicine* 8: 47-52.

Leuchtgens, H. (1993). *Crataegus* special extract WS 1442 in NYHA II heart failure. A placebo controlled randomized double-blind study. *Forschritte den Medizin* 111: 352-354.

Mavers, W.H. and Hensel, H. (1974). Veranderungen der lokalen myokarddurchblutung nach oraler gabe eines Crataegusextraktes bei nichtnarkotisierten hunden [Changes in local myocardial blood flow following oral administration of a *Crataegus* extract to non-anesthetized dogs]. *Arzneimittel Forschung/Drug Research* 24: 783-785.

Moerman, D.E. (1998). *Native American Ethnobotany* (pp. 183-184). Portland, OR: Timber Press, Inc.

Murakami, C., Myoga, K., Kasai, R., Ohtani, K., Kurokawa, T., Ishibashi, S., Dayrit, F., Padolina, W.G., and Yamasaki, K. (1993). Screening of plant constituents for effect on glucose transport activity in Ehrlich ascites tumor cells. *Chemical and Pharmaceutical Bulletin* 41: 2129-2131.

Murray, M. (1995). *The Healing Power of Herbs*. Rocklin, CA: Prima Publishing.

Nasa, Y., Hashizume, H., Ehsanul Hoque, A.N., and Abiko, Y. (1993). Protective effect of Crataegus extract on the cardiac mechanical dysfunction in isolated perfused working rat heart. *Arzneimittel Forschung/Drug Research* 43: 945-949.

Newall, C.A., Anderson, L.A., and Phillipson, J.D. (1996). *Herbal Medicines: A Guide for Health Care Professionals* (pp. 157-159). London, England: Pharmaceutical Press.

O'Conolly, M., Jansen, W., Bernhöft, G., and Bartsch, G. (1986). Behandlung der nachlassenden herzleistung. Therapie mit standardisiertem Crataegus-extrakt im höheren lebensalter [Treatment of decreasing cardia performance (NYHA stages I to II) in advanced age with standardized Crataegus extract]. *Fortschritte der Therapie* 104:805-808.

Rajendran, S., Deepalakshmi, P.D., Parasakthy, K., Devaraj, H., and Devaraj, S.N. (1996). Effect of tincture of *Crataegus* on the LDL-receptor activity of hepatic plasma membrane of rats fed an atherogenic diet. *Atherosclerosis* 123: 235-241.

Rakotoarison, D.A., Gressier, B., Trotin, F., Brunet, C., Dine, T., Luyckx, M., Vasseur, J., Cazin, M., Cazin, J.C., and Pinkas, M. (1997). Antioxidant activities of polyphenolic extracts from flowers, in vitro callus and cell suspension cultures of *Crataegus monogyna*. *Pharmazie* 52: 60-64.

Rogers, K.L., Grice, I.D., and Griffiths, L.R. (2000). Inhibition of platelet aggregation and 5-HT release by extracts of Australian plants used traditionally as headache treatments. *European Journal of Pharmaceutical Sciences* 9: 355-363.

Schlegelmilch, R. and Heywood, R. (1994). Toxicity of *Crataegus* (hawthorn) extract (WS 1442). *Journal of the American College of Toxicology* 13: 103-111.

Schmidt, U., Kuhn, U., Ploch, M., and Hubner, W.D. (1994). Efficacy of the hawthorn *(Crataegus)* preparation LI 132 in 78 patients with chronic congestive heart failure defined as NYHA functional class II. *Phytomedicine* 1: 17-24.

Schulz, V., Hänsel, R., and Tyler, V.E. (2001). *Rational Phytotherapy. A Physician's Guide to Herbal Medicine*, Fourth Edition (pp. 117-118). New York, NY: Springer-Verlag.

Schüssler, M., Fricke, U., Nikolov, N., and Holzl, J. (1991). Comparison of the flavonoids occurring in *Crataegus* species and inhibition of 3',5'-cyclic adenosine monophosphate phosphodiesterase. *Planta Medica* 57 (Suppl. 2): A133 (poster).

Schwinger, R.H.G., Pietsch, M., Frank, K., and Brixius, K. (2000). *Crataegus* special extract WS 1442 increases force of contraction in human myocardium cAMP-independently. *Journal of Cardiovascular Pharmacology* 35: 700-707.

Semm, K. (1952). [The action of *Crataegus* alone and in combination with *Digitalis purpurea, Digitalis lanata, Adonis vernalis,* and *Convallaria majalis* upon the heart of the guinea pig]. *Arzneimittel Forschung/Drug Research* 2: 562-567.

Shanthi, S., Parasakthy, K., Deepalakshmi, P.D., and Devaraj, S.N. (1994). Hypolipidemic activity of tincture of *Crataegus* in rats. *Indian Journal of Biochemistry and Biophysics* 31: 143-146.

Tauchert, M., Ploch, M., and Hübner, W.D. (1994). Wirksamkeit des weiß-dornextraktes LI 132 im vergleich mit Captopril: Multizentrische doppelblindstudie bei 132 patienten mit herzinsuffizienz im stadium II nach NYHA [Effectiveness of the hawthorn extract LI 132 compared with the ACE inhibitor Captopril: Multicenter double-blind study with 132 NYHA stage II heart failure patients]. *Munchener Medizinische Wochenschrift* 136(Suppl. 1): S27-S33.

Tauchert, R., Gildor, A., and Lipinski, J. (1999). High-dose *Crataegus* (hawthorn) extract WS 1442 for the treatment of NYHA class II heart failure patients. *Herz* 24: 465-474.

Trunzler, V.G. and Schuler, E. (1962). Vergleichende studien über wirkung eines *Crataegus*-extraktes, ven digitoxin, digoxin und δ–strophanthin am isolierten warmbluterherzen [Comparative studies on the effects of a *Cataegus* extract, digitoxin, digoxin and δ–strophanthin in isolated warm blooded hearts]. *Arzneimittel Forschung/Drug Research* 12: 198.

Tu, G., Fang, Q., Guo, J., Yuan, S., Chen, C., Chen, J., Chen, Z., Cheng, S., Jin, R., Li, M., et al. (Eds.) (1992). *Pharmacopoeia of the People's Republic of China,* English Edition (p. 69). Guangzhou, China: Guangdong Science and Technology Press.

Vibes, J., Lasserre, B., Gleye, J., and Declume, C. (1994). Inhibition of thromboxane A_2 biosynthesis in vitro by the main components of *Crataegus oxyacantha* (hawthorn) flower heads. *Prostaglandins, Leukotrienes and Essential Fatty Acids* 50: 173-175.

Weng, W.L., Zhang, W.Q., Liu, F.Z., Yu, X.C., Zhang, P.W., Liu, Y.N., Chi, H.C., Yin, G.X., and Huang, M.B. (1984). Therapeutic effect of *Crataegus pinnatifida* on 46 cases of angina pectoris—A double-blind study. *Journal of Traditional Chinese Medicine* 4: 293-294.

Weiss, R.F. (1988). *Herbal Medicine.* Beaconsfield, England: Beaconsfield Publishers.

Werbach, M.R. and Murray, M.T. (1994). *Botanical Influences on Illness: A Sourcebook of Clinical Research.* Tarzana, CA: Third Line Press.

Wicke, R.W. (1994). *Traditional Chinese Herbal Science: Herbs, Strategies, and Case Studies.* Hot Springs, MT: Rocky Mountain Herbal Institute.

Yao, D., Zhang, J., Chou, L., Bao, X., Shun, Q., and Qi, P. (Eds.) (1996). *A Coloured Atlas of the Chinese Materia Medica Specified in Pharmacopoeia of the People's Republic of China* (p. 34). Hong Kong: Joint Publishing (H.K.) Co., Ltd.

Zapfe jun, G. (2001). Clinical efficacy of Crataegus extract WS 1442 in congestive heart failure NYHA class II. *Phytomedicine* 8: 262-268.

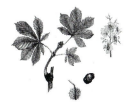

$\mathcal{H}orse\ \mathcal{C}hestnut$

BOTANICAL DATA

Classification and Nomenclature

Scientific name: *Aesculus hippocastanum* L.

Family name: Hippocastanaceae

Common names: horse chestnut, chestnut, robkastanie, marronier d'Inde (Dobelis, 1986)

Description

Horse chestnut *(Aesculus hippocastanum)* probably originated in the Himalayas or northern Persia from where the tree was imported to Europe by Turkish merchants in the 1500s (Bombardelli et al., 1996). Today, the tree grows throughout the United States, Europe, and in most countries worldwide. Horse chestnut is often found as an ornamental in parks, along boulevards, and in gardens. The fruits are tough and leathery, slightly larger than golf balls, and contain one to three seeds (nuts). Horse chestnut is a large deciduous tree that reaches a height of 39 m and is recognizable by its smooth gray bark which becomes scaly with age. The leaves are dark green above and light green below, born on long stalks in an opposite arrangement, with palmately compound leaflets up to 23 cm long. The showy yellow or red-spotted creamy-white flowers are born May through June on erect 20-38 cm terminal clusters resembling candelabras. The flowers are somewhat bilateral, sometimes staminate, with five sepals that are free or fused into a tube. The flowers have four to five petals and are unequal and clawed, with five to eight stamens and three ovary chambers (with generally two ovules per chamber). The prickly green seedpods are produced in autumn when they split open to release one to three large, shiny seeds (nuts) (Dobelis, 1986; Hickman, 1993; Bombardelli et al., 1996).

HISTORY AND TRADITIONAL USES

The name *hippocastanum* derives from the Greek words *castanon* for chestnut and *ippos* for horse. It is not clear whether the name became used from the similarity of the seeds to horse eyes or from use of the seeds to treat broken-winded horses. *Aesculus* is Latin for a type of oak having edible thorns, even though the thorns of horse chestnut are not edible (Bombardelli et al., 1996). Horse chestnut has many historical uses, for example, for the preparation of gunpowder, as an ornamental, and in manufacturing packing cases, furniture, and cutlery. Native Americans leached the mashed nuts for many days before using the meal to make breads. In addition, the powder of the seeds and branches served as a fish intoxicant. Medicinally, horse chestnut has been used to alleviate congestion, backache, and neuralgia and for the treatment of hemorrhoids (and other rectal complaints), arthritis, rheumatism (Duke, 1985; Werbach and Murray, 1994; Steele, 1995; Reynolds et al., 1996), sprains, sports injuries, and tendonitis. Horse chestnut extracts are used in Europe in topical preparations including cosmetics, hand creams, and lotions. Leaf preparations have been used to treat phlebitis, eczema, and varicose veins (D'Amelio, 1999; Reynolds et al., 1996).

CHEMISTRY

Terpenoid Compounds

The saponin escin (also aescin), which is a mixture of triterpene saponins, is the main pharmacological constituent of horse chestnut seeds, twigs, sprouts, and leaves (Mete Kockar et al., 1994). Escin has shown anti-inflammatory and antiedemic activities (Steele, 1995; Bruneton, 1995) and is used in numerous topical ointments and oral preparations as proprietary products designed for treatments of peripheral vascular diseases (Schulz et al., 2001). In high doses, various escin derivatives occurring in horse chestnut seed have shown hypoglycemic activity in glucose-loaded rats, but not in normal rats (Yoshikawa et al., 1998; Matsuda et al., 1998). The two primary glycosides in this mixture have aglycons that are derivatives of protoaescigenin acylated by acetic acid at the position of C-22 and by either angelic or tiglic acids at C-21 (Uberti et al., 1989). Escin exists in two essential forms as α-escin and β-escin, the later made up of over 30 components that derive from protoaescigenin and barringtogenol, occurring in the ratio 8:2 (Bombardelli et al., 1996). Higher contents of escin were found in the seeds of *A. indica* Colebr. (13.4%) than *A. hippocastanum* (9.5%), both growing in London, England (Srijayanta et al., 1999). However, escin usually constitutes up to 10% of the weight of the herbal drug (Uberti et al., 1990).

Other Constituents

A saponified extract of the seeds showed the presence of various fatty acids including arachidic, myristic, stearic oleic, and lauric acids. Palmitic acid was found in greatest quantity (Srijayanta et al., 1999). Horse chestnut seed oil contains 65-70% oleic acid. Other constituents include phenolic acids, coumarins, the coumarin derivative aesculin, hydrocarbons such as squalene and nonacosane, and cyclitols (Stankowic et al., 1987; Duke, 1985). Aesculin, extracted from the bark of horse chestnut, is used in preparations for the treatment of peripheral vascular diseases, hemorrhoids, cosmetics designed to ameliorate aging skin (Bombardelli et al., 1996), and in tanning preparations, in which the aglycone, esculetin, is also used (D'Amelio, 1999). Overall, the seeds contain 3% water, 3% ash, 11% crude protein, 5% oil, and 74% carbohydrates (Stankowic et al., 1987; Duke, 1985).

THERAPEUTIC APPLICATIONS

The primary therapeutic applications of horse chestnut are: (1) for the treatment of venous insufficiency; (2) for the treatment of inflammatory conditions; and (3) as an antiedemic. Horse chestnut is also indicated as a veinotonic and for reducing capillary permeability to minimize varicose veins (Werbach and Murray, 1994). The German Commission E monograph on horse chestnut refers to a standardized powder extract of the seeds containing 16-20 triterpene glycosides in the form of anhydrous escin. This extract is listed as appropriate for use in the treatment of "complaints found in pathological conditions of the veins of the legs (chronic venous insufficiency); for example, pains and a sensation of heaviness in the legs, nocturnal systremma (cramps in the calves), pruritus, and swelling of the legs" (Blumenthal et al., 1998, p. 149).

Another area of application for horse chestnut is in cosmetics or skin care products. Horse chestnut derivatives, such as escin, cholesterol-escin complex, and glycolic soft and dry horse chestnut extracts (HCEs), have been used in various cosmetic applications with formulations including antiedemic, astringent, and decongestive preparations (Proserpio et al., 1980). The seed extract in a concentration of 0.25%-0.5% has found use in hand creams, slimming products, and lotions and has been used in the treatment of hemorrhoids, strains, sports injuries, tendonitis, and cellulitis. Formulators have used the leaves for topical applications in swellings, varicose veins, eczema, and phlebitis, while the aglycone of esculin, esculetin, is an ingredient used in tanning formulations. Owing to UVB-absorbing activity, esculin has been employed in tanning preparations (D'Amelio, 1999).

PRECLINICAL STUDIES

Horse chestnut is used internally and topically to ameliorate venous insufficiency (congestive edema), inflammation, and the discomfort of hematomas. Researchers hold that saponins are the constituents responsible for the effectiveness of horse chestnut in these applications, although the mechanisms remain unclear. Owing to the presence of saponins in horse chestnut, it is thought to have significant cosmetic applications (Proserpio et al., 1980; Yamahara et al., 1979). Horse chestnut may prevent the enzymatic degradation of glycosaminoglycans, which would help to explain its efficacy in reducing capillary permeability (Proserpio et al., 1980).

Cardiovascular and Circulatory Functions

Peripheral Vascular Functions

Hyaluronic acid has been described as the major constituent of an extravascular matrix that envelopes capillary walls. The enzyme hyaluronidase degrades hyaluronic acid, leading to increased capillary permeability and subsequent loss of plasma from endothelial walls, which is a cause of edema typically found in venous insufficiency. Facino et al. (1995) reported that, tested in vitro, escin (300 μM) inhibited hyaluronidase activity by 93% and less from accordingly smaller doses. The IC_{50} was approximately 150 μM. Facino et al. considered this to be a weak inhibitory activity compared to the results produced by escin in animals, in which it caused remarkable antiexudative, veinotonic, and vasculotropic activities. They emphasized that greater concentrations of escin are able to penetrate the perivascular matrix in topical preparations used in vivo than those which inhibited hyaluronidase in vitro. The authors noted that topical applications involve much higher concentrations and formulation with topical vehicles which allow greater perivascular delivery (Facino et al., 1995).

Guillaume and Padioleau (1994) reported that an HCE (Veinotonyl 75, 70% escin) caused a dose-dependent contraction of isolated canine saphenous veins, an action that continued for over 5 h. The extract increased venous pressure of normal and pathological veins (stenosed eight days prior) and femoral venous flow pressure and thoracic lymphatic flow. Besides veinotonic activity, the extract showed evidence of vasculotropic activity by decreasing cutaneous capillary hyperpermeability and increasing vascular resistance in guinea pigs. In rats, the extract reduced experimental inflammation and edemas. The veinotonic activity of the extract was further demonstrated in vivo and in vitro with dogs and canine venous preparations. The results indicate that the extract (200-400 mg/kg, p.o.) possesses activities which act synergistically to affect venous and lymphatic insufficiencies, degradation of capillary and interstitial connective tissue, and some antioxidant activity.

Endocrine and Hormonal Functions

Hypothalamic and Pituitary Functions

Hiai et al. (1981) examined the effects of β-escin on adrenocortical function in rats. Because saponins from ginseng *(Panax ginseng)* have been found to stimulate the pituitary axis in rats, the study was designed to determine whether the saponin escin had any similar effects. Administered to rats, escin (5 mg/kg i.p.) caused a significant and dose-dependent increase in plasma corticosterone and glucose levels and a significant decrease in immunoreactive insulin levels. From oral administration (250 mg/kg), plasma glucose showed some increase and corticosterone showed a significant increase from 100 mg/kg p.o. and more so from the higher dose. These results were consistent with the idea that β-escin acted on the adrenal-pituitary axis to induce plasma adrenocorticotropin secretion, which induced corticosterone secretion. Escin has shown antiexudative and antigranulomatous activity, which might be explained by the induction of corticosterone secretion. Hiai et al. (1981) suggest that β-escin may also stimulate the release of epinephrine.

Immune Functions; Inflammation and Disease

Cancer

Antiproliferative activity. Tumor-inhibiting activity was found in vitro from sapogenols hippocaesculin and barringtogenol-C21-angelate, derived from a methanolic extract of horse chestnut seeds. Against human nasopharyngeal carcinoma 9-KB, the ED_{50} of hippocaesculin was 3.6 μg/mL, while that of barringtogenol-C21-angelate was 3.0 μg/mL (Konoshima and Lee, 1986).

Infectious Diseases

Viral infections. Escin inhibited the infectivity of influenza virus in vitro. At its estimated maximum tolerated concentration (12.5 μg/mL), escin inhibited influenza A_2 (Japan 305) by 92%. By comparison, the anti-influenza agent amantadine inhibited the same strain of influenza by 98% at a concentration of 25 mg/mL, 1/4 of its estimated maximum tolerated concentration (Rao and Cochran, 1974).

Inflammatory Response

A significant inhibition of acetic acid- and histamine-induced increased vascular permeability was shown by Matsuda et al. (1997) in rats administered from escins Ia, Ib, IIa, and IIb (50-200 mg/kg p.o.). Escins Ib, IIa, and IIb showed significant inhibitory activity against a serotonin-induced increase in vascular permeability (50-200 mg/kg p.o.), and caused a significant inhibition of compound 48/80-induced scratching behavior in mice. Escin Ia showed comparatively weaker activity in all these tests, although it is often referred to as the representative form of escin. In the carrageenan-induced edema test in rat hind paws, escin Ia (200 mg/kg p.o.) caused a significant inhibition of edema at hour one, but no inhibition from hours three through five. Escin Ib in the same dosage significantly inhibited the edema from hours one through five and escins IIa and IIb from hours one and two and less so from hours three through five. Based on their findings and a comparison of escin structures, Matsuda and colleagues were led to propose that structurally, 21- and 22-acyl groups in escins are essential for the various activities they found, and that the activities were more intensified from escins with a 21-angeloyl group than from a 21-tigoyl group.

CLINICAL STUDIES

Cardiovascular and Circulatory Disorders

Peripheral Vascular Disorders

Capillary edema. Horse chestnut seed extract (HCSE) is the most extensively prescribed oral treatment in Germany for venous edema (Schulz et al., 2001). The effects of horse chestnut on venous function in humans have been attributed to its ability to reduce vascular permeability and its effect on the hypothalamic-pituitary axis. It may also reduce the histamine response of inflammation. Past studies, referred to by Calabrese and Preston (1993), indicate that a 2% escin ointment penetrates the subcutis and muscle below. In one study, hematoma was induced in 70 volunteers by subcutaneous injection of the subjects' own blood. Tenderness was determined by a measure of pressure on the center of the hematoma at first indication of pain by the volunteer, and was taken by a calibrated tonometer. Thirty-four subjects were given escin and 36 placebo. After the hematoma induction and treatment, the active treatment group gave the first report of pain which was at a significantly higher mean-adjusted tonometric pressure than the placebo group for every time point. The differences in measured pain between the two groups remained significant even after the results were adjusted for variables of height, weight, age, and gender. These results indicated that the escin gel significantly reduced tenderness in the induced hematoma.

In a randomized double-blind, placebo-controlled crossover trial in 20 varicosis patients, Steiner (1990) tested a standardized HCE in the treatment of edema (Retardkapsel, Hersteller Klinge Pharmas, Munich, 10-60 mg dextrin plus 240-290 mg seed extract standardized to contain 50 mg escin/

300 mg capsule). Significant results compared to placebo ($p < 0.05$) were found from a dosage of one capsule b.i.d. for two weeks.

Marshall and Dormandy (1987) conducted a randomized double-blind controlled study of horse chestnut in 19 healthy subjects. After the subjects took a 15-h flight from Europe to Japan, edema of the ankle and foot was significantly less ($p < 0.05$) in those who had taken a HCE (300 mg b.i.d. for ten days) before embarking on the flight and until the flight landed, compared to subjects taking placebo. In the placebo group, no change was seen at 3 h of flight, but from 14 h a swelling of the ankles and heels of about 60 mL occurred. For those taking the extract, swelling was prevented completely. The extract (Venostasin retard) was standardized to contain 50 mg triterpene glycosides/300 mg capsule.

Rudofsky et al. (1986) reported a significant improvement in extravascular volume ($p < 0.001$) in 39 patients treated with HCE (300 mg Venostasin b.i.d. for 28 days) in a double-blind placebo-controlled trial with two parallel groups. Subjective complaints, such as itching, leg fatigue, pain, and feelings of tension also improved ($p < 0.05$); however, no improvement was found in venous capacity and drainage compared to placebo when measuring legs in an elevated position, and the circumference of ankles and calves showed no difference compared to placebo.

Bisler et al. (1986) assessed the effect of an encapsulated HCE (Venostasin) in 22 patients in a randomized, placebo-controlled, crossover double-blind trial. The extract was standardized to contain 50 mg escin/300 mg extract. A dose of 300 mg b.i.d. produced a significant inhibitory effect ($p < 0.001$) on edema formation via a decrease in transcapillary filtration of 22% after 3 h, which improved symptoms relating to edema in venous diseases of the legs. However, the reduction in intravascular volume of 5% from Venostasin compared to placebo was not significant.

In a placebo-controlled, double-blind crossover study in 95 patients treated with HCE (Venostasin, 300 mg b.i.d. for 20 days), Friederich et al. (1978) reported significant results compared to placebo in the amelioration of edema ($p < 0.05$), pain ($p < 0.01$), and spasms in the calves ($p < 0.01$).

Neiss and Böhm (1976) studied the effect of HCE (Venostasin, 300 mg b.i.d. for 20 days) in a placebo-controlled, double-blind crossover study in 887 patients. Significant benefits were found compared to placebo in edema, including reduction of pain (each $p < 0.01$), itching, and leg fatigue (each $p < 0.05$), but not leg cramp.

Venous insufficiency. A criteria-based review of 13 clinical trials of extracts of horse chestnut in the treatment of chronic venous insufficiency by Pittler and Ernst (1998) concluded that the extract is equipotent to reference medicines and more effective than placebo in providing relief from subjective symptoms and objective signs of the condition. While calling for "more rigorous" randomized controlled trials to confirm the effectiveness of the extract in long-term therapy, Pittler and Ernst further concluded that the evidence implies that extract of horse chestnut seed can be used safely and effectively for short-term therapy of chronic venous insufficiency symptoms.

Greeske and Pohlmann (1996) conducted a case-observation study involving over 800 general practitioners in Germany and over 5,000 of their patients diagnosed with chronic venous insufficiency who received treatment with HCE (Venostasin). Physicians reported complete disappearance or marked improvement in all symptoms: leg swelling, pain, itching, tension, tiredness, and tendency to edema.

Ottillinger and Greeske (2001) compared the outcomes of two multicenter trials of an oral horse chestnut seed extract (Venostasin, Klinge Pharma GmbH, Munich, Germany), one previously unpublished conducted in 355 patients with chronic venous insufficiency (CVI) grade II ($n = 284$) and grade IIIa ($n = 71$), and one published trial (Diehm et al., 1996, reviewed next) in 240 patients with grade I CVI. Both trials were conducted using a placebo control, randomization, and a two-week washout period. The new trial in more advanced CVI included 142 patients who openly received treatment with a compression stocking without a placebo control group. After 16 weeks of treatment with the extract (50 mg b.i.d.), no clear advantage was seen over the compression stocking treatment, which was superior to placebo ($p < 0.001$), whereas the extract was not. Comparing the two protocols, however, the extract was superior ($p = 0.018$), and although improvements in subjective symptoms between the two treatment groups were not significantly different, quality-of-life scores also showed the extract treatment to be superior. Better response in terms of volume reduction of leg swelling was seen in the grade II patients than in the grade III CVI patients treated with the extract, whereas use of compression stocking showed better results in the grade III patients. The incidence of adverse events between the two treatment groups showed no significant difference and none were of a serious nature. Among them, gastrointestinal complaints were more common in the extract group (15% versus 7%, respectively, $p = 0.09$) and consisted of abdominal cramps or pain, vomiting, nausea, gastroenteritis, diarrhea, and vomiting. In addition, there were a few cases of dry mouth ($n = 3$) and constipation ($n = 2$). The researchers concluded that for treating CVI in its early stages the extract may provide sufficient amelioration of the disease, provided that no permanent damage to the wall structures of the veins has been incurred. In advanced stages of CVI, horse chestnut seed extract may close gaps in the venular endothelium, which would provide some reduction of edema but not to the extent provided by compression stockings.

Diehm et al. (1996) conducted a placebo-controlled, partially blinded, randomized, three-armed parallel study in 240 patients diagnosed with venous insufficiency to compare efficacies between orally administered dried

HCSE (50 mg escin b.i.d.), the use of leg compression stockings (class II), and placebo. After 12 weeks, the lower leg volume of the HCSE group decreased by 43.8 mL ($p = 0.005$); it decreased by 46.7 mL in the compression group ($p = 0.002$); in the placebo group, the volume increased by 9.8 mL. The superior reduction in edema indicated that HCSE was a viable and effective alternative therapy for patients with venous insufficiency and comparably effective ($p = 0.001$) to treatment with the leg compression stocking.

Lohr et al. (1986) conducted a placebo-controlled, double-blind crossover study of HCE (Venostasin 300 mg b.i.d. for 56 days) in 74 patients with chronic venous insufficiency in two parallel groups. Significant improvements compared to placebo were found in leg volume (determined by leg circumference and water plethysmography) and in subjective complaints (each $p < 0.01$).

Kreysel et al. (1983) compared serum levels of glycosaminoglycan hydrolases in varicose patients and healthy subjects following a hypothesis that proteoglycans have a key function in capillary fragility and permeability, owing to their role as part of the "interendothelial cement" of capillaries. Proteoglycans also serve in the regulation of collagen biosynthesis and stabilization. Far higher levels of these hydrolases were found in varicose patients compared to healthy subjects (arylsulphatase +121.7%; β-N-acetylglucosaminidase +63.5%; and β-glucuronidase +70.0%). A subsequent 21-day, placebo-controlled double-blind study in 15 patients diagnosed with varicosis (internal saphenous vein stages II and III) found patients treated with HCE (Venostasin 300 mg t.i.d.) had significantly decreased ($p < 0.01$) serum levels of all three glycosaminoglycan hydrolases (ca. 30%), an effect already significant at days 3 through 5 in the active treatment group.

Although today horse chestnut is contraindicated in pregnancy (Steele, 1995) and should probably be avoided during lactation (see Safety Profile: Pregnancy and Lactation), a placebo-controlled, double-blind crossover study of HCE (Venostasin, 300 mg b.i.d. for 28 days) in 13 women with pregnancy-related varicose veins and seven with chronic venous insufficiency found significant improvements in leg volumes and subjective complaints (each $p < 0.01$) (Steiner and Hillemanns, 1986).

Digestive, Hepatic, and Gastrointestinal Disorders

Hemorrhoids

Pirard et al. (1976) conducted a placebo-controlled trial of escin in the treatment of acute symptomatic hemorrhoids. Patients received placebo ($n = 34$) or escin ($n = 38$) in the form of film-coated tablets (40 mg t.i.d.) for up to two months. On average, patients reported improvements in symptoms after six days of treatment. The majority of patients (81.6%) treated with escin reported improvement compared to 32.4% of those who received placebo. Endoscopic examinations at baseline, after two weeks and after the treatment period, revealed that 94.8% of the patients in the escin group who had bleeding improved versus 61.8% in the placebo group. Among those with swelling at baseline in the escin group, significantly more (86.9%) improved compared to the placebo group (38.3%, $p < 0.01$).

Integumentary, Muscular, and Skeletal Disorders

Skin Disorders

In a randomized placebo-controlled trial in 43 women volunteers (mean age 38.7) with cellulitis, Curri et al. (1989) tested an ointment containing 2% of a complex of escin, β-sitosterol, and phosopholipids in the form of a phytosomal product. Among the subjects, 16 (37.2%) presented with cellulitis (panniculopathy) of the thighs and glutea, 13 (30%) with cellulitis of the thighs, and the remainder with cellulitis affecting the thighs, knees, glutea, and abdomen. Once a day for 30 days, the ointment was gently massaged on the area affected (about 1 g/30 days). The researchers reported significant improvements in the complex ointment group compared to the placebo (vehicle only) group in lipoedema ($p < 0.04$), the intensity of skin flaccidity ($p < 0.0001$), abnormal plicability ($p < 0.03$), skin pastiness ($p < 0.004$), pale and cold skin ($p < 0.004$), provoked pain ($p < 0.004$), and spontaneous pain ($p < 0.04$). No cases of erythema or irritation were found resulting from the ointment. Following various tests, the researchers concluded that the treatment afforded improvements to tissue microcirculation of adipose and skin tissues, a concomitant increase in capillary blood flow, and a decrease in stasis and edema. No such results were found in the placebo group. A further short-term study in 20 women (ages 17-64) with cellulitis of the breasts required a different preparation owing to ethical reasons in treatments of breast disease. They used a commercially available ointment containing the same complex to which was added low molecular weight components of hyaluronic acid (5%), ruscogenins (1%, derived from butcher's broom, *Ruscus aculeatus*), hawthorn extract (1%, *Crataegus oxycantha*), and bilberry extract (0.9%, *Vaccinium myrtillus*). Again, the researchers reported significant results as measured by microvascular patterns which they found comparable to the improvements seen in the first study. No signs of irritations or erythema were found as a result of the ointment despite the more delicate skin of the breast (Curri et al., 1989).

Metabolic and Nutritional Functions

Pharmacokinetics

Pharmacokinetic studies of horse chestnut products in humans ($n = 9$) have to date shown considerable variations in the bioavailability of escin, both from one product to the next and from one batch to the next of the same product. The problem appears to be the absence of a reliable and effective method to determine the variability of escin and individual saponin fractions in these products (Loew et al., 2000).

DOSAGE

The usual oral dosage in clinical studies is 50 mg of escin twice to three times daily. Commercial extracts are usually standardized to 16% triterpene glycosides, calculated as escin. Recommended doses are the equivalent of 50 mg escin, two to three times daily (300 to 900 mg of a 16% extract). Topical gels are standardized to contain 2% escin.

The German Commission E monograph on horse chestnut refers to a standardized powder extract of the seeds containing 16-20 triterpene glycosides in the form of anhydrous escin. The dosage is 250-312.5 mg b.i.d. "in delayed release form," corresponding to 100 mg escin (Blumenthal et al., 1998). In the form of controlled-release extracts, tolerability is noted to be high (Schulz et al., 2001).

A provisional note in the German Commission E monograph advises practitioners that in all cases they must continue physician-prescribed treatments, including the use of supportive elastic stockings, leg compresses, and the application of cold water (Blumenthal et al., 1998).

SAFETY PROFILE

The genus *Aesculus* is considered toxic (Steele, 1995). Toxic reactions from ingestion of the raw seed and other plant parts underscore the importance of using only standardized products of horse chestnut, where careful control of dose is more assured. Doses of 100 mg esculin, corresponding to 250-313 mg horse chestnut extract b.i.d. in a "delayed release form," as specified by the German Commission E monograph, are associated with relatively few adverse effects (see Side Effects). Encounters with other forms of the plant have generated numerous reports of toxicity, including death. From the years 1985 to 1994, reports of toxicity from ingestion of the seed or other parts of the plant in the United States amounted to 340 cases in which the effect was moderate, and in 16 cases minimal. Thirty cases involved gastrointestinal symptoms (throat irritation, nausea, vomiting, and diarrhea), and one case reported drowsiness. No cases of serious toxicity were reported and in the majority of instances no toxic effects occurred. For another 2,374 instances of exposure to the plant reported to toxicology centers in the United States during this same period, no effect or a nontoxic effect not definitely linked to horse chestnut occurred (Maytunas et al., 1997). Children are especially sensitive and may be poisoned from the ingestion of 1% of their body weight (Duke, 1985). Of all the cases reported, close to half were in children younger than a year through five years and they occurred during the autumn when the seeds ripen (Maytunas et al., 1997). Horse chestnut poisoning in children has resulted from ingesting the seeds, or consuming a "tea" prepared from the twigs and leaves. Accordingly, horse chestnut is known as a toxic plant and is classified by the FDA as an unsafe herb. According to one author, children should never be exposed to internal or topical applications (Steele, 1995). Toxicity is attributable to the glucoside esculin, which in sufficient concentrations in humans causes the dilation of the pupils, stupor, diarrhea, vomiting, weakness, muscle twitching, paralysis, and lack of coordination. A method of preparing the seeds to eliminate toxicity was apparently known to American Indians who roasted the seeds before peeling and mashing them. Before consumption, the mash was leached in water for "several days" (Nagy, 1973). Ethnobotanical investigation of the efficacy of their detoxification method would be of interest.

Contraindications

Newall et al. (1996) state that horse chestnut is contraindicated in patients with either hepatic or renal impairment. Two cases of suspected toxic nephropathy were reported (Grasso and Corvaglia, 1976) that were thought probably to have resulted from ingesting high amounts of escin (Newall et al., 1996). Patients receiving high doses of escin intravenously (540 µg/kg) developed acute renal failure (Reynolds et al., 1996). However, clinical studies using whole horse chestnut extract found no signs of worsening of renal impairment in patients who had renal impairment, and no signs of development of renal impairment in patients with normal renal function (Sirtori, 2001). In an apparently unusual case report, a 37-year-old male patient with no history of liver disease developed hepatic injury 60 days after intramuscular injection of an extract of horse chestnut flowers (Venoplant, 65 mg) that he received prior to treatment of a pathological fracture of a brachial bone. Since 1967 the European product has been used in Japan for the treatment of inflammation after trauma or surgery. This was the first instance of hepatic injury attributed to the extract ever reported in the literature. Otherwise, the incidence of adverse effects from the extract was low in Japan and consisted of mild nausea, vomiting, urticaria, and, only rarely, general spasm and shock (Takegoshi et al., 1986).

Drug Interactions

Newall et al. (1996) caution that binding of drugs may be possible owing to the saponin contents of horse chestnut, since they bind to plasma proteins. In animal experiments, escin showed a 50% binding to plasma protein (Rothkopf et al., 1977).

A case of acute renal insufficiency was reported to be the result of a drug interaction in a patient treated with gentamicin in addition to β-escin (Voigt and Junger, 1978).

Pregnancy and Lactation

Horse chestnut is considered toxic at high doses and is contraindicated during pregnancy (Steele, 1995).

No information regarding the safety of horse chestnut during lactation is reported, but its toxicity in children indicates that it should be avoided (see Special Precautions).

Side Effects

Isolated cases of nausea, stomach discomfort, and itching are known (Schulz et al., 2001). Due to its saponin constituents, for some individuals horse chestnut may irritate the gastrointestinal tract (Newall et al., 1996). Controlled-release preparations are reported to have less of a tendency to upset the stomach when the dosage of extract is 250-313 mg b.i.d. providing the dose is equivalent to 100 mg escin (Schulz et al., 2001).

Special Precautions

HCE should not be applied to broken skin (Anonymous, 1987).

Aflatoxins, which are known to be potent carcinogens, have been identified in some cosmetic products containing horse chestnut (Steele, 1995).

Children are very sensitive to the toxins in horse chestnut and should never be exposed to internal or topical applications (Steele, 1995). Horse chestnut poisoning in children has resulted from ingesting the seeds or consuming a "tea" prepared from the twigs and leaves. Toxicity is attributable to the glucoside esculin, which in sufficient concentrations in humans causes dilation of the pupils, stupor, diarrhea, vomiting, weakness, muscle twitching, paralysis, and lack of coordination.

The bark and leaves contain the coumarins fraxin, scopolin, and aesculetin (Miller and Murray, 1998), which may preclude their use in bleeding disorders or in combination with anticoagulant medications. The bark, fruit pericarp, and buds contain the coumarins esculin and fraxin, along with their aglycones esculetin and fraxetin. However, these components are not found in horse chestnut seeds (Bombardelli et al., 1996).

Horse chestnut pollen is a frequent cause of allergic sensitization in children living in urban areas where the tree is more common (Popp et al., 1992).

The honey made from California buckeye is reportedly toxic (Steele, 1995).

Toxicology

Toxicity in Animal Models

In mice, rats, and guinea pigs, the oral LD_{50} of horse chestnut seed ranges from 134 to 720 mg/kg (Newall et al., 1996). However, the German Commission E reported that the oral LD_{50} in mice was 990 mg/kg; in rats 2,150 mg/kg, with no signs of toxicity from 400 mg/kg; 130 mg/kg in dogs; and in rabbits 1,530 mg/kg (Blumenthal et al., 1998).

REFERENCES

Anonymous (1987). The horse chestnut. *Medi Herb Newsletter* (December): 1.

Bisler, H., Pfeifer, R., Kluken, N., and Pauschinger, P. (1986). Effect of horse-chestnut seed extract on transcapillary filtration in chronic venous insufficiency. *Deutsche Medizinische Wochenschrift* 111: 1321-1329.

Blumenthal, M., Busse, W.R., Goldberg, A., Gruenwald, J., Hall, T., Riggins, C.W., and Rister, R.S. (Eds.) (1998). *The Complete German Commission E Monographs*. Boston, MA: Integrative Medicine Communications.

Bombardelli, E., Morazzoni, P., and Griffini, A. (1996). *Aesculus hippocastanum* L. *Fitoterapia* 67: 483-511.

Bruneton, J. (1995). *Pharmacognosy, Phytochemistry, and Medicinal Plants*. Paris: Lavoisier.

Calabrese, C. and Preston, P. (1993). Report of the results of a double-blind, randomized, single dose trial of a topical 2% escin gel versus placebo in the acute treatment of experimentally induced hematoma in volunteers. *Planta Medica* 59: 394-397.

Curri, S.B., Bombardelli, E., Della Loggia, R., Del Negro, P., and Tubaro, A. (1989). Topical anti-inflammatory activity of complexes of aescin and sterols with phospholipids. Part II. Anti-oedema properties in the treatment of panniculopathies of the thighs and breast. *Fitoterapia* 60 (Suppl.): 45-53.

D'Amelio, F.S. (1999). *Botanicals: A Phytocosmetic Desk Reference* (pp. 128-129). Boca Raton, FL: CRC Press.

Diehm, C., Trampsich, H.J., Lange, S., and Schmidt, C. (1996). Comparison of leg compression stocking and oral horse chestnut seed extract therapy in patients with chronic venous insufficiency. *Lancet* 347: 292-294.

Dobelis, I.N. (Ed.) (1986). *The Magic and Medicine of Plants*. Pleasantville, NY: Pegasus.

Duke, J.A. (1985). *CRC Handbook of Medicinal Herbs*. Boca Raton, FL: CRC Press.

Facino, R.M., Carini, M., Stefani, R., Aldini, G., and Saibene, L. (1995). Antielastase and anti-hyaluronidase activities of saponins and sapogenins from *Hedera helix, Aesculus hippocastanum,* and *Ruscus aculeatus*: Factors contributing to their efficacy in the treatment of venous insufficiency. *Archiv der Pharmazie* 328: 720-724.

Friederich, H.C., Vogelsberg, H. and Neiss, A. (1978). Ein beitrag zur bewertung von intern wirksamen venenpharmaka [A report on the internal usefulness of venous pharmaceuticals]. *Zeitschrift fur Hautkrankheiten* 53: 369-374.

Grasso, A. and Corvaglia, E. (1976). Due casi di sospetta tubulonefrosi tossica da escina [Two cases of suspected toxic tubulonephrosis due to escine]. *Gazzetta Medica Italiana* 135: 581-584.

Greeske, K. and Pohlmann, B.K. (1996). Roßkastaniensamenextrakt – ein wirksames therapieprinzip in der praxis. Medikamentöse therapie der chronisch venösen insuffizienz [Horse chestnut seed extract—An effective therapy principle in general practice: Drug therapy of chronic venous insufficiency]. *Fortschritte der Medizin* 114: 196-200.

Guillaume, M. and Padioleau, F. (1994). Veinotonic effect, vascular protection, anti-inflammatory and free radical scavenging properties of horse chestnut extract. *Arzneimittel-Forschung/Drug Research* 44: 25-35.

Hiai, S., Yokoyama, H., and Oura, H. (1981). Effect of escin on adrenocorticotropin and corticosterone levels in rat plasma. *Chemical Pharmaceutical Bulletin* 29: 490-494.

Hickman, J.C. (Ed.) (1993). *The Jepson Manual: Higher Plants of California*. Berkeley, CA: University of California Press.

Konoshima, T. and Lee, K.H. (1986). Antitumor agents, 82. Cytotoxic sapogenols from *Aesculus hippocastanum. Journal of Natural Products* 49: 650-656.

Kreysel, H.W., Nissen, H.P., and Enghoffer, E. (1983). A possible role of lysosomal enzymes in the pathogenesis of varicosis and the reduction in their serum activity by Venostasin®. *Vasa* 12: 377-382.

Loew, D., Schrödter, A., Schwankl, W., and März, R.W. (2000). Measurement of the bioavailability of aescin-containing extracts. *Methods and Findings in Experimental and Clinical Pharmacology* 22: 537-542.

Lohr, E., Garanin, G., Jesau, P., and Fischer, H. (1986). Ödemprotektive therapie bei chronischer veneninsuffizienz mit ödemneigung [Edema preventative therapy in chronic venous insufficiency with a tendency to edema formation]. *Munchener Medizinische Wochenschrift* 128: 579-581.

Marshall, M. and Dormandy, J.A. (1987). Oedema of long distance flights. *Phlebol* 2: 123-124.

Matsuda, H., Li, Y., Murakami, T., Ninomiya, K., Yamahara, J., and Yoshikawa, M. (1997). Effects of escins Ia, Ib, IIa, and IIb from horse chestnut, the seeds of *Aesculus hippocastanum* L., on acute inflammation in animals. *Biological and Pharmaceutical Bulletin* 20: 1092-1095.

Matsuda, H., Murakami, T., Li, Y., Yamahara, J., and Yoshikawa, M. (1998). Mode of action of aescins Ia, IIa and E,Z-senegin II on glucose absorption in gastrointestinal tract. *Bioorganic and Medicinal Chemistry* 6: 1019-1023.

Maytunas, N., Krenzelok, E., Jacobsen, T., and Aronis, J. (1997). Horse chestnut (*Aesculus* sp.) ingestion in the United States: 1985-1994. *Journal of Toxicology. Clinical Toxicology* 35: 527-528 (abstract).

Mete Kockar, O., Kara, M., Kara, S., et al. (1994). Quantitative determination of escin. A comparative study of HPLC and TLC-densitometry. *Fitoterapia* 65: 439-443.

Miller, L.G. and Murray, W.J. (1998). Specific toxicological considerations of selected herbal products. In L.G. Miller and W.J. Murray (Eds.), *Herbal Medicinals: A Clinician's Guide* (pp. 307-322). Binghamton, NY: Pharmaceutical Products Press.

Nagy, M. (1973). Human poisoning from horse chestnuts. *Journal of the American Medical Association* 226: 213 (letter).

Neiss, A. and Böhm, C. (1976). Zum wirksamkeitsnachweis von roßkastaniensamenextrakt beim varikösen symptomenkomplex [The effectiveness of horse chestnut extract in symptoms of varicosity]. *Munchener Medizinische Wochenschrift* 118: 213-216.

Newall, C.A., Anderson, L.A., and Phillipson, J.D. (1996). *Herbal Medicines: A Guide for Health-Care Professionals* (pp. 166-167). London: The Pharmaceutical Press.

Ottillinger, B. and Greeske, K. (2001). Rational therapy of chronic venous insufficiency—Chances and limits of the therapeutic use of horse-chestnut seed extract. *MBC Cardiovascular Disorders* 1: 5. Available on the Web at: <http://www.biomedcentral.com/1471-2261/1/5>.

Pirard, J., Gillet, P., Guffens, J.M., and Defrance, P. (1976). Etude en double aveugle du Reparil en proctologie [A double-blind study of Reparil in proctology]. *Revue Medicale de Liege* 31: 343-345.

Pittler, M.H. and Ernst, E. (1998). Horse-chestnut seed extract for chronic venous insufficiency: A criteria-based systematic review. *Archives of Dermatology* 134: 1356-1360.

Popp, W., Horak, F., Jager, S., Reiser, K., Wagner, C., and Zwick, H. (1992). Horse chestnut *(Aesculus hippocastanum)* pollen: A frequent cause of allergic sensitization in urban children. *Allergy* 47: 380-383.

Proserpio, G., Gatti, S., and Genesi, P. (1980). Cosmetic uses of horse chestnut extracts, of escin, and of the cholesterol/escin complex. *Fitoterapia* 51: 113-128.

Rao, S.G. and Cochrane, K.W. (1974). Antiviral activity of triterpenoid saponins containing acylated β-amyrin aglycones. *Journal of Pharmaceutical Sciences* 63: 471-473.

Reynolds, J.E.F., Parffitt, K., Parsons, A.V., and Sweetman, S.C. (Eds.) (1996). *Martindale. The Extra Pharmacopoeia,* Twenty-First Edition (p. 1670). London: Royal Pharmaceutical Society.

Rothkopf, M., Vogel, G., Lang, W., and Leng, E. (1977). Animal experiments on the question of the renal toleration of the horse chestnut saponin aescin. *Arzneimittel-Forschung* 27: 598-605.

Rudofsky, G., Neiss, A., Otto, K., and Seibel, K. (1986). Ödemprotektive wirkung und klinische wirksamkeit von roßkastaniensamenextrakt im doppleblindversuch [Edema protective effect and clinical efficacy of horse chestnut extract in a double-blind study]. *Phlebologie und Proktologie* 15: 47-54.

Schulz, V., Hänsel, R., and Tyler, V.E. (2001). *Rational Phytotherapy: A Physician's Guide to Herbal Medicine,* Fourth Edition (pp. 158-168). Berlin, Germany: Springer-Verlag.

Sirtori, C.R. (2001). Aescin: Pharmacology, pharmacokinetics and therapeutic profile. *Pharmacological Research* 44: 183-193.

Srijayanta, S., Raman, A., and Goodwin, B.L. (1999). A comparative study of the constituents of *Aesculus hippocastanum* and *Aesculus indica. Journal of Medicinal Food* 2: 45-50.

Stankowic, S.K., Bastic, M.B., and Jovanovic, J.A. (1987). Ontogenetic distribution of hydrocarbons in horse chestnut seed (*Aesculus hippocastanum* L.). *Herba Polonica* 33: 3-8.

Steele, N.M. (Ed.) (1995). Chestnut. *The Lawrence Review of Natural Products* (February).

Steiner, M. (1990). Untersuchung zur ödemvermindernden und ödemprotektiven wirkung von roßkastaniensamenextrakt [Examination of the edema reducing and edema protective effect of a horse chestnut seed extract]. *Phlebologie und Proktologie* 19: 239-242.

Steiner, M. and Hillemanns, H.G. (1986). Unterschung zur ödemprotektiven eines venentherapeutikums [Investigations of the edema protective action of a venous therapeutic agent]. *Munchener Medizinische Wochenschrift* 31: 551-552.

Takegoshi, K., Tohyama, T., Okuda, K., Suzuki, K., and Ohta, G. (1986). A case of Venoplant-induced hepatic injury. *Gastroenterologia Japonica* 21: 62-65.

Uberti E., Martinelli, E.M., and Pifferi, G. (1990). TLC-densitometric analysis of aescin in ointments. *Fitoterapia* 61: 57-60.

Voigt, E. and Junger, H. (1978). [Acute post-traumatic renal failure following therapy with antibiotics and β-aescin]. *Anaesthetist* 28: 81-83.

Werbach, M.R. and Murray, M.T. (1994). *Botanical Influences on Illness: A Sourcebook of Clinical Research*. Tarzana, CA: Third Line Press.

Yamahara, J., Takagi, Y., Sawada, T., Fujimura, H., Shirakawa, K., Yoshikawa, M., and Kitagawa, I. (1979). Effects of crude drugs on congestive edema. *Chemical Pharmaceutical Bulletin* 27: 1464-1468.

Yoshikawa, M., Murakami, T., Yamahara, J., and Matsuda, H. (1998). Bioactive saponins and glycosides. XII. Horse chestnut. (2): Structure of escins IIIb, IV, and VI and isoescins Ia, Ib, and V, acylated polyhydroxyoleanene triterpene oligoglycosides, from the seeds of horse chestnut tree (*Aesculus hippocastanum* L., Hippocastanaceae). *Chemical and Pharmaceutical Bulletin* 46: 1764-1769.

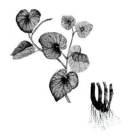

$\mathcal{K}ava$

BOTANICAL DATA

Classification and Nomenclature

Scientific name: *Piper methysticum* Forster f.

Family name: Piperaceae (pepper family)

Common names: kava, kava-kava, kawa, áva, áwa, yaqona

Description

Piper methysticum was first classified by J.G.A. Forster who joined Captain James Cook's second expedition to the South Seas (1772-1775) as a botanist along with his father, J.R. Forster, and A. Sparrman (Smith, 1943). The term *Piper methysticum* means "intoxicating pepper," *methysticum* being the Latin transcription of the Greek *methustikos,* which means "intoxicating drink" (Singh and Blumenthal, 1997).

Having only male flowers and being devoid of seeds and fruit, *Piper methysticum* is always cultivated and does not reproduce sexually. It is likely that the species originated from semidomesticated clones of a wild progenitor, *Piper wichmannii,* which is native to Vanuatu, the Solomon Islands, and New Guinea (Lebot and Lévesque, 1989). *Piper methysticum* is an attractive, slow-growing perennial that can attain heights of over 3 m. It has a knotty, thick stump, often containing holes or cracks created by the partial destruction of the parenchyma. A fringe of filiform lateral roots up to 3 m long extends from the thickened root. The roots consist of a multitude of ligneous fibers that are more than 60% starch; the rootstock color varies from white to dark yellow, depending on the concentration of psychoactive kavalactones that are concentrated in a lemon-yellow resin. Monopodial stems (averaging 22 in number, with up to ten internodes) with sympodial branches arise from the stump. The leaves are sparse, thin, single, whole, heart-shaped, alternate, petiolate, and long (8-25 cm); they are borne in petioles 2-6 cm in length, with three main veins that extend to the tips, deciduous, often pubescent on the underside and occasionally on the upper surface. The bases of the petioles and the stipules are enclosed in a caducous (easily shed) amplexicaul (sessile with base of petioles surrounding the stem) sheath. The first inflorescences appear at two to three years of age in the form of irregular spadices. Senescent plants range in age from 15-30 years, although 100-year-old specimens, with root masses of over 100 kg, have been reported. The root mass of kava weighs about 1 kg on average at an age of 11 months; the first inflorescences appear at two to three years of age in the form of irregular spadices (Johnston, 1997).

The term kava, kava-kava, and its variants reflect the vernacular names used for the plant and the beverage prepared from it throughout Polynesia. In parts of Polynesia, e.g., Hawaii, Tahiti, and the Marquesas, the initial K is often dropped to yield variants such as áva or áwa. The terms are related to Polynesian words describing the various properties of food and drink, such as bitter, sour, sharp, pungent, acidic, acrid, etc. (Singh and Blumenthal, 1997).

In Fiji, the plant and its beverage are known as "yangona" or "yagona," and sometimes "gona." Although apparently entirely related to the Polynesian terms, these vernacular names denote both "beverage" and "bitter" (Singh and Blumenthal, 1997). In addition to these vernacular names, which have widespread usage throughout the region of kava's distribution, *Piper methysticum* and its derivative beverages have numerous local names in parts of Polynesia where its use is common; Lebot et al. (1997) list over 37 names used in New Guinea and approximately 35 local names used in Vanuatu.

HISTORY AND TRADITIONAL USES

The journal of Captain James Cook from his South Seas Voyage of 1768 reported that kava-kava was used ceremonially in the form of an intoxicating beverage which reduced anxiety and fatigue and from overindulgence caused stupefaction and dizziness (Lebot et al., 1997). Kava is a relaxing, mildly psychoactive beverage prepared from the root of *Piper methysticum,* which is widely cultivated throughout the South Pacific, from Hawaii to New Guinea. The root is used in the preparation of a recreational beverage known by a variety of local vernacular names (e.g., kava, yagona, or áwa) and occupies a prominent position in the social, ceremonial, and daily life of Pacific Island peoples; kava may be fairly described as the social lubricant that facilitates the smooth running of business and daily life in the South Pacific (Lebot et al., 1997; Singh and Blumenthal, 1997).

In Hawaii, kava has long been used in the indigenous treatment of asthma. Ethnic Hawaiians have the highest mortality rate from asthma of any ethnic group in Hawaii (Hope et al., 1993). Kava has also been used in Hawaiian traditional medicine to treat urinary tract infections and as a tranquilizer (Locher et al., 1995) to induce sleep and relaxation and counteract fatigue. It was also used by the Hawaiians for weight loss ("excessive fat") and to treat rheumatism. Elsewhere in Polynesia, the root beverage has been used in traditional medicine to treat chronic cystitis, gonorrhea (Singh, 1992 in Singh and Blumenthal, 1997), bladder and kidney problems, coughs and cold, and sore throat. Fijian mothers have ingested a decoction of the pounded roots to prevent conception (Cambie and Ash, 1994), and the leaves placed inside the vagina are traditionally believed to provoke abortion. The root beverage prepared by mastication is used in Polynesia to prevent infections and to treat pulmonary pains, female puberty problems including menstrual problems, dysmenorrhea, migraine in "women's sicknesses," headaches, general weakness, sleeping problems, and "chills" (Lebot et al., 1997).

In the late 1800s, kava was extensively used in Germany to treat urinary problems (Singh and Blumenthal, 1997), whether as a diuretic, a genitourinary antiseptic (Anonymous, 1988), or to "dry up secretions." It was also used to induce sleep. After the development of chemical drugs for these applications, the use of kava in Germany collapsed (Degener, 1946). Until recently, kava had little economic importance, being primarily an indigenous beverage that was prepared and used locally. Other than this local use, kava has long been utilized in European phytomedicine as a sedative, tranquilizer, muscle relaxant, and treatment for menopausal symptoms, and urinary tract and bladder disorders. Few of these applications have been substantiated by well-designed clinical trials (Lehmann et al., 1996; Lindenberg and Pitule-Schodel, 1990; Warnecke, 1991).

Currently, over 17 phytopharmaceutical products derived from kava are available on the European market (Kilham, 1996). The plant is the subject of a therapeutic monograph in Germany (Blumenthal et al., 1998), while in the United States it is sold as a dietary supplement under the provisions of the Dietary Supplement Health and Education Act of 1994 (Blumenthal, 1994). In the United States, kava tinctures and other types of kava preparations have been sold in health food stores and ethnic markets for some time; however, it has been only within the past five to six years that kava has become widely incorporated into the mainstream of herbal products.

A wide variety of kava morphotypic cultivars exist; in traditional usage, consumers of kava recognize that beverages prepared from different cultivars can differ markedly in their psychotropic effects. Kava beverages can be weak or strong, produce euphoria or relaxation, or induce sleep; some varieties induce headaches and nausea (Lebot et al., 1997). These differing effects are thought to result from the differing proportions and amounts of psychotropic kavalactones present in the different cultivars (Lebot and Lévesque, 1989; Dinh et al., 2001); a number of different chemotypes have been characterized based on the differing levels and ratios of the major kavalactones (Lebot and Lévesque, 1989).

CHEMISTRY

Nitrogenous Compounds

Alkaloids

Pipermethysticine, an alkaloid specific to *P. methysticum,* has been isolated from its leaves (Smith, 1979). Reports of alkaloids in the rootstock have not been confirmed and, as alkaloids are not present in the lipid soluble fraction, it appears unlikely that alkaloids are implicated in the psychotropic actions of kava; they may, however, contribute to some of the activities measured in aqueous fractions (Lebot et al., 1997).

Phenolic Compounds

Flavonoids

Three flavokavins designated A, B, and C were isolated from kava rootstock (Duve, 1976; Dutta et al., 1976). Pinostrobin and 5-7-dimethoxyflavanone were recently identified in a methanolic extract of the rootstock (Wu et al., 2001).

Terpenoid Compounds

The active, psychotropic constituents of kava are the kavalactones; aryl-ethylene-α-pyrone derivatives having the general structure shown in Figure 1.

The "A" ring can have some degree of substitution (hydrogen, hydroxyl, methoxyl, or methylenedioxy); the ethyl moiety can possess a vinyl unsaturation or can be saturated; and the "C" lactone ring can have one or two double bonds. Approximately 18 kavalactones have been isolated and chemically characterized; however, only six are considered major constituents and the variation in psychotropic activity of kava is probably due to the varying amounts and proportions of these components (Shulgin, 1973; Duve, 1981; Lebot et al., 1997; Lechtenberg et al., 1999; Dinh et al., 2001; Hänsel, 1964). The structures of the six major kavalactones are shown in Figure 1. Kava pyrones (dihydro-5,6-dehydrokavain and 5,6-dehydrokavain) have also been detected in the leaves of *Alpinia zerumbet* (Pers.) Burtt. & Smith, a member of the ginger family (Zingiberaceae) used in traditional medicine in Brazil to control hypertension and as a diuretic (Kuster et al., 1999).

Other Constituents

Piper methysticum contains ketones, including cinnamalketone, methylene dioxy-3,4-cinnamalketone, and an alcohol, dihydrokavain-5-ol (Leung and Foster, 1996). It is not known what contribution these constituents make, if any, to the psychoactive effects of kava.

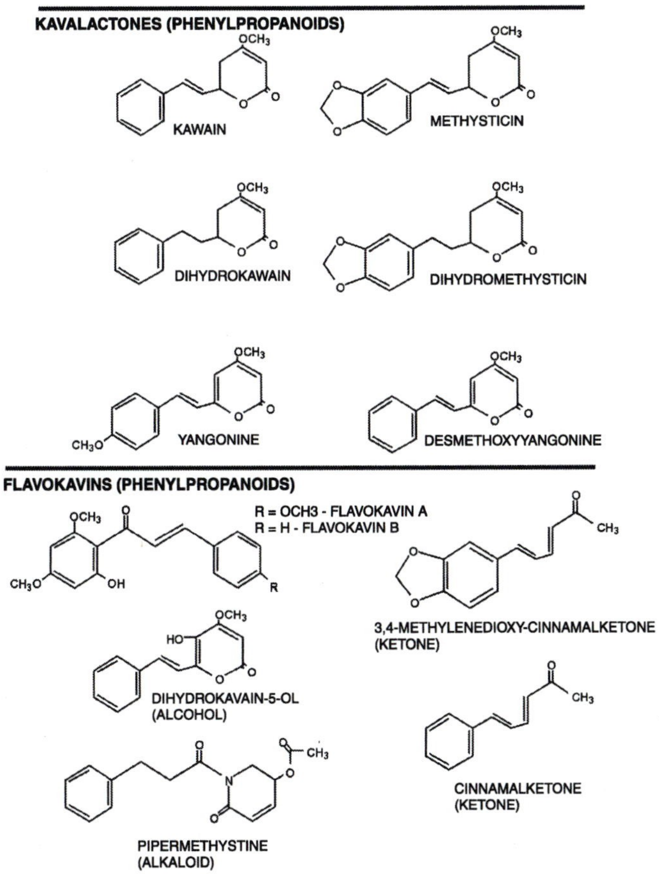

FIGURE 1. Major Isolated Constituents of Kava *(Piper methysticum)*

Kava contains minerals, including potassium, magnesium, calcium, sodium, aluminum, iron, and silica; sugars, including saccharose, maltose, fructose, and glucose; and over 15 amino acids. Nutritional analyses of the rootstock indicate that it contains 43% starch, 20% fiber, 12% water, 3.2% sugars, 3.6% proteins, 3.2% minerals, and 3-20% kavalactones (depending on plant age and cultivar) (Leung and Foster, 1996).

THERAPEUTIC APPLICATIONS

Current medical applications of standardized kava extracts in Europe are found mainly in treatments of nervous tension and anxiety. In Germany, these extracts are approved as over-the-counter (OTC) products for restlessness, stress, and nervous anxiety (Blumenthal et al., 1998).

PRECLINICAL STUDIES

In view of the potential medical applications of kavalactones as anxiolytics, anticonvulsants, analgesics, and neuroprotectants, it is surprising how little is known about their pharmacological properties and mechanisms of action at the molecular level.

Immune Functions; Inflammation and Disease

Infectious Diseases

Microbial infections. Kava is traditionally used as an antibacterial agent, particularly for urinary tract infections (Locher et al., 1995); however, in vitro studies do not support this usage, as a variety of pathogenic and nonpathogenic Gram-positive and Gram-negative bacteria will readily grow on media containing kavalactones. Some of the pyrones, however, display fungistatic activities against a wide variety of fungi, some of which are pathogenic to humans (Hänsel et al., 1966; Hänsel, 1968). A water extract of the stem has shown moderate inhibitory activity against the growth of *Epidermophyton floccosum* (Locher et al., 1995).

Inflammatory Response

The isolated kavalactone, (+)-kavain, inhibited arachidonic-acid (AA)-stimulated aggregation in human platelets, and also inhibited adenosine triphosphate (ATP)-induced exocytosis, cyclooxygenase activity, and thromboxane synthetase activity. In platelet preparations, application of (+)-kavain 5 min before AA dose-dependently diminished aggregation, ATP release, and synthesis of TXA_2 and PGE_2 (IC_{50} values of 78, 115, 71, and 86 µmol/L, respectively). The similarity of IC_{50} values indicated that cyclooxygenase was the primary target, suppressing the generation of TXA_2 which reduces aggregation of platelets and exocytosis of ATP via binding to TXA_2 receptors (Gleitz et al., 1997). In order of most to least potent in vitro inhibition of COX-I, the constituents responsible have so far been identified as flavokawain B (77% inhibition), cinnamic acid bornyl ester (66%), 5-7-dimethoxyflavanone (42%), pinostrobin (36%), and bornyl ester of 3,4-methylene dioxy cinnamic acid (16%). By comparison, prescription and over-the-counter non-steroidal anti-inflammatory drugs (NSAIDS) showed weaker activity. Aspirin, naproxen, Celebrex, ibuprofen, and Vioxx produced inhibition rates of 78%, 63%, 47%, 30%, and 23%, respectively. COX-II inhibition was strongest from flavokawain B, (19%), cinnamic acid bornyl ester (19%), and bornyl ester of 3,4-methylene dioxy cinnamic acid (18%). The researchers concluded that these findings may lend credence to the use of kava among the indigenous peoples of Polynesia for treating inflammatory conditions (Wu et al., 2001).

Integumentary, Muscular, and Skeletal Functions

Muscular Functions

Singh (1983) investigated the mechanisms underlying kava's muscle-relaxing actions using mouse and frog muscle preparations using a suspension of finely powdered kava stem. His results indicated that kava causes muscle relaxation by a direct action on muscle contractility rather than by interference with neuromuscular transmission. In the twitch-tension experiments, little difference existed between concentrations required to block directly and indirectly stimulated muscle. Blockade of twitches was poorly reversed by either calcium or neostigmine, i.e., prejunctionally by antagonizing blockade produced by compounds such as magnesium, and postjunctionally in reverse blockade produced by compounds such as tubocurarine, respectively. Intracellular recording supported this conclusion. Tests indicated that the kava suspension had little or no effect on neurotransmitter release and that it reduces postjunctional sensitivity. The suspension also caused a marked prolongation of miniature end-plate potentials (MEPPs) and end-plate potentials (EPPs) in a manner similar to that of other local anesthetics, such as lignocaine. This suggests that kava affects receptor ion channels. Blockade of receptor ion channels in the muscle membrane could result in a decrease in action potential conduction and hence in muscle contractility. In the frog muscle, the kava suspension slowed the rate of rise and then prolonged the rate of fall of the action potential, and blocked the electrical excitability of the membrane. Such effects are consistent with an action on ion channels similar to that of other local anesthetics.

Martin et al. (2000) hypothesized that because kava has been used in traditional medicine in the treatment for asthma, and kavain had previously shown smooth muscle-relaxant activity, kavain would relax airway smooth muscle. Their in vitro experiments with murine airway smooth muscle (contracted tracheal ring preparations) showed that this was indeed the case, with kavain inhibiting contraction and inducing relaxation of the tissues. Kavain diminished the maximal contractile response to voltage-operated calcium channel activation and to muscarinic receptor activation. In rings precontracted with carbachol, the IC_{50} of kavain was 177 μM and less in rings precontracted with potassium chloride (59.6 μM). As for the mechanisms involved in the mediation of the smooth muscle-relaxant activity by kavain, the researchers ruled out nitric oxide and concluded that prostaglandin pathways were unlikely to be involved.

Metabolic and Nutritional Functions

Pharmacokinetics

Rasmussen et al. (1979) characterized the urinary metabolites of several kavalactones, namely, dihydrokavain, kavain, methysticin, 7,8-dihydroyangonin, and yangonin in the rat. Approximately half the dose of dihydrokavain (400 mg/kg p.o.) was collected in the urine 48 h after administration, about two-thirds of which was hydroxylated metabolites (three mono- and three dihydroxylated derivatives) with p-hydroxydihydrokavain the most abundant. The remaining third consisted of metabolites formed by scission of the 5,6-dihydro-α-pyrone ring and included hippuric acid. Lower amounts of urinary metabolites were collected following kavain (400 mg/kg p.o.), with both hydroxylated and ring-opened metabolites being detected. No metabolites were detected from kavain at 100 mg/kg i.p. Methysticin gave rise to only small amounts of metabolites, formed by demethylation of the methylenedioxyphenyl moiety. Urinary metabolites of 7,8-dihydroyangonin and yangonin were formed via O-demethylation. No ring-opened metabolites were found. The researchers speculated that the extremely low solubility in water of the kavapyrones would be expected to reduce their absorption and could account for the variable and low extent of metabolism observed.

Duffield and co-workers (1989) characterized human urinary metabolites of kava using chemical ionization-gas chromatography/mass spectrometry (CI-GC/MS). Seven major kavalactones were identified in human urine, as well as several minor constituents. Metabolic transformations included reduction of the 3,4 double bond and/or demethylation of the 4-methoxy group of the a-pyrone ring system. Demethylation of the 12-methoxy substituent in yangonin or, alternatively, hydroxylation at C12 of desmethoxyyangonin, was observed. In contrast to the rat, no dihydroxylated metabolites or products of ring opening of the 2-pyrone ring system were observed in human urine. The researchers concluded that the analytical methods could be readily applied to determine whether individuals have recently consumed kava.

Using gas chromatography/mass spectrometry (GC/MS) and deuterated internal standards, Keledjian et al. (1988) measured the uptake into mouse brain of four kavalactones present as major components of kava resin: dihydrokavain, kavain, desmethoxyyangonin, and yangonin (100 mg/kg i.p.). At 5 min, dihydrokavain and kavain attained maximum concentrations in the brain (64.7 ± 13.1 and 29.3 ± 0.8 ng/mg wet brain tissue, respectively) and were rapidly eliminated. Desmethoxyyangonin and yangonin had poorly defined brain maxima (10.4 ± 1.5 and 1.2 ± 0.3 ng/mg tissue, respectively) and were slowly eliminated from brain tissue. From crude kava resin (120 mg/ kg i.p.), brain concentrations of kavain and yangonin increased markedly (two and 20 times, respectively) relative to their concentrations when injected individually. In contrast, dihydrokavain and desmethoxy-yangonin remained at the percentage incorporated into brain tissue established by i.p. injection of the compounds individually.

It was difficult to establish tolerance to the liposoluble components of kava in mice (Duffield and Jamieson, 1991). The aqueous extract (50 mg/kg i.p. for three days) was able to elicit tolerance to a subsequent test injection (150 mg/kg) that was close to the ED_{50}. Since tolerance was observed at the first test dose, it was assumed to be physiological tolerance. Kava resin (liposoluble) decreased spontaneous motility and caused a loss of muscle control. A minimally effective daily dose of kava resin (100 mg/kg) over seven weeks failed to elicit tolerance to a weekly test dose of 166 mg/kg. When the daily dose of resin was increased to 150 mg/kg b.i.d., partial tolerance to the test doses occurred within three weeks, but very little further tolerance was observed over an additional two weeks. In an attempt to induce behavioral (learned) tolerance, daily injections of the resin (166 mg/kg i.p.) for three weeks failed to produce tolerance.

Neurological, Psychological, and Behavioral Functions

Neurotoxicity/Neuroprotection

Backhauss and Krieglstein (1992) investigated the neuroprotective effects of kava and its constituents, kavain, dihydrokavain, methysticin, dihydromethysticin, and yangonin, on cerebral ischemic damage in mice and rats. Kava extract was administered orally, while individual kava-lactones were administered i.p. Effects were compared with the anticonvulsant memantine. Kava extract (150 mg/kg p.o., 1 h prior to ischemia), methysticin, and dihydromethysticin (10 and 30 mg/kg i.p., 15 min prior to ischemia) significantly diminished the infarct area in mouse brains and the infarct volume in rat brains. The effects of the kava extract and both compounds were comparable to memantine (20 mg/kg i.p., 30 min prior to ischemia). All other compounds tested failed to reduce the infarct area in mouse brains. The researchers concluded that kava extract exhibited neuroprotective activity, probably mediated by the constituents methysticin and dihydromethysticin.

Receptor- and Neurotransmitter-Mediated Functions

Many of the extant studies have focused on the pharmacological activity of one or more isolated kavalactones (Grunze et al., 2001). For example, Gleitz and colleagues (Gleitz, Friese, et al., 1996; Gleitz, Beile, et al., 1996) investigated the activity of (+/–)-kavain, a synthetic kavalactone, on voltage-dependent Ca^{2+} and Na^+ ion channels in synaptosomes prepared from rat cerebral cortex. They reported that (+/–)-kavain dose-dependently inhibited the release of calcium, sodium, and glutamate from 4-aminopyridine-stimulated synaptosomes. The compound also weakly displaced binding (Ki = 2mM) of [^{3}H]-batrachotoxin but not [^{3}H]-saxitoxin. Grunze et al. (2001) found kavalactones exhibit weak antagonistic activity on Na+ currents and pronounced antagonistic activity on L-type Ca^{2+} channels. (+/–)-Kavain showed no inhibition of long-term potentiation, indicating a lack of cognitive side effects. However, a kava extract (uncharacterized, Krewel Meuselbach GmbH, Eitorf, Germany) was active. Although this in vitro finding is indicative of potential cognitive side effects, such effects require confirmation in animals and humans.

Others have examined the interactions of kava extracts and individual kavalactones on $GABA_A$, $GABA_B$, and benzodiazepine receptors. Jussofie et al. (1994) examined the effects of kava extracts on $GABA_A$ receptors labeled with [^{3}H]-muscimol in different regions of rat brain; kava extract enhanced the binding of [^{3}H]-muscimol in the hippocampus, amygdala, and medulla oblongata, an effect due to an increase in the density of [^{3}H]-muscimol binding sites, rather than a change in the affinity. Inclusion of pentobarbital or hexobarbital produced synergetic rather than additive effects. By contrast, Davies et al. (1992) observed only weak interactions of kavalactones and kava resin on binding to $GABA_A$ receptors, no effect on binding to $GABA_B$ receptors, and weak effects only on [^{3}H]-diazepam-labeled binding sites. In animal studies, Davies et al. (1992) reported similar results ex vivo with kavalactones (i.p.) and in binding studies in which kavalactones failed to influence in vivo CNS binding of the benzodiazepine receptor ligand, [^{3}H]-Ro15-1788.

Binding of kava extracts to neuroreceptors was examined by Dinh et al. (2001) using methanolic extracts of the roots and leaves of four different cultivars of kava. The leaf extracts displayed more potent binding inhibition than the root extracts to $GABA_A$ receptors (IC_{50} 3 µg/mL versus 5-87 µg/mL), and also far more potently inhibited binding to dopamine D_2, histamine (H_1 and H_2), and opioid (γ and δ) receptors (IC_{50}s 1-100 mg/mL versus $100 \geq$ g/L), regardless of a generally lower concentration of kavalactones compared to the root. However, neither the root nor leaf extracts showed anything but weak binding to benzodiazepine and serotonin receptors (5-HT_6 and 5-HT_7), and the leaf extracts of the individual cultivars showed marked differences in binding activities for each of the receptors. These results indicate the presence of active substances in the leaves, which remain to be elucidated.

Kavain and dihydromethysticin were shown to decrease the amplitude of field potential changes in guinea pig hippocampus slices extracellularly treated with the serotonin agonist ipsapirone (Bayer AG, Leverkusen, Germany), an experimental antidepressant and anxiolytic agent. The effect was dose dependent and significant in a range of concentrations corresponding to previously estimated steady-state/therapeutic concentrations of kava pyrones (50-150 μmol/L). After 45 min the effect was completely reversible. The results of the experiment indicate that dihydromethysticin and kavain may elicit anxiolytic effects through modulation of serotonin$_{1A}$ receptors (Walden et al., 1997). Serdarevic et al. (2001) examined the acute effects of a kava extract (LI 158, 30% kavalactones) on the neurotransmitter levels of mice. Administered at doses of 250 and 500 mg/kg p.o., only the higher dose produced a significant decrease in dopamine levels and although it appeared to cause an insignificant decrease in serotonin levels, levels of the serotonin metabolite 5-hydroxyindolacetic acid (5HIAA) levels were significantly enhanced. Norepinephrine (NE) levels remained unchanged, as did levels of homovanillic acid (HVA), and 3,4-dihydroxyphenyl-acetic acid (DOPAC). By comparison, an extract of St. John's wort (LI 160) had no effect on NE levels, caused a significant increase in brain levels of HVA, DOPAC, and 5HIAA, and also slightly decreased dopamine levels, again, only from the higher dose. These results indicate that compared to the St. John's wort extract, the kava extract is only a weak antidepressant and/or modifier of brain neurotransmitter concentrations in the mouse.

Reversible inhibition of human platelet MAO-B derived from healthy volunteers was shown by Uebelhack et al. (1998) both from a kava extract (Krewel Meuselbach, GmbH, Eitorf, Germany, 67.6% kava pyrones) and synthetic kava pyrones. In intact platelets, kava pyrones methysticin and desmethoxyyangonin were effective inhibitors of MAO-B, inhibiting activity by 49% and 58%, respectively. Kavain and dihydrokavain were weakly active (MAO-B inhibition 12% and 22%, respectively). The kava extract produced an IC_{50} of 24 μM, which was a lower concentration than the IC_{50} of either desmethoxyyangonin (28.1 μM) or methysticin (39.5 μM), twice as potent as the tricyclic antidepressant imipramine, and equipotent to the MAO-A inhibitor brofaromine and the tricyclic antidepressant amitriptyline. In disrupted platelets, methysticin and desmethoxyyangonin were more potent inhibitors of MAO-B than tricyclic antidepressants and brofaromine. Comparative tests with deprenyl showed a nearly complete restoration of MAO-B activity from methysticin and the kava extract after incubation for 10 min, indicating that their effect is both reversible and short acting. Unpublished results of a clinical study found MAO-B activity reduced by 26% to 34% in three patients receiving kava pyrones (Antares brand, 120, 120-240 mg daily for 21-28 days). The researchers called for further studies in order to determine the contribution of MAO-B inhibition by kava extract and kava pyrones to anxiolytic activity.

Baum et al. (1998) found that in rats, kava extract (20 mg/kg i.p.) caused a significant increase in extraneuronal levels of dopamine ($p = 0.024$), and that higher doses resulted in greater increases (e.g., 120 mg/kg i.p.; $p = 0.0001$). Yet concentrations of DOPAC, a dopamine metabolite, were not affected, from dosages of less than 220 mg/kg i.p. Curiously, approximately half the animals also showed an increase in extracellular 5-hydroxytryptamine (or 5-hydroxy-3-indoleacetic acid), while the remaining rats showed either no change or a decrease in levels. Various kava pyrones also produced dopaminergic effects, with D,L-kavain increasing levels of dopamine for 8 h from a single dose (30 mg/kg i.p.), and yangonin reducing levels (120 mg/kg i.p.). Baum and colleagues concluded that the dopaminergic neuron-activating effect of kava extract demonstrated in rats appears to having a ceiling, which is likely owing to the potent dopamine-antagonist activity of yangonin, a relatively minor constituent of kava extract. They also concluded that the presence of yangonin could serve to "prevent the abuse of high doses of the extract" and that because of the activity-reducing effect of yangonin on neurons containing dopamine, ingesting high doses of kava extract will inhibit euphoric actions beyond those already produced. Whether such effects are produced from oral dosages remains to be determined.

Kava extract and a synthetic kavalactone, D,L-kavain, have shown synergistic actions on sedation in the mouse (Capasso and Calignano, 1988). Extracts of kava containing 7% kavapyrones administered to mice in combination with D,L-kavain (in a ratio of 1:0.12, 10 mL/kg i.p.) significantly reduced their spontaneous mobility. By contrast, 200 mg of D,L-kavain alone failed to cause a significant sedative reaction, and higher doses of kava extract alone (> 50 mg/kg i.p.) were needed to elicit a reduction in motility similar to that of the combination treatment. Neither kava extract alone (100 mg/kg i.p., 7 mg/kg kavapyrones) or D,L-kavain (12 mg/kg i.p.) were effective in reducing amphetamine-induced (s.c.) hypermotility, but the combination of extract and D,L-kavain at these doses caused hypermotility to be significantly reduced by 60.2%.

It has long been known that chewing the root produces a numbing effect on the tongue (Hänsel, 1968). Jamieson and Duffield (1990a) assessed the analgesic effects of kava extracts and kavalactones in mice. Both the aqueous and lipid-soluble extracts of kava displayed antinociceptive activity, as did 4/8 kavalactones assayed. The active lipid soluble fraction (150 mg/kg i.p.) markedly increased the tail-flick response latency (from 8 s to 40-50 s), while the aqueous extract (250 mg/kg i.p.) increased response latency from about 10-19 s. Purified kavalactones were available in limited amounts, so it was not possible to establish dose-response relationships. Instead, these compounds were tested at varying doses determined to be approximately equivalent based on a subjective assessment of the degree of sedation and loss of motor control and muscle tone. Of the compounds tested, kavain, dihydrokavain, methysticin, and dihydromethysticin showed the most potent analgesic properties. Peak analgesic effects were similar in all compounds, but the time course of action differed markedly. Thus, compared to saline-treated controls, dihydrokavain (150 mg/kg i.p.) displayed peak analgesia on tail-flick reaction time at 10 and 15 min after injection; kavain-treated mice (300 mg/kg i.p.) showed significant effects 10 and 70 min after injection; dihydromethysticin-treated animals (275 mg/kg i.p.) displayed significant differences from controls at 10 and 210 min after injection; and methysticin-treated animals (360 mg/kg i.p.) showed significant analgesia at 10 and 30-240 min, and hyperanalgesia at 330-360 min. Kava resin (200 mg/kg p.o.) significantly reduced acetic acid-induced writhing. The resin was not administered i.p. because of difficulties with the saline-cremefor vehicle by this route. The aqueous extract was inactive on oral administration but dramatically reduced writhing from 250 mg/kg i.p., 55 min before acetic acid. Treatment with naloxone, an opiate antagonist, failed to block the analgesic effects of the lipid-soluble and aqueous-soluble extracts, indicating that the antinociceptive effects of kava extract are not mediated via opiate receptors.

CLINICAL STUDIES

The bulk of clinical investigations on the human psychopharmacology of kava extracts and its constituents have focused on their anxiolytic properties. Standardized kava extract products cause brain wave changes similar to those of antianxiety drugs but do not produce tolerance or dependence. Other studies have investigated the effect of kava on cognitive functions and have addressed the interactions between kava and ethanol.

Immune Disorders; Inflammation and Disease

Cancer

Cancer prevention. Steiner (2000) examined the cancer incidence rates of the Pacific Islands from the 1980s and the most accurate records of kava consumption for the same areas and period; Steiner found a correlation between rates of kava consumption in the male population and their cancer incidence suggestive of a cancer chemopreventive effect of kava. The correlations were based on male consumption rates of kava because they are known to be more consistent than for women in the Pacific Islands and because the percentage of women and men who consume kava is largely unknown. The highest rates of cancer on the islands were found where the rate of kava consumption was lowest, and vice versa. In New Caledonia, where the rate of yearly kava consumption was only 0.6 kg/person, the cancer incidence in the 1980s was 182/100,000 males. In Fiji, the rate of cancer per 100,000 males was 75 and the consumption of kava was 2.8 kg/person per year. In Vanuatu, the incidence of cancer was the lowest in all of Polynesia (70.9/100,000 males) and the yearly rate of kava consumption was the highest (6.7 kg/person). In areas of Polynesia where kava consumption is now uncommon (Hawaii, New Zealand, and French Polynesia), the incidence of cancer is normal among the indigenous people. The countries with the highest rates of kava consumption (Fiji, Vanuatu, and Western Samoa) also showed lower rates of cancer among the males than among the females. Steiner is of the opinion that kava causes men to consume less tobacco and that this accounted for the difference in cancer incidence.

Neurological, Psychological, and Behavioral Disorders

Psychological and Behavioral Disorders

Anxiety. Pittler and Ernst (2000) conducted a meta-analysis and systematic review of trials on the efficacy of kava extract in the treatment of anxiety. Out of 14 double-blind, randomized controlled trials, seven met their inclusion criteria (Kinzler et al., 1991; Lehmann, 1998; Singh et al., 1997; Volz and Kieser, 1997; Warnecke, 1991; Warnecke et al., 1990). From those, the researchers concluded that the data suggest kava extract is efficacious as a symptomatic treatment for anxiety compared with placebo, that it is relatively safe, and that more rigorous inquiries into the risk-benefit relation of the treatment are warranted (Pittler and Ernst, 2000). Malsch and Kieser (2001) reported that administration of a kava extract (WS 1490) at increasing daily doses (50-300 mg p.o. for 36 days) in 40 outpatients of either sex (ages 21-75) tapering off benzodiazepines over a period of two weeks caused a further lessening of symptoms of anxiety compared to placebo. The trial was randomized, placebo-controlled, and double-blinded, with parallel treatment groups and included an intention-to-treat analysis. The patients had been diagnosed and treated for simple phobia ($n = 11$), generalized anxiety disorder ($n = 13$), and social phobia ($n = 14$). No significant side effects were found compared to placebo from the kava extract. The only side effects noted were attributable to benzodiazepine withdrawal. The researchers concluded that kava extract can be safely and efficaciously used to help anxiety patients replace treatment with benzodiazepines.

Volz and Kieser (1997) conducted a six-month, double-blind clinical study with kava extract (WS 1490, 300 mg daily, equivalent to 210 mg kavalactones daily) in 100 outpatients who were diagnosed according to the DSM-III-R criteria with tension, anxiety, and excitation. The randomized, placebo-controlled multicenter study was restricted to patients aged 18 or older diagnosed with a Hamilton Anxiety Scale (HAM-A) score of greater than 18, all of whom had adaptation disorders, agoraphobia, generalized anxiety, or a simple form of social phobia. HAM-A subscores provided secondary variables for psychic anxiety and for somatic anxiety, and the Clinical Global Impression scale (CGI), the sensitivity scale (Bf-S), and the Hopkins Symptoms Checklist (SCL-90-R) provided further target variables. After two months, patients in the kava group showed significant changes compared to their baseline readings at the start of the study ($p = 0.055$), and at the end the results were even more significant ($p = 0.0015$). Volz and Kieser reported that tolerance was excellent and that in the scores of anxiety, compulsivity, and depression, the kava extract produced clearly significant benefits. Although scores on the sensitivity scale were not as clear, the HAM-A subscores for both psychic anxiety and somatic anxiety were significantly improved.

Lehmann et al. (1996) conducted a placebo-controlled double-blind study of kava extract in patients with anxiety syndromes not due to mental disorders in a group of 29 patients (kava extract WS 1490 Laitan, 100 mg, t.i.d. or a placebo preparation). Therapeutic efficacy was assessed at one, two, and four weeks of treatment with the Hamilton Anxiety Scale, the Adjectives Check List, and the Clinical Global Impression Scale. The HAM-A scale, which scores overall anxiety symptomatology, revealed a significant reduction in anxiety in the kava group versus the control group after one week; the differences between the groups increased over the course of the study. Subscales of the HAM-A scale measuring "mental anxiety" and "somatic anxiety" showed similarly significant reductions. The Adjectives Check List, a self-assessment scale, is subdivided into groups measuring performance-oriented activation, general deactivation, extra-introversion, general well-being, emotional irritation, and anxiety/depression. Under this measure compared to placebo, performance-activation increased markedly with kava, while self-assessed anxiety/depression was significantly reduced. The other subscales showed no change. Under the Clinical Global Impression (CGI) scale, a physician-assessed scale which measures the severity of disease, symptoms decreased more significantly in the kava-treated group—rated at four (only slightly ill), versus six (markedly ill) in the majority of the placebo group. After treatment, 15 patients in the kava group were rated as no longer ill or only slightly ill versus only five patients in the placebo group. No adverse drug reactions were observed during the course of treatment, and the use/risk index was judged as good. The researchers concluded that WS 1490 was suitable for general practitioners to use in treating anxiety, tension, and excitedness.

Woelk et al. (1993) compared the efficacy and tolerance of a kava extract (WS 1490, 100 mg 3 t.i.d.) to bromazepam (3 mg t.i.d.) and oxazepam (5 mg t.i.d.) in a six-week randomized reference–substance-controlled double-blind study in 172 outpatients (ages 18-65) diagnosed with anxiety, tension, and agitation of nonpsychotic origin. The encapsulated medications were indistinguishable in size, color, taste, odor, and form. Although six tests were used to assess the outcome, the main target of the study was a change in the HAM-A score, which was over 18 in all the patients at the start of the trial. According to the CGI scale, on average, 80% of the patients had moderate to clear illness for up to six months. Active treatment commenced following a one-week no-medication washout phase. The results showed a drop in the HAM-A score in each medication group during the first week and until the end of the treatment period at week six. No significant difference was evident between the three groups when HAM-A scores were compared, although physician assessments indicated bromazepam was less effective than either the kava extract or oxazepam, and the improvements in anxiety were "mild to clear" in most patients in all three groups. According to the CGI, 19% of the kava group were markedly improved, compared to 17% in the bromazepam group and 20% in the oxazepam group. A "comprehensive" improvement was seen in 3% of the kava and bromazepam groups compared to 5% in the oxazepam group, and a mild improvement was found in 23% of the kava group, 27% of the bromazepam group, and 25% of the oxazepam group. No improvement was found in 10% of the kava and the bromazepam groups, compared to 2% of the oxazepam group. According to the Erlanger Scale for anxiety, aggression, and tension (EAAS), scores changed during the six-week treatment period by –10 in the kava group, –11 in the oxazepam group, and –13 in the bromazepam group. The slightly greater improvement in anxiety in the latter group was attributed primarily to improvements in somatic anxiety in week six. The physicians judged the three different treatments to be of comparably low risk. Based on the results of this study and those of previous controlled investigations, Woelk and colleagues (1993) concluded that the kava extract should be considered as an option in the treatment of anxiety, agitation, and tension of nonpsychotic origin.

Kinzler et al. (1991) studied the short-term effect of kava extract (WS 1490) on anxiety syndrome not resulting from psychotic disorders in 58 patients composed of men and women ages 18-60. The randomized, double-blind, placebo-controlled clinical trial ran for four weeks with a dosage of one capsule (100 mg) t.i.d., or matching placebo. The main inclusion criteria was a Hamilton Anxiety Scale (HAM-A) of more than 18 points and this was used as the main target variable in the outcome. All drugs that could affect the outcome were excluded from the trial and any patients taking such medications complied with a minimum passage of five half-life periods per drug prior to starting the trial. Exclusion criteria included, among others, suicidal tendencies, endogenous depression, dementia syndrome, schizophrenic forms of psychoses, organic psychoses, psychopathy, severe diseases affecting the circulatory system, heart, liver, lungs, or kidneys, neoplasma, and pregnancy. Mean Hamilton scores taken after one week showed a difference between the two groups, with the kava extract group showing a lower score in contrast to placebo. The researchers reported that the difference was statistically significant ($p < 0.01$) at the three examination intervals. In the Hamilton subscale for psychic anxiety, the median score after the four-week treatment had dropped by nearly half in the kava group versus 20% in the placebo group. The Hamilton subscore for somatic anxiety also showed a drop of nearly 50% versus nearly 10% in the placebo group. These group differences were statistically significant ($p < 0.01$). In both the median values of self-evaluated activity related to achievement and anxiety/depression, the decrease was more progressive in the kava group compared to the placebo, and a statistically significant result occurred in the group differences ($p < 0.05$). Although in other aspects of the Adjectives Check List no difference was seen between kava and placebo, the Clinical Global Impression scale (CGI) evaluating severity of illness also showed a greater decrease in the kava group. After 28 days, only four members of the kava group showed "slight illness" whereas most of the placebo group remained "clearly ill." At the end of the trial, 15 patients in the kava group showed no illness or slight illness versus five in the placebo group. By the trial end, four patients had dropped out from the kava group while two left the placebo group for reasons deduced as more likely incidental than owing to adverse effects, of which none were reported during the treatment period. The researchers concluded that their study helped to confirm that the kava extract shows "good tolerability" and that it can be applied in the treatment of anxiety syndrome "in general practice" (Kinzler et al., 1991).

In a placebo-controlled, double-blind clinical trial, Lindenberg and Pitule-Schodel (1990) compared the efficacy of D,L-kavain (Neuronika) and oxazepam in 38 outpatients, men and women (ages 18-60), diagnosed with anxiety associated with psychosomatic or neurotic disturbances. Anxiety Status Inventory (ASI) scores were at least 40 and among them, 25 patients were abusers of illicit drugs. Medications were allowed that posed no effect on neurotic or psychosomatic symptoms and would not interfere with the activity of D,L-kavain. The treatments consisted of 200 mg D,L-kavain t.i.d. plus two capsules of placebo/day, or one capsule of placebo plus one capsule of oxazepam (10 mg) daily for 28 days. Anxiolytic effectiveness was assessed by the ASI and the Self-Rating Anxiety Scale (SAS) of Zung. According to the ASI results, the test substances were equivalent in the nature and potency of their anxiolytic actions. Attending physician assessments showed good results for 45% and "very good" results for 55% of the D,L-kavain patients. For the oxazepam patients, the results were 29% and 71%, respectively. No adverse reactions were observed in either treatment group. In discussing these results, the researchers mention the fact that because D,L-kavain has been shown in animal studies to be "practically nontoxic," their findings are especially encouraging because suicidal use of this agent would not pose the same risk of benzodiazepine toxicity.

Receptor- and Neurotransmitter-Mediated Functions

Münte et al. (1993) investigated the effects of kava extract WS 1490, oxazepam, and placebo on behavior and event-related potentials (ERPs) in a word-recognition memory task structured as a double-blind crossover study in 12 healthy volunteers. Subjects received either placebo, kava extract WS 1490 (200 mg t.i.d. for five days prior to the study), or oxazepam (15 mg on the day before the testing, 75 mg on the day of testing). In the word-recognition test, oxazepam elicited a pronounced slowing of reaction time and a reduction in the number of correct responses, while from kava a nonsignificant increase in the number of correct responses was observed. The behavioral indices indicated a greatly impaired performance after oxazepam and an enhanced memory performance following kava. In the ERP measurements, the task was to identify within a list of visually presented words those shown for the first time and those repeated. Oxazepam was associated with a significantly decreased recognition rate, while kava caused a slightly increased recognition rate. The ERPs to the new words were virtually identical under the placebo treatment, but the correctly recognized old words showed an enhanced positivity compared to placebo. Thus, the old/new effect was largest in the kava condition, which was also associated with the best recognition behavior. Münte and colleagues (1993) reported that differences in the ERP patterns indicated a deficiency in the generation of an internal code for the word stimuli in the case of oxazepam, and in the case of kava an influence on later stages related to conscious recollection.

Prescott et al. (1993) assigned 24 subjects (11 male, 13 female) to receive a mixture of kava and fruit juice (500 mL of a 0.2 g/mL infusion mixed with 500 mL fruit juice) or fruit juice alone who were then subjected to various measurements of cognitive performance, physiological functions, and mood. Subjects receiving kava reported subjective feelings of intoxication, which was also reflected in a higher level of body sway. However, a high degree of individual variation in feelings of intoxication occurred which the investigators attributed to variations in the content of active kavalactones as well as to variations in the range of body weights in the subjects. Although in the cognitive performance tests a tendency toward impaired functions in the group receiving kava occurred (Sternberg memory scanning task, simple reaction times, choice reaction times, tracking, and divided attention), the results were not statistically significantly different compared to placebo, a failure attributed to an inadequate sample size. No differences were found between the kava and the control group in measurements of various physiological parameters, including respiration rate, heart rate, blood pressure, or stress levels, suggesting but not confirming that these measures were not influenced by the kava.

Saletu and co-workers (1989) investigated the encephalotropic and psychotropic effects of synthetic kavain compared to the benzodiazepine clobazam in a placebo-controlled double-blind study in 15 healthy volunteers. Subjects received, at weekly intervals, randomized doses of either placebo, 200, 400, or 600 mg kavain, or 30 mg clobazam as reference compound. Kavain induced pharmaco-EEG changes consisting of a dose-dependent increase of Delta, Theta, and Alpha-1 activity, while Alpha-2, Beta activity, and the centroid of the total activity decreased. These results indicated a sedative effect, which differed from that of Clobazam. Clobazam produced a decrease of Delta, Theta, Alpha 1, and Alpha 2 and an increase of Beta activity, while the centroid was accelerated. At the lowest dose (200 mg p.o.), kavain induced a decrease of Delta and Beta activity, an increase of Alpha activity and of total power, and showed vigilance-promoting effects. Psychometric investigations also showed clear differences between the two compounds. Kavain at all three doses produced a significant improvement in intellectual performance (Pauli test), attention, concentration, reaction time, and motor speed; opposite findings were observed after clobazam. At the lowest dose (200 mg p.o.), kavain produced improvements in variables such as drive, wakefulness, affectivity, mood, and well-being compared to placebo, while 600 mg kavain produced sedation, as did 30 mg clobazam. Time efficacy measurements demonstrated a pharmacodynamic peak in the first to second hour for kavain and a second peak at the eighth hour; clobazam produced a maximal central effect in the first hour, declining thereafter and showing a second peak at the sixth hour. Topographically, most encephalotropic effects after kavain were found in the frontal areas, and after clobazam in the central and parietal areas. Evaluations of pulse, blood pressure, and side effects showed good tolerability of both compounds, with 30 mg clobazam producing more sedation than kavain (Saletu et al., 1989).

Russell et al. (1987) assessed the effects of a low dose of kava on alertness; speed of access of information from long-term memory was assessed in nine healthy Caucasian volunteers, using a low dose (30 g kava root infused in water, final volume 250 mL) and a high dose (1 g/kg kava in 500 mL water). Subjects were instructed to indicate by pressing a key as quickly as possible without making errors whether a pair of letters displayed on a screen were the same or different. Software controlled the presented stimuli, time intervals, measured reaction times, and feedback on time and errors, with warning times of 60, 100, 200, 500, and 1,000 milliseconds. Neither the low nor the high doses of kava had any discernable effect on the speed with which information was accessed from long-term memory or on the time and course of alertness, and kava did not bring about a general slowing of response. The researchers concluded that in this experimental paradigm, kava had no apparent effect on cognitive functions; they suggested that due to its lack of impact on human performance, kava is preferable to alcohol as a beverage to be consumed on social occasions (Russell et al., 1987).

Reproductive Disorders

Menopause

In a randomized double-blind study, Warnecke (1991) assessed the efficacy of WS 1490 in a group of 20 female patients experiencing climacteric-related (menopausal) symptomatology in comparison to a placebo-treated control group. Patients received a kava extract (WS 1490, 100 mg t.i.d. for eight weeks) or a placebo. The HAM-A overall scale of anxiety was used for assessment and revealed a significant difference between the treatments. After one week of treatment, the HAM-A score decreased by 50% in the kava group compared to the placebo group ($p < 0.001$). By week eight the difference was still significant ($p < 0.0005$). Other parameters, such as depressive mood (DSI), subjective well-being (patient diary), severity of disease (CGI), and climacteric symptomatology (Kupperman Index and Schneider Scale) demonstrated a high level of efficacy of the kava extract in treating psychosomatic and neurovegetative symptoms, which was also associated with "very good tolerance of the preparation." Climacteric discomfort indicated in patient-reported changes (Kupperman Index) were "slight to moderate" before treatment and absent in the kava group after four weeks. The descriptive difference between placebo and kava extract in this score was significant ($p < 0.01$). Side effects reported by four patients in the placebo group and six in the kava group (tremors, fatigue, restlessness, and stomach pressure) were judged unlikely due to the kava extract. As for dropouts, by weeks six and seven, seven had left the placebo group, two from the kava group, all of whom complained that the treatment they received provided no benefit. De Leo et al. (2001) reported similar results in a randomized placebo-controlled study in 40 women diagnosed with menopausal anxiety (18 surgical menopause and 22 physiological menopause) who were treated concomitantly with hormone replacement therapy and a kava extract (100 mg/day for six months). The kava extract (uncharacterized), which contained 55% kavain, caused a more significant reduction in the HAM-A score ($p < 0.05$) than HRT, which was noticeable after therapy for three and six months.

DOSAGE

In traditional contexts, average daily intakes of kavalactones are often considerably in excess of the amounts recommended in European phyto-medicines. Since the kavalactone content of various cultivars consumed in traditional beverages can vary widely, it is difficult to arrive at a reliable figure for the average daily intake of a Pacific Islander accustomed to use of the beverage. In Fiji, a coconut shell of kava (approximately 100 mL) contains approximately 250 mg of kavalactones, and it is not uncommon for two or three shells' worth to be consumed over the course of an evening. In Vanuatu, however, the kava employed is considerably more potent, and a 100 mL serving may contain up to 1,000 mg of kavalactones (Kilham, 1996). Lebot confirms this estimate for Vanuatan kava (Lebot et al., 1997).

The majority of clinical studies have utilized a standardized kava root extract containing 70% kavalactones, with a customary dose of 100 mg t.i.d. in capsules providing a total of 210 mg kavalactones per day. This dose is effective for most anxiolytic applications, while somewhat higher doses may be used for sedation (up to 600 mg kavalactones) (Dentali, 1997). In the United States, kava root extracts have commonly been standardized to contain 30% to 40% kavalactones, with a suggested daily dosage of 150-750 mg, or 50-250 kavalactones/day (Flynn and Roest, 1995). More recently, the American Herbal Products Association (AHPA) issued recommendations stating that daily intake should not exceed 210 mg kavalactones. Erring on the side of caution, the German Commission E recommended a somewhat lower amount: only 60-120 mg kavalactones per day (in the treatment of stress, restlessness, and anxiety) and not for longer than three months "without medical advice" (Blumenthal et al., 1998). However, this dosage was based on the use of a thin-layer chromatography (TLC) method to measure kavalactone content. By HPLC methods, which have largely replaced the TLC method, the equivalent amounts are approximately 95-190 mg kavalactones (Gaedcke, 2000).

By one estimate, and despite their poor solubility in water, 60-120 mg of the main kavalactones is approximately half the amount found in a "standard bowl" of the traditional kava drink prepared from 100 g of the powdered root. In this instance, the beverage was found to contain about 240 mg of the main kavalactones/100 mL (Duve and Prasad, 1984). Whitton (2001) calculated that a water extract of kava root contained 2.97% kavalactones; an ethanol or acetone extract, 100%; and a 25% ethanol extract, 15%.

A number of different chemotypes have been characterized based on the differing levels and ratios of the major kavalactones (Lebot and Lévesque, 1989; Lebot et al., 1999). Therefore, because kava extract products may have differing effects depending on the proportions of individual kavalactones present from the source chemotype plant used, particular extract products tested in clinical trials offer the most assurity of efficacy and safety.

SAFETY PROFILE

A postmarketing surveillance study of kava extract conducted in Europe in 1992 involved over 3,000 patients who received a dosage equivalent to 120-240 mg/day and 105 mg kavalactones. Adverse reactions occurred in 2.3% of patients (Pittler and Ernst, 2000). An observational study of 4,049 patients who had taken a standardized kava extract (70% kavalactones) at a dosage of 105 mg/day for a period of seven weeks found the incidence of "objectionable side effects" was 1.5% (61 patients) (Schulz et al., 2001).

Kavalactones are relatively nontoxic, as indicated by the fact that efficacious doses are in the 100-600 mg range, but quantities of kava beverage equivalent to several grams of kavalactones are commonly consumed in traditional context. Therefore, it is unlikely that acute toxicity would be approached, even with excess use. The question of possible long-term toxicity resulting from excess use is another matter, as indicated by the study of Mathews et al. (1988). It may be for these reasons that the German Commission E recommended that continuous use of kava should not exceed three months (Blumenthal et al., 1998).

Contraindications

Anxiety is frequently accompanied by depression; under some circumstances (e.g., in the female climacteric) the anxiolytic actions of kava may help to alleviate depression (Warnecke, 1991). However, the German Commission E contraindicates kava for "endogenous depression" (Blumenthal et al., 1998). This precaution may be traced to the sedative effect in rodents of certain kavalactones (dehydrokavain and dihydromethysticin) and kava resin, and to the antiserotonin activity displayed by the resin and certain kavalactones (demethoxyyangonin and dihydromethysticin) in isolated rat uterus. Levels of endogenous serotonin in the brains of rats administered dihydromethysticin or water-soluble fractions of the root (i.p.) showed no change up to one hour after (Buckley et al., 1967). It remains that the water-soluble constituents of kava root are scarcely known (Lebot et al., 1997) and that whereas after seven weeks administration of kava resin (100 mg/kg i.p.), which largely contains kavalactones, physiological tolerance in mice was absent, tolerance did develop in mice administered a kavalactone-free water extract (50 mg/kg i.p.) after three days (Duffield and Jamieson, 1991).

Drug Interactions

According to the German Commission E monograph on kava (Blumenthal et al., 1998) and *The Botanical Safety Handbook* (McGuffin et al., 1997), the effects of kava may become potentiated if it is taken with alcohol, barbiturates, or other psychopharmacological agents. In view of the potential for adverse interactions and an incomplete understanding of the pharmacology of kavalactones, this caution is probably justified.

Numerous herbal combination products formulated with kava extract are available in Europe. For example, Reynolds (1996) lists proprietary products containing saw palmetto, horsetail, hydrangea, and kava (bladder discomfort), artichoke and kava (biliary disorders/dyspepsia), corn silk and kava (bladder discomfort), valerian, hops, passion flower, and kava (nervous disorders), yarrow and kava (anxiety/nervous tension), passion flower and kava (sleep disorders), and a product containing St. John's wort and kava for menopausal disorders, dystonia, migraine, nocturnal enuresis, hypertension, and psychiatric disorders. Brown (1997) comments that central nervous system-affecting herbs such as St. John's wort, passion flower, and valerian have not been clinically tested in combination with kava extracts and is of the opinion that such combinations be avoided.

In Germany, Strahl et al. (1998) reported a case of recurring necrotizing hepatitis, confirmed with a liver biopsy, in a woman aged 39 who had taken kava extract. Along with the extract (providing 60 mg of kavalactones), which also contained St. John's wort, she was taking a synthetic antidepressant (paroxetine, 20 mg/day) plus ethinylestradiol and desogestrel. Although she had a history of acute hepatitis with recurrences, metabolic, autoimmune, and viral causes were eliminated in the investigation; when she stopped taking the herbal supplements, her liver function "quickly became normal." Strahl et al. (1998) concluded that because the recovery of normal liver function was so rapid after cessation of the herbal preparation, it was the most plausible cause of the recurrence of acute hepatitis.

In Italy, Donadio et al. (2000) reported a case of myoglobinuria in a male weight trainer (age 29) who had recently returned to weight training with "mild and progressive" exercises after a two-year break and was taking an herbal product containing kava (100 mg), guaraná (500 mg), and *Ginkgo biloba* (200 mg) per 1 g flacon. Although tests ruled out an underlying myopathy, they showed abnormally high levels of myoglobin (10,000 ng/mL) (normal 0-90 ng/mL) and blood creatine kinase. Renal complications were absent despite the dark coloration of his urine; after discontinuing use of the product, the "diffuse severe muscle pain" he experienced gradually subsided over a period of six weeks. The researchers believe it is probable that this case was the result of a combination of neuromuscular blocking and dopamine antagonistic effects of kava and methylxanthine effects of guaraná acting in concert. Although admitting that other etiologies beside the use of the herbal product may be involved, they based this theory on the fact that in high doses, methylxanthines (such as caffeine, theophylline, and theobromine found in guaraná, *Paullinia cupana* Kunth) can cause myoglobinuria and induce contraction of muscles, and that antidopaminergic agents may cause a myoglobinuria-associated disorder known as neuroleptic malignant syndrome.

A possible case of toxicity from an additive effect of kava and the benzodiazepine alprazolam was reported by Almeida et al. (1996) in which a 54-year-old man became semicomatose. In addition to his regular medications of terazosin (an α-adrenergic blocker), cimetidine (a histamine$_2$ receptor antagonist), and alprazolam, the patient had been taking a kava product as a "natural tranquilizer" for three days. He insisted that he had followed the recommended dosage for the kava supplement and alprazolam. He was admitted to a hospital in a disorientated and lethargic state, and in several hours became "more alert." Tests showed a negative alcohol level and vital signs were normal. Cartledge (2001) reported adverse reactions in a 52-year-old female patient taking flunitrazepam after she added kava for three weeks. Thirty-six hours after stopping the kava, she developed a confused state and was admitted to the hospital where she presented with a disoriented state, irritability, agitation, and was wearing her dress inside out. With treatment (diazepam 5 mg and droperidol 10 mg each, b.i.d.) complete resolution of symptoms followed after 48 hours.

In a placebo-controlled double-blind study in 20 healthy volunteers, Herberg (1993) examined the effect of a standardized kava extract (WS 1490, 100 mg, t.i.d. over eight days) on various performance-related parameters alone and in combination with ethanol (0.05% blood alcohol concentration). The kava extract showed no negative multiplicative effects in combination with alcohol. On the contrary, in the concentration test on the fourth day, the kava extract plus ethanol-treated group performed significantly better than the ethanol only-treated group, indicating that the kava extract may counteract some of the performance-related deficits attributable to alcohol. These results are consistent with another study (Münte et al., 1993) in which kava extract was found to enhance word recognition and event-related potentials in a learning/memory test, while the benzodiazepine oxazepam reduced both parameters.

The results of the study by Herberg (1993) are in some contrast to those of a randomized placebo-controlled study by Foo and Lemon (1997) who used a crude kava extract. They examined the effects of combining kava with alcohol and compared it to a social dose of alcohol (0.75 g/kg), kava

(1 g/kg), or a placebo on cognitive and visuomotor performance and subjective measures of intoxication and impairment. The kava extract was prepared using a middle-grade kava powder from Fiji to which 500 mL of water was added and, after straining, yielded about 350 mL of kava liquid. Unsweetened orange juice was added to the test preparations of kava plus alcohol, kava alone, and alcohol alone. Forty subjects (20 men and 20 women) participated in a series of four trials. The results showed that the kava beverage alone had little if any effect on measured or perceived competence and that when combined with alcohol the kava beverage potentiated measured and perceived impairment caused by alcohol alone. In the visual search test, the kava and alcohol combination decreased performance even further; in the divided attention test, the combination produced a significantly larger decrease in performance compared to those taking the kava preparation alone. In the digit symbol coding test, both kava alone and combined with alcohol produced a negative effect. Self-reported levels of intoxication were increased when alcohol was combined with kava and unchanged when kava was taken alone. Alcohol alone had a negative effect on coordination, cognition, and sedation, which was potentiated when alcohol was combined with kava. However, the kava alone had no effect on sedation, intoxication, willingness to drive, or cognition. The researchers noted that feelings of minor to moderate intoxication were absent in those taking the kava preparation, which was in contrast to an earlier report by Prescott et al. (1993) and probably the result of a lower concentration of kava in the present study (Foo and Lemon, 1997).

A positive interaction between alcohol and kava resin on sleeping times in mice has been noted (Jamieson and Duffield, 1990b). In these experiments, kava resin suspended in 5% cremefor-EL in saline was administered at doses ranging from 200 to 700 mg/kg p.o. alone or in combination with ethanol (3.5 g/kg or 4 g/kg i.p.). Both kava resin and ethanol, administered separately, dose dependently increased sleeping time. Ethanol (4 g/kg i.p.) significantly potentiated the sleeping time induced by 300 mg/kg p.o. of kava resin alone—a dose that increased the toxicity of ethanol at 4 g/kg i.p., as it proved lethal to 3/6 mice in this dosage group. Combinations of resin and ethanol at higher doses were not tested, as ethanol alone was lethal at doses higher than 5 g/kg i.p. Similarly, ethanol caused a dose-dependent increase in the sleeping time of mice treated with kava resin. Combinations of ethanol and kava resin (1 g/kg i.p. and 350 or 450 mg/kg p.o., respectively) did not alter the sleeping times; however, at 350 mg/kg p.o. combined with 2 or 3 g of ethanol, it caused progressively greater prolongations of the mean sleeping time. Combinations of kava resin (450 mg/kg p.o.) and ethanol (2g/kg i.p.) were lethal to 3/5 mice, but kava resin alone was nonlethal at 600 mg/kg p.o. Thus, combinations of kava resin and ethanol produced very large increases in sleeping time resulting from relatively small increments in dose (e.g., a dose of 3 g/kg i.p. of ethanol, ineffective alone, caused a tenfold prolongation of sleeping time, equivalent to about 600 mg/kg of kava resin alone, when combined with kava resin in a minimally effective dose of 350 mg/kg p.o.). Similar small increments in the dose of ethanol greatly exacerbated its toxicity as measured by lethality. While 1.5 g/kg i.p. of ethanol combined with 450 mg/kg p.o. kava resin produced no significant prolongation of the sleeping time, 2.0 g/kg i.p. ethanol plus the same dose of kava resin was lethal in 3/5 mice (Jamieson and Duffield, 1990b).

The doses of kava resin used by Jamieson and Duffield (1990b) were, however, considerably greater than those commonly ingested, even by heavy users of kava. Among Aborigine populations in Darwin, Australia, heavy users consume approximately 440 grams of dried root per week, corresponding to 40-70 g of resin. Taking the larger of these numbers and converting to a daily dose, heavy users ingest approximately 10 g of resin daily, or 133.3 mg/kg per day, assuming an average body weight of 75 kg (Lebot et al., 1997).

Pregnancy and Lactation

The use of kava is contraindicated in pregnancy and lactation, according to the German Commission E monograph (Blumenthal et al., 1998). The *Botanical Safety Handbook* (McGuffin et al., 1997) also states that it should not be used by pregnant or lactating women. However, no specific documentation of use during pregnancy or lactation exists. Pharmacokinetic information indicated limited absorption of some kava constituents with both agonist and antagonist dopamine effects with intraperitoneal administration of kava constituents (see Pharmacokinetics). Ethnobotanical information indicates avoidance of kava to maintain fertility or during pregnancy but no conclusion regarding lactation can be made. Gutmanis (1976) provides some details of traditional use of kava and reproductive health in old Hawaii. In this society, high-ranking women did participate in kava drinking. Kava leaves were stuffed into the vagina to induce miscarriage. Gutmanis clearly states that women avoided any kava use immediately upon becoming pregnant, but is silent on whether breast-feeding women also followed a restriction of use (Gutmanis, 1976). According to conventional wisdom in other kava-drinking societies, kava renders women sterile and was used as an abortifacient. Laboratory investigations of kava on the fertility of male rats indicated no effects (Dam-Bakker et al., 1958). One authority posits that traditional prohibitions against the drinking of kava by women likely have more to do with the preservation of male privilege than with any pharmacological properties of the ingested drug (Lebot et al., 1997). However, traditional use to control fertility reflects that women used or avoided kava with their own agendas. There is insufficient information to reliably predict effects of kava use on infant or milk supply during lactation, although these potential risks should be assessed in light of known risks of addiction or infant sedation from alternative anxiety treatments, such as benzodiazepines. Use of kava during breast-feeding is known anecdotally (Personal communication, Humphrey, 2001). No reports of adverse effects are documented.

Side Effects

Up to about the year 2000 in Germany, approximately 60 adverse reactions to preparations containing kava were reported, the majority of which affected "the skin or central nervous system" (Schmidt and Boehncke, 2000). The German Commission E monograph on kava notes that allergic skin reactions, distinct from kava dermopathy described previously, may occur rarely (Blumenthal et al., 1998).

Heavy usage of kava can cause dermopathy, a peculiar scaly eruption of the skin which is apparently completely reversible with cessation of kava use. This dermopathy was noted by members of Cook's Pacific expeditions and can still be observed today in Pacific Islanders who consume excessive quantities of kava beverage (Norton and Ruze, 1994; Barguil et al., 2001). The causes of kava dermopathy remain unknown. It has been proposed that it is due to: a reduction of "glandular secretions"; the accumulation of flavopigments or kavalactones; chronic allergic dermatitis; a photosensitivity reaction; niacin deficiency; or interference in cholesterol metabolism (Norton and Ruze, 1994). With the exception of niacin deficiency, to date none of these hypotheses have been tested. In a double-blind placebo-controlled trial, Ruze (1990) used nicotinamide to supplement the diet of 29/200 kava drinkers in the Tonga islands who had severe kava dermopathy. Because their skin condition did not improve, she concluded that the condition is not attributable to niacin deficiency. Norton and Ruze (1994) noted that a similar reversible ichthyosis is associated with lipid-lowering agents such as triparanol (Winkelmann et al., 1963) and that early clinical studies with dihydromethysticin (300-800 mg/day) were observed to cause an exfoliative dermatitis not unlike that found in Polynesia among heavy users of kava beverage. Kava dermopathy is a side effect of heavy usage and is unlikely to constitute a significant risk factor for the doses commonly used in phytotherapy.

In Germany, a case was reported of an acute systemic, hematogenous allergic contact dermatitis following ingestion of a kava extract (Antares). In photopatch tests the patient showed a positive reaction to D,L-kavain (Süss and Lehmann, 1996). Also in Germany, Schmidt and Boehncke (2000) reported a delayed-type hypersensitivity reaction in a 36-year-old woman to a kava extract (Antares) after a dosage of 120 mg/day for three weeks. She presented with the complaint of severe itching and showed a "generalized erythema" with papules and a few wheals on her torso. The rash rapidly cleared after treatment with antihistamines and corticosteroids; however, the itching continued for several weeks. Later, she was tested with patch prick tests using the European standard series. While these tests gave negative results, a patch test using the kava extract gave a strongly positive result within a day (at 1:1 and 1:100 dilution), at which point eczematous changes in the skin were observed at the site of the earlier prick test. However, negative patch tests were obtained in ten control subjects from a 1:1 dilution of the extraction.

Two other cases of skin eruptions in patients taking kava extracts were reported in Germany by Jappe et al. (1998). A woman age 53, who had taken a kava extract for three weeks, presented with plaques and papules on her face which later appeared on her arms and dorsal and ventral thorax. Tests were negative for antiextractable nuclear antibody and antinuclear titers, but a biopsy showed "prominent infiltrate in the reticular dermis." A patch test with kava extract showed a positive reaction whereas in 20 adults who served as a control group the test was negative. The other case was that of a 70-year-old man who had taken kava extract for two to three weeks, along with yohimbine, allopurinol, furosemide, mesterolone, and spironolactone. After several hours' exposure to sunlight he developed itching and later erythematous, infiltrated plaques on the face and dorsal and ventricular thorax. Negative results were obtained in tests for antiextractable and antinuclear antibody titers, direct immunoflorescence, photopatch, and basophil cellular antigen stimulation. Following a biopsy, the authors found that a lymphocytic infiltrate was destroying lower infundibula and sebaceous glands and that the infiltrating cells were CD4 negative and CD8 positive. When serial dilutions of the suspect drugs were subjected to a lymphocyte-transformation test, only the kava extract produced a significant proliferation.

In a preliminary study, Mathews et al. (1988) examined the potential adverse effects of kava in 39 Australian Aborigines ages 16 and older who drank traditional kava beverage in a community that had banned the consumption of alcohol. Among those who abstained from kava, hepatic γ-glutamyltransferase (γ-glutamyl transpeptidase) (GMT) activity was found to be less often raised and to a far less extent than those of kava users. The majority of the subjects were "heavy" (310 g/week) and "very heavy" users (440 g/week). Female users ($n = 16$) showed elevated GMT in the heavy and very heavy user groups (139 and 126 U/L respectively), but at about half or less the GMT activity levels found in the male users ($n = 19$), whether they were "occasional," "heavy," or "very heavy" users (77, 312, and 251 U/L, respectively). Only one man out of the four "occasional" users (100 g/week) showed elevated GMT activity (77 U/L), whereas the two women showed normal levels. Confounding these findings, hepatitis B surface antigen was detected in 41% of the men and in 15% of the women and half the men showed antibody to HBsAg as did 78% of the women. Mathews and colleagues deduced that exposure to the virus was more than 90% in the men and women and that the men had a far higher carrier rate compared to the women; however, elevated GMT was just as frequent in HBsAg carriers as in others and users of kava showed no difference in frequency of HBsAg or anti-HBsAg compared to nonusers (Mathews et al., 1988).

Owing to limitations of the study by Mathews et al. (1988), it is not known whether the association of a higher incidence of elevated GMT activity in males versus female kava users is due to a culturally more prevalent use of kava among the males. Any association of kavalactones with elevated GMT activity is also speculative; we do not know the levels of kavalactones that the aborigines consumed. To date, only one clinical trial of kava extract has measured GMT levels and these were of menopausal women ages 45-60 in Germany. No abnormal GMT levels were found after an eight-week treatment period from a dosage of 100 mg t.i.d. of an extract standardized to contain 70% kavalactones (Warnecke, 1991). In an attempt to shed some light on this matter, a study of kava drinkers in New Caledonia by Barguil et al. (2001) focused on heavy users who were not taking medications and abstained from alcohol. Two women and 19 men described as heavy kava drinkers (8 g kavalactones/week for the past five years with a mean of 4.55 units/day on 5.9 days of the week) were given blood and urine tests for kavalactones, in addition to coagulation, hematological, and biochemical tests. The only abnormal reading of any significance ($p = 0.08$) was slightly increased levels of GMT in one woman and six of the men who showed a mean GMT value of 81.5 U/L, which is fairly above normal (< 43 U/L). Nearly half of the study participants showed ichtyosis (47%) but no other clinical signs. Barguil and colleagues noted that in their own observations of acute adverse reactions from kava use, which have resulted in allergic edema, sub- and fulminant hepatitis, they occurred in subjects who were light kava drinkers or in those taking medications, which suggested an immunoallergic reaction.

In Switzerland, Escher et al. (2001) reported a case of fulminant hepatic failure (hepatitis) in a patient taking a kava extract (Schwabe, Switzerland, Laitan) for the treatment of "slight" anxiety. The patient was a man age 50 who did not consume alcohol and was taking no other medications. After experiencing fatigue for four months, dark urine, and a "tanned" complexion, he visited his doctor because of jaundice. His only other medical complaint had been mild anxiety which for two months was treated with kava extract (three to four capsules/day providing 210-280 kavalactones). The maximum recommended dose was three capsules/day. The patient was admitted to the hospital following liver function tests that showed greatly elevated levels of GMT (γ-glutamyltransferase 691 IU/L; normal range 9-35 IU/L), conjugated and total bilirubin (279.2 μmol/L; normal range 6.8-25), an alkaline phosphatase level of 430 (normal range 30-125), a 70-fold increase in levels of ALT (alanine aminotransferase), and a 60-fold increase in levels of AST (aspartate aminotransferase). Tests were negative for various viruses (Epstein-Barr, HIV, hepatitis A, B, C, and E, and cytomegalovirus). An ultrasonographic scan revealed that the size of his liver was only slightly increased and had no signs of portal vein thrombosis or ascites. Two days later, he required intubation after developing stage-IV encephalopathy and in another two days received a liver transplant. His old liver showed extensive portal and lobular infiltration of neutrophils and lymphocytes, atrophy, and "extensive and severe hepatocellular necrosis." The authors concluded that the association with kava extract was supported by the exclusion of viral causes, the histological findings, and the chronology of the liver failure (Escher et al., 2001).

Since the publication of the foregoing case, about 30 other reports of adverse effects on the liver have been reported in Europe in patients taking concentrated extracts (ethanol or acetone) of kava root (American Herbal Products Association, 2002; Russman et al., 2001; Russmann and Helbling, 2001; Kraft et al., 2001; Keller, 2001). Four patients required liver transplants; one patient died; and six had liver failure. At the time of this writing, the cases, however rare, were still being evaluated. None involved traditional kava drinks, kava tinctures, or raw kava root. Dosages ranged from as little as 60-240 mg/day, and in at least half the cases the patients were taking medications that are known to cause hepatic side effects (e.g., paracetamol, hormonal ovulation inhibitors, cisaprid, celecoxib, pramino) (Keller, 2001).

Special Precautions

In response to the recent ongoing evaluation of potential hepatotoxic effects associated with the use of concentrated kava extracts in Europe, the American Herbal Products Association (2001) has issued a number of special considerations for consumers of dietary supplements containing kava:

1. Stop using kava if taking alcoholic beverages or OTC or prescription drugs.
2. Consult a health care practitioner before taking kava on any regular basis.
3. Stop taking kava and obtain medical attention upon any symptoms of jaundice (dark urine, fever, nausea, yellow discoloration of the eyes, etc.).

The German Commission E monograph on kava (Blumenthal et al., 1998) and *The Botanical Safety Handbook* (McGuffin et al., 1997) both caution against exceeding the recommended dosage of kava and against continuous usage exceeding three months without receiving medical advice.

Some authors caution against driving or operating heavy equipment when taking kava (Blumenthal et al., 1998; McGuffin et al., 1997).

Owing to the possibility that the sedative effects of anesthetics could be potentiated by kava, Ang-Lee et al. (2001) suggested that its use be discontinued at least a full day (24 h) before surgery.

Schelofsky et al. (1995) reported four case studies of patients in Germany who displayed symptoms indicative of a possible dopamine antagonism due to kava extracts. One patient had a history of acute dystonic reactions when treated with promethacin and fluspirilen for anxiety. In these instances, biperiden, an anti-Parkinson's agent, immediately relieved the symptoms. Some years later, the same patient presented at the hospital with an acute attack of involuntary neck extension and forceful upward deviation of the eyes, which had begun 90 min after his initial intake of a standardized kava extract (Laitan, 100 mg). The symptoms subsided spontaneously within about 40 min. Another patient, a 23-year-old woman who had been taking a kava extract (Laitan) for anxiety, presented with involuntary oral and lingual dyskinesia, tonic rotation of the head, and painful twisting movements of the trunk. She was given 2.5 mg biperiden i.v. and the symptoms disappeared immediately. No history of any other drug exposure during the preceding months was recorded. A 63-year-old woman taking a kava extract (Kavasporal forte, 150 mg t.i.d.) for anxiety presented in the emergency room with sudden onset of oral and lingual dyskinesia after four days of kava treatment. Biperiden (5 mg i.v.) immediately stopped the dyskinesia. The researchers reporting these case studies suggest caution in the use of kava due to the potential for extrapyramidal side effects. Although most of their cases involved young adults, they emphasized that special care should be taken in giving kava to elderly patients (Schelofsky et al., 1995). It has been suggested that these cases may be instances of cholinergic hypersensitivity (Nöldner and Chatterjee, 1999). From the foregoing, it may also be inferred that since biperiden is an anticholinergic used in the treatment of Parkinson's disease, the use of kava extract would be cautioned in this disease. There is now one case report of a 45-year-old woman who developed persistent and severe symptoms of Parkinson's disease after a matter of days of taking kava to treat anxiety. Because she had a family history of "essential tremor," the reporting physicians suggested that kava may cause severe Parkinson's symptoms in people with a genetic susceptibility to the disease (Meseguer et al., 2002).

The German Commission E also mentions that accommodative disturbances have occurred in patients taking kava (e.g., enlargement of the pupils and oculomotor equilibrium disturbances) (Blumenthal et al., 1998). The effect of kava on ocular functions was assessed in a single male subject (Garner and Klinger, 1985). Kava was reported to reduce the near point of accommodation, increase pupil diameter, decrease the near point of convergence, and disturb oculomotor balance. No changes were noted in stereoacuity, refractive error, or visual acuity. The authors speculated that the effects could be most readily explained by a cocaine-like effect on the ocular muscles (kava has local anesthetic properties), and/or a sedative or depressant effect on the central nervous system.

Toxicology

Toxicity in Animal Models

For kava extract, an LD_{50} of 250 mg/kg i.p. in rats was reported by Edwards et al. (1998), who noted that others have reported an LD_{50} of 450 mg/kg. Edwards et al. (in press) administered a powder extract of kava containing at least 30% kavalactones to 60-day-old male rats for seven consecutive days. At a dosage of 200 mg/kg i.p. there were no deaths. At 300 mg/kg i.p. the rate of mortality was 40%, and 100% from a dosage of 400 mg/kg i.p. administered on day three. Compared to controls, cognitive impairment (radial arm maze test for memory) was significant ($p > 0.05$) after 200 mg/kg i.p. for seven days but not at 100 mg/kg i.p. and not after two days at either dose. Increased liver GMT activity and excessive weight loss was evident in kava-treated rats compared to controls after dosages of either 100, 150, 200, or 300 mg/kg i.p. for seven days. The authors caution that definitive results in these tests will require further studies and that oral dosages of kava extract would provide a more accurate model of the effects of human consumption.

REFERENCES

Almeida, J.C. and Grrimsley, E.W. (1996). Coma from the health food store: Interaction between kava and alprazolam. *Annals of Internal Medicine* 125: 940-941.

American Herbal Products Association (2002). Kava information from the AHPA Executive Committee, January 14. Available online at: <http://www.ahpa.org/kavaexe.html>.

Ang-Lee, M.K., Moss, J., and Yuan, C.S. (2001). Herbal medicines and perioperative care. *Journal of the American Medicine Association* 286: 208-216.

Anonymous (1988). Kava. *Lancet* II: 258-259.

Backhuass, C. and Krieglstein, J. (1992). Extract of kava *(Piper methysticum)* and its methysticin constituents protect brain tissue against ischemic damage in rodents. *European Journal of Pharmacology* 215: 265-269.

Barguil, Y., Mandeau, A., Genelle, B., Derycke, T., Merzeau, C., Mouquet-Leeman, C., Barny, S., Duhet, D., and Cabalion, P. (2001). Kava and gamma-glutamyltransferase increase: Hepatic enzyme induction of liver function alteration. *British Medical Journal* (March 21): Available online at: <http://www.bmj.com/cgi/eletters/322/7279/139#12160>.

Baum, S.S., Hill, R., and Rommelspacher, H. (1998). Effect of kava extract and individual kavapyrones on neurotransmitter levels in the nucleus accumbens of rats. *Progress in Neuro-psychopharmacology and Biological Psychiatry* 22: 1105-1120.

Blumenthal, M. (1994). Congress passes dietary supplement health and education act of 1994: Herbs to be protected as supplements. *HerbalGram* 32 (Fall): 18.

Blumenthal, M., Busse, W.R., Goldberg, A., Gruenwald, J., Hall, T., Riggins, C.W., and Rister, R.S. (Eds.) (1998). *The Complete German Commission E Monographs* (pp. 156-157, 484). Austin, TX: American Botanical Council.

Brown, D.J. (1997). Kava kava clinical monograph. *Townsend Letter for Doctors and Patients* (July)168: 166-167.

Buckley, J.P., Furgiuele, A.R., and O'Hara, M.L. (1967). Pharmacology of kava. In Efron, D.H., Holmstedt, B., and Kline, N.S. (Eds.), *Ethnopharmacological Search for Psychoactive Drugs* (pp. 141-151). Washington, DC: Government Printing Office, U.S. Dept. of Health and Welfare, Publ. No. 1645.

Cambie, R.C. and Ash, J. (1994). *Fijian Medicinal Plants* (pp. 239-240). Australia: CSIRO.

Capasso, A. and Calignano, A. (1988). Synergism between the sedative actions of kava extract and D,L-kawain. *Acta Therapeutica* 14: 249-256.

Cartledge, A. (2001). Kava and benzodiazepines—worsening withdrawal. *British Medical Journal* (March 21). Available online at: <http://www.bmj.com/cgi/eletters/322/7279/139#12160>.

Dam-Bakker, A.W., van de Groot, A.P., and Luyken, R. (1958). Influence of wati *(Piper methysticum)* on the fertility of male rats. *Tropical and Geographical Medicine* 10: 68-70.

Davies, L.P., Drew, C.A., Duffield, P., Johnston, G.A., and Jamieson, D.D. (1992). Kava pyrones and resin: Studies on GABA-A, GABA-B and benzodiazepine binding sites in rodent brain. *Pharmacology and Toxicology* 71: 120-126.

De Leo, V., la Marca, A., Morgante, G., Lanzetta, D., Florio, P., and Petraglia, F. (2001). Evaluation of combining kava extract with hormone replacement therapy in the treatment of postmenopausal anxiety. *Maturitas* 29: 185-188.

Degener, O. (1946). *Flora Hawaiiensis, or The New Illustrated Flora of the Hawaiian Islands,* Second Edition. Honolulu, HI: Otto Deneger.

Dentali, S. (1997). *Herb Safety Review—Kava: Piper methysticum* Forster f. (Piperaceae). Boulder, CO: Herb Research Foundation.

Dinh, L.D., Simmen, U., Bueter, K.B., Bueter, B., Lundstrom, K., and Schaffner, W. (2001). Interaction of various *Piper methysticum* cultivars with CNS receptors in vitro. *Planta Medica* 67: 306-311.

Donadio, V., Bonsi, P., Zele, I., Monari, L., Liguori, R., Vetrugno, R., Albani, F., and Montagna, P. (2000). Myoglobinuria after ingestion of extracts of guarana, *Ginkgo biloba* and kava. *Italian Journal of Neurological Sciences* 21: 124 (letter).

Duffield, A.M., Jamieson, D.D., Lidgard, R.O., Duffield, P.H., and Bourne, D.J. (1989). Identification of some human urinary metabolites of the intoxicating beverage kava. *Journal of Chromatography* 475: 273-281.

Duffield, P.H. and Jamieson, D.D. (1991). Development of tolerance to kava in mice. *Clinical and Experimental Pharmacology and Physiology* 18: 571-578.

Dutta, C.P., Roy, L.P.K., Chatterjee, A., and Roy, D.N. (1976). Chemical investigation of *Piper methysticum* Forst. (Piperaceae). Structure and synthesis of flavokawain-C. Part 5 of studies on the genus *Piper. Journal of the Indian Chemical Society* 55: 932-934.

Duve, R.N. (1976). Highlight of the chemistry and pharmacology of yaqona, *Piper methysticum. Fiji Agricultural Journal* 38: 81-84.

Duve, R.N. (1981). Gas-liquid chromatographic determination of major constituents of *Piper methysticum. Analyst* 106: 160-165.

Duve, R.N. and Prasad, J. (1984). Efficacy of extraction of constituents in the preparation of yaqona beverage. Part 2: Major active constituents. *Fiji Agricultural Journal* 46: 11-16.

Edwards, J., La Grange, L., Wang, M., Reid, C., Benally, G., Charley, A., James, P., and Gonzales, L. (in press). The impact of chronic kava (*Piper methysticum* Forst.) administration on γ-glutamyl transpeptidase activity, weight loss, and memory in rats. *Journal of Herbal Pharmacotherapy* 1.

Edwards, J., Wang, M., Pecore, N., and La Grange, L. (1998). The LD_{50} of kavalactones from *Piper methysticum* in rats. *FASEB Journal* 12: A464 (abstract).

Escher, M., Desmeules, J., Giostra, E., and Mentha, G. (2001). Hepatitis associated with kava, a herbal remedy for anxiety. *British Medical Journal* 322 (Jan. 20): 139.

Flynn, R. and Roest, M. (1995). *Your Guide to Standardized Herbal Products* (p. 52). Prescott, AZ: One World Press.

Foo, H. and Lemon, J. (1997). Acute effects of kava, alone or in combination with alcohol, on subjective measures of impairment and intoxication and on cognitive performance. *Drug and Alcohol Review* 16: 147-155.

Gaedcke, F. (2000). Pharmaceutical characterization of kava-kava extracts and their formulations. In 3rd International Congress on Phytomedicine, October 11-13, 2000, Munich, Germany, Abstracts. *Phytomedicine* 7(Suppl. 2): 28 (abstract SL-49).

Garner, L.F. and Klinger, J.D. (1985). Some visual effects caused by the beverage kava. *Journal of Ethnopharmacology* 13: 307-311.

Gleitz, J., Beile, A., and Peters, T. (1996). (+/–)-Kavain inhibits veratridine-activated voltage-dependent Na(+)-channels in synaptosomes prepared from rat cerebral cortex. *Neuropharmacology* 34: 1133-1138.

Gleitz, J., Beile, A., Wilkens, P., Ameri, A., and Peters, T. (1997). Antithrombotic action of the kava pyrone (+)-kavain prepared from *Piper methysticum* on human platelets. *Planta Medica* 63: 27-30.

Gleitz, J., Friese, J., Beile, A., Ameri, A., and Peters, T. (1996). Anticonvulsive action of (+/–)-kavain estimated from its properties on stimulated synaptosomes and Na+ receptor sites. *European Journal of Pharmacology* 315: 89-97.

Grunze, H., Langosch, J., Schirrmacher, K., Bingmann, D., von Wegerer, J., and Walden, J. (2001). Kava pyrones exert effects on neuronal transmission and transmembraneous cation currents similar to established mood stabilizers—a review. *Progress in Neuro-Psychopharmacology and Biological Psychiatry* 25: 1555-1570.

Hänsel, R. (1964). Therapie mit phytopharmaka [Therapy with phytopharmaceuticals]. *Deutsche Apotheker Zeitung* (Stuttgart) 104: 459.

Hänsel, R. (1968). Characterization and physiological activity of some kava constituents. *Pacific Science* 22: 293-313.

Hänsel, R., Weiss, D., and Schmidt, B. (1966). Fungistatisch wirkung der kawadroge und ihrer inhalfstoffe. *Planta Medica* 14: 1-9.

Herberg, K.W. (1993). [Effect of kava special extract WS 1490 combined with ethyl alcohol on safety-relevant performance parameters]. *Blutalkohol* 30: 96-105.

Hope, B.E., Massey, D.G., and Fournier-Massey, G. (1993). Hawaiian materia medica for asthma. *Hawaii Medical Journal* 52: 160-166.

Humphrey, S. (2001). Sheila Humphrey, RN, BSc, ICBLC, personal communication with INPR, September.

Jamieson, D.D. and Duffield, P.H. (1990a). The antinociceptive actions of kava components in mice. *Clinical and Experimental Pharmacology and Physiology* 17: 495-508.

Jamieson, D.D. and Duffield, P.H. (1990b). Positive interaction of ethanol and kava resin in mice. *Clinical and Experimental Pharmacology and Physiology* 17: 509-514.

Jappe, U., Franke, I., Reinhold, D., and Gollnick, H.P. (1998). Sebotropic reaction resulting from kava-kava extract therapy: A new entity? *Journal of the American Academy of Dermatology* 38: 104-106.

Johnston, E. (1997). Personal communication to Dennis McKenna. Ed Johnston is owner/operator of the Alia Point 'Awa Nursery in Pepe'ekeo, Hawaii.

Jussofie, A., Schmiz, A., and Hiemke, C. (1994). Kavapyrone enriched extract from *Piper methysticum* as modulator of the GABA binding site in different regions of rat brain. *Psychopharmacology* 116: 469-474.

Keledjian, J., Duffield, P.H., Jamieson, D.D., Lidgard, R.O., and Duffield, A.M. (1988). Uptake into mouse brain of four compounds present in the psychoactive beverage kava. *Journal of Pharmaceutical Sciences* 77: 1003-1006.

Keller, K. (2001). *Clinical Assessment Report. Hepatotoxicity of Kava-Kava Extract*. Bonn, Germany: Budesinstitut für Arzneimittel und Medizinprodukte [Federal Institute for Drugs and Medical Devices]. Draft report.

Kilham, C. (1996). *Kava: Medicine Hunting in Paradise*. Rochester, VT: Park Street Press.

Kinzler, E., Krömer, J., and Lehmann, E. (1991). Wirksamkeit eines kava-spezialextraktes bei patienten mit angst-, spannungs-, und errgungszuständen nichtpsychotischer genese. Doppelblind-studie gegen plazebo über 4 wochen [Clinical efficacy of a kava extract in patients with anxiety syndrome. Double-blind placebo-controlled study over 4 weeks]. *Arzneimittel-Forschung/Drug Research* 41: 584-588 (translation).

Kraft, M., Spahn, T.W., Menzel, J., Senninger, N., Dietl, K.H., Herbst, H., Domschke, W., and Lerch, M.M. (2001). Fulminantes leberversagen nach einnahame des pflanzlichen antidepressivums kava-kava [Fulminant liver failure after administration of the herbal antidepressant kava-kava]. *Deutsche Medizinische Wochenschrift* 126: 970-972.

Kuster, R.M., Mpalantinos, M.A., de Hollanda, M.C., Lima, P., Brand, E.T., and Parente, J.P. (1999). GC-MS determination of kava-pyrones in *Alpinia zerumbet* leaves. *Journal of High Resolution Chromatography* 22: 129-130.

Lebot, V., Johnston, E., Zheng, Q.Y., McKern, D., and McKenna, D.J. (1999). Morphological, phytochemical, and genetic variation in Hawaiian cultivars of 'awa (*Piper methysticum,* Piperaceae). *Economic Botany* 53: 407-418.

Lebot, V. and Lévesque, J. (1989). The origin and distribution of kava (*Piper methysticum* Forst. F., Piperaceae): A phytochemical approach. *Allertonia* 5: 223-281.

Lebot, V., Merlin, M., and Lindstrom, L. (1997). *Kava: The Pacific Elixir*. Rochester, VT: Healing Arts Press.

Lechtenberg, M., Quandt, B., Kohlenberg, F.J., and Nahrstedt, A. (1999). Qualitative and quantitative micellar electrokinetic chromatography of kavalactones from dry extracts of *Piper methysticum* Forst. and commercial drugs. *Journal of Chromatography* A 848: 457-464.

Lehmann, E. (1998). Wirkung von kava: Kava bei akuter angst [Effect of kava: Kava during acute anxiety]. *Synopsis* 2: 59-64.

Lehmann, E., Kinzler, E., and Friedemann, J. (1996). Efficacy of a special kava extract *(Piper methysticum)* in patients with states of anxiety, tension, and excitedness of non-mental origin—A double-blind placebo-controlled study of four weeks treatment. *Phytomedicine* 3: 113-119.

Leung, A.Y. and Foster, S. (1996). *Encyclopedia of Common Natural Ingredients Used in Foods, Drugs and Cosmetics*. New York: John Wiley and Sons, Inc.

Lindenberg, D. and Pitule-Schodel, H. (1990). D,L-kavain im vergleich zu oxazepam bei angstzuständen: Doppelblindstudie zur klinischen wirksamkeit [D,L-kavain in comparison with oxazepam in anxiety states: Double blind clinical trial]. *Fortschritte der Medizin* 108: 31-34 (translation).

Locher, C.P., Burch, M.T., Mower, H.F., Berestecky, J., Davis, H., Van Poel, B., Lasure, A., Vanden Berghe, D.A., and Vlietinck, A.J. (1995). Antimicrobial activity and anticomplement activity of extracts obtained from selected Hawaiian medicinal plants. *Journal of Ethnopharmacology* 49: 23-32.

Malsch, U. and Kieser, M. (2001). Efficacy of kava-kava in the treatment of nonpsychotic anxiety, following pretreatment with benzodiazepines. *Psychopharmacology* 157: 277-283.

Martin, H.B., Stofer, W.D., and Eichinger, M.R. (2000). Kavain inhibits murine airway smooth muscle contraction. *Planta Medica* 66: 601-606.

Mathews, J.D., Riley, M.D., Fejo, L., Munoz, E., Milns, N.R., Gardner, I.D., Powers, J.R., Ganygulpa, E., and Gununuwawuy, B.J. (1988). Effects of the heavy usage of kava on physical health: Summary of a pilot survey in an Aboriginal community. *Medical Journal of Australia* 148: 548-555.

McGuffin, M., Hobbs, C., Upton, R., and Goldberg, A. (1997). *American Herbal Products Association's Botanical Safety Handbook* (pp. 86-87). Boca Raton, FL: CRC Press.

Meseguer, E., Taboada, R., Sanchez, V., Mena, M.A., Campos, V., and Garcia De Yebenes, J. (2002). Life-threatening parkinsonism induced by kava-kava. *Movement Disorders* 17: 195-196.

Münte, T.F., Heinze, H.J., Matzke, M., and Steitz, J. (1993). Effects of oxazepam and an extract of kava roots *(Piper methysticum)* on event-related potentials in a word recognition task. *Neuropsychobiology* 27: 46-53.

Nöldner, M. and Chatterjee, S.S. (1999). Inhibition of haloperidol-induced catelepsy in rats by root extracts from *Piper methysticum* F. *Phytomedicine* 6: 285-286.

Norton, S.A. and Ruze, P. (1994). Kava dermopathy. *Journal of the American Academy of Dermatology* 31: 89-97.

Pittler, M.H. and Ernst, E. (2000). Efficacy of kava extract for treating anxiety: Systematic review and meta-analysis. *Journal of Clinical Psychopharmacology* 20: 84-89.

Prescott, J., Jamieson, D., Emdur, N., and Duffield, P. (1993). Acute effects of kava on measures of cognitive performance, physiological function, and mood. *Drug and Alcohol Review* 12: 49-58.

Rasmussen, A.K., Scheline, R.R., Solheim, E., and Hänsel, R. (1979). Metabolism of some kava pyrones in the rat. *Xenobiotica* 9: 1-16.

Reynolds, J.E.F. (Ed.) (1996). *Martindale: The Extra Pharmacopoeia,* Twenty-First Edition. London, England: Royal Pharmaceutical Society.

Russell, P.N., Bakker, D., and Singh, N.N. (1987). The effects of kava on alerting and speed of access of information from long-term memory. *Bulletin of the Psychonomic Society* 25: 236-237.

Russmann, S., Escher, M., Stoller, R., and Lauterburg, B.H. (2001). Hepatotoxicity of kava *(Piper methysticum)*-containing herbal drugs: Recent cases in Switzerland and investigations regarding the mechanism. *Naunyn-Schmiedebergs Archives of Pharmacology* 363(4 Suppl.): R131.

Russmann, S. and Helbling, A. (2001). Kava hepatotoxicity. *Annals of Internal Medicine* 135: 68-69 (letter).

Ruze, P. (1990). Kava-induced dermopathy: A niacin deficiency? *Lancet* 335: 1442-1445.

Saletu, B., Grünberger, J., and Linzmaye, L. (1989). EEG-brain mapping, psychometric and psychophysiological studies on central effects of kavain—A kava plant derivative. *Human Psychopharmacology* 4: 169-190.

Schelofsky, L., Raffauf, C., Jendroska, K., and Poewe, W. (1995). Kava and dopamine antagonism. *Journal of Neurology, Neurosurgery and Psychiatry* 58: 639-640 (letter).

Schmidt, P. and Boehncke, W.H. (2000). Delayed-type hypersensitivity reaction to kava-kava extract. *Contact Dermatitis* 42: 363-364.

Schulz, V., Hänsel, R., and Tyler, V.E. (2001). *Rational Phytotherapy: A Physician's Guide to Herbal Medicine,* Fourth Edition (p. 84). New York: Springer-Verlag.

Serdarevic, N., Eckert, G.P., and Müller, W.E. (2001). The effects of extracts of St. John's wort and kava kava on brain neurotransmitter levels in the mouse. *Pharmacopsychiatry* 34(Suppl. 1): S134-S136.

Shulgin, A.T. (1973). The narcotic pepper: The chemistry and pharmacology of *Piper methysticum* and related species. *Bulletin on Narcotics* 25: 59-74.

Singh, N.N., Ellis, C.R., Best, A.M., Eakin, K., Parsons, C., and Sharp, I. (1997). Evidence on Kavatrol (effectiveness reducing daily stress and anxiety in adults: Study results). Unpublished. Corresponding author: N.N. Singh, Dept. of Psychiatry, Medical College of Virginia, Virginia Commonwealth University, Richmond, VA, USA 23298-0489.

Singh, Y.D. and Blumenthal, M. (1997). Kava: An overview. *HerbalGram* 39 (Spring): 34-55. Special review reprinted and updated from an original article by Singh, Y.D. (1992), Kava: An overview, *Journal of Ethnopharmacology* 37: 13-45.

Singh, Y.N. (1983). Effects of kava on neuromuscular transmission and muscle contractility. *Journal of Ethnopharmacology* 7: 267-276.

Smith, A.C. (1943). Notes on the Pacific species of *Piper*. Part 2 of studies of Pacific Island plants. *Journal of the Arnold Arboretum* 14: 347-361.

Smith, R.M. (1979). Pipermethystine: A novel pyridone alkaloid from *Piper methysticum* (cultivated in the South Pacific as a drug plant and a beverage plant). *Tetrahedron Letters* 5: 437-439.

Steiner, G.G. (2000). The correlation between cancer incidence and kava consumption. *Hawaii Medical Journal* 59: 420-422.

Strahl, S., Ehret, V., Dahm, H.H., and Maier, K.P. (1998). Nekrotisierende hepatitis nach einnahme pflanzlicher heilmittel [Necrotising hepatitis after taking herbal medication]. *Deutsche Medizinische Wochenshrift* 123: 1410-1414.

Süss, R. and Lehmann, P. (1996). Hämatogenes kontaktekzem durch pflanzliche medikamente am beispiel des kavawurzel-extraketes [Hematogenous allergic contact dermatitis from kava, an herbal product]. *Hautarzt* 47: 459-461.

Uebelhack, R., Franke, L., and Schewe, H.J. (1998). Inhibition of platelet MAO-B by kava pyrone-enriched extract from *Piper methysticum* Forster (kava-kava). *Pharmacopsychiatry* 31: 187-192.

Volz, H.P. and Kieser, M. (1997). Kava-kava extract WS 1490 versus placebo in anxiety disorders: A randomized placebo-controlled 25-week outpatient trial. *Pharmacopsychiatry* 30: 1-5.

Walden, J., von Wegerer, J., Winter, U., and Berger, M. (1997). Actions of kavain and dihydromethysticin on ipsapirone-induced field potential changes in the hippocampus. *Human Psychopharmacology* 12: 265-270.

Warnecke, G. (1991). Psychosomatische dysfunction im weiblichen klimakterium: Klinische wirksamkeit und verträglichkeit von kava–extrakt WS 1490 [Neurovegetative dystonia in the female climacteric: Studies on the clinical efficacy and tolerance of kava extract 1490]. *Fortschritte der Medizin* 109: 119-122.

Warnecke, G., Pfaender, H., Gerster, G., and Gracza, E. (1990). Wirksamkeit von kawa-kawa-extrakt beim klimakterischen syndrom [Effect of kava-kava extract on the menopausal syndrome]. *Zeitschrift fur Phytotherapie* 11: 81-86.

Whitton, P. (2001). Are standardized extracts truly herbal medicine? *British Medical Journal* (March 21): Available online at: <http://www.bmj.com/cgi/eletters/322/7279/139#12160>.

Winkelmann, R.K., Perry, H.O., Achor, R.W.P., and Kirby, T.J. (1963). Cutaneous syndromes produced as side effects of triparanol therapy. *Archives of Dermatology* 87: 372-377.

Woelk, H., Kapoula, O., Lehrl, S., Schröter, K., and Weinholz, P. (1993). A comparison of kava special extract WS 1490 and benzodiazepines in patients with anxiety. *Zeitschrift für Allgemeinmedizin* 69: 271-277 (translation in *The Healthnotes Review of Complementary and Integrative Medicine* 6: 265-270, 1999).

Wu, D., Nair, M.G., and DeWitt, D.L. (2001). Novel compounds from *Piper methysticum* Forst (Kava Kava) roots and their effect on cyclooxygenase enzyme. *Journal of Agricultural and Food Chemistry* 50: 701-705.

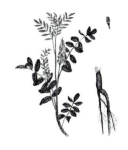

$\mathcal{L}icorice$

BOTANICAL DATA

Classification and Nomenclature

Scientific name: *Glycyrrhiza glabra* L.

Family name: Fabaceae

Common names: licorice, licorice root (English), gan cao (sweet herb), ou gan cao (common European licorice or *Glycyrrhiza glabra*) (Chinese), kanzo (Japanese) (*Glycyrrhiza uralensis*), Russian licorice (*Glycyrrhiza glabra* L. var. *glandulifera*), Spanish licorice (*G. glabra* var. *typica*) (Foster and Chongxi, 1992)

Description

Glycyrrhiza are perennial subshrubs or herbs with alternate pinnate leaves and whitish-violet or, rarely, yellow flowers. *Glycyrrhiza glabra* occurs in dry open areas, grassy plains, and wild deserts where the soil is alkaline and salty, mainly in the Mediterranean region. The roots, which are cylindrical and branching, are used. Stems growing beneath the ground can reach 1.8 m or more from the main plant, and they send forth shoots creating secondary plants after two years. The cultivated plant is harvested for its root after four years of growth. With removal of the bark, the root is used in the manufacture of licorice and in this form is regarded in China as being of superior quality. In China, *G. uralensis* Fischer et D.C. is the main species used medicinally, although the root of *G. glabra* is widely used and cultivated today. With the exception of Scandinavia, *G. glabra* is cultivated and naturalized in most European countries and northwest China (Foster and Chongxi, 1992).

HISTORY AND TRADITIONAL USES

With a 3,000-year history of use as a medicinal plant, licorice root *(G. glabra)* is one of the most ancient herbal medicines known and the subject of extensive studies (Bradley, 1992). The name *glycyrrhiza* is of Greek origin and means "sweet root." The root was mentioned by Pliny as useful as a carminative and expectorant, while Theophrastus recorded its uses in lung diseases, dry cough, and asthma (Anonymous, 1989). Hippocrates employed an ointment containing licorice root and Napoleon traveled with chests of licorice to relieve stomach pains during his battles. Extensive cultivation in northern England and Bavaria occurred during the sixteenth century (Foster and Chongxi, 1992). Later, modern texts gave its main use as a flavorant in the preparation of bitter-tasting cold and cough remedies (Anonymous, 1989).

Following World War II, a time when antacids were in short supply, Dutch physician E. F. Revers noticed the local popularity of a proprietary medicine containing licorice among patients with gastrointestinal problems. Following up on the purported benefits, research indicated that the ingredient licorice was indeed effective. He established the Western use of licorice for stomach ulcers when he prescribed a paste of licorice to patients for peptic ulcers. The paste was later improved in Europe for the treatment of gastric ulcers (Tewari and Trembalowicz, 1968; Larkworthy and Holgate, 1975).

Licorice root is used most extensively in Chinese herbal formulas (Foster and Chongxi, 1992). The root is recognized in traditional Chinese medicine (TCM) as a sweet, "mild" herb that helps to regulate stomach functions, tonifies the vital energy or "qi," invigorates "spleen" activity, and harmonizes herbal formulas to which it is added. TCM also recognizes the root as an antipyretic, an anti-inflammatory, a detoxicant, a lung demulcent, an expectorant, and a corrective adjuvant. Principal uses in TCM include treatment of cough, peptic ulcer, palpitations, skin ulcers, and stomachaches of psychogenic origin (Chang and But, 1986). The *Pharmacopoeia of the People's Republic of China* (Tu et al., 1992) specifies uses of the dried root and rhizome of *G. glabra* stir-fried in honey in the treatment of weakness and lassitude; arrhythmia; cough; sores and carbuncles; shortness of breath and cardiac palpitation; and spasmodic pain located in the limbs, epigastrium, and abdomen. The *Pharmacopoeia* notes that honey-processed licorice root is frequently used for "reducing the toxic or drastic action of other drugs" and that it acts to moderate the actions of other drugs (Tu et al., 1992).

Current European and Chinese texts list licorice root as: an expectorant, in the treatment of bronchitis, catarrh, coughs, and hoarseness (Bradley, 1992); pulmonary, in the treatment of tuberculosis (Chang and But, 1986); anti-inflammatory in duodenal and gastric ulcers for sore throat and mouth (locally), arthritis, rheumatism (Bradley, 1992), and allergies (Hsu et al., 1986); an ophthalmic against keratitis (Chang and But, 1986); a demulcent in chronic gastritis, epigastric distension, flatulence, poor digestion; an adjuvant in chronic gastritis, belching (Bradley, 1992), and peptic and duodenal ulcer (Chang and But, 1986); an adrenocorticotropic in adreno-corticoid insufficiency (Bradley, 1992) and Addison's disease, in mild cases; a hormonal in treating anterior pituitary insufficiency (postpartum) and improving hormone function (Chang and But, 1986); and a hepatic in the treatment of chronic, viral (Foster and Chongxi, 1992), and infectious hepatitis (Chang and But, 1986).

CHEMISTRY

Carbohydrates

Polysaccharides

Glycyrrhizan GA is a unique polysaccharide structure isolated from the root of *Glycyrrhiza glabra* var. *glandulifera*. It is largely composed of arabinose (54.6%) and galactose (30.2%), contains ten other sugar units, and has an estimated molecular mass of 85,000. The structure of glycyrrhizan GA, a neutral polysaccharide, is that of an α-(1,5)-linked L-arabino-β-(3,6)-branched D-galactan type of polysaccharide. Polysaccharides of similar structure occur in the medicinal plants *Echinacea purpurea* (cell culture), *Calendula officinalis* (flowers), and the roots of *Panax notoginseng* (Shimizu et al., 1991).

Phenolic Compounds

Flavonoids

More than 30 flavonoids are found in the root of *Glycyrrhiza glabra* (Bradley, 1992), and the elucidation of flavonoids in the species is ongoing (Kitagawa et al., 1994). Spanish and Russian species show a different profile of phenolics compared to flavonoids in Chinese licorice (Fukai et al., 1996). The main flavonoids of past pharmacologic interest are the flavonones liquiritigenin and liquiritin, and the chalcones isoliquiritigenin (4,2',4'-trihydroxychalcone) and isoliquiritin (Vaya et al., 1997; Chang and But, 1986). Liquiritigenin forms five conjugates in vivo. In rats, these are largely metabolized in the liver and kidney (Shimamura et al., 1993). *Glycyrrhiza glabra* roots also contain glycyrrhisoflavone (Hatano et al., 1989); the licochalcones A and B, glabrene, and glabridin (Okada et al., 1989); the major isoflavan in licorice root extract (11.6%) (Vaya et al., 1997); and other isoflavans: hispaglabridins A and B, 3'-hydroxy-4'-*O*-

methylglabridin, and 4'-*O*-methylglabridin (Kinoshita et al., 1996). Other flavonoid constituents of *G. glabra* include pinocembrin, glepidotins A and B (Mitscher et al., 1983), and the isoflavone formononetin (Vaya et al., 1997).

Phenylpropanoids

Licorice root contains licocoumarone (Hatano et al., 1989) and other coumarins: herniarin, licobenzofuran, umbelliferone (El Shayeb and Mabrouk, 1984), and kaempferol 3-*O*-methyl ether (Hatano et al., 1989).

Terpenoid Compounds

Triterpenes

The principle active constituents of licorice root are the anti-inflammatory triterpenic glycoside saponins, glycyrrhizin (glycyrrhizic acid or glycyrrhizinic acid) and glycyrrhetinic acid (glycyrrhitic acid). Both constituents have been extensively studied for pharmacological activity (Chang and But, 1986). In the West, licorice root was shown to cause a deoxycortisone-like activity in normal patients (MacKenzie et al., 1990). Structurally, glycyrrhetinic acid is similar to hydrocortisone (Teelucksingh et al., 1990).

The constituent glycyrrhizin is used as a sweetening agent in liquors, candies, chocolates, chewing gum, beer, and in the confection known as "licorice" (Cantelli-Forti et al., 1994). Glycyrrhizin occurs as salts of potassium, iron, barium, ammonia, and calcium (Chang and But, 1986). The principal sweet compound in licorice, glycyrrhizin (18β-glycyrrhizin), has 50 times the sweetness of sucrose. Amounts in the root are calculated to be from as little as 2% (Bradley, 1992) to as much as 24% (Wang et al., 1994).

Other Constituents

Numerous other constituents have been identified in licorice root including various common plant constituents, such as ferulic acid, sinapic acid, biotin, β-sitosterol, amino acids, sterols, sugars (5% to 15%), bitter principles, asparagine (1% to 2%), and starch (20%) (Kitigawa et al., 1994; Hatano et al., 1989; Chang and But, 1986; Bradley, 1992; Hiraga et al., 1984).

PRECLINICAL STUDIES

Cardiovascular and Circulatory Functions

Hypertension

Due to pulmonary hypertensive activity (Ruszymah et al., 1995), glycyrrhetinic acid, the aglycone of glycyrrhizin, has previously been used in the treatment of essential hypotension. Other diseases for which it has often been applied include Addison's disease and neurodermatitis (Ishida et al., 1989).

Digestive, Hepatic, and Gastrointestinal Functions

Gastric Functions

Administered orally in rats (10 mg/kg), the chalcone isoliquiritigen exhibited significant preventive activity against chemically induced ulcers, inhibiting their formation by up to 77% (Yamamoto et al., 1992). Glycyrrhetinic acid (200 mg/kg p.o.) inhibited stress-induced ulcer formation in mice by a much as 33% (Yano et al., 1989).

Hepatic Functions

In the Orient, glycyrrhizin is often used to treat chronic hepatitis (Ishida et al., 1989). The hepatoprotective effect of licorice was examined in male rats against carbon tetrachloride-induced acute hepatotoxicity, which served as a model of acute viral hepatitis. Using roots obtained from Egypt, researchers simply soaked them in cold water (1:2 w/v) for a day and then freeze-dried the licorice-water produced. At dosages of 10, 25, and 50 mg/ kg per day p.o. for ten consecutive days in separate dosage groups of CCl_4-treated rats, the licorice extract was tested as a 24-h posttreatment and as a 24-h pretreatment. Compared to CCl_4-treated controls, both the pre- and posttreatment groups showed significant reductions in liver enzymes (serum transaminases), alkaline phosphatase, and increases in hepatic albumin, globulin, and total protein at all three doses (each $p < 0.01$ in each parameter tested), and the hepatoprotective effect was dose dependent (Al-Qarawi et al., 2001).

Metabolites of glycyrrhizin have shown antihepatotoxic activity. In order of decreasing potency, these are: glycyrrhetinic acid, 3-*epi*-18β-glycyrrhetinic acid, glycyrrhizin, and 3-dehydro-18β-glycyrrhetinic acid (Kiso et al., 1984). In rat hepatocytes, the antihepatotoxic activity of glycyrrhetinic acid and glycyrrhizin appears to parallel their absorbability (Nose et al., 1993). Glycyrrhizin inhibited venom phospholipase A_2-induced release of acid phosphatase in rat liver lysosomes, suggesting a biomembrane stabilizing activity (Shiki et al., 1986).

Endocrine and Hormonal Functions

Reproductive Hormone Interactions

Glycyrrhetinic acid, the metabolite of glycyrrhizin, was found to inhibit testosterone production in vitro at a low concentration (10 μg/ml) and may account for the accidental finding of a reputedly effective traditional Chinese medical formula for patients with high levels of serum testosterone (Sakamoto et al., 1985).

In various in vitro assays for estrogenic activity, a methanolic extract of licorice root showed no significant binding to either estrogen receptors (ERα and ERβ) and only weak estrogenic activity in Ishikawa cells; the extract only weakly stimulated the expression of the progesterone receptor, failing to induce alkaline phosphatase activity; and it only weakly induced the expression of the estrogen-sensitive gene (*pS2*) in the S30 breast cancer cell line (Liu et al., 2001). However, in a radioreceptor assay, licorice showed strong in vitro estrogen-binding activity to the estrogen receptor of the human breast cancer cell line, MCF-7 (compared to 150 other plants used as herbs, foods, and spices). Whereas no estrogen- or progestin-binding activity was found from either glycyrrhizin or glycyrrhetinic acid, deglycerinized licorice (DGL) was found to hold a high degree of estrogen-binding activity, indicating that the progestin and estrogen activity of licorice is not attributable either to glycyrrhizin or glycyrrhetinic acid but to other constituents (Zava et al., 1998).

The isoflavan glabridin (11% w/w of an alcoholic extract of *G. glabra* roots) (Vaya et al., 1997) is a likely candidate and bears structural resemblance to estradiol. Glabridin exhibited in vitro estrogen-like activity and acted as an estrogen receptor agonist in human breast cancer cells (T47D cells) with an ED_{50} (~5 μM) similar to that of genistein from soybeans and other phytoestrogens. Further evidence of an estrogenic action was found in prepubertal female rats. Glabridin produced an increase in the wet weight of the uterus (200 μg/rat by injection) and induced immediate early creatine kinase B in skeletal, cardiovascular (2.5 mg/rat), and uterine tissues (25 μg/rat). Comparable effects were found from estradiol (5 μg) (Tamir et al., 2000).

In spayed mice, glycyrrhizin showed estrogenic action when administered by injection, concomitantly with 0.1 μg estradiol-17β. Glycyrrhizin at 1,000:1 estradiol-17β decreased uterine weight (antiestrogenic activity) but at 1 mg (10,000:1) had no estrogenic effect. In spayed rats, glycyrrhizin showed biphasic estrogenic activity; antiestrogenic activity at a ratio of 1,000:1 and 500:1 estradiol-17β, and estrogen-stimulatory activity at 5,000:1, but only with estradiol-17β (Kumagai et al., 1967).

Sakamoto and Wakabayashi (1988) examined the effects of glycyrrhizin (4.5 mg/kg per day p.o.); its main metabolite, glycyrrhetinic acid (4.5 mg/kg per day p.o.); and licorice root extract (45 mg/kg per day p.o.) on testosterone production in male rats after a 20-day treatment period. In Leydig cells stimulated with luteinizing hormone (LH), glycyrrhetinic acid or glycyrrhizin caused a significant decrease in basal testosterone production, the effect of glycyrrhetinic acid (90% inhibition of testosterone in vitro from 10 µg/mL) being much stronger than glycyrrhizin. Without LH stimulation, basal testosterone release was inhibited by approximately 40% from administration of either compound and by licorice root extract. In microsomal fractions of rat ovarian and testicular tissue, both compounds inhibited androstenedione conversion to testosterone, indicating that they inhibit 17β-hydroxysteroid dehydrogenase activity. 17β-hydroxysteroid dehydrogenase is an enzyme that catalyzes conversion of androstenedione to become testosterone.

In young animals, glycyrrhetinic acid and glycyrrhizin have shown estrogen-inhibitory activity that affected uterine growth. The activity was also found after removal of adrenal glands or ovaries. In a high dosage, however, glycyrrhizin potentiated estrogen activity (Chang and But, 1986).

Paolini et al. (1999) demonstrated that at high dosages, glycyrrhizin or licorice root extract (240 and 480 mg/kg p.o. and 3.138 and 6.276 mg/kg p.o., respectively for four days) administered to male rats as part of their diet suppressed testosterone 16α-hydroxylase activity by 51.4% from the higher dose of licorice extract, and from the respective doses of glycyrrhizin by 31.6% and 65%. The higher dosage of licorice extract corresponded to a human dose of approximately 25 g/day.

Immune Functions; Inflammation and Disease

Cancer

Chemopreventive activity. Niwa et al. (1999) examined the effect of short-term (two weeks) and long-term (30 weeks) dietary administration of licorice root extract (0.625% of the diet) on mouse endometrial carcinogenesis. In the short-term experiment, the extract-fed mice showed decreased levels of estradiol-17β-induced oncoproteins compared to the controls. In the long-term experiment in which a tumor-inducing chemical was administered (*N*-methyl-*N*-nitrosourea, or MNU, i.v.), the licorice extract-fed mice showed a significant decrease in the incidence of malignant lesions, uterine endometrial atypical hyperplastic lesions, and uterine weights. The researchers suggest that estradiol-17β-related endometrial carcinogenesis is inhibited in mice by way of suppression of estrogen-induced c-fos/jun-expressions, most likely by phytoestrogenic constituents of licorice root. They also note that expression of c-jun has been used as an indicator in the prognosis of human endometrial carcinomas and elevated expression of c-fos/jun expression has been reported in hamster kidney tumors induced by estrogen.

For these reasons, the researchers concluded that licorice root represents a promising means of preventing endometrial cancer in humans.

The major isoflavan in licorice root, glabridin, inhibited the in vitro growth of estrogen-negative human breast cancer cells (MDA-MB-468 cells) in a fashion distinguishable from that of tamoxifen. Although at low concentrations it bound to human estrogen receptors (~0.1-10 μM) and stimulated growth of estrogen-positive human breast cancer cells (T47D cells), at higher concentrations (≥ 25 μM) glabridin potently inhibited their growth (to levels of control cells) independent of these receptors. The growth-inhibitory concentration of glabridin is similar to that of genistein from soybeans and resveratrol from grape skins (Tamir et al., 2000).

Cultured mammary glands of mice exposed to the carcinogen DMBA (dimethylbenz[*a*]anthracene) followed by TPA (12-*O*-tetradecanoylphorbol 13-acetate) developed lesions. But when the cultured glands were treated with glycyrrhetinic acid prior to or simultaneously with the carcinogens, initiation of lesion growth was significantly inhibited, by 50% to 60% (Mehta and Moon, 1991).

The human carcinogenesis-initiating arylamines become carcinogenic through acetylation by *N*-acetyltransferase (NAT). Colorectal cancer and occupational bladder cancer in humans have been linked to acetylation, and higher levels of NAT activity have been associated with greater sensitivity to arylamine-induced mutagenesis. At various concentrations, glycyrrhizic acid showed a dose-dependent in vitro inhibition of NAT activity in *Heliobacter pylori* cultures obtained from 24 patients. From a concentration of 8 mM, NAT activity was significantly inhibited by 52% in cytosols, and by 48% in intact bacteria at a pH of 7.5, which is similar to that of the human intestine. Inhibition was still significant at a concentration of 2 mM ($p < 0.05$). The concentration of 8 mM is a dose of approximately 0.672 mg glycyrrhizic acid (Chung, 1998). Glycyrrhizic acid (8 mM) also inhibited DNA adduct formation in human colon tumor cells (adenocarcinoma cell line colo 25) (Chung et al., 2000).

Cytotoxicity

Isoliquiritigenin has also shown in vitro cytotoxic activity against human gastric cancer (MGC-803) cells in vitro (Ma et al., 2001) and a polyphenol glycoside (β-hydroxy-DHP, also found in *Rosa cymosa*) isolated from the root of *Glycyrrhiza glabra* has recently shown in vitro activity against leukemia (HL-60) and breast tumor cells (MCF-7 and T47D) (Rafi et al., 2001).

Immune Functions

Immunopotentiation. The polysaccharide glycyrrhizan GA showed more significant phagocytic activity (i.p.) in mice than several other polysaccharides previously isolated from *Glycyrrhiza uralensis* (Shimizu et al., 1991). Without cytotoxicity, glycyrrhizic acid has both an inhibiting activity on immature lymphocyte growth and a stimulating activity on interleukin-2 (IL-2) production/IL-3 receptor expression in vitro (Zhang et al., 1995); improved resistance in thermally injured mice to *Herpes simplex* 1 infection (Utsunomiya et al., 1995); enhanced production of interferon-γ in human peripheral lymphocyte-macrophage cultures by concanavalin A; and increased protein and RNA but decreased DNA synthesis in lymphocytes (Shinada et al., 1986).

Infectious Diseases

Fungal infections. Licorice root powder has also shown inhibitory activity against the growth of aflatoxin-producing *Aspergillus flavus* in liquid culture. The root powder inhibited the formation of aflatoxin at every concentration tested (0.1% to 10%). Aflatoxin formation was reduced by from 37.45% to 16% compared to the control. However, growth of *A. flavus* mycelia appeared to be stimulated at a concentration of 0.1% root powder, which decreased with increasing amounts of the added root powder (El Shayeb and Mabrouk, 1984). As much as streptomycin, glycycoumarin and licocoumarone inhibit the growth of some bacteria *(Bacillus subtilis, Staphylococcus aureus,* and *Streptococcus mutans).* They were also active against a number of fungi and yeasts for which streptomycin is inactive: *Aspergillus niger, Rhizopus formosaensis, Candida utilis, Pichia nakazawae,* and *Saccharomyces cerevisiae* (Demizu et al., 1988).

Microbial infections. The alcohol extract of licorice root has shown in vitro growth-inhibitory activity against *E. coli, Entamoeba histolytica, Mycobacterium tuberculosis, Staphylococcus aureus,* and *Trichomonas.* Against *S. aureus,* glycyrrhetinic acid potentiated the growth-inhibitory activity of the alkaloid berberine, a major constituent of goldenseal *(Hydrastis canadensis),* and promoted the formation of fibrosis in test tuberculosis lesions (Chang and But, 1986). Licochalcones A and B, glabrene, and glabridin have shown in vitro antimicrobial activity against Gram-positive *Bacillus subtilis* and *Staphylococcus aureus.* The in vitro antimicrobial potency of glabridin and licochalcone A was comparable to that of streptomycin. Against fungi and yeasts to which streptomycin was inactive *(Aspergillus niger, Candida utilis,* and *Saccharomyces cerevisiae),* glabridin showed significant in vitro antimicrobial activity (Okada et al., 1989). The constituent flavanone glabranin is weakly active in vitro against *Mycobacterium smegmatis* and *S. aureus* (Mitscher et al., 1983).

Using 22 strains of *Heliobacter pylori* obtained from 24 patients, Chung (1998) found dose-dependent growth-inhibitory activity from glycyrrhizic acid in vitro. Growth inhibition reached 90% from a concentration of 16 mM and at a concentration of 2 mM, glycyrrhizic acid inhibited growth of *H. pylori* by as much as 36%. Glycyrrhizic acid at a concentration of 8 mM in vitro, which is a dose of approximately 0.672 mg, growth of *Heliobacter pylori* obtained from human patients was inhibited from 62% to 76%.

Viral infections. Glycyrrhisoflavone (Hatano et al., 1989), glycyrrhizin (Hattori et al., 1989), and licopyranocoumarin (Hatano et al., 1989) have shown activity against HIV in vitro.

Inflammatory Response

Glycyrrhizin has shown a wide range of corticosteroid-like activities when injected in animals and humans (Chang and But, 1986). Glycyrrhizin has shown prostaglandin synthesis inhibition similar to that of cortisone (Ohuchi et al., 1981; Okimasu et al., 1983). Note that this is in contrast to the antiulcer agents DGL and carbenoxolone, which show little or no prostaglandin inhibition ex vivo (Bennett et al., 1985).

The flavonone isoliquiritigenin inhibits 5-lipoxygenase formation in vitro, which may partly account for the anti-inflammatory activity of licorice root. The flavonoids licochalcones A and B potently inhibit leukotriene biosynthesis in human neutrophils in vitro and reduce cytosolic free calcium concentrations (Kimura and Okuda, 1988). In mice, isoliquiritin (i.p.) showed a 50-fold greater inhibition of adjuvant-induced chronic inflammation than licorice extract. Isoliquiritin showed potent activity against granuloma angiogenesis and fluid exudation in the pouches of mice. Although granuloma formation was not inhibited by the flavonoid, effects were similar to those of the root extract (Kobayashi et al., 1995).

A platelet aggregation inhibitory coumarin named GU-7 displays various activities, including the inhibition of intracellular calcium increase, platelet phosphodiesterase activity, and the increase of intraplatelet cAMP concentration (Tawata et al., 1990).

Metabolic and Nutritional Functions

Antioxidant Activity

Isoflavans glabridin, and hispaglabridins A and B (Haraguchi et al., 2000; Vaya et al., 1997) are major antioxidant compounds in licorice root. An acetone extract of licorice roots (10 mg/L) inhibited oxidation of LDL obtained from healthy volunteers by 32% to 41%. Isoflavans isolated from the extract (30 μM) inhibited LDL oxidation by 65% to 85% with glabridin showing the most potent activity (75% to 85%). Glabridin at a concentration of 10 μM inhibited peroxidation of LDL cholesterol by 51% to 65% (measured using TBARS and lipid peroxidation) whereas vitamin E was inactive (Vaya et al., 1997). In vitro lipid peroxidation of rat liver mitochondria was also inhibited by isoflavans isolated from *G. glabra* roots. Against NADH-dependent lipid peroxidation, 3'-hydroxy-4'-*O*-methylglabridin was most potent, providing complete inhibition at a concentration of 1 μM (equivalent to butylated hydroxytuluene at 10 μM), followed by hispaglabridin A (8 mM), hispaglabridin B, 4'-*O*-methylglabridin, and glabridin (each at 30 μM) (Haraguchi et al., 2000).

The coumarin constituent licocoumarone is a potent antioxidant and quenches active oxygen (Demizu et al., 1988). Antioxidant activity from *Glycyrrhiza glabra* var. *glandulifera* against the oxidation of lard at 100°C was largely attributed to the flavonoids, licochalcones A and B, which were comparable in potency to vitamin E (Okada et al., 1989).

Hyaluronidase activation and histamine release is potently inhibited in vitro by the flavonone isoliquiritigenin. These activities may help to account for the clinical use of *Glycyrrhiza glabra* (Kagegawa et al., 1992) and glycyrrhizin in Japan for the treatment of allergies (Hikino, 1985). By catalyzing the formation of uric acid, xanthene oxidase induces gout. The enzyme is also known for causing oxidative damage in tissues by superoxide free radicals. Several flavonoids from licorice root showed inhibitory activity in vitro against xanthine oxidase (glycyrrhisoflavone and licochalcones A and B), although they were weaker than the gout remedy allopurinol (Hatano et al., 1989).

Glycyrrhizin (10 mg/kg p.o.) normalized renal levels of creatinine to those of controls and at 2.5 mg/kg p.o. suppressed urea nitrogen levels in rats when administered prior to ischemia-reperfusion. Activities of antioxidant enzymes catalase and GSH-Px in the left kidneys of rats treated with glycyrrhizin (2.5 or 10 mg/kg p.o.) showed a marked elevation compared to untreated controls; however, their levels were still not as high as those of normal controls and glycyrrhizin significantly decreased the renal activity levels of an important antioxidant enzyme, superoxide dismutase (SOD) (Yokozawa et al., 1999/2000).

Glycyrrhiza uralensis, the main species used medicinally in Chinese medicine (Foster and Chongxi, 1992), contains a recently isolated phenolic (tetrahydroxymethoxychalcone) exhibiting greater radical-scavenging activity against the DPPH radical (1,1-diphenyl-2-picrylhydrazyl radical) than licochalcone B. Scavenging of the DPPH radical is commonly used as a model for lipid free radicals (Hatano et al., 1997).

Respiratory and Pulmonary Functions

Bronchial Functions

The demulcent and expectorant activity of licorice root is attributable to glycyrrhizin, which stimulates mucus secretion in the trachea (Bradley, 1992).

CLINICAL STUDIES

Digestive, Hepatic, and Gastrointestinal Disorders

Gastric Disorders

Ulcers. Since carbenoxolone (synthetic glycyrrhetinic acid) was reported effective in the treatment of mouth ulcers and Herpes simplex infection, Das et al. (1989) instructed 20 patients with mouth ulcers to gargle and use deglycyrrhinated licorice (DGL) as a mouthwash q.i.d. for seven days using 200 mL warm water containing 200 mg dissolved DGL powder. Treatment commenced from two to five days following the occurrence of mouth ulcers. Fifteen of the patients reported 50% to 75% diminishment of pain in the first 24 h. By 72 h, the ulcers had completely healed with no apparent side effects.

Unlike the synthetic form of glycyrrhetinic acid (carbenoxolone), which is also used to treat stomach ulcers, deglycyrrhinated licorice (DGL) does not cause side effects of electrolyte and fluid imbalance, edema, increased blood pressure, or hyperkalemia (Tewari and Trembalowicz, 1968). DGL contains no more than 3% natural glycyrrhizin (Larkworthy and Holgate, 1975).

In a controlled study, 874 patients with chronic duodenal ulcers were given either DGL (Caved-S), cimetidine, antacids, or geranylferensylacetate. For 91% of the patients, all ulcers were healed in 12 weeks and the rate of healing between the groups showed no significant difference. In the numbers of relapsing patients, however, a noticeable difference existed between the treatment groups: DGL (8.2%), cimetidine (12.9%), antacids (16.4%), and geranylferensylacetate (15.5%) (Kassir, 1985). Caved-S (tablets) is a proprietary formulation containing powdered black licorice (380 mg), frangula bark (30 mg), sodium bicarbonate (100 mg), magnesium carbonate (200 mg), bismuth sunitrate (100 mg), and aluminum hydroxide (100 mg) (Tewari and Trembalowicz, 1968).

Morgan et al. (1982) found a 14% rate of relapse in 56 gastric ulcer patients treated with cimetidine (400 mg at bedtime) or DGL (Caved-S, 760 mg, b.i.d. between meals) as maintenance therapy for one year following the healing of gastric ulcers using the same agents. The researchers also reported that in 100 gastric ulcer patients on either agent—cimetidine (200 mg t.i.d. plus 400 mg at bedtime) or DGL (760 mg between meals t.i.d.)— the percentages of healed ulcers after six and 12 weeks were similar in both groups. They recommended surgery for patients who still had unhealed ulcers after 12 weeks.

Patients in a double blind, placebo-controlled crossover study received aspirin alone (325 mg, t.i.d.) or tablets containing aspirin plus DGL (325 mg and 175 mg, respectively per tablet, t.i.d.). Two periods of treatment lasted five days each. The researchers reported 20% less blood loss in the stools of patients on aspirin plus DGL and suspected that even less blood loss would be gained with a higher dosage of DGL (Rees et al., 1979).

DGL (Caved-S tablet) was compared to cimetidine in a randomized double-blind trial in patients with duodenal (DU) and gastric ulcers (GU). Endoscopic examination at the end of the fourth week of treatment revealed a significant healing of DU in patients on either medication, but ulcers were smaller in the group on cimetidine (1 g/day). At that point, endoscopic examination showed that ulcers were healed in 64% of the group receiving DGL (5 g/day), while in those on cimetidine 93% had healed. Maintenance therapy was administered in a second randomized, though open, treatment. At the second month, the relapse rate following healing was greater in the DGL group (42.8%) receiving maintenance therapy (3 g daily) than in those receiving cimetidine (400 mg/bedtime) maintenance therapy (12.8%). At the end of four months, no relapsed cases occurred in either group (D'Imperio et al., 1978).

The same investigators conducted a double-blind trial in gastric ulcer patients randomly assigned to the same doses of DGL. At the end of the fourth week, 57% of those on DGL and 57% of those on cimetidine showed healed ulcers. D'Imperio and colleagues concluded that although both therapies were effective against DU, cimetidine provided more complete and rapid healing, better diminishment of attendant inflammation and pain, and less relapse than DGL (D'Imperio et al., 1978).

In a double-blind placebo-controlled study of DGL in 48 patients with duodenal ulcers and six with gastric ulcers, Tewari and Trembalowicz (1968) found that gastric ulcer patients showed extensive healing. They noted a marked improvement of symptoms in the DU cases in four weeks. Side effects were minimal and radiological examinations showed a spasmolytic action of DGL in every case, whereas in patients on antacids alone no evidence of spasmolytic activity existed. The dosage employed was two tablets, t.i.d.

Hepatic Diseases

Hepatitis. Uncontrolled studies of licorice root in China claim success against infectious hepatitis. A decoction of the root administered orally (15 to 20 mL t.i.d.) for ten to twenty days is reported to have diminished hepatic pain within eight days, markedly reduced hepatomegaly in nine days, and, within ten days, a negative reading in urinary bile pigments was found (Chang and But, 1986).

A retrospective study on the long-term use of a standardized licorice root extract, Greater Neo-Minophagen C (SNMC), in Japanese patients diagnosed with hepatitis C found a chemopreventive effect in the form of a decreased incidence of hepatocellular carcinoma (Arase et al., 1997). SNMC is a common treatment for hepatitis C in Japan as a means to ameliorate altered levels of serum alanine aminotransferase (ALT). SNMC is made up of an aqueous extract of licorice root (as 0.2% glycyrrhizin), 2.0% glycine, and 0.1% cysteine dissolved in physiologic saline. Results were compared in 84 subjects receiving SNMC to 109 patients not receiving the preparation (100 mL/day i.v. for 8 weeks, followed by the same dose two to seven times per week for a median period of 10.1 years). Serum ALT levels decreased to within the normal range (6-50 IU) in 35.7% of cases taking SNMC compared to 6.4% of those not receiving SNMC ($p = 0.0001$). Side effects were observed in 10.7% of the SNMC group in the form of hypokalemia. Serum potassium levels did not decrease below 3 mEq/mL, and daily administration of spironolactone (150 mg) brought potassium levels back to within normal. Increased blood pressure occurred in 3.6% of the SNMC group and was also corrected using spironolactone (150-300 mg/day). No patient discontinued SNMC because of side effects. Deaths occurred in 9.5% in the SNMC group as a result of liver failure in one patient, progressed hepatocellular carcinoma in four, and from other causes in three patients. In the non-SNMC group, 17.4% died, including five from other diseases, progressed hepatocellular carcinoma in 13, and in one case from liver cirrhosis. The ten-year rates of hepatocellular carcinoma in hepatitis C patients of 3% and 13% (stages I, II, and III) in patients receiving SNMC were higher than in patients receiving lymphoblastoid interferon-α, but patients on SNMC showed considerably fewer side effects and the treatment is much less expensive (Arase et al., 1997). Improved treatment modalities for hepatitis C are urgently needed.

Endocrine and Hormonal Disorders

Hypothalamic and Pituitary Functions

In the treatment of postpartum anterior pituitary insufficiency, ten cases are reported to have responded completely from a decoction of licorice root and ginseng (Chang and But, 1986).

Immune Disorders; Inflammation and Disease

Infectious Diseases

Microbial infections. Against pulmonary TB, responses were reported with a combination of licorice preparations and conventional drug therapies for TB. The dosage used was 18 g of root decocted in 150 mL water t.i.d. (Chang and But, 1986).

Integumentary, Muscular, and Skeletal Disorders

Muscular Disorders

Researchers in China reported marked improvement in three to six days treatment (10-15 mL licorice root extract) in 241/254 cases of gastric muscle spasm (Chang and But, 1986).

Skin Diseases

In China, purpura was treated with uncured licorice root (30 g morning and afternoon). Remissions were found in a mean of 6.2 days, which were without relapse after 8-12 weeks (Chang and But, 1986).

Saxena et al. (1965), in an open-label preliminary clinical study, reported success in using licorice root to treat pemphigus, a chronic, relapsing, and sometimes fatal skin disease characterized by bulbous lesions. Licorice root powder (3 g t.i.d. with water for adults and half dosage for children under 8) showed benefits in three male and three female patients (ages 2-25) being successfully maintained with prednisolone. Taking licorice, five of these patients were able to substantially reduce their dosage of prednisolone without the lesions reerupting (Saxena et al., 1965).

Patients with intractable eczema treated with a topical ointment containing glycyrrhetinic acid showed marked improvement in 75% of cases. Only 2% showed a mild improvement. In a further comparative study of the ointment and cortisone, Evans (1958) found 83% improved on cortisone and 93% improved on the ointment.

Metabolic and Nutritional Disorders

Pharmacokinetics

The human intestinal flora converts glycyrrhizin into glycyrrhetinic acid (18β-glycyrrhetinic acid), • 3-*epi*-18β-glycyrrhetinic acid, and • 3-dehydro-18β-glycyrrhetinic acid (Kiso et al., 1984). More recently it was shown that the metabolites of glycyrrhizin (p.o.) in the stomach flora of rats are 3β-hydroxyglycyrrhetic acid, 3-oxo-hydroxyglycyrrhetic acid, and 3α-hydroxyglycyrrhetic acid; however, whether 3β-hydroxyglycyrrhetic acid is metabolized from glycyrrhizin via stomach contents in vivo is unknown (Akao, 1997).

Glycyrrhetinic acid administered orally to rats and human volunteers displayed practically the same low bioavailability and detectability in plasma over various intervals up to 36 h as glycyrrhizin (Cantelli-Forti et al., 1994). Twelve hours following oral administration in germ-free rats, glycyrrhizin was completely converted to glycyrrhetinic acid, which showed up in plasma after 9.3 h. The parent compound, glycyrrhizin, required 19.9 h (Takeda et al., 1996).

Protein binding of glycyrrhetinic acid in human serum albumin after oral administration of glycyrrhizin is over 99.9% (Ishida et al., 1988). In rats, the large intestine appears to be the main site of formation and absorption of glycyrrhetinic acid (Wang et al., 1994). The oral bioavailability of glycyrrhetinic acid is naturally increased by hydrophilic components of licorice root extract (Wang et al., 1995).

Metabolites of glycyrrhetinic acid by rat liver homogenates include 3-oxo-18β-glycyrrhetic acid, 22α-hydroxy-18β-glycyrrhetic acid, and 24-hydroxy-18β-glycyrrhetic acid (Akao et al., 1990).

Neurological, Psychological, and Behavioral Disorders

Neurodegenerative Disorders

Retinopathies. In China, out of 60 cases of keratitis (herpetic, conjunctive, and fascicular), application of extract drops (10% to 30% extract) into the eyes t.i.d. or q.i.d. daily appeared to cause remission in 56 cases in two to seven days. An 8% to 12% suspension of glycyrrhetinic acid was reported to be equally effective (Chang and But, 1986).

DOSAGE

Bradley's *British Herbal Compendium* (1992) gives a dosage for dried licorice root of 1-5 g t.i.d. whether in decoction or infusion. In the liquid extract form recognized by the *British Pharmacopoeia,* the dosage suggested is 2-5 mL t.i.d. For DGL extract, the dosage given is 0.4-1.6 g t.i.d., with high dosages not recommended for longer than four to six weeks (Bradley, 1992).

In France, the officially recognized dosage of licorice root infusion is a maximum of 8 g/24 h, which is given the equivalency of glycyrrhizin at 3 mg/24 h. All dosages are to be considered with regard to other sources of licorice in the diet, including confections (Bradley, 1992).

The German Commission E monograph on licorice root approves an average daily dose of 5-15 g, calculated as equivalent to glycyrrhizin at 200-

600 mg. In the form of succus liquiritae, the dosage given in treating catarrh is 0.5-1.0 g daily, and in gastric or duodenal ulcers, 1.5-3.0 g daily. In the absence of medical advice, administration of licorice root is not to exceed four to six weeks (Blumenthal et al., 1998). The maximum allowable daily dose of glycyrrhizin as flavoring is 100 mg (Bradley, 1992).

Because alcohol in the extract aggravates ulcers, some doctors in China recommend the powdered root at a dosage of 2.5-5.0 g t.i.d. for three to four weeks (Chang and But, 1986).

The content of glycyrrhizin in licorice root ranges from 1% to 24%, although the range is usually 6% to 14%. Commercial health products have been found to range from 0.30-47.1 mg/g (Chandler, 1997). Herbal products in the United States are known to be standardized to contain 12% glycyrrhizin (Flynn and Roest, 1995); however, most commercial extracts of licorice root are glycyrrhizin acid- and glycyrrhetinic acid-free.

In trials using capsules of DGL, encapsulation appears to have adversely affected favorable outcomes, whereas trials using DGL tablets found significant results compared to placebo (e.g., Feldman and Gilat, 1971); those using capsules have repeatedly shown poor results in different studies (Engqvist et al., 1973; Nussbaumer et al., 1977; Balakrishnan et al., 1978; Bardhan et al., 1978). Also, chewable tablets of DGL taken 20 min before meals produced better results than if taken after meals (Feldman and Gilat, 1971).

In the *British Pharmacopoeia,* the dosage for DGL extract is 0.4-1.6 g t.i.d., with high dosages not recommended for longer than four to six weeks (Bradley, 1992). DGL is standardized to contain no more than 3% natural glycyrrhizin (Larkworthy and Holgate, 1975).

SAFETY PROFILE

In the United States, licorice root is given the status of a generally recognized as safe (GRAS) food item (Bradley, 1992).

Prolonged or excessive intake of licorice may cause pulmonary or systemic hypertension (Ruszymah et al., 1995).

Contraindications

Licorice root is contraindicated in patients with hypokalemia, renal insufficiency, hypertension, chronic hepatitis, pregnancy, cholestatic liver diseases, liver cirrhosis (De Smet, 1993), chronic liver inflammation (Bradley, 1992), incipient kidney failure, and in thyroid, overweight, and cardiac patients (Anonymous, 1995). Because glycyrrhetinic acid causes sodium retention (MacKenzie et al., 1990), high doses would not be recommended in patients on a salt-restricted diet. Owing to the mineralocorticoid-like action of glycyrrhetinic acid (MacKenzie et al., 1990), licorice root may be contra-indicated in hypercortisolemia patients (Farese et al., 1991).

At a dosage of 7 g/day for seven days in young men (ages 22-24), a commercial extract of licorice (Saila, Bologna, Italy) was reported to cause serum 17-hydroxyprogesterone levels to significantly increase and testosterone levels to significantly decrease (each $p < 0.001$), as measured four days after the last dose. The results demonstrated that licorice extract can inhibit the activity of enzymes (17 alpha-hydroxylase: 17,20-lyase [P450 17] and 17β-hydroxysteroid dehydrogenase) that catalyze the conversion of 17-hydroxyprogesterone to androstenedione (Armanini et al., 1999). However, two attempts by Josephs et al. (2001) to replicate the results of Armanini et al. (1999) failed, an outcome which they attributed to probable errors in the statistical methods used by Armanini and colleagues to evaluate their results. Therefore, warnings of licorice being contraindicated in men with sexual dysfunction, such as decreased libido, would be premature. Previous research demonstrated that, in vitro, licorice blocked the action of 17β-hydroxysteroid dehydrogenase, an enzyme that catalyzes conversion of androstenedione to become testosterone (Sakamoto and Wakabayashi, 1988).

Drug Interactions

Licorice root can cause potassium loss leading to increased sensitivity to digitalis glycosides. Loss of potassium can increase in patients on thiazide and potassium-sparing diuretic agents (e.g., amiloride, spironolactone, or triamterine). Licorice root can interfere with regulation of blood pressure-lowering medications that act by decreasing water and sodium retention. Due to a mineralocorticoid effect, licorice root is not recommended for patients on corticoid treatment or cardiac glycosides (Bradley, 1992).

Glycyrrhetinic acid has been shown to potentiate the activity of hydrocortisone in human lung tissue, but glycyrrhizin has not. In healthy men, and similarly in patients with polyarteritis nodosa and rheumatoid arthritis, glycyrrhizin (p.o.) increased plasma concentrations of prednisolone (i.v.) and inhibited prednisolone metabolism. Taken at the same time with nitrofurantoin, deglycyrrhizinated licorice increased the bioavailability of the agent by more than 50%, and yet decreased tendency to emesis and nausea. With furosemide, chronic ingestion of licorice has been associated with acute renal failure. Glycyrrhizin may have synergistic activity with insulin, possibly causing disturbances in electrolytes and suppressing aldosterone and renin (Chandler, 1997).

MAO inhibition from a number of licorice root constituents in vitro indicates that the herb might potentiate MAO-inhibiting medications (Tanaka et al., 1987; Hatano et al., 1991) (see Special Precautions).

Glycyrrhetinic acid potentiated the activity of hydrocortisone in the skin by inhibiting the metabolism of cortisol to its inactive form, cortisone.

Mixed with a hydrocortisone acetate solution and applied to the skin of human volunteers, glycyrrhetinic acid significantly potentiated the vaso-constrictor activity of hydrocortisone acetate, whereas the compound alone had no such effect and hydrocortisone alone showed a flat activity response (Teelucksingh et al., 1990).

In an in vitro study, a commercially available ethanolic extract of licorice root *(G. glabra)* was shown to inhibit significantly the drug metabolizing enzyme P450 3A4 (CYP3A4). With an IC_{50} of 1.83% of the extract full strength, it was ranked as relatively high in potency among 21 other com-mercial plant extracts and in the order of red clover *(Trifolium pratense),* Echinacea roots *(E. purpurea* and *E. angustifolia),* chamomile *(Matricaria chamomilla),* and ginkgo *(G. biloba)* (Budzinski et al., 2000).

Pregnancy and Lactation

Licorice root has been contraindicated in pregnancy (Bradley, 1992; McGuffin et al.,1997; Blumenthal et al., 1998). A recent survey of licorice use in the diet of pregnant women documented an increased incidence of early birth but with no negative impact on birth weight. In a study on the ef-fects of licorice candy consumption by 1,049 women and their healthy in-fants, researchers in Finland found that babies born to mothers who were heavy consumers of licorice (equivalent to $\geq$ 500 mg glycyrrhizin/week) were twice as likely to be born early (before 38 weeks) (mean 2.52 days); however, they showed no significant difference in birth weight (Strandberg et al., 2001). Licorice has been found to have estrogenic activity, sufficient to increase uterine weight in animals. The likely constituent of activity is glabridin, not glycyrrhizin (see Reproductive Hormone Interactions). In India licorice root is considered a galactogogue (Bingel and Farnsworth, 1994). Chang and But (1986) note postpartum licorice use for treating what they describe as anterior pituitary insufficiency, presumably a galactogogue intent. In a study of basal prolactin levels and response to TRH stimulation, Le Moli et al. (1999) found long-term use of licorice was associated with significantly lower basal and stimulated prolactin levels in nonlactating women and in men. As with most other herbs, studies on licorice use have not been conducted on lactating women. The phytoestrogenic effects of lic-orice may offer a mode of action explaining reputed galactogogue action; many other galactogogue herbs have documented phytoestrogenic activity. No reports of adverse reactions during lactation are documented. Insuffi-cient information is available to predict the nature of lactation modulation that could occur. However, *Glycyrrhiza*-containing licorice candy, a com-mon foodstuff in Europe and Canada, is not known to alter lactation.

Side Effects

Most commercial extracts of licorice root are glycyrrhizin acid- and gly-cyrrhetinic acid-free. Research has shown that glycyrrhizin by itself or in drugs, candy, or drinks is not as safe as licorice root (Cantelli-Forti et al., 1994).

In normal doses, licorice candy, herbal preparations of licorice, or bever-ages containing licorice are not thought to represent any significant risk of health damage (Ruszymah et al., 1995). However, in 20% of people, licorice root long-term ingestion in high doses or in small oral doses produced side effects of hypokalemia, headache, spastic numbness, hypertension, weak limbs, dizziness, and edema (Chang and But, 1986), or so-called "minerol-corticoid excess." Based on published accounts of adverse events, a safe oral dose of licorice for healthy individuals providing a safety factor of ten was estimated to be the equivalent of ingesting 10 mg of glycyrrhizic acid per day or 5 g of licorice/day if the glycyrrhizin content is 0.2% (Stormer et al., 1993). This safe level was much lower than the acceptable daily intake (ADI) of 200 mg/day provided by the Dutch Nutrition Council in 1988 (van Gelderen et al., 2000). Following a randomized double-blind study in women ages 19-40 years, van Gelderen et al. (2000) have proposed a no-effect level of 2 mg glycyrrhizic acid per kg body weight/day and that for an ADI providing a safety factor of ten, the amount would be 0.2 mg/ kg per day or 12 mg/day for a healthy individual weighing 60 kg. Their study was conducted in healthy female volunteers ($n = 39$) because a previous dose-finding pilot study also randomized and double-blind, found that women appeared to be more sensitive to the minerolcorticoid excess effects of glycyrrhizic acid.

Mineralocorticoid excess is normally found from excessive licorice intake in people with a congenital deficiency of 11β-hydroxysteroid dehydrogenase, an enzyme system that converts active forms of corticosterone and cortisol to their respectively inactive forms (11-dehydrocorticosterone and cortisone). Licorice root, glycyrrhizin, or glycyrrhetinic acid caused suppression of this enzyme (MacKenzie et al., 1990). The inhibition is mediated through the glucocorticoid receptor, not the mineralocorticoid receptor (Whorwood et al., 1993). Therefore, among individuals deficient in these enzymes, plasma cortisol half-life may be prolonged. In those cases and for people who have taken an excess of licorice, a remedial response is found from treatment with spironolactone (MacKenzie et al., 1990). Increased potas-sium intake to counteract hypokalemia has been suggested for people taking licorice root, as well as monitoring of electrolytes and blood pressure (Farese et al., 1991; MacKenzie et al., 1990).

Over a period of ten years, five cases of transient visual loss/aberrations were documented in patients who had consumed 113 to 907 g of licorice candy. The authors propose that the effect is due to vasoconstrictive activity of licorice constituents, glycyrrhetinic acid, and carbenoxolone (synthetic glycyrrhetinic acid) (Dobbins and Saul, 2000).

A recent case was reported of a 64-year-old man who developed dyspnea upon exertion, fatigue, orthopnea, and pulmonary edema after eating about 1,000 g of black licorice Twizzlers (Hershey brand) over a period of three days (Chamberlain and Abolnik, 1997). Hypertension encephalopathy associated with chronic ingestion of licorice candy in low doses was reported in two cases by Russo et al. (2000). The patients were males, one age 42 and the other age 46. One patient had consumed 50 g/day (providing 100 mg glycyrrhizic acid) and the other about 40 g/day. Both required drug treatments in addition to discontinuing the use of licorice candy. The elevated blood pressure remained high even after intravenous urapidil and potassium were administered to the older man and labetalol was administered to the younger man. After two weeks, blood pressure was sufficiently normalized in the younger man to allow his discharge; both patients showed normalized blood pressure at follow-up four months later.

Several other instances of congestive heart failure associated with candy licorice have been reported (Chamberlain and Abolnik, 1997). In the Netherlands, two cases of hypertension, raised renal cortisol levels, and hypokalemia were reported in which the subjects had consumed licorice-flavored chewing gums in low doses. The authors noted that the gums contained considerable concentrations of glycyrrhizinic acid (10% in BenBits Cool Mint, a.k.a. Sorbits, and 8% to 12% in Stimorol Sugar Free), which amounted to a dose of 120 mg/day and 50 mg/day in the two respective patients. One patient who was taking chlorithiazide for pretibial edema denied ingesting any licorice. The correct diagnosis was nearly overlooked (Klerk et al., 1997).

Reversible side effects from glycyrrhizin intake are rare at dosages below 100 mg/day but are common at amounts of 400 mg/day or more (Stormer et al., 1993; van der Zwan, 1993). Side effects from glycyrrhizin may occur from greater than 100 mg/day or from licorice root at greater than 3 g daily taken for longer than six weeks. Either substance may cause hypertension, water and sodium retention, hypokalemia, and renin-aldosterone system suppression mediated by a pseudo-aldosterone action of the constituent glycyrrhetinic acid (Farese et al., 1991; MacKenzie et al., 1990).

Glycyrrhetinic acid in healthy volunteers (500 mg daily for seven days; equivalent to 200 g of licorice candy/day) caused a mineralocorticoid-like action, urinary potassium and plasma sodium to significantly increase, and plasma potassium to significantly fall. Marked suppression of the renin-angiotensin-aldosterone axis occurred and a significant fall in plasma aldosterone took place (MacKenzie et al., 1990). However, patients on glycyrrhizin whose normal diet was high in potassium and low in sodium, including patients with angina and high blood pressure, showed no pseudo-aldosterone side effects (Baron et al., 1969).

Special Precautions

Individuals with renal diseases or cardiovascular problems should be cautioned about licorice intake. Licorice root must also be used with caution in the elderly (Chang and But, 1986).

Although MAO inhibition remains to be shown from in vivo studies of licorice root, liquiritigenin and isoliquiritigenin were identified as in vitro substrate competitive inhibitors of monoamine oxidase (MAO). Isoliquiritigenin (IC_{50} = 17.3 mM) was a more potent inhibitor of oxidative deamination by MAO than harman HCL (IC_{50} = 742 mM), a standard MAO inhibitor. Liquiritigenin (IC_{50} = 742 mM) was much weaker (Tanaka et al., 1987). Other less active in vitro MAO-inhibiting flavonoids in licorice root include genistein, glycyrrhisoflavone, and glicoricone. The triterpene glycyrrhizin was also active. Coumarins isolated from licorice root can inhibit MAO—the strongest being licocoumarone, which showed inhibitory activity at a concentration slightly higher than that of harman HCL. Less active coumarins isolated from licorice root are licofuranone and licopyranocoumarin (Hatano et al., 1991).

In a recent unique case report, a man, age 32, without any previous history of allergies, developed an allergic reaction (nasal congestion, cough, sneezing, and moderate dyspnea) to licorice root after four years of working in a liqueur factory where he handled large quantities of the root. Tests showed that he had far higher levels of specific IgE for licorice than for any other plant material he handled in the factory or common aeroallergens (Gonzalez-Gutierrez et al., 2000).

Toxicology

Mutagenicity

Glycyrrhiza glabra root extract, glycyrrhizin, and glycyrrhetinic acid all showed antimutagenic activity (Zani et al., 1993).

Toxicity in Animal Models

Paolini et al. (1999) caution that at repeated high oral doses, licorice extract or glycyrrhizin (3.138 and 6.276 mg/kg and 240 and 480 mg/kg, respectively) administered to rats of either sex as part of their diet for four days caused changes in CYP isozymes in liver microsomes indicating potentially tumorigenic effects (unrelated to genotoxicity) of the kind found in association with the induction of CYP isoforms, such as those caused by aflatoxins, dioxins, polycyclic aromatic hydrocarbons, halogenated hydrocarbons, olefins, and activating aromatic amines. The researchers comment that the induction of CYP-associated monooxygenases (typical phase-I activating enzymes) by glycyrrhizin or licorice root extract raises serious doubts as to the usefulness of licorice as a chemopreventive supplement, despite the fact that the doses tested were much higher than those used in phytotherapy. The higher dosage of licorice extract corresponded to a human dose of approximately 25 g/day.

Most commercial extracts of licorice root are glycyrrhizin acid- and glycyrrhetinic acid-free.

REFERENCES

Akao, T. (1997). Localization of enzymes involved in metabolism of glycyrrhizin in contents of rat gastrointestinal tract. *Biological and Pharmaceutical Bulletin* 20: 122-126.

Akao, T., Aoyama, M., Akao, T., Hattori, M., Imai, Y., Namba, T., Tezuka, Y., Kikuchi, T., and Kobashi, K. (1990). Metabolism of glycyrrhetic acid by rat liver microsomes, II. *Biochemical Pharmacology* 40: 291-296.

Al-Qarawi, A.A., Abdel-Rahman, H.A., and El-Mougy, S.A. (2001). Hepatoprotective activity of licorice in rat liver injury models. *Journal of Herbs, Spices and Medicinal Plants* 8: 7-14.

Anonymous (1989). Licorice. *Lawrence Review of Natural Products* (July): 1-3.

Anonymous (1995). Botanical toxicology. *Protocol Journal of Botanical Medicine* 1: 147-158.

Arase, Y., Ikeda, K., Murashima, N., Chayama, K., Tsubota, A., Koida, I., Suzuki, Y., Saitoh, S., Kobayashi, M., and Kumada, H. (1997). The long term efficacy of glycyrrhizin in chronic hepatitis C patients. *Cancer* 79: 1594-1500.

Armanini, D., Bonanni, G., and Palermo, M. (1999). Reduction of serum testosterone in men by licorice. *New England Journal of Medicine* 341: 1158 (letter).

Balakrishnan, V., Pillai, M.V., Raveendran, P.M., and Nair, C.S. (1978). Deglycyrrhizinated liquorice in the treatment of chronic duodenal ulcer. *Journal of the Association of Physicians of India* 26: 811-814.

Bardhan, K.D., Cumberland, D.C., Dixon, R.A., and Holdsworth, C.D. (1978). Clinical trial of deglycyrrhizinised liquorice in gastric ulcer. *Gut* 19: 779-782.

Baron, J., Nabarro, J.D.N., Slater, J.D.H., and Tuffley, R. (1969). Metabolic studies, aldosterone secretion rate, and plasma renin after carbenoxolone sodium as biogastrone. *British Medical Journal* 2: 793-795.

Bennett, A., Melhuish, P.B., and Stamford, I.F. (1985). Carbenoxolone and deglycyrrhized liquorice have little or no effect on prostanoid synthesis by rat gastric mucosa ex vivo. *British Journal of Pharmacology* 86: 693-695.

Bingel, A.S. and Farnsworth, N.R. (1994). Higher plants as potential sources of galactogogues. In Wagner, H., Hikino, H., and Farnsworth, N.R. (Eds.), *Economic and Medicinal Plant Research,* Vol. 6 (pp. 1-54). New York, NY: Academic Press.

Blumenthal, M., Busse, W.R., Goldberg, A., Gruenwald, J., Hall, T., Riggins, C.W., and Rister, R.S. (Eds.) (1998). *The Complete German Commission E Monographs* (pp. 161-162). Austin, TX: American Botanical Council.

Bradley, P.R. (Ed.) (1992). *British Herbal Compendium*, Vol. 1 (pp. 145-148). Bournemouth, Dorset, England: British Herbal Medicine Association.

Budzinski, J.W., Foster, B.C., Vandenhoek, S., and Arnason, J.T. (2000). An in vitro evaluation of human cytochrome P450 3A4 inhibition by selected commercial herbal extracts and tinctures. *Phytomedicine* 7: 273-282.

Cantelli-Forti, G., Maffei, F., Bugamelli, F., Hrelia, P., Bernardi, M., D'Intino, P., Maranesi, M., and Raggi, M.A. (1994). Interaction of licorice on glycyrrhizin pharmacokinetics. *Environmental Health Perspectives* 102(Suppl.): 65-68.

Chamberlain, J.J. and Abolnik, I.Z. (1997). Pulmonary edema following a licorice binge. *The Western Journal of Medicine* 167: 184-185.

Chandler, R.F. (1997). *Glycyrrhiza glabra.* In De Smet, P.A.G.M., Keller, K., Hänsel, R., and Chandler, R.F. (Eds.), *Adverse Effects of Herbal Drugs,* Vol. 3 (pp. 67-87). Berlin, Germany: Springer-Verlag.

Chang, H.M. and But, P.P.H. (Eds.) (1986). *Pharmacology and Applications of Chinese Materia Medica,* Vol. 1 (pp. 304-317). Hong Kong: World Scientific.

Chung, J.G. (1998). Inhibitory actions of glycyrrhizic acid on arylamine *N*-acetyltransferase activity in strains of *Helicobacter pylori* from peptic ulcer patients. *Drug and Chemical Toxicology* 21: 355-371.

Chung, J.G., Chang, H.L., Lin, W.C., Wang, H.H., Yeh, C.C., and Hung, C.F. (2000). Inhibition of *N*-acetyltransferase activity and DNA-2-aminofluorene adducts by glycyrrhizic acid in human colon tumour cells. *Food and Chemical Toxicology* 38: 163-172.

Das, S.K., Das, V., Gulati, A.K., and Singh, V.P. (1989). Deglycyrrhizinated liquorice in aphthous ulcers. *Journal of the Association of Physician of India* 37: 647.

de Klerk, G.J., Nieuwenhuis, M.G., and Beutler, J.J. (1997). Hypokalaemia and hypertension associated with use of liquorice flavoured chewing gum. *British Medical Journal* 314: 731-732.

De Smet, P.A.G.M. (Ed.) (1993). *Adverse Effects of Herbal Drugs,* Vol. 2 (p. 46). New York: Springer-Verlag.

Demizu, S., Kajiyama, K., Takahashi, K., Hiraga, Y., Yamamoto, S., Tamura, Y., Okada, K., and Kinoshita, T. (1988). Antioxidant and antimicrobial constituents of licorice: Isolation and structure elucidation of a new benzofuran derivative. *Chemical and Pharmaceutical Bulletin* 36: 3474-3479.

D'Imperio, N., Piccari, G.G., Sarti, F., Soffritti, M., Spongano, S.K., Benvenuti, C., and Dal Monte, P.R. (1978). Double-blind trial in duodenal and gastric ulcers. *Acta Gastro-Enterologica Belgica* 41: 427-434.

Dobbins, K.R. and Saul, R.F. (2000). Transient visual loss after licorice ingestion. *Journal of Neuroophthalmology* 20: 38-41.

El Shayeb, N.M.A. and Mabrouk, S.S. (1984). Utilization of some edible and medicinal plants to inhibit aflatoxin formation. *Nutrition Reports International* 29: 273-282.

Engqvist, A., Von Feilitzen, F., Pyk, E., and Reichard, H. (1973). Double-blind trial of deglycyrrhizinated liquorice in gastric ulcer. *Gut* 14: 711-715.

Evans, F.Q. (1958). The rational use of glycyrrhetinic acid in dermatology. *British Journal of Clinical Practice* 12: 269-279.

Farese, R.V., Biglieri, E.G., Shackleton, C.H.L., Irony, I., and Gomez-Fontes, R. (1991). Licorice-induced hypermineralcorticoidism. *New England Journal of Medicine* 325: 1223-1227.

Feldman, H. and Gilat, T. (1971). A trial of deglycyrrhizinated liquorice in the treatment of duodenal ulcer. *Gut* 12: 449-451.

Flynn, R. and Roest, M. (1995). *Your Guide to Standardized Herbal Products* (pp. 55-56). Prescott, AZ: One World Press.

Foster, S. and Chongxi, Y. (1992). *Herbal Emissaries: Bringing Chinese Herbs to the West* (pp. 112-121). Rochester, VT: Healing Arts Press.

Fukai, T., Tantai, L., and Nomura, T. (1996). Isoprenoid-substituted flavonoids from *Glycyrrhiza glabra. Phytochemistry* 43: 531-532.

Gonzalez-Gutierrez, M.L., Sanchez-Fernandez, C., Esteban-Lopez, M.I., Sempere-Ortells, J.M., and Diaz-Alperi, P. (2000). Allergy to anis. *Allergy* (Copenhagen) 55: 195-196.

Haraguchi, H., Yoshida, N., Ishikawa, H., Tamura, Y., Mizutani, K., and Kinoshita, T. (2000). Protection of mitochondrial functions against oxidative stresses by isoflavans from *Glycyrrhiza glabra. Journal of Pharmacy and Pharmacology* 52: 219-223.

Hatano, T., Fukuda, T., Miyase, T., Noro, T., and Okuda, T. (1991). Phenolic constituents of licorice. III. Structures of glicoricone and licofuranone, and inhibitory effects of licorice constituents on monoamine oxidase. *Chemical and Pharmaceutical Bulletin* 39: 1238-1243.

Hatano, T., Tagaki, M., Ito, H., and Yoshida, T. (1997). Phenolic constituents of liquorice. VII. A new chalcone with a potent radical scavenging activity and accompanying phenolics from liquorice. *Chemical and Pharmaceutical Bulletin* 45: 1485-1492.

Hatano, T., Yasuhara, T., Fukuda, T., Noro, T., and Okuda, T. (1989). Phenolic constituents of licorice. II. Structures of licopyranocoumarin, licoarylcoumarin and glisoflavone, and inhibitory effects of licorice phenolics on xanthine oxidase. *Chemical Pharmaceutical Bulletin* 37: 3005-3009.

Hattori, T., Ikematsu, S., Koito, A., Matsushita, S., Maeda, Y., Hada, M., Fujimaki, M., and Takatsuki, K. (1989). Preliminary evidence for inhibitory effect of glycyrrhizin on HIV replication in patients with AIDS. *Antiviral Research* 11: 255-262.

Hikino, H. (1985). Recent research on Oriental medicinal plants. In Wagner, H., Hikino, H., Farnsworth, N.R (Eds.), *Economic and Medicinal Plant Research*, Vol. 1 (pp. 53-61). London, England: Academic Press.

Hiraga, Y., Endo, H., Takahashi, K., and Shibata, S. (1984). High-performance liquid chromatographic analysis of licorice extracts. *Journal of Chromatography* 292: 451-453.

Hsu, H.Y., Chen, Y.P., Shen, S.J., Hsu, C.S., Chen, C.C., and Chang, H.C. (Eds.) (1986). *Oriental Materia Medica: A Concise Guide* (p. 533). Long Beach, CA: Oriental Healing Arts Institute.

Ishida, S., Ishikawa, T., and Sakiya, Y. (1988). Binding of glycyrrhetinic acid to rat serum albumin, human serum, and human serum albumin. *Chemical and Pharmaceutical Bulletin* 36: 440-443.

Ishida, S., Sakiya, Y., Ichikawa, T., and Awazu, S. (1989). Pharmacokinetics of glycyrrhetic acid, a major metabolite of glycyrrhizin, in rats. *Chemical and Pharmaceutical Bulletin* 37: 2509-2513.

Josephs, R.A., Guinn, J.S., Harper, M.L., and Askari, F. (2001). Liquorice consumption and salivary testosterone concentrations. *Lancet* 358: 1613-1614 (letter).

Kagegawa, H., Matsumoto, H., and Satoh, T. (1992). Inhibitory effect of some natural products on the activation of hyaluronidase and their anti-allergic actions. *Chemical and Pharmaceutical Bulletin* 40: 1439-1442.

Kassir, Z.A. (1985). Endoscopic controlled trial of four drug regimens in the treatment of chronic duodenal ulcer. *Irish Medical Journal* 78: 153-156.

Kimura, Y. and Okuda, H. (1988). Effects of chalcones isolated from licorice roots on leukotriene biosynthesis in human polymorphonuclear neutrophils. *Phytotherapy Research* 2: 140-145.

Kinoshita, T., Kajiyama, K., Hiraga, Y., Takahashi, K., Tamura, Y., and Mizutani, K. (1996). Isoflavan derivatives from *Glycyrrhiza glabra* (licorice). *Heterocycles* 43: 581-588.

Kiso, Y., Yohkin, M., Hikino, H., Hattori, M., Sakamoto, T., and Namba, T. (1984). Mechanism of antihepatotoxic activity of glycyrrhizin. I. Effect of free radical generation and lipid peroxidation. *Planta Medica* 50: 298-302.

Kitigawa, I., Chen, W.Z., Hori, K., Harada, E., Yasuda, N., Yoshikawa, M., and Ren, J. (1994). Chemical studies of Chinese licorice-roots. I. Elucidation of five new flavonoid constituents from the roots of *Glycyrrhiza glabra* L. collected from Zinjiang. *Chemical and Pharmaceutical Bulletin* 42: 1056-1062.

Kobayashi, S., Miyamoto, T., Kimura, I., and Kimura, M. (1995). Inhibitory effect of isoliquiritin, a compound in licorice root, on angiogenesis in vivo and tube formation in vitro. *Biological and Pharmaceutical Bulletin* 18: 1382-1386.

Kumagai, A., Nishino, K., Shimomura, A., Kin, T., and Yamamura, Y. (1967). Effect of glycyrrhizin on estrogen action. *Endocrinologia Japanonica* 14: 34-38.

Larkworthy, W. and Holgate, P.F.L. (1975). Deglycyrrhizinated liquorice in the treatment of chronic duodenal ulcer: A retrospective endoscopic survey of 32 patients. *Practitioner* 215: 787-792.

Le Moli, R., Endert, E., Fliers, E., Mulder, T., Prummel, M.F., Romijn, J.A., and Wiersinga, W.M. (1999). Establishment of reference values for endocrine tests. II: Hyperprolactinemia. *Netherlands Journal of Medicine* 55: 71-75.

Liu, J., Burdette, J.E., Xu, H., Gu, C., van Breemen, R.B., Bhat, K.P., Booth, N., Constantinou, A.I., Pezzuto, J.M., Fong, H.H., et al. (2001). Evaluation of estrogenic activity of plant extracts for the potential treatment of menopausal symptoms. *Journal of Agricultural and Food Chemistry* 49: 2472-2479.

Ma, J., Fu, N.Y., Pang, D.B., Wu, W.Y., and Xu, A.L. (2001). Apoptosis induced by isoliquiritigenin in human gastric cancer MGC-803 cells. *Planta Medica* 67: 754-757 (letter).

MacKenzie, M.A., Hoefnagels, W.H.L., Jansen, R.W.M.M., Benraad, T.J.H., and Kloppenborg, P.W. (1990). The influence of glycyrrhetinic acid on plasma cortisol and cortisone in healthy young volunteers. *Journal of Clinical Endocrinology and Metabolism* 70: 1637-1642.

McGuffin, M., Hobbs, C., Upton, R., and Goldberg, A. (1997). *American Herbal Products Association's Botanical Safety Handbook* (p. 58). Boca Raton, FL: CRC Press.

Mehta, R.G. and Moon, R.C. (1991). Characterization of effective chemopreventive agents in mammary gland in vitro using an initiation-promotion protocol. *Anticancer Research* 11: 593-596.

Mitscher, L.A., Rao, G.S.R., Khanna, I., Veysoglu, T., and Drake, S. (1983). Antimicrobial agents from higher plants: Prenylated flavonoids and other phenols from *Glycyrrhiza lepidota*. *Phytochemistry* 22: 573-576.

Morgan, A.G., McAdam, W.A.F., Pacsoo, C., and Darnborough, A. (1982). Comparison between cimetidine and Caved-S® in the treatment of gastric ulceration, and subsequent maintenance therapy. *Gut* 23: 545-551.

Niwa, K., Hashimoto, M., Morishita, S., Yokoyama, Y., Mori, H., and Tamaya, T. (1999). Preventive effects of *Glycyrrhizae radix* extract on estrogen-related endometrial carcinogenesis in mice. *Japanese Journal of Cancer Research* 90: 726-732.

Nose, M., Ito, M., Kamimura, K., Simizu, M., and Ogihara, Y. (1993). A comparison of the antihepatotoxic activity between glycyrrhizin and glycyrrhetinic acid. *Planta Medica* 60: 136-139.

Nussbaumer, U., Landolt, M., Röthlisberger, G., Akovbiantz, A., Keller, H., Weber, E., Blum, A.L., and Peter, P. (1977). Postoperative steressblutung: Unwirksame prophylaxe mit einem pepsininhibitor und einem glycyrrhizinsaurefreinen sussfolzextrakt [Postoperative stress bleeding: Prophylaxic action of a pepsin inhibitor, deglycyrrhizinated licorice, and a sulfate extract]. *Schweizerische Medizinische Wochenschrift* 107: 276-279.

Ohuchi, K., Kamada, Y., Levine, L., and Tsurufuji, S. (1981). Glycyrrhizin inhibits prostaglandin E_2 production by activated peritoneal macrophages from rats. *Prostaglandins and Medicine* 7: 457-463.

Okada, K., Tamura, Y., Yamamoto, M., Inoue, Y., Takagaki, R., Takahashi, K., Demizu, S., Kajiyama, K., Hiraga, Y., and Kinoshita, T. (1989). Identification of antimicrobial and antioxidant constituents from licorice of Russian and Xinjiang origin. *Chemical and Pharmaceutical Bulletin* 37: 2528-2530.

Okimasu, E., Moromizato, Y., Watanabe, S., Sasaki, J., Shiraishi, N., Morimoto, Y.M., Miyahara, M., and Utsumi, K. (1983). Inhibition of phospholipase A_2 by glycyrrhizin, an anti-inflammatory drug. *Acta Medica Okayama* 37: 385-391.

Paolini, M., Barillari, J., Broccoli, M., Pozzetti, L., Perocco, P., and Cantelli-Forti, G. (1999). Effect of liquorice and glycyrrhizin on rat liver carcinogen metabolizing enzymes. *Cancer Letters* 145: 35-42.

Rafi, M.M., Vastano, B.C., Zhu, N., Ho, C.T., Ghai, G., Rosen, R.T., Gallo, M.A., and DiPaola, R.S. (2001). Novel polyphenol molecule isolated from licorice root (*Glycyrrhiza glabra*) induced apoptosis, G2/M cell cycle arrest, and Bcl-2 phosphorylation in tumor cell lines. *Journal of Agricultural and Food Chemistry* 50: 677-684.

Rees, W.D.W., Rhodes, J., Wright, J.E., Stamford, L.F., and Bennett, A. (1979). Effect of deglycyrrhinated liquorice on gastric mucosal damage by aspirin. *Scandinavian Journal of Gastroenterology* 14: 605-607.

Russo, S., Mastropasqua, M., Mosetti, M.A., Persegani, C., and Paggi, A. (2000). Low doses of liquorice can induce hypertension encephalopathy. *American Journal of Nephrology* 20: 145-148.

Ruszymah, B.H.I., Nabishah, B.M., Aminuddin, S., and Khalid, B.A. (1995). Effects of glycyrrhizic acid on right atrial pressure and pulmonary vasculature in rats. *Clinical and Experimental Hypertension* 17: 575-579.

Sakamoto, K., Murabe, K., Watanabe, M., Aburada, M., and Hosoya, E. (1985). Inhibitory effect of glycyrrhetinic acid on testosterone production. *Japanese Journal of Pharmacology* 39(Suppl.): 101p (abstract 02E1600).

Sakamoto, K. and Wakabayashi, K. (1988). Inhibitory effect of glycyrrhetinic acid on testosterone production in rat gonads. *Endocrinologia Japonica* 35: 333-342.

Saxena, R.C., Gupta, R.N., Gupta, G.P., and Bhargava, K.P. (1965). A clinical trial of *Glycyrrhiza glabra* in pemphigus. *Journal of the Indian Medical Profession* (December): 5575-5576.

Shiki, Y., Ishikawa, Y., Shirai, K., Saito, Y., and Yoshida, S. (1986). Effect of glycyrrhizin on lysosomes labilization by phospholipase A_2. *American Journal of Chinese Medicine* 14: 131-137.

Shimamura, H., Suzuki, H., Hanano, M., Suzuki, A., and Sugiyama, Y. (1993). Identification of tissues responsible for the conjugative metabolism of liquiritigenin in rats: An analysis based on metabolite kinetics. *Biological and Pharmaceutical Bulletin* 16: 899-907.

Shimizu, N., Tomoda, M., Satoh, M., Gonda, R., and Ohara, N. (1991). Characterization of a polysaccharide having activity on the reticuloendothelial system from the stolon of *Glycyrrhiza glabra* var. *glandulifera*. *Chemical and Pharmaceutical Bulletin* 39: 2082-2086.

Shinada, M., Azuma, M., Kawai, H., Sazaki, K., Yoshida, I., Yoshida, T., Suzutani, T., and Sakuma, T. (1986). Enhancement of interferon-γ production in glycyrrhizin-treated human peripheral lymphocytes in response to concanavalin A and to surface antigen of hepatitis B virus (42241). *Proceedings of the Society for Experimental Biology and Medicine* 181: 205-210.

Stormer, F.C., Reistad, R., and Alexander, J. (1993). Glycyrrhizic acid in liquorice—Evaluation of health hazard. *Food and Chemical Toxicology* 31: 303-312.

Strandberg, T.E., Jarvenpaa, A.L., Vanhanen, H., and McKeigue, P.M. (2001). Birth outcome in relation to licorice consumption during pregnancy. *American Journal of Epidemiology* 153: 1085-1088.

Takeda, S., Ishihara, K., Wakui, Y., Amagaya, S., Maruno, M., Akao, T., and Kobashi, K. (1996). Bioavailability study of glycyrrhetic acid after oral administration of glycyrrhizin in rats; relevance to the intestinal bacterial hydrolysis. *Journal of Pharmacy and Pharmacology* 48: 902-905.

Tamir, S., Eizenberg, M., Somjen, D., Stern, N., Shelach, R., Kaye, A., and Vaya, J. (2000). Estrogenic and antiproliferative properties of glabridin from licorice in human breast cancer cells. *Cancer Research* 60: 5704-5709.

Tanaka, S., Kuwai, Y., and Tabata, M. (1987). Isolation of monoamine oxidase inhibitors from *Glycyrrhiza uralensis* roots and the structure-activity relationship. *Planta Medica* 53: 5-8.

Tawata, M., Yoda, Y., Aida, K., Shindo, H., Sasaki, H., Chin, M., and Onaya, T. (1990). Antiplatelet action of GU-7, a 3-arylycoumarin derivative, purified from *Glycyrrhizae radix*. *Planta Medica* 56: 259-263.

Teelucksingh, S., Mackie, A.D.R., Burt, D., McIntyre, M.A., Brett, L., and Edwards, C.R. (1990). Potentiation of hydrocortisone activity in skin by glycyrrhetinic acid. *Lancet* 335 (May 5): 1060-1063.

Tewari, S.N. and Trembalowicz, F.C. (1968). Some experience with deglycyrrhizinated liquorice in the treatment of gastric and duodenal ulcers with special reference to its spasmolytic effect. *Gut* 9: 48-51.

Tu, G., Fang, Q., Guo, J., Yuan, S., Chen, C., Chen, J., Chen, Z., Cheng, S., Jin, R., Li, M., et al. (Eds.) (1992). *Pharmacopoeia of the People's Republic of China* (pp. 165-166). Guangzhou, China: Guangdong Science and Technology Press.

Utsunomiya, T., Kobayashi, M., Herndon, D.N., Pollard, R.B., and Suzuki, F. (1995). Glycyrrhizin (20 β-carboxy-11-oxo-30-norolean-12-en-3 β-yl-*O*-β-D-glucopyranuronosyl-α-D-glucopyranosiduronic acid) improves the resistance of thermally injured mice to opportunistic infection of *Herpes simplex* virus type 1. *Immunology Letters* 44: 59-66.

van der Zwan, A. (1993). Hypertension encephalopathy after liquorice ingestion. *Clinical Neurology and Neurosurgery* 95: 35-37.

van Gelderen, C.E.M., Bijlsma, J.A., van Dokkum, W., and Savelkoul, T.J.F. (2000). Glycyrrhizic acid: The assessment of a no effect level. *Human and Experimental Toxicology* 19: 434-439.

Vaya, J., Belinky, P.A., and Aviram, M. (1997). Antioxidant constituents from licorice roots: Isolation, structure elucidation and antioxidative capacity toward LDL during its oxidation. *Free Radical Biology and Medicine* 23: 302-313.

Wang, Z., Kurosaki, Y., Nakayama, T., and Kimura, T. (1994). Mechanism of gastrointestinal absorption of glycyrrhizin in rats. *Biological and Pharmaceutical Bulletin* 17: 1399-1403.

Wang, Z., Nishioka, M., Kuosaki, Y., Nakayama, T., and Kimura, T. (1995). Gastrointestinal absorption characteristics of glycyrrhizin from *Glycyrrhiza* extract. *Biological and Pharmaceutical Bulletin* 18: 1238-1241.

Whorwood, C.B., Shepphard, M.C., and Stewart, P.M. (1993). Licorice inhibits 11β-hydroxysteroid dehydrogenase messenger ribonucleic acid levels and potentiates glucocorticoid hormone action. *Endocrinology* 132: 2287-2292.

Yamamoto, K., Kagegawa, H., Ueda, H., Matsumoto, H., Sudo, T., Miki, T., and Satoh, T. (1992). Gastric cytoprotective anti-ulcerogenic actions of hydroxychalcones in rats. *Planta Medica* 58: 389-391.

Yano, S., Harada, M., Watanabe, K., Nakamaru, K., Hatakeyama, Y., Shibata, S., Takahashi, K., Mori, T., Hirabayashi, K., Takeda, M., et al. (1989). Anti-ulcer activities of glycyrrhetinic acid derivatives in experimental gastric lesion models. *Chemical and Pharmaceutical Bulletin* 37: 2500-2504.

Yokozawa, T., Liu, Z.W., and Chen, C.P. (1999/2000). Protective effects of Glycyrrhizae radix extract and its compounds in a renal hypoxia (ischemia)-reoxygenation (reperfusion) model. *Phytomedicine* 6: 439-445.

Zani, F., Cuzzoni, M.T., Daglia, M., Benvenuti, S., Vampa, G., and Mazza, P. (1993). Inhibition of mutagenicity in *Salmonella typhimurium* by *Glycyrrhiza glabra* extract, glycyrrhizinic acid, 18α- and 18β-glycyrrhetinic acids. *Planta Medica* 59: 502-507.

Zava, D.T., Dollbaum, C.M., and Blen, M. (1998). Estrogen and progestin bioactivity of foods, herbs, and spices. *Proceedings of the Society for Experimental Biology and Medicine* 217: 369-378.

Zhang, Y.H., Kato, M., Isobe, K.I., Hamaguchi, M., Yokochi, T., and Nakashima, I. (1995). Dissociated control by glycyrrhizin of proliferation and IL-2 production of murine thymocytes. *Cellular Immunology* 162: 97-104.

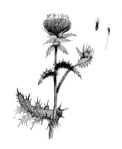

Milk Thistle

BOTANICAL DATA

Classification and Nomenclature

Scientific name: *Silybum marianum* (L.) Gaertner; synonyms: *Carduus marianus* L.; *Cnicus marianus, C. benedictus.*

Family name: Asteraceae (Compositae)

Common names: milk thistle, variegated thistle, wild artichoke; in older texts, referred to as Mary thistle, St. Mary thistle, Marian thistle, lady's thistle, holy thistle (Bone, 1996; Foster, 1990; Anonymous, 1985); Mariendistelfrüchte (German) (Blumenthal et al., 1998)

Description

The *Silybum* genus contains two species: *S. marianum* (L.) Gaertner and *S. eburneum*. Both species are indigenous to the Mediterranean region, although Kashmir is considered the native home of *S. marianum* (Morazzoni and Bombardelli, 1995).

Silybum marianum is a persistent herbaceous annual or biennial easily recognized by its stout thistle, reddish-purple flowers, large prickly leaves with milky white zones, and tubular-shaped flowers that terminate in sharp pines (Anonymous, 1985). The glabrous stem varies widely in height (20-150 cm high) and the upper part of the stem is erect and branched. The large and glabrous white-veined leaves have a distinct spiny margin. The brownish-colored fruits are hard skinned and shiny, average 6-8 mm in length, and display a white silk-like pappus at the apex (Morazzoni and Bombardelli, 1995).

In many regions, milk thistle *(S. marianum)* is a widespread wayside herb. Throughout Europe and North America, milk thistle is often found in wastelands, along roadsides, and on cultivated ground. The distribution of

S. marianum ranges from the sea to submountainous areas, where it grows in altitudes up to 700-1,100 m (Morazzoni and Bombardelli, 1995). European colonists reportedly transported the herb to the New World from Britain (Pickering, 1879, in Foster, 1990), and it has since become naturalized in the eastern United States, California, and parts of Canada. Milk thistle also grows in India, China, South America, Mexico, Australia, and Africa (Foster, 1990; Anonymous, 1985). Milk thistle has very few predators and matures in less than one year, flourishing best on well-draining soils and in sunny areas (Foster, 1990).

HISTORY AND TRADITIONAL USES

Silybum marianum is an edible plant; despined, the leaves are eaten much the same way as artichokes. The seeds, when roasted, can be brewed as a coffee substitute. Historically, the flavorful leaves and roots of this species were eaten as foods and occasionally employed in medicinal preparations (Morazzoni and Bombardelli, 1995). In Europe, milk thistle was cultivated in gardens both as a vegetable and an ornamental plant (Foster, 1990)

The genus name *Silybum* is from the Greek *sillybon*: a tuft or pendant. The oldest known mention of *Silybum* as a medicinal plant was by legendary Greek physician Dioscorides, who coined the name to describe a thistle with white-blotched leaves. He prescribed the roots of *S. marianum* as an emetic, and with the leaves he made a decoction to treat snakebites (Morazzoni and Bombardelli, 1995; Foster, 1990; Hobbs, 1984).

Bingel and Farnsworth (1994) list galactogogue use of the seed in England and the root or seed in Italy. John Evelyn wrote "Disarmed of its prickles and boiled, it is worthy of esteem, and thought to be a great breeder of milk and proper diet for women who are nurses" (Grieve, 1980, p. 797). To followers of the Doctrine of Signatures, the white blotches on the leaves would likely indicate its utility as a galactogogue. One legend relates that while nursing the infant Jesus, the Virgin Mary spilled a drop of her breast milk on the leaves, which forever after gave them their characteristic white veins. Still other legends appear to stem from an older, pre-Christian goddess myth when milk thistle was called Venus thistle and was dedicated to the Norse goddess Freya (Morazzoni and Bombardelli, 1995).

In the fourth century B.C., Theophrastus spoke of *S. marianum,* as did Dioscorides and Pliny in the first century A.D. During the middle ages, herbalists used several different parts, including the root and aerial parts, to treat swellings and erysipelas. The nineteenth-century British herbalist, Culpeper, recommended *S. marianum* for melancholy diseases, which at that time would include liver or bile-related diseases (including obstructions of the liver and spleen). Hobbs (1984) recounts that Culpeper used an infusion of the fresh root and seeds to treat jaundice.

In the United States, the eclectic physicians of the late nineteenth and early twentieth centuries prescribed remedies made from *S. marianum* for varicose veins, menstrual-related pelvic congestion, and congestion of the liver, spleen, and kidneys (Hobbs, 1984). Topical application of the decoction was claimed to be of benefit in treating cancer (Grieve, 1980). For these and other diseases, a tincture taken in a dose of five drops was prescribed by naturopathic doctors. Tinctures made from the seeds are still used to treat liver ailments, including jaundice, gallstones, peritonitis, hemorrhage, bronchitis, and varicose veins (Anonymous, 1985; Schauenberg and Paris, 1974). In France, the fruits, roots, and leaves of *S. marianum* are employed in remedies for a variety of related complaints: chronic constipation associated with jaundice, bile stones, hepatitis, and steatosis. Decoctions and tinctures of the fruits are thought to have therapeutic effects on the circulatory system, particularly hemorrhoids, varicose veins, hay fever, asthma, and nettle rash. In Italy, the fruits are used in treatments of hepatic complications such as oliguresis and hypotension. In Germany and Hungary, decoctions and tinctures are used against cholangiopathies, bile stones, and liver problems. In Greece, various plant parts are used to make remedies for varicose veins, cholelithiasis, duodenal ulcer, amenorrhea, and hepatic-related chronic constipation (Morazzoni and Bombardelli, 1995). Several thistles have been traditionally used in herbal remedies for liver ailments; however, only *S. marianum* contains silymarin, a complex of flavonoid-like compounds with demonstrable therapeutic effects (Hobbs, 1984).

Milk thistle is widely recommended today by physicians in Europe as both a protective and restorative agent for liver damage resulting from hepatitis, alcoholism, cirrhosis, and damage due to pharmaceutical drugs, anesthetics, and *Amanita* mushroom poisonings. In addition, the silymarin complex is prescribed by many European practitioners for various symptoms of subclinical liver diseases linked to environmental toxins. Among the various symptoms of environmental liver disorders that silymarin reportedly mitigates are: low energy postprandial sleepiness, depression, irritability, headaches, allergies, poor digestion, and acne (Foster, 1990; Hobbs, 1984; Morazzoni and Bombardelli, 1995).

CHEMISTRY

Lipid Compounds

The lipid fraction comprises 20% to 30% of fruits; of this, 52% to 53% is linoleic acid. In the saponifiable fraction, β-sitosterol has also been identified (Morazzoni and Bombardelli, 1995).

Phenolic Compounds

Flavonoids

The seeds contain the flavonoids quercetin, taxifolin, and dehydro-kaempferol (Morazzoni and Bombardelli, 1995; Hobbs, 1984).

Lignans

Flavonolignans in the plant, generally called silymarin, are the main active constituents. Flavonolignan-like substances found in the seeds include dehydrosilybin, desoxysilydianin (silymonin), silyhermin, neosilyhermin, silandrin, and silybinome (Awang, 1993; Rumyantseva, 1991; Wagner et al., 1974). The seeds contain the highest concentrations of silymarin. Higher quantities are typically found in specimens from southern, subtropical areas (Hobbs, 1984).

Silymarin is an umbrella term coined in 1968 by Wagner and colleagues to describe the entire group of active flavonolignan principles found only in the seeds of *S. marianum*. Silymarin consists of three isomers: silibinin (formerly silybin), silydianin, and silycristin (a.k.a. silidianin and silicristin, respectively). (Silybin is replaced with silibinin throughout this text.) Silibinins a and b are diastereoisomers (Tittel and Wagner, 1977; Wagner et al., 1974). The primary flavonolignan in the silymarin complex, silibinin a, consists of a benzodioxane grouping derived from the coupling of taxifolin with coniferyl alcohol (Morazzoni and Bombardelli, 1995).

Gas-liquid chromatographic analysis of extracts of *S. marianum* yielded 2,3-dehydrosilybin, as well as silibinin oligomers and dehydrodiconiferyl alcohol (Wagner et al., 1974). Three other flavonolignans (3-deoxy-flavonones) have been identified. In addition, studies show that the presence and concentration of active principles can vary by geographical region. For example, white-blooming varietal species of *S. marianum* have yielded new compounds: silymonin (3-deoxy-silydianin) and silyandrin (3-deoxy-isosilybin) (Morazzoni and Bombardelli, 1995).

THERAPEUTIC APPLICATIONS

Over the past four decades, researchers in Europe have conducted myriad scientific studies on the therapeutic properties of *S. marianum*. Extracts of the seeds have been shown to protect liver cells from damage stemming from chronic and acute hepatitis (Bode et al., 1977), cirrhosis of the liver, and toxins such as solvents, alcohol, and drugs (Flora et al., 1998). Silymarin, the complex of active compounds isolated from the seeds (mainly silibinin, isosilibinin, silidianin, and silicristin), exhibits both protective and restorative effects on fatty degeneration of the liver and on other hepatic complications (Morazzoni and Bombardelli, 1995).

PRECLINICAL STUDIES

Cardiovascular and Circulatory Functions

Cholesterol and Lipid Metabolism

Krecman et al. (1998) studied the cholesterol modulating effects of silymarin and silibinin in female rats fed a high cholesterol diet (10% lard and 1% cholesterol, both w/w of the feed for 19 days). The treatment groups consisted of those receiving no supplement, those receiving either silymarin or silibinin, and rats given feed containing either supplement plus probucol, an antioxidant cholesterol-lowering drug. At a dietary concentration of 0.5% and 1.0% (0.33 and 0.66 mg/kg per day, respectively), silymarin caused a significant decrease in liver cholesterol levels and a significant increase in liver glutathione (each $p < 0.05$), an endogenous antioxidant. Only at 1.0% of the diet did probucol cause a significant increase in liver glutathione levels; however, no decrease occurred in liver cholesterol levels (Krecman et al., 1998).

Probucol as 0.5% to 1.0% of the diet caused a significant decrease in high density lipoprotein cholesterol (HDL_c) and subfractions of HDL_a and HDL_b, whereas silymarin at the same concentrations caused both HDL_c and its subfractions to increase significantly to normal levels. At 0.1% to 1.0% of the diet, both substances caused significant decreases in serum total cholesterol, low density lipoprotein cholesterol (LDL_c), and very low density lipoprotein cholesterol ($VLDL_c$) ($p < 0.05$). Comparative studies with dietary silibinin, silymarin, probucol, and unsupplemented control rats showed much the same results, except that silibinin (45% of silymarin) was not as effective as silymarin; possibly owing to comparatively weaker bioavailability. However, at inhibiting *tert*-butyl hydroperoxide-induced lipoperoxidation, silibinin showed a tendency to be stronger than either silymarin or probucol, although in this test none of the treatments produced activity that reached statistical significance (Krecman et al., 1998).

Nassuato et al. (1983) found no decrease in serum cholesterol levels in male rats administered silibinin (100 mg/kg per day i.p. for seven days), although biliary cholesterol concentrations were decreased.

Hypertension

Silibinin, as part of the feed of rats (300 mg/kg p.o. for eight to twelve days) with acute coronary artery occlusion and spontaneous hypertension, lowered blood pressure, reduced the incidence of postocclusion arrhythmias following acute coronary occlusion, and decreased mortality. Despite the high dosage of silymarin employed, the authors speculated that it might be useful in reducing the mortality of hypertensive patients with acute myocardial infarction and ventricular hypertrophy (Chen et al., 1993). Silybin also decreased the severity of necrosis associated with in vitro ischemia reperfusion of rat liver tissue. Silymarin presumably achieved this effect by lowering the amount of cytosolic enzymes that leaked from the liver cells (Wu et al., 1993).

Digestive, Hepatic, and Gastrointestinal Functions

Hepatic Functions

Silymarin and its main component, silibinin, exhibit hepatoprotective activity against a wide range of toxins injurious to the liver. These include carbon tetrachloride, galactosamine, ethanol, paracetamol, *Amanita phalloides* mushroom toxin, thioacetamide, and microcystin-LR from certain strains of the blue-green algae *Microcystis aeruginosa* (Morazzoni and Bombardelli, 1995). Blossoms of the algae in the freshwaters of temperate zones pose a biohazard to animals and humans (Hermansky et al., 1991). In Canada, several blue-green algae products sold as health supplements were found to contain dangerous levels of microcystin (Health Canada, 1999). While significantly decreasing serum enzymes in mice and rats induced by this highly hepatotoxic heptapeptide, silymarin also completely eliminated pathological changes and lethal effects of the toxin. Intravenous administration appears to produce greater protective effects against microcystin-LR (Mereish et al., 1991) than intraperitoneal administration (Hermansky et al., 1991).

Liver-protectant activity of silymarin has been demonstrated against chronic administration of heavy metals and several drugs, poisons of lanthamden (from lanthanum), sulphur acetamide, and the hepatotoxic virus FU3 of cold-blooded animals (Bone, 1996). These noxious agents induce hepatotoxicity through the formation of free radicals—specifically, causing lipid peroxidation, the chain reaction initiated by these unstable free radicals in the presence of unsaturated fatty acids on cell membranes. Furthermore, silymarin has shown dose-dependent activity against peroxidation in liver microsomes of the rat (Bosisio et al., 1992) and inhibits xanthine oxidase (IC_{50} of 27.58 μM), serum levels of which dramatically increase in patients during the early stages of viral hepatitis. Xanthine oxidase levels also cause a measure of brain injury and brain edema (Sheu et al., 1998).

In vitro and in vivo investigations have shown that silymarin promotes protein synthesis (Sonnenbichler and Zetl, 1986; Sonnenbichler and Pohl, 1980; Sonnenbichler et al., 1998). In animal models, the ability of silymarin to stimulate protein synthesis was judged to be a primary mechanism through which silymarin regenerated hepatocytes in damaged livers (Sonnenbichler and Zetl, 1986). During the repair phase of damaged liver tissue, silymarin stimulated the activity of an RNA polymerase that synthesizes ribosomal RNA and accelerates the formation of ribosomes in isolated hepatocytes—processes critical for protein synthesis (Hobbs, 1984).

Ethyl alcohol and paracetamol are known to cause liver damage primarily through depletion of glutathione levels. This depletion is one of the major mechanisms through which liver damage occurs. In rats treated with ethyl alcohol and paracetamol, silymarin and silibinin exert a hepatoprotective effect by elevating glutathione levels (Valenzuela et al., 1985). Silymarin treatment (200 mg/kg i.p.) significantly raised the level of glutathione and oxidized hepatocellular glutathione over control rats (vehicle only). At three days, liver, duodenum, intestine, and stomach from the silymarin-treated rats showed a 50% increase in total glutathione and glutathione/oxidized glutathione levels compared to the control group. A further elevation in glutathione levels was observed six days later in the treatment group. In addition, the ratio of reduced glutathione/oxidized glutathione improved. The researchers found no alterations in animal body weight or in food intake (Valenzuela et al., 1989).

In isolated hepatocytes of experimentally intoxicated rats (NADPH and ADP/Fe^{2+} induced), silibinin was more effective than silychristin and silydianin in blocking the release of cytosol enzymes (Bosisio et al., 1992). The protective activity of silymarin appears to involve the inhibition of other cytosol enzymes, including alanine amino transferase (ALT/GPT) and lactic dehydrogenase (LDH) (Hikino et al., 1984). These enzymes can alter the integrity of the cell membrane; they may even cause cell death. Intoxication with various noxious agents, including ethanol and ethionine, blocks phospholipid synthesis on the microsomal membrane of rat livers. Studies have shown that silymarin is capable of counteracting the inhibition of phospholipid synthesis (Castigli et al., 1977).

Silymarin compounds have been employed for their therapeutic benefits in cases of poisoning from *Amanita phalloides,* the deathcap mushroom. This fungus contains two potentially lethal cyclopeptides: phalloidine, a highly virulent toxin that disrupts the outer membrane of liver cells; and α-amanatine. Either compound can be fatal after 3-5 h. α-amanatine enters the nucleus of the cell where it blocks the activity of RNA polymerase-II, an enzyme crucial to the synthesis of messenger-RNA and ultimately crucial to protein synthesis (Hobbs, 1984). Silymarin apparently exerts its protective effects by occupying the binding sites on cell membrane receptors and possibly altering and stabilizing the outer membrane of the hepatocyte to resist penetration from the toxin (Munter et al., 1986). One of the clinical results is a decrease in the blood level of urea (Vogel et al., 1975). Silymarin also accelerated the regeneration rate of rat livers damaged by α-amanatine (Vogel and Temme, 1969; Vogel et al., 1975).

In morphological and biochemical studies, silymarin appeared to mitigate liver damage in rabbits receiving long-term administration of toxic drugs, such as indomethacin, isoniazid, tolbutamide, and clofibrate (Bone, 1996). Silymarin also ameliorated in vitro damage to rat hepatocytes caused by various toxicants, including erythromycin estolate, tricyclic antidepressants, and *tert*-butyl hydroperoxide, as measured by intracellular enzyme leakage and morphological alterations (Davila et al., 1989).

An in vitro study suggested that silymarin is cytoprotective against acetaminophen-induced toxicity in human hepatoblastoma Hep G2 and human epidermoid A431 cells (Shear et al., 1995). In rats administered acetaminophen (500 mg/kg i.p.), the acetaminophen-induced increase in serum levels of GOT and GPT was significantly ameliorated by silibinin (50 mg/kg i.v.). Acetaminophen also caused liver glutathione levels to decrease, whereas treatment with silibinin plus acetaminophen significantly inhibited the depletion (Garrido et al., 1989).

Against cyclosporine (CsA)-induced toxicity in rats (30 mg/kg i.p. per day), silibinin treatment 30 min prior (5 mg/kg i.p.) significantly decreased the CsA-induced elevation of total malondialdehyde ($p < 0.05$), indicating a significant decrease in lipid peroxidation caused by CsA. In a group of female rats administered both CsA and silibinin (30 mg/kg i.p. plus 5 mg/kg i.p., respectively) followed by CsA (30 mg/kg i.p.), a significant increase occurred in levels of cytochrome P-450 in liver microsomes ($p < 0.05$) compared to a placebo-treated control group and a CsA-only treatment group. This result suggested a pathway through which silibinin exerted its effect on the biotransformation of CsA. In other parameters, silibinin showed no protective effects against CsA. Compared to the placebo group, the glomerular filtration rate of both the CsA-only group and the CsA-plus silibinin group was significantly decreased ($p < 0.001$), yet no significant difference was found between the CsA-plus silibinin and the CsA-only groups in levels of creatine, urea, and total protein of the rats (Zima et al., 1998).

Silymarin may attenuate pruritus in women with intrahepatic cholestasis during pregnancy but shows no benefit to alterations in biochemistry characteristic of the disease (Reyes and Simon, 1993).

Animal studies indicate that silymarin (90 mg/day) may ameliorate, prevent, or correct damage to the liver in pregnant women taking estroprogestins and in women taking birth control pills (Martines et al., 1979).

Anticholestatic Activity

In test animals, silibinin countered cholestasis (i.e., suppression of bile flow) induced by paracetamol and ethynylestradiol (Shukla et al., 1991). In rats, silymarin lowered biliary cholesterol and phospholipid concentrations (anticholestatic) (50 mg/kg i.p. for seven days) without affecting the bile flow. Compared to the control group, the test rats showed no changes in biliary parameters. At double the dose for seven days, silibinin lowered biliary cholesterol and phospholipid concentrations more than (60.9% and 72.9%, respectively) the control group (Nassuato et al., 1991). Although silibinin had no effect on total liver cholesterol levels, in vitro studies revealed that silibinin produced a dose-dependent inhibition of the rat liver microsomal enzyme, 3-hydroxy-3-methlglutaryl-CoA (HMG-CoA) reductase (at concentrations of 0.5-8 mg/kg). Nassuato and colleagues concluded that silibinin may decrease biliary cholesterol concentrations at least partly by reducing the synthesis of cholesterol in the liver.

Endocrine and Hormonal Functions

Carbohydrate Metabolism; Antidiabetic Activity

Schönfeld et al. (1997) studied the effect of silibinin on pancreatic functions of male rats treated with CsA. Silibinin had no effect on glucose concentrations, whether administered alone (50, 100, or 200 mg/kg i.p.) or combined with CsA (10 mg/kg p.o.). Silibinin had no effect on the body weight of the animals and no effect on CsA concentrations. Against CsA-induced inhibition of amylase, however, silibinin in a high dose (200 mg/kg i.p.) was found to restore amylase secretion to normal. When the two agents were combined, silibinin attenuated the inhibited secretion of amylase. Silibinin inhibited the glucose-stimulated release of insulin in vitro while showing no such effect in vivo. Schönfeld and colleagues concluded, therefore, that silibinin may cause insulin secretion to decrease without causing blood-glucose levels to increase—a combination, they suggested, that may be advantageous in the treatment of non-insulin-dependent diabetes yet without the serious adverse effects posed by drugs such as metformin. In conclusion, they found silibinin prevented toxicity to the exocrine pancreas caused by CsA and suggested that it may protect the organ against other toxins, including alcohol.

Reproductive Hormone Interactions

Silbinin has shown competitive binding activity for the estradiol receptor (derived from pork uteri) and was found to influence only ribosomal RNA synthesis (Sonnenbichler and Zetl, 1988).

Genitourinary and Renal Functions

Renal Toxicity

Sonnenbichler et al. (1999) studied the in vitro nephroprotective and proliferative influence of the main flavanolignans of milk thistle against the toxicity of paracetamol (= acetaminophen) and chemotherapy agents vincristin and cisplatin on two nonmalignant kidney cell lines from the African green monkey (epitheloid BSC-1 cells and fibroblast-like Vero cells). At 10 μM, silibinin hemisuccinate increased the growth of the Vero cells by 14% after three days; after five days, the increase was still as high as 12%. Higher concentrations (up to 40 μM) caused further increases in growth stimulation (up to 23%), but at 60 μM the stimulation ceased and at 100 μM the rate of growth decreased, as did DNA biosynthesis, whereas 20 μM increased DNA synthesis of the Vero cells by 19%. Similar results were found from silibinin on protein biosynthesis, indicating that unlike its effect on liver cells, metabolism of silibinin does not occur in kidney cells. Dose responses in BSC-1 cells were much the same as those in Vero cells, with concentrations greater than 60 μM inhibiting cell growth and lower concentrations stimulating growth. In tests with other flavanolignans of milk thistle cells, isosilibinin and silidianin inhibited cell growth of the Vero cells by 10% and 6%, respectively, at the same concentration (20 μM) that silicristin or pure silibinin increased cell growth (14% and 16%, respectively). Similar results were obtained in tests on protein synthesis and on LDH (lactate dehydrogenase) activity of the Vero cells exposed to these flavanolignans. Addition of silibinin hemisuccinate (20 μM or 40 μM) before or after damage to the Vero cells induced by paracetamol, cisplatin, or vincristin produced protectant and restorative effects, as shown by amelioration of the reduced protein biosynthesis, inhibited cellular proliferation, and inhibition of LDH activity caused by the test agents. Greatest amelioration was found against paracetamol-induced damage: administration of silibinin hemisuccinate beforehand produced a relative improvement in Vero cell integrity of 22% to 33% and applied after paracetamol caused a relative improvement of cellular integrity of 16% to 26%. Relative improvements against cisplatin-induced damage were 20% to 26% with silibinin hemisuccinate applied before and 26% and 28% with application after damage, and 10% to 22% applied before and 6% to 16% applied after vincristin.

Gaedeke et al. (1996) demonstrated that in large doses, silibinin (200 mg/kg i.v.) completely or partly ameliorated the deleterious effects of cisplatin (5 mg/kg i.v.) on the kidney functions of rats yet showed no effect on kidney function by itself. Protective effects were found from silibinin against cisplatin-induced alterations to proximal and glomerular tubular function as well as to their morphology. The cisplatin-induced decrease in creatinine clearance and the increase in proteinuria induced by cisplatin were completely prevented by silibinin when administered as a one-hour pretreatment. Gaedeke and co-workers concluded that silibinin may show nephroprotectant activity in clinical applications.

As a pretreatment in rats administered cisplatin, silibinin caused a significant inhibition of tubular cell excretion of brush-border magnesium and enzymes. However, the excretion of urinary magnesium and serum levels of magnesium were not affected by the silibinin pretreatment. Whereas cisplatin caused a significant decrease in the rate of creatinine clearance, animals administered silibinin before cisplatin showed no significant change. The researchers concluded that their data could be used as a basis for conducting a randomized clinical study on silibinin as a potential antinephrotoxic agent in testicular cancer patients undergoing treatment with cisplatin (Bokemeyer et al., 1996).

Rats treated with gentamicin sulphate (100 mg/kg per day i.p. for 28 days) that received silymarin (Madaus Co.) as a pretreatment (15 mg/kg per day p.o. six times/day for 28 days) and concomitant treatment showed significantly less nephrotoxicity than controls not treated with silymarin. Similar results were found in a third group treated only concomitantly. Statistically significant benefits, compared to the group not treated with silymarin, included less lethargic animals, less weight loss, and reduced mortality ($p < 0.01$). The pretreatment also reduced excretion of urinary NAG (N-acetyl-β-glucosaminidase) and protein ($p < 0.01$), lessened the decrease in creatinine clearance ($p < 0.01$), and lowered kidney tissue levels of gentamicin ($p < 0.05$). Also, comparatively fewer myelin-like bodies were visible in kidney sections of rats treated with silymarin (Chan and Ng, 1989).

Immune Functions; Inflammation and Disease

Cancer

Antiproliferative activity. The in vitro inhibitory activity of silymarin on androgen-independent human prostate carcinoma DU145 cells appears to be the result of arresting cell-growth initiating factors, such as the epidermal growth factor receptor (erbB1) pathway (Bhatia and Agarwal, 2001). Silymarin inhibited transforming growth factor-α (TGF-α)-mediated activation of the pathway to highly significant degrees when precultured in androgen-independent human prostate cancer cells, indicating the potential for arrest of carcinogenesis. The overexpression of the epidermal growth factor receptor (erbB1) in these cancer cells, in addition to their synthesis and secretion of TGF-α, in turn interacts with erbB1 to allow autonomous growth in a vicious circle of feedback, leading to increased and continual growth of prostate carcinoma. From doses of 75 and 100 μg/mL, silymarin exhibited, respectively, 90% and 100% inhibition of human prostate tumor cell growth. The use of an androgen-independent tumor cell line in these experiments was predicated upon the fact that prostate cancer, while at first an androgen-dependent event, can eventually progress to regrowth of tumors that are not dependent on male hormones and therefore not susceptible to androgen-derpivation therapies used to treat the initial occurrence of prostate cancer

(Zi, Grasso, et al., 1998). In further studies, Zi et al. (2000) found that silibinin inhibited the proliferation of the androgen-independent prostate cancer cell line PC-3 by 54% to 74% at "pharmacologically achievable" concentrations (0.02-20 μM). Evidence showed that the inhibition of cell growth involved an increase in secretion and gene expression of insulin-like growth factor-binding protein (IGFBP-3) and the inhibition of the peptide growth factor, IGF (insulin-like growth factor).

Silymarin caused a time- and dose-dependent complete in vitro inhibition of human breast carcinoma (MDA-MB 468) anchorage-dependent cell growth at a concentration of 50 and 75 μg/mL ($p < 0.0001$). At 25 mg/mL, tumor cell growth was time-dependently inhibited by close to 50% ($p < 0.001$) (Zi, Feyes, et al., 1998).

In an anticarcinogenic assay, silymarin caused a significant inhibition of tumor cell colony formation, inhibiting the number of colonies by 23% from 5 μg/mL to as much as 94% from 75 μg/mL. At a high concentration (50 μg/mL), silymarin induced G1 arrest of the cell-cycle progression of the breast cancer cells. G1 expression in cancer cells allows their uncontrolled growth. A dose- and time-dependent induction of Cip1/p21 protein expression in breast carcinoma cells was evident from silymarin in doses of 10-75 μg/mL. Zi, Feyes, et al. (1998) concluded that the strong anticarcinogenic activity of silymarin in vitro could be the result of the highly significant increase in the level of Cip1/p21 protein expression, which could lead to a decrease in G1 cyclins.

Scambia et al. (1996) reported a dose-dependent in vitro antiproliferative effect from silibinin on the growth of MCF-7 doxorubicin-resistant breast cancer cells (IC_{50} 24 μM), cisplatin-resistant and parental human ovarian cancer cells (A2780) (IC_{50} 12-14 μM), and, more potently, the human ovarian carcinoma cell line OVCA 433 (IC_{50} 4.8 μM). Silibinin increased the G0-G1 phase of the cell cycle while concomitantly decreasing the S and G2-M phases. Silibinin also competitively bound with nuclear type-II estrogen binding sites of serous ovarian carcinoma cells. Silibinin acted synergistically in potentiating the antiproliferative effects of cisplatin and doxorubicin against cisplatin-resistant human ovarian cancer cells, parental human ovarian cancer cells (A2780), and MCF-7 doxorubicin-resistant breast cancer cells. Apparently, silibinin altered the resistance of the tumor cells to the anticancer agents. In addition, silibinin (4-7.4 μM) displayed antiproliferative activity on primary human ovarian tumors. Scambia and colleagues noted that at the concentrations producing a dose-dependent antiproliferative effect on the tumor cells studied (0.1-20 μM), silibinin could be given orally and achieve the same concentrations. They were prompted to investigate the antiproliferative activity of silibinin in part because it can better cross the intestinal barrier when complexed with phosphatidylcholine.

Phase I clinical studies in patients with ovarian cancer receiving silibinin were already underway.

Bhatia et al. (1999), after nearly six years of investigating the potential anticarcinogenic and cancer chemopreventive activity of silymarin, compared the in vitro growth-inhibitory effects of pure silibinin to silymarin in human ectocervical carcinoma cells (A431), human prostate carcinoma (LNCaP cells, androgen-independent and -dependent, and DU145 cells), and human breast carcinoma (MCF-7 cells, estrogen-independent and -dependent, and MDA-MB468 cells). At 100 μM concentration in each of the tumor cell lines, silymarin and silibinin both produced significant and comparable inhibition of tumor cell growth; cervical carcinoma cells were the exception, in that cell death occurred with a 50% reduction in cell viability from silibinin and 70% from silymarin after five days of treatment. DNA synthesis in the tumor cell lines was also comparable between silymarin and silibinin (53% to 81%) and, again, statistically significant compared to the vehicle control. In the case of human prostate carcinoma cells (LNCaP), however, silibinin produced a statistically significantly greater inhibition (74% inhibition of DNA synthesis) than silymarin (about 70%). Bhatia and colleagues conclude that silibinin is primarily responsible for the anticarcinogenic and cancer chemopreventive activity of silymarin and plan to conduct more extensive studies toward developing silibinin as an agent with these properties against "different human cancers."

Chemopreventive activity. Intestinal bacteria are a source of β-glucuronidase, an enzyme linked to colon cancer in rats and humans. It has been suggested that the enzyme may be linked to liver cancer. Kim et al. (1994) found that rats at high risk of developing colon cancer fed a synthetic β-glucuronidase inhibitor showed a decreased risk for the cancer. Silymarin and silibinin (0.8 mg/mL) noncompetitively inhibited rat liver microsomal β-glucuronidase in vitro by 53% and 50%, respectively. Silymarin and silibinin were also shown to inhibit β-glucuronidase in a human colon cancer patient and a healthy subject. Both compounds inhibited *E. coli* and 2 β-glucuronidase-positive bacteria derived from human feces. Serum β-glucuronidase activity in rats after treatment with carbon tetrachloride (CCl_4) increased 1.8-fold. β-Glucuronidase activity was decreased by silymarin or silibinin (30 mg/kg p.o. daily for four days) by 30% and 22%, respectively, compared to the control, and as a pretreatment by 28% and 22%, respectively, compared to the control (Kim et al., 1994).

Katiyar et al. (1997) reported that ultraviolet B (UVB)-induced tumors in hairless mice were inhibited by as much as 40% from a topical treatment with silymarin (9 mg/application). The 100% incidence of tumors induced by phorbol ester and promoted by UVB was reduced by 60% and their multiplicity was reduced by 90%. More significant results were found using the two-stage initiation-promotion carcinogenesis model, which utilizes a more carcinogenic toxin (7,12-dimethylbenz[a]anthracene) followed by UVB as a tumor promoter. In this experiment (complete carcinogenesis), the 100% incidence of tumors was reduced to 25%, and while tumor volume was reduced by 97% per mouse, silymarin also reduced tumor multiplicity by 92%. Further tests revealed that silymarin caused significant inhibition of skin edema, UVB-induced sunburn, catalase activity depletion, formation of apoptotic cells, and the induction of ornithine decarboxylase (ODC) and cyclooxygenase (COX) activities, including ODC mRNA expression. These results indicated that silymarin possesses potent protective activities against various stages of UVB-induced carcinogenesis. The researchers concluded that together these results warrant testing of silymarin in humans for protective activity against solar radiation-induced skin cancers of the nonmelanoma type (Katiyar et al., 1997).

Tumor necrosis factor-alpha (TNF-α), an endogenous promoter of tumor cells and a critical factor in tumor promotion in animal models using carcinogens such as 12-O-tetradecanoylphorbol 13-acetate (TPA) and okadaic acid (OA), was inhibited by silymarin when applied topically on mouse skin before applying either OA or TPA. Silymarin inhibited highly to completely TNF-α mRNA expression induced by either tumor promoter. Thus, silymarin exhibits chemopreventive activity against tumor promotion caused by TNF-α (Zi et al., 1997). However, when incubated with rat Kupffer cells, silibinin showed no effect on TNF-α formation (Dehmlow, Murawski, et al., 1996).

Epidermal growth factor receptor (EGFR)-mediated cell signaling induced by promoters of skin tumors, as well as by UVB radiation and oxidative stress, has also been implicated in mouse skin as a promoting factor in skin cancer (Ahmad et al., 1998). Following very high rates of protection by silymarin against tumors induced by skin tumor-promoting factors (Mukhtar and Agarwal, 1996; Chatterjee et al., 1996), Ahmad and co-workers (1998) investigated its effect on EGFR activation. In vitro studies showed that silymarin inhibits EGFR activation in cells and very significantly inhibits EGFR kinase activity. Silymarin produced a significant and time- and dose-dependent inhibition of cell growth and DNA synthesis in human epidermoid carcinoma cells (A431). Silymarin (50, 75, and 100 µg/mL) produced a highly significant modulation of cell-cycle progression in human epidermoid carcinoma cells (A431), leading the researchers to conclude that silymarin exerts its chemopreventive action by way of impairing EGFR signaling—in turn, resulting in a perturbed cell-cycle progression, inhibition of cell growth, and ultimately cell arrest. DNA synthesis in the tumor cells was significantly inhibited by 42% by silymarin (10 µg/mL, $p < 0.001$) and by 78% from a higher concentration (50 µg/mL, $p < 0.0001$). Tumor cell (A431) growth was inhibited by 85% from silymarin at the same dose in vitro ($p < 0.0001$). Cytotoxic effects on the tumor cell line were evident only at 75 µg/mL from treatments lasting as long as four and five days. The researchers commented that collectively these results indicate a possible future role of silymarin as a chemopreventive against skin tumor initiation (Ahmad et al., 1998).

The effects of silymarin on radiation toxicity were studied in the liver, spleen, and bone marrow tissue of rats. A high postradiation dosage of silymarin (700 mg/kg p.o. b.i.d. for 14 days) antagonized genetic damage provoked by γ-radiation. Silymarin caused liver concentrations of RNA and DNA to increase. The 20% to 30% increase in both nucleic acids in the spleen was significant compared to the controls, after only a seven-day treatment with silymarin. Similar results were found in the bone marrow contents of RNA and DNA from seven-day and 14-day treatments with silymarin (Hakova and Misurova, 1993).

Bokemeyer et al. (1996) demonstrated that at nontoxic concentrations, in combination with cisplatin or without, silibinin had no interfering effect on the in vitro cytotoxicity of cisplatin against human testicular tumor cells. Similar results were found with silibinin and 4-hydroperoxy-ifsofamide. The authors also showed that the cisplatin-induced (5 mg/kg i.v.) increase in plasma levels of urea was not seen in rats pretreated with silibinin (200 mg/kg i.v.).

Inflammatory Response

In several experiments, silymarin showed a dose-dependent inhibition of activities involved in inflammation, including histamine release from rat serosal mast cells (Fantozzi et al., 1986), histamine release from human basophilic leukocytes (Miadonna et al., 1987), and activation of human T-lymphocytes (Meroni et al., 1988).

The antiedematous effect of silymarin (silymarin Phytosome) was studied in male mice with topical croton oil-induced dermatitis of the ears. Topical treatment with silymarin complexed with a synthetic phospholipid (distearoylphosphatidylcholine), which increased skin permeation, significantly ameliorated croton oil-induced ear edema. At the same dose (0.5 μM /ear), silymarin alone was clearly less effective, reducing edema by 13.9% compared to 88.9% from the silymarin-phospholipid formulation, and from indomethicin by 75.1%. Myeloperoxidase activity measured at 12 and 24 h postadministration (0.5 μM/ear) showed no reduction in the silymarin-treated mice, whereas the silymarin-phytosome group showed significant reductions at both times (32.4% and 38.3%, respectively) compared to untreated controls. Macrophage-induced chemoluminescence in vitro was also significantly reduced by the formulation, indicating a decrease in free radicals produced by stimulated leukocytes (Bombardelli et al., 1991).

Ischemia-reperfusion-induced gastric injury in male rats was ameliorated by pretreatment with silymarin. Significantly fewer and less severe ulcers were found in silymarin-pretreated rats from dosages of 10, 25, 50, and 100 mg/kg p.o., inhibiting ulceration by as much as 89.45% from the highest dose. Mucosal myeloperoxidase (MPO) activity, increased by the ischemia-reperfusion-induced gastric injury, was used to measure neutrophilic polymorphonuclear leukocyte (neutrophil) infiltration. In an activated state, neutrophils are a source of various cytotoxic proteins, including lactoferrin, MPO, and proteases. Silymarin pretreatment (50 and 100 mg/kg p.o.) significantly reduced the mean ulcer index ($p < 0.05$ and $p < 0.005$, respectively) and produced a significant though not dose-dependent reduction in mucosal MPO levels ($p < 0.05$), indicating a decrease of after-injury PMN leukocyte infiltration into the gastric wall (de la Lastra et al., 1995).

Silymarin inhibited chemoluminescence (CL) without significantly influencing the phagocytic, chemotactic, and photoabsorption activities of PMNs. Immunopotentiating activity can be measured in vitro in macrophage models. In one study, preincubation of PMNs with silymarin resulted in a dose-dependent inhibition of phagocytic activity as measured by CL. Furthermore, superoxide anion production (cytochrome C reduction assay) was not affected by the preincubation, nor was cell viability (Minozio et al., 1988).

Silibinin in particular increased the motility of polymorphonuclear leukocytes (PMNs) immobilized by various toxic agents in vitro (Kalmar et al., 1990). Silymarin inhibited leukocyte accumulation responsible for inflammation in carrageenan-induced paw edema in rats (De La Puerta et al., 1996).

Catalase, a hydrogen peroxide scavenger, exhibited an inhibition of luminol-enhanced CL similar to that of silibinin. However, incubation of the PMNs with catalase and silibinin in combination did not show an additive inhibitory effect. It has been suggested that the inhibiting activity by silibinin of luminol-enhanced CL from stimulated PMNs may occur through inhibition of hydrogen peroxide (Minozio et al., 1988).

Dehmlow, Erhard, et al., (1996) proposed that the ability of silibinin to selectively inhibit leukotriene formation by rat liver Kupffer cells partly explains its hepatoprotective effects and found that it took less silibinin to inhibit leukotriene B_4 formation in human liver phagocytic cells than in rat liver phagocytic cells (Kupffer cells). At 10 µmol/L, silibinin inhibited LTB_4 by 66.3% in human cells versus only 19.4% in rat cells. Silibinin also caused a significant inhibition of the 5-lipoxygenase pathway, and at amounts reached in human plasma (0.4-1.3 µmol/L) (Dehmlow, Erhard, et al., 1996) from the common clinical dose (240 mg) (Dehmlow, Murawski, et al., 1996).

Gupta et al. (1999) reported significant anti-inflammatory activity from silymarin (25-100 mg/kg p.o.) against papaya latex-induced inflammation as a model of established arthritis in male rats. Pretreatment of the rats with silymarin produced inhibition rates of 20.49% to 26.22%. Against adjuvant-induced developing arthritis, rats treated with silymarin the day before and for 14 days of adjuvant treatments showed significant inhibition of paw edema from silymarin at doses of 12.5 or 25 mg/kg per day p.o., which produced inhibition rates of 23.73% and 31.64%, respectively. In the model of established arthritis, however, the effect of 25 mg/kg p.o silymarin against inflammation was less pronounced (20.49% inhibition). The researchers propose that the difference owes to the free-radical scavenging activity of silymarin, which inhibits enzymatic peroxidation, in turn, inhibiting the formation of leukotrienes and prostaglandins involved in the development of arthritic conditions.

Metabolic and Nutritional Functions

Antioxidant Activity

Locher et al. (1998) showed that silibinin causes a significant inhibition of auto-oxidation of human LDL cholesterol in vitro and suggested the possibility of using silibinin as a preventive and therapeutic in atherosclerosis. However, the antioxidant effect found was from concentrations of silymarin tenfold higher than plasma concentrations detected in human volunteers following ingestion of silibinin (Weyhenmeyer et al., 1992). Although much higher concentrations of silibinin are required to scavenge free radicals than are achieved in human plasma from clinical doses, it may be that local concentrations of silibinin in vivo are higher, in which case the free-radical scavenging effect would become important. Otherwise, this aspect of silibinin in heptoprotection is questionable (Dehmlow, Erhard, et al., 1996).

The liver-protecting properties of silymarin are widely attributed to the antioxidant, free-radical scavenging abilities of the flavonolignan complex. Silymarin, particularly silibinin, appear to intercept the process of lipid peroxidation on microsomes in the liver. Phenolic groups of silymarin and silibinin can react with oxygen and hydroxylic free radicals, thus rendering them more stable and less reactive with compounds in hepatic microsomes (Mira et al., 1987).

Hepatotoxicity can be induced by carbon tetrachloride, thallium, ethanol, paracetamol, and other agents that cause free-radical formations in the lipid layers of the membranes of liver cells. Lipid peroxidation refers to the chain reaction initiated by these unstable free radicals in the presence of unsaturated fatty acids on cell membranes. Silymarin, and in particular silibinin, serve as scavengers of both free radicals and reactive oxygen species (ROS). Both have been shown to enhance the antioxidant capabilities of hepatocytes by interrupting free-radical reactions (Valenzuela et al., 1989).

Several groups of investigators have demonstrated that silibinin can block lipid peroxidation in microsomes and mitochondria of rat livers (Bindoli et al., 1977; Valenzuela et al., 1986; Valenzuela and Guerra, 1986).

Silymarin and silibinin inhibited lipid peroxidation on hepatic microsomes and in mitochondria of rats by interacting with iron in the peroxidating system (Bindoli et al., 1977; Valenzuela et al., 1986; Valenzuela and Guerra, 1986). However, this inhibition is probably not due to a simple chelating effect on the iron, as in the case of the true flavonoids (Bindoli et al., 1977; Cavallini et al., 1978).

In numerous experiments, silymarin reduced the activity of enzymes (e.g., monoxygenases) involved in lipid peroxidation (Lettéron et al., 1990) and blocked other adverse mechanisms linked to in vitro lipid peroxidation. Silymarin protected erythrocytes from hemolysis and inhibited the formation of methemoglobin. When erythrocytes and lymphocytes taken from patients with liver disease were incubated with silymarin, superoxide dismutase (SOD) activity was enhanced, suggesting that silymarin exerts its antioxidant effects by increasing the activity of SOD, a key enzyme involved in scavenging free radicals (Muzes et al., 1991). At a concentration within the parameters of clinical use, silymarin (Legalon) was shown to significantly increase SOD activity when incubated with human erythrocytes from healthy donors (Altorjay et al., 1992).

Gyorgy et al. (1992) studied the effect of silibinin as a pretreatment (25 mg/kg i.p. daily for 14 days) on the protection of liver microsomes following γ-irradiation of rats. As measured by malondialdehyde (MDA) levels (indicating peroxidation of membrane lipids) and by levels of post-γ-irradiation drug-metabolizing enzymes, pretreatment with silibinin produced a substantial inhibition of degradation in both indices.

Dehmlow, Murawski, et al. (1996) showed that silibinin is a strong scavenger of hypochlorite produced by phorbol-12-myristate-13-acetate (PMA)-activated human granulocytes (IC_{50} 7 μM), but that its effect against superoxide radicals in these cells is rather weak. Silibinin strongly inhibited leukotriene B_4 (LTB_4) formation by human granulocytes produced by human granulocytes (IC_{50} 15 μM) but proved a weak inhibitor of the cyclooxygenase pathway. Significant results were also found from silibinin against the formation of leukotrienes by human granulocytes (IC_{50} 14.5 μM); however, much higher concentrations were needed to inhibit prostaglandin E_2 (PGE_2) formation by human monocytes (IC_{50} 45 μM), thromboxane-2 formation by human thrombocytes (IC_{50} 69 μM), and 6-K-$PGF_{1\alpha}$ formation by human omentum endothelial cells (IC_{50} 52 μM). The researchers concluded that the inhibition of hypochlorite production could account for a considerable amount of the cytoprotective effect of silibinin (Dehmlow, Murawski, et al., 1996).

Hypochlorite figures prominently in inflammatory reactions and is a cytototoxic agent known to disturb protein functions and to oxidize suflhydryl groups, even at low concentrations. Hypochlorite is also a potent antimicrobial produced by neutrophils. Dehmlow, Murawski, et al. (1996)

noted that the ability of silibinin to inhibit hypochlorite production as well as the 5-lipoxygenase pathway in concentrations within the range of plasma concentrations (0.4-1.3 μM) from a typical clinical oral dose of 240 mg indicates that silibinin may do more than protect hepatic cells; it may also exhibit cellular protective effects in other tissues and organs.

CLINICAL STUDIES

Cardiovascular and Circulatory Disorders

Effects on Cholesterol and Lipid Metabolism

Nassuato et al. (1991) conducted a placebo-controlled trial of silymarin (Legalon, 420 mg p.o. daily for 30 days) in 15 cholecystectomized and four gallstone patients in which they examined changes in biliary lipid composition. Concentrations of biliary cholesterol were significantly reduced in both groups compared to placebo ($p < 0.02$); however, total bile salts and phospholipids showed an insignificant increase. Prior animal studies combined with the clinical trial results led the researchers to conclude that the effect by silibinin of reducing biliary cholesterol levels in vivo may owe to a decrease in cholesterol synthesis of the liver, possibly by inhibiting HMG-Co-A reductase activity, which they reported to be a dose-dependent effect of silibinin in vitro, but not in vivo; liver microsomes of rats treated with silibinin (100 mg/kg i.p. daily for seven days) showed no significant difference in HMG-CoA reductase activity compared to control rats.

Digestive, Hepatic, and Gastrointestinal Disorders

Hepatic Diseases

In a recent review, Flora et al. (1998) lamented the poor quality of clinical trials of milk thistle in the treatment of hepatic conditions; the majority involve small numbers of patients, liver diseases of varying severity and etiology, inconsistencies in the usage of alcohol by subjects, poorly defined endpoints, inconsistent employment of control groups, and in most trials lack of due consideration to the ability of the liver to repair when offending toxins, such as alcohol, are discontinued.

Cirrhosis. Lang, Nekum, Deak, et al. (1990) conducted a four-week randomized double-blind placebo-controlled study of milk thistle extract (Legalon, 140 mg p.o. t.i.d.) in 60 cirrhosis patients (mean age 44.7 years) with a mean duration of alcohol consumption of 8.6 years. The main purpose of the trial was to examine the antioxidant and immunological effects of the extract (reviewed under Immunomodulation). The patients were diagnosed with mild compensated alcoholic cirrhosis, histologically confirmed by micronodular cirrhosis. Results were compared to placebo and a second active treatment group was administered Aica-P (Chinoin, Budapest, 200 mg p.o. t.i.d.), an antioxidant hepatoprotectant agent derived from imidazol. Both active agents caused a marked improvement in hepatic functions, whereas no change of any significance was found in the placebo group. In the silymarin group, bilirubin (SEBI), aspartate aminotransferase (AST), and alanine aminotransferase (ALT) levels, which were moderately elevated at the start of the trial, had all normalized ($p < 0.05$, $p < 0.01$, and $p < 0.02$, respectively). Previous markedly elevated baseline γ-glutamyl transferase (GGT) levels showed a significant decrease ($p < 0.05$) compared to placebo. In the Aica-P group, SEBI and ALT levels showed no significant change, but AST and GGT significantly decreased ($p < 0.01$ and $p < 0.05$, respectively) compared to placebo. Lang, Nekum, Deak, and colleagues (1990) determined that these improvements were not the result of reduced alcohol intake. A similar study by Lang, Nekum, Gonzales-Cabello, et al. (1990) found practically identical results in 40 patients diagnosed with alcoholic cirrhosis of the liver.

Ferenci et al. (1989) conducted a two-year, double-blind, placebo-controlled clinical trial on cirrhosis of the liver in 91 alcoholic and 79 nonalcoholic patients. Patients in the treatment group were given an oral dose of 200 mg 70% silymarin extract t.i.d. At the conclusion of the study, patients who received silymarin had a 23% mortality rate compared to a 33% rate in the placebo group. The silymarin-treated group had a cumulative survival rate of 58%, while the placebo group had a rate of only 38%.

Further analysis revealed that silymarin was more efficacious in the treatment of milder (Child Class A) cases of alcohol cirrhosis. For example, in a four-week, double-blind controlled study, silymarin (420 mg p.o. daily) administered to patients with mild liver disease helped reduce undesirable elevations in blood levels of liver enzymes. Among the favorable effects produced by silymarin were: normalization of serum transaminases, sulphabromphthalein (BSP) retention, lowered SGPT (serum level of glutamic-pyruvic transaminase) and SGOT (serum level of glutamic-oxalacetic transaminase) activity, as well as decreased serum concentrations of total and conjugated bilirubin (Salmi and Sarna, 1982).

The results of other investigations imply that silymarin improves hepatic function in alcoholic patients without adverse side effects (Fintelmann and Albert, 1980; Feher et al., 1989; Ferenci et al., 1989; Trinchet et al., 1989; Bunout et al., 1992; Vailati et al., 1993; Grungreiff et al., 1995), and counters alcohol-induced liver damage when administered prior to alcohol consumption (Salmi and Sarna, 1982).

Hepatitis. The therapeutic efficacy of silymarin in acute and chronic hepatitis has been the subject of over 300 investigations (Foster, 1996). Controlled trials on biochemical and morphological function in human livers indicate that silymarin accelerates liver repair. Hepatic restoration has been reported following improvements in pathological liver function parameters. These include significant decreases in SGOT ($p < 0.10$), SGPT ($p < 0.05$), gamma-glutamyl-transpeptidase (γ-GT) ($p < 0.05$), and bilirubin in 66 patients with liver toxicity of various origins in a double-blind, placebo-controlled clinical trial (Fintelmann and Albert, 1980).

In a 25-month, double-blind, crossover clinical trial, patients with chronic active hepatitis initially received either 420 mg silymarin daily or 600 mg ursodeoxycholic acid (UDCA) daily. Patients in both groups showed significant declines in serum levels of several liver enzymes (SGPT, SGOT) and those receiving UDCA had a significant reduction in γ-GT levels. Galactose elimination capacity and antipyrine clearance did not deteriorate in either treatment group, suggesting stabilization of a functional liver mass. In the crossover phase of this study, patients were either given a combined treatment of silymarin and UDCA or taken off all therapy. The combined therapy showed no advantage over either silymarin or UDCA administered as a single treatment. In patients who discontinued therapy, the activity of serum liver enzymes worsened when compared to the favorable improvements of each treatment administered separately (Lirussi and Okolicsanyi, 1992).

In a statistical analysis of a randomized, double-blind clinical study (Berenguer and Carrasco, 1977), Scheiber and Wohlzogen (1978) disputed the advantage of silymarin over placebo (20 patients, placebo or silymarin as Legalon, 420 mg p.o. daily for 12 months). The treatment with silymarin was reported to result in a statistically significant reversal of pathological hepatic changes in patients with chronic hepatitis of diverse origins. Among the specific hepatopathological events reported to have shown improvement were intralobular mesenchymal reactions and parenchymatous changes associated with chronic cirrhosis (Berenguer and Carrasco, 1977).

Hepatoxicity. In a review of double-blind studies on milk thistle extractives, Hikino and Kiso (1988) discussed numerous laboratory and clinical studies showing the therapeutic benefits of silymarin in protecting the liver from toxic agents. Biochemical studies suggested that silymarin achieves its liver-protecting effect through flavonolignans in the silymarin complex which stabilize the cell membrane and stimulate protein synthesis. Simultaneously, silymarin accelerated the regeneration of hepatocytes in damaged liver tissue. These three activities in concert were presumed to account for the overall therapeutic effect of the flavonolignans in a host of liver problems.

In a double-blind study, silymarin was reported to be efficacious against hepatopathies in 60 female patients who had been taking psychopharmaceutical drugs such as phenothiazines or butrophenones for at least five years. Silymarin (800 mg p.o. daily for 90 days) produced a significant decline in malondialdehyde (MDA) levels compared to those of the control group, even in those who continued to take the psychoactive agents (Palasciano et al., 1994).

In an open-label trial, 975 patients ages 15-89 were given 140 mg of a standardized 70% milk thistle extract p.o., b.i.d. or t.i.d. for 12 weeks. All patients had liver damage due to various causes, with the majority (63.3%) resulting from ethanol. Ultrasound and biopsy confirmed the diagnosis of fatty liver in 570 patients. Of these, 143 had fatty liver hepatitis and 214 had hepatic cirrhosis. With the exception of two patients who discontinued therapy because of adverse reactions (diarrhea and a pruitic skin rash), all subjects completed the study. Sixteen patients who finished the regimen reported a side effect of loose stools. Laboratory analysis showed a reduction in the mean levels of serum liver enzymes and a normalization of total bilirubin concentration. SGOT dropped from 46.0 µg/L to 28.8 µg/L; SGPT declined from 48.0 µg/L to 31.0 µg/L; and γ-GT fell from 112.0 µg/L to 60.6 µg/L (Grungreiff et al., 1995).

In a study of 2,169 patients with toxic liver damage administered silymarin orally for eight weeks (264 ± 103 mg/day), Frerick et al. (1990) reported that patients improved or showed normalized clinical and biochemical readings. Over 82% of the patients experienced improvements in subjective complaints of tiredness, upper abdominal pressure, poor appetite, nausea, and itching.

Silymarin was administered to 49 workers who had been exposed to toluene and/or xylene vapors on the job for five to twenty years. All showed low blood platelet counts and abnormal liver function. After taking silymarin for 30 days (140 mg t.i.d. p.o.), the treatment group ($n = 30$) showed a significant improvement in liver and hematological laboratory tests compared to the control group ($n = 19$) even as they continued to work in the toxic environment (toluene concentration 33 mg/m^3; xylene 115-220 mg/m^3). Compared to the control group, the silymarin group showed a rise in platelet counts as well as improvements in parameters of leukocytosis, relative lymphocytosis, serum γ-GT, ALT, and AST. For ten of the silymarin-treated group who complained of headaches, after the 30-day treatment they no longer had the problem. Distention of the abdomen, the most frequently reported complaint ($n = 13$), also ceased after the silymarin treatment (Szilard et al., 1988).

The effect of long-term treatment with silymarin on hepatopathological changes in 19 mostly schizophrenic patients (ages 32-65) taking chlorpromazine with or without benzodiazepine was investigated in a comparative study by Saba et al. (1976). Evident liver damage was not ameliorated with prior standard treatments in these patients. Silymarin (70 mg p.o. t.i.d. for six months) was compared to standard treatments in another group of 18 similar patients with liver damage also resulting from long-term treatment with psychopharmaceuticals. Comparative analysis of 15 patients from each group indicated that silymarin provided far better improvements than conventional agents by improving SGOT and SGPT, bilirubin, alkaline phosphatase, and protein levels. In many cases, values returned to normal. The researchers concluded that their study confirmed the hepatoprotective effects of silymarin in ameliorating iatrogenic toxicity and without interruption of treatments.

Fintelmann (1973) reported that compared to controls, the use of silymarin in postoperative gallstone patients appeared to ameliorate the toxicity of narcotics used in their anesthesia and decreased levels of serum cholinesterase. Compared to the control group ($n = 32$), patients who received silymarin before and after surgery ($n = 51$) showed no excessive change in liver enzymes. Best results were seen from oral doses of 140 mg administered t.i.d.

In a case report, Invernizzi et al. (1993) reported good results from silymarin in a 34-year-old female patient receiving antiblastic agents for acute promyelocytic leukemia. Treatment was interrupted on numerous occasions owing to raised liver transaminase levels from the agents. Treated with silymarin (800 mg/day p.o.) along with 6-mercaptopurine (6-MP) and methotrexate (MTX) as maintenance therapy for four months, her serum levels of ALT, AST, and γ-GT stayed within normal levels, and bilirubin showed an initial increase and then fell to levels below her baseline, whereafter she stopped all treatment and remained healthy. A prospective study to validate the concomitant use of silymarin in similar clinical applications was then in progress.

Amanita *poisoning.* The ingestion of *Amanita phalloides* mushrooms can be fatal because they contain phalloidine, one of the most rapidly absorbed and toxic liver poisons known. As little as 50 g or three mushrooms can kill a human. Phalloidine and the α-amanatins, the second toxin in the deathcap mushroom, disrupt normal liver and kidney function. The toxins are eliminated through the bile and then continually reabsorbed by the intestines, setting in motion a vicious cycle. In over 50% of human cases of *Amanita* poisoning, death usually occurs within three to five days after the mushroom is ingested. Besides *Amanita phalloides, A. virosa,* and *A. verna* are also known to be fatal (Sabeel et al., 1995).

Research by Sabeel et al. (1995) suggests that silymarin taken either alone or in combination with penicillin is potentially beneficial to patients poisoned by *Amanita.* The researchers describe a treatment for *Amanita* poisoning that they evaluated over a period of 15 years in 41 patients with various degrees of poisoning (18 women and 23 men). Every patient showed improvement and most of those with moderate and severe *Amanita* poisoning remained without sequalae after their hospital discharge. The longest hospitalization periods lasted 13 ± 2 days in those with severe *Amanita* mushroom poisoning. This treatment would appear to be superior to previous detoxification methods, which have shown mortality rates of 10% to

12% and even 30% to 90%. The treatment consisted of the following measures: penicillin i.v.; charcoal hemoperfusion combined with hemodialysis; oral lactulose and activated charcoal; a protein-free, carbohydrate-rich meal; electrolyte and fluid replacement; upon admission, in some cases, thioctic acid i.v.; in 22 patients, silibinin (20 mg/kg i.v. daily in four divided doses), with the other interventions over 24 h except during hemodialysis.

Hruby et al. (1983) reported that liver damage was prevented in 17/18 patients who received silymarin in a mean dosage of 33 mg/kg i.v. daily as part of a combined treatment within 48 h after consuming *Amanita phalloides*. In two cases, silymarin was administered in single doses of 1.4 and 4.2 g p.o.

Immune Disorders; Inflammation and Disease

Immune Functions

Immunomodulation. To examine the antioxidant and immunomodulatory effects of a milk thistle extract (Legalon), Lang, Nekum, Deak, et al. (1990) conducted a four-week randomized double-blind placebo-controlled study in 60 patients (mean age 44.7 years) diagnosed with mild compensated alcoholic cirrhosis, histologically confirmed by micronodular cirrhosis. The mean duration of alcohol consumption was 8.6 years. The treatment groups consisted of a placebo group (vehicle-treated), a silymarin group (140 mg p.o. t.i.d.), and an Aica-P group (Chinoin, Budapest, 200 mg t.i.d.). Aica-P, or amino-imidazol-carboxamid-phosphate, is an antioxidant hepatoprotectant agent derived from imidazol. Among their findings, both the silymarin group and the Aica-P showed significant decreases in the T-suppressor (CD8+) cell population ($p < 0.05$ and $p < 0.01$, respectively), a marked enhancement of lectin-induced lymphoblast transformation rates (each $p < 0.01$), and a significant decrease in natural killer (NK) cell activity from either silymarin ($p < 0.02$) or Aica-P ($p < 0.05$), compared to placebo. Antibody-dependent, cell-mediated cytotoxicity was significantly decreased in the silymarin group ($p < 0.05$) but not in the Aica-P group, while spontaneous lymphocytotoxicity was significantly decreased in both treatment groups ($p < 0.02$ and $p < 0.05$, respectively) compared to placebo. In addition, four of the patients in the silymarin group showed a normalization of their initially low T-cell numbers. The treatments were well tolerated and no side effects were seen in any of the groups (Lang, Nekum, Deak, et al., 1990).

Infectious Diseases

Viral infections. A multicenter trial of silymarin conducted over 38 months in 200 alcoholics diagnosed with proven liver cirrhosis found no side effects from a dosage of 150 mg t.i.d. in capsules (Parés et al., 1998).

The placebo-controlled, double-blind randomized trial found that silymarin had no effect on survival or the clinical course of liver cirrhosis in these patients; however, among 75 patients who tested positive for hepatitis-C virus, none died in the silymarin group, whereas four died in the placebo group, although this result failed to attain statistical significance. In discussing the overall negative results, the researchers surmised that silymarin may not be as beneficial in chronic cases of liver cirrhosis as in milder, earlier stages of the disease in patients who are able to abstain completely from alcohol (Parés et al., 1998).

Buzzelli et al. (1993) conducted a pilot placebo-controlled, double-blind trial in 20 patients diagnosed with chronic active hepatitis B and C. The patients were treated with silymarin in the form of a complex with phosphatidylcholine (IdB1016, Inverna della Beffa S.p.A., Milan, Italy) in a dosage equivalent to 480 mg of silibinin/day (two 120 mg capsules b.i.d. for seven days, 2 h before breakfast and dinner). The researchers reported that the preparation had favorable effects on histopathological parameters, including indices of hepatocellular necrosis and hepatic fibrosis. Significant decreases were seen in serum ALT, AST, GGT, and total bilirubin, but not in plasma malondialdehyde (MDA) in this short trial (Buzzelli et al., 1993). The authors of a pilot study of IdB1016 in eight patients with hepatitis B or C and in three cases with both infections reported that after two months of treatment the patients showed significant changes in liver function: a 36% decrease in serum MDA levels, an increase of 15% in galactose elimination capacity, and a decrease in AST and ALT levels of 17% and 16%, respectively. Decreases in bilirubin (9%) and GGT (10%) were only slight, however. The treatment was well tolerated at one capsule between meals, each capsule equivalent to 120 mg silibinin (Moscarella et al., 1993).

The effect of silymarin in children ages three to nine diagnosed with acute viral hepatitis was investigated in a comparative clinical study by Mingrino et al. (1979). The researchers acknowledged that the disease is usually of less severity and with a shorter duration in children than in adults. A population of 16 boys and 14 girls with acute viral hepatitis treated during a preceding year with multivitamin preparations were compared to a matched group (disease duration, sex, and age) administered silymarin: 100 mg p.o. b.i.d. until normal or near-normal serum transaminases were reached. Silymarin treatment was limited to children admitted to the clinic with acute infective hepatitis within 15-20 days of disease onset and within four days of jaundice onset. Two patients in the silymarin group tested positive for hepatitis B antigen versus four in the multivitamin group, yet their serum transaminase and total bilirubin showed no significant differences from the other patients in either group. Thirty days after commencing silymarin, mean SGOT levels had decreased from 276.2 to 34.4 U/mL, and mean SGPT decreased from 592.7 U/mL to 58.7 U/mL compared to baseline and remained at these levels. The comparison group not receiving silymarin showed a respectively slower rate of decrease in mean SGOT and SGPT (58.7 U/mL and 73.1 U/mL, respectively). Mingrino and co-workers acknowledged that in benign, acute viral hepatitis, SGPT and SGOT levels become normal again eight weeks from the time of jaundice onset, even without treatment. However, the faster normalization in their levels in children treated with silymarin compared to the controls indicated that damage from hepatic necrosis was limited. No side effects were found. Renal function, total protein, alkaline phosphatase, bilirubin levels, and the prothrombin index, which were all normal at the start, remained so throughout the study.

Shortened treatment time was reported in a three-week, randomized, placebo-controlled double-blind study of 57 patients with acute hepatitis A or B infection. From an oral dose of silymarin (70 mg t.i.d. for ≥ 3 weeks), patients showed significantly lower mean levels of bilirubin, AST, and ALT than controls, and significantly more patients treated with silymarin showed normalized AST (82% versus 52%) and bilirubin (40% versus 11%). However, silymarin appeared to have no effect on HBsAg patient immune reaction (Magliulo et al., 1978).

Integumentary, Muscular, and Skeletal Disorders

Dermatitis

In a placebo-controlled study, 20 volunteers received a topical silymarin preparation (silymarin-Phytosome), made by complexing silymarin with a synthetic phospholipid (distearoylphosphatidylcholine), or placebo. Following tests for tolerability that showed no sensitizing or irritant effects from the preparation (aqueous gel containing 5% silymarin-Phytosome), subjects were irradiated with ultraviolet light (1.5 Rad for 4 min) to produce erythema then immediately treated. Compared to the placebo group, the silymarin-phospholipid group showed a reduction in skin redness of 24%, as measured subjectively and by Minolta Chromameter (Bombardelli et al., 1991).

Metabolic and Nutritional Disorders

Antioxidant Activity

In a six-month double-blind study of silymarin (Legalon, 420 mg/day) in the treatment of 36 patients with chronic alcoholic liver disease, Gyorgyi et al. (1990) found both erythrocyte and lymphocyte SOD activity significantly enhanced ($p < 0.001$ and $p < 0.01$, respectively) and a restoration of lymphocyte SOD expression in the silymarin group compared to the placebo group and to their low baseline readings. Silymarin markedly increased glutathione peroxidase activity and serum levels of free SH groups (each $p < 0.05$) compared to placebo, while significantly decreasing serum levels of MDA ($p < 0.02$). A similar result was reported by Muzes et al. (1990) in patients given 20 mg silymarin/day (Legalon) who showed increased levels of superoxide dismutase (SOD) in both red and white blood cells compared to a control group, and by Feher et al. (1990) who reported that erythrocytes from alcoholic cirrhosis patients previously administered silymarin (140 mg Legalon, t.i.d. for 30 days) showed a significantly increased expression of SOD by lymphocytes and erythrocytes and lymphocyte SOD activities compared to a placebo-control group.

Pharmacokinetics

Total bioavailability of silibinin, the main active flavonolignan constituent of milk thistle seed extract, is acknowledged as poor (Savio et al., 1998). In one study, silibinin, the main component of silymarin, was found to reach a plasma concentration of only 0.4-1.3 µmol/L in vivo (Dehmlow, Erhard, et al., 1996). Research has shown that on average, only 10% of plasma silibinin following oral administration of silymarin (Legalon) in men is found in unconjugated form (Weyhenmeyer et al., 1992).

A comparative analysis of the pharmacokinetics of single oral doses of three milk thistle extractives administered orally to postoperative cholecystectomy patients found significant differences in biliary excretion rates. Following silymarin (120 mg, as an equivalent of silibinin), the amount of silibinin (free and conjugated) recovered in bile after 48 h was 3% of the dose administered. Following silipide (120 mg, as an equivalent of silibinin), also known as IdB1016 (a "lipophilic silybin [silibinin]-phosphatidylcholine complex"), the amount of free and conjugated forms of silibinin recovered in bile after 48 h amounted to 11% of the dose (Schandalik et al., 1992).

Studies showed that the pharmacokinetic parameters of silymarin in cirrhotic patients and healthy subjects were nearly equal (Morazzoni and Bombardelli, 1995). In six healthy male volunteers given single doses of silibinin in the form of silymarin (Legalon 140, 102, 253, 203, and 254 mg), the elimination half-life of total silibinin was about 6 h. Approximately 5% of each tested dose was excreted into the urine in the form of total silibinin (at a renal clearance rate of about 30 mL/min). Even with the highest dosage of five capsules/day (254 mg each), no adverse effects occurred. At this dosage, the peak plasma concentration of total silibinin isomers reached 2 mg/L (Weyhenmeyer et al., 1992).

An open clinical study (randomized, two-way, balanced crossover trial) of a commercially available silibinin-phosphatidylcholine complex (1:2 ratio) in healthy men and women (ages 18-45) found a threefold higher level of silibinin following ingestion of a softgel (C_{max} 710 ng/mL plasma) versus ingestion of the same complex in a hard capsule (C_{max} 193.46 ng/mL plasma), and in less than half the time (Savio et al., 1998).

Silibinin complexed with soybean phosphatidylcholine (IdB1016) was reported to show a terminal half-life in healthy volunteers of less than 4 h. An oral dose of 120 mg t.i.d. (measured as an equivalent of 360 silibinin) afforded on average 4.6 times greater bioavailability of silibinin than silymarin in the same equivalent dosage, as measured by plasma silibinin levels at ten intervals. In a separate experiment, healthy male volunteers were administered IdB1016 every 12 h (120 mg as an equivalent of silibinin) for eight consecutive days. Plasma silibinin levels showed no significant pharmacokinetic difference compared to the single dose, while conjugated plasma silibinin showed on average about four times the levels of silibinin in free form, indicating that the vast majority of silibinin in systemic circulation shows up in conjugated form (Barzaghi et al., 1990).

Investigations on cholecystectomy patients have provided data on the pharmacodynamic properties of silymarin at different doses. A study of 11 patients showed that silibinin (150 mg t.i.d.) does not accumulate in the bile. Biliary excretion took place within two days with silibinin detected in the bile for up to 72 h (Lorenz et al., 1984). In one investigation, the biliary concentration of silibinin was 20% to 40%, and elimination took about 24 h to complete (Flory et al., 1980). When a relatively low dose of 140 mg silymarin (silibinin: 60 mg) was given to cholecystectomy patients, maximum silibinin concentrations were found in bile. This contrasted with lower silibinin concentrations and lower renal excretion in patients administered a higher dose of silymarin (560 mg silymarin; silibinin 240 mg). At the dose of 140 mg, serum concentrations of silibinin were 100 times higher than those observed from the higher dose (Lorenz et al., 1984).

Mascher et al. (1993) developed an analytical method for the detection of silibinin diastereomers in the plasma of humans following oral intake of silibinin or silymarin.

DOSAGE

A typical dosage of milk thistle extract is 200-400 mg of a 70% silymarin standardized concentrate, standardized according to silibinin. For the raw herb, many practitioners recommend a medium dosage of 12-15 g per day in the treatment of various hepatic disorders. This quantity of raw plant material corresponds to 200-400 mg silibinin (Blumenthal et al., 1998). In a human clinical study, a daily dosage of 420 mg of silibinin produced therapeutic benefits in patients with mild compensated alcoholic cirrhosis (Lang, Nekum, Deak, et al., 1990). This dose would correspond to a daily intake of 600 mg/day of a 70:1 extract of *S. marianum.*

A clinical study in children ages three to nine used a daily dosage of silymarin of 100 mg b.i.d. for 30 days (Mingrino et al., 1979).

SAFETY PROFILE

Clinical research indicates that dosages up to 360 mg (equivalent to silibinin) t.i.d. for 21 days are well tolerated (Marena and Lampertico, 1991). Milk thistle is considered exceptionally safe, since the acute toxicity is quite low. The fact that all parts of the plant have been used for centuries as foods, apparently without provoking adverse reactions, supports the safety of milk thistle for oral consumption (Foster, 1990).

In both animal and human studies, seed extracts have been shown to be devoid of significant adverse side effects (Foster, 1990; Der Marderosian and Liberti, 1988; Anonymous, 1985). Long-term clinical trials have not generated any evidence of toxicity or teratogenic effects (Bone, 1996). However, several isolated cases of a mild laxative effect have been reported (Blumenthal et al., 1998), as have several isolated instances of seeming adverse reactions to milk thistle. In one case, a man, age 83, was subsequently found to have thrombocytopenia and any association with milk thistle to his condition was uncertain. In another case, a woman reported insomnia, nausea, listlessness, and abdominal pains following ingestion of milk thistle. In a further case, a woman, age 57, taking prescription medications (amitriptyline and ethinylestradiol), complained of watery diarrhea, nausea, vomiting, sweating episodes, weakness, colicky abdominal pain, and collapse after taking an Australian milk thistle product (Microgenics Herbals Milk Thistle Vegicaps). When she stopped taking the product, her symptoms ceased. Upon taking a capsule some weeks later, they returned in a "violent reaction." Extensive examination of the patient revealed nothing abnormal. The most likely explanation for her reactions was that something other than milk thistle was responsible (ADRAC, 1999).

Children ages three through nine administered silymarin (100 mg b.i.d. for 30 days) showed no side effects. No signs of dyspepsia or renal function were found; total protein, alkaline phosphatase, bilirubin levels, and the prothrombin index remained normal throughout the study (Mingrino et al., 1979).

Contraindications

There are no known contraindications or cautions for milk thistle and silibinin in therapeutic doses (Bone, 1996; Blumenthal et al., 1998).

Drug Interactions

No adverse reactions have been reported for milk thistle when administered in combination with other medications, except for rare cases of a mild laxative effect (Blumenthal et al., 1998).

Alcohol showed no accelerated elimination in healthy male and female subjects administered a single dose of silibinin (1,050 mg p.o.) and brandy or vodka to reach a blood alcohol content of 1-1.5 mg/mL (Varga et al., 1991).

Silibinin potentiated the in vitro activity of the anticancer agents doxorubicin and cisplatin against human breast and human ovarian cancer cells (Scambia et al., 1996).

In a model of altered liver hemodynamics in rats used to mimic liver atrophy following portacaval shunt, the increased aspirin metabolism (200 mg/kg p.o.) that usually follows from oral administration was ameliorated following silymarin (1,500 mg/kg p.o.) (Favari et al., 1997). When coadministered with silymarin (50 mg/kg p.o.), the reduced bioavailability of aspirin (i.p.) in rats with carbon tetrachloride-induced liver cirrhosis was completely countered (Mourelle and Favari, 1988).

Allain et al. (1999) reported that in Alzheimer's disease patients with mild to moderate dementia treated for the first time with tacrine (Cognex, 40-80 mg/day), milk thistle extract (Legalon, 420 mg/day) caused no impairment of tacrine's cognitive effects of the drug and showed a tendency to reduce cholinergic and gastrointestinal side effects of the drug compared to placebo plus tacrine.

Venkataramanan et al. (2000) examined the effect of silymarin on hepatic drug-metabolizing enzymes in cultures of human hepatocytes. In the MTT assay, silymarin (0.5 mM) caused a significant decrease in mitochondrial respiration. At 0.1 mM, activity of the CYP3A4 enzyme was significantly reduced by silymarin (−50%) and completely reduced at a higher concentration (0.25 mM). Taken together, these effects suggest that silymarin has the potential to impede the hepatic metabolism of some drugs if taken at the same time. Budzinski et al. (2000) reported that a commercial ethanolic extract of milk thistle was moderately inhibitory of CYP3A4.

Pregnancy and Lactation

The *Lawrence Review of Natural Products* states that long-term safety in pregnant or lactating women has not been conclusively demonstrated for milk thistle (Anonymous, 1985); this statement must be considered an equally true yet clinically irrelevant observation for most medications and almost all herbs. Milk thistle is not considered a toxic plant (Hale, 2000) and has been used for centuries as a food and as a galactogogue (see History and Traditional Uses). Neither the German Commission E (Blumenthal et al., 1998) nor the *American Herbal Products Association's Botanical Safety Handbook* (McGuffin et al., 1997) list any contraindication for fruit (seed) preparations during pregnancy or lactation. Silibin has been found to have competitive binding activity for the estradiol receptor (Sonnenbichler and Zetl, 1988). Silymarin probably transfers to human milk to some extent, but its incomplete oral availability (23%-47%) would limit entry and further absorption by the infant (Hale, 2000). Galactogogue use is traditional and anecdotal reports of use are known, though no scientific study during lactation is available. No adverse effects are known for lactation, though the possibility of an undesired increase in milk supply or letdown may exist.

Side Effects

No side effects are known for *S. marianum* preparations except for isolated cases of a mild laxative effect from some formulations sold in Germany (Blumenthal et al., 1998). An observational study of 2,160 patients taking a silymarin preparation sold in Germany reported that 1% experienced side effects, mostly transient gastrointestinal symptoms (Schulz et al., 2001). In an open-label trial in which adult patients were given 280-420 mg of a standardized 70% milk thistle extract over 12 weeks, two patients discontinued therapy because of adverse reactions (diarrhea and a pruitic skin rash), and 16 patients who finished the regimen reported a side effect of loose stools. All 975 patients had liver damage due to various causes before entering the study, the majority (63.3%) resulting from ethanol, and all but two patients completed the trial (Grungreiff et al., 1995).

Special Precautions

None known.

Toxicology

In Vitro Toxicity

In tests for cytotoxicity to liver cells (HepG2), silymarin caused no decrease in cell viability, as indicated by an absence of lactate dehydrogenase-release. The researchers found a depletion of reduced glutathione levels, which reached 10% to 30% of control cell levels—a finding that remains to be explained (Duthie et al., 1997).

Mutagenicity

In vitro DNA double-stranded breaks caused by reactive oxygen species generated by bleomycin and doxorubicin hydrochloride were inhibited by silymarin (Yu and Anderson, 1997). The possibility of cell-growth inhibition, cytotoxicity, and DNA damage of silymarin on isolated human lymphocytes and cultured human colon, liver, and epithelial cells was examined by Duthie et al. (1997).

At concentrations of 0-2500 μM dissolved in DMSO, silymarin caused no increase in DNA damage to human liver cells (HepG2) above those of untreated cell levels. Human colon cells (Caco-2) showed no DNA damage from silymarin either. However, DNA break frequency was increased in epithelial cells (HeLa) by silymarin at approximately 100 μM and more. In the Comet assay (single gel electrophoresis), normal human lymphocytes taken from nonsmoking healthy males (ages 35-50) showed increased genotoxicity when incubated with silymarin at concentrations above 10 mM. In testing silymarin for inhibition of cell growth in stimulated human lymphocytes and in HeLa cells, growth began to show inhibition at approximately 10 μM concentration; however, no cytotoxic effects on the lymphocytes were seen at 250 μM silymarin. No increase in levels of damaged pyrimidine bases compared to the endogenous control was seen from silymarin in human lymphocytes of HeLa cells, indicating that oxidative damage to DNA was not induced by silymarin. The researchers noted that if circulating levels of silymarin do not reach beyond the levels used in their experiments, genotoxic effects in human cells may not be physiologically found in humans (Duthie et al., 1997).

At high concentrations in the Comet assay, silymarin produced antigenotoxic effects. Silymarin reduced DNA damage to human sperm when combined with either of two kinds of food mutagens: 2-amino-3-methyl-imidazo-4,5-*f*) quinoline, or IQ, and 3-amino-1-methyl-5H-pyrido (4,3-b) indole, or Trp. Both agents are known to cause mutagenic activity in the Ames test; in the Comet assay they produce DNA strand breakage. Silymarin in the same high concentration range (100-500 μM) also reduced DNA damage to human peripheral lymphocytes; yet at low concentrations in peripheral lymphocytes, it exacerbated the genotoxicity of the food mutagens (Anderson et al., 1997). In the same concentration range, silymarin showed only antimutagenic effects in the Comet assay with human sperm (Anderson et al., 1998).

Obviously, in vivo studies will be necessary to determine realistically any mutagenic effects of silymarin, which, like other plant-derived, putative antimutagens, may be expected to show different results in different assays, with or without different mutagens, and in different concentrations (Ferguson, 1994).

Toxicity in Animal Models

The LD_{50} values of silibinin (as sodium hemisuccinate) administered i.v. to test animals were 1,010 mg/kg in mice, 873 mg/kg in male and female rats (Desplaces et al., 1975), and 300 mg/kg in rabbits.

In adult albino mice, no mortalities were found in either sex administered oral doses of *S. marianum* seeds in the form of petroleum ether, ethanol, or distilled water extracts in dosages of from 500-2,000 mg/kg (Pandey and Shrivastava, 1990). Oral doses of silymarin administered to mice (20 g/kg) and to dogs (1,000 mg/kg) failed to produce mortality or any signs of adverse effects (Hahn et al., 1968).

Oral doses of 1,000 mg/kg silymarin per day administered to rats for 15 days failed to produce any adverse effects in the test animals. Similarly, no evidence of adversity was seen in long-term tests (16-22 weeks) in which rats were administered oral doses of 100 mg/kg silymarin per day (Hahn et al., 1968).

No toxic effect on embryos has been demonstrated in animal experiments (Foster, 1990).

Animal studies of IdB1016 for acute and subacute toxicity showed the preparation was safe up to an oral dosage of 20 g/kg per day (Marena and Lampertico, 1991).

REFERENCES

Adverse Drug Reaction Advisory Committee (ADRAC) (1999). An adverse reaction to the herbal medication milk thistle *(Silybum marianum)*. *Medical Journal of Australia* 170: 218-219.

Ahmad, N., Gali, H., Javed, S., and Agarwal, R. (1998). Skin cancer chemopreventive effects of a flavonoid antioxidant silymarin are mediated via impairment of receptor tyrosine kinase signaling and perturbation in cell cycle progression. *Biochemical and Biophysical Research Communications* 248: 294-301.

Allain, H., Schuck, S., Lebreton, S., Srenge-Hesse, A., Braun, W., Gandon, J.M., and Brissot, P. (1999). Aminotransferase levels and silymarin in de novo Tacrine-treated patients with Alzheimer's disease. *Dementia and Geriatric Cognitive Disorders* 10: 181-185.

Altorjay, I., Dalmi, L., Sari, B., Imre, S., and Balla, G. (1992). The effect of silibinin (Legalon®) on the free radical scavenger mechanisms of human erythrocytes in vitro. *Acta Physiologica Hungarica* 80: 375-380.

Anderson, D., Basaran, N., Dobrzynska, M.M., Basaran, A.A., and Yu, T.W. (1997). Modulating effects of flavonoids on food mutagens in human blood and sperm samples in the Comet assay. *Teratogenesis, Carcinogenesis, and Mutagenesis* 17: 45-58.

Anderson, D., Dobrzynska, M.M., Basaran, N., Basaran, A., and Yu, T.W. (1998). Flavonoids modulate Comet assay responses to food mutagens in human lymphocytes and sperm. *Mutation Research* 402: 269-277.

Anonymous (1985). The milk thistles. *Lawrence Review of Natural Products* 6 (January): 1-3.

Awang, D.V.C. (1993). Milk thistle. *Canadian Pharmaceutical Journal* 126: 403-404, 422.

Barzaghi, N., Crema, F., Gatti, G., Pifferi, G., and Perucca, E. (1990). Pharmacokinetic studies on IdB 1016, a silybin-phosphatidylcholine complex, in healthy human subjects. *European Journal of Drug Metabolism and Pharmacokinetics* 15: 333-338.

Berenguer, J. and Carrasco, D. (1977). Ensayo doble ciego de silimarina frente a placebo en el tratamiento de hepatopatias crónicas de diversa génesis [A double-blind study of silymarin against a placebo in the treatment of chronic hepatopathies of diverse origin]. *Munchener Medizinische Wochenschrift* 119: 240-260.

Bhatia, N. and Agarwal, R. (2001). Detrimental effect of cancer preventive phytochemicals silymarin, genistein and epigallocatechin 3-gallate on epigenetic events in human prostate carcinoma DU145 cells. *Prostate* 46: 98-107.

Bhatia, N., Zhao, J., Wolf, D.M., and Agarwal, R. (1999). Inhibition of human carcinoma cell growth and DNA synthesis by silibinin, an active constituent of milk thistle: Comparison with silymarin. *Cancer Letters* 147: 77-84.

Bindoli, A., Cavallini, L., and Siliprandi, N. (1977). Inhibitory action of silymarin on lipid peroxide formation in rat liver mitochondria and microsomes. *Biochemical Pharmacology* 26: 2405-2409.

Bingel, A.S. and N.R. Farnsworth (1994). Higher plants as potential sources of galactogogues. In Wagner, H., Hikino, H., and Farnsworth, N.R. (Eds.), *Economic and Medicinal Plant Research,* Vol. 6 (pp. 1-54). New York: Academic Press.

Blumenthal, M., Busse, W.R., Goldberg, A., Gruenwald, J., Hall, T., Riggins, C.W., and Rister, R.S. (Eds.) (1998). *The Complete German Commission E Monographs* (pp. 169-170, 563-565). Austin, TX: American Botanical Council.

Bode, J.C., Schmidt, V., and Durr, H.K. (1977). Zur behandlung der akuten virushepatitis mit silymarin? Ergebnisse einer kantrollierten studie [Silymarin for the treatment of acute viral hepatitis? Report of a controlled trial]. *Medizinische Klinik* (Munich) 72: 513-518.

Bokemeyer, C., Fels, L.M., Dunn, T., Voigt, W., Gaedeke, J., Schmoll, H.J., Stolte, H., and Lentzen, H. (1996). Silibinin protects against cisplatin-induced nephrotoxicity without compromising cisplatin or ifosfamide anti-tumour activity. *British Journal of Cancer* 74: 2036-2041.

Bombardelli, E., Spelta, M., Della Loggia, R., Sosa, S., and Tubaro, A. (1991). Aging skin: Protective effect of silymarin-Phytosome®. *Fitoterapia* 62: 115-122.

Bone, K. (1996). *Silybum marianum. MediHerb* 2: 22-23.

Bosisio, E., Benelli, C., and Pirola, O. (1992). Effect of the flavanolignans of *Silybum marianum* L. on lipid peroxidation in rat liver microsomes and freshly isolated hepatocytes. *Pharmacological Research* 25: 147-154.

Budzinski, J.W., Foster, B.C., Vandenhoek, S., and Arnason, J.T. (2000). An in vitro evaluation of human cytochrome P450 3A4 inhibition by selected commercial herbal extracts and tinctures. *Phytomedicine* 7: 273-282.

Bunout, D., Hirsch, S., Petermann, M., de la Maza, M.P., Silva, G., Kelly, M., Ugarte, G., and Iturriaga, H. (1992). [Controlled study of the effect of silymarin on alcoholic liver disease]. *Revista Medica de Chile* 120: 1370-1375.

Buzzelli, G., Moscarella, S., Giusti, A., Duchini, A., Marena, C., and Lampertico, M. (1993). A pilot study on the liver protective effect of silybin-phosphatidylcholine complex (IdB1016) in chronic active hepatitis. *International Journal of Clinical Pharmacology, Therapy, and Toxicology* 31: 456-460.

Castigli, E., Montanini, I., Roberti, R., and Porcellati, G. (1977). The activity of silybin on phospholipid metabolism of normal and fatty liver in vivo. *Pharmacological Research Communications* 9: 59-69.

Cavallini, L., Bindoli, A., and Siliprandi, N. (1978). Comparative evaluation of antiperoxidative action of silymarin and other flavonoids. *Pharmacological Research Communications* 10: 133-136.

Chan, M.K. and Ng, W.L. (1989). Silymarin ameliorates gentamicin nephrotoxicity. In Bach, P.H. and Lock, E.A. (Eds.), *Nephrotoxicity. In vitro to In vivo. Animals to Man* (pp. 201-206). New York: Plenum Press.

Chatterjee, M.L., Agarwal, R., and Mukhtar, H. (1996). Ultraviolet B radiation-induced DNA lesions in mouse epidermis: An assessment using a novel ^{32}P-posylabelling technique. *Biochemical and Biophysical Research Communications* 229: 590-595.

Chen, H., Chen, S., Zhang, T.H., Tian, H.C., Guan, Y., and Su, D.F. (1993). Protective effects of silybin and tetrandine on the outcome of spontaneously hypertensive rats subjected to acute coronary artery occlusion. *International Journal of Cardiology* 41: 103-108.

Davila, J., Lenhern, A., and Acosta, D. (1989). Protective effect of flavonoids on drug-induced hepatotoxicity in vitro. *Toxicology* 57: 267-286.

de la Lastra, C.A., Martin, M.J., Motliva, E., Jimenez, M., La Casa, C., and Lopez, A. (1995). Gastroprotection induced by silymarin, the heptoprotective principle of *Silybum marianum* in ischemia-reperfusion mucosal injury: Role of neutrophils. *Planta Medica* 61: 116-119.

De La Puerta, R., Martinez, E., Bravo, L., and Ahumada, M.C. (1996). Effect of silymarin on different acute inflammation models and on leukocyte migration. *Journal of Pharmacy and Pharmacology* 48: 968-970.

Dehmlow, C., Erhard, J., and de Groot, H. (1996). Inhibition of Kupffer cell functions as an explanation for the hepatoprotective properties of silibinin. *Hepatology* 23: 749-754.

Dehmlow, C., Murawski, N., and de Groot, H. (1996). Scavenging of reactive oxygen species and inhibition of arachidonic acid metabolism by silibinin in human cells. *Life Sciences* 58: 1591-1600.

Der Marderosian, A. and Liberti, L. (1988). *Natural Product Medicine: A Scientific Guide to Foods, Drugs, Cosmetics*. Philadelphia, PA: George F. Stickley Co.

Desplaces, A., Choppin, J., Vogel, G., and Trost, W. (1975). The effects of silymarin on experimental phalloidine poisoning. *Arzneimittel-Forschung/Drug Research* 25: 89-96.

Duthie, S.J., Johnson, W., and Dobson, V.L. (1997). The effect of dietary flavonoids on DNA damage (strand breaks and oxidized pyrimidines) and growth in human cells. *Mutation Research* 390: 141-151.

Fantozzi, R., Brunelleschi, S., Rubino, A., Tarli, S., Masini, E., and Mannaioni, P.F. (1986). FLMP-activated neutrophils evoke histamine release from mast cells. *Agents and Actions* 18: 155-158.

Favari, L., Soyto, C., and Mourelle, M. (1997). Effect of portal vein ligation and silymarin treatment on aspirin metabolism and disposition in rats. *Biopharmaceutics and Drug Disposition* 18: 53-64.

Feher, J., Deak, G., Muzes, G., Lang, I., Niederland, V., Nekam, K., and Karteszi, M. (1989). [Hepatoprotective activity of silymarin (Legalon) therapy in patients with chronic alcoholic liver disease]. *Orvosi Hetilap* 130: 2723-2727.

Feher, J., Lang, I., Nekam, K., Gergeley, P., and Muzes, G. (1990). In vivo effect of free radical scavenger hepatoprotective agents on superoxide dismutase (SOD) activity in patients. *Tokai Journal of Experimental and Clinical Medicine* 15: 129-134.

Ferenci, P., Dragosics, B., Dittroch, H., Frank, H., Benda, L., Lochs, H., Meryn, S., Base, W., and Schneider, B. (1989). Randomized controlled trial of silymarin treatment in patients with cirrhosis of the liver. *Journal of Hepatology* 9: 105-113.

Ferguson, L.R. (1994). Antimutagens as cancer chemopreventive agents in the diet. *Mutation Research* 307: 395-410.

Fintelmann, V. (1973). Postoperatives verhalten der serumcholinesterase und anderer leberenzyme [Postoperative behavior of serum cholinesterase]. *Medizinische Klinik* 68: 809-815.

Fintelmann, V. and Albert, A. (1980). Nachweis der therapeutischen wirksamkeit von Legalon bei toxischen lebererkrankungen im doppelblindversuch [The therapeutic activity of Legalon in toxic hepatic disorders demonstrated in a double blind trial]. *Therapiewoche* 30: 5589-5594.

Flora, K., Hahn, M., Rosen, H., and Benner, K. (1998). Milk thistle *(Silybum marianum)* for the therapy of liver disease. *The American Journal of Gastroenterology* 93: 139-143.

Flory, P.J., Krug, G., Lorenz, D., and Mennicke, W.H. (1980). [Studies on elimination of silymarin in cholecystectomized patients]. *Planta Medica* 38: 227-237.

Foster, S. (1990). *Milk Thistle*. Austin, TX: American Botanical Council.

Foster, S. (1996). *Herbs for Your Health*. Loveland, CO: Interweave Press.

Frerick, H., Kuhn, U., and Strenge-Hesse, A. (1990). Silymarin—ein phytopharmakon zur behandlung von toxischen leberschäden [Silymarin is a phyto pharmacon used for the therapy of toxic liver damages]. *Der Kassenarzt* 33/34: 36-41.

Gaedeke, J., Fels, L.M., Bokemeyer, C., Mengs, U., Stolte, H., and Lentzen, H. (1996). Cisplatin nephrotoxicity and protection by silibinin. *Nephrology, Dialysis, Transplantation* 11: 55-62.

Garrido, A., Fairlie, J., Guerra, R., Campos, R., and Valenzuela, A. (1989). The flavonoid silybin ameliorates the protective effect of ethanol on acetaminophen hepatotoxicity. *Research Communications in Substances of Abuse* 10: 193-196.

Grieve, M. (1980). *A Modern Herbal* (p. 797). New York: Penguin Books.

Grungreiff, K., Albrecht, M., and Strenge-Hesse, A. (1995). Nutzen der medikamentösen lebertherapie in der hausärtztlichen praxis [The value of drug therapy for liver disease in general practice]. *Medizinische Welt* 46: 222-227.

Gupta, O.P., Sing, S., Bani, S., Sharma, N., Malhotra, S., Gupta, B.D., Banerjee, S.K., and Handa, S.S. (1999). Anti-inflammatory and anti-arthritic activities of silymarin acting through inhibition of 5-lipoxygenase. *Phytomedicine* 7: 21-24.

Gyorgy, I., Antus, S., Blazovics, A., and Foldiak, G. (1992). Substituent effects in the free radical reactions of silybin: Radiation-induced oxidation of the flavonoid at neutral pH. *International Journal of Radiation Biology* 61: 603-609.

Gyorgyi, M., Gyorgy, D., Istvan, L., Kristof, N., Vilmos, N., and Janos, F. (1990). Silymarin (Legalon) kezéles hatása idült alkoholos májbetegek antioxidáns védorendszerére és a lipid peroxidációra (kettos vak protokoll). *Orvosi Hetilap* 131: 863-866.

Hahn, G., Lehmann, H., Kurten, M., Uebel, H., and Vogel, G. (1968). Zur pharmakologie und toxikologie von silymarin, des antihepatotoxischen wirkprinzipes aus *Silybum marianum* (L.) Gaertn. [On the pharmacology and toxicology of silymarin, an antihepatotoxic active principle from *Silybum marianum* (L.) Gaertn]. *Arzneimittel-Forschung/Drug Research* 18: 698-704.

Hakova, H. and Misurova, E. (1993). The effect of silymarin and Gamma radiation on nucleic acids in rat organs. *Journal of Pharmacy and Pharmacology* 45: 910-912.

Hale, T. (2000). *Medications and Mother's Milk* (pp. 454-455). Amarillo, TX: Pharmasoft Medical Publications.

Health Canada (1999). Warning: Toxins may be present in blue-green algae products. *Health Canada Online,* May 5. Accessed at <http://www.hc-sc.gc.ca/english/archives/warnings/99_69e.htm>.

Hermansky, S.J., Stohs, S.J., Eldeen, Z.M., Roche, V.F., and Mereish, K.A. (1991). Evaluation of potential chemoprotectants against microcystin-LR hepatotoxicity in mice. *Journal of Applied Toxicology* 11: 65-74.

Hikino, H. and Kiso, Y. (1988). Natural products for liver disease. In Wagner, H., Hikino, H., and Farnsworth, N.R. (Eds.), *Economic and Medicinal Plant Research,* Vol. 2 (pp. 39-72). London: Academic Press.

Hikino, H., Kiso, Y., Wagner, H., and Fiebig, M. (1984). Antihepatotoxic actions of flavolignans from *Silybum marianum* fruits. Part 16. Tohoku University series on liver-protective drugs. *Planta Medica* 50: 248-250.

Hobbs, C. (1984). *Milk Thistle: The Liver Herb,* Second Edition. Capitola, CA: Botanica Press.

Hruby, K., Fuhrmann, M., Csomos, G., and Thaler, H. (1983). Pharmakotherapie der knollenblatterpilzvergiftung mit silibinin [Pharmacotherapy of *Amanita phalloides* poisoning with silybin]. *Wiener Klinische Wochenschrift* 7: 225-231.

Invernizzi, R., Burnuzzi, S., Ciani, D., and Ascari, E. (1993). Silymarine during maintenance therapy of acute promyelocytic leukemia. *Haematologica* 78: 340-341 (letter).

Kalmar, L., Kadar, J., Somogyi, A., Gergely, P., Csomos, G., and Feher, J. (1990). Silibinin (Legalon-70) enhances the motility of human neutrophils immobilized by formyl-tripeptide, calcium ionophore, lymphokine and by normal human serum. *Agents and Actions* 29: 239-246.

Katiyar, S.K., Korman, N.J., Mukhtar, H., and Agarwal, R. (1997). Protective effects of silymarin against photocarcinogenesis in a mouse skin model. *Journal of the National Cancer Institute* 89: 556-566.

Kim, D.H., Jin, Y.H., Park, J.B., and Kobashi, K. (1994). Silymarin and its components are inhibitors of β-glucuronidase. *Biological and Pharmaceutical Bulletin* 17: 443-445.

Krecman, V., Skottova, N., Walterova, D., Ulrichova, J., and Simanek, V. (1998). Silymarin inhibits the development of diet-induced hypercholesterolemia in rats. *Planta Medica* 64: 138-142.

Lang, I., Nekam, K., Deak, G., Muzes, G., Gonzales-Cabello, R., Gergely, P., Csomos, G., and Feher, J. (1990). Immunomodulatory and hepatoprotective effects of in vivo treatment with free radical scavengers. *International Journal of Gastroenterology* 22: 283-287.

Lang, I., Nekam, K., Gonzalez-Cabello, R., Muzes, G., Gergely, P., and Feher, J. (1990). Hepatoprotective and immunological effects of antioxidant drugs. *Tokai Journal of Experimental and Clinical Medicine* 15: 123-127.

Lettéron, P., Labbe, G., Degott, C., Berson, A., Fromenty, B., Delaforge, M., Larrey, D., and Pessayre, D. (1990). Mechanism for the protective effects of silymarin against carbon tetrachloride-induced lipid peroxidation and hepatotoxicity in mice. Evidence that silymarin acts both as an inhibitor of metabolic activation and as a chain-breaking antioxidant. *Biochemical Pharmacology* 39: 2027-2034.

Lirussi, F. and Okolicsanyi, L. (1992). Cytoprotection in the nineties. Experience with ursodeoxycholic acid and silymarin in chronic liver disease. *Acta Physiologica Hungarica* 80: 363-367.

Locher, R., Suter, P.M., Weyhenmeyer, R., and Vetter, W. (1998). Inhibitory action of silibinin on low density lipoprotein oxidation [Hemmende wirkung von silibinin auf die oxidation von low density lipoprotein]. *Arzneimittel-Forschung/Drug Research* 48: 236-239.

Lorenz, D., Lucker, P.W., Mennicke, W.H., and Wetzelsberger, M. (1984). Pharmacokinetic studies with silymarin in human serum and bile. *Methods and Findings in Experimental and Clinical Pharmacology* 6: 655-661.

Magliulo, E., Gagliardi, B., and Fiori, G.P. (1978). Zür wirkung von silymarin bei der behandlung der akuten virushepatitis [Results of a double blind study on the effect of silymarin in the treatment of acute viral hepatitis, carried out at two medical centers]. *Medizinische Klinik* 73: 1060-1065.

Marena, C. and Lampertico, M. (1991). Preliminary clinical development of silipide: A new complex of silybin in toxic liver disorders. *Planta Medica* 57 (Suppl. 2): A124-A125 (poster).

Martines, G., Piva, M., Copponi, V., and Cagnetta, G. (1979). La silimarina in gravidanza e nel trattamento contraccettivo ormonale. Relievi ematochimici ed ultrastrutturali su modello sperimentale [Silymarin in pregnancy and during hormonal contraceptive treatment. Blood chemistry and ultrastructural findings in the experimental model]. *Archivo per le Scienze Mediche* (Torino) 136: 433-454.

Mascher, H., Kikuta, C., and Weyhenmeyer, R. (1993). Diastereomeric separation of free and conjugated silibinin in plasma by reversed phase HPLC after specific extraction. *Journal of Liquid Chromatography* 16: 2777-2789.

McGuffin, M., Hobbs, C., Upton, R., and Goldberg, A. (1997). *American Herbal Products Association's Botanical Safety Handbook* (p. 107). Boca Raton, FL: CRC Press.

Mereish, K.A., Bunner, D.L., Ragland, D.R., and Creasia, D.A. (1991). Protection against microcystin-LR-induced hepatotoxicity by silymarin: Biochemistry, histopathology, and lethality. *Pharmaceutical Research* 8: 273-277.

Meroni, P.L., Barcellini, W., Borghi, M.O., Vismara, A., Ferraro, G., Clani, D., and Zanussi, C. (1988). Silybin inhibition of human T-lymphocyte activation. *International Journal of Tissue Reactions* 10: 177-181.

Miadonna, A., Tedeschi, A., Leggieri, E., Lorini, M., Froldi, M., and Zanussi, C. (1987). Effects of silybin on histamine release from human basophil leukocytes. *British Journal of Clinical Pharmacology* 24: 747-752.

Mingrino, F., Tosti, U., Anania, S., Buglioni, M.C., and Viola, F. (1979). Studio clinicio sill'zione terapeutica della silimarina nell'epatite infettiva acuta dell'inf [A clinical investigation into the therapeutic effects of silymarin in acute infective hepatitis in children]. *Minerva Pediatrica* 31: 451-460 (translation).

Minozio, F., Venegoni, E., Ongari, A., Ciani, D., and Capsoni, F. (1988). Modulation of human polymorphonuclear leukocyte function by the flavonoid silybin. *International Journal of Tissue Reactions* 10: 223-231.

Mira, M., Azeedo, M.S., and Manso, C. (1987). The neutralization of hydroxyl radical by silybin, sorbinil and bendazac. *Free Radical Research Communications* 4: 125-129.

Morazzoni, P. and Bombardelli, E. (1995). *Silybum marianum (Carduus marianus)*. *Fitoterapia* 66: 3-42.

Moscarella, S., Giusti, A., Marra, F., Marena, C., Lampertico, M., Relli, P., Gentilini, P., and Buzzelli, G. (1993). Therapeutic and antilipoperoxidatant effects of silybin-phosphatidylcholine complex in chronic liver disease: Preliminary results. *Current Therapeutic Research* 53: 98-102.

Mourelle, M. and Favari, L. (1988). Silymarin improves metabolism and disposition of aspirin in cirrhotic rats. *Life Sciences* 43: 201-207.

Mukhtar, H. and Agarwal, R. (1996). Skin cancer chemoprevention. *Journal of Investigative Dermatology Symposium Proceedings* 1: 209-214.

Munter, K., Mayer, D., and Faulstich, H. (1986). Characterization of a transporting system in rat hepatocytes: Studies with competitive and non-competitive inhibitors of phalloidin transport. *Biochimica et Biophysica Acta* 860: 91-98.

Muzes, G., Deak, G., Lang, I., Nekam, K., Gergely, P., and Feher, J. (1991). Effect of the bioflavonoid silymarin on the in vitro activity and expression of superoxide dismutase (SOD) enzyme. *Acta Physiologica Hungarica* 78: 3-9.

Muzes, G., Deak, G., Lang, I., Nekam, K., Niederland, V., and Feher, J. (1990). Silymarin (Legalon) kezeles hatasa idult alkoholos majbetegek antioxidans vedorendszerere es a lipid peroxidaciora (kettos vak protokoll) [Effect of silymarin (Legalon) therapy on the antioxidant defense mechanism and lipid peroxidation in alcoholic liver disease. A double blind study]. *Orvosi Hetilap* 131: 863-866.

Nassuato, G., Iemmolo, R., Lirussi, F., Orlando, R., Giacon, L., Venuti, M., Strazzabosco, M., Csonos, G., and Okolicsanyi, L. (1983). Effect of silybin on biliary lipid composition in rats. *Pharmacological Research Communications* 15: 337-346.

Nassuato, G., Iemmolo, R., Strazzabosco, M., Lirussi, F., Deana, R., Francesconi, M.A., Muraca, M., Passera, D., Fragasso, A., Orlando, R., et al. (1991). Effect of silibinin on biliary lipid composition: Experimental and clinical study. *Journal of Hepatology* 12: 290-295.

Palasciano, G., Portincasa, P., Palmieri, V., Ciani, D., Vendemiale, G., and Altomare, E. (1994). The effect of silymarin on plasma levels of malondialdehyde in patients receiving long-term treatment with psychotropic drugs. *Current Therapeutic Research* 55: 537-545.

Pandey, G.P. and Shrivastava, D.N. (1990). Phytochemical and acute toxicity studies of *Silybum marianum* and *Wedelia calendulacea*. *Indian Veterinary Journal* 67: 773-776.

Parés, A., Planas, R., Torres, M., Caballeria, J., Viver, J.M., Acero, D., Panes, J., Rigau, J., Santos, J., and Rodes, J. (1998). Effects of silymarin in alcoholic patients with cirrhosis of the liver: Results of a controlled, double-blind, randomized and multicenter trial. *Journal of Hepatology* 28: 615-621.

Pickering, C. (1879). *Chronological History of Plants*. Boston, MA: Little, Brown and Co.

Reyes, H. and Simon, F.R. (1993). Intrahepatic cholestasis of pregnancy: An estrogen-related disease. *Seminars in Liver Disease* 13: 289-301.

Rumyantseva, Z.N. (1991). The pharmacodynamics of hepatoprotectants derived from blessed milk thistle *(Silybum marianum)*. *Vrachebnoe Delo* 5: 15-19.

Saba, P., Galeone, F., Salvadorini, F., Guarguaglini, M., and Troyer, C. (1976). Effetti terapetutici della silimarina nelle epatopatie croniche indotte da psicofarmaci [Therapeutic action of silymarin on chronic hepatopathies caused by psychopharmaceuticals]. *Gazzetta Medica Italiana* 135: 236-251 (translation).

Sabeel, A.I., Kurkus, J., and Lindholm, T. (1995). Intensive hemodialysis and hemoperfusion treatment of *Amanita* mushroom poisoning. *Mycopathologica* 131: 107-114.

Salmi, H. and Sarna, S. (1982). Effect of silymarin on chemical, functional and morphological alterations of the liver: A double-blind controlled study. *Scandinavian Journal of Gastroenterology* 17: 517-521.

Savio, D., Harrasser, P.C., and Basso, G. (1998). Softgel capsule technology as an enhancer device for the absorption of natural principles in humans: A bioavailability cross-over randomized study on silybin. *Arzneimittel-Forschung/Drug Research* 48: 1104-1106.

Scambia, G., De Vincenzo, R., Raneletti, F.O., Panici, P.B., Ferrandina, G., D'Agnostino, G., Fattorossi, A., Bombardelli, E., and Mancuso, S. (1996). Antiproliferative effect of silybin on gynaecological malignancies: Synergism with cisplatin and doxorubicin. *European Journal of Cancer* 32A: 877-882.

Schandalik, R., Gatti, G., and Perucca, E. (1992). Pharmacokinetics of silybin in bile following administration of silipide and silymarin in cholecystectomy patients. *Arzneimittel-Forschung/Drug Research* 42: 964-968.

Schauenberg, P. and Paris, F. (1974). *Guide to Medicinal Plants.* New Canaan, CT: Keats Publishing.

Scheiber, V. and Wohlzogen, F.X. (1978). Analysis of a certain type of 2×3 tables, exemplified by biopsy findings in a controlled clinical trial. *International Journal of Clinical Pharmacology and Biopharmacy* 16: 553-535.

Schönfeld, J., Weisbrod, B., and Müller, M.K. (1997). Silibinin, a plant extract with antioxidant and membrane stabilizing properties, protects exocrine pancreas from cyclosporin A toxicity. *Cellular and Molecular Life Sciences: CMLS* 53: 917-920.

Schulz, V., Hänsel, R., and Tyler, V.E. (2001). *Rational Phytotherapy: A Physician's Guide to Herbal Medicine,* Fourth Edition (pp. 261-264). New York: Springer-Verlag.

Shear, N., Malkiewicz, I., Klein, D., Koren, G., Randoe, S., and Neuman, M.G. (1995). Acetaminophen-induced toxicity to human epidermoid cell line A431 and hepatoblastoma cell line Hep G2, in vitro, is diminished by silymarin. *Skin Pharmacology* 8: 279-291.

Sheu, S.Y., Lai, C.H., and Chiang, H.C. (1998). Inhibition of xanthine oxidase by purpurogallin and silymarin group. *Anticancer Research* 18: 263-268.

Shukla, B., Visen, P.K., Patnaik, G.K., and Dhawan, B.N. (1991). Choleretic effect of picroliv, the hepatoprotective principle of *Picrorhiza kurroa. Planta Medica* 57: 29-33.

Sonnenbichler, J. and Pohl, A. (1980). Untersuchungen zum wirkungsmechanismus von silybin. IV. Struktur-wirkungsbeziehungen [Mechanism of silybin action. IV. Structure-action relationship]. *Hoppe-Seyler's Zeitschrift für Physiologische Chemie* 361:1757-1761.

Sonnenbichler, J., Scalera, F., Sonnenbichler, I., and Weyhenmeter, R. (1999). Stimulatory effects of silibinin and silcristin from the milk thistle *Silybum marianum* on kidney cells. *Journal of Pharmacology and Experimental Therapeutics* 290: 1375-1383.

Sonnenbichler, J. Sonnenbichler, I., and Scalera, F. (1998). Influence of the flavonolignan silibinin of milk thistle on hepatocytes and kidney cells. In Lawson, L.D. and Bauer, R. (Eds.), *Phytomedicines of Europe: Chemistry and Biological Activity* (pp. 263-277). ACS Symposium Series 691. Washington, DC: American Chemical Society.

Sonnenbichler, J. and Zetl, I. (1986). Biochemical effects of the flavonolignane silibinin on RNA, protein and DNA synthesis in rat livers. In Cody, V., Middleton, E. Jr., and Harborne, J.B. (Eds.), *Plant Flavonoids in Biology and Medicine: Biochemical, Pharmacological and Structure-activity Relationships* (pp. 319-331). New York: Alan R. Liss.

Sonnenbichler, J. and Zetl, I. (1988). Specific binding of a flavonolignane derivative to an estradiol receptor. In Cody, V., Middleton, E. Jr., and Harborne, J.B. (Eds.), *Plant Flavonoids in Biology and Medicine. II. Biochemical, Cellular, and Medicinal Properties* (pp. 369-374). New York: Alan R. Liss.

Szilard, S., Szentgyorgyi, D., and Demeter, D. (1988). Protective effect of Legalon in workers exposed to organic solvents. *Acta Medica Hungarica* 45: 249-256.

Tittel, G. and Wagner, H. (1977). [High-performance liquid chromatographic separation of silymarins and their determination in a raw extract of *Silybum marianum* Gaertn.]. *Journal of Chromatography* 135: 499-501.

Trinchet, J.C., Coste, T., Levy, V.G., Vivet, F., Duchatelle, V., Legendre, C., Gotheil, C., and Beaugrand, M. (1989). Traitement de l'hepatite alcoolique par la silymarine. Une etude comparative en double insu chez 116 malades [A randomized double-blind trial of silymarin in 116 patients with alcoholic hepatitis]. *Gastroenterologie Clinique et Biologique* 13: 120-124 (abstract).

Vailati, A., Arista, I., Sozze, E., Milani, F., Inglese, V., Galenda, P., Bossolo, P.A., Ascari, E., Lampertico, M., Comis, S., et al. (1993). Randomized open study of the dose-effect relationship of a short course of IdB 1016 in patients with viral or alcoholic hepatitis. *Fitoterapia* 64: 219-228.

Valenzuela, A., Aspillaga, M., Vial, S., and Guerra, R. (1989). Selectivity of silymarin on the increase of the glutathione content in different tissues of the rat. *Planta Medica* 55: 420-442.

Valenzuela, A. and Guerra, R. (1986). Differential effect of silybin on the Fe^{2+}-ADP and t-butyl hydroperoxide-induced microsomal lipid peroxidation. *Experientia* 42: 139-141.

Valenzuela, A., Guerra, R., and Videla, L. (1986). Antioxidant properties of the flavonoids silybin and (+)cyanidanol-3: Comparison with butylated hydroxyanisole and butylated hydroxytoluene. *Planta Medica* 19: 438-440.

Valenzuela, A., Lagos, C., Schmidt, K., and Videla, L.A. (1985). Silymarin protection against hepatic lipid peroxidation induced by acute ethanol intoxication in the rat. *Biochemical Pharmacology* 34: 2209-2212.

Varga, M., Buris, L., and Fodor, M. (1991). Der einflß von antihepatotoxischem silibinin auf die alkoholelimination beim menschen [Ethanol elimination in man under the influence of hepatoprotective silibinin]. *Blutalkohol* 28: 405-408.

Venkataramanan, R., Ramachandran, V., Komoroski, B.J., Zhang, S., Schiff, P.L., and Strom, S.C. (2000). Milk thistle, a herbal supplement, decreases the activity of CYP3A4 and uridine diphosphoglucuronosyl transferase in human hepatocyte cultures. *Drug Metabolism and Disposition* 28: 1270-1273.

Vogel, G. and Temme, I. (1969). Die curative antagonisierung des durch phalloidin hervorgerufenen leberschadens mit silymarin als modell einer antihepatotoxischen therapie [Curative antagonism of phalloidin induced liver damage with silymarin as a model of an antihepatotoxic therapy]. *Arzneimittel-Forschung/Drug Research* 19: 613-615.

Vogel, G., Trost, W., Braatz, R., Odenthal, K.P., Brusewitz, G., Antweiler, H., and Seeger, R. (1975). Untersuchungen zu pharmakodynamik, angriffspunkt und wirkungsmechanismus von silymarin, dem antihepatotoxischen prinzip aus *Silybum marianum* (L.) Gaertn. [Pharmacodynamics, site and mechanism of action of silymarin, the antihepatotoxic principle from *Silybum marianum* (L.) Gaertn. 1. Acute toxicology or tolerance, general and specific (liver) pharmacology]. *Arzneimittel-Forschung/Drug Research* 25: 82-89.

Wagner, H., Diesel, P., and Seitz, M. (1974). Zur chemie und analytik von silymarin aus *Silybum marianum* Gaertn. [The chemistry and analysis of silymarin from *Silybum marianum* Gaertn.]. *Arzneimittel-Forschung/Drug Research* 24: 466-471.

Wagner, H., Horhammer, L., and Munster, R. (1968). On the chemistry of silymarin (silbin), the active principle of the fruits from *Silybum marianum* (L). Gaertn. (*Carduus marianus* L.). *Arzneimittel-Forschung/Drug Research* 18: 688-696.

Weyhenmeyer, R., Mascher, H., and Birkmayer, J. (1992). Study on dose-linearity of the pharmacokinetics of silibinin diastereomers using a new stereospecific assay. *International Journal of Clinical Pharmacology, Therapy and Toxicology* 30: 134-138.

Wu, C.G., Chamuleau, R.A., Bosch, K.S., and Frederiks, W.M. (1993). Protective effect of silymarin on rat liver injury induced by ischemia. *Virchow B9s Archiv B, Cell Pathology Including Molecular Pathology* 64: 259-263.

Yu, T.W. and Anderson, D. (1997). Reactive oxygen species-induced DNA damage and its modification: A chemical investigation. *Mutation Research* 379: 201-210.

Zi, X., Feyes, D.K., and Agarwal, R. (1998). Anticarcinogenic effect of a flavonoid antioxidant, silymarin, in human breast cancer cells MDA-MB 468: Induction of G_1 arrest through an increase in Cip1/p21 concomitant with a decrease in kinase activity of cyclin-dependent kinases and associated cyclins. *Clinical Cancer Research* 4: 1055-1064.

Zi, X.L., Grasso, A.W., Kung, H.J., and Agarwal, R. (1998). Flavonoid antioxidant, silymarin, inhibits activation of erbB1 signaling and induces cyclin-dependent kinase inhibitors, G_1 arrest, and anticarcinogenic effects in human prostate carcinoma DU145 cells. *Cancer Research* 58: 1920-1929.

Zi, X., Mukhtar, H., and Agarwal, R. (1997). Novel cancer chemopreventive effects of a flavonoid antioxidant silymarin: Inhibition of mRNA expression of an endogenous tumor promoter TNFα. *Biochemical and Biophysical Research Communications* 239: 334-339.

Zi, X., Zhang, J., Agarwal, R., and Pollak, M. (2000). Silibinin up-regulates insulin-like growth factor-binding protein 3 expression and inhibits proliferation of androgen-independent prostate cancer cells. *Cancer Research* 60: 5617-5620.

Zima, T., Kameníkova, L., Janebová, M., Buchar, E., Crkovska, J., and Tesar, V. (1998). The effect of silibinin on experimental cyclosporine nephrotoxicity. *Renal Failure* 29: 471-479.

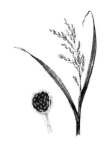

Red Yeast Rice

BOTANICAL DATA

Classification and Nomenclature

Scientific name: *Monascus purpureus* Went.

Family name: Monascaceae (Ascomycotina)

Common names: red yeast rice, red rice, red leaven, beni-koji (Japanese), hung-chu, hong qu, angkak, zhitai (Chinese)

Description

Monascus purpureus is a strain of *M. ruber* van Tieghen, a destructive mold that grows on starch and silage (Went, 1895; Juzlova, Martinkova, et al., 1996) and exists naturally in dairy products. The yeast causes fermentation of cellobiose, maltose, fructose, and glucose, but does not ferment cane sugar (Ying et al., 1987). *Monascus purpureus* is distinguished by its ascospores. These are usually spherical, being 5 μM in diameter, or ovoid (6 × 5 μM). At the early stages, the young part of the mycelium is white. However, it rapidly changes to a rich pink and later to a distinctly yellow-orange color, reflecting the increasing acidity of the medium and the production of yellow-orange hyphae. A deep crimson color is found at the substratum as the culture ages (Went, 1895; Juzlova, Martinkova, et al., 1996).

HISTORY AND TRADITIONAL USES

Red yeast rice (*Monascus purpureus* Went.) is traditionally prepared by fermenting boiled nonglutinous rice with red wine mash, natural juice of *Polygonum* grass, and alum water. In reality, red yeast rice (RYR) is composed of two organisms, *M. purpureus* and a yeast—the former being capable of breaking down rice starch into simple sugar, while the latter renders further conversion into alcohol possible. In practice, the fungus is cultivated on rice and the mycelium develops rapidly until the rich crimson pigment has permeated the grains completely, giving the product its characteristic red color. The whole mass is then ground to a powder (Sung, 1966).

RYR has been used for centuries in the making of rice wine, as a food preservative for maintaining the color and taste of fish and meat, and for its medicinal properties. The use of this food product can be traced as far back as 800 A.D. during the T'ang dynasty. The ancient Chinese pharmacopoeia, *Ben Cao Gang Mu-Dan Shu Bin Yi,* published during the Ming dynasty (1368-1644), contains a complete and detailed description of the preparation of this product and its use as a food and medicinal (Sung, 1966; Stuart, 1979). In this treatise, RYR is described as a nonpoisonous product useful for the treatment of indigestion and diarrhea, anthrax, bruised muscles, hangovers, colic dyspepsia in children, postpartum problems, for improving blood circulation, and for promoting the health of the spleen and stomach. It is also mentioned as a component of several herbal preparations for the treatment of indigestion, diarrhea, heart pains, and abdominal pains (Stuart, 1979; Liu and Bau, 1980). In the Yuan dynasty work by Wu Rui, *Materia Medica for Daily Use,* RYR is stated to eradicate "blood stasis to permit movement of medicine," to "counteract miasma from mountain mists," and to heal bruises and cuts and "other injuries." In the Yuan dynasty work by Zhu Zhien-Xiang, *Supplements on Developments of Herb Medicine,* RYR is recorded as a substance that "mollifies dyspepsia, invigorates blood circulation and spleen function and warms stomach." It was also used to "cure" dysentery. During the Ming dynasty, Li Shih-chen wrote of RYR in his *Compendium of Materia Medica,* stating that it "cures women's menoxenia and continuous bleeding after childbirth," for which it was to be taken with wine (Ying et al., 1987).

Today, RYR is still used in traditional Chinese medicine (TCM) and in powdered form as a food coloring in Asia and in Chinese communities in North America, most commonly for coloring fish, alcoholic beverages, and cheeses (Patakova-Juzlova et al., 1998). Considerable interest has been shown in using *M. purpureus* as a nitrite/nitrate substitute for the preservation of meats (Fink-Gremmels et al., 1991) and as a potential replacement for synthetic food dyes (Juzlova, Martinkova, et al., 1996). European manufacturers of meat products have recently popularized its use in coloring sausages and salami (Patakova-Juzlova et al., 1998). It is interesting to note that a century ago in Asia the yeast was used as a "food disinfectant" (Went, 1895).

In 1976, Professor Akira Endo of Japan and co-workers reported the discovery of mevastatin, a fungal metabolite isolated from the cultures of *Penicillium citrinum* and *P. brevicompactin* (Endo et al., 1976; reviewed in

Alberts et al., 1989). Mevastatin was found to be an unusually potent inhibitor of the enzyme 3-hydroxy-3-methylglutaryl coenzyme A reductase (HMG-CoA reductase). This enzyme, the third in a 21-step biosynthetic sequence, is the rate-limiting step in the synthesis of cholesterol. As such it represents a pivotal target for regulating the levels of this lipid. Consequently, the discovery of this powerful, naturally occurring inhibitor provided both a new direction for the management of serum cholesterol and the inspiration for the subsequent development of a new class of effective cholesterol-lowering agents.

Endo later reported the discovery of another potent HMG-CoA reductase inhibitor from a strain of *Monascus*. Initially designated monacolin K (Endo, 1979), this compound was subsequently found to be identical to mevinolin. Today, these naturally occurring fungal metabolites and related compounds inspired by these discoveries (e.g., simvastatin and pravastatin) play a prominent role in the management of hypercholesteremia, a significant risk factor for coronary artery disease (for reviews, see Alberts et al., 1989; Grundy, 1988). Mevinolin has since been found to occur in other species of fungi, including the edible oyster mushroom *(Pleurotus ostreatus)* (Gunde-Cimerman et al., 1993).

Until recently, the nutritional and medicinal properties of RYR were not fully appreciated by the Western world. However, spurred by a renewed interest in natural remedies, recent biochemical and pharmacological studies have identified RYR as a beneficial dietary supplement for maintaining a healthy balance of cholesterol and related lipids in the body.

CHEMISTRY

Lipid Compounds

RYR may contain large quantities of mono-, di-, and polyunsaturated fatty acids (>125 mg/g extract) (Juzlova, Rezanka, et al., 1996). The beneficial effects of unsaturated fatty acids on cardiovascular health are widely recognized (Ensminger et al., 1994); however, analysis of a commercially available RYR powder (MPU Company, Beijing, China) showed only 2.8% fatty acids, comprising only saturated (mainly palmitic, stearic, and arachidic) and 1.43% unsaturated fatty acids (mainly linoleic, oleic, and linolenic) (Ma et al., 2000).

Terpenoid Compounds

RYR contains mevinolin and related monacolins, which in most cases occur in the amounts of around 0.4% w/w rice. Analysis of a commercial RYR powder product, prepared using traditional methods and a proprietary strain of *M. purpurea* (MPU Company, Beijing, China), revealed that monacolin K was present in far greater quantity than other monacolins, including dihydro, dehydro, and hydroxy acid forms of monacolin K and monacolin L; the latter two accounting for 90% of the "total monacolin fraction" (Ma et al., 2000) (see Figure 1).

Analyses of nine different proprietary RYR preparations sold as dietary supplements in the United States revealed a great degree of variation in monacolin content, which ranged from 0% to 0.58% w/w. Per-capsule amounts of monacolin K varied from 0.15 mg to 3.37 mg (Heber et al., 2001).

Other Constituents

Other constituents of the mixture include sugar (starch), crude proteins, amino acids, phytosterols (β-sitosterol, campesterol, and stigmasterol), isoflavone and its glycoside, saponins, trace elements (Xie and Duan, 1996), and various red pigments (Blanc et al., 1995). Polyketide pigments in RYR include ankaflavin, monascidin, monascorubramine, monascorubrine, and citrinin, a mycotoxin found in some strains of *M. purpureus* (Ma et al., 2000). In one analysis, seven out of nine proprietary RYR products sold in the United States as dietary supplements contained some amount of citrinin (0.47 to 11.82 µg/capsule) (Heber et al., 2001) (see Special Precautions).

R = CH3 = Monacolin K
R = H = ML236B

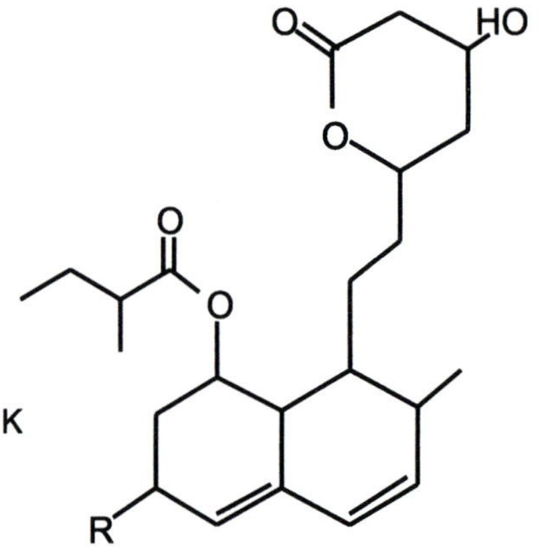

HMG Co-A Reductase Inhibitors from
Monascus purpureus (M. ruber)

FIGURE 1. Major Constituent of Red Yeast Rice

PRECLINICAL STUDIES

Cardiovascular and Circulatory Functions

Cholesterol and Lipid Metabolism

In rabbits fed a diet of 25% casein, a model of endogenous hyperlipidemia, serum cholesterol increased from 1.81 mmol/L to 7.51 mmol/L within 60 days (Li et al., 1998). When these animals were subsequently treated with Xuezhikang (a concentrated extract of *M. purpureus* yeast rice) for 30 days while maintaining the casein diet, total serum cholesterol (TC) and LDL cholesterol (LDL-c) were reduced in a dose-dependent fashion. At the highest dose of 800 mg/kg per day, RYR reduced TC and LDL-c levels by 59% and 44%, respectively. Moreover, this treatment also decreased the TC:HDL-c ratio from 18.9:1 to 6.5:1, although HDL cholesterol levels remained unchanged. By comparison, mevinolin at a daily dose of 8 mg/kg reduced TC by 52% and the TC:HDL-c ratio to 8.9:1.

Rabbits maintained on a hyperlipidemia-inducing diet for 60 days developed a ninefold increase in TC, a threefold increase in triglycerides (TG), and a twofold increase in both HDL-c and LDL-c. The addition of RYR to this diet for 40 days dose-dependently blunted the increase in TC and TG levels. At 400 and 800 mg/kg per day, TC and TG levels were reduced by 32% and 43%, respectively, relative to pretreatment levels. The treatment also caused a twofold reduction in the TC:HDL-c mean ratio and a significant decrease in the liver:body weight ratio. (Rabbits fed a fat-rich diet showed increased liver weights and liver:body weight ratios.) At autopsy, treatment with the RYR was found to have reduced the formation of atheromatous plaques in the aorta. A control group of rabbits fed the same hyperlipidemic diet plus capsules containing mevinolin (8 mg/kg per day p.o.) showed similar improvements compared to controls in liver:body weight ratios, decreases in TC and TG levels and reduction in the TC:HDL-c mean ratio (Li et al., 1998).

In a third study (Li et al., 1998), exogenous hyperlipidemia was induced in the quail after two weeks on a diet of cholesterol, lard, and soy oil. Total cholesterol, triglycerides, and LDL-c levels increased fivefold to ninefold in the quail compared to baseline. The addition of RYR (100, 200, or 400 mg/ kg per day) to this diet caused a dose-dependent reduction in TC and TG. However, LDL-c levels were decreased only from the highest dose and HDL-c levels were unaffected. Mevinolin (4 mg/kg per day p.o.) decreased LDL-c, TC, and TG, and had no effect on HDL-c.

Kritchevsky et al. (1998) maintained rabbits on either a normal diet or a semipurified atherogenic diet containing 0.2% cholesterol. In addition, rabbits receiving the atherogenic diet were given either no treatment, lovastatin (2.16 mg/kg per day), or one of two doses of RYR (0.4 or 1.35 mg/kg per day). After six months, total serum cholesterol and triglyceride levels in those animals receiving the atherogenic diet increased 14-fold and three-fold, respectively. However, with lovastatin or RYR treatment, these increases were significantly blunted. Similarly, visual examination of aortas at necropsy showed that lovastatin inhibited atherosclerosis by 87%. RYR suppressed atherosclerosis by 36% at the low dose and by 67% at the high dose, clearly displaying dose dependence.

Wang et al. (2000) conducted a similar study in hypertriglyceridemic rats, induced with the condition by feeding them a diet containing high amounts of fructose. For six months, groups of rats were fed either a basic 30% fructose-containing diet, the basic diet plus a RYR powder (*Monascus* species not divulged) at 2% of the feed, or the basic diet plus lovastatin (250 mg/kg); another control group was fed a basal diet; a fifth group was fed a basal diet containing 2.0% of the RYR powder. The results showed that regardless of the diet and supplement added, no significant difference in body or food intake was evident in the five groups of rats; 100% of the animals survived. Also no significant effects on superoxide dismutase activity occurred in the serum of rats fed the basal diet plus RYR (BD-RYR) compared to the basal diet group. The activity of lipoprotein lipase in adipose tissue showed some increase, and epididymal adipose tissue weight showed some decrease in the BD-RYR group—though not significantly so compared to the basal diet and the 30% fructose group. The activity of hepatic lipase in the liver of the BD-RYR groups showed a significant increase ($p < 0.05$) compared to the basal diet group, whereas no increase took place in the 30% fructose-fed group. The researchers note that increased hepatic lipase activity is associated in humans with a predisposition to a faster rate of developing atherosclerosis. Serum triglyceride levels in the group fed the 30% fructose-RYR diet showed a highly significant decrease ($p < 0.005$) compared to rats on the same diet without 2.0% RYR; however, liver triglyceride levels showed no significant change, nor in the group fed 30% fructose-lovastatin compared to the control group. Liver cholesterol levels in the 30% fructose-RYR diet group were the same as those in the rats fed a basal diet plus 2.0% RYR while the decrease in liver cholesterol levels was significant ($p < 0.05$) in the group that received lovastatin in their diet compared to the 30% fructose-fed group.

Digestive, Hepatic, and Gastrointestinal Functions

Hepatic Functions

RYR powder made with *Monascus anka* was examined for potential hepatoprotectant activity in male rats by Aniya et al. (1998). The rats were randomly assigned to three groups: a control group treated with 30% dimethyl sulfoxide solution i.p.; a group treated with acetaminophen (180 mg/kg i.p.) dissolved in 30% dimethyl sulfoxide which was administered 24 h after administration of 3-methylchoranthrene (25 mg/kg i.p.), an inducer of cytochrome P450; and a group that would receive acetaminophen (180 mg/kg i.p.) plus RYR powder (4 mL/kg i.p.) dissolved in water (1 g/4 mL), 1 h and 15 h prior to treatment with acetaminophen. The results showed that pretreatment with the RYR powder significantly inhibited acetaminophen-induced toxicity to the livers of the rats. Without RYR as a pretreatment, serum levels of GSH S-transferase increased to 2,106% of the control rats. With RYR, the increase was only 1,061% ($p < 0.01$). Serum AST (aspartate aminotransferase) activity increased in the acetaminophen-treated rats by 598% of the control rats, whereas RYR-pretreated rats showed an increase in AST of 249% of the control rats. Cytosolic glutathione S-transferase (GST) of the rats treated with acetaminophen was decreased to 53% of the control level, and glutathione (GSH) peroxidase was decreased to 46% of the control. Pretreatment with RYR slightly increased GSH peroxidase to 55% of control levels and cytosolic GST to 65% of the control. However, the increase in microsomal GST and microsomal GSH by acetaminophen to 176% and 126% of the control, respectively, was not ameliorated by RYR pretreatment. The content of liver GSH, which was nearly depleted by acetaminophen, was also not affected by RYR. Although acetaminophen did not affect liver microsomal aniline hydroxylase activity, RYR administered alone caused a significant decrease in activity to 85% of the control, although serum and liver enzyme activities showed no change and lipid peroxidation showed a slight though insignificant decrease. Aniya et al. (1998) investigated this activity by examining the effect of RYR on cytochrome P450 activity in vitro and reported a dose-dependent inhibition of aniline hydroxylase. The researchers concluded from this that the inhibition may in fact be beneficial for the prevention of acetaminophen-induced injury to the liver because the acetaminophen-derived reactive metabolite NAPQI (*N*-acetyl-*p*-benzoquinone imine) causes liver toxicity via the cytochrome P450 system. The authors explain that NAPQI causes liver toxicity by covalently binding to liver proteins and by generating reactive oxygen species by reacting with a ferrous-oxyform of cytochrome P450, or by activating neutrophils and macrophages (Aniya et al., 1998).

Immune Functions; Inflammation and Disease

Cancer

Chemopreventive activity. In a study of the effect of *Monascus* pigment on tumor promotion in mice, Yasukawa et al. (1996) reported that the addition of *Monascus* pigment (derived from *M. anka,* a red yeast widely used as a food coloring in Japan and Asia) to the drinking water of mice (0.1% and 0.02%) dose-dependently reduced the incidence of skin tumor formation following a single topical exposure to the carcinogen DMBA (7,12-dimethylbenz[a]anthracene) (50 mg), and subsequently promoted by twice-weekly topical applications (1 mg) of the tumor promoter TPA (12-*O*-tetradecanoylphorbol-13-acetate). The untreated group produced 10.5 tumors/mouse at the end of the twentieth week, while those given 0.1% and 0.02% *Monascus* pigment had 3.6 and 4.4 tumors per mouse, respectively. This represented a reduction in tumor formation of 66% and 58% respectively, compared to the mice receiving only DMBA plus TPA.

Another group of Japanese investigators (Izawa et al., 1997) tested the effects of *Monascus* pigments on the mutagenicity of selected heterocyclic amines in the Ames assay. Although not mutagenic, both the red and yellow pigments inhibited the mutagenicity of the food mutagens, including Tryp-P-2(NHOH) (3-hydroxyamino-1-methyl-5H-pyrido[4,8-*b*]indole), a primary metabolite of several direct-acting (i.e., not requiring metabolic activation) mutagens. Both the red and yellow pigments inhibited Tryp-P-2(NHOH) mutagenicity more than 50% at a concentration of less than 0.1 mg/mL. *Monascus* yellow strongly inhibited the mutagenicity of metabolically activated (MeIQ) at 0.1 mg/mL, while *Monascus* red was less active against this metabolite, inhibiting mutagenicity less than 50% at a concentration greater than 1.0 mg/mL. *Monascus* red showed similar activity against activated IQ (2-amino-3-methylimidazo[4,5-*f*]quinoline), a food mutagen, but showed slightly stronger activity against activated cooked-meat extract. In further mechanistic studies, these researchers reported that incubation of *Monascus* red or yellow pigments with the food mutagen Tryp-P-2(NHOH) accelerated its spontaneous degradation, as measured by HPLC and UV/visible spectrophotometry. *Monascus* red was more than twice as active as *Monascus* yellow in accelerating the degradation of the carcinogen. The concentrations of the pigments remained unchanged during the course of the incubation (Izawa et al., 1997). However, the fermentation of red yeast on rice and other grains may render these pigments inactive by conversion to complexes with amino acids, and their concentrations may not reach sufficient levels to be effective in this form (Martinkova et al., 1995, 1999).

Metabolic and Nutritional Functions

Antioxidant Activity

Aniya et al. (1998) assayed RYR powder made with *Monascus anka* for antioxidant activity using the lipid-soluble radical DPPH (1,1-diphenyl-2-picrylhydrazyl) to measure free-radical scavenging activity in vitro. The RYR powder (50 μL) dose-dependently scavenged the radical and inhibited lipid peroxidation at various dilutions. The dosage of 4 mL/kg used in the acetaminophen toxicity study above was determined based on the concentration showing 50% DPPH scavenging activity. Antioxidant activity from

RYR remains to be shown in vivo. Wang et al. (2000) reported that with an RYR powder as part of the diet (2.0%) of rats with hypertriglyceridemia, no effect on superoxide dismutase activity was evident after six months.

CLINICAL STUDIES

Cardiovascular and Circulatory Disorders

Effects on Cholesterol and Lipid Metabolism

In recent years, at least 34 separate clinical studies (17 controlled and 17 open label) in China and the United States have assessed the efficacy of *M. purpureus* RYR as a cholesterol-lowering agent. The results of these studies are consistent with those obtained in the preclinical evaluation.

In a double-blind, placebo-controlled, randomized clinical study, Heber et al. (1999) evaluated the efficacy and safety of an *M. purpureus* extract (Cholestin, Pharmanex, Inc.) as a dietary supplement in an otherwise healthy American population with untreated hyperlipidemia. (As of 2001, Pharmanex, Inc. has replaced red yeast rice in Cholestin sold in the United States with policosanol, a cholesterol-lowering substance extracted from beeswax [Pharmanex, 2001].) The study also sought to separate the effects of diet from those of the extract. The study involved 83 subjects: 46 males and 37 females, ages 34-78; TC 204-338 mg/dL; LDL 128-277 mg/dL; TG 55-246 mg/dL; HDL 30-95 mg/dL. The subjects were given either placebo or the extract (2.4 g/day) and instructions to maintain a diet providing 30% of calories from fat, less than 10% saturated fat and less than 300 mg of dietary cholesterol. After eight weeks, levels of TC in the RYR extract group decreased by 18% ($p < 0.001$) while those in the placebo group remained unchanged. The extract group also showed reductions in the LDL and TG levels. However, HDL levels did not change significantly. Since no differences could be detected in the dietary intake of the two groups, the researchers concluded that the lowering of cholesterol levels in the RYR group could not be attributed to dietary factors. Consistent with previous studies, no serious adverse effects were observed in this study. Liver and kidney function tests also revealed no abnormalities (Heber et al., 1999).

Another major prospective, double-blind, placebo-controlled, randomized clinical trial involved 152 subjects: mean age, 55 years; TC 250 mg/dL and/or TG 200 mg/dL (Shen et al., 1996). After discontinuing cholesterol-lowering medications for at least four weeks, patients were given either a placebo or zhitai capsules (an early, nonconcentrated form of *Monascus purpureus* RYR) twice a day for two months. Patients maintained a normal lifestyle during the study. After eight weeks, total cholesterol was reduced by 19% compared to 1.5% in the placebo group. Triglycerides were reduced by 36% in the zhitai group compared to 10% in the placebo group, and LDL was reduced by 27% with no change in the placebo-treated group. The zhitai group also showed a 17% increase in HDL; the placebo group was unaffected.

In an interesting development, when the zhitai group was divided into three subpopulations based on the extent of hyperlipidemia, the results showed that the effect of zhitai treatment was greater at the higher levels of serum TC and TG (or lower levels of HDL). For instance, in the three subpopulations wherein pretreatment HDL levels were 0.91, 0.91-1.16, and > 1.16 mmol/L, posttreatment levels showed increases of 5%, 24% and 75%, respectively. No adverse effects were reported in this study. Standard biochemical evaluation of liver and kidney function and other biochemical testing revealed no abnormalities. EEG examinations were also normal (Shen et al., 1996).

DOSAGE

The traditional dosage of RYR in Chinese medicine is usually 6-9 g/day (Liu and Bau, 1980). The recommended dose of a proprietary RYR extract (Cholestin) is 1.2 g b.i.d.

SAFETY PROFILE

Contraindications

RYR is contraindicated for individuals who are hypersensitive or allergic to rice or yeast.

Drug Interactions

RYR contains the HMG-CoA reductase inhibitor mevinolin; therefore, the concurrent use of other cholesterol-lowering medications may result in additive or supra-additive effects on the levels of serum lipids. Patients taking cholesterol-lowering medications should consult a physician before taking RYR-containing products.

Grapefruit juice taken concomitantly with HMG-CoA reductase inhibitors has been shown to cause their serum levels to increase approximately five- to 20-fold; therefore, in general, grapefruit juice should be avoided by individuals taking HMG-CoA reductase inhibitors (Kantola et al., 1998).

Pregnancy and Lactation

Cholesterol is an essential component of cell membranes, and thus a critical ingredient for proper fetal and infant development. Currently, anticholesterol drugs are not recommended for use by pregnant or lactating women. Pregnant and breast-feeding women have normally elevated cholesterol and triglycerides levels, making diagnosis of hypercholesteremia unreliable during pregnancy or at least 9 months postpartum. For patients with primary hypercholesterolemia, discontinuing use of lipid-lowering agents during pregnancy and lactation is not expected to change therapeutic outcomes (Hale, 2000).

Side Effects

In clinical trials, only a few mild side effects have been associated with the administration of *M. purpureus* RYR. These include heartburn, abdominal flatulence, and dizziness. In addition, the product may exacerbate preexisting gastritis. The frequency of these effects is extremely low (less than 2%) (Wang et al., 1995).

Special Precautions

Some individuals may be allergic to RYR. In a case report, an atopic, 26-year-old male butcher experienced a severe anaphylactic response after handling RYR powder and subsequently showed a strongly positive reaction to skin prick testing with the RYR diluted in water and to cultured *M. purpureus*. No reaction was elicited in healthy controls. The patient also showed positive reactions in the cellular antigen stimulation test after exposure to cultured *M. purpureus* and the RYR. In the RAST test, investigators found *M. purpureus*-specific IgE antibodies (Wigger-Alberti et al., 1999).

The liver plays a pivotal role in regulating cholesterol and lipoprotein metabolism. Cholesterol-lowering drugs like HMG-CoA inhibitors exert their actions by targeting enzymes in the liver. Because of the presence of mevinolin in RYR, long-term users of this product should consider undergoing periodic monitoring of liver function (Wang et al., 1995). Individuals with preexisting liver disorders should consult their physician before use of RYR preparations.

RYR preparations containing the deydroisocoumarin mycotoxin citrinin—a potent naturally occurring antibiotic formerly known as monascidin A—should be avoided unless the content is sufficiently low enough not to cause toxicity (Blanc et al., 1995). Citrinin is more commonly known to be produced by species of *Penicillium (P. citrinum, P. expansum, P. viridicatum)* (Bilgrami et al., 1988; Ciegler et al., 1977; Wu et al., 1974) and was isolated as an antimicrobial from *Pythium ultimum* Thom (Endo and Kuroda, 1976).

In animal studies, citrinin has shown teratogenic (Ciegler et al., 1977), growth-retarding (Carlton and Tuite, 1969, 1970; Ambrose and De Eds, 1964), nephrotoxic, hepatotoxic activity (Bilgrami et al., 1988; Arai and Hibino, 1983), and hypolipidemic activity (Endo and Kuroda, 1976). Administered to mice before meals, citrinin (50 ppm of a 0.25 mL solution/mouse p.o. for 120 days) caused serious kidney and liver damage (Bilgrami et al., 1988).

Citrinin and two different commercial *Monascus* red yeast rice products originating from China and sold in Europe showed mutagenic activity in the *Salmonella*-hepatocyte assay when strain TA-98 was applied, but not in the standard Ames test (*Salmonella*-microsome assay with or without S9 mix), indicating that citrinin needs to undergo complex transformation in cells before it can produce mutagenicity. Levels of citrinin in 12 different commercial products varied widely, from 0.2 to 17.1 µg/g. Only the two commercial products containing the highest levels of citrinin (8.4 and 17.1 µg/g) showed mutagenic activity (Sabater-Vilar et al., 1999).

The amount of citrinin detected in a noncommercial *Monascus purpureus* dried, fermented rice powder was reported to be 100 mg/kg (Blanc et al., 1995). In commercially available samples of RYR sold in the United States, seven out of nine products analyzed contained citrinin (0.47 to 11.82 µg/capsule) (Heber et al., 2001).

Other toxins that may occur in *M. purpureus* mycelium are oligoketides (monascorubrin, rubropunctatin, monascin, and ankaflavin), which have shown in vitro embryotoxic and teratotoxic effects (in chicken embryos), and in vitro immunosuppressant activity (in mouse T splenocytes) (Martinkova et al., 1999). However, a RYR produced using *M. purpureus* CCM 8152 caused no toxicity in chicken embryos at 100 mg/embryo (Martinkova et al., 1995).

REFERENCES

Alberts, A.W., MacDonald, J.S., Till, A. E., and Tobert, J.A. (1989). Lovastatin. *Cardiovascular Drug Reviews* 7: 89-109.

Ambrose, A.M. and De Eds, F. (1964). Some toxicological and pharmacological properties of citrinin. *Journal of Pharmacology and Experimental Therapeutics* 88: 173-186.

Aniya, Y., Yokomakura, T., Yonamine, M., Nagamine, T., and Nakanishi, H. (1998). Protective effect of the mold *Monascus anka* against acetaminophen-induced liver toxicity in rats. *Japanese Journal of Pharmacology* 78: 79-82.

Arai, M. and Hibino, T. (1983). Tumorigenicity of citrinin in male Fischer 344 rats. *Cancer Letters* 17: 281-287.

Bilgrami, K.S., Sinha, S.P., and Jeswal, P. (1988). Nephrotoxic and hepatotoxic effects of citrinin in mice *(Mus musculus)*. *Proceedings of the Indian National Science Academy* (Part B) B54: 35-37.

Blanc, P.J., Laussac, J.P., Le Bars, J., Le Bars, P., Loret, M.O., Pareilleux, A., Prome, D., Prome, J.C., Santerre, A.L., and Goma, G. (1995). Characterization of monascidin from *Monascus* as citrinin. *International Journal of Food Microbiology* 27: 201-213.

Carlton, W.W. and Tuite, J. (1969). Toxicosis in miniature swine induced by corn cultures of *Penicillium viridicatum*. *Toxicology and Applied Pharmacology* 14: 636.

Carlton, W.W. and Tuite, J. (1970). Mycotoxicosis induced in guinea pigs and rats by corn cultures of *Penicillium viridicatum*. *Toxicology and Applied Pharmacology* 16: 345-361.

Ciegler, A., Vesonder, R.F., and Jackson, L.K. (1977). Production of patulin and citrinin from *Penicillium expansum*. *Applied and Environmental Microbiology* 33: 1004-1006.

Endo, A. (1979). Monacolin K, a new hypocholesterolemic agent produced by a *Monascus* species. *Journal of Antibiotics* 32: 852-854.

Endo, A. and Kuroda, M. (1976). Citrinin, an inhibitor of cholesterol synthesis. *Journal of Antibiotics* (Tokyo) 29: 841-843.

Endo, A., Kuroda, M., and Tusija, Y. (1976). ML-336, ML-236B and ML-236C, new inhibitors of cholesterogenesis produced by *Penicillium citrinum*. *Journal of Antibiotics* 29: 1346-1348.

Ensminger, A.H., Ensminger, M.E., Konlande, J.E., and Robson, J.R.K. (Eds.) (1994). *Foods and Nutrition Encyclopedia,* Second Edition. Boca Raton, FL: CRC Press.

Fink-Gremmels, J., Dresel, J., and Leistner, L. (1991). Einstaz von *Monascus*-extrakten als nitrat-alternative bei fleischerzeugnissen [Use of *Monascus* extracts as an alternative to nitrite in meat products]. *Fleischwirtschaft* 71: 329-331.

Grundy, S.M. (1988). HMG-CoA reductase inhibitors for treatment of hypercholesterolemia. *New England Journal of Medicine* 319: 24-33.

Gunde-Cimerman, N., Plemenitas, A., and Cimerman, A. (1993). *Pleurotus* fungi produce mevinolin, an inhibitor of HMG CoA reductase. *FEMS Microbiology Letters* 113: 333-338.

Hale, T. (2000). *Medications and Mother's Milk* (pp. 407-408). Amarillo, TX: Pharmasoft Medical Publications.

Heber, D., Lembertas, A., Lu, Q.Y., Bowerman, S., and Go, V.L.W. (2001). An analysis of nine proprietary Chinese red yeast rice dietary supplements: Implications of variability in chemical profile and contents. *Journal of Alternative and Complementary Medicine* 7: 133-139.

Heber, D., Yip, I., Ashley, J., Elashoff, D.A., Elashoff, R.M., and Go, V.L. (1999). Cholesterol-lowering effects of a proprietary Chinese red-yeast-rice dietary supplement. *American Journal of Clinical Nutrition* 69: 231-236.

Izawa, S., Harada, N., Watanabe, T., Kotokawa, N., Yamamoto, A., Hayatsu, H., and Arimoto-Kobayashi, S. (1997). Inhibitory effects of food coloring agents derived from *Monascus* on the mutagenicity of heterocyclic amines. *Journal of Agricultural and Food Chemistry* 45: 3980-3984.

Juzlova, P., Martinkova, L., and Kren, V. (1996). Secondary metabolites of the fungus *Monascus:* A review. *Journal of Industrial Microbiology* 16: 163-170.

Juzlova, P., Rezanka, T., Martinkova, L., and Kren, V. (1996). Long-chain fatty acids from *Monascus purpureus*. *Phytochemistry* 43: 151-153.

Kantola, T., Kivistö, K.T., and Neuvonen, P.J. (1998). Grapefruit juice greatly increases serum concentrations of lovastatin and lovastatin acid. *Clinical Pharmacology and Therapeutics* 63: 397-402.

Kritchevsky, D., Li, C., Wei, W., and Wang, Y. (1998). Influence of *Monascus purpureus*-fermented rice (red yeast rice) on experimental atherosclerosis in rabbits. *FASEB Journal* 12: A206.

Li, C., Zhu, Y., Wang, Y., Zhu, J.S., Chang, J., and Kritchevsky, D. (1998). *Monascus purpureus*-fermented rice (red yeast rice): A natural food product that lowers blood cholesterol in animal models of hypercholesterolemia. *Nutrition Research* 18: 71-81.

Liu, B. and Bau, Y.S. (1980). *Fungi Pharmacopoeia (Sinica)* (pp. 8-10). Oakland, CA: The Kinoko Company.

Ma, J., Li, Y., Ye, Q., Li, J., Hua, Y., Ju, D., Zhang, D., Cooper, R., and Chang, M. (2000). Constituents of red yeast rice, a traditional Chinese food and medicine. *Journal of Agricultural and Food Chemistry* 48: 5220-5225.

Martinkova, L., Juzlova, P., and Vesely, D. (1995). Biological activity of polyketide pigments produced by the fungus *Monascus*. *Journal of Applied Bacteriology* 79: 609-616.

Martinkova, L., Patakova-Juzlova, P., Kren, V., Kucerovat, Z., Havlicek, V., Olsovsky, P., Hovorka, O., Rihova, B., Vesely, D., Vesela, D., et al. (1999). Biological activities of oligoketide pigments of *Monascus purpureus*. *Food Additives and Contaminants* 16: 15-24.

Patakova-Juzlova, P., Rezanka, T., and Viden, I. (1998). Identification of volatile metabolites from rice fermented by the fungus *Monascus purpureus* (an-kak). *Folia Microbiologica* 43: 407-410.

Pharmanex (2001). <http://www.pharmanex.com>. Accessed September 2001.

Sabater-Vilar, M., Maas, R.F.M., and Fink-Gremmels, J. (1999). Mutagenicity of commercial *Monascus* fermentation products and the role of citrinin contamination. *Mutation Research* 444: 7-16.

Shen, Z., Yu, P., Sun, M., Chi, J., Zhou, Y., Zhu, X., Yang, C., and He, C. (1996). [A prospective study on zhitai capsule in the treatment of primary hyperlipidemia]. *National Medical Journal of China* 76: 156-157 (translation).

Stuart, G.A. (1979). *Chinese Materia Medica—Vegetable Kingdom* (pp. 233-234). Taipei, Taiwan: Southern Materials Center Inc.

Sung, Y.H. (1966). Yeasts. In Sun, E-Tu Zen and Sun, Shiou-Chuan, *T'ien-Kung K'ai-wu. Chinese Technology in the Seventeenth Century* (translation) (pp. 292-294). University Park, PA: Pennsylvania State University Press.

Wang, I.K., Lin-Shiau, S.Y., Chen, P.C., and Lin, J.K. (2000). Hypotriglyceridemic effect of anka (a fermented rice product of *Monascus* sp.) in rats. *Journal of Agricultural and Food Chemistry* 48: 3183-3189.

Wang, J., Su, M., Lu, Z., Kou, W., Chi, J., Yu, P., and Wang, W. (1995). [Clinical trial of extract of *Monascus purpureus* (red yeast) in the treatment of hyperlipidemia]. *Chinese Journal of Experimental Therapeutics for Prepared Chinese Medicine* 1: 1-5 (translation).

Went, F.A.F.C. (1895). *Monascus purpureus* le champignon de l'ang-quac une nouvelle thélébolée. *Annales des Sciences Naturelles. Botanique et Biologie* 8: 1-18.

Wigger-Alberti, W., Bauer, A., and Elsner, P. (1999). Anaphylaxis due to *Monascus purpureus*-fermented rice (red yeast rice). *Allergy* 54: 1330-1331.

Wu, M.T., Ayres, J.C., and Koehler, P.E. (1974). Production of citrinin by *Penicillium viridicatum* on country-cured ham. *Applied Microbiology* 27: 427-428.

Yasukawa, K., Takahashi, M., Yamanouchi, S., and Takido, M. (1996). Inhibitory effect of oral administration of *Monascus* pigment on tumor promotion in two-stage carcinogenesis in mouse skin. *Oncology* 53: 247-249.

Ying, J., Mao, X., Ma, Q., Zong, Y., and Wen, H. (1987). *Icones of Medicinal Fungi from China* (p. 9). Beijing, China: Science Press.

Xie, S. and Duan, Z. (1996). [Xuezhikang capsule regulates blood lipids with high efficacy: An overview of its preparation, pharmacology, toxicology, and results of clinical trials]. *Chinese Medical News* 11: 13-14 (translation).

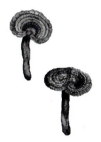

Reishi

BOTANICAL DATA

Classification and Nomenclature

Scientific name: *Ganoderma lucidum* (W. Curt.: Fr.) Karst.

Family name: Aphyllophoromycetideae (Polyporaceae)

Common names: reishi, sachitake, mannentake (ten-thousand-year mushroom) (Japan), ling zhi (China), youngzi (Korea) (Mayzumi et al., 1997; Chang and Buswell, 1999), good omen plant, herb of spiritual potency, miraculous chih (Liu and Bau, 1980)

Description

Ganoderma lucidum is a wood-rotting fungus with a corky interior that occurs in a shelf-like form on the sides of trees and stumps from which it digests lignin, cellulose, and hemicellulose (Adaskaveg and Gilbertson, 1994). Growing from the tops of stumps or submerged logs, reishi can form a longer stem (stipe) and a cap (pileus). The cap then appears in the shape of a lotus leaf. Concentric furrows or rings meet at the top of the stem and the cap often appears shiny (lucidum), usually reddish-orange or reddish-brown, with a white underside when mature. The stem is blackish-brown (Steyaert, 1972). The spores are brown, oval, dimpled, rounded at the base, and narrowly rounded at the top. The spore wall has several layers (Adaskaveg and Gilbertson, 1988) and the spore print is brown (Lincoff, 1981).

Ganoderma lucidum occurs in most parts of the world (Hobbs, 1995). In North America, the exceptions are the western plains and central Rocky Mountains (Adaskaveg and Gilbertson, 1988). In Europe, *G. lucidum* grows on hardwoods and favors oaks (*Qercus* spp.) (Gilbertson and Ryvarden, 1986). It starts to appear in early autumn on fir, spruce, beech, birch, alder, ash, oak, and in some regions pine and larch. By October to November, when the pore layer turns from white to brownish and the cap loses its luster, *G. lucidum* is commonly attacked by insects and then rots (Petersen, 1987). Old plum trees are believed to be particularly susceptible to the fungus in Japan (Matsumoto, 1979), where cultivated reishi forms well on Japanese species of oak and apricot (Mayzumi et al., 1997). In China, *G. lucidum* is found on logs, stumps of broad-leaved trees, and occasionally on conifers. It commonly causes heart-rot disease in Chinese hemlock *(Tsuga chinensis)* (Liu and Bau, 1980) and appears in the northern latitudes between 4°N and 25°N. Here, it prefers temperate climes with a comparatively low amount of rain and grows best on deciduous trees in open forests under indirect sunlight (Zhao and Zhang, 1994).

The artificial cultivation of reishi began in the 1970s and rapidly developed in China during the 1980s (Chang and Buswell, 1999). Cultivation involves warm temperatures and humid conditions, usually indoors. Methods include inoculated short log sections (20 cm) buried to their tops in sand in greenhouses, long logs (120 cm) inoculated with the fungus and left outdoors, and oak sawdust culture in plastic bags in temperature-controlled greenhouses. The size of the cap and stem varies according to growing conditions. Under ideal conditions, cultivated reishi can reach a large size. Younger specimens typically have caps 16 cm wide with stems about half that size, while older growths have stems 15 cm long and caps 25 cm wide (Mayzumi et al., 1997). Genetic analytical methods for differentiation of *Ganoderma* species from other members of the *G. lucidum* complex of fungi (e.g. *G. tsugae* Murr.) in commercial preparations has been proposed by Hseu et al. (1996).

HISTORY AND TRADITIONAL USES

In Central Europe, *G. lucidum* is noted for its beauty in color and shape as a dried object displayed on the mantle during the Christmas season (Petersen, 1987). However, in China, *G. lucidum* has been cherished for over 2,000 years as a longevity-promoting herbal tonic (Chang and Buswell, 1999; Jones, 1996). According to Hikino (1991), "the most important elixirs in the Orient" have been ginseng *(Panax ginseng* C.A. Meyer) and the fruit bodies of reishi. Since the Yuan (Mongol) dynasty (A.D. 1280-1368), representations of reishi have been rendered on everything from belt buckles to carpets, furniture, jade, and paintings (Wasson, 1968). When Pei Sung dynasty (A.D. 1004-1007) Emperor Chen Sung ordered all reishi to be handed in to the royal palace, a count of 10,000 was recorded (Kobayasi, 1983). In Japan, the mushroom was hung in the hallways of homes as a symbol to ward off evil, and it was carried by brides into their new homes for use should any "grave" matters ensue in the new family (Matsumoto, 1979).

Emperor Kenso (A.D. 487) created a Department of "Good Herb" when reishi was found growing in the Imperial courtyard. In the year A.D. 726 Emperor Shomo ordered all the poets in the land to compete in writing a poem about reishi, and 112 participated. In 1803 in Japan, Lord Shimazu Shigehide ordered the local Buddhist temple monks (Sohan) to devote time to collecting reishi (Kobayasi, 1983), probably as a means of paying their taxes. As recently as the 1950s, wild specimens have been offered to China's leaders in Taiwan and on the mainland (Chang and Buswell, 1999).

Fascination with *Ganoderma* began under the name of *ling chih,* later transliterated *reishi* in Japanese. The fungus first appeared in the Chinese literature during the Han dynasty (B.C. 206-A.D. 220). The Emperor Wu associated a growth of the fungus in an inner chamber of the Imperial palace (Dubs, 1944) with a plant of immortality, known simply as the chih plant or chih fungus (Wasson, 1968). In the Forbidden City in Beijing, a large metal-covered wooden carving of a nine-capped *Ganoderma* fungus apparently commemorates the event to this day (Chilton, 1996). A century earlier, Emperor Shih-huang had searched in vain for such a plant, records of which were certainly known to Emperor Wu. He became so enthralled with the "miraculous" growth that he set prisoners free throughout the empire, and commanded that an ox and wine be given to every 100 families. He also ordered that an ode be written to record the phenomena ("Song of the Fungus of Immortality Room") (Dubs, 1944), which is believed to be the first ever written about a fungus or mushroom. This event helped to seal the association between a plant of immortality or longevity and the chih fungus we know today as reishi. A century later, the Han dynasty chronicler Pan Ku wrote a poem using the term *ling chih* (Dubs, 1944; Wasson, 1968). However, the association between the original chih fungus and *Ganoderma lucidum* had clearly derived from legends of an earlier mysterious chih fungus or chih plant of immortality recorded in India. Indeed, versions of the Indian legends concerning it are found later in almost identical form in the Chinese literature in reference to what would remain ling chih (reishi) (Wasson, 1968), while the identity of the true chih plant or fungus of immortality remains in dispute (Flattery and Schwartz, 1989).

Reverence for *Ganoderma* as a life-enhancing herbal medicine can be traced through the centuries in China and Japan (Kobayasi, 1983; Matsumoto, 1979), where the chih plant of immortality has long been associated with Taoist writings (Bretschneider, 1895). The philosopher Wang Ch'ung, writing in the first century, stated that the Taoists dosed "themselves with the germ of gold and jade, [ate] the finest fruit of the purple polypore [Polyporaceae] fungus," and that in so doing "their bodies are lightened" (Schafer, 1967). The purple polypore may have been a reference to *Ganoderma japonicum* (Fr.) Lloyd (a.k.a. *G. sinensis,* family Polyporaceae), which is used to this day in

Chinese medicine and bears a dark purplish-brown to black color (Jones, 1996, 1998).

Medical uses of reishi in ancient China included the treatment of "a knotted and tight chest," increasing "intellectual capacity," correcting "forgetfulness," promoting agility, and lengthening the life span (Li, 1933; Yang, 1998). Contemporary medical uses of cultivated reishi in China parallel these ancient uses (Mayzumi et al., 1997). They include treatment of: neurasthenia, debility from prolonged illness, insomnia, anorexia, dizziness, chronic hepatitis, hypercholesterolemia, mushroom poisoning (antidote), coronary heart disease, hypertension, prevention of altitude sickness (Chang and But, 1986; Ying et al., 1987), treatment of "deficiency fatigue," carcinoma, and bronchial cough in the elderly (Hsu et al., 1986). Chinese research on *Ganoderma* during the past decade has focused on much the same uses, whether in the fields of antiaging/life prolongation, brain ischemia/reperfusion injury, chronic viral hepatitis, male sexual dysfunction, hypercholesterolemia, immunological function in the elderly, chemotherapy-induced toxicity, narcotic-induced immunosuppression, anticarcinogenic and antitumor activity, and immunostimulation. However, with so many questions concerning the identity of active constituents and mechanisms of activity still unanswered (Liu, 1999), the incomplete pharmacological knowledge of reishi remains as much a part of its mystery as its legendary uses in the past.

CHEMISTRY

Carbohydrates

Polysaccharides

Polysaccharides in reishi include ganoderans B and C (Hikino et al., 1989, 1985; Tomoda et al., 1986) and various β-1,3-D-glucopyranan polysaccharides with β-1,6-D-glycosyl branched chains and a few 1,4-linked glycosyl units (Sone et al., 1985).

Nitrogenous Compounds

Nucleotides and Nucleosides

Nucleosides in reishi include adenosine (Shimizu et al., 1985) and 5-deoxy-5' methylsulphinyladenosine (Kawagishi et al., 1993).

Terpenoid Compounds

Triterpenes

At least 119 different triterpenes have been identified in *G. lucidum* (reviewed in Kim and Kim, 1999), with researchers in Korea reporting 137 (Chang and Buswell, 1999). The majority are bitter tasting and largely occur as ganoderic acids (Kim and Kim, 1999). A new triterpenoid, named ganosporeric acid A, was recently isolated from the ether-soluble fraction of the spores (Chen and Yu, 1999), while Min et al. (2000) reported the isolation of six new lanostane-type triterpenes, also from the spores (ganoderic acids γ, δ, ε, ζ, η, and θ). Preliminary studies indicate that the spores contain considerably higher contents of ganoderic acids than other parts of the fungus and that triterpene composition of the fruit body varies from one growing area to the next (Min et al., 1999). The spores also contain triterpene lactones (Chen and Yu, 1999).

Other Constituents

Reishi also contains ergosterol (Subramanian and Swamy, 1961), sterols (Kac et al., 1984), amino acids, soluble protein (Tseng and Lay, 1988; Jong and Birmingham, 1992), oleic acid (Tasaka, Akagi, et al., 1988), cyclooctasulfur (Tasaka, Mio, et al., 1988), an ergosterol peroxide (5,8-epidioxy-5α,8α-ergosta-6,22*E*-dien-3β-ol) (Mizushina, Watanabe, et al., 1998), and the cerebrosides (4*E*,8*E*)-N-D-2'-hydroxystearoyl-1-*O*-β-D-glucopyranosyl-9-methyl-4-8-sphingadienine, and (4*E*,8*E*)-N-D-2'-hydroxypalmitoyl-1-*O*-β-D-glucopyranosyl-9-methyl-4-8-sphingadienine (Mizushina, Hanashima, et al., 1998).

THERAPEUTIC APPLICATIONS

Reishi is used in contemporary traditional Chinese medicine (TCM) in the treatment of a list similar to its traditional uses: neurasthenia, debility from prolonged illness, insomnia, anorexia, dizziness, chronic hepatitis, hypercholesterolemia, coronary heart disease, hypertension (Chang and But, 1986; Ying et al., 1987), "deficiency fatigue," carcinoma, and bronchial cough in the elderly (Hsu et al., 1986). More recently, reishi has become recognized as an alternative adjuvant in the treatment of hepatitis B, diabetes, carcinoma, and leukemia (Teow, 1995; Chang and But, 1986). Clinical studies to date lack the controls needed to make a scientific assessment of the efficacy of reishi in a given application, a situation expected to change soon with increasing international interest from Western-trained scientists.

PRECLINICAL STUDIES ·

Cardiovascular and Circulatory Functions

Cholesterol and Lipid Metabolism

The powdered mycelium of reishi, at 5% of the diet of spontaneously hypertensive rats for four weeks, caused plasma total cholesterol to significantly decrease (by 18.6%) compared to controls. Total liver triglyceride and total liver cholesterol levels were also significantly lower in the reishi-fed group (by approximately 46% and 56%, respectively) (Kabir et al., 1988).

Hypertension

A water extract of the mycelium administered to rats and rabbits (3-30mg/kg i.v.) produced significant hypotensive effects, an activity the researchers suggested is secondary to the primary effect that suppresses sympathetic outflow of the central nervous system (Lee and Rhee, 1990). The powdered mycelium of reishi, at 5% of the diet of spontaneously hypertensive rats for four weeks caused systolic blood pressure to lower by a significant amount (approximately 10 mm Hg) without causing a significant difference in the heart rate (Kabir et al., 1988).

Digestive, Hepatic, and Gastrointestinal Functions

Hepatic Functions

Against carbon tetrachloride-induced liver toxicity in rats, a water extract of reishi (1 g/kg i.p.) failed to improve the morphology of the liver but significantly lowered SGOT (serum level of glutamic-oxalacetic transaminase) and SGPT (serum level of glutamic-pyruvic transaminase) activities (Lin et al., 1993). A similar study found significant inhibition of SGOT and SGPT from a water extract of reishi in rats (30 mg/kg i.p., 45.85% inhibition; 100 mg/kg i.p., 65.89% inhibition). Serum lactic dehydrogenase activity was also significantly lowered by the extract in the same dosages (Lin et al., 1995). Pretreatment of female rats with a freeze-dried, water-soluble extract of reishi (200 mg/kg p.o. three or six times a day) significantly protected against carbon tetrachloride-induced hepatotoxicity. Plasma levels of ALT (alanine transaminase) in the reishi pretreatment group showed a significantly lower level of increase compared to the control group treated with carbon tetrachloride (CCL_4) alone.

Based on the popular notion strongly asserted in TCM that reishi promotes good health in old age, Ng et al. (1993) examined the effects of a water extract of reishi in accordance with the oxidative stress hypothesis as a model of aging. The extract was prepared by allowing the dried fruit body to soak in double-distilled water before heating at 60ºC for five hours to obtain a water-soluble extract with a yield of 7%-10% (w/w). The extract was then freeze-dried before administration to the rats for three or six days at a dosage of 200 mg/kg p.o. prior to intragastric administration of CCL_4. As a preventive agent against CCL_4-induced free radical damage to the tissues of the rats, reishi proved significantly and equally effective at either the three- or six-day pretreatment; reduced glutathione levels in hepatic tissue were significantly protected from depletion in the groups administered reishi as a pretreatment, compared to the control group treated with CCl_4 without reishi pretreatment. No statistically significant increases in hepatic Cu,Zn-superoxide dismutase or glutathione reductase activities were found from the pretreatment, although they clearly showed a tendency to be much higher compared to untreated control groups. However, controls administered the reishi extract without subsequent administration of CCL_4 showed no change in hepatic antioxidant parameters (Ng et al., 1993).

Using a model of alcohol-induced free radical- and oxidative stress-associated liver damage in male mice, Shieh et al. (2001) studied the potential hepatoprotective effect of a concentrated water decoction of reishi fruit bodies (1 g/mL w/v of extract based on the weight of the dried fruit body) which was freeze-dried into powder form before administration. The mice received treatment with either 95% ethanol (0.1 mL p.o.), the reishi decoction 30 min prior to receiving ethanol, or the decoction without subsequent ethanol. Reishi at dosages of 10, 25, and 50 mg/kg p.o. in separate groups of mice produced dose-dependent and inhibition of lipid peroxidation in the liver of mice not treated with ethanol (lipid peroxidation-induced malonic dialdehyde formation), which was significantly greater than controls at the two higher doses (20.19% and 22.54% inhibition, respectively). In mice pretreated with the decoction, ethanol-induced lipid peroxidation was significantly inhibited at all three doses (43.2%, 46.2%, and 74.9%, respectively).

Kim et al. (1999) reported that polysaccharides from *G. lucidum* showed more potent in vitro glutathione S-transferase-inducing activity than polysaccharides from *Aloe barbadensis* Miller, shiitake mushroom *(Lentinula edodes),* or the fungus *Trametes versicolor* (= *Coriolus versicolor*).

An extracellular polymer derived from a submerged mycelial culture of reishi (*G. lucidum* WK-003) exhibited hepatoprotective effects in male rats treated with CCl_4. Compared to rats treated only with CCl_4, those pretreated with the mycelial exopolymer dissolved in saline (20 mg/kg p.o. q.i.d.) showed 31% lower levels of serum GPT (glutamate-pyruvate transaminase) ($p < 0.01$) and although not reaching statistical significance, 73% lower levels of serum GOT (glutamate-oxaloacetate transaminase). Here, Song et al. (1998) commented that serum GPT levels provide a more sensitive index of hepatic cell damage than GOT.

A protein-bound polysaccharide isolated from reishi mycelium produced antifibrotic activity in rats with liver failure (5 mg/day p.o. for 28 days). The compound improved the morphology of the liver, produced a significant inhibition of cell destruction, and significantly lowered liver collagen levels and serum levels of AST (aspartate transaminase), ALT, total bilirubin, and ALP (alkaline phosphatase) (Park et al., 1997).

Endocrine and Hormonal Functions

Diabetes

A water extract of reishi reduced the increase in blood glucose and blood insulin levels in rats (50 mg p.o.) following the oral glucose test. Following adrenaline (i.v.) or oral glucose in rats, reishi inhibited increases in blood glucose without raising blood insulin levels (Kimura et al., 1988). Glycans (ganoderans B and C) from reishi have shown significant hypoglycemic activity in mice (Hikino et al., 1989, 1985; Tomoda et al., 1986).

Genito-urinary and Renal Functions

Renal Functions

Shieh et al. (2001) reported that pretreatment of male mice with a hot water decoction of the fruit body (concentrated to 1 g/mL of extract based on the weight of the dried fruit body) caused a significant reduction in ethanol-induced (0.1 mL p.o.) lipid peroxidation as measured by formation of malonic dialdehyde. The effect was dose dependent and was found from 30 min pretreatments with the decoction at doses of 10, 25, and 50 mg/kg p.o. (38.9%, 49.5%, and 52.6% inhibition, respectively). In mice not subsequently treated with ethanol, the reishi decoction produced significant inhibition of lipid peroxidation at doses of 25 and 50 mg/kg p.o. (22.84% and 25.31% inhibition, respectively).

Immune Functions; Inflammation and Disease

Cancer

Antiproliferative activity. A hot-water extract of reishi (10 mg/kg i.p. for ten days) inhibited the growth of sarcoma 180 tumors in mice by 99%, and 67% of the mice showed complete tumor regressions (Maruyama et al., 1989). A polysaccharide (β-1,3-glucan) from the liquid growing medium of reishi mycelium (PLM) and one from a hot-water extract of the fruit body (PHW) inhibited tumor growth (sarcoma 180) in mice. At dosages of 10 mg/kg per day i.p. for ten days, the polysaccharides produced tumor inhibition rates of 97.9% (PHW) and 91.6% (PLM). Complete tumor regressions were found in 80% of mice treated with PHW and in 71% of mice treated with PLM (Sone et al., 1985).

Chemopreventive activity. Lee et al. (1998) identified ganoderic acids A and C as inhibitors of farnesyl protein transferase, thereby providing important lead compounds for the development of antagonists of Ras-dependent cell transformation, which promote tumor growth. However, compounds identified in garlic showed more potent activity (Lee et al., 1998).

A feeding study in mice compared the tumor incidence-inhibiting effects of various natural supplements, including reishi. When added in large amounts to the normal feed of mice destined to develop a high incidence of lung tumors, reishi (25% of the diet) inhibited tumor incidence by 82.2%. This rate was higher than that of ascorbic acid (37.5% from 10 mg/mL of drinking water), soybean lecithin (71.2% from 25 mg/mL of drinking water), caffeine (54% from 2 mg/day), fresh red ginseng *(Panax ginseng)* extract (58% from 1 mg/mL of drinking water), carrots (500 mg/g of diet), spinach (25% of diet), β-carotene (500 mg/g of diet), sesame seeds (5% of diet), or 13-cis retinoic acid (240 mg/kg of diet) (Yun et al., 1995).

From an extract of reishi fruit bodies, Mizushina, Hanashima, et al. (1998) identified a mixture of two cerebrosides as among the strongest selective inhibitors of replicative DNA polymerases in vitro. The cerebrosides were identified as (4*E*,8*E*)-N-D-2'-hydroxystearoyl-1-*O*-β-D-glucopyranosyl-9-methyl-4-8-sphingadienine and (4*E*,8*E*)-N-D-2'-hydroxypalmitoyl-1-*O*-β-D-glucopyranosyl-9-methyl-4-8-sphingadienine. Dose-dependent inhibition of replicative polymerases was shown from the cerebroside mixture, with strongest activity shown against α-type polymerase (IC_{50} 12 μg/mL) from animals or mushrooms. However, very weak activity was found against rat DNA polymerase β activity and moderate inhibition (IC_{50} 57 μg/mL) was found against δ-type polymerase activity from cherry salmon *(Oncorhynchus masou)*, which contain DNA polymerase δ almost identical to that of humans (Mizushina, Hanashima, et al., 1998). These researchers also reported the identity of an ergosterol peroxide in the fruit bodies of reishi (5,8-epidioxy-5α,8α-ergosta-6,22*E*-dien-3β-ol) that selectively enhanced the inhibiting activity of linoleic acid against mammalian DNA polymerases. Linoleic acid was also identified as the major polymerase inhibitory compound in reishi, though not as active as the ergosterol peroxide that also occurs in coral, sea hare, sponge, and tunicate. In the presence of the ergosterol peroxide (0.25 μM), little linoleic acid (10 μM and less) was required to inhibit almost completely rat DNA polymerase β (pol. β); by itself, the concentration of linoleic acid required for near complete inhibition was eight times greater (Mizushina, Watanabe, et al., 1998).

Reishi fruit bodies collected in the forests of France were entered into a screening program for potential chemopreventive compounds derived from plants. In cultured murine hepatoma (Hepa lclc) cells, a chloroform extract of the specimen induced NAD(P)H:quinone oxireductase activity, doubling the activity of the drug metabolizing enzyme at a concentration of 16.1 µg/mL. Researchers isolated active inducing constituents in the form of two new lanostane triterpenes. Compound 1 doubled the inducing activity of the enzyme in the hepatoma cells at a concentration of 3.0 µg/mL, while compound 2 proved less active, even at a concentration of 20 µg/mL. Compound 1 was also found in greater quantity in the dried fruit body (0.02%) than compound 2 (0.015%) (Ha et al., 2000).

Cytotoxicity. Toth et al. (1983) reported that ganoderic acids U, V, W, X, Y, and Z isolated from the cultured mycelium exhibited in vitro cytotoxic activity against hepatoma cells grown in culture. Min et al. (2000) compared the in vitro cytotoxic activity of triterpenes isolated from the spores of reishi in mouse lung carcinoma (LLC) cells and mouse sarcoma (Meth-A) cells, using adriamycin as the positive control. The effective doses at which 50% of the cells were killed (ED_{50}) by individual triterpenes isolated from the spores were found for 14 triterpenoids previously known to occur in reishi, along with six ganoderic acid triterpenes isolated from the spores for the first time, designated ganoderic acids γ, δ, ϵ, ζ, η, and θ (gamma, delta, epsilon, zeta, eta, and theta). Against the LLC tumor cell line, greatest cytotoxic activity was found from the ganoderic alcohol, lucidumol A, ganoderiol F, and ganodermanontriol (ED_{50} 2.3, 6.0, and 9.6 µg/mL, respectively). Against the Meth-A tumor cell line, greatest activity was shown by ganodermanondiol, lucidumol A, ganoderiol F, ganodermanontriol, ganoderic acid θ, and lucidumol B (ED_{50} 3.4, 4.2, 4.4, 5.4, 5.7, and 8.5 µg/mL, respectively). The anticancer agent adriamycin showed an ED_{50} of 0.15 µg/mL against LLC cells and 0.01 µg/mL against Meth-A cells. The remaining ganoderic acids were either very weakly active or inactive.

However, Wu et al. (2001) found significant in vitro cytotoxic activity against hepatic tumor cell lines (Hep G2, Hep G2,2,15) and a leukemic tumor cell line (P388) from the triterpenes ganoderic acid E, lucidenic acid A, and lucidenic acid N.

Immune Functions

Immunopotentiation. The mycelium of reishi has shown a rather high rate of anticomplementary activity (31.5%) which was comparable to that of *Cordyceps* spp. (31.1%), and the shiitake mushroom *(Lentinula edodes)* (31.7%) (Jeong et al., 1990). From the spores of reishi fruit bodies, Min et al. (2001) isolated three terpenoids that showed potent in vitro anticomplementary activity against the classical pathway of the complement system. Ganoderiol F was especially active (IC_{50} 4.8 µM) while ganodermanontriol and ganodermanondiol were weaker (IC_{50}s 17.2 µM and 41.7 µM, respectively).

A water extract of reishi administered to mice (1 g/kg p.o. daily for nine days) produced a significant increase in the carbon clearance value of macrophages (11.9 ± 3.5). Administration of the same extract i.p. (250 mg/kg daily for four days) produced a carbon clearance value of 6.6 ± 2.8, which was significantly higher than the respective control group (3.8 ± 2.0) (Yang et al., 1992).

After exposure to a water-soluble polysaccharide fraction of reishi (PSG), the conditioned medium from pure monocytes-macrophages produced anti-tumor cytokines (TNF-α and interferon-γ) that acted synergistically against the growth of human leukemia cells (U937 and HL-60). Whereas the polysaccharide fraction showed no such activities, the conditioned medium induced 40% to 45% of the leukemia cells to undergo differentiation, becoming mature monocytic cells with surface antigens expressing CD68 and CD14. In both leukemic cell lines, the conditioned medium also induced apoptosis (in HL-60 by 38.3 ± 4.5%, and in U937 by 44.5 ± 3.8%). In addition, macrophages and T-lymphocytes showed enhanced production of cytokines. Compared to control macrophages, those exposed to the water-soluble polysaccharide fraction (100 μg/mL) produced a marked 29-fold greater increase in interleukin-6 (IL-6), a 9.8-fold greater increase in tumor necrosis factor-alpha (TNF-α), and a 5.1-fold higher level of IL-1β. T-lymphocytes exposed to the polysaccharide fraction (50 μg/mL) released about double the levels of interferon-gamma (INF-γ) (Wang et al., 1997).

Lieu et al. (1992) reported that the optimal concentration of a water-soluble polysaccharide fraction of reishi for differentiation-inducing activity in U937 leukemia cells was 50 mg/mL, which they judged to be low.

Immunoprotection. A polysaccharide-bound peptide isolated from reishi showed in vitro (Lu and Lin, 1994a) and in vivo antagonizing effects against the immunosuppressive effects of morphine. Morphine-dependent mice administered peptide-bound polysaccharides (PBP) of reishi (50 mg/kg i.g. daily for four days) showed complete restoration of immunological activities, including macrophage functions of cytoxicity (against tumor cells), phagocytosis, and secretion of TNF and IL-1. Following PBP, B-cell- and T-cell-mediated responses suppressed by morphine were completely restored, even exceeding normal levels (Lu and Lin, 1994b).

Infectious Diseases

Microbial infections. An aqueous extract of reishi strongly inhibited the in vitro growth of *Heliobacter pylori* but had very weak activity against *H. pylori* urease (Kim et al., 1996).

An aqueous extract of reishi showed strong in vitro growth-inhibitory activity against *Micrococcus luteus* ATCC 9341 (MIC, 0.75 mg/mL), *Escherichia coli* ATCC 25922 (MIC, 1.75 mg/mL), and *Klebsiella pneumoniae* ATCC 10031 (MIC, 1.25 mg/mL) (Yoon et al., 1994).

Viral infections. Min et al. (1999) identified triterpenes in the spores and fruit bodies of reishi that showed activity against HIV-1 protease activity. The most active constituent was ganoderic acid β (IC_{50} 20 μM). A hot-water extract of the fruit body inhibited the virus-induced cytopathic effect of *Herpes simplex* virus-1 and -2 (HSV-1 and -2) in vitro by 50% at concentrations of 1.510 mg/mL and 1.790 mg/mL, respectively. In the antiherpetic activity assay, which consisted of measuring the inhibition of plaque formation produced by these viruses, a dose-dependent inhibition was shown by the hot-water extract. The effective concentrations at which 50% of plaque formation produced by HSV-1 and -2 was inhibited (EC_{50}) were respectively 580 μg/mL and 590 μg/mL. By comparison, the antiviral agent acyclovir inhibited the plaque formation of HIV-1 and HIV-2 at EC_{50}s of 0.6 and 0.9 μg/mL, respectively (Eo et al., 1999b).

Antiherpetic activity was reported from an acidic protein-bound polysaccharide (APBP) composed of about 40.6% polysaccharide and 7.80% protein, which was isolated from the hot-water extract of artificially grown reishi purchased at a local health food store in Korea (Eo et al., 2000). APBP showed potent in vitro activity against plaque formation caused by HSV-1 (EC_{50} 300 μg/mL) and HSV-2 (EC_{50} 440 μg/mL) (Eo et al., 1999a). APBP combined with interferon-alpha (INF-α) inhibited in vitro plaque formation at still lower concentrations. Against HSV-1, a synergistic effect was observed with INF-α whereas in combination with interferon-gamma (INF-γ) an antagonistic effect was found. However, against HSV-2, either interferon was synergistic with the polysaccharide. The researchers concluded that the polysaccharide may be of use as a potential treatment for herpes and, as an agent used in combination with inherently toxic antiviral agents, it may allow the use of lower dosages without compromising antiviral activity (Kim et al., 2000).

Oh et al. (2000) investigated the antiviral activity of APBP in HSV-1 and -2, finding their respective 50% effective concentrations (EC_{50}) against growth of viruses in cultured Vero cells at 300 and 440 μg/mL by plaque reduction assay. When APBP was combined with antiherpetic agent acyclovir, synergistic activity was evident in both HSV-1 and -2. In the plaque reduction assay, the combination was significantly greater than acyclovir alone ($p < 0.01$) compared to virus-treated control cells. At a ratio of APBP:acyclovir of 1000:1, the EC_{50} in the plaque reduction assay of HSV-1 formation was 134.20 μg/mL, which was considerably less than the value obtained from the polysaccharide alone (EC_{50} 300 μg/mL). The synergistic effect of the combination was also apparent in HSV-2 (EC_{50} 125.56 μg/mL). With APBP combined with another antiherpetic agent, vidarabine (200:1), the synergistic effect was even stronger against HSV-1 (EC_{50} 138.83 μg/mL); however, the combination proved antagonistic in HCV-2.

The mechanisms of antiherpetic activity of APBP remain largely unknown. Eo et al. (2000) showed that although the polysaccharide failed to produce interferon-inducing activity in vitro, a concentration of 90 μg/mL inhibited attachment of HSV-2 to Vero cells by up to 50%, and that for HSV-1 the dose required was not much more (50% cytotoxic concentration or CC_{50}, 100 μg/mL). These concentrations were also shown to inhibit the penetration of the herpes viruses into the Vero cells, presumably through a binding mechanism.

Inflammatory Response

A water extract of reishi administered to rats at a high dose (2 g/kg, s.c.) inhibited carrageenan-induced inflammation by 58.6% (Lin et al., 1993).

A water-soluble fraction of reishi has shown significant inhibitory action against platelet aggregation in vitro (Shimizu et al., 1985). A protease isolated from an extract of liquid-cultured mycelium of reishi has shown fibrinolytic activity in vitro. Fibrinolytic agents such as streptokinase and urokinase are used in the treatment of proximal venous thrombi in cases of iliofemoral thrombosis and cases of established pulmonary emboli. In human plasma, the protease exhibited anticoagulant activity. From a concentration of 0.22 μM, the protease prolonged the thrombin time by a factor of three compared to the control. The anticoagulant effect of the protease appeared to be thrombin specific. It inhibited thrombin and also hydrolyzed fibrin. The researchers speculated that the anticoagulant effect of the protease may be the result of a competitive inhibition of the interaction of thrombin with fibrinogen (Choi and Sa, 2000). Ganodermic acid S (GAS), a major triterpene identified in the cultured mycelium (Shiao and Lin, 1987), appears also to contribute to platelet aggregation-inhibitory activity and has shown high solubility in human platelet membranes in vitro. At low concentrations (< 20 μM), GAS exhibited a concentration- and time-dependent inhibitory activity against in vitro platelet aggregation induced by adenosine diphosphate-fibrinogen, collagen, and thrombin (Wang et al., 1991). GAS was more potent against thromboxane B_2-induced platelet aggregation in vitro than either collagen- or thrombin-induced aggregations (Su et al., 1999a, 1999b). At 7.5 μM, GAS was also shown to potentiate in vitro prostaglandin $E_1(PGE_1)$-induced inhibition of collagen-induced platelet aggregation and at 4 μM, potentiated levels of cyclic AMP in PGE_1-induced platelets (Su et al., 2000).

Metabolic and Nutritional Functions

Aging and Senescence; Longevity Enhancement

A water extract of reishi significantly prolonged the life span of male and female fruit flies (by 17.8% and 16.6%, respectively) (Yang et al., 1992). Others have shown that a water extract of reishi significantly prolongs the maximum, median, and mean life span of fruit flies and significantly increases mating activity (Li et al., 1993).

Endurance-enhancing and antihypoxic activity was seen in mice administered an aqueous extract of reishi (60-240 mg/kg, p.o.) (Yang and Wang, 1995). Using an aging model in mice (induced with D-galactose, 40 mg/kg s.c. daily for 28 days), Liu (1999) reported that a reishi extract (125, 250, and 500 mg/kg p.o. daily for 28 days) markedly prevented D-galactose-induced increases in tail hydroxyproline content and brain MAO-B activity.

Antioxidant Activity

Whole body γ-irradiated male mice administered a water extract of reishi in continuous high dosage (400 mg/kg for 35 days, route not stated) showed a greater degree of recovered immunocompetence than a control group given the experimental drug Krestin (PSK) (Chen et al., 1995). The latter is a fungus-derived (*Trametes versicolor* = *Coriolus versicolor*) crude polysaccharide immunomodulator used clinically in Japan as an adjuvant in cancer therapies (Sakagami and Takeda, 1993).

Free-radical scavenging activity was shown in vitro from a water extract of reishi (IC_{50} 0.2 µg/mL). At a low concentration (0.1 mg/mL), superoxide radicals were inhibited by 41.8%, and by 95.7% and 99.9% from higher concentrations (1.0 mg/mL and 10.0 mg/mL, respectively) (Yang et al., 1992). Others have shown that at higher concentrations, a water extract of reishi inhibited superoxide activity (IC_{50} 0.66 mg/mL) and hydroxyl radical activity (IC_{50} 12.66 mg/mL) (Lin et al., 1995). Antioxidant activity is attributed to various triterpenes in reishi (Zhu et al., 1999).

Neurological, Psychological, and Behavioral Functions

Neurotoxicity/Neuroprotection

Despite ancient records that assert reishi increases "intellectual capacity" and corrects "forgetfulness" (Li, 1933; Yang, 1998), to date few studies have focused on its neurological effects. A water-soluble extract of reishi administered to rats (25 mL/kg p.o. t.i.d.) prior to experimentally induced cortical infarction produced cerebroprotective effects, protecting superoxide dismutase (SOD) and Na+K+-ATPase activity (Xia et al., 1996). In preliminary in vitro studies on the neuronal activities of an aqueous extract of the cultured mycelia of reishi, researchers found a number of potential neuroprotective activities. In cultures of rat pheochromocytoma (PC12) cells, the extract (5 to 100 mg/mL) failed to cause any cytotoxic effect. On the contrary, in cells destined to perish by apoptosis, the rate of death was reduced by the extract from 60% to 15%. In further experiments, it was shown that the extract (50 mg/mL) induced neuronal differentiation of the PC12 cells and induced expression of neurofilaments that constitute major neuronal proteins which make up the neuronal skeleton. PC12 cells treated with the extract (50 and 100 mg/mL) also showed activation of the MAP (mitogen-activated protein) kinases Erk1, Erk2 (ras/extracellular signal-regulated kinases 1 and 2), and CREB (cyclic AMP-response element binding protein), the latter being of current interest in the field of learning and memory processes in which CREB signaling plays an important role. These findings raise the possibility that reishi may possess neuromodulating activity on various signaling pathways, some possibly related to memory and learning, and neuroprotective effects that would prevent neuronal apoptosis (Cheung et al., 2000).

Receptor- and Neurotransmitter-Mediated Functions

Rats allowed free access to a diluted water extract of reishi (31.4 ± 1.7 mL/day for seven days) showed a significant 8.5% increase in paradoxical sleep, which increased to 11.9% during a seven-day withdrawal. They also showed a significant 6.5% increase in deep sleep, known as nocturnal slow wave sleep (SWS) while on reishi water, but not during the light phase. During withdrawal from the reishi drinking water, SWS increased 11.1%. The researchers note that their study was predicated on the basis of reports that people habitually using a decoction of the fungus had sometimes claimed sleepiness (Inoue and Honda, 1988).

Koyama et al. (1997) found a significant 55.6% antinociceptive activity from a high dose of a chloroform extract of reishi (300 mg/kg s.c.) administered prior to acetic acid in mice. Ganoderic acids A, B, G, H, and C6 were identified as the active constituents, with ganoderic acid H showing the most significant ($p < 0.001$) antinociceptive activity (64.1% inhibition from 3 mg/kg s.c.). Acetylsalicylic acid served as the positive control and showed comparable inhibition (65.1%) at a dose of 100 mg/kg s.c. Ganoderic acid B was the second most significantly active triterpene ($p < 0.01$), producing an inhibition rate of 48.3% from 5 mg/kg s.c.

Respiratory and Pulmonary Functions

Allergies and Asthma

A methanol extract of reishi has shown histamine release-inhibitory activity in rat mast cells (Kohda et al., 1985). A water extract of reishi tested in models of experimental allergy in rats (500 mg/kg p.o.) showed activity against serum sickness nephritis; reishi improved blood pressure, kidney glomeruli, and the amount of protein excreted in urine. In mice, reishi inhibited ear swelling in a model of contact dermatitis (100 mg/kg p.o., 39.6% inhibition; 500 mg/kg p.o., 56.7% inhibition). In a model of asthma in guinea pigs, reishi (500 mg/kg p.o.) ameliorated the incidence of respiratory disorders (Nogami et al., 1986).

CLINICAL STUDIES

Clinical research of reishi has largely been conducted in China in the form of open-label studies. By Western medical standards, the results of these studies are essentially anecdotal. As such, these inquiries may serve only as suggestions for future inquiries.

Cardiovascular and Circulatory Disorders

In open-label studies, researchers in China reported benefits in coronary heart disease patients given a 20% reishi syrup (10 mL t.i.d.). Out of 92 patients, over half claimed improvements in sleep and appetite, 65% claimed fewer symptoms of shortness of breath and tachycardia, and 72% reported relief from chest pain. In hyperlipidemic patients, the syrup was reported to have substantially lowered LDL cholesterol and total cholesterol in 14/15 of the cases. A study with a reishi alcohol extract (tincture) in 39 angina pectoris patients found 18 apparently cured, 17 improved, and four unresponsive to the treatment. Abnormal ST-T waves were reported to have been eliminated (Dharmananda et al., 1986).

Thrombosis, Hemostasis, and Embolism

In an open-label study, antisclerotic and antiatherogenic activity was reported in men with coronary heart disease (CHD) treated with a reishi extract (1.5 g p.o. in a single dose). Results were compared with age- and weight-matched controls. In cultivated human aortic intimal cells, the blood serum from untreated CHD patients caused cholesterol to accumulate. Following administration of reishi, researchers reported that the activity was reduced by 30% to 41% and remained at significantly lower levels 5 h later (Ryong et al., 1989).

In an open-label study, a water-soluble extract of reishi administered to healthy volunteers and atherosclerotic patients (1,000 mg p.o. t.i.d. for 14 days) was reported to produce a significant inhibition of platelet aggregation. In addition, the weight and length of thrombi from the atherosclerotic patients was significantly reduced following the course of reishi (Tao and Feng, 1990).

Hypertension

Jin et al. (1996) conducted a double-blind, placebo-controlled clinical study of reishi in 54 patients (20 females and 34 males, average age 58.60 ± 8.20 years) with primary stage-II hypertension who had not responded to previous drug treatments (captopril 25 mg t.i.d. or nimodipine 20 mg t.i.d.). In the group administered reishi extract tablets (two tablets b.i.d. or 220 mg/day), systemic blood pressure significantly improved in 82.5%, with capillary and arterial blood pressure showing significant improvements in as little as 14 days. No changes of any significance were found in the placebo group.

A controlled, comparative clinical study of reishi extract tablets (240 mg six times a day for six months) was conducted in 53 hypertensive patients: 12 with mild hypertension, 12 with essential hypertension, and the normotensive controls. Blood pressure was significantly lowered in the essential hypertensives but not in the mildly hypertensive or normotensive subjects. No side effects of any kind were noticed in any of 21 hematological and biochemical tests over the course of the study. At the end of the study, systolic blood pressure had decreased in 57.5% of the essential hypertensives by approximately 11.3%, and in 60% diastolic BP had decreased by approximately 7.3% (Kanmatsuse et al., 1985).

Digestive, Hepatic, and Gastrointestinal Disorders

Hepatic Diseases

Hepatitis. In a three-month, open-label clinical study of eight cases of hepatitis B given reishi powder extract (2 g p.o. t.i.d.), patients showed significant decreases in serum bilirubin, SGOT, and SGPT, and in every case seroconverted to HBs antibody from HBs antigen (Teow, 1995). A recent controlled study in China in patients with chronic viral hepatitis compared the effects of a "reishi tea powder" (2 g t.i.d. for 60 days) taken by 100 patients to a group of 50 patients receiving vitamin C, ATP (adenosine triphosphate), and a Coenzyme A mixture (dosage not specified). SGPT levels returned to normal in both treatment groups in about 60 days; however, normalization occurred in ten days in the reishi group and in 20 days in the other treatment group (Liu, 1999).

Endocrine and Hormonal Disorders

Diabetes

A two-month open label, comparative clinical study of a reishi powder extract (1 g t.i.d.) in eight diabetic patients (four with NIDD and four with IDDM) found hypoglycemic effects comparable to those found in controls administered insulin (100 IU/mL for 60 days) or oral hypoglycemic agents (250 mg/day for 60 days) (Teow, 1995).

Immune Disorders; Inflammation and Disease

Cancer

Chemotherapy adjunct treatments. Kupin (1992) conducted an open-label comparative study with a 1:10 diluted reishi extract (1.5 g p.o. b.i.d. for 36 days before breakfast and supper) in 48 patients with advanced stage carcinomas (renal, gastric, and breast carcinomas). The patients were concomitantly administered chemo- and radiotherapy. Compared to normal controls, immune cell counts of those who had initially low or abnormally high indices showed normal indices following reishi. Immunocompromised patients given reishi showed increased levels of CD4/CD8 ratio and T-cell counts, and lowered levels of T-suppressor cell counts; however, no effect was found in any immune indices in normal controls given reishi. Radio- and chemotherapy intolerance was reduced in the cancer patients on reishi, and leukopenia from the treatments was completely ameliorated. A quick restoration of the CD4/CD8 ratio and of T-cell counts lowered by chemotherapy was shown following reishi, and no side effects occurred from the extract in the patients or the normal controls. Subjects on reishi showed improved vigor and appetite. In those undergoing surgery and receiving reishi extract, recovery was faster and wound healing was improved (Kupin, 1992). Similar results were reported by Teow (1995) in a smaller study of cancer patients (nasopharyngeal carcinoma stage III and acute myeloblastic leukemia patients) given chemo- and radiotherapies who received a reishi extract (3 g p.o. t.i.d. seven days prior to the therapies and for three months after). Teow reported that the cancers remained in remission eight months later.

Immunomodulation

Cellular immune response. Liu (1999) reported that added to peripheral mononuclear cells from the blood of elderly people in vitro, reishi caused interferon and IL-2 production to increase markedly. Subsequently, in an open study, Liu reported that after 30 elderly subjects (average 65.1 years of age) given a 30-day course of reishi (1.5 g p.o. t.i.d.) showed improved cellular immune function. After the treatment, production of interferon and interleukin-2 (IL-2) were significantly increased.

Metabolic and Nutritional Disorders

Fatigue and Debility

An open-label, comparative clinical study of reishi extract (dosage not stated) in 37 cases of debility and weakness (insomnia, bad memory, tiredness, palpitation) found the values for debility and weakness lowered by 56.3% after four to six weeks. The lymphoid transformation rate had increased, and levels of IL-2, complement C3, and immunoglobulin G were reported to be higher after the course of reishi (Yang and Wang, 1996).

Neurological, Psychological, and Behavioral Disorders

Neurotoxicity/Neuroprotection

An open-label, comparative study of reishi extract (approximately 1,000 mg/day) in 900 soldiers traveling to an altitude of 15,500 feet in Tibet found 94.1% free from vomiting and 82.4% free from headaches in the oxygen-poor environment. The results were significant compared to the rate of altitude sickness (77.2% to 83%) in soldiers without some preventive medication. A concurrent study in 976 soldiers on reishi extract showed 83.7% experienced no headaches and 96.1% no vomiting during the journey (Hunan Institute of Pharmaceutical Industry, 1979).

Receptor- and Neurotransmitter-Mediated Functions

In a case study, reishi powder extract (17:1) was used in the treatment of postherpetic neuralgia caused by *Herpes zoster* (shingles) (Hijikata and Tamada, 1998). No drugs used to treat postherpetic neuralgia, such as nonsteroidal anti-inflammatory drugs (NSAIDs) or acyclovir, were permitted during the treatment. In the case of a 58-year-old woman, skin lesions from an earlier infection with *H. zoster* had cleared, but the severe pain that remained was unresolved with NSAIDs. She reported a dramatic decrease in pain after four days of taking reishi and ceased treatment after six weeks (2.13 g p.o. t.i.d. before meals and after in the case of stomach discomfort). Her pain returned during a cold with high fever, whereupon she resumed reishi for one month and found the pain completely gone. More than four years later she reported that the pain had not returned. Similar results were reported by subjects with outbreaks of *H. zoster* and postherpetic pain who used the same dosage and double the dosage in more severe pain. In all these cases, the pain eventually did not return after two weeks to ten months treatment with reishi. The researchers speculated that the effect of reishi could be due to an immunological action allowing inactivation of reactivated *H. zoster* virus (Hijikata and Tamada, 1998).

Reproductive Disorders

Sexual Dysfunctions (Male)

Liu (1999) related that in a recent open-label study in China, 60 men with decreased "sexual ability" reported improvement after one month of drinking a decoction prepared from the fruit bodies of a related species, *Ganoderma japonicum* (Fr.) Lloyd (100-150 mL from 6 g of fruit body/day after lunch). No improvement was reported by four patients; a slight improvement was reported by 17; 25 claimed marked improvement; and 14 reported they were cured. Liu added that other drugs were not taken during the treatment with reishi.

DOSAGE

- Fruit body: 1.5-9 g (Hsu et al., 1986); 3-15 g (Liu and Bau, 1980)
- Fruit body powder extract (typically 4:1): 1.5-9 g/day in divided doses (Teow, 1996); or 300 mg to 2 g/day in divided doses of a 16:1 extract standardized to 12.5% polysaccharides and 4% triterpenes
- Decocted fruit body: minimal effective dose approximately 300 mg (Chang, 1995)
- Mushroom poisoning: decoction of dried fruit body, 200 g (Ying et al., 1987)
- Health maintenance: fruit body decoction, 0.5-1 g/day (Chang, 1995)
- Chronic health problems (e.g., fatigue, stress, autoimmune conditions): fruit body decoction, 2-5 g/day (Chang, 1995)
- Serious illnesses: fruit body decoction, 5-10 g/day (Chang, 1995)

SAFETY PROFILE

Contraindications

None known.

Drug Interactions

Because reishi potentiates the immune system, caution is advised for those receiving immunosuppressive therapies.

The inhibition of platelet aggregation by reishi (Shimizu et al., 1985; Tao and Feng, 1990) may present an additive effect in those taking blood thinning medications such as daily aspirin or warfarin.

Synergistic antimicrobial activity was shown with an aqueous extract of reishi in combination with cefazolin against *Klebsiella oxytoca* ATCC 8724 and *Bacillus subtilis* ATCC 6633. Additive effects were observed with cefazolin against *Bacillus anthracis* ATCC 6603, *Staphylococcus aureus* ATCC 25923, *Escherichia coli* ATCC 25922, and *Salmonella typhi* ATCC 6509 (Yoon et al., 1994).

Pregnancy and Lactation

No specific information regarding pregnancy or lactation was found. Reishi is known to absorb heavy metals (see Special Precautions).

Side Effects

Habitual use of a decoction of *Ganoderma sinensis* (a.k.a. *Ganoderma japonicum* [Fr.] Lloyd) may cause sleepiness (Inoue and Honda, 1988). In oral dosages of 1.5-9 g/day, some patients, when initially taking a powder extract of reishi, have experienced temporary symptoms of sleepiness, thirst, rashes, bloating, frequent urination, abnormal sweating, and a loose stool (Teow, 1996). Large oral doses of vitamin C (6-12 g/day) taken at the same time as reishi powder extract (2-10 g/day) reportedly counteracted loose stools (Jones, 1996).

Special Precautions

Some individuals with allergies may show allergic respiratory reactions to reishi (Horner et al., 1993). When sensitization to *Ganoderma lucidum* was reported among the atopic population of Delhi, India, researchers found a corresponding increase in spore levels of reishi in the rainy season (July to September 1995) with exacerbated symptoms of asthma and rhinitis in 11% ($n = 19$) of 172 nasobronchial allergy patients studied. In all, 17.44% reacted positively to intradermal skin testing with an extract of the fruit bodies of *G. lucidum,* and 28.48% reacted positively to an extract of the spores. Over 80% of these positive patients showed elevated serum levels of reishi-specific IgE against both the fruit body and spore extract. The researchers concluded that over 28% of the population of Delhi have been sensitized to *G. lucidum* (Singh et al., 1995). The researchers note that the problem is international.

In China, Japan, Korea, and Malaysia, cultivators of reishi have been known to enrich the growth substrate with germanium in the belief that it possesses health-inducing qualities (Tong et al., 1994; Tong and Chong,

1996; Lim and Choi, 1991; Mizuno et al., 1988). Since a number of toxic reactions have been reported in the literature from people taking germanium-
enriched supplements (Tao and Bolger, 1997; Becker et al., 1996), reishi
should be analyzed for heavy metals and germanium content if sourcing
from the Orient. In addition, since reishi accumulates atmospheric radioactive cesium (137Cs) and may serve as a bioindicator for cesium pollution
(Tran Van and Le Duy, 1991), sourcing reishi from areas where 137Cs levels are low or negligible is advisable. Boiling mushrooms in water appears
to lower concentrations of 137Cs by about 50% (Grueter, 1971).

Toxicology

Toxicity in Animal Models

The aqueous extract of reishi administered to mice (5 g/kg p.o. for 30
days) produced no changes in body weight, organ weight, or hematological
parameters. The polysaccharide fraction at the same dosage produced no lethal or serious effects (Kim et al., 1986). Reishi produced no changes in the
estrus cycles of ovariectomized mice from a dosage of 10 g/kg p.o. and no
increase in the weight of levator cavernosa and testicles in male mice from
the same dosage. The LD_{50} in mice of the reflux percolate was 38.3 ± 1.048
g/kg i.g. No organ toxicity was found in rabbits from a syrup preparation of
reishi (progressively dosed with 4-140 mL/kg p.o. daily for ten days), nor in
dogs (2 mL/kg and 4 mL/kg p.o. daily for 10 days). An alcoholic extract (1.2
and 12 g/kg i.g. daily for 30 days) produced no signs of toxicity in young
rats in ECG, major organs, hepatic function, growth, or development. Toxic
reactions were absent in dogs administered an alcoholic extract (12 g/kg i.g.
daily for 15 days and at 24 g/kg i.g. daily for 13 days); however, they did display lethargy (Chang and But, 1986).

To test the toxicity of wild reishi, fruit bodies harvested in a rural area of
Hong Kong were prepared as a freeze-dried extract powder (yield, 1 g/20 g
of freeze-dried fruit bodies and 50 mL of extract solution/100 g of freeze-
dried fruit bodies). Examining acute toxicity, male mice were administered
the extract solution (0.9259 g/kg) at a dosage equivalent to one commonly
recommended by manufacturers of commercial concentrated extracts. No
evidence of acute toxicity was found, nor were serum contents of urea,
GOT, or GPT significantly different compared to controls. Subchronic toxicity was measured after 14 days administration of the extract solution.
None of the mice perished and all lived to the end of the assay period. No
signs of abnormality in terms of behavior or clinically were found. The only
difference compared to controls was a steady increase in body weight starting from the second day of administration. During the second week of administration, body weight gain became variable with 20% of the mice showing a decrease in body weight. However, in the end, significant differences

in body weight compared to the control were not evident. No abnormalities were found in histological examinations of livers and kidneys, organ weights (liver, kidney, heart, lung, and spleen), or organ/body weight ratios compared to the control. Tested for genotoxic activity, the extract showed no evidence of causing chromosomal breakage, nor did it protect the mice against induced DNA breakage caused by a mutagen (ethyl methanesulphonate) (Chiu et al., 2000).

REFERENCES

Adaskaveg, J.E. and Gilbertson, R.L. (1988). Basidiospores, pilocystidia, and other basidiocarp characters in several species of the *Ganoderma lucidum* complex. *Mycologia* 80: 493-507.

Adaskaveg, J.E. and Gilbertson, R.L. (1994). Wood decay caused by *Ganoderma* species in the *G. lucidum* complex. In Buchanan, P.K., Hseu, R.S., and Moncalvo, J.M. (Eds.), *Ganoderma: Systematics, Phytopathology and Pharmacology* (pp. 79-93). Proceedings of Contributed Symposium 59A,B, 5th International Mycological Congress, Vancouver, B.C., August 14-21, 1994. Taipei, Taiwan: Applied Microbiology Dept., National Taiwan University.

Becker, B.N., Greene, J., Evanson, J., Chidsey, G., and Stone, W.J. (1996). Ginseng-induced diuretic resistance. *Journal of the American Medical Association* 276: 606-607.

Bretschneider, E. (1895). *Botanicum Sinicum*. Part III (pp. 418-419). Shanghai, China: Kelly and Walsh, Limited.

Chang, H.M. and But, R.P. (Eds.) (1986). *Pharmacology and Applications of Chinese Materia Medica,* Vol. 1 (pp. 642-653). Singapore: World Scientific.

Chang, R. (1995). Effective dose of *Ganoderma* in humans. In Buchanan, P. K., Hseu, R.S., and Moncalvo, J.M. (Eds.), *Ganoderma: Systematics, Phytopathology and Pharmacology, Proceedings of Contributed Symposium* (pp. 117-121). 59A,B, 5th International Mycological Congress, Vancouver, B.C., August 14-21, 1994. Taipei, Taiwan: Applied Microbiology Dept., National Taiwan University.

Chang, S.T. and Buswell, J.A. (1999). *Ganoderma lucidum* (Curt.: Fr.) P. Karst (Aphyllophoromycetideae)—A mushrooming medicinal mushroom. *International Journal of Medicinal Mushrooms* 1: 139-146.

Chen, R.Y. and Yu, D.Q. (1999). Studies on the triterpenoid constituents of the spores of *Ganoderma lucidum* (Curt.: Fr.) P. Karst. (Aphyllophoromycetideae). *International Journal of Medicinal Mushrooms* 1: 147-152.

Chen, W.C., Hau, D.M., and Lee, S.S. (1995). Effects of *Ganoderma lucidum* and Krestin on cellular immuno-competence in γ-ray-irradiated mice. *American Journal of Chinese Medicine* 23: 71-80.

Cheung, W.M., Hui, W.S., Chu, P.W., Chiu, S.W., and Ip, N.Y. (2000). Ganoderma extract activates MAP kinases and induces the neuronal differentiation of rat pheochromocytoma PC12 cells. *FEBS Letters* 486: 291-296.

Chilton, J. (1996). Personal communication with Kenneth Jones. Jeff Chilton is president of North American Reishi, Ltd. July.

Chiu, S.W., Wang, Z.M., Leung, T.M., and Moore, D. (2000). Nutritional value of *Ganoderma* extract and assessment of its genotoxicity and anti-genotoxicity using comet assays of mouse lymphocytes. *Food and Chemical Toxicology* 38: 173-178.

Choi, H.S. and Sa, Y.S. (2000). Fibrinolytic and antithrombotic protease from *Ganoderma lucidum. Mycologia* 92: 545-552.

Dharmananda, S., Chen, F.T., and Weissmann, G. (1986). Herbal foods in Asia: Role in the prevention and treatment of cardiovascular diseases. In Watson, R. (Ed.), *Nutrition and Heart Disease,* Vol. II (pp. 96-97). Boca Raton, FL: CRC Press.

Dubs, H.H. (1944). *The History of the Former Han Dynasty by Pan Ku, Vol. II* (pp. 91, 239). Baltimore, MD: Waverly Press, Inc.

Eo, S.K., Kim, Y.S., Lee, C.K., and Han, S.S. (1999a). Antiherpetic activities of various protein bound polysaccharides isolated from *Ganoderma lucidum. Journal of Ethnopharmacology* 68: 175-181.

Eo, S.K., Kim, Y.S., Lee, C.K., and Han, S.S. (1999b). Antiviral activities of various water and methanol soluble substances isolated from *Ganoderma lucidum. Journal of Ethnopharmacology* 68: 129-136.

Eo, S.K., Kim, Y.S., Lee, C.K., and Han, S.S. (2000). Possible mode of antiviral activity of acidic protein bound polysaccharide isolated from *Ganoderma lucidum* on herpes simplex viruses. *Journal of Ethnopharmacology* 72: 475-481.

Flattery, D.S. and Schwartz, M. (1989). *Hoama and Harmaline: Near Eastern Studies Vol. 21.* Berkeley, CA: University of California Press.

Gilbertson, R.L. and Ryvarden, L. (1986). *North American Polypores.* Oslo, Norway: Gungiflora.

Grueter, H. (1971). Radioactive fission product 137Cs in mushrooms in W. Germany during 1963-1970. *Health Physics* 20: 655-666.

Ha, T.B.T., Gerhäuser, C., Zhang, W.D., Ho-Chong-Line, N., and Fourasté, I. (2000). New lanostanoids from *Ganoderma lucidum* that induce NAD(P)H: quinone oxidoreductase in cultured Hepalclc7 murine hepatoma cells. *Planta Medica* 66: 681-684 (letter).

Hijikata, Y. and Tamada, S. (1998). Effect of *Ganoderma lucidum* on postherpetic neuralgia. *American Journal of Chinese Medicine* 26: 375-381.

Hikino, H. (1991). Traditional remedies and modern assessment: The case of ginseng. In Wijesekera, R.O.B. (Ed.), *The Medicinal Plant Industry* (pp. 149-166). Boca Raton, FL: CRC Press.

Hikino, H., Ishiyama, M., Suzuki, Y., and Konno, C. (1989). Mechanisms of hypoglycemic activity of ganoderan B: A glycan of *Ganoderma lucidum* fruit bodies. *Planta Medica* 55: 423-428.

Hikino, H., Konno, C., Mirin, Y., and Hayashi, T. (1985). Isolation and hypoglycemic activity of ganoderans A and B, glycans of *Ganoderma lucidum* fruit bodies. *Planta Medica* 51: 339-340.

Hobbs, C. (1995). *Medicinal Mushrooms: An Exploration of Tradition, Healing, and Culture,* Second Edition. Santa Cruz, CA: Botanica Press, Inc.

Horner, W.E., Helbling, A., and Lehrer, S.B. (1993). Basidiomycete allergens: Comparison of three Ganodermataceae species. *Allergy* (Copenhagen) 48: 110-116.

Hseu, R.S., Wang, H.H., Wang, H.F., and Moncalvo, J.M. (1996). Differentiation and grouping of isolates of the *Ganoderma lucidum* complex by random amplified polymorphic DNA-PCR compared with grouping on the basis of internal transcribed spacer sequences. *Applied and Environmental Microbiology* 62: 1354-1363.

Hsu, H.Y., Chen, Y.P., Shen, S.J., Hsu, C.S., Chen, C.C., and Chang, H.C. (Eds.) (1986). *Oriental Materia Medica: A Concise Guide* (pp. 640-641). Long Beach, CA: Oriental Healing Arts Institute.

Hunan Institute of Pharmaceutical Industry, No. 201 Research Group (1979). [A spot survey on the prevention of acute unadapted symptoms at plateau with *Ganoderma*]. *Chinese and Traditional Drugs* 6:29-31.

Inoue, S. and Honda, K. (1988). Sleep-promoting effects of a bracket fungus, *Fomes japonicus*. In Koella, W.P. and Obal, F. (Eds.), *Sleep '86* (pp. 338-339). New York: Gustav Fischer Verlag.

Jeong, H., Lee, J.W., and Lee, K.H. (1990). Studies on the anticomplementary activity of Korean higher fungi. *Korean Journal of Mycology* 18: 145-148.

Jin, H., Zhang, G., Cao, X., Zhang, M., Long, J., Luo, B., Chen, H., Qian, S., Mori, M., and Wang, Z. (1996). Treatment of hypertension by linzhi combined with hypotensor and its effects on arterial, arteriolar and capillary pressure microcirculation. In Niimi, H., Xiu, R.J., Sawada, T., and Zheng, C. (Eds.), *Microcirculatory Approach to Asian Traditional Medicine: Strategy for the Scientific Evaluation, Excerpta Medica, International Congress Series* 1117 (pp. 131-138). Amsterdam, NY: Elsevier.

Jones, K. (1996). *Reishi: Ancient Herb for Modern Times,* Second Edition. Seattle, WA: Sylvan Press, Inc.

Jones, K. (1998). Reishi mushroom: Ancient medicine in modern times. *Alternative and Complementary Therapies* 4 (August): 256-266.

Jong, S.C. and Birmingham, J.M. (1992). Medicinal benefits of the mushroom *Ganoderma*. *Advances in Applied Microbiology* 37: 101-134.

Kabir, Y., Kimura, S., and Tamura, T. (1988). Dietary effect of *Ganoderma lucidum* mushroom on blood pressure and lipid levels in spontaneously hypertensive rats (SHR). *Journal of Nutrition and Science of Vitaminology* 34: 433-438.

Kac, D., Barbieri, G., Falco, M.R., Seldes, A.M., and Gros, E.G. (1984). The major sterols from three species of Polyporaceae. *Phytochemistry* 23: 2686-2687.

Kanmatsuse, K., Kajiwara, N., Hayashi, K., Shimogaichi, S., Fukinbara, I., Ishikawa, H., and Tamura, T. (1985). [Studies on *Ganoderma lucidum*. I. Efficacy against hypertension and side effects]. *Yakugaku Zasshi* 105: 942-947.

Kawagishi, H., Fukuhara, F., Sazuka, M., Kawashima, A., Mitsubori, T., and Tomita, T. (1993). 5'-deoxy-5'-methylsulphinyladenosine, a platelet aggregation inhibitor from *Ganoderma lucidum*. *Phytochemistry* 32: 239-241.

Kim, D.H., Bae, E.A., Jang, I.S., and Han, M.J. (1996). Anti-*Heliobacter pylori* activity of mushrooms. *Archives of Pharmacal Research* 19: 447-449.

Kim, H.S., Kacew, S., and Lee, B.M. (1999). In vitro chemopreventive effects of plant polysaccharides (*Aloe barbadensis* Miller, *Lentinus edodes*, *Ganoderma lucidum* and *Coriolus versicolor*). *Carcinogenesis* 20: 1637-1640.

Kim, H.W. and Kim, B.K. (1999). Biomedicinal triterpenoids of *Ganoderma lucidum* (Curt.: Fr.) P. Karst. (Aphyllophoromycetideae). *International Journal of Medicinal Mushrooms* 1: 121-138.

Kim, M.J., Kim, H.W., Lee, Y.S., Shim, M.J., Coi, E.C., and Kim, B.K. (1986). Studies on safety of *Ganoderma lucidum*. *Korean Journal of Mycology* 14: 49-59 (abstract).

Kim, Y.S., Eo, S.K., Oh, K.W., Lee, C.K., and Han, S.S. (2000). Antiherpetic activities of acidic protein bound polysaccharide isolated from *Ganoderma lucidum* alone and in combinations with interferons. *Journal of Ethnopharmacology* 72: 451-458.

Kimura, Y., Okuda, H., and Arichi, S. (1988). Effect of extracts of *Ganoderma lucidum* on blood glucose level in rats. *Planta Medica* 54: 290-294.

Kobayasi, Y. (1983). *[Historical and Ethnological Mycology]*. Tokyo, Japan: Hirokawa Publishing Company.

Kohda, H., Tokumoto, W., Sakamoto, K., Fujii, M., Hirai, Y., Yamasaki, K., Komoda, Y., Nakamura, H., Ishihara, S., and Uchida, M. (1985). The biologically active constituents of *Ganoderma lucidum* (Fr.) Karst. Histamine release-inhibitory triterpenes. *Chemical and Pharmaceutical Bulletin* 33: 1367-1374.

Koyama, K., Imaizumi, T., Akiba, M., Kinoshita, K., Takahashi, K., Suzuki, A., Yano, S., Horie, S., Watanabe, K., and Naoi, Y. (1997). Antinociceptive components of *Ganoderma lucidum*. *Planta Medica* 63: 224-227.

Kupin, V. (1992). A new biological response modifier—*Ganoderma lucidum*—and its application in oncology. In *The 4th International Symposium on Ganoderma lucidum* (pp. 36-39). Hyatt Regency Hotel, June 10, 1992, Seoul, Korea, Program and Abstracts. Seoul, Korea: Seoul National University.

Lee, S., Park, S., Oh, J.W., and Yang, C. (1998). Natural inhibitors for protein prenyltransferase. *Planta Medica* 64: 303-308.

Lee, S.Y. and Rhee, H.M. (1990). Cardiovascular effects of mycelium extract of *Ganoderma lucidum*: Inhibition of sympathetic outflow as a mechanism of its hypotensive action. *Chemical and Pharmaceutical Bulletin* 38: 1359-1364.

Li, H., Wang, X., Jiang, M., Zhang, P., Peng, H., and Mori, M. (1993). Effects of ling zhi on sex vitality and longevity in *Drosophila melanogaster*. In Zhu, S. and

Mori, M. (Eds.), *The Research on Ganoderma lucidum* (Part One) (pp. 289-294). Shanghai, China: Shanghai University Press.

Li, S.C. (1933). *Pen T'sao Kang Mu* [The great pharmacopoeia]. Shanghai: Shang Wu Printer.

Lieu, C.W., Lee, S.S., and Wang, S.Y. (1992). The effect of *Ganoderma lucidum* on induction of differentiation in leukemic U937 cells. *Anticancer Research* 12: 1211-1216.

Lim, U.K. and Choi, K.S. (1991). [The study of chemical component on *Ganoderma lucidum*]. *Seoul National University Journal of Agricultural Sciences* 16: 109-114.

Lin, J.M., Lin, C.C., Chen, M.F., Ujiie, T., and Takada, A. (1995). Radical scavenger and antihepatotoxic activity of *Ganoderma formosanum, Ganoderma lucidum* and *Ganoderma neo-japonicum*. *Journal of Ethnopharmacology* 47: 33-41.

Lin, J.M., Lin, C.C., Chiu, H.F., Yang, J.J., and Lee, S.G. (1993). Evaluation of the anti-inflammatory and liver-protective effects of *Anoectochilus formosanus, Ganoderma lucidum* and *Gymnostemma pentaphyllum* in rats. *American Journal of Chinese Medicine* 21: 59-69.

Lincoff, G. H. (1981). *The Audubon Society Field Guide to North American Mushrooms* (pp. 460-461). New York: Chanticleer Press/Alfred A. Knopf.

Liu, B. and Bau, Y.S. (1980). *Fungi Pharmacopoeia (Sinica)* (pp. 170-172). Oakland, CA: Kinoko Company.

Liu, G.T. (1999). Recent advances in research of pharmacology and clinical applications of *Ganoderma* P. Karst. species (Aphyllophoromycetideae) in China. *International Journal of Medicinal Mushrooms* 1: 63-67.

Lu, Z.W. and Lin, Z.B. (1994a). Antagonistic effect of *Ganoderma* polysaccharides peptide against immunosuppression of morphine. In *'94 International Symposium on Ganoderma Research* (p. 82). October 24-26, 1994, Beijing Medical University, Beijing, China, Program and Abstracts.

Lu, Z.W. and Lin, Z.B. (1994b). Antagonistic effects of *Ganoderma* polysaccharides peptide on inhibition of immune response caused by repetitive in vivo treatments of morphine. In *'94 International Symposium on Ganoderma Research* (p. 83). October 24-26, 1994, Beijing Medical University, Beijing, China, Program and Abstracts.

Maruyama, H., Yamazaki, K., Murofushi, S., Konda, C., and Ikekawa, T. (1989). Antitumor activity of *Sarcodon aspratus* (Berk.) S. Ito and *Ganoderma lucidum* (Fr.) Karst. *Journal of Pharmacobio-Dynamics* 12: 118-123.

Matsumoto, K. (1979). *The Mysterious Reishi Mushroom*. Santa Barbara, CA: Woodbridge Press.

Mayzumi, F., Okamoto, H., and Mizuno, T. (1997). Cultivation of reishi *(Ganoderma lucidum)*. *Food Reviews International* 13: 365-382.

Min, B.S., Gao, J.J., Hattori, M., Lee, H.K., and Kim, Y.H. (2001). Anticomplement activity from the spores of *Ganoderma lucidum*. *Planta Medica* 67: 811-814.

Min, B.S., Gao, J.J., Nakamura, N., and Hattori, M. (2000). Triterpenes from the spores of *Ganoderma lucidum* and their cytotoxicity against meth-A and LLC tumor cells. *Chemical and Pharmaceutical Bulletin* 48(7): 1026-1033.

Min, B.S., Nakamura, N., Miyashiro, H., Bae, K.W., and Hattori, M. (1999). Triterpenes from the spores of *Ganoderma lucidum* and their inhibitory activity against HIV-1 protease. *Chemical and Pharmaceutical Bulletin* 46: 1607-1612.

Mizuno, T., Ohtahara, S., and Li, S. (1988). [Mineral composition and germanium content of several medicinal mushrooms]. *Bulletin of the Faculty of Agriculture, Shizuoka University* 38: 37-46.

Mizushina, Y., Hanashima, L., Yamaguchi, T., Takemura, M., Sugawara, F., Saneyoshi, M., Matsukage, A., Yoshida, S., and Sakaguchi, K. (1998). A mushroom fruiting body-inducing substance inhibits activities of replicative DNA polymerases. *Biochemical and Biophysical Research Communications* 249: 17-22.

Mizushina, Y., Watanabe, I., Togashi, H., Hanashima, L., Takemura, M., Ohta, K., Sugawara, F., Koshino, H., Esumi, Y., Uzawa, J., et al. (1998). An ergosterol peroxide, a natural product that selectively enhances the inhibitory effect of linoleic acid on DNA polymerase β. *Biological and Pharmaceutical Bulletin* 21: 444-448.

Ng, P.C., Kong, Y.C., Ko, K.M., Ko, K.M., So, C.M., and Yick, P.K. (1993). Antioxidant activity of *Ganoderma lucidum*: Protective effects on carbon tetrachloride-induced hepatotoxicity. *Acta Horticulturae* 332: 219-225.

Nogami, M., Ito, M., Kubo, M., Takahashi, M., Kimura, H., and Matsuike, Y. (1986). [Studies on *Ganoderma lucidum*. VII. Anti-allergic effect. (2)]. *Yakugaku Zasshi* 106: 600-604.

Oh, K.W., Lee, C.K., Kim, Y.S., Eo, S.K., and Han, S.S. (2000). Antiherpetic activities of acidic protein bound polysaccharide isolated from *Ganoderma lucidum* alone and in combinations with acyclovir and vidarabine. *Journal of Ethnopharmacology* 72: 221-227.

Park, E.U., Ko, G., Kim, J., and Sohn, D.H. (1997). Antifibrotic effects of a polysaccharide extracted from *Ganoderma lucidum,* glycyrrhizin, and pentoxifylline in rats with cirrhosis induced by biliary obstruction. *Biological and Pharmaceutical Bulletin* 20: 417-420.

Petersen, J. (1987). *Ganoderma* of Northern Europe. *The Mycologist* 21 (Part 2): 63-67.

Ryong, L.R., Tertov, V.V., Vasil'ev, A.V., Tutel'yan, V.A., and Orekhov, A.N. (1989). Antiatherogenic and antiatherosclerotic effects of mushroom extracts revealed in human aortic intima cell culture. *Drug Research and Development* 17: 109-117.

Sakagami, H. and Takeda, M. (1993). Diverse biological activity of PSK (krestin), a protein-bound polysaccharide from *Coriolus versicolor* (Fr.) Quel. In Chang, S.T., Buswell, J.A., and Chiu, S. (Eds.), *Mushroom Biology and Mushroom Products* (pp. 237-245). Proceedings of the First International Conference on

Mushroom Biology and Mushroom Products, August 23-26, 1993, The Chinese University of Hong Kong. Hong Kong: The Chinese University Press.

Schafer, E.H. (1967). *Ancient China* (p. 63). New York: Time-Life Books.

Shiao, M.S. and Lin, L.J. (1987). Two new triterpenes of the fungus *Ganoderma lucidum. Journal of Natural Products* 50: 886-890.

Shieh, Y.H., Liu, C.F., Huang, Y.K., Yang, J.Y., Wu, I.L., Lin, C.H., and Lin, S.C. (2001). Evaluation of the hepatic renal-protective effects of *Ganoderma lucidum* in mice. *American Journal of Chinese Medicine* 29: 501-507.

Shimizu, A., Yano, T., Saito, Y., and Inada, Y. (1985). Isolation of an inhibitor of platelet aggregation from a fungus, *Ganoderma lucidum. Chemical and Pharmaceutical Bulletin* 33: 3012-3015.

Singh, A.B., Gupta, S.K., Pereira, B.M.J., and Prakash, D. (1995). Sensitization to *Ganoderma lucidum* in patients with respiratory allergy in India. *Clinical and Experimental Allergy* 25: 440-447.

Sone, Y., Okuda, R., Wada, N., Kishida, E., and Misaki, A. (1985). Structures and antitumor activities of the polysaccharides isolated from fruiting body and the growing culture of mycelium of *Ganoderma lucidum. Agricultural and Biological Chemistry* 49: 2641-2653.

Song, C.H., Byung, K.Y., Kyung, S.R., Dong, H.S., Park, E.J., Go, G.I., and Kim, Y.H. (1998). Hepatoprotective effect of extracellular polymer produced by submerged culture of *Ganoderma lucidum* WK-003. *Journal of Microbiology and Biotechnology* 8: 277-279.

Steyaert, R.L. (1972). Species of *Ganoderma* and related genera mainly of the Bogor and Lieden Herbaria. *Persoonia* 7: 55-118.

Su, C., Shiao, M., and Wang, C. (1999a). Differential effects of ganodermic acid S on the thromboxane A_2-signaling pathways in human platelets. *Biochemical Pharmacology* 58: 587-595.

Su, C., Shiao, M., and Wang, C. (1999b). Predominant inhibition of ganodermic acid S on the thromboxane A_2-dependent pathway in human platelets response to collagen. *Biochemica et Biophysica Acta* 1437: 223-234.

Su, C., Shiao, M., and Wang, C. (2000). Potentiation of ganodermic acid S on prostaglandin E(1)-induced cyclic AMP elevation in human platelets. *Thrombosis Research* 99: 135-145.

Subramanian, S.S. and Swamy, M.N. (1961). Ergosterol from *Ganoderma lucidum. Journal of Scientific and Industrial Research* (India) 20B: 29.

Tao, J. and Feng, K.Y. (1990). Experimental and clinical studies on inhibitory effect of *Ganoderma lucidum* on platelet aggregation. *Journal of Tongji Medical University* 10: 240-243.

Tao, S.H. and Bolger, P.M. (1997). Hazard assessment of germanium supplements. *Regulatory Toxicology and Pharmacology* 25: 211-219.

Tasaka, K., Akagi, M., Miyoshi, M., Mio, M., and Makino, T. (1988). Anti-allergic constituents in the culture medium of *Ganoderma lucidum*. I. Inhibitory effect of oleic acid on histamine release. *Agents and Actions* 23: 153-156.

Tasaka, K., Mio, M., Izushi, K., Akagi, M., and Makino, T. (1988). Anti-allergic constituents in the culture medium of *Ganoderma lucidum*. (II). The inhibitory effect of cyclooctasulfur on histamine release. *Agents and Actions* 23: 157-160.

Teow, S.S. (1995). The therapeutic value of *Ganoderma lucidum*. In Buchanan, P.K., Hseu, R.S., and Moncalvo, J.M. (Eds.), *Ganoderma: Systematics, Phytopathology and Pharmacology, Proceedings of Contributed Symposium 59A, B, 5th International Mycological Congress* (pp. 105-113). Vancouver, B.C., Aug. 14-21, 1994, Taipei, Taiwan, Republic of China: National Taiwan University.

Teow, S.S. (1996). Effective dosage of *Ganoderma* nutriceuticals in the treatment of various ailments. In *1996 Taipei International Ganoderma Research Conference,* Abstracts, Taipei International Convention Center, Taipei, Taiwan, August 14-15, 1996, paper 2-2. Taipei, Taiwan: National Taiwan University.

Tomoda, M., Honda, R., Kasahara, Y., and Hikino, H. (1986). Glycan structure of ganoderans B and C, hypoglycemic glycans of *Ganoderma lucidum* fruit bodies. *Phytochemistry* 25: 2817-2820.

Tong, C.C. and Chong, P.J. (1996). Mycelial growth and germanium uptake by four species of *Ganoderma*. *Pertanika Journal of Tropical Agricultural Science* 19: 171-174.

Tong, C.C., Khoong, S.L., and Lee, C.K. (1994). Germanium uptake by the fruiting bodes and mycelium of the fungus *Ganoderma lucidum*. *Asian Food Journal* 9: 69-72.

Toth, J.O., Luu, B., and Ourisson, G. (1983). Les acides ganoderiques T à Z: triterpenes cytotoxiques de *Ganoderma lucidum* (Polyporacée) [The ganoderic acids T to Z: Cytotoxic triterpenes of *Ganoderma lucidum* (Polyporaceae)]. *Tetrahedron Letters* 24: 1081-1085.

Tran Van, L. and Le Duy, T. (1991). Linchi mushrooms as biological monitors for 137Cs pollution. *Journal of Radioanalytical and Nuclear Chemistry* 155: 451-458.

Tseng, T.C. and Lay, L.L. (1988). Studies on *Ganoderma lucidum* IV. Identification of strains by chemical compositions in mycelial extracts. *Botanical Bulletin of Academia Sinica* 29: 189-199.

Wang, C.N., Chen, J.C., Shiao, M.S., and Wang, C.T. (1991). The inhibition of human platelet function by ganodermic acids. *Biochemical Journal* 277: 189-197.

Wang, S.Y., Hsu, M.L., Hsu, H.C., Tzeng, C.H., Lee, S.S., Shiao, M.S., and Ho, C.K. (1997). The antitumor effect of *Ganoderma lucidum* is mediated by cytokines released from activated macrophages and T lymphocytes. *International Journal of Cancer* 70: 699-705.

Wasson, R.G. (1968). *Soma: Divine Mushroom of Immortality* (pp. 80-92). Los Angeles, CA: Harcourt Brace Jovanovich, Inc.

Wu, T.S., Shi, L.S., and Kuo, S.C. (2001). Cytotoxicity of *Ganoderma lucidum* triterpenes. *Journal of Natural Products* 64: 1121-1122.

Xia, Y., Hu, C., and Dong, W. (1996). The prophylactic protective mechanism of EGL on the cerebral ischemic damage in rat. *Journal of Neurochemistry* 67(Suppl.): S22, abstract D.

Yang, Q.Y. and Wang, M.M. (1995). The effect of *Ganoderma lucidum* extract against fatigue and endurance in the absence of oxygen. In Buchanan, P.K., Hseu, R.S., and Moncalvo, J.M. (Eds.), *Ganoderma: Systematics, Phytopathology and Pharmacology, Proceedings of Contributed Symposium 59A,B, 5th International Mycological Congress* (pp. 101-104). Vancouver, B.C., August 14-21, 1994. Taipei, Taiwan, China: National Taiwan University.

Yang, Q.Y. and Wang, M.M. (1996). The anti-aging effects of *Ganoderma* essence. In 1996 *Taipei International Ganoderma Research Conference,* Taipei International Convention Center (TICC), August 15-15, 1996, Abstracts, Special Lecture.

Yang, Q.Y., Xi, H.T., and Qin, D.A. (1992). The experiments on the *Ganoderma lucidum* extract for its anti-aging and invigorating effects. In *The 4th International Symposium on Ganoderma lucidum* (pp. 40-45). Hyatt Regency Hotel, Seoul, Korea, Program and Abstracts, June 10, 1992.

Yang, S.Z. (1998). *The Divine Farmer's Materia Medica: A Translation of the Shen Nong Ben Cao Jing.* Boulder, CO: Blue Poppy Press.

Ying, J., Mao, X., Ma, Q., Zong, Y., and Wen, H. (1987). *Icones of Medicinal Fungi from China* (p. 145). Beijing, China: Science Press.

Yoon, S.Y., Eo, S.K., Kim, Y.S., Lee, C.K., and Han, S.S. (1994). Antimicrobial activity of *Ganoderma lucidum* extract alone and in combination with some antibiotics. *Archives of Pharmacal Research* (Seoul) 17: 438-442.

Yun, T.K., Kim, S.H., and Lee, Y.S. (1995). Trial of a new medium-term model using benzo[a]pyrene induced lung tumor in new born mice. *Anticancer Research* 15: 839-846.

Zhao, J.D. and Zhang, X.Q. (1994). Importance, distribution and taxonomy of Ganodermataceae in China. In Buchanan, P.K., Hseu, R.S., and Moncalvo, J.M. (Eds.), *Ganoderma: Systematics, Phytopathology and Pharmacology, Proceedings of Contributed Symposium 59A,B, 5th International Mycological Congress* (pp. 1-2). Vancouver, B.C., August 14-21, 1994. Taipei, Taiwan, China: National Taiwan University.

Zhu, M., Chang, Q., Wong, L.K., Chong, F.S., and Li, R.C. (1999). Triterpene antioxidants from *Ganoderma lucidum*. *Phytotherapy Research* 13: 529-531.

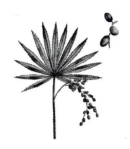

Saw Palmetto

BOTANICAL DATA

Classification and Nomenclature

Scientific name: *Serenoa repens* (Bartram) Small; synonym: *Sabal serrulata* (Michaux) Nutall ex Schultes (Blumenthal, 1997); previously named *Sabal serrulatum* Roem & Schult., *Serenoa serrulata* (Michaux) Hook f. (Vogel, 1970); *Brahea serrulata* (Michaux) H. Wendl.; *Chamaerops serrulata* (Michaux) H. Wendl.; *Corypha repens* Bartram; and others (Bennett and Hicklin, 1998)

Family name: Arecaceae

Common names: saw palmetto, palmetto scrub (Pizzorno and Murray, 1993), American dwarf (Koch and Biber, 1994), dwarf palmetto, Sabal japa (Vogel, 1970), Sabal (McGuffin et al., 1997), and cabbage palm (Anonymous, 1994)

Description

Serenoa repens, the sole member of the genus (Bennett and Hicklin, 1998), is an evergreen palm indigenous to Florida, South Carolina, and the West Indies, with spiny, ascending leaves arranged in a fan shape consisting of 18-24 segments. It grows to heights of 2 m or more and the leaves measure 1 m in width. In Florida, saw palmetto commonly occurs in pine forests. The genus name *Serenoa* was given in honor of Serenoa Watson of Harvard University, and *repens* is descriptive of the creeping growth of the plant (Bennett and Hicklin, 1998). According to Bailey (1939, 1949), the name *saw palmetto* was given in reference to the stiff palm-shaped leaves that are attached to petioles of up to 1.5 m in length covered with sharp, tough, recurved teeth such as those of a saw.

The stems grow horizontally and the trunk is usually horizontal too. Although of rare occurrence, if growing upright the trunk can reach heights of 7.6 m. The flowers are axillary, small, white, and numerous. From April to June, they appear on branches of shorter length than the leaves. The green or yellowish-green fruits ripen in September and October (Vines, 1960; Bailey, 1939, 1949). The berries, known as *bayas negras* by the locals (Harnischfeger and Stolze, 1989), are drupes reminiscent of olives. Deep reddish-brown and bluish-black when ripe, they reach a size of approximately 1.2 cm in length and 0.6 cm in width (Pizzorno and Murray, 1993; Bailey, 1939, 1949; Vines, 1960).

Saw palmetto also grows in Central America (Stenger et al., 1982), the Mediterranean region of southern Spain, North Africa (Weiss, 1996), Louisiana (Bailey, 1939, 1949), and Texas (Anonymous, 1994). Saw palmetto berries are harvested in Georgia, Alabama, and south and central Florida (Foster, 1997). During the late 1940s, saw palmetto covered an estimated 10% of the land surface of Florida (Bennett and Hicklin, 1998).

HISTORY AND TRADITIONAL USES

The Mayas used the roots and leaves of *Sabal japa* to make an infusion to treat abdominal pain and dysentery. The crushed root served as a poultice to treat sores on the breasts of men. The Mayas made a decoction of the inner trunk for the same purposes, which was also applied as a poultice on ulcers and taken as treatment for insect bites and snakebites. The Hoama Indians crushed the roots of dwarf palm *(Sabal adamsonii)* to obtain a juice they applied to sore eyes, even though it was known to produce a burning sensation. A decoction of the roots served as a treatment for kidney problems, while the dried root was given in cases of high blood pressure and the sensation of swimming in the head. The Alabama Indians employed the roots in a decoction with bramble *(Smilax glauca)* in the treatment of stomach problems and applied the mixture topically on broken back bones and back injuries (Vogel, 1970).

Saw palmetto provides cover or food for over 61 species of reptiles, 27 species of mammals, 100 species of birds, and 25 amphibian species. In Florida, the berries are a food source for bears, foxes, raccoons, gopher tortoises, feral hogs, waterfowl, and fishes. For white-tail deer, the berries constitute an important food source in the fall and winter. During the 1950s, it was said that cows feeding on the berries gave more, richer milk than could be produced from any other feed. In Europe, oil cakes made from the residue of the seeds and fruit were fed to livestock. Earlier, it was claimed that the berries fattened animals quicker than those fed either flax or rapeseed (Bennett and Hicklin, 1998).

The seeds were used as a food by American Indians and later the berries became an aromatic ingredient of cognac (Duke, 1985). Saw palmetto berries served as one the most important foods for pre-Columbian Indians of Florida, and they were eaten by sixteenth-century settlers from Spain. Their export to Europe began in 1602. At the turn of the nineteenth century, a soft drink sold in Miami known as "Metto" was made from the berry juice mixed with carbonated water. The taste of the berries was described by some early settlers to Florida as abhorrent. Seminole Indians warned against eating a serving of more than five berries at once, claiming that too many would cause the mouth to burn. Today, the Seminoles make a drink from the juice to which sugar is added (Bennett and Hickman, 1998). The branches served early settlers as material for brooms and baskets, and hats were made from the branches in Bermuda (Vogel, 1970). The fibrous roots have served in the manufacture of scrub brushes and the root pulp in the manufacture of wall board and for cartridge plugs during World War II. The dried petioles have been used by indigenous peoples of Florida to make ritual baskets used to sift corn, baskets for collecting medicinal plants, baskets for selling to tourists, and Seminole Indian dolls. These and numerous other recorded uses of saw palmetto by the Indians of Florida are reviewed by Bennett and Hicklin (1998).

During the late 1800s, Hale (1898) recorded numerous medicinal uses of the berries: rheumatism, anti-inflammatory/anticatarrhal, ozena, antitumor, alcoholism, headaches, neuralgia, anemia, alopecia, poor appetite, poor digestion, breast enlarging, breast atrophy, ovarian atrophy, asthma, bronchitis, laryngitis, respiratory congestion, respiratory infections, whooping cough, diarrhea, dysentery, dysmenorrhea, leukorrhea, cystitis, infections of the urinary tract, gonorrhea, male impotence, dysuria, urinary incontinence, irititis, prostate gland enlargement, afflictions of the reproductive organs, testicular atrophy, and sexual stimulant (Bennett and Hicklin, 1998, citing Hale, 1898). Both American Indians and the early eclectic and naturopathic physicians prescribed the berries in treating diseases of the genitourinary tract. For men, the berries were prescribed for relieving membrane irritations of the prostate and genitourinary tract and for increasing testicle function. In women, the berries were prescribed in treatments of the breasts. Taken long term, they were said to increase breast size (Pizzorno and Murray, 1993). Many herbalists of the day claimed the berries were an aphrodisiac (Pizzorno and Murray, 1993; Duke, 1985). As an aphrodisiac, the berries were said to quickly increase the flesh and strength of glandular tissue and for that reason were prescribed in the treatment of underdeveloped breasts and testes. One reference lists the berries as stimulating to the uterus, ovaries, testicles, prostate, and bladder, as well as being an aphrodisiac. Other attributes of the berries mentioned include: in folk medicine stimulant, diuretic, sedative, tonic, rejuvenating, and extremely nourishing. They were particularly noted for their efficacy in the treatment of the common cold, especially in alleviating irritations of the mucous membranes of the sinus, throat, and upper respiratory tract (Duke, 1985). The berries were listed in the *U.S. Pharmacopoeia* and *National Formulary* as an "official" drug during the period from 1906 to 1950, but after World War II they fell into disuse (Tyler, 1994; Blumenthal, 1997). In 1926, the twenty-sixth edition of the *United States Dispensatory* listed saw palmetto as an herbal remedy with a history of being particularly recommended for the treatment of enlarged prostate in elderly men (Foster, 1997); in 1900 and 1910, saw palmetto was listed among the official herbal medicines in the *U.S. Pharmacopoeia* (Boyle, 1991). Saw palmetto is currently being seriously considered for reentry into the *U.S. Pharmacopoeia* (Bennett and Hicklin, 1998).

CHEMISTRY

Carbohydrates

Saponifiable Lipids

The oil content of the berries is approximately 1.5% (Duke, 1985). Pharmacological studies of the total lipid extract and saponifiable extract of saw palmetto (Gutierrez, Garcia de Boto, et al., 1996; Gutierrez, Hidalgo, et al., 1996; Sultan et al., 1984) suggest that the lipophilic fraction consisting of fatty acids and sterols is the putative active constituent (Pizzorno and Murray, 1993); liposterolic extracts of the berries are standardized for oral use in human benign prostatic hypertrophy (BPH) (Blumenthal, 1997). With the probable exception of β-sitosterol, which occurs in saw palmetto in lower amounts (0.25%) (Niederprum et al., 1994) than found in everyday foods (Wagner et al., 1981), the putative active fraction of sterols in the supercritical CO_2 extract consists of the following: campesterol (0.063%), stigmasterol (0.024%), lignoceryl alcohol (0.003%), heaxacosanol (0.018%), L-octacosanol (0.190%), and triacontanol (0.027%) (Breu et al., 1992).

Lipid Compounds

Fats

Up to 75% of the total lipid fraction of the fruits consists of free fatty acids (Kloss, 1966). The other 25% of the fraction consists of neutral substances (Jommi et al., 1988). The content of fatty acids in the fatty acid fraction of a supercritical CO_2 extract of saw palmetto fruits is as follows: oleic acid (31.82%), lauric acid (28.64%), myristic acid (11.09%), palmitic acid (8.89%), linoleic acid (5.02%), stearic acid (2.70%), capric acid (1.76%), caproic acid (0.64%), and linolenic acid (0.59%). Other fatty acids in the extract are tridecanoic and undecanoic acid. The supercritical CO_2 extract itself consists of 0.17% fatty alcohols, 93.73% fatty acids, and 0.36% sterols (Niederprum et al., 1994). Variations in the amounts of these fatty acids occur, as evident in a more recent analysis of a supercritical CO_2 extract of the fruits—differences that may owe both to the raw material analyzed and the settings used to make the extract. An ethanolic extract of the fruits showed somewhat different amounts of the same fatty acids, most notably with greater concentrations of caproic (2.15% versus 1.39%) and oleic acids (34.84% versus 29.96%) and lesser amounts of linoleic (3.36% versus 6.42%) and capric acid (1.78% versus 2.74%) compared to the CO_2 extract (Ganzera et al., 1999).

Other Constituents

The fatty acid fraction of the fruits also contains cycloartenol, 24-methylene-cycloartenol, lupeol, long chain alcohols (farnesol and phytol), and polyprenolic alcohols (Jommi et al., 1988). The whole fruits contain 6% pectin, 10% sugars (sorbitol, fructose, and glucose), zinc (0.52 mg/100 g dry weight), phosphorus (1,620 mg/100 g dry weight), 0.9 calories/g, and 2.9% ash (Pedersen, 1994). They consist of about 16% flesh, 10% seed casing, 38% seed, and 36% skin (Harnischfeger and Stolze, 1989). In addition, carotenoids were found, which lend a strong orange color to the berry extracts (Griebel and Bames, 1916). Anthranilic acid in alcohol extracts of the fruits were found by Hänsel et al. (1964, 1966), and Hiermann (1989) isolated flavonoids. Wagner and Flachsbarth (1981) and Wagner et al. (1981, 1984, 1985) identified a number of polysaccharides. Shimada et al. (1997) found two monoacylglycerides. In an ether extract of the trunk and petiole, Pearl et al. (1959) detected acetovanillone, vanillin, vanillic acid, syringic acid, p-hydroxybenzaldehyde, and in the trunk extract found a considerable amount of p-hydroxybenzoic acid (> 80%). Ferulic acid and p-cumaric acid were found only in the trunk material.

THERAPEUTIC APPLICATIONS

Based on a selective review of the scientific literature on saw palmetto from 1977-1996 (Weissbach et al., 1977; Stenger et al., 1982; Tarayre et al., 1983; Smith et al., 1986; Breu et al., 1992; Niederprum et al., 1994; Koch and Biber, 1994; Carraro et al., 1996), ailments for which it may have therapeutic value include

- benign prostatic hypertrophy (BPH)
- urinary tract inflammation in men
- nocturia in men

- increased urinary frequency in men
- reduced caliber and force of urination in men
- painful urination in men
- bladder irritations in men
- urethral irritations in men

PRECLINICAL STUDIES

Endocrine and Hormonal Functions

Adrenal Functions

Against the backdrop of numerous proposed mechanisms of saw palmetto in the treatment of BPH, including 5α-R inhibition, sex hormone-binding globuline, and inhibition of lipoxygenase and cyclooxygenase, Goepel et al. (1999) emphasized that these mechanisms have failed to be demonstrated as therapeutically operative. Since most of the agents in wide use for the treatment of lower urinary tract symptoms "suggestive of benign prostatic obstruction" are α_1-adrenoreceptor antagonists (e.g., alfuzosin, doxazosin, prazosin, tamulosin, terazosin), Goepel and co-workers tested saw palmetto extract for the same activity. Other phytopharmaceutical substances used in the treatment of BPH, such as β-sitosterol, extracts of medicinal pumpkin (*Curcurbita pepo* L.), and stinging nettle (*Urtica dioica* L.) were also tested. Pumpkin seed powder and pumpkin seed extract oils showed no significant inhibition of the α_1-adrenoreceptor antagonist [^{3}H] prazosin in its binding to cloned human prostatic α_1-adrenoreceptors (up to a concentration of 0.1%), and five different extracts of stinging nettle showed only very weak activity (a maximum of 14% inhibition at 100 μg/mL). In the same test, β-sitosterol from three sources failed to show any significant inhibition at up to 10 mM. In sharp contrast, every saw palmetto oil they tested (TAD Pharma, Hoyer, Sanofi Winthrop, and Dr. Willmar Schwabe) and two powder extracts (SmithKline Beecham) tested showed almost complete inhibition of [^{3}H]prazosin binding to cloned human prostatic α_1-adrenoreceptors. The two powder extracts showed a maximum inhibition of [^{3}H]prazosin binding of 74 ± 4% from 125 μg/mL, and the other 59 ± 17% from 160 μg/mL. Their half-maximal inhibitory concentrations were approximately 60 μg/mL (Goepel et al., 1999). However, despite this positive in vitro activity, in a placebo-controlled, double-blind, four-way crossover study in healthy young men, three different saw palmetto extracts (320 mg p.o.) failed to produce α_{1A}-adrenoreceptor antagonistic activity (Goepel et al., 2001).

Reproductive Hormone Interactions

One of the main pharmacological activities of saw palmetto berries is inhibition of 5α-reductase (5α-R), the enzyme that catalyzes the conversion of testosterone to 5α-dihydrotestosterone (DHT). An accumulation of DHT in the prostate is believed to contribute to enlargement or hyperplasia of the gland (Koch and Biber, 1994). Additional interest in 5α-R inhibitors stems from the observation that DHT also plays a significant role in male pattern baldness, resistant acne, and idiopathic hirsuitism (Tenover, 1991; Liang and Liao, 1992).

Stenger et al. (1982) demonstrated a significant antiandrogenous effect ($p < 0.001$) in seminal vesicles and ventral prostate glands of male mice administered a liposterolic extract of the berries (PA 109, 300 mg p.o. daily for 13 days). In castrated male rats, the same extract (200 mg p.o. daily for six days) produced highly significant antiandrogenous activity without resistance to anabolizing effects. From concomitant administration of testosterone propionate, no changes were found in the weight of adrenal glands, spleen, and thymus, and no changes occurred in body weight. When tested against gonadotropin, the saw palmetto extract counteracted organ weight increases of the seminal vesicles, preputial glands, and the prostate, but not the adrenal glands or the thymus. Further tests in vitro and in vivo demonstrated an affinity of the extract for receptors in the prostate of rats, and inhibition of endogenous and exogenous androgenic stimulation of the prostate.

Screened in an in vitro assay using human foreskin fibroblasts, the liposterolic extract significantly inhibited the conversion of testosterone to dihydrotestosterone (DHT); antiandrogenic activity was observed only from high, unphysiological concentrations of the extract in vitro (Sultan et al., 1984). Similarly, Carilla et al. (1984) noticed that the liposterolic extract could inhibit binding of synthetic androgen to the cyctostolic receptor of the rat prostate in a competitive manner, which appeared to be the result of a direct interaction with prostate androgen receptors.

Duker et al. (1989) studied receptor binding and enzyme-inhibitory activities of an alcoholic extract of saw palmetto in human genital skin fibroblasts. They reported a substantial 50% inhibition of 5α-R from a 0.005% solution of the extract in dry form. Contrary to the liposterolic extract (Sultan et al., 1984) the alcohol extract caused no inhibition of androgen binding. In further tests, Duker and colleagues demonstrated that active substances from the alcoholic extract can penetrate through human genital skin fibroblasts. Inhibition of 5α-R activity reached 50% from a 0.01% solution of the extract in dried form. Extracting the fruits using a solvent of low polarity (petroleum ether) produced an extract "highly enriched" with an active principle, which they left undefined. The researchers explained that even though they could find no receptor binding "principle," the extract exerted some influence on tissues responsive to DHT, though seemingly without affecting testosterone-sensitive tissue.

Rhodes et al. (1993) compared the 5α-R inhibiting activity of a liposterolic extract of saw palmetto with that of finasteride (Proscar), a 5α-R-inhibiting drug approved by the FDA for the treatment of BPH. Using human prostate cells from patients with benign prostatic hyperplasia, an in vitro assay with radiolabeled testosterone showed finasteride (IC_{50} 1.0 ng/mL) to be 5,600 times more active than the saw palmetto extract (IC_{50} 5,600 ng/mL). Applying the ratio of activity found in vitro, they calculated a theoretically effective oral dose for rats as 560 mg/day, and then more than tripled it to 1,800 mg/day. Tests showed no activity on the growth of rat prostate. Other oral tests of the extract in rats with one and two times the human dose showed no 5α-reductase inhibitory activity, nor any antiandrogenic activity. Finasteride significantly inhibited testosterone-stimulated growth of rat prostate glands, but not DHT-stimulated growth of the prostate, which was consistent with the previously known activity of finasteride. The researchers noted that their results were not consistent with those of Sultan et al. (1984) or Carilla et al. (1984); the latter researchers, using exceptionally high in vitro doses of the extract (ID_{50}s equivalent to 268 μg/mL and 1,528 μg/mL, respectively), did demonstrate inhibition of 5α-R binding to human foreskin fibroblasts (Rhodes et al., 1993).

In further efforts to define 5α-R inhibition from a saw palmetto liposterolic extract, Niederprum et al. (1994) used incubated human genital skin fibroblast enzyme with labeled testosterone. To derive the active components of the extract, which were found to be free fatty acids, they used activity-guided fractionation. The nonsaponifiable fraction, which would hold triterpenes, sterols, and fatty alcohols, showed no 5α-R inhibitory activity, nor did anthranilic acid. Inhibition of 5α-R was shown to be dependent upon the chain length of the individual straight chain saturated fatty acids but only to a certain limit. Whereas they found no inhibitory activity from stearic, palmitic, margaric, caprylic, nonanoic, or caproic acids, in order of greater to lesser strength, the most significant inhibition of 5α-R was shown from linoleic (IC_{50} 0.8 mg/L), linolenic (IC_{50} 1.0 mg/L), tridecanoic (IC_{50} 1.3 mg/L), and lauric acid (IC_{50} 1.6 mg/L), which were more potent than the total saw palmetto extract (IC_{50} 44.7 mg/L). By contrast, weak inhibitors were oleic acid (IC_{50} 4.4 mg/L) and undecanoic acid (IC_{50} 3.5 mg/L). Active inhibitors of 5α-R with IC_{50}s soluble within the range in water were linolenic, tridecanoic, lauric, and undecanoic acids (Niederprum et al., 1994).

An ethanolic extract of the berries was studied in vitro by Weisser et al. (1996), who determined the active fatty acids in assays for 5α-R inhibition in the epithelium and stroma of incubated human BPH tissue. They reported no activity from the hydrophilic fraction containing polysaccharides, amino acids, and carbohydrates. The nonsaponifiable fraction, which contained mostly β-sitosterine and other sterols, showed only weak inhibitory activity of 5α-R in BPH stroma (15%) and epithelial cells (10%). In concentrations of 2 mM, the most active constituents were once again found in the free fatty acids, especially lauric acid with 51% and 42% inhibitory activity in stroma and epithelial cells, respectively, and myristic acid with 43% and 34% inhibitory activity in the same cells, respectively. Oleic acid (5% and 0%) and palmitic acid (2% and 0%) in the same respective assays showed only weak activity, while the ethanol extract of the berries showed more activity in the respective BPH cells (29% and 45%, with an IC_{50} of 500 µg/mL). In whole prostate homogenates, the IC_{50} was 2,200 µg/mL. A maximal inhibition of 5α-R was found with lauric acid at 0.2 mM, with inhibitory activity starting from 0.02 mM. Finally, the identities of the main fatty acids found in the ethanol extract were in accordance with the earlier findings of Kloss (1966) as oleic, myristic, palmitic, and lauric acids—collectively, over 90% of the total fatty acids present in the ethanol extract (Weisser et al., 1996).

Niederprum et al. (1994) explained that 5α-R as a membrane-bound enzyme is known to stabilize conformations through specific lipid environments, and may therefore be "influenced by free fatty acids." However, as common components of the Western European diet, the 5α-R-inhibitory fatty acids they found in saw palmetto are dwarfed by the amounts regularly ingested in foods. They speculated that the efficacy of saw palmetto liposterolic extracts may have been due to the fact that the fatty acids in the fruit are largely free fatty acids, whereas the majority of the free fatty acids known are mostly esterfied. They further speculated that in the unesterfied state as found in saw palmetto, free fatty acids may be more efficiently or readily taken up by the intestines. They noted that among the total lipids in BPH tissue, a substantial amount are free fatty acids (11.3 ± 1.4%), which may undergo changes that influence the lipid environment of 5α-R, in turn, producing another kind of enzyme activity (Niederprum et al., 1994). Five years later, 5α-R-inhibitory activity would become less of an issue when Goepel et al. (1999) reported that despite repeated testing, this mechanism had never been demonstrated as clinically operative.

Bayne et al. (1999), using a novel coculture model of BPH, examined the in vitro effects of a saw palmetto liposterolic (hexane) extract (Permixon) on changes in cell morphology. The in vitro model exhibits prostate-specific antigen (PSA), androgen receptors, and the two isoforms of α-R, and employs human BPH tissue (Bayne et al., 1998). At an in vitro concentration based on the recommended dosage and plasma concentration found in patients treated with the liposterolic extract (Permixon, 10 µg/mL), Bayne et al. (1999) found 5α-R types I and II were significantly inhibited (55.9% and 60.7%, respectively). Compared to the untreated prostatic fibroblast and epithelial cells, the intracellular (but not cellular) and mitochondrial membranes of the saw palmetto-treated prostate fibroblast and epithelial cells were disrupted, suggesting that the extract induced apoptotic activity and inhibited 5α-R types I and II by way of disrupting their enzyme environment. Prostate fibroblast and epithelial cell growth were not affected by the therapeutic concentration; a cytotoxic response was found only from concentrations of at least 25 μg/mL. Bayne and colleagues reported that PSA excretion by epithelial cells was unaffected by the therapeutic concentration, despite stimulating the cells with testosterone, and that contrary to the findings of others using unphysiologically high concentrations of saw palmetto extract, androgen receptor binding was not inhibited. In further in vitro studies using the same proprietary extract (Permixon), Bayne et al. (2000) reported that in cultures of epithelial and fibroblast cells of the testes, prostate, eididymis, kidneys, breast, and skin, the extract (10 μg/mL) caused the apoptotic index to increase by 35% in prostate stromal cells and by 12% in fibroblasts of the prostate epithelium, but by only 3% in skin fibroblast and not at all in the other cell cultures. 5α-R types I and II isoenzymes were inhibited by the extract but only in the prostate cells.

Immune Functions; Inflammation and Disease

Cancer

Cytotoxicity. Monoacylglycerides (1-monolaurin and 1-monomyristicin) derived from an ethanol extract of the berry powder have shown significant though moderate in vitro antitumor activity against human renal carcinoma (A-498) and human pancreatic carcinoma (PACA-2) cells. Antitumor activity against the human prostate adenocarcinoma cell line PC-3 was marginal, and the most potent activity was found from 1-monomyristicin against human pancreatic carcinoma (PACA-2) cells (ED_{50} 1.87 μg/mL) (Shimada et al., 1997).

Immune Functions

Immunopotentiation. Wagner and colleagues identified a number of polysaccharides from the berries that showed immunostimulating activity (Wagner and Flachsbarth, 1981; Wagner et al., 1981, 1984, 1985). A 4:1 water extract of the fruit produced an increase in phagocytosis activity of 36% from a concentration of 0.001% in vitro (Wagner et al., 1984). In mice, the polysaccharide fraction (10 mg/kg i.p.) produced a much higher carbon clearance value (3.8163) than Siberian ginseng (*Eleutherococcus senticosus,* 2.9040), Echinacea (*Echinacea purpurea,* 2.2152), and nine other different medicinal plant extracts (Wagner et al., 1985).

Inflammatory Response

Prior to the importance placed on 5α-R inhibition, it was assumed that the beneficial effects of saw palmetto extracts in BPH were largely due to antiedematous effects. To test the extract for antiedematous effects, Stenger et al. (1982) administered a liposterolic extract of saw palmetto to rats (5 g/kg p.o. followed by dextran i.p.). Compared to control rats receiving an equal dosage of olive oil, the saw palmetto extract produced significant antiedematous activity, indicating an inhibition of vascular phase inflammation. From doses of 1 g/kg p.o. and more, the extract also inhibited dextran-induced hypoaggregation of platelets in rats, and histamine-induced capillary fragility was inhibited by the extract when administered one hour before histamine.

Tarayre et al. (1983) used a liposterolic (hexane) extract of saw palmetto (1 mL/kg p.o. for five days) compared to controls treated with olive oil to test for activity against centrifuge-produced edema in mice. Saw palmetto extract exhibited no significant effects at 1 mL/kg (29%), but at 3 mL/kg p.o. the reduction of edema was significant (81%). In carrageenan-induced edema in rats, no significant inhibition of edema was found even with highest dose (10 mL/kg p.o.), a failure the researchers ascribed to an inherent lack of platelet cyclooxygenase activity by the extract. In dextran-induced edema in rats, a dose of 5 mL/kg p.o. one hour before the induced reaction significantly inhibited edema. Also, in passive IgE-dependent cutaneous anaphylactic shock reaction in rats, the extract (10 mL/kg p.o. administered 30 min beforehand) caused a significant inhibition of 34%. In the same dosage, the extract significantly reduced capillary permeability elicited by bradykinin and serotonin (maximally after 3 h). A further test of the extract in ultraviolet-induced erythema in guinea pigs found a significant reduction in the intensity of erythema from a one-hour prior dose of the extract (1 mL/kg p.o. in the 1-h exposure, and from 5 mL/kg p.o. in a 2-h exposure).

Breu et al. (1992) tested the in vitro antiphlogistic activity of a supercritical CO_2 extract of saw palmetto fruits (Talso, SG 291). The extract exhibited a dual inhibitory action: active on the 5-lipoxygenase pathway (IC_{50} 18.0 μg/mL) and the cyclooxygenase pathway (IC_{50} 28.1 μg/mL).

Integumentary, Muscular, and Skeletal Functions

Connective Tissue Functions

Using prostate tissues obtained from BPH patients, Paubert-Braquet et al. (1998) examined the in vitro antiproliferative activity of a saw palmetto liposterolic extract (Permixon) on the cell-proliferating effect of basic fibroblast growth factor (b-FGF, a growth factor identified in human prostate tissues), and on epidermal growth factor (EGF)-induced cellular proliferation of the prostatic tissue. The extract showed significant basal cell antiproliferative activity, but only on less than half of the specimens at the highest concentration tested (30 μg/mL). At 10 μg/mL and at 30 μg/mL, the saw palmetto extract showed a significant inhibition of b-FGF-induced proliferation of the human prostate tissues ($p < 0.01$) and a more modest inhibition of EGF-induced cell proliferation ($p < 0.05$) at the highest concentration (30 μg/mL). In comparison, the positive control, lovastatin, caused a pronounced inhibition of basal cell proliferation, b-FGF-induced proliferation ($p < 0.01$), and EGF-induced proliferation ($p < 0.001$).

In further tests, the researchers examined the antiproliferative activity of the unsaturated fatty acid fraction of the saw palmetto extract (UFA). From 1-30 ng/mL, no effect was found on basal-cell proliferation, and a modest and insignificant effect on b-FGF-induced proliferation was found. In one test in which a dramatic proliferation of BPH cells induced by b-FGF occurred, the UFA fraction caused a marked inhibition at 1, 10, and 30 μg/mL, reducing growth levels to those of the basal cell value ($p < 0.001$, compared to b-FGF-induced cell proliferation alone); however, the effect of the UFA fraction on basal-cell proliferation was minimal and in each case the effect of lovastatin was comparatively far more pronounced.

In a separate experiment, the main components of the saw palmetto extract and the extract itself were found to inhibit both b-FGF-induced and basal-cell growth of the DU145 prostate cell line. The researchers concluded that the beneficial effects of the saw palmetto extract as an inhibitor of EGF- and b-FGF-induced proliferation of human BPH prostate cells in cultures may explain the beneficial effects of the extract seen in BPH patients (Paubert-Braquet et al., 1998).

Muscular functions

In aorta, bladder, and uterus tissues, norepinephrine-induced smooth muscle contractions were dose-dependently inhibited in rat tissues ex vivo by the total lipid extract (EC_{50} 0.53 ± 0.05 mg/mL) and the total saponifiable extract (EC_{50} 0.5 ± 0.04 mg/mL) of saw palmetto. The maximum inhibition reached over 90% with either preparation from concentrations of 0.1 to 1 mg/mL. Against acetylcholine-induced contractions in rat urinary bladder tissues, both fractions (0.3-1 mg/mL) antagonized the contractions in a dose-dependent manner. Lower EC_{50} values were found in potassium chloride-induced smooth-muscle contractions than in norepinephrine-induced contractions of smooth-muscle tissue (Gutierrez, Garcia de Boto, et al., 1996); the possible involvement of α_1-adrenoreceptor-antagonizing activity was not determined (Goepel et al., 1999).

From in vitro tests of a lipidic extract of saw palmetto (free fatty acid content of 80% to 90%), Gutierrez, Garcia de Boto, et al. (1996) deduced that the spasmolytic effect of the extract may be due in part to interference with the mobilization of intracellular calcium and Na^+/Ca^{++} exchanger activation, and that the mediator may be cAMP. They also suggested that protein synthesis represents yet another part of the spasmolytic action of the extract.

Neurological, Psychological, and Behavioral Functions

Receptor- and Neurotransmitter-Mediated Functions

Vacher et al. (1995) tested the liposterolic extract of saw palmetto for prolactin-interfering activity in Chinese hamster ovary cells, which are devoid of 5α-R activity. Prolactin is a pituitary hormone that, like 5α-R, affects the growth of the prostate gland. The researchers explained that prolactin may stimulate prostate growth by itself or in conjunction with androgens, and that it may increase receptor levels of nuclear androgen. The saw palmetto extract (1 µg/mL) dose- and time-dependently reduced prolactin signal transduction in Chinese hamster ovary cells, and a high concentration (10 µg/mL) completely blocked the effects of prolactin. The action was due to prolactin-induced intracellular calcium-ion release; the saw palmetto extract inhibited K^+ conductance, thereby blocking Ca^{2+} influx. The researchers concluded that the most likely explanation for this action was that the saw palmetto extract acted directly on the K^+ channel, although several steps in the prolactin signal transduction pathway were also inhibited by the extract: inhibition of Ca^+-dependent K^+ channels; reduction of prolactin-stimulated Ca^+ influx; reduction of Ca^+ mobilization "from intracellular stores"; and inhibition of prolactin-stimulated protein kinase C activity of the liposterolic extract. Noting that prolactin alone is known to be involved in breast cancer and autoimmune diseases and that research has shown K^+ channel inhibitors interrupt cell growth, Vacher and co-workers pointed out that these actions of the extract may have implications in other disease conditions involving intracellular calcium, K^+ channels, and prolactin.

Van Coppenolle et al. (2000) compared the effects of saw palmetto extract (Permixon) to finasteride in models of hyperprolactinemia in intact and castrated male rats treated with implants containing either 5α-dihydrotestosterone or testosterone. Antiprolactinic activity in the prostate was evident from the saw palmetto extract but was absent in rats treated with finasteride.

Reproductive Functions

Prostate Functions

An uncharacterized extract of saw palmetto failed to significantly decease the weight or volume of enlarged prostate glands of dogs ($n = 20$) diagnosed with moderate to severe BPH, either from a dosage of 1,500 or

300 mg/day p.o. for 91 days. Since these doses were, respectively, equivalent to 50 mg/kg and 10 mg/kg, they were far in excess of those found clinically useful in humans (calculated at 4 mg/kg per day). The researchers also point out that unlike humans with BPH, it is uncommon for dogs to have an attendant decrease in the peak urine flow rate and an increase in residual volume (Barsanti et al., 2000).

CLINICAL STUDIES

Reproductive Disorders

Prostate Functions

The following selection of clinical studies is fairly representative of the trials of saw palmetto extracts that have largely been conducted with small numbers of patients diagnosed with BPH, a disorder estimated to affect 65% or more of men age 55 or older (Berry et al., 1984). The clinically relevant mechanism(s) of saw palmetto extract in BPH remain(s) to be established. Clinical trials of saw palmetto in combination with other herbs used to treat BPH (e.g., Marks et al., 2000) are not discussed.

In a comprehensive review of the evidence for saw palmetto for the treatment of BPH, Gerber (2000), commented that although objective and subjective benefits are suggested by meta-analyses and placebo-controlled trials, firm conclusions on the effectiveness of saw palmetto are constrained by the fact that the majority of them contain methodological flaws, were of short duration, and used small numbers of patients. Therefore, Gerber concluded that placebo-controlled trials in large numbers of patients would be required to determine the efficacy of saw palmetto.

Critical and systematic reviews of saw palmetto extracts in the treatment of BPH have arrived at much the same conclusions. A systematic review by Wilt et al. (1998) concluded that although the data are limited by short-term studies, variable study designs, extract preparations, and outcomes, they do suggest improvements in urological symptoms and urinary flow. Compared to finasteride, the results were similar, yet with fewer adverse events. Wilt and colleagues concluded that the determination of "long-term effectiveness and ability to prevent BPH complications" (Wilt et al., 1998, p. 1608) requires further research using standardized extracts of saw palmetto.

In a critical review of the research on saw palmetto, Bone (1998) noted that Descotes et al. (1995) specifically recruited from placebo nonresponders in their patient selection. Bone concluded that similar to the elusive mechanism of saw palmetto as a treatment for BPH, the cause of BPH itself remains inconclusively known, which renders the problem more understandable. He believes that although the evidence for saw palmetto has yet to become incontrovertible, it is sufficient enough to justify the use of saw palmetto in the treatment of mild to moderate cases of BPH (Bone, 1998).

Lowe and Ku (1996) noted that in the trials to date there were inconclusive evaluations of efficacy owing to problems of short treatment (usually a three-month duration), inclusion/exclusion criteria, and the lack of uniformity in symptom scores and analyses. They pointed out that contrary to the majority of placebo-controlled trials on BPH agents such as finasteride, doxazosin, and terazosin, which all found relatively high rates of improvements in the placebo groups, clinical studies of saw palmetto had more often than not reported no improvements from placebo. Therefore, they advised caution in regarding the results reported in the majority of clinical studies on saw palmetto, even though six of the seven double-blind studies to date had reported improvements, subjective and objective (Lowe and Ku, 1996).

Gerber et al. (2001) reported significant improvement in men with lower urinary tract symptoms administered an extract of saw palmetto (160 mg b.i.d., Nutraceutical, Ogden, Utah) standardized to contain 85% to 95% sterols and fatty acids. The clinical trial in 85 men age 45 or older diagnosed according to an International Prostate Symptom Score (IPPSS) of at least eight was randomized, double blind, and placebo controlled with a run-in period of one month. Patients were excluded if they had previously been treated with an alpha blocker within the past month, finasteride, saw palmetto, other alternative therapies, prostate surgery, or if they had any history of urethral stricture disease or prostate cancer. After a treatment period lasting six months, the men who received the saw palmetto extract showed twice the decrease in mean symptom score found in the placebo group (4.4 versus 2.2). No significant improvements compared to placebo were found in peak urinary flow rates, sexual function, or the quality-of-life score, which, however, increased more than in the placebo group (0.7 versus 0.3). The only side effects reported by those in the saw palmetto group were from a patient who complained of mild gastric distress and another who experienced diarrhea.

Weisser et al. (1997) conducted a prospective, randomized, double-blind placebo-controlled trial of saw palmetto extract in a high dosage (Strogen, IDS 89, 640 mg t.i.d. for three months) in 18 patients diagnosed with BPH. Following prostatectomy, tissues obtained from the patients were used to assess effects on BPH tissue enzyme activities for indications of effects on androgen metabolism. However significant, the changes found were at most moderate and their clinical significance to BPH was doubtful.

Braeckman, Bruhwyler, et al. (1997) conducted a multicenter single-blind, parallel, randomized, controlled design study of a critical CO_2 saw palmetto extract (Prostaserene) in 132 patients diagnosed with symptomatic BPH. Their purpose was to determine the therapeutic equivalence between a once-daily and a twice-daily dosage of the extract and its safety and efficacy. Patients were blinded as to the dosage received. Data analyses were performed only on patients showing a mictional volume of at least 100 mL at all visits, an international prostate symptom score (IPSS) of 12-24, a maximum age of 75, residual urinary volume of < 100, and a serum prostate-specific antigen (PSA) concentration of ≤ 10 ng/mL. Among the exclusion criteria were those individuals on any previous treatment for BPH, indications of surgical intervention, tumors or infections of the urinary tract, and those who were previously subjected to endoscopy of the lower urinary tract. The dosages compared were 160 mg b.i.d. and a single 320-mg dose daily for 360 days. The results of the intent-to-treat analysis showed that the two dosage groups were comparable in terms of evolution of the treatment according to the IPSS, and either dosage was significantly effective in modifying the score from day 30 until the end of the 360-day treatment period ($p < 0.0001$), in the end showing a 60% improvement in the score. This score included factors of prostatic volume decrease ($p < 0.0001$ from day 90 on), the maximum flow rate increase ($p < 0.0001$ from day 30), and the mean flow rate increase (days 30 and 180, $p < 0.01$; days 90 and 360, $p < 0.0001$). After the treatment, prostatic volume had improved 12%, the maximum flow rate by 22%, and the mean flow rate by 17%. Measurements of residual volume in the two groups showed the most significant decrease on day 30 ($p < 0.0001$), no significant decrease on day 90, and significant decreases on days 180 and 360 ($p < 0.01$ and $p < 0.05$, respectively). After day 360, the residual urinary volume showed an improvement of 16%. However "clinically nonsignificant," it is interesting to note that a statistically significant increase occurred ($p < 0.05$) in PSA levels in both groups from six months onward. The researchers concluded that the treatment was both "safe and effective" for BPH-associated mictional problems in patients with mild to moderate (grade I-II BPH) forms of the condition in either of the dosages tested, and that at six months the treatment was relatively comparable to results found in a six-month study with a hexane (liposterolic) extract of saw palmetto by Carraro et al. (1996). An equal number of patients in both groups reported side effects ($n = 8$), which appeared most often (75%) in the form of symptoms related to the course of the condition of BPH rather than to the treatment with the extract. The percentage of satisfied patients in the two groups was 83% and 88% for the 160 mg b.i.d. and 320 mg/day groups, respectively (Braeckman, Bruhwyler, et al., 1997).

With the purpose of confirming the safety and efficacy of a saw palmetto extract (Prostaserene, 160 mg b.i.d. for three months), Braeckman, Denis, et al. (1997) conducted a double-blind, randomized placebo-controlled trial in 238 patients diagnosed with mild to moderate symptoms of BPH. Nine patients withdrew or could not be reached for follow-up in the first month, leaving 229 patients for the safety evaluation. Efficacy was evaluated with data from 205 patients after 24 failed to meet the necessary inclusion criteria of BPH. The results showed that saw palmetto extract was superior to placebo in significantly decreasing urgency, dysuria (each $p < 0.01$), nocturia, and pollakisuria (each $p < 0.05$). Also, a higher number of patients in the saw palmetto group no longer experienced perineal heaviness (53.5%) compared to the placebo group (34.4%). Significant differences in symptoms of BPH were also found in saw palmetto patients after 60 days of treatment ($p < 0.05$). After 90 days of treatment, the differences were more significant ($p < 0.01$) in favor of saw palmetto. Nine patients reported side effects in the placebo group (8.3%) compared to 11 (9.1%) in the saw palmetto group, a difference of no statistical significance. Side effects probably related to the treatments also showed no significant difference between the two groups: two cases of allergic reactions and two of gastrointestinal complaints in the placebo group (3.7%), versus one each of fatigue, sexual, and gastrointestinal symptoms in the saw palmetto group (2.5%).

Carraro et al. (1996) studied a hexane extract of saw palmetto (Permixon) in a six-month, double-blind, randomized equivalence trial with finasteride (Proscar) in 1,098 patients (age 50 years and older) with moderate symptoms of BPH. Patients took the saw palmetto extract in the usual dosage (160 mg morning and evening) and finasteride in a dosage of 5 mg (mornings only). In general, symptoms were relieved with either agent in approximately 2/3 of cases, but some significant differences were found. An improved peak urinary flow rate was found in several more patients in the finasteride group (39%) than the saw palmetto group (36%). In residual volume, a significantly greater decrease occurred in the finasteride group compared to the saw palmetto group. Prostate volume was reduced in both groups, with the saw palmetto group showing a reduction of 7% versus a significantly greater 16% in the finasteride group. Serum levels of PSA were significantly lower at the end of the trial in the finasteride group but showed no change in the saw palmetto group. During the trial, seven patients on saw palmetto had acute urinary retention versus three on finasteride. The number of patients who withdrew from the trial was also greater in the saw palmetto group ($n = 86$) than in the finasteride group ($n = 61$). Conversely, among those in the finasteride group, a statistically significant number reported sexual function had deteriorated compared to those in the saw palmetto group. In the quality-of-life scores, saw palmetto improved the rate by 38% and finasteride by 41%. In the end, however, Carraro et al. (1996) concluded that both treatments were equally effective in the treatment of BPH.

Grasso et al. (1995) compared saw palmetto (160 mg b.i.d. for three weeks) to the α-adrenergic antagonist alfuzosin (2.5 mg t.i.d. for three weeks) in the treatment of 63 patients (ages 50-80) diagnosed with BPH in a double-blind, randomized parallel-groups study in which safety was also compared. Using the Boyarsky rating scale for urinary improvements, alfuzosin was superior to saw palmetto in the total score of reducing symptoms. With the exception of urgency, in which the number of patients who improved was almost identical in either treatment group (alfuzosin 25.0% versus saw palmetto 25.8%), greater numbers of patients treated with alfuzosin showed improvements in daytime frequency (68.7% versus 51.6%), nocturia (68.7% versus 64.5%), quality of stream (43.7% versus 25.9%), sensation of incomplete voiding (43.7% versus 35.5%), and hesitancy (46.8% versus 35.5%). Patient assessment of the increase in quality of micturition was significantly different between the two groups ($p < 0.0001$), also in favor of alfuzosin. The number of patients with a greater than 25% increase in peak flow rates compared to baseline was also noticeably greater in the alfuzosin group compared to the saw palmetto group (71.8% versus 48.4%). Grasso and colleagues reported that with the exception of one patient in the saw palmetto group who complained of mild pruritus which cleared up without treatment, no other complaints of side effects were noted, and heart rate, diastolic BP, and systolic BP showed no change related to either of the treatments.

Descotes et al. (1995) sought to reduce the high rate of placebo effect witnessed in a previous study of saw palmetto extract (Permixon) (Smith et al., 1986) by selecting symptomatic BPH patients already shown to be nonresponders to placebo. The short-term, double-blind, placebo-controlled multicenter study in 176 nonresponders to placebo consisted of an initial single-blind phase of selecting patients who showed less than a 30% improvement in their peak urinary flow rate from saw palmetto extract (Permixon, 160 mg b.i.d. for 30 days). The second phase consisted of randomly assigning the selected 176 men to the double-blind treatment with either placebo or the saw palmetto extract for 30 days using the same dose as the initial phase. All subjects were outpatients diagnosed with stage I or II (mild to moderate) BPH who two weeks before their entry had stopped all previous treatments. Hormonal therapies were stopped two months before patient entry. After the 30-day treatment, Descotes and his team found a respectively higher number of patients on saw palmetto extract compared to placebo with ameliorated symptoms of BPH: improvement in dysuria (31.3% versus 16.1%); daytime urinary frequency (11.3% versus 2.9% reduction); and significant in both groups (32.5%, $p = 0.0001$ versus 17.7%, $p = 0.0004$), a decrease in nocturnal urinary frequency ($p = 0.03$ versus placebo). Compared to baseline, the increase in the mean peak urinary flow rate was very significant in the saw palmetto (28.9%, $p < 0.0001$) but not significant in the placebo group (8.5%). Compared to placebo, the increase was also significant ($p = 0.04$). As for physician and patient global assessments of the treatments, the differences between the two groups were not significant, nor was patient assessment of tolerability as good (96.1% versus 98.9% for placebo). A closer examination of tolerability in the saw palmetto group revealed no instances of sexual dysfunction and only a single case in which treatment was discontinued because of complaints of symptoms (depression, fatigue, and upset stomach). The researchers commented that a six-month study would better allow the treatment to be assessed for therapeutic benefit (Descotes et al., 1995).

Braeckman, Denis, et al. (1997) reported the results of a multicentered placebo-controlled, double-blind randomized trial of a supercritical CO_2 extract of saw palmetto (Prostaserene, Indena, 160 mg p.o. b.i.d. for three months). After the treatment of 238 patients with mild to moderate BPH (229 evaluated for safety and 205 evaluated for efficacy), Braeckman and co-workers found statistically significant improvements in BPH symptoms of hesitancy, urgency, pollakisuria, dysuria, and nocturia, and the residual urinary volume and quality-of-life score, but not in urinary flow rates and prostatic volume. At the end of three months, favorable subjective evaluations of the saw palmetto treatment were highly significant, as were the physician evaluations ($p < 0.001$). Side effects probably related to the saw palmetto treatment occurred in only 2.5% of the patients (fatigue, sexual, and gastrointestinal), versus 3.7% of the placebo group (allergic reactions and gastrointestinal). Although nine patients were lost to follow up, the benefit of knowing the reasons was not provided by the researchers.

Rhodes et al. (1993) conducted a seven-day placebo-controlled clinical trial comparing finasteride (Proscar, 5 mg/day) with a saw palmetto extract (Permixon, 160 mg b.i.d.) or placebo in 32 male volunteers in good health. Using the normal prescribed dosages of each agent, they reported no significant changes in serum testosterone levels between any of the three groups, except at days 3 and 6 in the finasteride patients compared to the saw palmetto patients. They also reported significant decreases in serum dihydrotestosterone (DHT) levels in the finasteride group from days 2 to 8, but no changes in DHT of any significance in the saw palmetto group on any day. Similarly, Strauch et al. (1994) compared the effect of saw palmetto (Permixon) to that of finasteride (Proscar) to determine 5α-R inhibitory activity in 32 healthy male volunteers (ages 20-30). The one-week open, randomized placebo-controlled study consisted of tests for serum DHT levels to assess 5α-R inhibition, and treatment with either saw palmetto (160 mg b.i.d.), finasteride (5 mg/day), or placebo. Serum testosterone levels showed no increases outside of the normal range in either the saw palmetto or finasteride group. Serum DHT levels showed no significant change or difference in the saw palmetto group compared to the placebo group, whereas in the finasteride group the levels showed a significant and sustained decrease. The researchers concluded that based on the lack of data regarding cellular alterations of androgen from saw palmetto and the results of their own study, the proprietary saw palmetto extract (Permixon) tested would be unlikely to alter the androgen-dependent physiology of the prostate by way of 5α-reductase inhibition (Strauch et al., 1994).

In 35 BPH patients never previously treated for BPH, Di Silverio et al. (1992) conducted a randomized, double-blind placebo-controlled trial of a saw palmetto extract (brand or source not stated, 160 mg b.i.d.) to investigate effects on estrogen receptors. They reported significant antiestrogenic activity upon estrogen receptors in prostatic tissue and a significant decrease in progesterone receptor concentration of the saw palmetto extract-treated patients versus the placebo group ($p < 0.01$). Thus, the saw palmetto extract appeared to inhibit androgen and estrogen from binding to their respective receptors in BPH tissue of patients treated with the extract.

Mattei et al. (1988) conducted a placebo-controlled double-blind study in 40 patients with BPH. Significant differences were found compared to placebo in nocturia, dysuria, and residual urine ($p < 0.05$) after three months of treatment with a saw palmetto extract (LG 166/S, Laboratori Guidotti S.p.A., Pisa, Italy, 160 mg b.i.d.). The change in residual urine was also significant compared to baseline in the active treatment group ($p < 0.01$).

Smith et al. (1986) performed a 12-week, placebo-controlled clinical trial of a saw palmetto extract (Permixon). Results were evaluated in 70 patients with BPH (ages 55-80) whose symptoms had been ongoing for between six months and 6.5 years. At the end of the trial, urinary flow rate was significantly improved in both groups of patients (2.5 cc/s, $p < 0.01$); however, no significant change occurred in the bladder residual volume in either group. Physician assessments found significant improvements in both groups in many symptoms but, compared to each other, the two groups were equivocal. After six months, a follow-up questionnaire revealed that 26 of the patients felt they were improved. One patient reported a relapse since going off the treatment, and the remaining patients felt they had maintained their improvement since the end of the trial and did not require surgery. Among them, 13 had received the placebo and 12 had received saw palmetto. Comparison of self-assessment data showed no significant difference in the improvements reported between the two groups, although during the trial a greater number of symptoms were reported improved by the placebo group than the saw palmetto group. Among the few reporting any side effects, one patient ceased taking the extract for a day due to dizziness, two extract patients quit the trial because of nausea and vomiting, one ceased the extract for a few days because of nausea, and one patient in the saw palmetto group reported increased libido after the second week of treatment (Smith et al., 1986).

Tasca et al. (1985) conducted a randomized, double-blind placebo-controlled trial of a liposterolic extract of saw palmetto in 27 patients (ages 49-81) with stage I and II prostatic adenomas. Taken in the usual recommended dosage of 160 mg b.i.d., after 30 days the placebo group showed positive results in 15.4% of cases versus 42.9% in the active treatment group. Only one case of gastric disturbance occurred in the active treatment group.

Champault et al. (1984) studied the effects of saw palmetto extract (Permixon) in a placebo-controlled, randomized prospective trial in 110 outpatients (ages 47-92) with BPH who were not in need of surgery. The selection criteria consisted of men who had a sufficient extent of prostatic adenoma to cause constant suffering as the result of either objective problems, such as a diminishing rate of micturition and postmicturitional residue, or functional problems, such as nocturnal and diurnal pollakisuria (too frequent urination) and dysuria, or both types of problems. Of the initial 110 patients, data on 94 were available for analysis. Following 30 days of treatment (160 mg b.i.d.), the mean number of nocturnal micturitions was reduced in the saw palmetto group by 46%, which was significantly different from the placebo-treated patients ($p < 0.001$). The reduction in dysuria was also significantly greater in the saw palmetto group, as was the rate of micturition ($p < 0.001$), which showed an increase in volume of 50%. In the placebo group no change in these parameters occurred. In the postvoid residue (PVR), a minor increase was noted in the placebo group after 30 days, while those on saw palmetto showed a significant decrease of 42% compared to baseline ($p < 0.001$). In subjective assessments of the treatment, the saw palmetto group reports scored significantly higher than the placebo group ($p < 0.001$). Physician assessments of the two groups also showed a highly significant difference in favor of the saw palmetto group, and the treatment was well tolerated.

Boccafoschi and Annoscia (1983) reported a significantly increased flow rate of 9.6-13.7 cc/s in a double-blind trial of a saw palmetto extract (Permixon, 320 mg/day for 60 days) in 22 patients diagnosed with prostatic adenomatosis. The PVR decreased from 63 cc to 36 cc in the saw palmetto group, whereas in the placebo group the tendency was toward a decrease in the PVR of 29 cc. Similarly, the flow rate improved in the placebo group by 1.9 cc/s and in the active treatment group by 2 cc/s.

In 30 BPH patients (ages 44-78), Emili et al. (1983) conducted a randomized, placebo-controlled double-blind trial of a saw palmetto liposterolic hexane extract (Permixon, 160 mg b.i.d. for 30 days). At the end of the study, significant differences compared to placebo were reported with improvements of strangury, residual urine, nocturia, dysuria, voiding rate, and the volume of the prostate. The flow rate showed an increase of 3.4 cc/s and the PVR decreased from 71 cc/s at the start of the trial to 36 cc/s after the saw palmetto treatment.

Open-label studies of saw palmetto extracts have largely reported the same favorable results found in placebo-controlled trials but remain suspect owing to the lack of a placebo control (Gerber et al., 1998; Braeckman,

Bruhwyler, et al., 1997; Bach and Ebeling, 1996; Vahlensieck et al., 1993; Casarosa et al., 1988; Carreras, 1987).

DOSAGE

The standardized liposterolic extract (85%-95% fatty acids and sterols) of saw palmetto is used in a dosage of 160 mg b.i.d. The dosage for the unprocessed berries is 10 g b.i.d. (Pizzorno and Murray, 1993), but anti-inflammatory/antiphlogistic effects are not expected from anything less than a liposterolic extract (Tyler, 1994).

SAFETY PROFILE

The Belgian government approves the use of saw palmetto as a prescription adjuvant in the treatment of BPH. In Germany, the Commission E approves the use of saw palmetto in nonprescription use for the relief of "symptoms associated with enlarged prostate" (Blumenthal et al., 1998, p. 201). In Sweden, the berries are simply given the status of a natural product; in the United States, saw palmetto is classified as a dietary supplement (Blumenthal, 1997), and previously by the FDA it was classified as an herb of undefined safety (Duke, 1985).

Ingestion of large amounts of saw palmetto berries is reported to cause diarrhea (Anonymous, 1994; Blumenthal, 1997).

Contraindications

No contraindications for saw palmetto are given by the German Commission E (Blumenthal et al., 1998).

Drug Interactions

No drug interactions are known (Blumenthal et al., 1998).

Pregnancy and Lactation

The *Lawrence Review of Natural Products* (Anonymous, 1994) and Blumenthal (1997) considered saw palmetto berries contraindicated for use during pregnancy and lactation, citing a lack of safety data and potential hormonal activity. The German Commission E monograph does not include pregnancy or lactation as a contraindication nor does it address female reproductive issues at all (Blumenthal et al., 1998), perhaps assuming women would not use saw palmetto. However, saw palmetto has been used as a treatment for conditions such as alopecia and polycystic ovarian syndrome

(PCOS)-related symptoms, and is reputed to increase breast size, so use by women must be anticipated (see History and Traditional Uses).

A recent animal study showed dose-dependent inhibition of norepinephrine-induced smooth-muscle contractions by saw palmetto extract in ex vivo rat uterine tissues (Goepel et al., 1999) (see Preclinical Studies: Adrenal Functions). Vacher et al. (1995) found antiprolactinemic activity in female hamsters. A saw palmetto extract (1 µg/mL) dose and time dependently reduced prolactin signal transduction in ovarian tissue. At high concentration (10 µg/mL), prolactin effects were completely blocked. In another study, comparing a saw palmetto extract (Permixon) and finesteride in male rats, Van Coppenolle et al. (2000) found evidence of antiprolactinemic activity in the prostate with saw palmetto extract, but not with finesteride (see Preclinical Studies: Receptor- and Neurotransmitter-Mediated Functions).

On the other hand, previous short-term toxicology studies with female animals have so far failed to show any negative reproductive effects, though studies of pregnant or lactating animals and offspring are lacking. Following oral dosing, no effect on the estrus cycle in mature female mice was found. In prepubescent mice, no estrogenic or progestational activity was detected after oral treatment for three days. After six days, there was no increase in uterine or ovarian weight. No change in pituitary function was found (Stenger et al., 1982) (see Toxicity in Animal Models). Clinical trials involving women appear to be completely lacking.

Saw palmetto berries have been a main source of food for some aboriginal cultures in North America. Ethnomedicinal use included a very wide range of conditions, including breast enlargement. Historic use by the Eclectic physicians included use specific to treating the breast; their writings included observations of breast enlargement with long-term use. The berries have also been used as galactogogues in animals, with reports of increased and richer milk in cows (see History and Traditional Uses).

Recommendations for use during pregnancy or lactation are not able to be guided by specific information at this time. Documented antiprolactin effects indicate caution, even though toxicology studies focused on fertility have failed to show negative effects at the doses used. Its traditional use as food and medicine give a positive impression. Studies of pregnant or lactating animals are lacking. Studies of women are completely lacking. No documented adverse effects during pregnancy or lactation are known.

Side Effects

No side effects of a significant nature have been reported in clinical trials of the berry extract (Pizzorno and Murray, 1993); however, headaches have been reported (Anonymous, 1994). The German Commission E reports an infrequent occurrence of cramping and nausea (Anonymous, 1996) and stomach problems (Blumenthal et al., 1998).

Special Precautions

Due to a lack of safety data, saw palmetto is not recommended for children (Anonymous, 1994).

The German Commission E suggests that patients using the herb for an enlarged prostate consult with their physician regularly because the berry extract may only treat symptoms of the condition (McGuffin et al., 1997).

Toxicology

Toxicity in Animal Models

No side effects were found in male Sprague-Dawley rats with oral doses of 10 mL/kg (Tarayre et al., 1983). Using a hexane extract of the berries, the acute oral LD_{50} in male rats was shown to be 54 mL/kg. In male mice, no fatalities occurred even from a dose of 50 mL/kg. No side effects were found in male Sprague-Dawley rats with oral doses of 10 mL/kg (Tarayre et al., 1983).

Stenger et al. (1982) demonstrated that the liposterolic extract of the berries (PA 109) at dosages of 100, 200, and 400 mg p.o. daily for three days had no effect on the estrus cycle in adult female mice. Administered to prepubertal female mice, the extract (100 and 200 mg p.o. daily for three days) produced no estrogenic or progestational activity. Female mice treated with extract (100 mg p.o. daily for six days) also showed no uterine hypertrophy; it was without effect on estradiol benzoate on the uterus; and it showed no effect on pituitary inhibition and no change in the weight of the uterus or the ovaries.

REFERENCES

Anonymous (1994). Saw palmetto. *Lawrence Review of Natural Products,* p. 2.

Anonymous (1996). Botanical toxicology. *The Protocol Journal of Botanical Medicine* 1: 227.

Bach, D. and Ebeling, L. (1996). Long-term drug treatment of benign prostatic hyperplasia—Results of a prospective 3-year multicenter study using *Sabal* extract IDS 89. *Phytomedicine* 3: 105-111.

Bailey, L. (1939). *The Standard Cyclopedia of Horticulture* (p. 3639). New York: Macmillan Co.

Bailey, L. (1949). *Manual of Cultivated Plants on the Continental United States and Canada* (p. 1116). New York: Macmillan Co.

Barsanti, J.A., Finco, D.R., Mahaffey, M.M., Fayrer-Hosken, R.A., Crowell, W.A., Thompson, F.N., and Shotts, E.B. (2000). Effects of an extract of *Serenoa repens* on dogs with hyperplasia of the prostate gland. *American Journal of Veterinary Research* 61: 880-885.

Bayne, C.W., Donnelly, F., Chapman, K., Bollina, P., Buck, C., and Habib, F.K. (1998). A novel co-culture model for benign prostatic hyperplasia expressing both forms of 5α-reductase. *Journal of Clinical Endrocrinology and Metabolism* 83: 206-213.

Bayne, C.W., Donnelly, F., Ross, M., and Habib, F.K. (1999). *Serenoa repens* (Permixon®): A 5α-reductase types I and II inhibitor—New evidence in a coculture model of BPH. *The Prostate* 40: 232-241.

Bayne, C.W., Ross, M., and Habib, F.K. (2000). Selectivity and specificity of actions of lipido-sterolic extract of *Serenoa repens* (Permixon) on prostate. *Journal of Urology* 164 (3, Part 1): 876-881.

Bennett, B.C. and Hicklin, J.R. (1998). Uses of saw palmetto (*Serenoa repens*, Arecaceae) in Florida. *Economic Botany* 52: 381-393.

Berry, S.J., Coffey, D.S., Walsh, P.C., and Ewing, L.L. (1984). The development of human benign prostatic hyperplasia with age. *Journal of Urology* 132: 474-479.

Blumenthal, M. (1997). *Popular Herbs in the U.S. Market: Therapeutic Monographs* (pp. 55-56). Austin, TX: American Botanical Council.

Blumenthal, M., Busse, W.R., Goldberg, A., Gruenwald, J., Hall, T., Riggins, C.W., and Rister, R.S. (Eds.) (1998). *The Complete German Commission E Monographs* (p. 201). Austin, TX: American Botanical Council.

Boccafoschi, C. and Annoscia, S. (1983). Confronto fra estratto di *Serenoa repens* e placebo mediate prova clinica controllata in pazienti con adnenomatosi prostatica. *Urologia* 50: 1257-1268.

Bone, K. (1998). Saw palmetto—A critical review. *European Journal of Herbal Medicine* 4: 15-24.

Boyle, W. (1991). *Official Herbs: Botanical Substances in the United States Pharmacopoeias 1820-1990* (pp. 46-47). East Palestine, OH: Buckeye Naturopathic Press.

Braeckman, J., Bruhwyler, J., Vandekerckhove, K., and Geczy, J. (1997). Efficacy and safety of the extract of *Serenoa repens* in the treatment of benign prostatic hyperplasia: Therapeutic equivalence between twice and once daily dosage forms. *Phytotherapy Research* 11: 558-563.

Braeckman, J., Denis, L., de Laval, J., Keuppens, F., Cornet, A., De Bruyne, R., De Smedt, E., Pacco, J., Timmermans, L., Van Vliet, P., et al. (1997). A double-blind, placebo-controlled study of the plant extract *Serenoa repens* in the treatment of benign hyperplasia of the prostate. *European Journal of Clinical Research* 9: 247-259.

Breu, W., Hagenlocher, M., Redl, K., Tittel, G., Stadler, F., and Wagner, H. (1992). Antiphlogistische wirkung eines mit hyperkritischem kohlendioxid gewonnenen sabalfrucht-extraktes [Anti-inflammatory activity of sabal fruit extracts prepared with supercritical carbon dioxide. In vitro antagonists of cyclooxygenase and 5-lipoxygenase metabolism]. *Arzneimittel-Forschung/Drug Research* 42: 547-551.

Carilla, E., Briley, M., Fauran, F., Sultan, C., and Duvilliers, C. (1984). Binding of Permixon®, a new treatment for prostatic benign hyperplasia, to the cytosolic androgen receptor in the rat prostate. *Journal of Steroid Biochemistry* 20: 521-523.

Carraro, J.C., Raynaud, J.P., Koch, G., Chisholm, G.D., Di Silverio, F., Teillac, P., Da Silva, F.C., Cauquil, J., Chopin, D.K., Hamdy, F.C., et al. (1996). Comparison of phytotherapy (Permixon®) with finasteride in the treatment of benign prostate hyperplasia: A randomized international study of 1,098 patients. *Prostate* 29: 231-240.

Carreras, J.O. (1987). Nuestra experiencia con extracto hexánico de *Serenoa repens* en el tratamiento de la hipertofia benigna de próstata [New experiences with a hexane extract of *Serenoa repens* in the treatment of benign hypertrophy of the prostate]. *Archivos Españoles de Urologia* 40: 310-313.

Casarosa, C., De Coscio, M.C., and Fratta, M. (1988). Lack of effects of a liposterolic extract of *Serenoa repens* on plasma levels of testosterone, follicle-stimulating hormone, and luteinizing hormone. *Clinical Therapy* 10: 585-588.

Champault, G., Bonnard, A.M., Cauquil, J., and Patel, J.C. (1984). Traitment médical de l'adénome prostatique—Essai control: PA 109 versus placebo chez cent dix patients [A controlled study: PA 109 versus placebo in one hundred and ten patients]. *Actualite Therapeutique, Annales d Urologie* (6), 407-410 (translation). See also Champault, G., Patel, J.C., and Bonnard, A.M. (1984). A double-blind trial of an extract of the plant *Serenoa repens* in benign prostatic hyperplasia. *British Journal of Clinical Pharmacology* 18: 461-462 (letter).

Descotes, J.L., Rambeaud, J.J., Deschaseaux, P., and Faure, G. (1995). Placebo-controlled evaluation of the efficacy and tolerability of Permixon® in benign prostatic hyperplasia after exclusion of placebo responders. *Clinical Drug Investigation* 9: 291-297.

Di Silverio, F., D'Eramo, G., Lubrano, C., Flammia, G.P., Sciarra, A., Palma, E., Caponera, M., and Sciarra, F. (1992). Evidence that *Serenoa repens* extract displays an antiestrogenic activity in prostatic tissue of benign prostatic hypertrophy patients. *European Urology* 21: 309-314.

Duke, J.A. (1985). *CRC Handbook of Medicinal Herbs* (p. 443). Boca Raton, FL: CRC Press.

Duker, E.M., Kopanski, L., and Schweikert, H.U. (1989). Inhibition of 5α-reductase activity by extracts from *Sabal serrulata*. *Planta Medica* 55: 587.

Emili, E., Lo Cigno, M., and Petrone, U. (1983). Resultati clinici su un nuovo farmaco nella terapia dell'ipertrofia della prostata (Permixon®) [Clinical results with a new drug in the therapy of hypertrophy of the prostate (Permixon)]. *Urologia* 50: 1042-1048.

Foster, S. (1997). Saw palmetto comes of age. *Business of Herbs* (May/June): 14-16.

Ganzera, M., Croom, E.M. Jr., and Khan, I.A. (1999). Determination of the fatty acid content of pumpkin seed, *Pygeum,* and saw palmetto. *Journal of Medicinal Food* 2: 21-27.

Gerber, G.S. (2000). Saw palmetto for treatment of men with lower urinary tract symptoms. *The Journal of Urology* 163: 1408-1412.

Gerber, G.S., Kuznetsov, D., Johnson, B.C., and Burstein, J.D. (2001). Randomized, double-blind, placebo-controlled trial of saw palmetto in men with lower urinary tract symptoms. *Urology* 58: 960-965.

Gerber, G.S., Zagaja, G.P., Bales, G.T., Chodak, G.W., and Conteras, B.A. (1998). Saw palmetto *(Serenoa repens)* in men with lower urinary tract symptoms: Effects on urodynamic parameters and voiding symptoms. *Urology* 51: 1003-1007.

Goepel, M., Dinh, L., Mitchell, A., Schafers, R.F., Rubben, H., and Michel, M.C. (2001). Do saw palmetto extracts block human α_1-adrenoceptor subtypes in vivo? *Prostate* 46: 226-232.

Goepel, M., Hecker, U., Krege, S., Rubben, H., and Michel, M.C. (1999). Saw palmetto extracts potently and noncompetitively inhibit human α_1-adrenoreceptors in vitro. *Prostate* 38: 208-215.

Grasso, M., Montesano, A., Buonaguldi, A., Castelli, M., Lania, C., Rigatti, P., Rocco, F., Cesana, B.M., and Borghi, C. (1995). Comparative effects of alfuzosin versus *Serenoa repens* in the treatment of symptomatic benign prostatic hyperplasia. *Archivos Españoles de Urologia* 48: 97-104.

Griebel, C. and Bames, E. (1916). Über eine zur aromatisierung des kognaks dienende palmfrucht [About a palm fruit used to aromatize cognac]. *Zeitschrift für Untersuchung der Nahrungs- und Genussmittel sowie der Gebrauchsgenstaende* 31: 282-290.

Gutierrez, M., Garcia de Boto, M.J., Cantabrana, B., and Hidalgo, A. (1996). Mechanisms involved in the spasmolytic effect of extracts from *Sabal serrulata* fruit on smooth muscle. *General Pharmacology* 27: 171-176.

Gutierrez, M., Hidalgo, A., and Cantabrana, B., (1996). Spasmolytic activity of a lipid extract from *Sabal serrulata* fruits: Further study of the mechanisms underlying this activity. *Planta Medica* 62: 507-511.

Hale, E.M. (1898). *Saw palmetto (Sabal serrulata, Serenoa serrulata): Its History, Botany, Chemistry, Pharmacology, Provings, Clinical Experience and Therapeutic Applications.* Philadelphia: Boericke and Taffel.

Hänsel, R., Rimpler, H., and Schopflin, G. (1964). Eine dunnschicht chromatographische untersuchung der sabalfruchte [A thin layer chromatographic examination of the sabal fruit]. *Planta Medica* 12: 169-172.

Hänsel, R., Schopflin, G., and Rimpler, H. (1966). Notiz uber das vorkommen von anthranilsaure in sabalfruchten *(Serenoa repens)* [A note on the occurrence of anthranilic acid in sabal fruits]. *Planta Medica* 14: 261-265.

Harnischfeger, G. and Stolze, H. (1989). *Serenoa repens*—die sagezahnpalme [*Serenoa repens*—The saw tooth dwarf palm]. *Zeitschrift für Phytotherapie* 10: 71-76.

Hatinguasi, P., Belle, R., Basso, Y., Ribet, J.P., Bauer, M., and Pouset, J.L. (1981). Composition de l'extrait hexanique de fruits de *Serenoa repens* Bartram [Composition of the hexane extract of the fruits of *Serenoa repens* Bartram]. *Travaux de la Societe de Pharmacie de Montpellier* 41: 253-262.

Hiermann, A. (1989). Über inhalstoffe von sabalfrüchten und prufung auf entzundünghemmende wirkung [About the contents of sabal fruits and their examination searching for an anti-inflammatory effect]. *Archiv der Pharmazie* 322: 111-114.

Jommi, G., Orsini, F., Sisti, M., and Verotta, L. (1988). Enantioselective synthesis of 3(S)-acetoxy-5(R)-hydroxycyclopent-1-ene by an enzymic transesterification in organic solvents. *Gazzetta Chimical Italiana* 118: 863-864.

Kloss, P. (1966). [Steam vaporizable constituents of pressed juice of *Sabal serrulatum* (Roem et Schutt)]. *Arzneimittel-Forschung/Drug Research* 16: 95-96.

Koch, E. and Biber, A. (1994). Pharmacological effects of *Sabal* and *Urtica* extracts as basis for a rational medication of benign prostatic hyperplasia. *Urologe* 34: 90-95 (translation).

Liang, T. and Liao, S. (1992). Inhibition of steroid 5α-reductase by specific aliphatic unsaturated fatty acids. *Biochemical Journal* 285: 557-562.

Lowe, F.C. and Ku, J.C. (1996). Phytotherapy in treatment of benign prostatic hyperplasia: A critical review. *Urology* 48: 12-20.

Marks, L.S., Partin, A.W., Epstein, J.I., Tyler, V.E., Simon, I., Macairan, M.L., Chan, T.L., Dorey, F.J., Garris, J.B., Veltri, R.W., et al. (2000). Effects of a saw palmetto herbal blend in men with symptomatic benign prostatic hyperplasia. *Journal of Urology* 163: 1451-1456.

Mattei, F.M., Capone, M., and Acconcia, A. (1988). Impeigo dell'estratto di *Serenoa repens* nel trattamento medico della ipertrofia prostatica benigna [*Serenoa repens* in the medical treatment of benign prostatic hypertrophy]. *Urologia* 55: 547-552.

McGuffin, M., Hobbs, C., Upton, R., and Goldberg, A. (Eds.) (1997). *American Herbal Products Association's Botanical Safety Handbook* (p. 107). Boca Raton, FL: CRC Press.

Niederprum, H.J., Schweikert, H.U., and Zanker, K.S. (1994). Testosterone 5α-reductase inhibition by free fatty acids from *Sabal serrulata* fruits. *Phytomedicine* 1: 127-133.

Paubert-Braquet, M., Cousse, H., Raynaud, J.P., Mencia-Huerta, J.M., and Braquet, P. (1998). Effect of the lipidosterolic extract of Serenoa repens (Permixon®) and its major components on basic fibroblast growth factor-induced proliferation of cultures of human prostate biopsies. *European Urology* 33: 340-347.

Pearl, I.A., Beyer, D.L., and Laskowski, D. (1959). Alkaline hydrolysis of representative palms. *Tappi* 42: 779-782.

Pedersen, M. (1994). *Nutritional Herbology: A Reference Guide to Herbs* (p. 153). Warsaw, IN: Wendell W. Whitman Company.

Pizzorno, J.E. and Murray, M.T. (1993). *A Textbook of Natural Medicine,* Vol. 1. Seattle, WA: Bastyr College Publications.

Rhodes, L., Primka, R.L., Berman, C., Vergult, G., Gabriel, M., Pierre-Malice, M., and Gibelin, B. (1993). Comparison of finasteride (Proscar®), a 5α-reductase inhibitor, and various commercial plant extracts in in vitro and in vivo 5α-reductase inhibition. *Prostate* 22: 43-51.

Shimada, H., Tyler, V.E., and McLaughlin, J.L. (1997). Biological active acylglycerides from the berries of saw-palmetto *(Serenoa repens)*. *Journal of Natural Products* 60: 417-418.

Smith, H.R., Memon, A., Smart, C.J., and Dewbury, K. (1986). The value of Permixon® in benign prostatic hypertrophy. *British Journal of Urology* 58: 36-40.

Stenger, A., Tarayre, J.P., Carilla, E., Delhon, A., Charveron, M., Morre, M., and Lauressergues, H. (1982). Étude pharmacologique et biochemique de l'extrait hexanique de *Serenoa repens* B (PA 109) [Pharmacological and biochemical study of the hexanoic extract of *Serenoa repens* B (PA 109)]. *Gazette Medical de France* 89: 2041-2048 (translation).

Strauch, G., Perles, P., Vergult, G., Gabriel, M., Gibelin, B., Cummings, S., Malbecq, W., and Malice, M.P. (1994). Comparison of finasteride (Proscar®) and *Serenoa repens* (Permixon®) in the inhibition of 5-Alpha reductase in healthy male volunteers. *European Urology* 26: 247-252.

Sultan, C., Teaza, A., Devillier, C., Carilla, E., Briley, M., Loire, C., and Descomps, B. (1984). Inhibition of androgen metabolism and binding by a liposterolic extract of *"Serenoa repens* B" in human foreskin fibroblasts. *Journal of Steroid Biochemistry* 20: 515-519.

Tarayre, J.P., Delhon, A., Lauressergues, H., Stenger, A., Barbara, M., Bru, M., Villanova, G., Caillol, V., and Aliagra, M. (1983). Action anti-oedemateuse d'un extrait hexanique de drups de *Serenoa repens* Batr. [Anti-edematous action of a hexane extract from *Serenoa repens* Bartr. drupes]. *Annales Pharmaceutiques Francaises* 41: 559-570 (translation).

Tasca, A., Barulli, M., Cavazzana, A., Zattoni, F., Artibani, W., and Pagano, F. (1985). Trattamento della sintomatologigia ostruttiva da adenoma prostatico con estratto di *Serenoa repens:* Studio clinico in doppio cieco *versus* placebo [Treatment of obstructive symptomatology in prostatic adenoma with an extract of *Serenoa repens:* Double-blind clinical study versus placebo]. *Minerva Urologica e Nefrologica* 37: 87-91 (translation).

Tenover, J.S. (1991). Prostates, pates, and pimples. *Endocrinology and Metabolism Clinics of North America* 20: 893-909.

Tyler, V.E. (1994). *Herbs of Choice: The Therapeutic Use of Phytomedicinals* (pp. 82-85). Binghamton, NY: The Haworth Press, Inc.

Vacher, P., Prevarskaya, N., Skryma, R., Audy, M.C., Vacher, A.M., Odessa, M.F., and Dufy, B. (1995). The lipidosterolic extract from *Serenoa repens* interferes with prolactin receptor signal transduction. *Journal of Biomedical Science* 2: 357-365.

Van Coppenolle, F., Le Bourhis, X., Carpentier, F., Delaby, G., Cousse, H., Raynaud, J.P., Dupouy, J.P., and Prevarskaya, N. (2000). Pharmacological effects of the lipidosterolic extract of *Serenoa repens* (Permixon®) on rat prostate hyperplasia induced by hyperprolactinemia: Comparison with finasteride. *Prostate* 43: 49-58.

Vines, R.A. (1960). *Trees, Shrubs and Woody Vines of the Southwest* (p. 1104). Austin, TX: University of Texas Press.

Vogel, V.J. (1970). *American Indian Medicine* (pp. 365-366). Norman, OK: University of Oklahoma Press.

von Vahlensieck, W., Volp, A., Lubos, W., and Kuntze, M. (1993). Benigne prostatahyperplaise—Behandlung mit sabalfrucht-extrakt [Benign prostatic hyperplasia—Treatment with sabal fruit extract. A treatment study of 1,334 patients]. *Fortschritte der Medizin* 111: 323-326.

Wagner, H. and Flachsbarth, H. (1981). A new antiphlogistic principle from *Sabal serrulata*, I. *Planta Medica* 41: 244-251.

Wagner, H., Flachsbarth, H., and Vogel, G. (1981). Über ein neues antiphlogistisches wirkprinzip aus *Sabal serrulata* II [A new antiphlogistic principle from *Sabal serrulata* II]. *Planta Medica* 41: 252-258 (translation).

Wagner, H., Proksch, A., Riess-Maurer, I., Vollmar, A., Odenthal, S., Stuppner, H., Jurcic, K., Le Turdu, M., and Fang, J.N. (1985). [Immunostimulating action of polysaccharides (heteroglycans) from higher plants. Preliminary communication]. *Arzneimittel-Forschung/Drug Research* 35: 1069-1075.

Wagner, H., Proksch, A., Reiss-Maurer, I., Vollmar, A., Odenthal, S., Stuppner, H., Jurcic, K., Le Turdu, M., and Heur, Y.H. (1984). [Immunostimulating action of polysaccharides (heteroglycans) from higher plants. Preliminary communication]. *Arzneimittel-Forschung/Drug Research* 34: 659-661.

Weiss, F.R. (1996). *Herbal Medicine* (pp. 249-250). Beaconsfield, England: Beaconsfield Publishers Ltd.

Weissbach, I., Wegner, G., and Schweikert, H.U. (1977). Konservative therapie der prostataerkrankungen [The conservative therapy of diseases of the prostate gland]. *Therapiewoche* 27: 6009-6021 (translation).

Weisser, H., Behnke, B., Helpap, B., Bach, D., and Krieg, M. (1997). Enzyme activities in tissue of human benign prostatic hyperplasia after three months' treatment with the *Sabal serrulata* extract IDS 89 (Strogen®) or placebo. *European Urology* 31: 97-101.

Weisser, H., Tunn, S., Behnke, B., and Krieg, M. (1996). Effects of *Sabal serrulata* extract IDS 89 and its subfractions on 5α-reductase activity in human benign prostatic hyperplasia. *Prostate* 28: 300-306.

Wilt, T.J., Ishani, A., Stark, G., MacDonald, R., Lau, J., and Mulrow, C. (1998). Saw palmetto extracts for treatment of benign prostatic hyperplasia. A systematic review. *Journal of the American Medical Association* 280: 1604-1609.

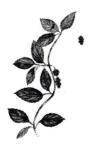

$\mathcal{S}chisandra$

BOTANICAL DATA

Classification and Nomenclature

Scientific name: *Schisandra chinensis* (Turcz.) Baillon, *Schisandra sphenanthera* Rehd. et Wils.

Family name: Schisandraceae (or Magnoliaceae)

Common names: schisandra, magnolia vine (Canada, England, United States), wuweizi (China), limonnik (Russia), omicha (Korea), gomishi (Japan)

Schisandra chinensis was first described as *Kadsura chinensis,* and later also as *Maximowiczia chinensis.* Both genera were renamed *Schisandra,* joining *S. coccinea,* an American species for which the genus was first described (Foster and Yue, 1992).

The name *Schisandra* is derived from the Greek *schizein,* meaning to cleave, and *andros,* or man, which refers to the split or separate anther cells of the stamen described of *S. coccinea* (Foster and Yue, 1992). In China, wuweizi is the most frequently used common name; however, beiwuweizi (fruit of *Schisandra chinensis*) is more accurate. The spellings *Schisandra* and *Schizandra* are both found in naming the genus and are used as common names; we therefore refer to *S. chinensis* as schisandra unless otherwise indicated. Other names include: *Fructus Schisandrae, Fructus Schisandrae chinensis,* and schizandraes (Wagner and Bauer, 1996; Foster and Yue, 1992). In Russia, Schisandra is called *limonnik,* referring to the lime fragrance of the crushed fruit. In Korea, the common name is *omicha* and in Japan, *gomishi* (Ikeya et al., 1979). In the United States and Canada, schisandra is the most frequently used common name.

Description

Introduced from Eastern Russia into European botanical gardens in the late 1850s, the common English name is magnolia vine or Chinese magnolia vine. Schisandra often grows in English and other Western European gardens as an ornamental. All species are native to eastern Asia except *Schisandra coccinea,* which occurs as a rare vine in the southeastern United States in Florida, Louisiana, Georgia, Arkansas, Tennessee, and North Carolina. The species used medicinally range over eastern portions of Siberia, the Sakhalin peninsula, Korea, Japan, and northeastern China. *Schisandra chinensis* (beiwuweizi), the species most commonly used in commerce, originates in Northern China and has red/violet-red fruit. *Schisandra sphenanthera* (nanwuweizi) has smaller and browner fruits and originates in Southern China (Foster and Yue, 1992).

Schisandra is a woody perennial vine with deciduous leaves and a stem 10-15 m in length (1.2-1.5 cm in diameter) known to wind around the trunks of trees. The attractive leaves are alternate, cuspidate, and elliptic, and are wedge shaped at their base (Hancke et al., 1999). The dioecious flowers are white, yellow, or reddish in color and have a pleasant fragrance. The spherical fruits are a brilliant scarlet when ripe and contain one to two yellow kidney-shaped seeds, which are used medicinally with the outer fruit (Foster and Yue, 1992). The fruits measure 5-7 mm in diameter when ripe and the hard yellow seeds are about 3.5 mm wide and 4.5 mm long. In China, the dried fruits are considered best when they are flat, large, and shiny with a purplish-red color and a wrinkled appearance (Yen, 1992). However, other authorities claim that bright red berries, large, oily, and shiny in appearance, are the best quality. When the fruits ripen from September to November, the receptacle takes on a distinctive cluster-like shape (pedicle), like that of a small bunch of grapes. The fruits smell like limes; the skin is sweet; the flesh is sour; and the seeds are pungent or hot/astringent. The overall effect, however, is salty—hence the name wuweizi, or "five-taste fruits" (Foster and Yue, 1992).

HISTORY AND TRADITIONAL USES

Schisandra was first cited in the *Shen Nong Ben Cao Jing* (The divine farmer's materia medica), which is thought to have been written more than 4,000 years ago. Here, the fruits of schisandra are noted for their usefulness in treating cough, emaciation and languor, taxation damage, boosting the essence of males, supplementing insufficiency, and fortifying yin. In eighteenth-century China, schisandra was used to treat impotence (Yang, 1997).

In current TCM use, schisandra is used mainly to treat asthmatic cough, dry mouth related to dehydration, spontaneous or night sweats, chronic diarrhea and dysentery, nocturnal emission, insomnia, amnesia, and palpitation (Chang and But, 1986). Official indications for the fruits in China include diabetes, frequent urination, night sweats, chronic cough, and shortness of breath (Tu et al., 1992). In the traditional medicine of China and Japan, schisandra is used as an antihepatotoxic, antidiabetic, antiasthmatic, antitussive, sedative, tonic, and to treat cholera (Wagner and Bauer, 1996). In southwest China, schizandra is widely employed to treat bone fractures, influenza, and snakebites (Huang, 1999).

Schisandra fruits are combined in many Chinese traditional medicines. For example, *sheng mai san,* a compound of *Schisandra chinensis, Panax ginseng* Meyer, and *Ophiopogon japonicus* (Thunb.) Ker-Gawl in a ratio of 1.5:1:3 (Zhu et al., 1988) is used to treat coronary heart disease (Li et al., 1996). Another compound formula *(pen zu yian nian bo zi ren yuan),* containing one part each of biota seeds (*Biota orientalis* Endl.) and the roots of *Panax ginseng* to three parts schisandra fruits, was used to treat amnesia, insomnia, palpitations, asthma, bronchitis, spermatorrhea, dry stools, constipation, and congestion; however, animal studies indicate that it may benefit memory registration, consolidation (Nishiyama et al., 1995), and retention (Nishiyama et al., 1996).

CHEMISTRY

The main active constituents have been identified as lignans; they have been variously named by Chinese, Russian, and Japanese scientists employing a nonstandardized terminology. This monograph generally uses botanical Latin-derived terminology over the competing Chinese or Japanese terms (see Table 1) The general term often used for the schisandra lignans is *schisandrins* (or *schizandrins*). Throughout the main body of this chapter, the updated chemical nomenclature, after Hancke et al., 1999, and Zhu, 1998, precedes the older equivalents used by the various researchers cited; e.g., gomisin A (= schisandrol B).

Lipid Compounds

Oils

The fruit contains 2%-3% essential oil (Zhu, 1998; Hancke et al., 1999) consisting of β-chamigrenal, α- and β-chamigrene, and citral. The fatty oil content of the total fruit is 38% (Zhu, 1998) and the fixed oil content of the seed is 30% to 33% (Yen, 1992).

TABLE 1. Schisandra Lignan Nomenclature

General Name for Schisandra Lignans (Schisandrins, Schizandrins)	Alternate Name
Schisantherin A (Ser A)	Gomisin C, wuweizu ester A, schisandrer A, schisander A, schizanhenol (Sal)
Schisantherin B (Ser B)	Gomisin B, wuweizu ester B, schisandrer B, schisander B
Schisantherin C	None known
Schisantherin D	None known
Schisantherin E	None known
Schisandrin A (Sin A)	Deoxyschisandrin, schizandrin A
Schisandrin B (Sin B/Sch B)	Schizandrin B
Schisandrin C (Sin C)	None known
Schisandrol A (Sol A)	Gomisin A, wuweizichum B, schisandrol, TJN-101, schizandrol A
Schisandrol B (Sol B)	None known
Gomisin D - N, S & T	None known
Angeloylgomisin	None known
Anwulignan	None known
Wulignan	None known
Epiwulignan	None known
Epischishisandron	None known
DDB	Synthetic schisandrin: dimethyl-4,4'-dimethoxy-5,6, 5', 6'-dimethylenediox biphenyl-2,2'-dicarboxylate
Schiarisanrin A	None known
Schiarisanrin B	None known
Schiarisanrin C	None known
Schiarisanrin D	None known

Source: Adapted from Wagner and Bauer, 1996.

Organic Acids

The fruits contain fumaric, citric, malic, and tartaric acids (Hancke et al., 1999).

Phenolic Compounds

Lignans

The lignans of schisandra are dibenzo-[*a,c*]-cyclooctene lignans. The seeds contain more than 30 different lignans, comprising about 7% to 19% of the total constituents, while they make up only about 2% of the fruit (Hancke et al., 1999). The stems contain from 1.3% to as high as 10% of these lignans (Hancke et al., 1999). Seeds from cultivated plants in Europe have shown a 2.76% lignan content, with schisandrin, gomisin N, and deoxyschizandrin occurring as the main lignans (Slanina et al., 1995). Others have shown that the amounts of lignans in the fruits vary according to time of harvest and that the major lignans are schisandrin (2% to 9%), schisandrin B (= γ-schisandrin) (1% to 5%), gomisin A (= schisandrol B) (0.7% to 3%), and deoxyschisandrin (0.2% to 1.1%). A more recent analysis of the dried fruits found the major constituents to be schisandrin, gomisin L_2, schisandrin C, gomisin L_1, schisanhenol, gomisin N, tigloylgomisin H, and gomisin A (= schisandrol B) (He et al., 1997).

Terpenoid Compounds

Nigranoic acid (3,4-secocycloarta-4(28),24-(Z)-diene-3,-26-dioic acid) (Wagner and Bauer, 1996).

Monoterpenes

Borneol, 1-8 cineol, citral, *p*-cymol, and α- and β-pinene (Wagner and Bauer, 1996).

Sesquiterpenes

Sesquicarene, (+)α-ylangene, chamigrenal, α- and β-chamigrene (Wagner and Bauer, 1996).

Other Constituents

Vitamins C and E, fumaric acid, stigmasterol, nordihyroguaiaretic acid (NDGA) (Wagner and Bauer, 1996), and citrostadienol (3β, 4α, 5α, 24Z)-4-methylstigmasta-7,24(28)-dien-3-ol, α_1-sitosterol (Lee et al., 1997). Major constituents of the leaves are (*E*)-cinnamic acid, kaempferol, quercetin (Sladkovsky et al., 2001), and β-carboline alkaloids (Tsuchiya et al., 1999).

THERAPEUTIC APPLICATIONS

By far, the most extensive data on schisandra supporting clinical application concerns hepatoprotective activities, especially in infectious or toxin-induced hepatitis, and as an aid for liver tissue regeneration after liver surgery/hepatectomy, and hepatitis.

In Chinese traditional medicine, schisandra is used mainly to treat asthmatic cough, dry mouth from dehydration, spontaneous or night sweating, nocturnal emission, chronic diarrhea, dysentery, insomnia, amnesia, palpitation, other nervous states (Chang and But, 1986), and to induce sedation (Yao et al., 1996). Bensky and Gamble (1990) list traditional uses for coughs, wheezing, diarrhea, nocturnal emission, spermatorrhea, leukorrhea, frequent urination, morning diarrhea, amnesia, and insomnia.

The evidence to date, obtained mostly from equestrian research, shows some potential of schisandra as an aid to athletic performance and recovery. Human studies indicate improved mental work, night vision, and other improvements in visual and tactile performance assessments, which have suggested the application of schisandra against symptoms such as fatigue (Hancke et al., 1994, 1996; Ahumada et al., 1989).

Anecdotal reports from China include the use of schisandra in the treatment of mild spastic paralysis resulting from stroke, as well as in cerebellar ataxia and Parkinson's disease. Use of a combination product in treating Meniere's disease may merit further investigation. Other uses of schisandra by doctors in China are as an antidote to morphine-induced respiratory depression, in treating prolonged labor, gastrointestinal (GI) bleeding, dysentery, infectious shock states, and symptoms of neurasthenia (headache, insomnia, dizziness, palpitations, and physical and mental fatigue) (Chang and But, 1986). More contemporary anecdotal accounts from China claim success in treating chronic fatigue syndrome with whole schisandra berries and ginseng (decoction of 150 g berries and 10 g ginseng rootlets), and the berries alone in treating menopausal syndrome (100 g taken daily as a decoction) (Leung, 1999).

PRECLINICAL STUDIES

The main pharmacological activities of schisandra were summarized by Wagner and Bauer (1996):

In vitro: antioxidant (Lu and Liu, 1992) and antibacterial (Chang and But, 1986)

In vivo: liver-protective; SGPT-lowering (Bensky and Gamble, 1990); anti-inflammatory in stomach and GI tract (Tang and Eisenbrand, 1992); stimulating lung function (Chang and But,

1986); "adaptogenic"; cardiovascular (systemic); uterine stimulant (Bensky and Gamble, 1990); neuroleptic; and anticonvulsant (Tang and Eisenbrand, 1992).

Although nearly all the work with isolated schisandrins has focused on gomisins B and C (= schisantherins A and B), deoxyschisandrin (= schisandrin A), schisandrins B and C, and/or schisandrin (= schisandrol A), extensive in vitro and in vivo investigations of various schisandra lignans have been performed. Overall, many of the observed hepatic effects are very similar to those of milk thistle *(Silybum marianum)* and appear to be based on similar mechanisms of action in the protection of hepatic and other vital tissues (Wagner and Bauer, 1996).

Cardiovascular and Circulatory Functions

Cardiotonic; Cardioprotection

Jung et al. (1997) showed that deoxyschisandrin (= schisandrin A) inhibited platelet activating factor (PAF) receptor binding in vitro; however, it was calculated to be 100 times less potent than ginkolide B from *Ginkgo biloba;* schisandrins B and C were even less potent. Li et al. (1996) reported that pretreatment of rats with a high dosage of a lignan-enriched extract of schisandra (800 mg/kg per day p.o. for three days) protected against myocardial injury in isolated perfused rat hearts. These effects were similar to a pretreatment benefit from α-tocopherol at the same dosage. The researchers related the benefit to previously demonstrated antioxidant effects of schisandra.

Cholesterol and Lipid Metabolism

Kwon et al. (1999) identified 12 lignans from schisandra that exhibited moderate acyl-CoA:cholesterol acyltransferase inhibitory activity in vitro, the most potent being gomisin N (IC_{50} 25 μM), one of the most abundantly occurring lignans in the fruits. Other active schisandra lignans were identified as gomisins K3 (IC_{50} 37 μM), L2 (IC_{50} 38 μM), A, B, J (IC_{50} 51 μM), angeloylgomisin H, benzoylgomisin O (IC_{50} 47 μM), schisandrin, schisantherin D, tigloylgomisin P, and wuweizisu (Kwon et al., 1999).

Digestive, Hepatic, and Gastrointestinal Functions

Gastric Functions

Salbe and Bjeldanes (1985) studied intestinal tissue from rats fed two-week dietary regimens of either a semisynthetic basal diet (control), a basal diet plus schisandra fruits 5%, or a basal diet plus 25% brussels sprouts or rat chow. One group of chow-fed rats received 20 mg of 3-methylcholanthrene/kg p.o. before sacrifice. Microsomal and cytosol fractions were examined for various enzyme activities, including assays of benzo[a]pyrene (BaP) metabolism. The largest increase in intestinal mixedfunction oxidase activity was seen in the toxin-treated group. In the tissue of schisandra-fed rats, an increase in cytochrome P-450 was not seen but induction was noted in the brussels sprouts and rat chow group. The production of aryl hydrocarbon hydroxylase (AHH) was inhibited in the schisandra group, whereas the activity of 7-ethoxycoumarin O-deethylase (ECD), epoxide hydratase (EH) and glutathione S-transferase (GST) were increased compared to the control. In assays of BaP metabolism, the smallest amounts of BaP-epoxide and BaP-quinones were produced in the brussels sprouts and schisandra groups, leading the researchers to suggest that both plants can mediate toxicity induced by ingested chemicals at the level of intestinal exposure.

In high doses in rats, schisandrin, and to a lesser extent gomisin A, inhibited stress-induced gastric ulceration by 74.4% and 51.3%, respectively (each 100 mg/kg p.o.). In pylorus-ligated rats, schisandrin also inhibited gastric juice secretion (100 mg/kg i.d.) whereas gomisin A was weakly active (Maeda et al., 1981). Conversely, when Hernandez et al. (1988) investigated the antisecretory and antiulcer activity of a schisandra fruit powder extract (4:1) in male rats, a single 30-min pretreatment (50 mg/kg i.p.) had no effect on cold-restraint stress-induced gastric ulcers, and none on gastric acid secretion.

Hepatic Functions

Numerous animal studies on the hepatoprotective activity of schisandra extracts or its constituents have reported improvements in survival rates and liver enzyme profiles. Despite the fact that the doses tested have often been far in excess of a human therapeutic dose of schisandra or a concentrated extract thereof, the results are promising and may lead to the development of a drug for the treatment or prevention of various diseases affecting the liver.

A standardized (2% schizandrins) dried extract of Chinese-grown *S. chinensis* fruit was used in a randomized placebo-controlled study of racehorses suffering from poor performance and persistently high levels of hepatic gamma-glutamyltransferase (GGT), hepatic and striated muscle enzyme GOT, and striated and cardiac muscle enzyme creatinine phosphokinase (CPK). Treatment or placebo was administered daily (3 g/day p.o.) for 14 days, with serum levels of these enzymes assayed on days 7 and 14. At both times, the results showed that the extract significantly reduced GGT, GOT, and CPK levels, and that by day 14 it had decreased indirect bilirubin levels. The researchers concluded that horses with high enzyme levels fundamentally suffered from hepatic and muscle damage, and that in those treated with the schisandra extract both kinds of tissues were recovering by day 14.

No evidence of improved racing performance was presented (Hancke et al., 1996).

Zhu et al. (2000) studied the restorative/therapeutic effect of a spray-dried powder extract of Schisandra seeds containing 84.1% dibenzocyclooctene derivatives (160 mg/kg i.g. at 8, 24, 32, and 48 h) in a model of liver impairment in male rats treated with CCl_4. After the last dose, antipyrine (80 mg/kg i.g.) was administered as a probe to gauge oxidative drug metabolism. The Schisandra-treated rats showed a dramatic 2.3-fold increase in hepatic cytochrome P-450 ($p < 0.01$) and a significant 1.5-fold increase in oxidative drug metabolism (according to the pharmacokinetics of antipyrene), compared to CCl_4-treated rats without schisandra.

Schisandra fruit extracts administered either before or following exposure of mice to carbon tetrachloride (CCl_4) decreased liver SGPT levels compared to untreated controls (Liu, 1977). Schisandrins B and C, gomisins A, B, and C (= schisandrol B, schisantherin B, and schisantherin A, respectively) were active, while deoxyschisandrin (= schisandrin A) and schisandrin (= schisandrol A) were not active against CCl_4 toxicity in vitro (Liu and Lesca, 1982; Bao et al., 1980). The seed extract showed more hepatoprotectant activity than the fruit extract (Bao et al., 1980). This heptoprotective activity was thought to be due to the induction of hepatic microsomal cytochrome P-450, with each lignan showing a varying profile of inductive effects that elude simple classification. Liu and Lesca (1982) concluded that the active schisandrins affect CCl_4 metabolism mediated by hepatic cytochrome P-450, which leads to decreased peroxidative damage and alkylation of lipids in membranes of the hepatic endoplasmic reticulum (see also Liu et al., 1981).

Kubo et al. (1992) reported that in rats administered gomesin A (50 mg/kg p.o.) prior to partial hepatectomy, hepatic DNA synthesis, the mitotic index, and levels of ornithine decarboxylase (ODC) and putresine were significantly enhanced. Increased ODC activity is considered an important biochemical event in the early stages of liver regeneration, and stimulation of ODC by gomesin A was interpreted as evidence of liver regeneration activity. Mizoguchi, Kawada, et al. (1991) reported that pretreatment of rats with a diet containing 0.06% gomisin C (= schisantherin A) for at least four weeks increased the survival rate in a model of acute liver failure (*Propionbacterium acnes* induced). Histological changes of the liver improved remarkably. Splenocyte reactivity to phytohemmagglutin and pokeweed mitogen as well as splenocyte interleukin-1 (IL-1) productivity were retained. The researchers suggested that oral administration of gomisin C may arrest the development of acute hepatic failure. In a model of immunologically induced acute hepatic failure in guinea pigs, Mizoguchi, Shin, et al. (1991) reported that gomisin C (10 or 50 mg/kg p.o.) significantly increased survival rates of the animals (by 60% and 75%, respectively) and significantly decreased serum transaminase levels (GOT and GPT).

Rats administered CCl_4 and gomisin C (= schisantherin A) as a pretreatment showed markedly reduced liver enzyme activities (GOT, GTP, LDH, T-BIL, and T-CHO). Other schisandrins showed positive but weaker effects. Similar positive effects were seen with gomisin C against the effects of other toxins (galactosamine, orotic acid). Gomisin C (50 mg/kg i.p.) countered CCl_4-induced decrease of indocyanin green secretion in rats showing reduced liver function, allowing bile flow and biliary output of electrolytes to maintain at near-normal levels. Gomisin C also enhanced DNA synthesis and cell division after partial hepatectomy. Ornithine decarboxylase as well as hepatic putrescine activity was enhanced in the early stages of regeneration (Maeda et al., 1985).

Mak and Ko (1997) reported that pretreatment with schisandrin B (0.875 μmol/kg per day p.o. for three days) protected streptozotocin-induced, short-term diabetic male rats against CCl_4 hepatotoxicity (0.2 mL/kg i.g.), as did pretreatment with insulin (4 U i.m. in the morning and 6 U i.m. in the evening for three days). The increase in plasma alanine aminotransferase (ALT) activity was inhibited from pretreatment with schisandrin B by 78%, and from insulin pretreatment by 92%. Schisandrin B pretreatment also resulted in a significant lowering of hepatic oxidized glutathione (GSSG) levels, and although it had no effect on the decreased level of reduced glutathione (GSH), it improved the ratio of GSH/GSSG and partly restored hepatic vitamin-C levels depleted by CCl_4. In contrast, insulin pretreatment completely restored the hepatic vitamin-C level. Both insulin and schisandrin B-pretreated rats showed significant increases in hepatic microsomal GST (glutathione S-transferase) activity compared to those treated with CCl_4 alone. Schisandrin B also prevented the increased activity in mitochondrial selenium-glutathione peroxidase (GPX) induced by CCl_4. As a treatment, rather than a pretreatment, schisandrin B (0.875 mmol/kg p.o. in a suspension of 0.5 mL olive oil daily for three days) increased hepatic mitochondrial glutathione reductase (GRD) activity in CCl_4-intoxicated diabetic rats and those not treated with CCl_4. Mak and Ko (1997) concluded that schisandrin B may useful in protecting the liver against toxicity from xenobiotics in diabetic states.

Suzuki et al. (1989) reported that gomisin C (= schisantherin A) (10^{-8} to 10^{-5} M) exhibited a cytoprotective effect on cell membranes of cultured rat hepatocytes against heat- or hypotonia-induced hemolysis and inhibited the influx of calcium ions into and the leakage of glutamic oxalacetic acid transferase (GOT) out of injured hepatic cells. Ohkura et al. (1990) demonstrated suppression of leukotriene B_4 (LTB_4) production with gomisin C in ex vivo rat macrophages; however, 5-lipoxygenase was unaffected. Gomisin C dose-dependently suppressed the release of arachidonic acid from guinea pig macrophages stimulated with fMet-Leu-Phe or calcium ionophore A23187, but the activity of phospholipase A_2 was not affected. The researchers suggested that gomisin C prevents the release of arachidonic acid, thus preventing LTB_4 production, and that gomisin C's previously demonstrated ability to stabilize cell membranes and suppress calcium influx may be the mechanisms by which arachidonic acid release and thus leukotriene production is avoided in liver-cell injury (Ohkura et al., 1990).

Liu et al. (1982) reported that schisandrins and DDB, an intermediate in the synthesis of schisandrin C (see Table 30.1), favorably affect rat liver microsomal monooxygenases and epoxide hydrolase. According to Liu (1985), schisandrins B and C, gomisin A (= schisandrol B) and DDB significantly increase rat liver cytochrome P-450 concentration, NADPH-cytochrome c reductase, benzphetamine, and aminopyrine demethylase activities, and strongly stimulate smooth endoplasmic reticular proliferation of rat liver cells. As part of their inducing effects, the schisantherins bind to cytochrome P-450 or trans-stilbene oxide, which induces cytochrome P-450.

Schisandrin B or DDB (1 mmol/kg per day p.o. for 3 days) prior to treatment of mice with CCl_4 suppressed the increase in ALT activity—schisandrin B more so than DDB. Schisandrin B also caused a significant decrease in plasma sorbital dehydrogenase activity, but DDB was inactive. Hepatic mitochondrial glutathione redox status and mitochondrial glutathione reductase activity of the CCl_4-treated and control mice pretreated with schisandrin B was significantly increased, whereas DDB increased these measurements only in control mice (Ip et al., 2000a). As pretreatment in mice against hepatic oxidative changes induced by menadione, schisandrin B (1 mmol/kg p.o. for three days) decreased plasma ALT activity by 78% and the level of hepatic malondialdehyde by 70%. In cultured rat hepatocytes isolated from the menadione-treated rats that received schisandrin B, researchers found that the rate of menadione elimination had increased, a change the researchers associated with a significant increase in DT-diaphorase activity in the hepatocytes of the mice pretreated with schisandrin B compared to controls (Ip et al., 2000b).

In a study on cAMP monophosphate phosphodiesterase (PDE), the schisandra constituent nordihyroguaiaretic acid (NDGA) proved a very potent inhibitor of cAMP PDE. NDGA noncompetitively inhibited cAMP PDE, displaying inhibition kinetics in Lineweaver-Burk plots that were similar to papaverine. The researchers concluded that NDGA and NDGA tetramethyl ether both inhibit cAMP PDE by a similar mechanism. The schisantherins were also tested and showed highly variable inhibitory effects. Gomisin C (= schisantherin A) inhibition kinetics showed a noncompetitive inhibition pattern in Lineweaver-Burk plots (Sakurai et al., 1992). Other in vitro studies demonstrating hepatoprotective effects of schisandra lignans are found in Hikino et al. (1984), Takeda et al. (1987), Ohtaki et al. (1994), and Ko et al. (1994).

Immune Functions; Inflammation and Disease

Cancer

Antiproliferative activity. In a two-stage carcinogenesis model in mouse skin, Yasukawa et al. (1992) found potent inhibition of 7,12-dimethyl-benz[*a*]anthracene (DMBA)-induced skin tumors (papillomas) from topical pretreatment with gomisin A (5 μmol) 30 min prior to treatment with 12-*O*-tetradecanoylphorbl-13-acetate (TPA) as a tumor promoter. Without gomisin A, 100% of the mice developed tumors, whereas only 50% receiving gomisin A developed tumors. The number of tumors per mouse was also inhibited by gomisin A. Without the gomisin A pretreatment, the average number per mouse was 19.8. With gomisin A the number was 85% less, or on average 3.0/mouse (Yasukawa et al., 1992).

Miyamoto et al. (1991) and Nomura et al. (1994) studied the antitumor activity of gomisin C (= schisantherin A) in rats. Phenobarbital (PB) was found to promote, while gomisin C (30 mg/kg per day p.o. for five weeks) suppressed proliferation and growth of 3'-MeDAB (3'-methyl-4-dimethyl-aminoazobenzene)-induced tumors. Miyamoto et al. (1995) focused on the tumor promoter role of BaP and deoxycholic acid (DCA) in the presence of 3'-MeDAB. Gomisin C (30 mg/kg per day p.o. for five weeks) was found to significantly inhibit the chemically induced tumors, even in the presence of the promoter chemicals. It was also found to inhibit the increase in serum bile acid concentration produced by DCA administration but had no influence on the effect of BaP on bile acids. The ability of gomisin C to inhibit the promoter effects of BaP appeared to be related to an enhancement of the metabolism and direct excretion of BaP.

Chemopreventive activity. Hendrich and Bjeldanes (1986) investigated the ex vivo hepatic carcinogen-metabolizing activity of an ethanol extract of schisandra as 5% of a basal diet of adult female and male mice. Results were compared to control mice fed a basal and a standard mouse-chow diet. Some differences in results were found between the males and the females on the schisandra diet. Liver weights in the males were 21% higher than the male basal group compared to 27% higher in the female mice compared to their corresponding basal diet group. In hepatic xenobiotic-metabolizing enzyme assays, liver fractions from the schisandra group showed significant increases in monooxygenase activities. Curiously, a significant increase in cytochrome *P*-450 was found in liver fractions from the female mice (1.6-fold), whereas the increase in the males was only slight (1.2-fold). In addition, cytostolic epoxide hydratase (EH) activity in the males showed no significant difference compared to control males fed the basal diet, while in the female mice the same activity was significantly (2.2-fold) higher than that of the basal group. Cytostolic GST activity in the male mice was significantly increased (24%) compared to the basal diet group, and the females showed a fivefold increase compared to their corresponding basal diet group.

Preneoplastic lesions in the livers of male rats treated with 3'-MeDAB (3'-methyl-4-dimethyl-aminoazobenzene) as part of their feed plus the lignan gomisin A (0.03% of feed) showed decreased levels of GST-P expression (glutathione-S-transferase placental form, a sensitive enzyme marker of preneoplastic liver lesions) and a decrease in the number and size of GST-P-positive foci compared to rats not administered gomisin A (Nomura et al., 1994).

Infectious Diseases

Microbial infections. Schisandra has shown inhibitory activity against *Mycobacterium tuberculosis* 607, a rapidly growing but nonvirulent strain, as well as other more virulent strains of this genus (Anonymous, 1988). In vitro activity was also shown by schisandra against *Bacillus, Anthracis, Staphylococcus aureus, S. albus, Salmonella paratyphi* A and B, *S. typhi, S. enteriditis, Klebsiella pneumoniae, Shigella dysentariae, S. dysentariae* variant, *Vibrio cholerae, Enterobacter aerogenes,* and *Proteus vulgaris.* Some activity was noted against *Pseudomonas aeruginosa* (Chang and But, 1986). NAPRALERT (1990) lists a Taiwanese study of a whole plant decoction as inactive against many of these organisms and showing weak activity against *Bordatella bronchiseptica.*

Parasitic infections. Chang and But (1986) noted that antiascaridic activity has been shown by schisandra. Rhee et al. (1982) tested a boiled-water extract of schisandra for anthelmintic activity against the Chinese liver fluke *Clonorchis sinensis,* which affects cats, dogs, and humans. Among 223 other traditional Korean medicines tested, schisandra was among three others as the most effective herbal medicines (i.e., *Aster tataricus* radix, *Platycodon grandifolum* radix, and *Polygala tenuifolia* herb). The researchers noted that since ancient times, schisandra has been one of the medicines used to treat symptoms of infection caused by Chinese liver fluke, such as hepatic dysfunction, hepatic cirrhosis, dilated belly, jaundice, and hepatic hypertrophy (Rhee et al., 1982).

Viral infections. In an in vitro model of hepatitis C virus (HCV) infection, Cyong et al. (2000) screened the effects of 11 herbs that make up a traditional herbal formula used in Japan in the treatment of hepatitis C (ninjinjin-yoei-to or Ginseng compositae formula) and found an extract of schisandra berries was the most active. In patients treated with the formula, the daily dosage of schisandra extract was only 225 mg. In the in vitro assay, a water extract of schisandra berries (10 μg/mL) markedly inhibited HCV infection in MOLT-4 cells, as did gomisin A, only more potently and dose dependently (0.01 to 10 μg/mL). In a model of immunologically induced acute hepatic failure in mice (by heat-killed *Propionibacterium acnes* i.v. followed by LPS i.p.), all the mice perished within 24 h. For the mice that also received gomisin A (40 or 80 μg/kg i.p.), however, 20% survived after 24 h.

Synthetic halogenated gomisin J derivatives have been of some interest to the development of drugs that potently inhibit cytopathological effects of HIV. The synthetic derivative showed an ED_{50} of 0.1-0.5 mM in human MT4 T-cells (Fujihashi et al., 1995).

Immune Functions

Immunopotentiation. The in vitro immunomodulating activity of a water extract of schisandra on murine spleen cells of mice was shown by Yoshida et al. (1997). However moderate, dilutions of the extract (1:40, 1:60, and 1:640) significantly enhanced normal mouse spleen-cell proliferation, yet showed no natural killer (NK) cell activity-inducing or cytotoxic T cell-inducing activity, and no effect on tumor necrosis factor (TNF) or interleukin-6 (IL-6) production by macrophages.

Since the activation of complement results in organ transplant rejection and a host of other conditions, including asthma, arthritis, lupus erythematosus, and atopic dermatitis, Lee et al. (1997) investigated the effect of schisandra fruits on complement. A potent anticomplementary activity from schisandra led to their isolation of citrostadienol as the active constituent. Citrostadienol, described as (3β, 4α, 5α, 24Z)-4-methylstigmasta-7,24(28)-dien-3-ol, $α_1$-sitosterol, exhibited potent anticomplementary activity on the classical pathway (LD_{50} of 4.6×10^{-8} M)—considerably higher than that of lipopolysaccharide, inulin, stigmasterol, β-sitosterol, or campesterol. The researchers concluded that citrostadienol may be useful in the treatment of the aforementioned diseases in which complement plays a significant role (Lee et al., 1997).

Immunosuppression. In contrast to the research showing immunopotentiating activity, others have evidence that the alcoholic extract of schisandra possesses immunosuppressive activity. In mice, the extract prolonged the survival of transplanted myocardium and showed a synergistic effect with immunosuppression (Zhu, 1998).

Inflammatory Response

A study of induced immunological liver damage in mice revealed that gomisin C (= schisantherin A) protected against the injury. Mortality was reduced, but infiltration of nonspecific inflammatory cells was not (Ohkura et al., 1987). A study of gomisin C (= schisantherin A) using three immunological liver-injury models in mice found the lignan was effective against liver injury. The researchers concluded that gomisin C had little effect against antibody formation and complement activation and that its hepatoprotective effects were more related to postinjury enzyme inhibition protecting the hepatocyte plasma membrane (Nagai et al., 1989). Another study of immunologically induced hepatic failure showed that gomisin C (= schisantherin A) (60 mg/kg per day p.o. for four to ten weeks) effectively improved histological changes in the guinea pig (Mizoguchi, Kawada, et al., 1991).

Against TPA-induced inflammation in mouse ears, pretreatments with either gomisin A (1.4 μmol/ear), schisandrin C (wuweizisu C) (2.4 μmol/ear), or gomisin J (4.4 μmol/ear) produced substantial inhibitions of inflammation, of 93%, 76%, and 55%, respectively. By comparison, quercetin was less potent (6.6 μmol/ear; 50% inhibition), as were caffeine and glycyrrhizin (Yasukawa et al., 1992).

Integumentary, Muscular, and Skeletal Functions

Muscular Functions

The effects of 15 schisandra lignans were studied on smooth muscle tissues in various animals (Suekawa et al., 1987). Contractions induced by prostaglandin $F_{2\alpha}$ and $CaCl_2$ in dog mesenteric artery tissue were inhibited by all 15 lignans. In addition, six lignans—notably gomisin J—inhibited epinephrine (NE)-induced contraction as well. In the anaesthetized dog, gomisin J (10 mg intra-arterially) produced an increase in coronary artery flow with an effect only slightly weaker than that of diltiazem, a calcium antagonist.

Ko et al. (1996) showed that in a high dosage (1.6 g/kg p.o. for three days), a lignan-enriched petroleum ether extract of the dried fruits as a pretreatment in female rats 24 h before exercise significantly protected the animals against exercise-induced (treadmill running) skeletal muscle damage ($p < 0.0005$), compared to exercised controls pretreated with the same dosage of vitamin E and untreated exercised animals. The researchers speculated that the protective effect of schisandra may be attributed to a significantly enhanced hepatic glutathione status ($p < 0.0005$), presumably providing a supply of glutathione that may serve to protect the muscles.

Metabolic and Nutritional Functions

Antioxidant Activity

Numerous studies of schisandra describe antioxidant effects (Liu and Xiao, 1994). Most relate to hepatic tissue functioning. Antioxidant effects, though less often studied specifically in other tissues, undoubtedly contribute to many of the effects described for other body systems affected by schisandra (Wagner and Bauer, 1996).

Zhang et al. (1995) reported that gomisin C (schisantherin A) reduces the production of reactive oxygen species by inhibiting neutrophil activity. Lin et al. (1990) found that gomisin C (schisantherin A) inhibited neutrophil activities in vitro in a dose-dependent manner. In rat neutrophils, chemotaxis, phagocytosis, and superoxide anion production were inhibited at 1, 10, and 100 μmol/L concentrations.

Li et al. (1990) reported that the scavenging effects of schizandrin C showed stronger scavenging effects on active oxygen radicals produced by stimulated human leukocytes than schisandrin B. Lin et al. (1990) studied the antioxidant properties of gomisin C (schisantherin A) by electron spin resonance (ESR) and spin trapping. Using human neutrophils, gomisin C scavenged oxygen radicals produced by tetradecanoylphorbol (TDPA). In Fenton reaction system experiments, the rate of hydroxyl radical inhibition was 34.4%. In the xanthin-xanthine oxidase and UV-irradiation of riboflavin system, gomisin C scavenged 26.1% and 21.9% of superoxide anion radicals, respectively. In all these studies, gomisin C was shown to be more potent as an antioxidant than vitamin E. However, Zhao et al. (1990) reported even stronger effects from schisandrin B and gomisin C (= schisantherin A) in the Fenton reaction. At equal concentrations (5×10^{-4}M), the rate of hydroxyl radical scavenging was 77% from schisandrin B, 63% from gomisin C, 56% from vitamin C, and 35% from vitamin E. Against superoxide radicals in the riboflavin/EDTA system, schisandrin B showed a higher rate of scavenging (46%) than gomisin C (14%) or vitamin E (23%) but not vitamin C (96%).

In experiments with rats, Lu and Liu (1991) reported that schisandrins B and C and gomisin C (= schisantherin A) were more potent than vitamin E at inhibiting vitamin C/NADPH-induced lipid peroxidation. Gomisin C and schisandrin B markedly reduced ethanol-induced malondialdehyde production. Evidence for superoxide anion formation-inhibition and free-radical scavenging (ESR study) activity by these lignans suggested strong antioxidant effects, especially with gomisin C and schisandrin B. Liu and Lu (1988) reported that whereas antioxidant activity was evident from 9 schisandrins in vitro and in vivo, Lu and Liu (1991) found that, overall, gomisin C was the most active.

Mak et al. (1996) compared schisandrin B to vitamin E (dl-α-tocopherol) against CCl_4-induced lipid peroxidation in female mice. After pretreatment with the agents (3 mmol/kg p.o. daily for three days), the mice received CCL_4 (0.1 mL/kg p.o.), which resulted in an increase in hepatic MDA of 40%, indicating that lipid peroxidation was enhanced. Plasma alanine aminotransferase (ALT) activity increased 869-fold, indicating severe damage to the liver. Compared to controls not treated with either agent, the vitamin E-pretreated mice showed no significant difference in either hepatic MDA or plasma ALT levels. In sharp contrast, the schisandrin B group compared to the CCL$_4$-treated controls showed a 115% protection against increased hepatic MDA ($p < 0.05$) and a 99% protection against the increase in plasma ALT activity ($p < 0.0001$). Even at 10% of the pretreatment dose for three days, schisandrin B caused a significant degree of protection against CCL$_4$-induced increases in hepatic MDA and plasma ALT, protecting the mice by 70% ($p < 0.05$) and 92% ($p < 0.0001$), respectively. Mak and colleagues surmised that the lack of in vitro pro-oxidant activity of schisandrin B against ferric chloride-induced oxidation of erythrocyte membranes versus the pro-oxidant activity of vitamin E in the same test, may have partly accounted for the difference in results. They added that administration of CCL$_4$ is known to increase the amount of hepatic iron in animals and that vitamin E is known to stimulate iron-induced lipid peroxidation (Mak et al., 1996).

Ip and colleagues (1995) reported that pretreating female mice with schisandrin B (= γ-schizandrin) (1 to 4 mmol/kg per day i.g. for three days) caused a dose-dependent increase in hepatic glutathione *S*-transferase (GST) and glutathione reductase (GRD), with down-regulation of glucose-6-phosphate dehydrogenase (G6PDH), selenium-glutathione peroxidase (GPX), and gamma-glutamylcysteine synthetase (GCS) activities, resulting in a beneficial effect on the hepatic reduced glutathione (GSH) antioxidant system, possibly through stimulation of GSH-related enzyme activities. When the mice were challenged with CCl$_4$, the beneficial effects of schisandrin B were clearly dose dependent. Dose-dependent hepatoprotection was associated with increased tissue levels of GSH and a corresponding decrease in the susceptibility of tissue homogenates to GSH depletion.

Ip and Ko (1996) compared the antioxidant effects of butylated hydroxytoluene (BHT) to those of schisandrin B at the same pretreatment dosage (3 mmol/kg p.o. t.i.d.) in female mice treated with the liver toxin CCl$_4$. Liver levels of reduced glutathione (GSH) increased in the schisandrin B-treated mice but decreased in the BHT-treated group. In the schisandrin B group, hepatic mitochondrial levels of GSH were sustained, whereas BHT provided no protective effects in the same assay; and while schisandrin B and BHT caused hepatic levels of vitamin C to reach levels found in the control mice not treated with CCl$_4$, only the schisandrin B group showed a sustained increase in the level of vitamin C. Since hepatic vitamin E levels were also sustained in the schisandrin B group, Ip and Ko concluded that the protection of hepatic levels of vitamin C and E against the oxidative stress of CCl$_4$ may be mediated in part through an inhibition of CCl$_4$ metabolism by the lignan and is likely an effect secondary to the enhancement of liver ascorbate redox status and hepatic glutathione by schisandrin B.

Wang et al. (1994) showed that gomisin C exerted an inhibitory effect on the respiratory burst of peripheral neutrophils from rats. They attributed the effect partly to inhibition of the release of intracellular stores of Ca^{2+} and partly to a suppressive activity on NADPH oxidase, which holds a key position in the respiratory burst pathway. The effect could not be attributed to the scavenging of superoxide radicals released from the neutrophils; however, gomisin C acted in the fashion of a "pure" superoxide scavenger by decreasing neutrophil consumption of superoxides. Superoxide dismutase showed no such effect.

Gomisin A has also received considerable attention as an antioxidant component of schisandra fruits. In vitro studies in rat liver cells demonstrated that gomisin A is not as potent at inhibiting CCl_4-induced free radical generation as vitamin E, nor against ascorbate/Fe^{2+}-induced lipid peroxidation (Kiso et al. 1985). As a pretreatment in rats subsequently treated with a high dose of acetaminophen as a liver toxin (750 mg/kg by gavage), gomisin A (50 mg/kg i.p.) significantly inhibited the toxin-induced increase in hepatic hydroperoxide content, serum aminotransferase activity, and the degree of hepatocyte necrosis and degeneration (Yamada et al., 1993).

Because hepatocyte growth factor (HGF) was shown to prevent damage to the liver from hepatotoxins, Shiota et al. (1996) examined the effect of gomisin A (50 mg/kg i.p.) on HGF in male rats as a pretreatment followed with a high dose of acetaminophen. HGF mRNA expression was induced in the group treated with gomisin A alone, but not in pretreated rats after treatment with acetaminophen, nor in rats treated only with acetaminophen. Although the researchers concluded that the role of HGF in the hepatoprotective activity of the lignan against acetaminophen-induced liver injury remains unknown, the induction of HGF by gomisin A may have other importance: HGF inhibits many kinds of tumor cells, stimulates liver regeneration and cell motility of keratinocytes, and induces DNA synthesis of renal tubular cells (Shiota et al., 1996).

Performance Enhancement

Hancke et al. (1994) demonstrated that a single dose of standardized schisandra extract administered 30 min prior to the exercising of racing horses significantly reduced their heart rate and respiratory frequency. Lactic acid levels were lower and glucose levels increased following exercise. The researchers suggested that these effects could be due to reduced synthesis of lactic acid in the muscles and/or stimulated gluconeogenesis in the liver. They noted other studies that showed improved gaseous exchange and oxygenation of tissues (Hancke et al., 1994). Others have disputed these effects, however (Chang and But, 1986).

A previous study reported the effect of schisandra on horse-racing performance in which the treatment group acted as its own control ($n = 30$). The horses were exercised in two sets of prescribed galloping. When the horses were treated with a single 48-g dose of schisandra 30 min before the exercise, the plasma concentration of lactate but not of glucose was found to be significantly reduced at 10 and 50 min postexercise. Treated horses showed a lower heart rate throughout the exercise period and a quicker recovery of normal respiratory frequency at 0 and 5 min postexercise. The researchers reported a statistically significant improvement in track time for the treatment groups and in individual comparison at 800-m distances (Ahumada et al., 1989). Others have reported increased swimming times in male albino mice administered a tincture of schisandra of at least 135% (Azizov and Seifulla, 1998).

Pharmacokinetics

The structural characteristics of the large number of metabolites found in the bile and urine of the rat from metabolism of schisandra were investigated by Ikeya et al. (1990). An in vitro study on the metabolic transformation of schisandrin in a rat liver microsomal fraction found virtually identical metabolites produced in vivo when rats were administered schisandrin (150 mg/kg i.p.). The major metabolites formed were identified by HPLC as 7,8-dihydroxy-2-demethyl-schisandrin and 7,8-dihydroxy-schisandrin, while 7,8-dihydroxy-3-demethyl-schisandrin was identified using MS, NMR, and UV spectral analyses and chromatographic comparison with the authentic compound (Cui and Wang, 1993).

Neurological, Psychological, and Behavioral Disorders

Neurotoxicity/Neuroprotection

Neurological effects of schisandra were studied in mice by Volicer et al. (1965). The crude extract (10-30 mg/kg p.o.) protected mice against the convulsive effects of metrazole and nicotine bitartrate when administered 30 min beforehand. No anticonvulsive effects were noted against strychnine. Other nicotine effects were potentiated at small doses and antagonized at large doses of schisandra extract, thus resembling methylphenidate in its actions. Volicer and co-workers reported that schisandra extract in a number of trials acted in ways similar to some peripheral cholinomimetic drugs, thereby suggesting a mechanism to explain the purported antifatigue effect of the berries. They also found that schisandrin B potentiated some reserpine effects, while chlorpromazine effects were unchanged.

Psychological and Behavioral Disorders

Cognitive functions. In a rat model of impaired memory and learning (cycloheximide-induced amnesia) employing a passive avoidance task, daily oral administration of a water-soluble fraction of schisandra (25 mg/kg for seven days) significantly reversed the step through latency shortened by cycloheximide, whereas hexane- and chloroform-soluble fractions of the fruit did not. A 50% alcoholic extract of the fruits also produced a significant reversal of the cycloheximide-induced latency at 250 and 750 mg/kg p.o., although the lower dose was more effective and equal in significance to that of the water-soluble extract ($p < 0.001$) (Hsieh et al., 2001).

Sleep disturbances. The effects of seven schisandrins on pentobarbital sleeping time (PST), determined as the interval between the loss and return of righting reflex in mice, was studied by Bao et al. (1980). The PST was significantly prolonged ($p < 0.01$) following a 60-min pretreatment dose of schizandrin B, schizandrin C, or gomisin A (= schisandrol B) (each 12.5 mg/kg p.o. or i.p.). Deoxyschisandrin (= schizandrin A) and schisandrin (= schizandrol A) were inactive while schizandrin C showed by far the strongest effect, p.o. or i.p. Neurological outcomes were to some extent related to the effect of schisandrins on liver drug metabolism of pentobarbital.

Ahumada et al. (1991) demonstrated that the crude extract of schisandra can produce a CNS-depressant effect in mice. A statistically significant increase in narcosis time was found to be sex and dose dependent when the mice were treated with pentobarbital (50 mg/kg i.p.) and the crude extract (10, 30, or 100 mg/kg i.p.) at the same time.

Receptor- and Neurotransmitter-Mediated Functions

At a dose of 10-30 mg/kg p.o., a crude petroleum ether extract of the berries affected the cholinergic system of rats. The convulsant threshold decreased and the excitatory activity of carbachol on rat intestines was potentiated. The antidiuretic effect of nicotine was also potentiated (Hancke et al., 1999).

Reproductive Disorders

Pregnancy and Labor Disorders

Schisandra has shown uterine stimulant properties in the pregnant, nonpregnant, or postpartum rabbit uterus (NAPRALERT, 1990). Chang and But (1986) noted that in vivo or in vitro, rhythmic contractions of nonpregnant, pregnant, and postpartum rabbit uterus could be induced by a 70% schisandra extract, fruit suspension, and a mixture of the fruit and fruit coat. The muscular tone of the uterus and the blood pressure were unchanged. The researchers surmised that these actions resembled oxytocin but not ergot (see Clinical Studies for a description of use during labor). A tincture of schisandra (30 mg/kg s.c.) administered to rabbits caused uterine tension and contractility to increase. A higher dose (100 mg/kg s.c.) caused a pronounced enhancement of uterine tension.

Endocrine receptor studies of schisandra appear to be lacking, despite various bits of information indicating possible hormone interactions, including traditional use in treating spermatorrhea, urinary frequency, and as a labor aid (NAPRALERT, 1990). Chang and But (1986) mention that in rodents schisandra antagonizes testosterone-induced adrenal atrophy and prevents changes caused by hydrocortisone.

CLINICAL STUDIES

Digestive, Hepatic, and Gastrointestinal Disorders

Hepatic Diseases

Hepatitis. Chang and But (1986) note that over 5,000 cases of various types of hepatitis have been treated with unspecified doses of schisandra in China. They recounted that of these cases, elevated liver enzymes were decreased in 84% to 97%, and the liver enzyme profile was normalized in 75% of patients. In cases of toxin-induced hepatitis, 83/86 cases were reported to have normalized in seven to twenty-eight days. Of these, it was reported that liver enzyme levels continued to drop after the treatment was discontinued.

Schisandra reduced elevated serum glutamic pyruvic transaminase (SGPT) in patients with chronic hepatitis. A study of the residue (called AEKFS or alcoholic extract of the kernel of *Fructus Schizandrae*) left after the preparation of *Fructus Schizandrae* syrup, found that it contained fractions that could lower SGPT. In one multicenter controlled study in three hospitals, 189 patients with chronic viral hepatitis and elevated SGPT levels were divided into a treatment group of 107 patients receiving 1.5 g of the crude material t.i.d., and a control group of 82 patients receiving a liver extract and a vitamin B complex. SGTP levels of 73 patients (68.2%) in the schisandra group fell to within normal limits accompanied by symptom improvement. No rebound effect was noted after treatment withdrawal. In the control group, SGPT levels had returned to normal in 36 out of 82 patients (43.9%); however, this required a longer treatment (eight weeks) than that of the schisandra group (four weeks). The improvement of other measures of liver function was also less pronounced (no details given in the controls). Reported side effects in the schisandra group were rare and only slight: 4/107 patients developed mild and transient nausea, headache, and stomachache. Other complaints, such as sleeplessness, fatigue, abdominal tension, and loose bowels, were reported to have been relieved in the treatment group (Liu, 1977).

Metabolic and Nutritional Disorders

Performance and Endurance Enhancement

Volicer et al. (1965) alluded to human clinical trials conducted in the Soviet Union by Levedev in the mid-1950s when schisandra was reported to
improve athletic performance in noncontrolled settings. Chang and But
(1986) noted that in human trials, schisandra increased tactile discrimination, quickened and strengthened reflexes, and improved work efficiency.
According to Hancke et al. (1999), these effects were obtained from the
seed powder in an oral dosage of 3 g/day.

Panossian et al. (1999) conducted a double-blind, randomized placebo-
controlled study in athletes administered a schisandra extract in which they
measured changes in blood levels of cortisol and saliva levels of nitric oxide
(NO) induced by heavy physical exercise. Another "adaptogenic" herb extract, *Byronia alba,* was compared. Athletes (109 weightlifters, wrestlers,
and boxers, ages not stated) were administered either schisandra extract tablets (standardized to contain 3.1 mg gamma-schisandrin and schisandrin per
91.1 mg tablet, b.i.d. for eight days), *B. alba* extract tablets (standardized to
contain 1 mg cucurbitacin R/tablet, two tablets/day for seven days), or
placebo. The athletes followed identical diets and training regimes. Prior to
administration of the extracts, the researchers found salivary levels of NO
increased in beginner athletes following heavy exercise, but not in the well-
trained top-level athletes. The researchers interpreted this as implying that
salivary NO "could be a measure of adaptation of an organism to heavy
physical exercise." They added that NO functions as a potent vasodilator
which increases blood flow and plays an important role in mediating the
"stress system," otherwise known as the neuroimmune complex. Large
amounts of NO are also produced during immunological reactions and as
part of the host defense mechanism. The results showed that compared to
placebo, either of the herbal extracts significantly increased basal concentrations of NO in the saliva of the athletes, which correlated with increased
extensions of physical performance versus placebo. Panossian and colleagues also found an increase in plasma levels of cortisol in the athletes
treated with either herbal extract versus placebo. In beginner athletes, treatment with either of the herbal extracts caused both cortisol and NO to increase under "chronic heavy physical exercise," whereas in well-trained
athletes the same herbal extracts caused cortisol to decrease compared to
before exercise, and NO to increase. The schisandra extract caused a significant increase in postexercise salivary NO in well-trained weightlifters
compared to placebo ($p < 0.05$), and in well-trained top-level athletes in
preexercise salivary NO levels compared to beginner athletes. The schisandra
extract also caused a significant ($p < 0.05$) increase in preexercise salivary
NO compared to placebo in well-trained boxers, weightlifters, and wrestlers

compared to placebo, and in well-trained boxers caused a significant increase in salivary NO compared to placebo, both preexercise and postexercise ($p < 0.05$).

Pharmacokinetics

Following oral administration of schisandrin (a lignan component of schisandra) in six healthy males (15 mg p.o.), using gas chromatography-mass spectrometry Ono and colleagues (1995) measured the plasma concentration. Schisandrin was measurable in the plasma for 8 h postadministration and from 0.5 to 2.0 h the average maximum plasma concentration of the lignan was 96.1 ± 14.1 ng/mL.

Neurological, Psychological, and Behavioral Disorders

The use of placebo in controlled studies is comparatively recent and still rare in China. Therefore, the following studies are mentioned for the purpose of stimulating possible further investigations.

Neurodegenerative Disorders

According to Chang and But (1986), Russian scientists described therapeutic effects of schisandra for mild spastic paralysis resulting from stroke when treatment was initiated within two to four days, and that the extract showed therapeutic effects when used in cerebellar ataxia and in Parkinson's disease. They also mention that in China researchers reported Ménière's disease was cured in 20 patients after four to five doses of schisandra in combination with *Ziziphus jujuba* var. *inermis*, *Angelica sinensis* root, and *Euphorbia longan* seeded fruit (Chang and But, 1986).

Psychological and Behavioral Disorders

Cognitive functions. In an open-label study in China, healthy young adult males taking schisandrin (5-10 mg/day p.o.) while performing tasks such as telegraphic transmissions, marathon running, and needle threading, were reported to show improved fine coordination, concentration, endurance, and sensitivity (Chang and But, 1986).

Neuroses. In China, an uncontrolled, comparative study was made of schisandra tincture (40% to 100%, 2.5 mL given two to three times/day for two to four weeks) in patients suffering from "insomnia, headache, dizziness, blurred vision, palpitation and nocturnal emission" (Chang and But, 1996, p. 205) judged to be of neurotic origin. Researchers claimed that the tincture produced complete alleviation of symptoms in 58.8%, and 17.8% of the patients improved. In one case, no effect was noted and 21.3% of the patients discontinued the treatment. No side effects were reported. The tincture was also claimed to have been helpful by reducing symptoms of hallucination, paranoia, and "neurosis" in psychotic patients (Chang and But, 1986).

Retinopathies. Bensky and Gamble (1990) and Chang and But (1986) have noted that schisandra extract is reported to increase visual acuity and visual fields in both normal and vision-impaired patients and to have improved night vision (Chang and But, 1986).

Reproductive Disorders

Pregnancy and Labor Disorders

Schisandra is believed to strengthen uterine rhythmic contractions and is used in traditional Chinese medicine to induce or promote prolonged labor (Bensky and Gamble, 1990). In China, a study in 80 women with prolonged labor administered a schisandra tincture (20-25 drops once an hour for three hours) reported good results in 72 cases. Of the other eight cases, uterine atony or tonic uterine contraction was noted (Chang and But, 1986).

DOSAGE

Foster and Yue (1992) give the traditional dose as 1.5-15 g. Yen (1992) gives the daily dosage as 1.5-3.0 g, and Zhu (1998) gives 1.5-6 g. A summary of doses used in clinical studies follows:

Hepatitis: 3-5, 20 mg tablets containing 1.5 g crude material, t.i.d.
Labor: 20-25 drops, wuweizi tincture three times once an hour
Neurasthenia: 40-100% wuweizi tincture, 2.5 mL given two to three times a day for two to four weeks
Infantile dysentery: 90% tincture containing 0.25-2 g crude extract administered at 30-40 drops or 0.5 g of extract (age or weight of infant/child not stated, nor dosing frequency)
Keshan disease: 40% wuweizu tincture, 30 drops for two to three courses, each course lasting ten days (Chang and But, 1986)

SAFETY PROFILE

No clinical reports of overdosage in humans have been found. CNS depression has been noted in animal studies only at near-lethal doses (see Toxicology: Toxicity in Animal Models). Bensky and Gamble (1990) describe overdose symptoms as restlessness, insomnia, and dyspnea.

Contraindications

Bensky and Gamble (1990) note that in TCM, schisandra is contraindicated in excess heat and in patients showing early signs of a rash or cough. Chang and But (1986) list epilepsy, excessive exercise, high blood pressure, increased intracranial pressure, mental excitement, and peptic ulcer as contraindications for schisandra.

Drug Interactions

Clinical information on concurrent use with medications is lacking. Chang and But (1986) note the use of schisandra in China as an antidote to morphine-induced respiratory depression. Therefore, it may be contraindicated in patients about to receive anesthesia. Drug interactions would be expected due to the documented effects of schisandra on liver (and gastric) enzymes that metabolize many drugs. Reserpine is potentiated by schisandra (Volicer et al., 1965) and cholinergic drug effects may also be potentiated in an additive fashion by schisandra. Possible adrenocorticomimetic effects may interact with or counter corticosteroid effects, although the decoction antagonized morphine (Chang and But, 1996). schisandra may also interact with calcium channel blockers, such as diltiazem (Suekawa et al., 1987), and is reported to prolong barbiturate-induced sleep and to have a potentiating effect upon the stimulating action of strychnine (Huang, 1999).

In rats, low doses of a petroleum ether extract of the fruit (10-30 mg/kg p.o.) showed cholinergic effects: potentiating the antidiuretic activity of nicotine, the excitatory activity of carbachol (on the intestines), and decreasing the convulsant threshold (Hancke et al., 1999).

As a pretreatment in mice, schisandra (50 mg/kg i.p.) caused significantly reduced sleeping times induced by sodium pentobarbital (50 mg/kg i.p.), ether (1-2 min exposure), and ethanol (5.2 g/kg i.p.) (each $p < 0.001$) compared to controls treated with vehicle plus the sleep-inducing agents (Hancke et al., 1986). Therefore, use of schisandra may be contraindicated prior to anesthesia in patients about to undergo surgery.

Pregnancy and Lactation

Clinical descriptions of use during pregnancy are lacking in regard to teratogenicity or other effects on the developing fetus. A standardized dry extract (2% schisandrin) of the berries produced no signs of fetotoxicity and had no effect on implantation and other measures of reproductive function (Hancke et al., 1999) (see Toxicology: Toxicity in Animal Models). Schisandra has shown uterine-stimulant properties in the pregnant, nonpregnant, or postpartum rabbit uterus (NAPRALERT, 1990). Chang and But (1986) found schisandra extract could induce rhythmic contractions without changing the muscular tone of the rabbit uterus or blood pressure, activities they characterized as more similar to oxytocin than ergot. However, these activities were inducible in both pregnant and nonpregnant uterine tissue. Endocrine receptor studies of schisandra are needed to clarify its mode of activity on the uterus (see Clinical Studies: Reproductive Disorders). Schisandra is believed to strengthen uterine rhythmic contractions and is used in Chinese traditional medicine to induce or promote labor (Bensky and Gamble, 1990). Chang and But (1986) mention that in one study, three administrations of a 70% tincture of schisandra in a dosage of 20-25 drops/hour was successfully used to treat prolonged labor in 72/80 cases. The nonresponding patients were diagnosed with tonic uterine contraction or uterine atonia.

The entry of schisandra constituents into breast milk is uncertain, but expected because of the chemical characteristics of the plant constituents. No adverse effects during lactation are documented. Schisandra may act as an oxytocic agent (Chang and But, 1986) and thus may have a stimulating effect on the milk ejection reflex (MER). This may or may not be a desirable effect for all nursing mothers. The noted effect of schisandra as an ovulation inducer suggests that use of the herb could conceivably produce unpredictable effects on lactation amenorrhea states.

Side Effects

Huang (1999) mentions that schisandra may in some cases cause dizziness or diarrhea, which may be eliminated by reducing the dosage. After a clinical trial of schisandra in China, Liu (1977) described the side effects of schisandra as being rare and only slight. Only 4/107 patients developed mild and transient nausea, headache, and stomachache. Chang and But (1986) list heartburn, acid indigestion, stomachache, and anorexia as side effects in some patients. The tincture is described as being very acidic, and many of these side effects may be related to the form and therefore the high acidity of the preparation.

Special Precautions

The acidity of some preparation forms may cause GI upset (see Drug Interactions).

Toxicology

Mutagenicity

In the presence of mutagens, such as benzo[a]pyrene (BaP) and aflatoxin B (AFB), increased cytochrome P-450 activity and a resultant increase in the metabolism of these substances was observed in mice administered schisandra. In vitro mutagenicity of AFB was found to increase with schisandra; however, in an in vivo study of chemicals that induce similar patterns of enzymes, schisandra showed reduced in vivo binding of AFB to DNA (Anonymous, 1988).

In the Ames assay for *Salmonella* mutagenicity, BP mutagenicity, and aflatoxin B_1 (AFB_1) mutagenicity, Hendrich and Bjeldanes (1986) reported that microsomes from male mice fed a 95% basal diet with 5% schisandra showed a significant increase in BP mutagenicity (2.5-fold) compared to a basal diet-only group, but not to a mouse chow-only group (2.4-fold increase). A corresponding test for female mice was not conducted. In AFB_1 mutagenicity, microsomes from the males in the schisandra group showed a 4.6-fold increase in mutagenicity compared to the basal group, whereas microsomes from female mice fed the schizandra-supplemented diet showed a 5.4-fold increase compared to their basal group. Even at a 50-fold lower amount of aflatoxin B_1, the microsomes showed significantly higher DNA binding (2.5-fold) to the toxin compared to the basal or the chow groups. This resulted despite the significant increases in GST, which decreases aflatoxin B_1 DNA binding and mutagenicity. The researchers mentioned that these in vitro results may represent greater exposures to the toxins than would occur in vivo, and that the increased mutagenicities may result from a small number of constituents in schisandra which affect monooxygenase activities (Hendrich and Bjeldanes, 1986).

Toxicity in Animal Models

The acute toxicity of schisandra is considered low (Bensky and Gamble, 1990; Chang and But, 1986). In mice, single high oral doses of crude extract (10-15 g/kg; petrol-ether "purified" extract diluted 1:10 in olive oil) resulted in dyspnea (labored breathing) in 15-60 min, and decreased activity followed by death one to two days later. Oral intake of the purified extract (2.8 g/kg) resulted in depression, dyspnea, ataxia, and death of all the mice within 1-3 h (Chang and But, 1986).

The toxic dose is reported to be in the order of 10-15 g/kg p.o. (Bensky and Gamble, 1990). An extract of the dried fruits (4:1) standardized to contain 2% schisandrins produced an oral LD_{50} in rats of ≥21 g/kg (Hancke et al., 1999). However, an oral LD_{50} of 5.1 g/kg for the ethanol extract was cited by Zhu (1998), and others report that 5 g/kg p.o. in rats was not lethal. An ethanolic extract given orally to mice (0.6 or 1.2 g/kg for ten days) resulted in mild toxic effects (decreased activity, piloerection, and apathy). Their body weight increased, yet blood/organ health was not affected (Chang and But, 1986).

A standardized dry extract (2% schisandrin) of the berries (4:1) administered to mice and rats at doses of 105 to 0.500 mg/kg p.o. daily produced no signs of fetotoxicity and had no effect on implantation and other measures of reproductive function (Hancke et al., 1999).

In Landrace piglets, a standardized dry extract (2% schisandrin) of the berries (4:1) fed for 90 days at doses of 0.07, 0.36, and 0.73 mg/kg had no effect on body weight, food intake, red blood cells, white blood cells, hematocrit, hemoglobin, or concentrations of urea, protein, glycemia, tri-glycerides, GGT, and GOT compared to controls. Organ tissues, including lungs, heart, liver, kidneys, intestine, gonads, and spleen showed no toxic effects from the doses of the standardized schisandra extract (Hancke et al., 1999).

Chang and But (1986) describe a study of schisandrin B in rats: a single oral dose of 2 g/kg was not fatal. Intragastric doses of 200 mg/kg for 30 days had no discernable toxic effects. In dogs, intragastric administration of 10 mg/kg per day for four weeks effected no toxic changes.

Maeda et al. (1985) reported mean LD_{50}s in mice for gomisin C (= schisantherin A) of 777 mg/kg p.o., 390 mg/kg i.p., and 500 mg/kg s.c. Maeda et al. (1981) reported the same mean LD_{50}s and respective routes of administration for gomisin A in mice. For schisandrin, the mean LD_{50}s were 1,448 mg/kg p.o., 518 mg/kg i.p., and 1,861 mg/kg s.c.

Bao et al. (1980) reported that in male mice no deaths were found at doses ≥ 500 mg/kg p.o. or i.p. of deoxyschisandrin (= schisandrin A) or schisandrins B or C; schisandrin (= schisandrol A) ≥ 250 mg p.o. or i.p.; gomisin A (= schisandrol B) ≥ 125 mg/kg p.o. or i.p.; schisantherin A (= schisandrer A) ≥ 500 mg/kg p.o. or i.p.; and schisantherin B (= schisandrer B) ≥ 125 mg/kg p.o. or i.p.

REFERENCES

Ahumada, F., Hermosilla, J., Hola, R., Pena, R., Wittwer, F., Wegmann, E., Hancke, J., and Wikman, G. (1989). Studies on the effect of *Schizandra chinensis* extract on horses submitted to exercise and maximal effort. *Phytotherapy Research* 3: 175-179.

Ahumada, F., Trincado, M.A., Arellano, J.A., Hancke, J., and Wikman, G. (1991). Effect of certain adaptogenic plant extracts on drug-induced narcosis in female and male mice. *Phytotherapy Research* 5: 29-31.

Anonymous (1988). Schizandra. *Lawrence Review of Natural Products* (June):1-2.

Azizov, A.P. and Seifulla, R.D. (1998). [The effect of Elton, Leveton, Phytoton, and Adapton on the working capacity of experimental animals]. *Eksperimentalnaia I Klinicheskaia Farmakologiia* 61: 61-63.

Bao, T.T., Liu, G.T., Song, Z.Y., Xu, G.F., and Sun, R.H. (1980). A comparison of the pharmacological actions of 7 constituents isolated from *Fructus Shizandrae*. *Chinese Medical Journal* 93: 41-47.

Bensky, D. and Gamble, A. (1990). *Chinese Herbal Medicine: Materia Medica.* Seattle, WA: Eastland Press.

Chang, H.M. and But, P. (Eds.) (1986). *Pharmacology and Applications of Chinese Materia Medica,* Vol. 1. (pp. 199-209). Singapore: World Scientific.

Cui, Y.Y. and Wang, M.Z. (1993). Aspects of schizandrin metabolism in vitro and in vivo. *European Journal of Drug Metabolism and Pharmacokinetics* 18: 155-160.

Cyong, J.C., Kim, S.M., Iijima, K., Kobayashi, T., and Furuya, M. (2000). Clinical and pharmacological studies on liver diseases treated with kampo herbal medicine. *American Journal of Chinese Medicine* 28: 351-360.

Foster, S. and Yue, Y. (1992). *Herbal Emissaries* (pp. 146-152). Rochester, VT: Healing Arts Press.

Fujihashi, T., Hara, H., Sakata, T., Mori, K., Higuchi, H., Tanaka, A., Kaji, H., and Kaji, A. (1995). Anti-human immunodeficiency virus (HIV) activities of halogenated gomisin J derivatives, new nonnucleoside inhibitors of HIV type 1 reverse transcriptase. *Antimicrobial Agents and Chemotherapy* 39: 2000-2007.

Hancke, J.L., Burgos, R.A., and Ahumada, F. (1999). *Schisandra chinensis* (Yurcz.) Baill. *Fitoterapia* 70: 451-471.

Hancke, J., Burgos, R., Caceres, D., Brunett, F., Durigon, A., and Wikman, G. (1996). Reduction of serum hepatic transaminases and CPK in sport horses with poor performance treated with a standardized *Schisandra chinensis* fruit extract. *Phytomedicine* 3: 237-240.

Hancke, J., Burgos, R., Wikman, G., Ewertz, E., and Ahumada, F. (1994). *Schizandra chinensis,* a potential phytodrug for recovery of sports horses. *Fitoterapia* 65: 113-118.

Hancke, J.L., Wikman, G., and Hernandez, D.E. (1986). Antidepressant activity of selected natural products. *Planta Medica* 52: 542-543 (poster).

He, X.G., Lian, L.Z., and Lin, L.Z. (1997). Analysis of lignan constituents from *Schisandra chinensis* by liquid chromatography—Electrospray mass spectrometry. *Journal of Chromatography* A 757: 81-87.

Hendrich, S. and Bjeldanes, L.F. (1986). Effects of dietary *Schizandra chinensis,* Brussels sprouts and *Illicium verum* extracts on carcinogen metabolism systems in mouse liver. *Food and Chemical Toxicology* 24: 903-912.

Hernandez, D.E., Hancke, J.L., and Wikman, G. (1988). Evaluation of the anti-ulcer and antisecretory activity of extracts of *Aralia elata* root and *Schizandra chinensis* fruit in the rat. *Journal of Ethnopharmacology* 23: 109-114.

Hikino, H., Kiso, Y., Taguchi, H., and Ikeya, Y. (1984). Antihepatotoxic actions of lignoids from *Schizandra chinensis* fruits. *Planta Medica* 50: 213-218.

Hsieh, M.T. and Liu, C.P. (1999). Effects of *Fructus Schisandrae* on cycloheximide-induced amnesia in rats. *Phytotherapy Research* 13: 256-257.

Hsieh, M.T., Wu, C.R., Wang, W.H., and Lin, L.W. (2001). The ameliorating effect of the water layer of *Fructus Schizandrae* on cycloheximide-induced amnesia in rats: Interaction with drugs acting at neurotransmitter receptors. *Pharmacological Research* 43: 17-22.

Huang, K.C. (1999). *The Pharmacology of Chinese Herbs,* Second Edition (pp. 255-257). Boca Raton, FL: CRC Press.

Ikeya, Y., Mitsuhashi, H., Sasaki, H., Matsuzaki, Y., Matsuzaki, T., and Hosoya, E. (1990). Studies on the metabolism of gomisin a (TJN-101). Structure determination of biliary and urinary metabolites in rat. *Chemical and Pharmaceutical Bulletin* 38: 136-141.

Ikeya, Y., Taguchi, H., Yosioka, I., and Kobayashi, H. (1979). The constituents of *Schizandra chinensis* Baill. I. Isolation and structure determination of 5 new lignans, gomisin A, B, C, F, and G, and the absolute structure of schizandrin. *Chemical and Pharmaceutical Bulletin* 27: 1383-1394.

Ip, S.P. and Ko, K.M. (1996). The crucial antioxidant action of schisandrin B in protecting against carbon tetrachloride hepatotoxicity in mice: A comparative study with butylated hydroxytoluene. *Biochemical Pharmacology* 52: 1687-1693.

Ip, S.P., Poon, M.K.T., Wu, S.S., Che, C.T., Ng, K.H., Kong, Y.C., and Ko, K.M. (1995). Effect of schisandrin B on hepatic glutathione antioxidant system in mice: Protection against carbon tetrachloride toxicity. *Planta Medica* 61: 398-401.

Ip, S.P., Yiu, H.Y., and Ko, K.M. (2000a). Differential effect of schisandrin B and dimethyl diphenyl bicarboxylate (DDB) on hepatic mitochondrial glutathione redox status in carbon tetrachloride intoxicated mice. *Molecular and Cellular Biochemistry* 205: 111-114.

Ip, S.P., Yiu, H.Y., and Ko, K.M. (2000b). Schisandrin B protects against menadione-induced hepatotoxicity by enhancing DT-diaphorase activity. *Molecular and Cellular Biochemistry* 208: 151-155.

Jung, K.Y., Lee, I.S., Oh, S.R., Kim, D.S., and Lee, H.K. (1997). Lignans with platelet activating factor antagonistic activity from *Schisandra chinensis* (Turcz.) Baill. *Phytomedicine* 4: 229-231.

Kiso, Y., Tohkin, M., Hikino, H., Ikeya, Y., and Taguchi, H. (1985). Mechanism of antihepatotoxic activity of wuweizisu C and gomisin A. *Planta Medica* 4: 331-334.

Ko, K.M., Ip, S.P., Poon, M.K.T., Wu, S.S., Che, C.T., Ng, K.H., and Kong, Y.C. (1994). Effect of a lignan-enriched *Fructus Schisandrae* extract on hepatic glutathione status in rats: Protection against carbon tetrachloride toxicity. *Planta Medica* 61: 134-137.

Ko, K.M., Mak, D.H.F., Li, P.C., Poon, M.K.T., and Ip, S.P. (1996). Protective effect of a lignan-enriched extract of *Fructus schisandrae* on physical exercise induced muscle damage in rats. *Phytotherapy Research* 10: 450-452.

Kubo, S., Ohkura, Y., Mizoguchi, Y., Matsui-Yuasa, I., Otani, S., Morisawa, S., Kinoshita, H., Takeda, S., Aburada, M., and Hosoya, E. (1992). Effect of gomisin A (TJN-101) on liver regeneration. *Planta Medica* 58: 489-492.

Kwon, B.M., Jung, H.J., Lim, J.H., Kim, Y.S., Kim, M.K., Kim, Y.K., Bok, S.H., Bae, K.H., and Lee, I.R. (1999). Acyl-CoA:cholesterol acyltransferase inhibitory activity of lignans isolated from *Schizandra*, *Machilus* and *Magnolia* species. *Planta Medica* 65: 74-76 (letter).

Lee, I.S., Oh, S.R., Jung, K.Y., Kim, D.S., Kim, J.H., and Lee, H.K. (1997). Anticomplementary activity and complete ^{13}C NMR assignment of citrostadienol from *Schizandra chinensis*. *International Journal of Pharmacognosy* 35: 358-363.

Leung, A.Y. (1999). Herb notes. *Leung's Chinese Herb News* (20): 3.

Li, P.C., Mak, D.H.F., Poon, M.K.T., Ip, S.P., and Ko, K.M. (1996). Myocardial protective effect of sheng mai san (SMS) and a lignan-enriched extract of *Fructus Schisandrae*, in vivo and ex vivo. *Phytomedicine* 3: 217-221.

Li, X.L., Zhao, B., Liu, G., and Xin, W.J. (1990). Scavenging effects on active oxygen radicals by schizandrins with different structures and configurations. *Free Radical Biology and Medicine* 9: 99-104.

Lin, T.J., Liu, G.T., Li, X.J., Zhao, B.L., and Xin, W.J. (1990). Detection of free radical scavenging activity of schisanhenol by electron spin resonance. *Acta Pharmacologica Sinica* 11: 534-539.

Liu, G.T. (1985). Hepato-pharmacology of *Fructus Schizandrae*. In Chang, H.H., Yeung, H.W., Tso, W.W., and Koo, A. (Eds.), *Advances in Chinese Medicinal Materials Research* (pp. 257-267). Singapore: World Scientific.

Liu, G.T. and Lu, H. (1988). Anti-oxidant activity of nine dibenzocyclooctene lignans isolated from *Schizandraes*, a Chinese medicinal plant. *Proceedings of the Society for Experimental Biology and Medicine* 188:521.

Liu, J. and Xiao, P.G. (1994). Recent advances in the study of antioxidative effects of Chinese medicinal plants. *Phytotherapy Research* 8: 445-451.

Liu, K.T. (1977). Studies on *Fructus Schizandrae chinensis*. Annex 12: Studies on *Fructus Schisandrae chinensis*. Plenary lecture, World Health Organization (WHO) seminar on the use of medicinal plants in health care, September, 1977, Tokyo, Japan. In *World Health Organization Regional Office for the Western Pacific. Final Report* (November, 1977) (pp. 101-112). Manila, Philippines.

Liu, K.T., Cresteil, T., Columelli, S., and Lesca, P. (1982). Pharmacological properties of dibenzo[a,c]cyclooctene derivatives isolated from *Fructus Schizandrae chinensis*. II. Induction of phenobarbital-like hepatic monooxygenases. *Chemico-Biological Interactions* 39: 315-330.

Liu, K.T., Cresteil, T., Provost, E.L., and Lesca, P. (1981). Specific evidence that schizandrins induce a phenobarbital-like cytochrome P-450 form separated from rat liver. *Biochemical and Biophysical Research Communications* 103: 1131-1137.

Liu, K.T. and Lesca, P. (1982). Pharmacological properties of debenzo[a,c]cyclooctene derivatives isolated from *Fructus Schisandrae chinensis*. III. Inhibitory effects on carbon tetrachloride-induced lipid peroxidation, metabolism and covalent binding of carbon tetrachloride to lipids. *Chemico-Biological Interactions* 41: 39-47.

Lu, H. and Liu, G.T. (1991). Effect of dibenzo[*a,c*]cyclooctene lignans isolated from *Fructus Schizandrae* on lipid peroxidation and antioxidative enzyme activity. *Chemico-Biological Interactions* 78:77-84.

Lu, H. and Liu, G.T. (1992). Anti-oxidant activity of dibenzocyclooctene lignans isolated from Schisandraceae. *Planta Medica* 58: 311-313.

Maeda, S., Sudo, K., Aburada, M., Ikeya, Y., Taguchi, H., Yoshioka, I., and Harada, M. (1981). [Pharmacological studies on Schizandra fruit. I. General pharmacological effects of gomisin A and schizandrin]. *Yakugaku Zasshi* 101: 1030-1041.

Maeda, S., Takeda, S., Miyamoto, Y., Aburada, M., and Harada, M. (1985). Effects of gomisin A on liver functions in hepatotoxic chemicals-treated rats. *Japanese Journal of Pharmacology* 38: 347-353.

Mak, D.H.F., Ip, S.P., Li, P.C., Poon, M.K., and Ko, K.M. (1996). Effects of schisandrin B and α-tocopherol on lipid peroxidation, in vitro and in vivo. *Molecular and Cellular Biochemistry* 165: 161-165.

Mak, D.H.F. and Ko, K.M. (1997). Alterations in susceptibility to carbon tetrachloride toxicity and hepatic antioxidant/detoxification system in streptozotocin-induced short-term diabetic rats: Effects of insulin and schisandrin B treatment. *Molecular and Cellular Biochemistry* 175: 225-232.

Miyamoto, K., Hiramatsu, K., Ohtaki, Y., Kanitani, M., Nomura, M., and Aburada, M. (1995). Effects of gomisin A on the promoter action and serum bile acid concentration in hepatocarcinogenesis induced by 3'-methyl-4-dimethylamino-azobenzene. *Biological and Pharmaceutical Bulletin* 18: 1443-1445.

Miyamoto, K., Wakusawa, S., Nomura, M., Sanae, F., Sakai, R., Sudo, K., Ohtaki, Y., Takeda, S., and Fujii, Y. (1991). Effects of gomisin A on hepatocarcinogenesis by 3'-methyl-4-dimethylaminoazobenzene in rats. *Japanese Journal of Pharmacology* 57: 71-77.

Mizoguchi, Y., Kawada, N., Ichikawa, Y., and Tsutsui, H. (1991). Effect of gomisin A in the prevention of acute hepatic failure induction. *Planta Medica* 57: 320-324.

Mizoguchi, Y., Shin, T., Kobayashi, K., and Morisawa, S. (1991). Effect of gomisin A in an immunologically-induced acute hepatic failure model. *Planta Medica* 57: 11-14.

Nagai, H., Yakuo, I., Aoki, M., Teshima, K., Ono, Y., Sengoku, T., Shimazawa, T., Aburada, M., and Koda, A. (1989). The effect of gomisin A on immunologic liver injury in mice. *Planta Medica* 55: 13-17.

NAPRALERT (1990). Database. Board of Trustees, University of Illinois. Department of Medicinal Chemistry and Pharmacognosy, Program for Collaborative Research in the Pharmaceutical Sciences.

Nishiyama, N., Chu, P.J., and Saito, H. (1996). An herbal prescription, S-113m, consisting of biota, ginseng and *Schizandra,* improves learning performance in senescence accelerated mouse. *Biological and Pharmaceutical Bulletin* 19: 388-393.

Nishiyama, N., Wang, Y.L., and Saito, H. (1995). Beneficial effects of S-113m, a novel herbal prescription on learning impairment model in mice. *Biological and Pharmaceutical Bulletin* 18: 1498-1503.

Nomura, M., Nakachiyama, T., Hida, T., Ohtaki, Y., Sudo, K., Aizawa, T., Aburada, M., and Miyamoto, K.I. (1994). Gomisin A, a lignan component of *Schizandra* fruits, inhibits development of preneoplastic lesions in rat liver by 3'-methyl-4-dimethylamino-azobenzene. *Cancer Letters* 76: 11-18.

Ohkura, Y., Misoguchi, Y., Morisawa, S., Takeda, S., Aburada, M., and Hosoya, E. (1990). Effect of gomisin (TJN-101) on the arachidonic acid cascade in macrophages. *Japanese Journal of Pharmacology* 52: 331-336.

Ohkura, Y., Mizoguchi, Y., and Sakagami, Y. (1987). Inhibitory effect of TJN-101 ((+)-(6S,7S,R-Biar)-5,6,7,8-tetrahydro-1,2,3,12-tetramethoxy-6,7-dimethyl-10,11-methy-lenedioxy-6-dibenzo[*a,c*]cyclooctenol) on immunologically induced liver injuries. *Japanese Journal of Pharmacology* 44: 179-185.

Ohtaki, Y., Nomura, M., Hida, T., Miyamoto, K., Kanitani, M., Aizawa, T., and Aburada, M. (1994). Inhibition of gomisin A, a lignan compound, of hepatocarcinogenesis by 3'-methyl-4-dimethylaminoazobenzene in rats. *Biological and Pharmaceutical Bulletin* 17: 808-814.

Ono, H., Matsuzaki, Y., Wakui, Y., Takeda, S., Ikeya, Y., Amagaya, S., and Maruno, M. (1995). Determination of schizandrin in human plasma by gas chromatography-mass spectrometry. *Journal of Chromatography* B, 674: 293-297.

Panossian, A.G., Oganessian, A.S., Ambartsumian, M., Gabrielian, E.S., Wagner, H., and Wikman, G. (1999). Effects of heavy physical exercise and adaptogens on nitric oxide content in human saliva. *Phytomedicine* 6: 17-26.

Rhee, J.K., Woo, K.J., Baek, B.K., and Ahn, B.J. (1982). Screening of the wormicidal Chinese raw drugs on *Clonorchis sinensis*. *American Journal of Chinese Medicine* 9: 277-284.

Sakurai, H., Nikaido, T., and Ohmoto, T. (1992). Inhibitors of adenosine 3',5'-cyclic monophosphate phosphodiesterase from *Schisandra chinensis* and the structure activity relationship of lignans. *Chemical and Pharmaceutical Bulletin* 40: 1191-1195.

Salbe, A.D. and Bjeldanes, L.F. (1985). The effects of dietary Brussels sprouts and *Schisandra chinensis* on the xenobiotic-metabolizing enzymes of the rat small intestine. *Food and Chemical Toxicology* 23: 57-65.

Shiota, G., Yamada, S., and Kawasaki, H. (1996). Rapid induction of hepatocyte growth factor mRNA after administration of gomisin A, a lignan component of *Schizandra* fruits. *Research Communications in Molecular Pathology and Pharmacology* 94: 141-146.

Sladkovsky, R., Solich, P., and Opletal, L. (2001). Simultaneous determination of quercetin, kaempferol and *(E)*-cinnamic acid in vegetative organs of *Schisandra chinensis* Baill. by HPLC. *Journal of Pharmaceutical and Biomedical Analysis* 24: 1049-1054.

Slanina, J., Taborska, E., Bochorakova, H., and Musil, P. (1995). Isocratic high-performance liquid chromatography of dibenzocyclooctadiene lignans from seeds of *Schisandra chinensis* Baill. *Scripta Medica* 68: 335-342.

Suekawa, M., Shiga, T., Sone, H., Ikeya, Y., Taguchi, H., Aburada, M., and Hosoya, E. (1987). [Effects of gomisin J and analogous lignan compounds in Schisandra fruits on isolated smooth muscles]. *Yakugaku Zasshi* 107: 720-726.

Suzuki, Y., Ohkura, Y., Takeda, S., and Hosoya, E. (1989). Effect of gomisin A (TJN-101) on membrane stability and calcium influx into hepatocytes. *Japanese Journal of Pharmacology* 49(Suppl.): 197 (abstract P-078).

Takeda, S., Arai, I., Kase, Y., Ohkura, Y., Hasegawa, M., Sekiguchi, Y., Sudo, K., Aburada, M., and Hosoya, E. (1987). Pharmacological studies on antihepatotoxic action of (+)-(6S,7S,R-Biar)-5,6,7,8-tetrahydro-1,2,3,12-tetramethoxy-6,7-di-methyl-10,11-methy-lenedioxy-6-dibenzo[a,c]cyclooctenol (TJN-101), a lignan component of Schisandra fruits. Influences of resolvents on the efficacy of TJN-101 in the experimental acute hepatic injuries. *Yakugaku Zasshi* 107: 517-524.

Tang, W. and Eisenbrand, G. (1992). *Chinese Drugs of Plant Origin*. Berlin: Springer-Verlag.

Tsuchiya, H., Shimizu, H., and Inuma, M. (1999). Beta-carboline alkaloids in crude drugs. *Chemical and Pharmaceutical Bulletin* 47: 4340-4443.

Tu, G., Fang, Q., Guo, J., Yuan, S., Chen, C., Chen, J., Chen, Z., Cheng, S., Jin, R., Li, M., et al. (Eds.) (1992). *Pharmacopoeia of the People's Republic of China* (pp. 82-83). Guangzhou, China: Guangdong Science and Technology Press.

Volicer, L., Janku, I., and Motl, O. (1965). The mode of action of *Schisandra chinensis*. In Chen, K.K., Mukerji, B., and Volicer, L. (Eds.), *Pharmacology of Oriental Plants* (pp. 29-38). New York: Pergamon Press Book, Macmillan Co.

Wagner, H. and Bauer, R. (1996). *Fructus Schisandrae—Wuweizi*. In *Chinese Drug Monographs and Analysis*, Vol. 1 (pp. 1-8). Kotzing/Bayer, Wald, Germany: Verlag für Ganzheitliche Medizin Dr. Erich Wühr GmbH.

Wang, J.P., Raung, S.L., Hsu, M.F., and Chen, C.C. (1994). Inhibition by gomisin C (a lignan from *Schizandra chinensis*) of the respiratory burst of rat neutrophils. *British Journal of Pharmacology* 113: 945-953.

Yamada, S., Murawaki, Y., and Kawasaki, H. (1993). Preventive effect of gomisin A, a lignan component of schizandra fruits, on acetaminophen-induced hepatotoxicity in rats. *Biochemical Pharmacology* 46: 1081-1085.

Yang, S.Z. (1997). *The Divine Farmer's Materia Medica: A Translation of the Shen Nong Ben Cao Jing* (p. 47). Boulder, CO: Blue Poppy Press, Inc.

Yao, D., Zhang, J., Chou, L., Bao, X., Shun, Q., Qi, P., Zheng, H., Zhang, J., Gao, S., Guo, J., et al. (1996). *A Coloured Atlas of the Chinese Materia Medica Specified in Pharmacopoeia of the People's Republic of China* (p. 78). Hong Kong, China: Joint Publishing (H.K.) Co., Ltd.

Yasukawa, K., Ikeya, Y., Mitsuhashi, H., Iwasaki, M., Aburada, M., Nakagawa, S., Takeuchi, M., and Takido, M. (1992). Gomisin A inhibits tumor promotion by 12-O-tetradecanoylphorbol-13-acetate in two-stage carcinogenesis in mouse skin. *Oncology* 49: 68-71.

Yen, K.Y. (1992). *The Illustrated Chinese Materia Medica: Crude and Prepared* (p. 151). Taipei, Taiwan: SMC Publishing Inc.

Yoshida, Y., Wang, M.Q., Liu, J.N., Shan, B.E., and Yamashita, U. (1997). Immunomodulating activity of Chinese medicinal herbs and *Oldenlandia diffusa* in particular. *International Journal of Immunopharmacology* 19: 359-370.

Zhang, E.J., Lin, T.J., and Qin, L. (1995). Effect of schisanhenol on function and surface shape of rat neutrophils. *Acta Pharmacologica Sinica* 16: 234-238.

Zhao, B.L., Li, X.J., and Liu, G.T. (1990). Scavenging effect of schizandrins on active oxygen radicals. *Cell Biology International Reports* 14: 99-109.

Zhu, M., Yeung, R.Y., Lin, K.F., and Li, R.C. (2000). Improvement of phase I drug metabolism with *Schisandra chinensis* against CCl_4 hepatotoxicity in a rat model. *Planta Medica* 66: 521-525.

Zhu, Y.P. (1998). *Chinese Materia Medica: Chemistry, Pharmacology and Applications* (pp. 653-657). Amsterdam, the Netherlands: Harwood Academic.

Zhu, Y., Yan, K., Wu, J., and Tu, G. (1988). Assay of lignans of *Schizandra chinensis* in sheng mai san by high performance liquid chromatography. *Journal of Chromatography* 438: 447-450.

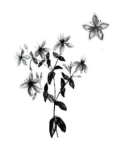

St. John's Wort

BOTANICAL DATA

Classification and Nomenclature

Scientific name: *Hypericum perforatum* L.

Family name: Guttiferae or Hypericaceae

Common names: St. John's wort (St. John's "herb"), Klamath weed, Hypericum (Hobbs, 1989), Johanniskraut (German), bassanti (Hindi), khoontir (Kashmir) (Gaind and Ganjoo, 1959)

Description

There are over 400 species of *Hypericum* distributed worldwide. The plants are glabrous, erect perennials with yellow, five-petaled flowers and sessile, opposite, ovate-linear leaves with translucent glands appearing as red dots. *Hypericum perforatum* blooms from June to September. It should not be confused with the ornamental ground-cover rose of Sharon (*H. calycinum*), commonly planted around buildings, in gardens, and parks. *Hypericum perforatum* is native to North Africa, the Azores, Madeira, West Asia, and Europe. In the United States, it is especially abundant in Northern California and Southern Oregon, an area from which it derives one of its common names, Klamath weed (Hobbs, 1989).

HISTORY AND TRADITIONAL USES

In the time of Galen and Hippocrates, the herb was used for wound healing, as a diuretic, as a treatment for neuralgic conditions such as sciatica and hip pain, and as an emmenagogue and a febrifuge, possibly for malarial fevers. Dioscorides wrote that the plant was good for burns, and Gerard in the

923

1600s wrote that no other herb was so efficacious in the treatment of deep wounds. Various authorities from the distant past used St. John's wort for treating depression and neuralgic disorders. Not surprisingly, it was believed to afford protection from evil spirits and demonic possession. In the early 1500s Paracelsus wrote that the herb could serve as an amulet to protect against apparitions and enchantments, and indeed one of its common names during the Middle Ages was "Devil's Scourge" (Hobbs, 1989). A Hebrew text from the fifteenth century shows a demon next to the herb named *fuga demonum* ("chase away the demon"), and an Italian herbal from the sixteenth century depicts the plant *erba ypericon* or *perforatta* curing a man with a demon flying away above him (Silberman, 1996). Linnaeus described the genus *Hypericum* and believed the origin of the name lay in the Greek words *eikon,* meaning a figure or image, and *yper,* meaning upper (Hobbs, 1989). Another interpretation of *Hypericum* is "over an apparition" (Duke, 1985), possibly in reference to herbal depictions of demons rendered above the herb. However, the original meaning of the name appears to have been lost in antiquity (Silberman, 1996; Hobbs, 1989).

Duke (1985) recounts its use as a dye plant producing a violet-red coloration to wool and silks, and when boiled with alum, a yellow color. He mentions records of its use in folk medicine in the treatment of ovarian carcinoma, uterine cancers, stomach cancers, and tumors of the lymph, adding that in the National Cancer Institute plant screening program of the 1960s the plant failed to show activity in the tumor screens then in use. Among its uses in herbal medicine, Duke cites a Russian application in bronchial asthma and numerous others: diarrhea, dysentery, neurasthenia, nervous depression, hysteria, chronic catarrh, rabies, worms, hemorrhage, and bladder problems, to name a few.

Moerman (1998) mentions use of the plant by the Cherokee Indians in an abortifacient formula, and as an emmenagogue, antidiarrheal, febrifuge (infusion), a treatment for sores, venereal disease (milky substance, possibly sap), hemostat for nosebleed (as snuff), snakebite remedy (root chewed and used as a poultice), and the root infusion as a wash to give infants strength. The Montagnais Indians decocted the plant for a cough medicine and the Iroquois used *H. perforatum* as a febrifuge and to prevent sterility.

CHEMISTRY

St. John's wort contains a wide variety of active constituents, including napthodianthrone derivatives, flavonoids, phloroglucinols, xanthones, and essential oils (Erdelmeier, 1998) (see Figure 1).

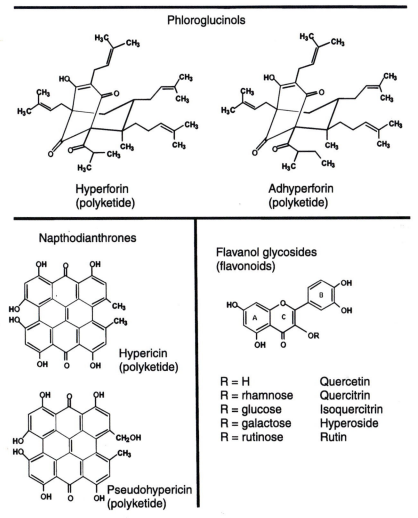

FIGURE 1. *Hypericum perforatum* L. (St. John's Wort): Representative Active Compounds

Terpenoid Compounds

The volatile components in St. John's wort include monoterpenes and sesquiterpenes. The major volatile compounds are 2-methyl-octane and α-pinene (Upton, 1997; Hobbs, 1989).

Phenolic Compounds

Polyphenolics

St. John's wort contains proanthocyanidins consisting of dimers, trimers, and higher polymers of catechin (procyanidins A2, B1, B2, B3, B5, B7, and C1) (Ploss et al., 2001), which comprise about 12% of the dried weight of the aerial portions of the plant (Upton, 1997) and of the total extract, usually a maximum of 20% (Erdelmeier, 1998).

Flavonoids

The following flavonols have been identified in the plant: kaempferol, luteolin, myricetin, quercetin, flavonol glycosides, quercitrin, isoquercitrin, hyperin/hyperoside, I3,II8-biapigenin, amentoflavone, leucoanthocyanidin, and rutin (Hansen et al., 1999; Kurth and Spreemann, 1998; Nahrstedt and Butterwick, 1997; Hobbs, 1989); however, Mártonfi et al. (2001) identified a rutin-free chemotype growing in Italy. Butterweck et al. (2000) isolated miquelianin (quercetin 3-*O*-glucuronide) and astilbin (taxifolin 3-*O*-rhamnopyranoside).

Phenylpropanoids

Caffeic, *p*-coumaric, ferulic, isoferulic, gentisic (Upton, 1997; Hobbs, 1989), and shikimic acids (Bilia et al., 2001) have also been reported.

Lipid Compounds

Polyketides (acetogenins)

The major napthodianthrones in St. John's wort are hypericin, pseudohypericin, isohypericin, and emodin-anthrone. In fresh material, protohypericin and protopseudohypericin are also present, and these are transformed by light into hypericin and pseudohypericin, respectively (Upton, 1997). Cyclopseudohypericin, an oxidation product of pseudohypericin, has also been reported and is partly responsible for the red color of St. John's wort extracts (Haberlein et al., 1992). The dried flowers can yield as much as 1.8% hypericin. Pseudohypericin concentrations are two to three times greater than hypericin concentrations (Upton, 1997). Tests of various commercially available extracts revealed amounts of between 0.171% and 0.355% hypericin, or from 47% to 165% of the concentrations stated on their labels (Constantine and Karchesy, 1999).

Phloroglucinols in St. John's wort are predominantly comprised of prenylated derivatives of hyperforin (2.0% to 4.5%) and adhyperforin (0.2% to 1.9%) (Upton, 1997; Hobbs, 1989) and are found only in the reproductive parts (about 2% in the flower, 4.4% in the ripe fruit, and 4.5% in the unripe fruit) (Maisenbacher and Kovar, 1992; Tekel'ová et al., 2000). However, traditional preparations such as teas and tinctures of St. John's wort contain little or no hyperforin (Meier, 2001). Furohyperforin, the major oxidation product of hyperforin, occurs in the aerial parts at about 5% of the hyperforin concentration (Verotta et al., 1999). In addition, oxepahyperforin (Verotta et al., 2000) and other oxidation analogues of hyperforin continue to be elucidated (Ming et al., 2001). Acylphloroglucinol-type compounds are the main compounds found in the fresh herb (Erdelmeier, 1998). Supercritical carbon dioxide (CO_2) extracts of the dried herb contain higher concentrations of hyperforin than other types of solvent extracts. Following prolonged storage, the hyperforin content of CO_2 extracts remained stable, whereas in other types of extracts it disappeared or gradually decreased. Tests of various commercially available solvent extracts revealed in some cases no hyperforin and in others amounts of between 1% and 5% (Chatterjee, Nölder, et al., 1998). Hyperforin and adhyperforin deteriorate rapidly upon exposure to air and light (Gray et al., 2000).

Other Constituents

Other compounds reported in St. John's wort include xanthones, carotenoids, β-sitosterol, pectin, fatty acids, amino acids, vitamin C, tannins (Duke, 1985), bisanthraquinone glycosides (Wirz et al., 2000), and in the stems and leaves, hydroperoxycadiforin (Rücker et al., 1995).

THERAPEUTIC APPLICATIONS

Most recent interest in St. John's wort has focused on its antidepressant effects; however, the herb has shown other activities, including wound-healing, antiviral activity, protein kinase C inhibition, coronary vasodilatory effects, induction of melatonin synthesis, analgesic, and hepatoprotective effects. Some of these findings are based on in vitro assays, in which cases the equivalent effective doses in humans have not been determined.

PRECLINICAL STUDIES

Cardiovascular and Circulatory Functions

Cardiotonic; Cardioprotection

A procyanidin fraction of St. John's wort enhanced coronary arterial flow in an isolated guinea pig perfusion in the same manner as procyanidins from hawthorn (*Crataegus* spp.). Procyanidin fractions antagonized histamine or prostaglandin F_{2d}-induced arterial contractions (Melzer et al., 1989, 1991).

Immune Functions; Inflammation and Disease

Cancer

Antiproliferative activity. Protein kinase C (PKC) has been implicated in the formation and proliferation of tumors. Hypericin inhibited the growth of glioma cell lines in vitro and induced glioma cell death due to inhibition of PKC, as measured by [^{3}H]-thymidine uptake. The glioma-inhibitory activity of hypericin was comparable to or greater than tamoxifen ($IC_{50} < 10$ versus 10 μmol/L, respectively). The activity was enhanced by approximately 13% from exposure of hypericin to visible light (Couldwell et al., 1994). When light activated, hypericin was shown to induce apoptosis in HL-60 promyelocytic cells in vitro (Mirossay et al., 2000).

Infectious Diseases

Microbial infections. A decoction of St. John's wort showed relatively weak in vitro activity against the growth of 40 clinical strains of aggregative and nonaggregative *Escherichia coli*. However, the hydrophobicity of 13 strains was significantly enhanced ($p < 0.04$) in the salt aggregation test, indicating that the ability of the strains to adhere to cell surfaces of the host may be compromised by St. John's wort (Türi et al., 1997).

Studies of the antimicrobial activity of the various plant parts in India (Gaind and Ganjoo, 1959) led to the isolation of an antibacterial principle named hyperforin (Schempp et al., 1999), which is currently recognized as an antidepressant principle of St. John's wort (Chatterjee, Nölder, et al., 1998; Chatterjee, Bhattacharya, et al., 1998). The inherent instability of hyperforin in its pure form obviated further studies of antimicrobial activity until an investigation by Schempp et al. (1999). Using the agar-dilution method, the researchers reported that hyperforin showed no antibacterial activity in concentration of 0.1-100 μg/mL in cultures of Gram-negative bacteria, and no activity against *Candida albicans*. Against Gram-positive bacteria, hyperforin inhibited the growth of all strains tested, including methicillin- and penicillin-resistant *Staphylococcus aureus* (1–100 μg/mL). The methicillin-resistant strain was also resistant to a number of penicillins and to cephalosporins, clindamycin, erythromycin, gentamicin, ofloxacin, and piperacillin/tazobactam. Against *Corynebacterium diptheriae* (E 6046), as little as 0.1 μg/mL was required to inhibit growth, and 1.0 μg/mL was needed to inhibit *Streptococcus agalactiae* B (D 595) and *S. pyogenes* A (E12449). Testing the toxicity of hyperforin on the viability of peripheral blood mononuclear cells, the researchers found little; cell viability after exposure to hyperforin at 100 µg/mL was reduced to 75%, to 80% at 10 µg/mL, and remained 100% at 1.0 µg/mL. The researchers concluded that their results lend support to the traditional use of St. John's wort in treating infected wounds (Schempp et al., 1999).

Viral infections. Hypericin has been proposed for use in decontaminating blood infected by a broad spectrum of pathogenic viruses (Lavie, Mazur, Lavie, and Meruelo, 1995). Hypericin and pseudohypericin inhibit the replication of a variety of encapsulated viruses, including herpes simplex types 1 and 2, HIV-1, murine cytomegalovirus, parainfluenza 3 virus, Sindbis virus, vesicular stomatitis virus, and equine infectious anemia virus (Serkedjieva et al., 1990; Yip et al., 1996; Wood et al., 1990; Weber et al., 1994; Lavie et al., 1990; Lavie, Mazur, Lavie, and Meruelo, 1995; Lavie, Mazur, Lavie, Prince, et al., 1995). Both compounds display antiviral activity that may involve a nonspecific association with viral and cellular membranes. Photoactivation of these compounds, leading to the formation of activated oxygen species, appears to participate in the inactivation of viral fusion and syncytia formation. However, this light-driven mechanism may limit therapeutic activity in vivo (Stevenson and Lenard, 1993). Hypericin, however, can form semiquinone radicals in the absence of light (Lavie, Mazur, Lavie, and Meruelo, 1995).

Inflammatory Response

Panossian et al. (1996) examined the effects of hypericin on the release of inflammatory mediators by human immune system cells. At low concentrations (IC_{50} 4-8 µM), hypericin significantly and dose-dependently inhibited the release of arachidonic acid (AA) and, as a result, of leukotriene B_4 (LTB_4). The authors found that hypericin strongly inhibited interleukin-1 alpha (IL-1α), possibly by way of inhibiting protein kinase C (PKC), as shown by Takahashi et al. (1989) at about the same concentration (0.1-10 µM). IL-1α is well known as a potent factor in mediating inflammation and fever, inducing acute-phase reaction, nitric oxide production, reactive oxygen intermediate leading to free-radical production, and activating B cells, eosinophils, natural killer (NK) cells, granulocytes, and T cells. However, an extract of St. John's wort proved far stronger than hypericin at inhibiting the release of IL-1α and of LTB_4. The researchers suggested that inhibition of these mediators results in a quelling of the inflammatory response (immunosuppression) and that, apparently besides hypericin, other active constituents are involved (Panossian et al., 1996).

NF-κB is a transcription factor involved in immunological and inflammatory responses. NF-κB is activated by physical stress (from UV light and gamma-radiation), oxidative stress from free radical-producing chemicals in the system (e.g., hydrogen peroxide), products of bacteria (e.g., lipopolysaccharide), viral products (e.g., double-stranded RNA), viruses (e.g., herpes simplex type 1, human herpes virus 6, hepatitis B, HIV, Epstein Barr), and various inflammatory cytokines, including interleukin-1 (IL-1), IL-2, LTB$_4$, tumor necrosis factor alpha (TNFα), and others (Baeuerle and Henkel, 1994). An investigation of the effect of St. John's wort on the NF-κB inflammation factor was conducted by Bork et al. (1999). Their in vitro experiments demonstrated that whereas a St. John's wort ethanolic extract (Schwabe) standardized to contain hyperforin and hypericin (5% and 0.15%, respectively) showed no activity at 200 μg/mL, hypericin at 2 μg/mL proved a potent inhibitor of TNFα-induced activation of NF-κB, and at a concentration comparable to that of a potent NF-κB inhibitor (parthenolide 5 μM) found in feverfew (*Tanacetum parthenium* [L.] Schulz Bip). Hypericin (2 μg/mL) also inhibited the transcription of interleukin-6 (IL-6) (an inflammatory cytokine), almost totally preventing the TNF-α-induced expression of IL-6. Hyperforin, however, showed no appreciable activity, even at 20 μg/mL (37.3 μM). The researchers therefore concluded that anti-inflammatory effects of St. John's wort extract preparations containing hypericin appear to be at least partly due to the inhibition of NF-κB.

Integumentary, Muscular, and Skeletal Functions

Skin Diseases

One of the oldest traditional uses of St. John's wort has been as a vulnerary (an herb used to promote wound healing). When orally administered to male albino rats, a tincture of the flowering tops and fresh leaves proved more effective than the topical application of another wound-healing herb, an undiluted tincture of marigold *(Calendula)* flowering tops and fresh leaves. Both preparations were prepared in the same manner and strength (1:10 parts 60% alcohol at a dose of 0.1 mL diluted to 1 mL in distilled water). In treating incision wounds, epithelization occurred in 15 days from the St. John's wort treatment (p.o. once daily for 10 days), and in 16.5 days in the marigold group treated topically for the same number of days. The rate in both groups was significantly superior to that of the untreated control group with epithelization in 23 days ($p < 0.001$). The breaking strength of the wounds was also greater in the St. John's wort group (396 g, $p < 0.001$) and the marigold group (351 g, $p < 0.01$) compared to the control group (270 g). In a 21-day treatment of excision wounds, wound contraction occurred at about the same time in all three groups, yet the researchers found better epithelization in the St. John's wort group than that in either the control or marigold group. In a ten-day treatment of dead space wounds, St. John's wort tincture alone was compared to the control group since topical treatments would affect the weight of the granuloma produced. Although a significant difference in granuloma weight was not found, the breaking strength of the dead space wounds was considerably greater

($p < 0.001$) in the St. John's wort group (423 g versus 252 g) (Rao et al., 1991).

Neurological, Psychological, and Behavioral Functions

Psychological and Behavioral Functions

Cognitive functions. Kumar et al. (2000) compared the cognitive function-enhancing effects of a standardized ethanolic extract of St. John's wort to those of the nootropic agent piracetam. Albino rats of either sex were administered the extract at 100 and 200 mg/kg p.o. for three days and compared to controls administered vehicle and a group administered an acute dose of piracetam (500 mg/kg i.p.). Significant effects of the St. John's wort extract were found in the following animal models of cognitive dysfunction compared to untreated controls: sodium nitrate- and scopolamine-induced amnesia (transfer latency antagonized at both doses); scopolamine-induced passive avoidance retention deficit (reversed deficit from 200 mg/kg); sodium nitrate- and scopolamine-induced increase in transfer latency in the elevated plus-maze (increased transfer latency significantly antagonized by either dose); active avoidance test (acquisition and retention facilitated by either dose); sodium nitrate- and scopolamine-induced conditioned avoidance response (both doses attenuated the retention deficits). The researchers concluded that although the St. John's wort extract was minimally effective at increasing learning acquisition in their tests, it did show a facilitatory effect on retention and on retention of acquired learning, indicating that it may be considered as a nootropic agent.

Khalifa (2001) found evidence of nootropic effects in male mice administered an extract of St. John's wort at doses equivalent to those used in the treatment of human patients with depression. Effects on memory retrieval were measured using a passive avoidance test in which latencies of action served as a measure of memory levels. Administered 30 min prior to the task, significant and dose-dependent increases in latencies were found at doses of 4 to 25 mg/kg i.p.; the highest dose equivalent to a human therapeutic dose of 1,800 mg/day. In the same test, these doses failed to produce increased latencies against scopolamine-induced amnesia (3.0 mg/kg administered 30 min prior to the St. John's wort extract)—a result in contrast to those of Kumar et al. (2000) who used much higher doses of St. John's wort. The same procedure was used to test the effects of various adrenergic, dopaminergic, and serotonergic antagonists on the memory retrieval-enhancing effect of St. John's wort extract. Dopaminergic antagonists (sulpiride and SCH 23390) caused no alterations in the effect of St. John's wort and had no effect on the measured response of the animals when either one was administered alone. Against individual adrenoreceptor antagonists (phentolamine and propranolol), the latency-increasing effect of St. John's wort was significantly reduced, yet either of the antagonists alone had no effect. Finally, against pretreatments of the mice with the serotonergic 5-HT$_{1A}$ receptor antagonist (–)-pindolol and a serotonergic 5-HT$_{2A}$ blocker, spiperone, the effect of St. John's wort was significantly decreased by (–)-pindolol, which had no effect when administered alone, yet the serotonergic receptor blocker spiperone had no effect alone or in combination with St. John's wort. The researchers explained that these results indicate that whereas the effect of St. John's wort on memory retrieval appears not to involve serotonergic 5-HT$_{2A}$ receptors or dopaminergic mechanisms, they may involve serotonergic 5-HT$_{1A}$ receptors and both α- and β-adrenergic receptors.

Klusa et al. (2001) reported significant memory-increasing activity in rats administered an ethanolic extract of St. John's wort (50 mg/kg p.o. daily for seven days) used in the manufacture of a commercial product (Neuroplant, Willmer Schwabe GmbH). The effective dose was equal to that of the antidepressant dose in the behavioral despair test. After nine days without treatment, the rats continued to show significant retention of learned responses despite discontinuation of training. In the same tests with hyperforin, the effective dose (1.25 mg/kg p.o. daily for seven days) was lower than that required for antidepressant activity (10-30 mg/kg p.o. per day). The researchers commented that an effective therapy for cognitive impairments related to depression or geriatric depression are presently unavailable.

Depression. Studies of St. John's wort extracts have repeatedly shown significant antidepressive effects in various animal models of depression (Bhattacharya et al., 1998; Butterweck et al., 1998; Chatterjee, Bhattacharya, et al., 1998, and references cited therein). The mechanisms responsible are as yet incompletely understood, as they are for standard antidepressants, and are clearly different from the latter in a number of activities. For example, unlike standard antidepressants, commercially available St. John's wort extracts exhibit an excitatory effect on hippocampal cells (Langosch et al., 2001); fail to show inhibiting activity on serotonergic neurons, serotonin metabolism, or turnover (Fornal et al., 2001); and without changing receptor affinity, up-regulate postsynaptic 5-hydroxytryptamine (5-HT$_{1A}$) and 5-HT$_{A2}$ receptors (Nathan, 1999).

The optimal doses of hypericin (9-28 µg/kg p.o.) and pseudohypericin (166 µg/kg p.o.) in the immobility test corresponded to the MAO inhibitor bupropion at a dose of 20 mg/kg p.o. (Butterweck et al., 1998). The suggestion, however, that the antidepressant action of St. John's wort is due to monoamine oxidase (MAO) inhibition, is no longer credited. St. John's wort is a weak MAO inhibitor in vitro (Müller et al., 1997; Bladt and Wagner, 1994) and in vivo (Yu, 2000). An exception may be a CO_2 extract of St. John's wort; a dosage of 1 mg/kg p.o. caused a significant increase of dopamine outflow in rats (Di Matteo et al., 2000). Alternative hypotheses are that

1. St. John's wort extracts inhibit catechol-O-methyl transferase (COMT), an enzyme that degrades catecholamine neurotransmitters (Upton, 1997);
2. they inhibit serotonin reuptake;
3. they inhibit serotonin receptor expression (Nathan, 1999); and
4. they reduce expression of the cytokine interleukin-6, which may cause depression in some people (Calapai et al., 2001).

St. John's wort extracts also inhibit GABA (γ-amino butyric acid) uptake and $GABA_A$ receptors in vitro at low concentrations (1 mg/mL and 3 μg/mL respectively) (Upton, 1997). Evidence suggests that GABAergic mechanisms may be implicated in depressive states (Petty et al., 1995), both unipolar (Petty et al., 1992) and bipolar (Petty et al., 1993). However, these possible mechanisms have yet to be demonstrated in vivo at pharmacologically relevant doses of St. John's wort extracts (Upton, 1997; Philippu, 2001; Kaehler et al., 1999). Similar in vitro inhibition of $GABA_A$ was found from an ethanolic extract of passionflower *(Passiflora incarnata)* (Simmen et al., 1999).

Simmen et al. (1999) speculated that other active constituents may well exist in the lipophilic hexane fraction and that a combination of the various receptor-binding activities may work synergistically to account for the antidepressant activity of the plant. Butterweck et al. (1998) found evidence to suggest that the solubility of hypericin and pseudohypericin is enhanced by procyanidins in the crude extract and that procyanidin B_2 was especially active. The presence of the procyanidins significantly increased the antidepressant activity of hypericin and pseudohypericin, as measured by immobility and swimming tests in rats. Solubility of hypericin was increased maximally by the crude procyanidin fraction at a ratio of 1:1 and 1:2. Butterweck et al. (2000) have since shown that flavonoid fractions from St. John's wort are significantly active in the forced swimming test (FST) when administered in acute treatments. Active constituents in these fractions were identified as miquelianin (quercetin 3-O-glucuronide) and isoquercitrin. However, in a chronic (12-day) treatment, antidepressant activity in the FST was significant compared to a control with imipramine (20 mg/kg p.o., $p < 0.01$), hyperoside ($p < 0.05$), and miquelianin ($p < 0.01$), but not isoquercitrin (each at 0.6 mg/kg p.o.).

Receptor- and Neurotransmitter-Mediated Functions

Perovic and Müller (1995) demonstrated that an extract of St. John's wort (LI 160) dose-dependently inhibited serotonin uptake in vitro in rat synaptosomes (IC_{50} 6.2 μg/mL), thereby allowing an increase in serotonin concentration at postsynaptic receptor sites. However, its mode of antidepressant action remains unknown. In vitro studies have since shown that crude extracts of St. John's wort nonselectively inhibit the uptake of dopamine, γ-aminobutyric acid (GABA), norepinephrine, and L-glutamate, but not by a mechanism common to standard antidepressants (Fornal et al., 2001).

Simmen et al. (1999) found that in vitro neuroreceptor-binding activities of St. John's wort extracts varied depending on the type of solvent used. An ethanolic extract of St. John's wort prepared from the whole plant minus the roots (Zeller AG, Romanshorn, Switzerland) weakly inhibited in vitro binding to κ-, δ- and μ-opioid, estrogen-α, and $GABA_A$ receptors expressed in Chinese hamster ovary cells (Semliki Forest virus expression system) and had no effect on serotonin receptors ($5-HT_6$ and $5-HT_7$). A methanolic extract prepared from the flowers and leaves was about ten times more potent as an inhibitor, however moderately active. Extracts of St. John's wort nonspecifically inhibited binding of the serotonin, neurokinin-1 (NK-1), and human ^{3}H-nociceptin receptors, whereas some fractions specifically inhibited binding to NK-1 and the serotonin receptors. Hexane-extracted fractions of St. John's wort showed by far the strongest inhibition of binding to both the opioid and serotonin receptors (1-4 μg/mL). Finally, hyperforin showed more potent inhibition of binding to the opioid and serotonin receptors (0.4-1.0 μM) than either pseudohypericin (1-10 μM) or hypericin (1 to (10 μM).

Kleber et al. (1999) demonstrated that, based on total hypericins, extracts of St. John's wort inhibit dopamine-β-hydroxylase at a lower IC_{50} than pure, commercially available hypericin (IC_{50} 0.1 μmol/L versus IC_{50} 21 μmol/L, respectively). The approximate 200-times-greater potency of the total hypericins implied that other constituents are responsible. Gobbi and collaborators (1999) raised the same possibility after demonstrating a lack of serotonin transporter inhibition in rat brain cortex and no significant changes in levels of rat brain 5-hydroxyindoleacetic acid after oral administration of St. John's wort extract on a scheduled basis. Their receptor binding experiments led them to further conclude that neither GABA, serotonin, nor benzodiazepine receptors are involved in the antidepressant effect of St. John's wort extracts since in each case IC_{50} values were above 5 μg/mL.

Work continues on determining the spectrum of receptors involved in the antidepressant activity of St. John's wort extracts and the active constituents responsible. Raffa (1998) screened hypericin against 30 reuptake or receptor sites. With the exceptions of high affinity binding to nonselective Sigma (σ) receptors, which are found in the limbic and other emotional-regulatory regions of the brain, and muscarinic acetylcholine receptor (mAChR) sites (48% and 49% inhibition, respectively), he found specific binding inhibited in less than 40% of the reuptake or receptor sites. Hypericin displayed only weak inhibiting activity for nicotinic acetylcholine receptor (nAChR) sites and no significant activity for central benzodiazepine, dopamine D_1, GABA, opioid, or adrenergic (α_1, α_2, or β_1) sites. Raffa noted that although a correspondence to the action to synthetic selective norepinephrine reuptake inhibitors (SNRIs) and selective serotonin reuptake inhibitors (SSRIs) is possible, in this regard St. John's wort appears too weak for these activity models to stand as the sole explanation of its action as an antidepressant.

In a study on the anxiolytic effects of a total extract of St. John's wort, Vandenbogaerde et al. (2000) found results that appear to contradict some of those of Raffa (1998). Rats administered the total extract exhibited increased locomotor activity in the open field test and anxiolytic effect was apparent in the light-dark test. The anxiolytic effect was blocked when the rats were pretreated with a benzodiazepine antagonist (flumazenil), thereby suggesting that the activation of benzodiazepine receptors may be involved in the anxiolytic effect. Tests with hypericin found a reduction in GABA-activated chloride currents, the opposite effect from pseudohypericin, and found from both compounds an inhibition of NMDA receptor activation. Yet neither compound showed any in vivo anxiolytic effect; nor did they increase locomotor activity.

Panocka and co-workers (2000) followed up on the finding of Raffa (1998), which showed that St. John's wort extract binds with high affinity to σ receptors, in part because these receptors may figure significantly in relief from behavioral despair in the forced swimming test. The anti-immobility effect of St. John's wort extract in rats (from 250 mg/kg i.p. t.i.d.) was completely suppressed by administration of a σ receptor antagonist (rimcazole) administered 30 min beforehand. A comparatively less pronounced suppression of the anti-immobility effect of St. John's wort was found from intracerebroventricular pretreatment with a serotonin-depleting agent (5,7-dihydroxytryptamine). Although pretreatment with either agent had no significant effect on ethanol intake of the rats administered St. John's wort, the researchers concluded that their results indicate the involvement of σ receptors in the antidepressant-like effect of the herb. Further studies using clinically relevant oral dosages of St. John's wort extracts will be needed to confirm this involvement.

Xanthones may also contribute to the antidepressant activity of St. John's wort. Commercial extracts were found to contain relatively small amounts of xanthones (1%-3%) whereas an Indian specimen contained 2%-4% xanthones. A xanthone-enriched fraction from this specimen was administered to rats (5 mg/kg p.o.), who showed significant activity in the forced swimming test and exhibited receptor binding inhibitory activities in the frontal cortex, suggesting up-regulation of benzodiazepine and serotonin receptors and down-regulation of dopamine D_2 receptors. Four trioxygenated xanthones isolated from the plant also exhibited significant antidepressant activity. A hyperforin-enriched fraction at the same dosage was equipotent to the xanthone-enriched fraction. When the two extracts were combined in suboptimal dosages of 2.5 mg each, they caused a significant antidepressant effect, which was slightly greater in extent than exhibited by either the hyperforin-enriched or the xanthone-enriched fraction (Muruganandam et al., 2000).

Wirz et al. (2000) identified two bisanthraquinone glycosides in a dry extract of St. John's wort aerial parts that showed moderate binding to corticotropin-releasing hormone receptors in vitro. Wirz and co-workers concluded that their concentration in the dry plant is too low to play anything more than a minor role in the antidepressant effect, even though the IC_{50} values were much greater than those of either hypericin or hyperforin. They add that the activity of these glycosides may partly explain the in vivo and in vitro observations by Thiele et al. (1993) of reduced levels of tissue corticosteroids in rats administered St. John's wort extracts. Also estimated to be of minor effect are several hyperforin analogues identified in the aerial parts of the plant, which showed greater than tenfold less activity in a serotonin reuptake inhibition assay compared to hyperforin (Verotta et al., 2000).

Because astrocytes act as regulators of neurotransmission by way of their own uptake systems and encircle synaptic terminals, Neary and Bu (1999) examined neurotransmission effects displayed by astrocytes exposed to St. John's wort extracts. The extracts caused a dose-dependent inhibition of serotonin and norepinephrine uptake, with norepinephrine uptake somewhat more potently inhibited than that of serotonin. They also examined the effect of two methanolic extract batches of St. John's wort (LI 160) on norepinephrine and serotonin transport into cultured astrocytes. Their results showed that whereas uptake sites for norepinephrine underwent a 4.5-fold reduction in apparent affinity for the neurotransmitter, maximal transport of serotonin decreased by 50%. The researchers deduced that the effect was not toxic since both serotonin and norepinephrine uptake could be restored after removal of the extract. They concluded that although the action of St. John's wort extract on these neurotransmitters is different, together they demonstrated an antidepressant activity of the herb.

Müller et al. (1998) showed that hyperforin potently inhibits synaptosomal serotonin, norepinephrine, and dopamine reuptake (IC_{50} 80-205 nmol/L), whereas hypericin proved to be a comparably weak reuptake inhibitor of all three neurotransmitters (IC_{50} >10,000 nmol/L). A methanolic extract of *Hypericum* showed only weak activity as an inhibitor of MAO-A or MAO-B, and a hyperforin-rich CO_2 extract was even weaker. The CO_2 extract, richer in hyperforin than the methanolic extract, behaved more like an antidepressant drug in that it potently inhibited norepinephrine and/or serotonin. Indeed, others have also shown evidence in support of hyperforin as the main active constituent in St. John's wort, with hypericin being secondary

(Dimpfel et al., 1998; Chatterjee, Bhattacharya, et al., 1998; Müller et al., 1998).

Kaehler et al. (1999) administered hyperforin (Dr. Willmer Schwabe GmbH, Karlsruhe, Germany) to male rats (10 mg/kg i.p.) to see what influence it might have on the concentration of extracellular neurotransmitters in the rat locus coeruleus, a pigmented area eminent in the superior angle of the brain floor. Injection alone had no influence on the rate at which the neurotransmitters were released. The concentration of extracellular norepinephrine was immediately increased and persisted for at least 150 min. At 30 min postinjection of hyperforin, the researchers observed a long-lasting and pronounced increase in concentrations of extracellular glutamate, an excitatory amino acid. However, concentrations of the inhibitory amino acids aspartate, arginine, serine, taurine, or GABA were not influenced. At 45 min postinjection of hyperforin, extracellular dopamine concentration showed an increase and a tendency to be enhanced until the experiment end. At 60 min, the concentration of serotonin showed a marked increase which also persisted until the experiment end, yet the extracellular amount of the main metabolite of serotonin, 5-hydroxyindolacetic acid (5-HIAA), was not influenced, although taurine showed an insignificant increase after about 3 h. Kaehler and co-workers concluded that their results conformed with those of prior in vitro studies which showed that hyperforin inhibits monoamine and glutamate uptake in synaptosomal preparations, and that in the rat locus coeruleus hyperforin can enhance extracellular concentrations of glutamate, dopamine, norepinephrine, and serotonin. However, unlike prior in vitro findings (citing Chatterjee, Bhattacharya, et al. 1998), hyperforin had no influence on the extracellular concentration of GABA in vivo. The researchers noted that the lack of influence by hyperforin on extracellular 5-HIAA suggests that it enhances the level of serotonin by inhibiting its presynaptic uptake rather than by increasing its turnover (Kaehler et al., 1999).

Singer et al. (1999) performed in vitro experiments in brain synaptosomes from female mice and platelets from nonmedicated humans in an effort to characterize the apparently unique serotonin reuptake inhibition mechanism of hyperforin. Unlike any other known antidepressant drug, in vitro studies demonstrated that hyperforin potently inhibits the uptake of not just serotonin, dopamine, and norepinephrine but also the synaptosomal uptake of glutamate and GABA. Furthermore, compared to tricyclic or SSRI antidepressants, hyperforin showed only weak inhibition of radiolabeled paroxetine binding in relation to its serotonin uptake activity. Unlike most antidepressant drugs, their tests indicated that hyperforin does not competitively bind to the serotonin binding site of the transporter molecule. Following the findings of others who demonstrated that the uptake of serotonin requires external sodium, they compared the mode of serotonin reuptake inhibition of the SSRI citalopram and the sodium ionophore monensin (a veterinary antiprotozoal, antifungal, and antibacterial agent) to that of hyperforin, speculating that it may also work by increasing sodium. Not only did hyperforin behave in a similar manner inasmuch as it increased sodium in human platelets at the concentration required for serotonin uptake to be inhibited, but the researchers discovered that hyperforin also shows activity at the human serotonin transporter. Singer and collaborators speculated that the antidepressant mechanism of hyperforin is one of elevating sodium, although not to an extracellular level (even at high concentrations), and that its effect on sodium is associated with a cellular ion-exchange mechanism which in turn inhibits serotonin uptake. The researchers noted that, if proven, hyperforin would represent the first substance known with potential use as a clinical antidepressant that works by influencing intracellular sodium (Singer et al., 1999). Studies on the role of specific sodium channels in the antidepressant activity of hyperforin are continuing (Wonnemann et al., 2000).

A preponderant number of in vitro and animal studies have shown that the main antidepressant constituent of commercial St. John's wort extracts is hyperforin (Müller et al., 2001; Gambarana et al., 2001; Eckert and Müller, 2001). At the same time, there are studies that show this may not apply to traditional preparations of the herb or all commercial extract preparations of St. John's wort.

Coleta et al. (2001) studied the effects of an aqueous extract of the aerial parts of St. John's wort in mice for antianxiety activity using the elevated plus maze, horizontal wire, and open-field tests. The plant was collected in the wild in Coimbra, Portugal; the extract was prepared according to traditional methods; and contents of total flavonoids, hypericins, and hyperforin were determined using published methods. Significant sedative effects were found from doses of 25, 50, and 100 mg/kg, and an anxiolytic effect was found from a dose of 5 mg/kg. Given the absence of hyperforin in the extract and the presence of hypericins (0.16%), Coleta and co-workers concluded that the anxiolytic effect of the traditional extract is not due to hyperforin.

In a study on neuroreceptor-binding activity of a hypercritical carbon dioxide and a hydromethanolic extract of St. John's wort, Gobbi et al. (2001) found that whereas the hydromethanolic extract interacted with $GABA_A$ receptors (5.5 µg/mL), at 10 µg/mL neither extract inhibited ligand binding at benzodiazepine, serotonin $5HT_6$ and $5HT_7$, neuropeptide Y1 or Y2, or sigma receptors, despite the relatively high concentration of hyperforin in the CO_2 extract (2.5 µg/mL). Although both extracts showed interactive activity with dopamine transporters, the effect was found only from high concentrations (12 µg/mL and 24.5 µg/mL, respectively). Tests using biapgenin, hyperforin, and hypericin showed that biapgenin inhibited only benzodiazepine receptor ligand binding (1 µg/mL), hyperforin (1 µg/mL) only dopamine transporters and then only from a higher concentration (5 μM) than that required for inhibition of dopamine reuptake in synaptosomes (0.8 μM), and that hypericin (1 μg/mL) failed to show any significant inhibitory effect on dopamine transporters, serotonin ($5HT_6$ and $5HT_7$), $GABA_A$, or benzodiazepine receptors. Hypericin did show inhibitory activity against ligand binding to sigma receptors and to neuropeptide Y1 and Y2 receptors (IC_{50}s 3-4 μM), but when the same experiment was performed in the dark the effects on sigma receptors substantially decreased and practically vanished on neuropeptide Y1 and Y2 receptors. However, even in the light the concentrations of hypericin required for activity were much higher than those attained in humans from effective antidepressant dosages of St. John's wort extracts, at least in the plasma. Whether higher concentrations are found in the brain remains to be determined. Gobbi and colleagues concluded that their in vitro study failed to show that extracts of St. John's wort exhibit significant effects on the brain receptors "potentially involved" in the antidepressant and anxiolytic effects of the herb, leaving open the question of other active constituents.

Kientsch et al. (2001) raised the question of hyperforin and hypericin as the putative main active constituents in a study on a commercial St. John's wort extract (Ze 117, Zeller Medical AG, Romanshorn, Switzerland) standardized to contain 0.2% hypericin. Effects of the extract were studied on serotonin (5-HT) and norepinephrine (NE) uptake inhibition and β-adrenoreceptor concentrations using rat brain slices. Ze 117 is a 50% ethanol extract standardized to contain total hypericins in a concentration of 1 mg per daily dosage (250 mg b.i.d.) and corresponds to 2-3.5 g of the crude herb. Clinical trials of the extract in mild to moderate depression showed efficacy in comparison to fluoxetine (20 mg/day, imipramine (150 mg/day) and placebo (Meier, 2001). Kientsch and co-workers found dose-dependent uptake inhibition of 5-HT and NE from Ze 117, much more so NE uptake (IC_{50} 1,010 μg/mL, corresponding to 4 μM hypericin, versus IC_{50} 54.6 μg/mL, respectively), which was inhibited about 20 times more than 5-HT and was comparable to the inhibition produced by the standard antidepressant desipramine. As for comparative efficacy on the uptake of NE and 5-HT, tests showed that the extract was equal to the standard antidepressants fluvoxamine, desipramine, and imipramine. When hypericin and hyperforin were run through the same tests, however, no inhibition of 5-HT or NE uptake into rat brain slices was evident, even at concentrations of 10^{-5} or 10^{-6}. At higher concentrations than these, hyperforin appeared to show toxicity. In a chronic exposure study, the extract also showed activity on the β-adrenoreceptor, which was down-regulated about as much as by desipramine (30-40%). The researchers note that down-regulation of β-adrenoreceptor is also found from chronic treatment using standard antidepressants and is associated with clinical improvement. In efforts to explain the discrepancy of their findings on hyperforin with those of others using synaptosomal preparations, the researchers pointed to possible differences in test models, purity of the compounds, pharmacokinetics, and pharmacodynamics. For hypericin, however, their results concurred with previous studies. The antidepressant action of Ze 117 therefore appears to involve the inhibition of NE uptake and β-adrenoreceptor down-regulation. Regardless of the fact that the extract contained no hyperforin, Kientsch and colleagues drew no conclusions as to the active principles involved because their results were found using the whole plant extract.

Ion modulating effects of St. John's wort constituents on rat neurons in vitro have shown that although hyperforin is clearly the most active, when it comes to an ethanolic extract multiple mechanisms and multiple other constituents may be involved, in particular biapigenin, quercitrin, and hyperosid (Krishtal et al., 2001).

Given that several studies have recently found antidepressant activity from hyperforin-free extracts of St. John's wort (Wonnemann et al. [2001] citing De Vry et al., 1999 and Butterweck et al., 1998), and that the constituents responsible for St. John's wort's antidepressant activity have yet to be fully elucidated, Wonnemann et al. (2001) conducted a further examination of the synaptosomal neurotransmitter uptake inhibitory activity of various constituents of St. John's wort, this time adding ten different commercial extracts of the herb. The extracts were tested for activity on synaptosomal uptake of dopamine, epinephrine, NE, GABA, L-glutamine, and serotonin, and their effects were checked for correlation to hyperforin content. The various constituents of St. John's wort, which were tested only for inhibition of L-glutamate, NE, and serotonin, comprised: adhyperforin, hyperforin, hypericin, hypericin and pseudohypericin, hyperoside, kaempferol, amentoflavone, biapigenin, isoquercitrin, quercitrin, quercetin, myricetin, oligomeric procyanidins, and rutin. The results showed that although the content of hyperforin in the commercial extracts correlated with the inhibition of the various neurotransmitters in all cases except for NE, hyperforin-free extracts showed weak to moderate inhibitory activity. Tests revealed that this activity was attributable to the content of adhyperforin, which showed strong activity in tests for synaptosamal uptake inhibition of L-glutamate, NE, and serotonin (Wonnemann et al., 2001). In other synaptosomal tests for monoamine uptake inhibition, adhyperforin was reported to be slightly more potent than hyperforin in NE, 5-HT, and dopamine uptake (Jensen et al., 2001). As for the various constituents, oligomeric procyanidins were weakly to moderately active. They showed more potent activity than adhyperforin in serotonin and NE uptake inhibition, but less potent activity in L-glutamate inhibition. The rest of the constituents were devoid of activity, leaving Wonnemann and colleagues (2001) to conclude that the antidepressant activities of these constituents found in animal models of depression must therefore be caused by other mechanisms.

Finally, in a recent study using a rat model of conditioned fear, Philippu (2001) reported that hyperforin (10 mg/kg i.p.) increased the release rates of dopamine and noradrenaline in the locus coeruleus, and increased extracellular concentrations of serotonin and L-glutamate, but not those of GABA. In the same tests, a hyperforin-free extract of St. John's wort (uncharacterized) increased the extracellular concentrations of NE and dopamine in the locus coeruleus, yet decreased extracellular levels of serotonin while having no effect on GABA or L-glutamate. Because the profile of activity differed from that of hyperforin, Philippu deduced that this may be an indication of other active constituents in the St. John's wort extract. He also concluded that because the hyperforin-free extract decreased extracellular concentrations of serotonin, as did conditioned fear in the rats, the use of St. John's wort extracts may be less beneficial than hyperforin.

CLINICAL STUDIES

Immune Disorders; Inflammation and Disease

Cancer

Cancer treatment. The photodynamic activation of hypericin has shown subsequent antitumor activity. Alecu et al. (1998) examined the topical use of hypericin as a photodynamic anticancer therapy in 19 patients with skin cancer: 11 patients (median age 66) diagnosed with basal cell carcinoma and eight patients (ages 39-72) with squamous cell carcinoma, five of whom had not received prior treatments for their cancer. Treatment consisted of intralesional (i.l.) injections of hypericin followed with irradiation using visible light (intensity, 24 mW/cm² at a dose of 86 J/cm² per session) to photoactivate hypericin. For ethical reasons, surgery was performed after the experimental therapy to remove residual tumor lesions and to make an assessment of possible impairments caused by the phototherapy. Among the squamous cell carcinoma patients, tumors were reduced by 33% after treatment with hypericin (40-100 µg hypericin i.l. three to five times/week for two to six weeks) and in one case the treatment appeared to cause complete remission. One female patient showed no tumor reduction after ten injections (540 µg hypericin) over 15 days into a tumor of the lower lip (30/20 × 10 mm in size). Analysis of the results showed that tumor reduction was dependent on initial tumor size and the dosage of hypericin administered. The analysis also revealed that in total 1,000 µg plus would be required in order for hypericin to reach acceptability as an alternative treatment for squamous cell carcinoma. Among the patients with basal cell carcinoma, treatment with hypericin (40-200 µg hypericin i.l., three to five times/week for two to six weeks) resulted in tumor reductions of less than 10% to as much as 100% (in two cases with complete remission). For all 11 patients, photodynamic treatment with hypericin represented their first therapy for cancer. All of these patients refused follow-up surgery and five months later showed no sign of the cancer remaining or recurring. In total, these patients received from 1,500-3,000 µg of hypericin. The only side effect observed was edema and erythema of a mild transient nature at the tumor site, which occurred in three patients in the basal cell carcinoma group and two in the squamous cell group. As the lesions healed, the researchers observed decrusting, inflammation, necrosis, and new epithelium formation, which covered the lesion. Although small, isolated groups of tumor cells remained in the dermis after healing, along with necrosis evidence suggested that lymphocytes had infiltrated the remaining tumor cells. The treatment appeared to be nontoxic and tumor selective, and it left no scarring (Alecu et al., 1998).

Infectious Diseases

Viral infections. St. John's wort extract (LI 160) may be of benefit in the treatment of herpes infections. In a prospective double-blind, placebo-controlled randomized trial in 110 patients with herpes genitalis, symptoms were significantly and equally reduced compared to placebo ($p < 0.0001$), including severity of episodes, size of area affected, and numbers of blisters. The treatment period lasted 90 days with an oral dosage of 300 mg t.i.d. and 600 mg t.i.d. on the days of herpes episodes. In a parallel trial of the same design and duration in 94 patients with herpes labialis, the results were reported to be of the same significance with equal alleviation of the same symptoms (Koytchev et al., 1999).

Immune Disorders

HIV/AIDS. Gulick et al. (1999) treated 30 HIV-positive patients, all of whom showed blood levels of CD4 cells of less than $350/mm^3$, with synthetic hypericin (VimRx Pharmaceuticals, Wilmington, DE, 0.25 or 0.5 mg/kg i.v. twice weekly or 0.25 mg/kg i.v. three times/week, or 0.5 mg/kg per day p.o. for eight weeks). Owing to phototoxic effects, only 14 patients completed the study. No significant change was found in CD4 cell counts, HIV p24 antigen levels, or HIV RNA copies; out of 23 patients available for evaluation, 11 developed severe cutaneous phototoxicity, including all who received oral hypericin.

Metabolic and Nutritional Disorders

Fatigue and Debility

In an open trial, Stevinson et al. (1998) administered a St. John's wort extract (Kira, Lichtwer Pharma, standardized to contain 300 µg hypericin/ 50 mg tablet) to 20 patients (17 females and 3 males ages 32-60) who complained to their doctors of fatigue but not depression. The outcome measured was perceived fatigue using a visual analogue scale (VAS). One subject dropped out due to experiencing dizziness. The 19 subjects remaining in treatment (50 mg t.i.d. for six weeks) appeared to produce no adverse events. Significant improvements compared to baseline were noted in those with borderline anxiety and borderline depression ($p < 0.05$), including significant improvements in the HAD (Hospital Anxiety and Depression) scale for anxiety ($p < 0.01$) and depression ($p < 0.01$). Among those with borderline depression, improvement in fatigue was observed in 7/9 subjects and in 3/10 subjects who were not depressed, according to HAD scores. VAS scores for fatigue correlated with scores from the HAD test for depression ($p < 0.01$) and were compared to baseline at the end of the study ($p < 0.01$). The results suggested that patients presenting with fatigue may have undiagnosed depression (Stevinson et al., 1998).

Pharmacokinetics

In healthy volunteers, the elimination half-life of hyperforin is approximately 9 h from a dose of 300 mg St. John's wort extract containing 5% hyperforin and about the same from doses of 600 mg and 900 mg. After repeated dosing of a 5% hyperforin, St. John's wort extract at the standard therapeutic dose (900 mg/day for eight days) in healthy young volunteers, hyperforin did not accumulate in plasma and the extract was well tolerated compared to placebo controls. The steady state plasma concentration of hyperforin from the repeated dosing was estimated to be approximately 100 ng/mL (Biber et al., 1998).

Staffeldt et al. (1994) estimated the elimination half-life of hypericin to be about 24 h in healthy male volunteers. St. John's wort extract LI 160 at a dosage of 300 mg t.i.d. for four days resulted in a mean maximal plasma level of hypericin of 8.5 ng/mL and a mean trough level of 5.3 ng/mL. In a follow-up to this report, a more complete study on the pharmacokinetics of hypericin (and pseudohypericin) by Kerb et al. (1996) found that from long-term treatment with the extract at the standard therapeutic dose of 300 mg t.i.d., the concentration of hypericin in plasma was up to 20 µg/L. After a single oral dose of the St. John's wort extract (LI 160 coated tablets) in healthy male volunteers, hypericin showed a lag time of 2 h before appearing in systemic circulation, whether from doses of 300, 900, or 1,800 mg (250, 750, or 1,500 µg hypericin).

Neurological, Psychological, and Behavioral Disorders

Psychological and Behavioral Disorders

Depression. Whiskey et al. (2001) conducted a systematic review and meta-analysis of 21 published randomized controlled trials of St. John's wort extracts in the treatment of depression and found the effects superior to placebo. The difference in their efficacy compared to standard tricyclic antidepressants was insignificant. However, owing to the fact that the majority of equivalence studies have not been of sufficient size to detect a difference in efficacy of < 20%, the matter of equivalence to standard antidepressants remains unresolved. The studies ranged in length from four to eight weeks and included patients with neurotic, mild and moderate, and major depression (Whiskey et al., 2001). A systematic review of English-language studies on St. John's wort in the treatment of depression by Gaster and Holroyd (2000) found 8/12 studies to be of sufficient methodological rigor for their evaluation. Only two of the eight trials selected for their systematic review were found to be without at least one significant flaw in methodology. They concluded that the evidence in favor of St. John's wort as an effective, safe, and well-tolerated agent in the treatment of mild to moderate depression was modest. In order to make an assessment of St. John's wort in the treatment of severe depression, they expressed the need for further studies.

A critical review of the extant data on St. John's wort extracts in the treatment of depression was presented by Benedetto Vitiello (1999) of the U.S. National Institutes of Mental Health. He noted that of 13 placebo-controlled studies with extracts of the herb, in ten of them St. John's wort extracts showed better results against depression than placebo and the number of responders (55%) was more than twice that of the placebo groups (22%). Of 16 placebo-controlled studies of the herb extract, he found only two used criteria applied in the United States which met those needed to diagnose major depression in the DSM-III, DSM-III-R, or DSM-IV (*Diagnostic and Statistical Manual of Mental Disorders,* American Psychiatric Association, 1980-1994). Of the 14 studies that did not meet these criteria, patients were included who met the *International Classification of Diseases* criteria (ICD) of the World Health Organization for reactive depression, neurotic depression, or adjustment disorder. He therefore concluded that even if test subjects showed improvements according to HAM-D scores, it remains to be shown whether St. John's wort extracts produce "clinically significant antidepressant effects in patients suffering not only from depressive symptomatology, but also from a depressive disorder." In further criticisms, Vitiello arrived at the following conclusions:

1. The majority of studies lasted only four weeks; sample sizes in the treatment arms were over 50 in only 4/16 studies; in two studies no response to placebo occurred, whereas in most clinical studies on antidepressants the placebo groups have shown responses in 30% to 60% of cases.
2. The active antidepressant constituents of the herb remain to be determined.
3. The extant clinical data remain unconvincing for the use of St. John's wort extracts in the treatment of clinical depression.

Kim et al. (1999) performed a meta-analysis of double-blind controlled studies of St. John's wort extracts in the treatment of depression dating from 1983 to March 1998. In their criteria for inclusion, the studies selected were limited to trials in which depression was defined by the DSM-IV, DSM-III-R, or by the ICD-10, with measured outcomes that used the Hamilton Depression Scale (HAM-D). A further criterion for inclusion was that the subjects treated had a similar socioeconomic background. Only six trials qualified, five of them lasting six weeks; all calculated efficacy based on rates of an intention to treat with rate ratios given for both the rate of change and the rate of response. Two of the qualifying studies were placebo-controlled and the other four compared St. John's wort extracts with tricyclic antidepressants (TCAs) (75 mg/day amitriptyline or imipramine, and 30 mg/day maprotiline). Doses of the extracts ranged from 200 mg/day to 900 mg/day, with most using the latter. Among their findings: patient dropout rates were significantly lower in the St. John's wort extract groups (12.6%) compared to the TCA-treated patient dropouts (16.2%); TCAs showed 1.7 times the likelihood of causing side effects than the St. John's wort extracts; compared to placebo, St. John's wort extracts showed 1.5 times the likelihood of improving depression. Kim et al. (1999) considered this rate of efficacy unconvincing for an effective antidepressant. Among their criticisms: any mention of the exclusion of patients with bipolar depression was at best scant; the dosages of the TCAs used were all subtherapeutic; the patients treated with TCAs showed higher response rates "than would have been expected," making questionable the assumption that St. John's wort extracts have a similar efficacy to TCAs; and the majority of treatments and diagnoses may have been performed by primary care practitioners who may have lacked the necessary skills to properly employ the HAM-D (citing Nielsen and Williams, 1980). Moreover, they commented that five of the trials were conducted in Germany, where psychiatric outcomes are influenced by cultural factors favoring less than "objective and standardized measures" (citing Kunze and Priebe, 1998); therefore, they could not rule out the possibility that the conduct of some of the studies may have been influenced by this as well. In the end, Kim et al. (1999) concluded that although their meta-analysis showed that the "effectiveness" of St. John's wort extracts "in the short-term treatment of mild to moderately severe depression" was similar to that of low-dose TCAs, they still had serious doubts in regard to the quality of the design of the clinical trials they analyzed.

Linde et al. (1996) conducted a systematic meta-analysis of 23 randomized clinical trials of St. John's wort extracts, including a total of 1,757 outpatients with mild to moderate depressive disorders. Fifteen studies were placebo-controlled, while the remaining eight compared St. John's wort with other drug treatments. Linde and colleagues calculated that St. John's wort preparations were 2.67 times more effective in the placebo-controlled trials and displayed a comparable efficacy to standard antidepressant medications (tricyclic antidepressants) in the comparative trials. Dropouts due to side effects were rare in the St. John's wort-treated groups (0.8%) compared to the drug-treated groups (3.0%). Side effects occurred in 19.8% of patients on St. John's wort extract and 52.8% of patients receiving standard antidepressants (tricyclics). The researchers identified key questions left unanswered by the clinical studies they had analyzed:

1. Is St. John's wort extract more effective for treating certain types of depressive states than others?
2. A need exists for longer-term, better-controlled comparative studies with standard antidepressants, which include formal, standard mechanisms for the assessment of side effects. Extant comparative studies indicate that St. John's wort extracts have fewer short-term side effects than tricyclic antidepressants, but data on long-term side effects are lacking.
3. Additional studies are needed to evaluate the effects of different St. John's wort preparations and dosages. (Linde et al., 1996)

In a review comparing the results of 25 controlled-therapy studies in a total of 1,592 patients, Harrer and Schulz (1994) concluded that the efficacy of St. John's wort extract versus placebo was clearly demonstrated in the treatment of mild to moderate depression. In comparative studies, responder rates were equivalent to those of synthetic antidepressants (imipramine, maprotiline, amitriptyline, desipramine, diazepam, bromazepan), but the side effects associated with St. John's wort extracts were generally less severe and more tolerable (Harrer and Schulz, 1994).

Over 25 double-blind clinical trials have been conducted to investigate the clinical efficacy of St. John's wort extracts in the treatment of mild to moderate depression. Some of the key studies are summarized below.

Osterheider et al. (1992) reported no significant benefits from St. John's wort in a double-blind placebo-controlled trial of a liquid extract in the treatment of 46 patients diagnosed with severe depression; however, Vorbach et al.

(1997), in a preliminary study on St. John's wort powder extract in the treatment of severe depressive episodes, reported encouraging results.

Vorbach et al. (1997) compared a relatively low dosage of imipramine (50 mg t.i.d. for six weeks) to a high dosage of St. John's wort extract (Lichtwer Pharma, LI 160, 600 mg t.i.d. for six weeks) in a multicenter, randomized, double-blind comparative study design (209 men and women ages 18-70), which followed a single-blind stage in which placebo responders were eliminated. The researchers found that although the treatments were comparable in reducing the HAM-D total score, St. John's wort extract was superior to imipramine because fewer patients reported adverse events (23% versus 41%), and these effects were comparatively fewer in number (37 versus 83). This result was found despite the high dosage of the extract. Global assessments (CGI scale) of efficacy showed improvements rated as very good/good in 61.2% of those in the St. John's wort group and 70.1% in the imipramine group, which closely corresponded with global evaluations by the patients. The researchers concluded that while the herbal extract "might" serve as an alternative to imipramine in the treatment of severe depressive episodes, additional studies are required before any definite assertion can be made in this regard (Vorbach et al., 1997).

Shelton et al. (2001) conducted a large-scale, randomized, double-blind, placebo-controlled multicenter trial of St. John's wort extract (Lichtwer Pharma GmbH, Berlin, Germany) in 200 outpatients with major depression, the first study of its kind in the United States. The patients (mean age 42.4 years) were diagnosed according to the HAM-D and the DSM-IV. Their average history of depression was over two years and at baseline they had a score of 20 or more in the HAM-D. The patients were not seeking an herbal treatment for their depression. At no cost to the subjects, all were provided "antidepressant treatment" for six months after they participated in the trial. Efficacy of the treatment was assessed using intention-to-treat analyses and the HAM-A (Hamilton Anxiety Scale), HAM-D, CGI-I, CG-S (physician-rated Clinical Global Impression-Improvement and -Severity, respectively), BDI (Beck Depression Inventory, self administered) and the GAF (Global Assessment of Function scale). After a one-week placebo run-in phase in which more susceptible placebo responders were eliminated, the dosage of placebo or St. John's wort was 300 mg t.i.d. for four weeks or more, and 400 mg t.i.d. if improvement after week 4 was insufficient. The treatment period was eight weeks and patients were allowed a sleep aid (zolipidem tartrate ≥ 10 mg/day) only during the first 21 days of the trial. Also allowed was ongoing psychotherapy if patients were already receiving this therapy for three months or more before baseline measurements were taken and if during the trial the frequency of psychotherapy remained the same. Among these were four in the St. John's wort groups and eight in the placebo group. The results showed no significant difference in outcome scores compared to placebo, nor among a subgroup of less severely depressed subjects ($n = 110$) with a HAM-D score of less than 22. The only significant difference in outcomes was a greater number of reported headaches (41%) in those receiving St. John's wort compared to placebo (25%). The researchers commented that subjects who have a preference for alternative medicine in their treatment "might have a different outcome" (Shelton et al., 2001). It remains, however, that based on the positive results in major depression obtained by Vorbach et al. (1997) with a higher dosage of St. John's wort extract (1,800 mg/day), the dosage used by Shelton and colleagues (900-1,200 mg/day) may well have been insufficient, a fact that Shelton and collaborators failed to mention.

Randomized double-blind studies have compared the effectiveness of St. John's wort extract LI 160 to maprotiline (Harrer et al., 1994) and imipramine (Vorbach et al., 1994, 1997). In these studies, positive responses in St. John's wort extract-treated subjects were comparable to those of the drug-treated subjects, but St. John's wort was better tolerated and elicited fewer side effects.

Woelk (2000) compared the efficacy and tolerability of St. John's wort extract (ZE 117, Bayer Vital, Leverkusen, Germany) to imipramine in the treatment of 324 outpatients (mean age midforties) diagnosed with mild to moderate depression according to the tenth edition of *International Classification of Diseases* (ICD-10). Fewer cases of moderate depression (135/324) than mild depression (189/324) were found, and 71% were women. The largest study to date of St. John's wort in the treatment of depression, the randomized, multicenter, double-blind, parallel group-design trial evaluated the results of a six-week treatment period using the HAM-D, patients' global impression scale, and the clinical global depression scale (CGI). The St. John's wort extract (standardized to contain 0.2% hypericin) was taken in a dosage of 250 mg b.i.d. and imipramine was taken at a dosage of 75 mg b.i.d. Although no significant difference was found between the treatments according to patients' global impression scores, mean CGI scores, or the HAM-D, the anxiety-somatization subscale of the HAM-D was significantly different in favor of the St. John's wort extract. Adverse events were reported by 63% of patients taking imipramine and 26% of patients taking the St. John's wort extract. Similarly, 16% of the patients taking imipramine withdrew from the trial, as did 3% of patients taking the St. John's wort extract. The most common adverse effect reported was dry mouth (8% of those taking ZE 117 and 25% of those taking imipramine). The conclusion reached by the trial conductors was that St. John's wort is better tolerated than imipramine and, although of equivalent therapeutic effect, St. John's wort may be more efficacious in relieving depression-associated anxiety than desipramine (Woelk, 2000).

Philipp et al. (1999) examined the safety and efficacy of a St. John's wort extract (Steiner Arzneimittel, Berlin, STEI 300; standardized to contain 2% to 3% hyperforin and 0.2% to 0.3% hypericin and pseudohypericin) in the treatment of moderate depression (ICD-10, codes F32.1 and F33.1). Their study was a randomized, double-blind, placebo-controlled, parallel group multicenter trial in 263 patients composed of 197 women and 66 men (ages 18-65). Results were compared in patients receiving treatment with the St. John's wort extract (350 mg t.i.d.), imipramine (100 mg/day; 50 mg, 25 mg, and 25 mg) or placebo (t.i.d.) for eight weeks. The three treatments were identical in taste and appearance. The results showed significant benefits from the St. John's extract compared to placebo on the HAM-D, the Zung self-rating depression scale, and the CGI scale, and that imipramine was comparable in efficacy to the St. John's wort extract. The response rates in the HAM-D scale at week eight were 63% (placebo), 76% (St. John's wort), and 66.7% (imipramine). The researchers note that in studies of synthetic antidepressants, at week six the response rates in the HAM-D scale is 0% to 70%, with placebo at 47%, and in previous studies on St. John's wort, 0% to 56%. The response rates in the CGI scale at week eight were 65.3% (placebo), 77% (St. John's wort), and 74.2% (imipramine). In the SF-36, the results from the standardized mental component scale showed quality of life was more improved from either St. John's wort or imipramine compared to placebo; however, improvement in the physical component scale was only evident from St. John's wort. In terms of safety, adverse events were reported by 19% of the placebo group, 22% of the St. John's wort group, and 46% of the imipramine group. No events of serious nature were reported except for one suicide attempt by a patient in the placebo group. The most frequently reported adverse event reported was dry mouth (13% in the placebo group, 7% in the St. John's wort group, and 38% in the imipramine group) (Philipp et al., 1999).

Harrer et al. (1999) became the first to publish a comparative clinical trial of St. John's wort extract and fluoxetine, reporting that the two treatments were equivalent in their effects against depression in elderly patients. The 149 patients (ages 60-80) diagnosed with mild to moderate depression (ICD-10) received tablets of fluoxetine (20 mg/day for six weeks), placebo, or coated tablets (Dysto-lux) of a dry extract of St. John's wort (LoHyp-57, Dr. Werner Loges and Co., GmbH, Winsen, Germany, 800 mg/day for six weeks). The extract was made from five to seven parts herb to one part ethanol (60% w/w) (Harrer et al., 1999) and contained hypericin ($\geq$ 53 mg/100 g extract) and hyperforin (6.5%) (Biller, 1999). In both moderate depressive and mild depressive episode patients, the randomized, double-blind, multicenter comparative study found remarkably similar scores in response rates and changes in symptoms (HAM-D, CGI, and patient self-assessment in the SDS scale) from both active medications. According to statistical calculations, the response rate was 72.2% for fluoxetine and 71.4% for the St. John's wort extract. More patients in the fluoxetine group (n = 16) withdrew from the trial than those in the St. John's wort group (n = 8), yet the reason of an adverse event was nearly equal between the groups (four versus five, respectively). A total of 12 patients in the St. John's wort group reported adverse effects that were probably or possibly related to the medication, versus 17 in the fluoxetine group. The four probable adverse effects in the extract group were each exclusive to four different patients: inner restlessness (moderate); racing heartbeat at night (severe); nausea (moderate); and headaches, vertigo, and stabbing chest pains (moderate). Eleven adverse events in the fluoxetine group were probably related to the medication and matched those known to occur in patients taking the drug. Of these, eight were severe effects reported individually by eight different patients: allergic eczema; persistent, recurring vertigo; palpitations, hand tremor; neck tension; previously absent trembling and inner restlessness; stomatitis and increased restlessness; nausea and more frequent headaches; and upper abdominal symptoms. The researchers point out that St. John's wort extract could be regarded as a better choice of treatment for elderly depressive patients because it has been shown not to impair driving ability, potentiate alcohol effects, and in no way adversely effects cognitive performance (Harrer et al., 1999). Since this trial, at least two studies have arrived at similar findings in patients whose mean age was the midforties; in the treatment of mild to moderate depression, St. John's wort extract was comparable in efficacy to fluoxetine (Schrader, 2000) and to sertraline (Brenner et al., 2000).

Lenoir et al. (1999) conducted a clinical study on the tolerability of a St. John's wort extract (Bioforce AG, Roggwil, Switzerland, Hyperiforce) prepared from the shoot tips of fresh plants, as well as its efficacy in 348 outpatients with mild to moderate depression. The results of the randomized, double-blind, multicenter, parallel group comparative study were measured using the HAM-D (17-item version) for the primary outcome, and the Depression Scale (DS), the Hospital Anxiety and Depression Scale (HADS), and the CGI scale. For six weeks, the patients took one tablet t.i.d. of standardized extracts of the fresh shoot tips providing three different daily doses of hypericin, providing either 1 mg hypericin/day (119 patients), 0.33 mg/day (115 patients), or 0.17 mg/day (114 patients). The results at the end of the treatment showed a relative HAM-D score reduction of about 50% for all the groups, with response rates for the respective groups of 68%, 65%, and 62% (n = 260).

Since adverse effects probably caused by the extracts were reported in only 2% (n = 7) of the patients (n = 348), Lenoir and colleagues (1999) concluded that the extract was well tolerated. The mean compliance of the patients was over 90%. Patients numbered 28 who withdrew before the trial ended owing to medical or other reasons, and 60 who deviated from the trial protocol. The researchers note that the response rates of 62% to 68% were better than those of 55% in clinical trials reviewed by Linde et al. (1996) and Volz (1997) in which St. John's wort extracts provided between 0.5 and 2.7 mg hypericin/day; the difference, they suggest, perhaps owes to their use of an extract made from the fresh shoot tips which contain a comparatively "higher concentration of constituents" (Lenoir et al., 1999). However, without repeated evidence of superior response rates from placebo-controlled trials of this preparation, their speculation remains to be tested.

In a six-week multicenter study by Laakmann et al. (1998), a St. John's wort hydroalcoholic extract (standardized to 0.5% hypericin) was compared to a placebo and to a hydroalcoholic extract standardized to contain 5% stabilized hyperforin. Male and female outpatients diagnosed as mildly to moderately depressed according to the DSM-IV ($n = 147$) participated in a randomized, double-blind placebo-controlled study, which ran for 42 days with an initial placebo run-in lasting three to seven days. Each of the three groups of patients received 300-mg tablets t.i.d. and were evaluated using scores obtained from HAM-D (17-item version), D-S (Depression Self-Rating Scale), and physician rating at days 0 and 42 with the CGI.

At day 42, HAM-D scores were significantly better in the group administered the hyperforin-standardized extract (HPSE) compared to the hypericin-standardized extract (HYSE) and to the placebo group. HAM-D scores in 49% of the HPSE group were 50% and lower compared to baseline, versus 32.7% lower in the HYSE group and 38.8% lower in the placebo group. In the D-S score at day 42, the placebo group showed a slightly better score than the HYSE group, and the HPSE group a better score than either of the other two groups. Compared to the placebo group, the D-S score was highly significant in favor of the HPSE group ($p < 0.001$). The responder rates in patients with more severe depression revealed a better response rate in the HPSE group (50%) than in either the HYSE (12.5%) or placebo group (25%). In the CGI score at day 42, patients on placebo showed moderate depression scores in 55.1% of cases, compared to a 30.6% score in the HPSE group and a 38.8% score in the HYSE group (Laakmann et al., 1998).

In evaluating safety, 23 adverse effects were reported in the placebo group, 24 in the HYSE group, and 17 in the HPSE group. The only adverse event reported by all three groups was bronchitis. Blood tests performed before and after the study for calcium, creatinine, erythrocytes, GOT, GPT, γ-GT, TSH basal, hemoglobin, platelets, and leukocytes revealed no significant changes in any of the treatment groups (Laakmann et al., 1998).

Schrader et al. (1998) conducted a prospective, randomized, multicenter, double-blind, placebo-controlled study of a St. John's wort extract (Zeller AG, Switzerland, ZE117 ethanolic extract standardized to contain 1 mg hypericin/500 mg) in 162 patients (ages 30-59) diagnosed with mild to moderate depression. Tablets of the extract (250 mg twice daily) or placebo were taken by 108 women and 54 men for six weeks, with 151 completing the study. HAM-D scores showed that 24% of those taking placebo achieved remission versus 82% of those taking the St. John's wort extract ($p < 0.001$). The 41% difference was comparable to efficacy results reported by others in placebo-controlled trials of St. John's wort extracts. CGI scores also showed a favorable outcome for the extract versus placebo in the assessment of change and therapeutic index, as did severity of illness and patient self-assessment (VAS) (each $p < 0.001$). In the assessment of sleep disorders in depression derived from the HAM-D scores, the extract-treated group showed significant improvement ($p < 0.001$) compared to baseline. As for adverse events, six were reported by the extract group and seven by the placebo group. The only adverse event reported in both groups was abdominal pain ($n = 2$ versus $n = 3$) (Schrader et al., 1998).

In a multicenter trial, Wheatley (1997) compared a St. John's wort extract (LI 160, 300 mg t.i.d. for six weeks) to a low dosage of amitriptyline (25 mg t.i.d.) after a three- to seven-day placebo run-in phase in 156 adult outpatients who met the DSM-IV criteria for mild to moderate depression. The results of the double-blind, randomized parallel group-designed study showed that the HAM-D score was significantly lower in favor of the amitriptyline group ($p < 0.05$) compared to the St. John's wort group, and more patients responded to amitriptyline (78%) than to the St. John's wort extract (60%). More patients reported adverse events in the amitriptyline group (64%) compared to the extract group (37%), significantly so for dry mouth and drowsiness (Wheatley, 1997). This trial has been criticized on the basis that the dose of amitriptyline used was not sufficient enough to show a significant difference in response compared to placebo (Shelton et al., 2001), a point noted by the researchers, who explained that the dose of amitriptyline used was about half that of the maximally recommended dose used in outpatients (Wheatley, 1997).

Hänsgen et al. (1994), in a double-blind, multicenter, placebo-controlled, randomized, crossover-design clinical trial of St. John's wort extract (LI 160, 300 mg t.i.d. for four weeks), reported significant improvements in HAM-D scores and the von Zerssen Depression Scale (each $p < 0.001$ compared to baseline measurements versus placebo). The patients ($n = 72$, ages 18-70) were diagnosed with mild to moderate depression (DSM-III-R). In 81% of the St. John's wort group, HAM-D scale responder rates were reduced by over 50% compared to baseline (from 21.8 to 9.3 points after), versus 26% in the placebo group. When switched to the active treatment during weeks five and six, the placebo group also showed a significant improvement. The extract was significantly superior to placebo after weeks two and after four weeks (both $p < 0.001$). Scores from the symptom evaluation questionnaire showed more significant effects in symptoms of anxiety/phobia, cardiovascular symptoms, and well-being in week four. Clinical Global Impressions compared to placebo revealed a greater reduction in the severity of symptoms in the extract group after four weeks. Symptomatic changes from the start of the trial to week four and their measurement by external and internal assessments showed a significant correlation ($p < 0.001$). Side effects were mild and occurred in one patient on the extract (sleep distur-   bance) and two in the placebo group (gastrointestinal complaints). A weakness of this trial was that patients knew they would be receiving the active treatment during two or more weeks.

Hübner et al. (1994) conducted a randomized, placebo-controlled double-blind study of St. John's wort extract (Lichtwer Pharma, GmbH, Jarsin 300, 300 mg t.i.d. for four weeks) in 89 patients (ages 20-64) diagnosed with relatively mild depression with somatic symptoms (most frequently, fatigue, sleep disturbances, heart palpitations, and lack of drive). Results were measured using HAM-D, CGI, and the von Zerssen Health Complaint Survey (B-L). Remarkably, no "relevant adverse effects" were found in any of the patients, and 70% were reported free of symptoms after four weeks, versus a responder rate of 47% in the placebo group. The researchers attributed the rather high rate of response in the placebo group as probably owing in part to their mild depression (Hübner et al., 1994). These responses were considerably higher than the average of 22.3% reported in trials of St. John's wort extracts (Linde et al., 1996).

Woelk et al. (1994) investigated the acceptance and effectiveness of a four-week treatment with a standardized St. John's wort extract (LI 160) in 3,250 patients (76% women and 24% men, ages less than 20 and up to 90) under the care of 623 practitioners. Forty-nine percent were mildly depressed patients, 46% moderately depressed, and 3% severely depressed. Symptoms normalized or improved in about 80% of the patients during the study, based on subjective reports. More objective measurements (e.g., the HAM-D scale) gave positive response rates of between 60% and 70%. These numbers were comparable to tricyclic and other standard antidepressants from which placebo response rates are about 30%. Undesirable side effects were mild (gastrointestinal disturbances, allergic reactions, tiredness, restlessness) and reported in only 2.4% of the patients. The rate of incidence compared favorably to those in a drug-monitoring study of 943 patients treated with fluoxetine (Prozac) in which 19% reported side effects, especially nausea, nervousness, dizziness, and headaches.

Seasonal affective disorder (SAD). St. John's wort extracts may help to stabilize seasonal mood changes in patients with seasonal affective disorder (SAD), with or without additional light therapy. Kasper (1997) conducted an open, randomized single-blind trial of St. John's wort extract (LI 160, 300 mg, t.i.d. for four weeks) in 20 patients diagnosed with SAD in which one group received phototherapy with bright white light while the other received dim light (3000 lux versus < 300 lux, respectively) at eye level for two h/day. The bright light source was adjusted to filter infrared and ultraviolet to protect the eyes, and in both groups patients were instructed to keep a distance from the light of 90 cm and to look at the light once/minute. The results showed a significant difference between the two patient groups in symptoms of SAD. For the bright light group the total HAM-D score dropped 72%, while in the dim light group the score fell 60%. Significant improvements in the HAM-D score were also found in the duration of time ($p < 0.001$), and for the whole group of patients symptoms showed highly significant decreases: bad temper ($p = 0.001$), despondency ($p = 0.001$), fatigue ($p = 0.0001$), and "desire for action" ($p = 0.0001$). No adverse effects were reported by patients in either group and a standardized ophthalmological examination for retinal side effects revealed none. Data from a comparably designed five-week trial of fluoxetine (20 mg/day) in SAD patients were obtained simultaneously and compared to the four-week trial of St. John's wort. Depression scores showed the same drop, but in the fluoxetine study side effects occurred, most notably agitation (Kasper, 1997).

Martinez et al. (1994), after a randomized single-blind study in 20 SAD patients, reported that although no indication of an additive effect was found, St. John's wort appeared to produce antidepressant activity in these patients. He encouraged larger trials to establish whether the benefits of the herbal extract might be "potentiated" from phototherapy in SAD in placebo-controlled trials.

Sleep disturbances. Since synthetic antidepressants commonly decrease REM (rapid eye movement), Sharpley et al. (1998) examined the effect of a St. John's wort extract on sleep using the polysomnogram in healthy volunteers in two single doses (Kira, Lichtwer Pharma, standardized to contain either 0.9 mg or 0.18 mg hypericin). In separate double-blind, placebo-controlled, balanced-order crossover-designed studies, one trial used the lower hypericin content extract in 11 volunteers (males and females ages 27-44), while the second used the higher concentration in ten volunteers (males and females ages 20-41). The results showed that either amount of hypericin in a single dose was effective in causing a significant decrease in REM, and, although numerically superior to placebo, the high dose was not statistically greater in efficacy compared to the low dose. The results also showed that unlike synthetic antidepressants (tricyclics, SSRIs, and MAOIs), REM sleep time was not decreased (Sharpley et al., 1998).

St. John's wort extracts also appear to improve sleep patterns in older individuals. A double-blind, placebo-controlled crossover study of St. John's wort extract (LI 160, 300 mg, t.i.d. for four weeks) was conducted in 12 volunteers (mean age 59.8 ± 4.8 years), all in good health. The results showed that sleep onset or sleep time was not altered by the extract; however, St. John's wort extract appeared to increase the proportion of the sleep cycle that the subjects spent in deep sleep, and slow-wave sleep showed an increase from a mean percentage of 1.5% to 6.0% (Schulz and Jobert, 1994).

DOSAGE

In the treatment of mild to moderate depression, clinical trials have utilized daily therapeutic doses of St. John's wort extract ranging from 300-900 mg/day (Harrer and Schulz, 1994), and in severely depressed patients, 1800 mg/day (Vorbach et al., 1997). LI 160, the extract favored in clinical trials, is standardized to contain 0.3% hypericin. The average daily dosage used in clinical trials is equivalent to about 2,000-4,000 mg of the crude herb (Reuter, 1998), although the hypericin content of commercial preparations can vary widely (Linde et al., 1996; Sloley et al., 2001; Wurglics et al., 2001). Most St. John's wort extracts are standardized according to hypericin content as this compound is a readily measurable, unique chemical marker and extracts standardized to 0.3% hypericin have been shown effective (Upton, 1997; Reuter, 1998).

More recently, hyperforin has become the topic of intense research as possibly the main active antidepressive constituent of the herb (Philippu, 2001; Müller et al., 2001; Gambarana et al., 2001; Franklin and Cowen, 2001; Eckert and Müller, 2001). St. John's wort extracts can now be standardized to a hyperforin content of 3% (Orth et al., 1999; Erdelmeier, 1998; Brown, 1998) to as much as 5% (Laakmann et al., 1998). However, in commercial St. John's wort preparations hyperforin concentrations have varied from 0.5% to 6% (Nathan, 1999) and evidence continues to show that other known and possibly unknown constituents may play a significant role in the antidepressant activity of St. John's wort extracts (Krishtal et al., 2001; Misane and Ögren, 2001; Coleta et al., 2001; Wonnemann et al., 2001; Kientsch et al., 2001).

SAFETY PROFILE

The common opinion of a number of reviewers is that St. John's wort extracts have few side effects and are well tolerated by most people (Woelk et al., 1994; Vorbach et al., 1994; Linde et al., 1996). A drug-monitoring study involving 3,250 patients treated with the most widely sold St. John's wort product in Germany found the frequency of adverse events was 2.43% (Woelk et al., 1994). Others have reported the incidence of adverse events in persons treated with St. John's wort preparations in Europe is 1% to 3% (Schulz, 2001). After a systemic review of the literature, however, Ernst et al. (1998) concluded that further research on St. John's wort is required to establish the safety of long-term use and whether it is as effective as conventional antidepressants.

Contraindications

Recent case reports strongly suggest that, like other antidepressants, St. John's wort extracts may exacerbate mania and other symptoms of bipolar depression in persons previously diagnosed or undiagnosed with this form of depression (Nierenberg et al., 1999; O'Breasail and Argouarch, 1998; Moses and Mallinger, 2000). Given that 25% of patients initially presenting with unipolar depression are in the majority of cases only correctly diagnosed with the bipolar form eight to ten years later (Nierenberg et al., 1999), special care must be taken to obtain a correct diagnosis before treating depression with St. John's wort extracts. Like other antidepressants, in some patients with panic disorder and unipolar depression, St. John's wort extracts may cause mania and hypomania, hostility, increased irritability, grandiose behavior, aggression racing "distorted" thoughts, agitation, and lowered need for sleep (O'Breasail and Argouarch, 1998).

St. John's wort extracts have yet to be studied in children with depression (Rey and Walter, 1998).

Two case reports are noted of schizophrenic patients who experienced psychotic relapses while taking St. John's wort. Use of the herb was only learned of by their physician after they improved following treatment with antipsychotic agents (Lal and Iskandar, 2000).

Due to its photosensitizing effects, patients receiving therapeutic ultraviolet light treatments have been advised to avoid taking St. John's wort extracts (Upton, 1997). A recent laboratory study found evidence suggesting that hypericin can damage ocular proteins, which could be indicative of cataract development (Johnston, 1999). However, in a study of SAD patients taking St. John's wort extract (LI 160, 300 mg t.i.d. for four weeks) who were exposed daily to bright light using a light box that filtered infrared and ultraviolet, no signs of ocular damage were found (Kasper, 1997). In a study of topical preparations of St. John's wort (ointment and oil containing 30 and 100 µg/100 mL, respectively), minimal erythema was found on the skin of volunteers exposed to simulated solar radiation. Although the evidence for severe phototoxicity from these topical preparations was absent, the researchers concluded that evidence of an increased tendency of photosensitivity could affect individuals with fair skin, diseased skin, or those exposed to the sun's rays for extended periods (Schempp et al., 2000). In a modified neutral red assay using a line of human keratinocytes (HaCaT cells), the constituent identified as mainly responsible for phototoxic effects of the herb is hypericin, although rutin also showed phototoxic activity (Wilhelm et al., 2001).

Drug Interactions

Animal studies have shown that St. John's wort extract can significantly prolong narcotic-induced sleeping times and antagonize the effects of reserpine (Okpanyi and Weischer, 1987). Hypericin, however, was reported to cause a reduction in barbiturate-induced sleeping times (Öztürk et al., 1992).

Agents for which concomitant use of St. John's wort extracts have been precautioned against include: MAOIs (Upton, 1997), OTC cold and flu medications, narcotics, alcoholic beverages, amphetamines, ma huang (*Ephedra* species containing ephedrine) (Chavez and Chavez, 1997), cyclosporin (Rey and Walter, 1998; Ruschitzka et al., 2000; Breidenbach, Kliem, et al., 2000; Breidenbach, Hoffmann, et al., 2000; Karliova et al., 2000), digoxin (Johne et al., 1999), phenprocoumon (Maurer et al., 1999), theophylline, *R*-warfarin, imipramine, clomipramine, clozapine, olanzapine (Nebel et al., 1999), paroxetine (Gordon, 1998), sertraline, nefazodone (Lantz et al., 1999), nevirapine (de Maat et al., 2001), indinavir, and other HIV protease inhibitors (Piscitelli et al., 2000), the photodiagnostic agent δ-aminolaevulinic acid (Ladner et al., 2001), oral contraceptives (Department of Health, 2000), cyclosporine (Barone et al., 2001), amscarine, etoposide (Peebles et al., 2001), and others.

An advisory on the potential of St. John's wort drug interactions was issued February 29, 2000, by the Committee on Safety of Medicines (CSM), an independent expert committee that provides the British government with advice on the effectiveness, quality, and safety of medicines. A summary of the advisory (Breckenridge, 2000) was followed by another from the British Department of Health (BDH) on March 1, 2000. Although primarily addressed to doctors and pharmacists, the BDH included a "Fact Sheet for the Public" providing examples of various prescription drugs taken concomitantly with St. John's wort and warned against immediately stopping the herb, lest the action of the prescription drug increase and cause side effects. Such individuals are advised by the BDH to consult with a physician for guidance on decreasing the dose of their prescriptions while discontinuing St. John's wort, and other remedial tactics. These individuals include anyone being treated for epilepsy or fits, chronic bronchitis, asthma, blood clots, or a heart condition (Department of Health, 2000).

For those taking oral contraceptives, the BDH advises to simply stop taking St. John's wort ("as it may stop your pill from working") and to mention the instance to one's physician or pharmacist upon the next visit. They give the same advice for patients taking prescription antimigraine and antidepressant medications and those being treated for HIV, except that for the latter the advice is to have viral loads checked after discontinuing St. John's wort. Similar advice is given by the CSM for warfarin (have INR checked and stop taking the herb), cyclosporin (check blood levels and stop taking the herb), anticonvulsants, digoxin, and theophylline (stop taking the herb and check blood levels of prescription drug) (Breckenridge, 2000). For those already taking prescription drugs who would like to take the herb, and for those taking St. John's wort who may then be given a prescription for a drug, the BDH advises that these individuals first discuss this with a doctor or pharmacist (Department of Health, 2000).

The list of drugs that the CSM advises against taking with St. John's wort (cyclosporin, digoxin, indinavir, oral contraceptives, theophylline, warfarin) is appended with drugs for which direct evidence is lacking for "important interactions," but which are likely to occur with concomitant use of the herb and could result in "serious adverse reactions": anticonvulsants (carbamazepine, phenobarbitone, phenytoin), HIV protease inhibitors (nelfinavir, ritonavir, saquinavir), HIV nonnucleoside reverse transcriptase inhibitors (efavirenz, vevirapine), triptans used against migraine (naratriptan, rizatriptan, sumatriptan, zolmitriptan), and SSRI antidepressants (fluoxetine, fluvoxamine, sertaline, citralopram, paroxetine) (Breckenridge, 2000).

Hypericin was believed not to have significant MAO inhibitory activity (Müller et al., 1997); however, Denke et al. (2000) found in vitro inhibition of dopamine-β-hydroxylase from hypericin (I_{50} 5 μM/L) and from pseudohypericin (I_{50} 3 μM/L). The IC_{50}s of various flavonoids in St. John's wort were in the order of 50 μM/L and higher (Denke et al., 2000). Still, the standard contraindications for patients receiving MAOIs and avoidance of tyramine-containing foods may not apply to St. John's wort extracts. What MAO activity the whole extract does have is quite low; St. John's wort extracts display only weak MAOI activity in vitro (Upton, 1997) and in vivo (Yu, 2000). An exception may be a critical carbon dioxide extract of St. John's wort; a dosage of 1 mg/kg p.o. caused a significant increase of dopamine outflow in rats (Di Matteo et al., 2000). A possible further exception may be extracts of St. John's wort with a relatively higher concentration of xanthones (Muruganandam et al., 2000) (see Receptor- and Neurotransmitter-Mediated Functions).

Considering its widespread use in Europe and a lack of reported side effects related to dietary factors in numerous human studies, it is unlikely that adverse interactions with tyramine-containing foods should apply (Upton, 1997). Reports of dietary factors causing MAOI-like interactions with St. John's wort extracts are unknown (Rey and Walter, 1998). However, the safest course is to consult your physician before taking a St. John's wort extract as a supplement, especially if you are receiving prescription medications for depression.

Markowitz et al. (2000) reported that CYP 3A4 and CYP 2D6 activity were not inhibited in seven normal volunteers (ages 24-32, four males and three females) when an extract of St. John's wort standardized to contain

0.3% hypericin (Solaray, Park City, UT, 300 mg p.o.) was coadministered with or without oral dextramethorphan (Benylin syrup, 30 mg) or alprazolam (1 or 2 mg) for three days, which the researchers admitted may not be long enough to detect an inductive effect from the extract on CYP 3A4.

Burstein et al. (2000) conducted a longer study of St. John's wort in healthy, nonsmoking volunteers (three women and five men, ages 24-43) to determine effects on steady state carbamazepine pharmacokinetics. Subjects took the carbamazepine for 14 days (100 mg b.i.d. for three days; 200 mg b.i.d. for the next three days; 400 mg daily for the next 28 days), followed by 14 days taking St. John's wort tablets (Hypericum Buyers Club, Los Angeles, CA, 300 mg t.i.d. with food) and concurrent intake of carbamazepine (100 mg/day). For 30 days prior to the treatment period, no drugs or foods were allowed that are considered to induce or inhibit cytochrome P-450-mediated drug metabolism, and none of the volunteers were lactating or pregnant. Blood sampling revealed that St. John's wort caused no increase in the clearance of carbamazepine. No significant differences were found in levels of carbamazepine compared to the period without the addition of St. John's wort in oral clearance, peak concentration, trough concentration, or area under the plasma concentration-time curve. Given that the main enzyme that metabolizes carbamazepine is CYP3A4, these findings were unexpected. Carbamazepine is also an inducer of CYP3A4, and as the researchers suggest, "St. John's wort may not be potent enough to alter a system that is already induced." Although they conclude that the results suggest carbamazepine and St. John's wort may be taken together by patients, they also note that one subject showed a 24% increase in oral clearance of the drug. This indicated that variability in drug-metabolizing enzyme activity varies from one individual to the next, and in the case of taking carbamazepine concomitant with St. John's wort, individuals would have to be monitored when they reported loss of effects or side effects not previously reported.

In an open-label study in eight HIV-negative, healthy adult volunteers, concomitant St. John's wort (standardized to contain 0.3% hypericin; tablets, 300 mg t.i.d. with meals for 14 days) decreased 8-h blood levels of the HIV protease inhibitor indinavir by an extrapolated 81%. The researchers stressed the danger of concomitant use of St. John's wort by individuals taking protease inhibitors to treat HIV, since less-than-optimal concentrations of these agents in HIV-positive individuals can quickly lead to HIV resistance (Piscitelli et al., 2000). Nonnucleoside reverse transcriptase inhibitors used in the treatment of HIV may also be affected by St. John's wort because they are also metabolized by CYP3A4 (Piscitelli et al., 2000; Lumpkin and Alpert, 2000).

A randomized, single-blind, placebo-controlled crossover study incorporating a two-week washout period examined the potential interaction of

St. John's wort extract (LI 160, 300 mg t.i.d. for ten days) with the oral anticoagulant phenprocoumon in 10 healthy male volunteers (ages 18-50). A single dose of phenprocoumon (12 mg) on day 11 resulted in a significant decrease in the plasma concentration of free phenprocoumon ($p = 0.007$). The researchers speculated that the drug interaction may have been caused by inhibited absorption of phenprocoumon or by an increase in the elimination of the drug caused by induction of CYP450 enzymes (Maurer et al., 1999).

A single-blind, placebo-controlled parallel group study was conducted in 25 volunteers to examine the possible interaction of St. John's wort with digoxin. After administration of digoxin for 5 d to achieve a steady state of the drug, volunteers received either St. John's wort extract (LI 160, 900 mg/ day) and digoxin or placebo and digoxin for ten days. The results showed a significant decrease in levels of digoxin in the group taking the drug along with the St. John's wort extract compared to the group taking a placebo plus digoxin ($p = 0.003$ for area under curve), which further decreased with continued administration of the St. John's wort extract. The researchers speculated that the effect might be explained by an induced increase in the activity of drug metabolizing enzymes or by an induction of drug transporters, and pointed their suspicions to flavonoids in St. John's wort rather than hypericin (Johne et al., 1999). A similar study using a randomized, double-blind, placebo-controlled parallel group design evaluated interactions of a St. John's wort powder extract (Lichtwer, Jarsin) and digoxin. After 14 days of comedication (900 mg/day plus a maintenance dose of digoxin), the 24 h AUC of digoxin showed a reduction of 24.6% compared to placebo (Uehleke et al., 2000). However, administration of either the fatty oil of St. John's wort (1.2 g/day, encapsulated), a tea prepared from the raw herb (two cups/day = 1.6 g), or the raw powdered herb in capsules (4 g/day) failed to cause any significant change in AUCs or trough levels compared to placebo.

The Medical Products Agency of Sweden cited eight reports they received of women who experienced intramenstrual bleeding after taking St. John's wort, most of them aged 23-31 and having used birth control pills for many years. In most cases, the abnormal bleeding took place a week after beginning St. John's wort. The researchers noted that inducers of the CYP3A4 isoenzyme, which participates in metabolizing steroids, is known to cause breakthrough bleeding (and a decrease in steroid levels) when combined with oral contraceptives. Seven cases in their files record a decreased anticoagulant effect of warfarin in association with the use of St. John's wort. After tests showed a decreased international normalization ratio (INR), warfarin dosages were increased or St. John's wort was discontinued before INR values returned to therapeutic levels (Yue et al., 2000).

Investigators at the Medical Products Agency (MPA) of Sweden recounted evidence indicating that St. John's wort can interfere with the metabolism of various prescription drugs, and "must not be used concomitantly with any medicinal product"—a warning the MPA has requested manufacturers of St. John's wort products include with patient information in all St. John's wort products. Their warning follows case reports provided by manufacturers of St. John's wort products in Sweden and studies finding that the herb increases activity of the hepatic cytochrome P450 enzyme system, which is involved in the metabolism of a long list of different kinds of drugs. They note that although in vitro studies have shown conflicting evidence of St. John's wort activating an isoenzyme of the P450 system known as CYP3A4, more recent research has shown that the same isoenzyme is induced in patients taking St. John's wort concomitant with the cough suppressant dextromethorphan (Yue et al., 2000).

It has been suggested that the altered metabolism of digoxin by St. John's wort may be due to some effect on the P-glycoprotein drug transport system rather than CYP3A4, since digoxin and other cardiac glycosides are not metabolized by the hepatic system (Pennachio, 2000). In vitro studies indicate that St. John's wort extracts cause hepatic cytochrome P450 activity to approximately double (Ernst, 1999). At clinically relevant, low in vitro concentrations, a methanolic extract of St. John's wort also caused significant induction of P-glycoprotein expression, a multidrug transporting enzyme (Perloff et al., 2001). Tests of 21 ethanolic herbal extract products sold in Canada for in vitro inhibitory activity on cytochrome P450 3A4 (CYP3A4) found about 66% showed significant inhibition of CYP3A4 at concentrations of less than 10% of their full-strength source preparations. Only three showed activity from a median inhibitory concentration of less than 1% "full strength"; an extract of St. John's wort (0.04%) was the second most potent after an extract of goldenseal (*Hydrastis canadensis,* 0.03% full strength). Cat's claw (*Uncaria tomentosa,* 0.79% full strength) appeared to be the third most potent inhibitor. However significant, these median CYP3A4-inhibitory concentrations were far greater than that of ketoconazole (7.18×10^{-4} mM). Hypericin was active with median inhibitory concentration of 0.33 mM. While acknowledging that in vivo studies are required to determine the relevancy of their results, the researchers noted the potential of their findings for herbal products that could increase the toxicity of conventional drugs when administered concomitantly, and for the use of herbal products that inhibit CYP3A4 as drug-sparing substances which could facilitate the use of lower dosages of expensive drugs taken concomitantly (Budzinski et al., 2000).

Obach (2000) investigated commercially available St. John's wort extracts in the United States and elucidated the constituents involved. Fractions containing hyperforin, hypericin, and the flavonoid I3,II8-biapigenin inhibited various P450 enzyme activities (CYP1A2, CYP2C9, CYP2C19, CYP2D6, CYP3A4) in vitro. The most potent competitive inhibition of CYP1A2, CYP2C9, and CYP3A4 was found from I3,II8-biapigenin. Hyperforin showed potent noncompetitive inhibition of CYP2D6 and potent competitive inhibition of CYP3A4 and CTP2C9 activities.

Wentworth et al. (2000) showed that St. John's wort activates the steroid X receptor, which in turn activates cytochrome P-450 gene expression. Hypericin was inactive, whereas hyperforin does this through coactivator recruitment and transactivation of steroid X. These results suggest that interactions of St. John's wort with drugs which are metabolized through the CYP3A pathway results from steroid X activation. The researchers suggest that in the future, St. John's wort extracts might be developed which lack this ability.

Moore et al. (2000) report that St. John's wort extracts and hyperforin are potent ligands for the pregnane X receptor, the murine counterpart of the steroid X receptor. The pregnane X receptor regulates the expression of cytochrome P450 (CYP) 3A4 monooxygenase. The researchers note that because St. John's wort extracts and hyperforin caused a marked induction of CYP3A4 expression in primary hepatocytes, and because this enzyme is involved in the metabolism of more than half of all drugs, it is likely that St. John's wort extracts interact with a far greater number of drugs than so far reported. Like Wentworth and colleagues (2000), Moore and colleagues suggest the possibility of developing St. John's wort extracts that do not activate the pregnane X receptor.

In vivo studies of St. John's wort on the P450 system are to date lacking. Dürr and co-workers (2000) examined the effect of a St. John's wort extract in male rats (LI 160, 1000 mg/kg by gavage for 14 days) and found a 3.8-fold increase in the expression of intestinal P-glycoprotein/Mdr1 and a 2.5-fold increase in the expression of hepatic CYP3A2. To study effects on hepatic drug-metabolizing enzymes and interactions with digoxin, they administered the extract to eight healthy men (ages 25-35) instructed to abstain from coffee, citrus fruits, medications, and alcohol for a minimum of five days prior to and during the study. During days in the clinic, they received no food for 10 h before testing. Prior to receiving St. John's wort, the pharmacokinetics of digoxin (0.5 mg p.o.) were determined in each subject along with an erythromycin breath test and the taking of intestinal biopsy specimens. The results showed that St. John's wort (LI 160, 300 mg t.i.d. after meals for 14 days) caused plasma levels of a subsequent dose of digoxin to decrease by 18%. Intestinal (duodenum) P-glycoprotein/MDR1 expression showed a 1.4-fold increase and intestinal CYP3A4 showed a 1.5-fold increase. Hepatic CYP3A4 showed a 1.4-fold increase in functional activity (^{14}C-erythromycin breath test). These results indicate that, in humans, St. John's wort is an inducer of both intestinal and hepatic CYP3A4 (Dürr et al., 2000). Other inducers of CYP3A4 are barbiturates, rifampicin, carbamazepine, and phenytoin (Glue and Clement, 1999). Drugs partly eliminated by the P-glycoprotein system include calcium channel blockers, lidocaine, doxorubicin, quinidine, amiodarone, and cyclosporine (Yu, 1999).

At the same time, several groups have reported a lack of effect from St. John's wort extracts on hepatic drug-metabolizing enzymes (cited in Schulz, 2001); in a study of seven healthy volunteers on cytochrome 2D6, 3A4, and P-450 activity using dextromethorphan and alprazolam probe methodologies (Markowitz et al., 2000); on intestinal P-glycoprotein (Mdr 1) in rats (Gerloff et al., 2000); on CYP3A4 in a study using dextromethorphan as a probe (Ereshewsky et al., 1999); and on CYP 1A2 using caffeine probe methodology (Gewertz et al., 1999). A more recent study in 12 healthy volunteers reported no effect on CYP isozymes from a single 900 mg dose of a widely used St. John's wort extract (Sundown Herbals, Boca Raton, FL) over eight hours, but after two weeks (300 mg t.i.d. with meals for 14-15 days) the metabolism of intravenous midazolam decreased by 20% and oral bioavailability was decreased by greater than 50%. Midazolam is metabolized by CYP3A, as are over 40% of prescription drugs. Coadministration of tolbutamide during the two-week treatment phase resulted in increased hypoglycemia and a 55% reduction in the bioavailability of the drug, indicating that St. John's wort altered metabolism of CYP3A enzymes which otherwise selectively and almost completely metabolize the drug. The St. John's wort extract was found to contain 11 ± 0.63 µg hyperforin and 840 $\pm$ 56 mg hypericin per 300 mg capsule (Wang et al., 2001).

Like St. John's wort, various tricyclic and SSRI antidepressants (e.g., amitripyline, imipramine, clomipramine, and Serzone, Prozac, Luvox, Wellbutrin/Zyban, respectively) are partly metabolized by and have been reported to inhibit the same isoenzyme (and other isoenzymes of the hepatic cytochrome P450 enzyme system) (Bhatia and Bhatia, 1997; Gillis et al., 1999). Case reports of possible antidepressant drug interactions with St. John's wort include patients taking paroxetine (Gordon, 1998), sertraline (Lantz et al., 1999), nefazodone (Lantz et al., 1999), and venlafaxine (Prost et al., 2000).

In the absence of large-scale case-control studies of St. John's wort extracts, the following summaries of case reports primarily serve as examples of the present inherent difficulty in evaluating the safety of St. John's wort in combination with prescription drugs.

Gordon (1998) reported a possible case of toxicity in a patient taking a St. John's wort extract with the SSRI paroxetine. The patient developed sedation and lethargy, which abated after the St. John's wort extract was discontinued. Lantz et al. (1999) reported four cases of elderly patients (ages 64-84) taking sertaline and one taking nefazodone for the treatment of depression who experienced side effects when St. John's wort extract was added to their medications and abated after it was discontinued. In one case, a man taking no other medications but sertraline (75 mg/day) and a St. John's wort extract (300 mg b.i.d.) experienced anxiety, nausea, and epigastric pain in three days on the combination. In another case, a woman taking nefazodone (100 mg b.i.d.) who added a St. John's wort extract (300 mg t.i.d.) to her regimen experienced profound nausea, restlessness, and vomiting within three days on the extract. Told to stop taking both substances, she chose instead to stop the nefazodone and continue with the St. John's wort extract (300 mg b.i.d.). Her symptoms improved gradually over a period of a week, and although she continued to show some mild to moderate symptoms of depression, she refused all prescription medications. The other cases that Lantz and colleagues recount experienced anxiety, irritability, confusion, headache, nausea, vomiting, dizziness, and feelings of restlessness within 2-4 d after taking St. John's wort extracts (300 mg two to three times/day) in addition to sertaline (50-75 mg/day) (Lantz et al., 1999).

During preoperative evaluation, surgery was rescheduled for a woman who informed hospital staff that she had taken St. John's wort extract for the past year. Because they believed St. John's wort extract could have SSRI and MAOI effects, as a precaution, surgery was delayed two weeks while the patient stopped the use of the herb to avoid any possibility of drug interactions with anesthetics (Murphy, 1999).

For depressive patients taking prescription antidepressants, it has been recommended that a washout period of at least two weeks pass before beginning St. John's wort extracts; in the case of SSRIs, a four- to five-week washout period is suggested (Moss, 1998). At least one physician in the United States has suggested that for patients wanting to change their antidepressant medication from an SSRI, an initial dosage of 300 mg/day of St. John's wort extract and half the dose of SSRI for the first week may be safely increased to 600 mg/day of the extract while tapering the dose of SSRI. In place of prescribing a tranquilizer in cases of anxiety during the transition, an extract of kava *(Piper methysticum)* is used (Roundtree, 1999). To our knowledge, this transition regimen has yet to be studied to determine safety and efficacy in a controlled trial.

The possibility of drug interactions of St. John's wort with cyclosporin are reported by a number of researchers (Mai et al., 2000; Karliova et al., 2000; Barone et al., 2000, 2001). The Australian Adverse Drug Reactions Advisory Committee recorded one case of a seeming drug interaction in a female patient in her twenties taking a St. John's wort extract in 1998 who showed a drop in cyclosporin levels of 25% (Rey and Walter, 1998). In Germany, 35 recipients of kidney and ten of liver transplants showed drops in blood levels of cyclosporin of 30% to 64% after taking St. John's wort. In at least two of these cases, transplanted patients experienced organ rejection episodes, which were attributed to the use of St. John's wort (Breidenbach, Kliem, et al., 2000; Breidenbach, Hoffmann, et al., 2000). In Switzerland, two cases of decreased cyclosporin concentrations were reported in heart transplanted patients taking St. John's wort who experienced acute heart transplant rejection. When St. John's wort was stopped, therapeutic plasma cyclosporin levels returned (Ruschitzka et al., 2000).

A case report of a probable drug interaction of St. John's wort with cyclosporin involved a 21-year-old woman who had received a pancreas and kidney transplant. For immunosuppression she was taking prednisone (10 mg/day) and cyclosporine (100 mg b.i.d.) plus clonidine (0.2 mg/day) to control blood pressure. She had stable levels of cyclosporine until she began taking St. John's wort (300-mg tablets standardized to contain 0.3% hypericin, one to two/day) for the purpose of raising her mood. Over a period of 30 days, her cyclosporin concentrations fell to 155 ng/mL and then fell to 97 ng/mL in the next three weeks. At this time, her serum amylase levels were significantly increased and the pain she was experiencing over her new pancreas indicated acute transplant rejection. Over a two-week period during which she received remedial care with antirejection drugs and an increased dosage of cyclosporin, her physicians learned of her self-medication with St. John's wort. During the next two-week period, her trough concentrations of cyclosporine achieved a maximum level (510 ng/mL), whereupon her dosage was adjusted to 100 mg twice daily to get concentrations back to the desired range. However, her serum amylase levels were still elevated and, owing to chronic rejection of the transplanted organs, she was returned to treatment with dialysis (Barone et al., 2000). A similar case report in Germany concerned severe acute organ rejection in a 63-year-old male liver transplant patient taking oral cyclosporin in addition to St. John's wort (900 mg b.i.d.). The researchers noted that his blood levels of cyclosporin immediately returned to normal after discontinuation of the herb and liver enzymes eventually returned to normal. Like the former case, levels of cyclosporin had to be increased and were adjusted down after use of St. John's wort was stopped (Karliova et al., 2000).

A "possible interaction" of St. John's wort extract with theophylline was reported (Nebel et al., 1999) in the case of a 42-year-old woman required to take a very high dose of theophylline (Theo-Dur, 800 mg b.i.d.) following her discharge from hospital to produce a steady state of 9.2 μg/mL. Yet, previous to hospitalization, 300 mg of theophylline b.i.d. was sufficient to stabilize her condition. Upon questioning, she revealed that for two months she had been taking 300 mg/day of a St. John's wort extract reported to contain 0.3% hypericin in addition to theophylline and her various other medications: prednisone, albuterol, triamcinolone acetonide (inhaled), potassium, furosamide, ibuprofen, morphine, valproic acid, zafirlukast, zolpidem, and amitriptyline. When on her own accord she discontinued the St. John's wort extract, as it was the sole new agent since the problem with theophylline concentrations arose, her concentrations seven days later measured 19.6 μg/ mL and her dosage of theophylline was consequently lowered. Nebel and colleagues offered the possible explanation that because hypericin and pseudohypericin resemble substances that affect hepatic enzymes, which allow theophylline to be cleared (i.e., CYP1A2 in particular, but also glutathione-S-transferase), St. John's wort extract may have been the culprit. Preliminary in vitro studies by the researchers showed that when hypericin (12.5 µM) was incubated with HepG2 human hepatoma cells, it caused the transcriptional enhancer sequence, called the xenobiotic response element (XRE), to be induced 1.8-fold compared to controls, as indicated by a standard method for gene inducibility (chloramphenicol acetyltransferase, or CAT). Although the literature suggested that plasma levels of 0.04-3.0 µM of hypericin are achieved, the researchers were not able to extrapolate their in vitro findings to the case in question. They advised that concomitant use of St. John's wort extracts with other CYP1A2 enzyme substrates, including the drugs R-warfarin, imipramine, clomipramine, clozapine, and olanzapine, may result in other cases of altered drug metabolism and should be cautioned against until more is known.

Pregnancy and Lactation

At least one naturopathic physician in the United States is of the opinion that St. John's wort extracts should not be taken during lactation or pregnancy (Brown, 1996). However, the German Commission E monograph does not contraindicate use during pregnancy or lactation (Blumenthal et al., 1998). The American Herbal Pharmacopoeia (Upton, 1997) notes that St. John's wort is considered slightly uterotonic and states concern for use during pregnancy. The monograph makes no statement about lactation. Most animal studies have shown no toxicity during pregnancy over a wide dose range, with the exception of one study (see Toxicology: Toxicity in Animal Models). There is one report of two women who took St. John's wort while pregnant without adverse events (Grush et al., 1998). No other reports of use during pregnancy were found.

St. John's wort is one of the few herbs where pharmacokinetic data exists, allowing a fuller examination of risk during lactation. Pharmacokinetic studies of hypericin, pseudohypericin, and hyperforin show serum levels in the ng/mL range (see Clinical Studies: Pharmacokinetics). Hale (2000), in a detailed lactation monograph on the herb, notes that although no characterization of constituent milk entry has yet been done, the constituents penetrate the blood-brain barrier poorly and thus are likely to penetrate the breast milk compartment poorly as well, as these compartments are similar. Given the relatively long half-life of hypericin (26.5 h), though, some milk entry would be expected. For postpartum depression, he notes that other antidepressant drugs are considered relatively safe during breast-feeding and are better characterized. The severity of the depression is the primary consideration for best treatment; St. John's wort is currently considered efficacious for mild to moderate depression only. Secondary to that, comparison of side effects of pharmaceutical agents versus St. John's wort are favorable for the herb, perhaps balancing the lack of definitive data on use during lactation. There are no documented adverse effects from use of St. John's wort during lactation. However, there are informal reports of increased milk flow with use. Given the report of uterotonicity, the herb may have an oxytocic effect on the breast, increasing the strength of the milk ejection reflex, though no studies exist to verify this. One mother reported that her four-month-old infant showed increased fussiness and choking at the breast after four days of maternal use of a standardized St. John's wort product (300 mg t.i.d., standardized to contain 0.3% hypericin), symptoms consistent with the development of an overactive milk ejection reflex and/or oversupply (personal communication, Humphrey, 2001). At one time in the United States, external application of the flowers was used to relieve severe engorgement; stimulation of the milk ejection reflex would make milk flow, softening "caked" breast (Bingel and Farnsworth, 1994).

Side Effects

The incidence of adverse events in observational studies with St. John's wort preparations is 1% to 3%. From use of Germany's leading St. John's wort product (Jarsin or Jarsin 300) between 1991 and 1999 the most commonly reported adverse events in reports made to the German ADR recording system were (based on 300 mg t.i.d. for six weeks): "allergic" skin reactions ($n = 27/95$); increased prothrombin times ($n = 16/95$) in patients receiving concomitant treatment with coumarin-based anticoagulant agents; gastrointestinal complaints (9/95); breakthrough bleeding in patients concomitantly using birth control pills ($n = 8/95$); reduced cyclosporin levels in recipients of organ transplants ($n = 7/95$); tingling paraesthesias ($n = 4/95$); and cardiovascular symptoms ($n = 3/95$). During this period, the estimated number of patients who used the product was 8,588,000 and since at least 4 million were women of childbearing age, it is estimated that breakthrough bleeding occurred in about 1/500,000. The incidence of "increased sensitivity to sunlight" (as "reversible skin reactions") was 1/100,000 (Schulz, 2001).

The most common side effects reported in an open study of 3,250 patients were gastrointestinal symptoms (0.6%), allergic reactions (0.5%), and fatigue (0.4%). A total of 2.43% of patients receiving St. John's wort extract reported side effects; an incidence that compared favorably to a drug monitoring study of 943 cases treated with a newer synthetic antidepressant, fluoxetine (Prozac), in which 19% of patients reported side effects, especially nausea, nervousness, dizziness, and headaches (Woelk et al., 1994).

The Australian Adverse Drug Reactions Advisory Committee has recorded few adverse effects from St. John's wort extracts (see also Drug Interactions). In 1998, they recorded the case of a woman, age 38, who experienced hyperesthesia and in another case, a woman, age 47, who experienced multiple side effects from the herb extract: dyspnea, headache, pain, nausea, hyperventilation, palpitations, tremor, flushing, mydriasis, and rhinitis (Rey and Walter, 1998). The latter symptoms appear to suggest an allergic reaction.

No negative influences on performance or ability to drive have been reported from St. John's wort extracts.

Sexual dysfunction is a known side effect from SSRIs but appears to be of extremely rare occurrence in the case of St. John's wort. A temporal association of sexual dysfunction with St. John's wort appears in a case report of a man, age 49, with a ten-year history of depression being treated with sertaline (100 mg/day). He complained of delayed ejaculation and a lack of erections; however, no evidence was found of neurological or vascular disease, and when he discontinued sertaline he reported that sexual function returned to normal after just three days. At his request, he was put on St. John's wort (two tablets b.i.d.). After one week he again experienced delayed orgasm and erectile dysfunction. He continued to take St. John's wort and was prescribed sildenafil (25 mg) for use one hour prior to sexual intercourse. The patient reported that his mood was improved even more than before and that his erections and intercourse were successful. The researcher notes that although he knew of other psychiatric patients taking St. John's wort, reports of sexual dysfunction were absent (Assalian, 2000).

Special Precautions

It is estimated that patients taking St. John's wort preparations should discontinue its use at least five days before undergoing surgery (Ang-Lee et al., 2001).

In cases of inadvertent overdosage of St. John's wort extracts, it is recommended to avoid exposure to bright sunlight or other sources of UVA/UVB (Upton, 1997). This precaution may be especially important in patients receiving photodiagnostics (Ladner et al., 2001). Other have cautioned that topical use of St. John's wort can lead to burning and subsequent scarring if the patient is exposed to direct sunlight following application (Upton, 1997; Lane-Brown, 2000).

A woman, age 35, taking the ground whole herb of St. John's wort (500 mg/day for four weeks) to treat mild depression developed acute neuropathy of the face, hands, legs, and arms following exposure to sunlight without developing signs of skin burn. Cold and light gusts of air at room temperature provoked a strong pain reaction in areas previously exposed to sunlight. Discontinuation of St. John's wort whole herb resulted in symptomatic improvements after three weeks and symptoms resolved during the following two months. The reporting physician (Bove, 1998) suspected the patient experienced demyelination of the cutaneous axions, partly because the recovery time course was consistent with a remyelination time period. It is believed that a potential for developing erythema exists for fair-skinned patients taking oral doses greater than 1,800 mg daily of a 0.3% hypericin extract who are exposed to ultraviolet light (UVA or UVB). This is approximately twice the efficacious dose used in treating depression. In one clinical trial with AIDS patients given 0.5 mg/kg (i.v.) of synthetic hypericin, transient facial pain and erythema developed on exposure to sunlight. These symptoms disappeared within a few days following discontinuation of the drug (Upton, 1997).

In one controlled clinical trial, patients received metered doses of UVA/UVB irradiation after receiving the LI 160 extract (0.24% to 0.32% total hypericin; 600 mg p.o. t.i.d.). After 15 days, a measurable increase in erythema could be detected. The dosage used was approximately twice the usual recommended therapeutic dose, and these individuals had blood levels of hypericin and pseudohypericin twice those seen in normal use of St. John's wort extracts for the treatment of depression. No other adverse effects were seen (Upton, 1997).

In HIV-positive patients treated with synthetic hypericin intravenously (VimRx Pharmaceuticals, Wilmington, DE, 0.25 or 0.5 mg/kg i.v. twice per week or 0.25 mg/kg i.v. three times per week), owing to phototoxic effects only 14 patients completed the study. Out of 23 patients the researchers could evaluate, 11 developed severe cutaneous phototoxicity, including all who received hypericin orally at 0.5 mg/kg per day for eight weeks (Gulick et al., 1999).

Toxicology

In Vitro Toxicity

Bernd et al. (1999) examined the phototoxic effects of a St. John's wort methanolic extract containing 0.3% hypericin-like compounds (A.S.A.C. Pharmaceutical A.I.E., Alicante, Spain) in cultured human keratinocytes. High amounts of the extract ($\geq$ 50 µg/mL), UVA (1 J/cm^2), or visible light (neon tubes for 3 h) irradiation produced definite toxic effects on the DNA synthesis of keratinocytes, but not with lower amounts of extract (< 50 mg/mL), and 4 h of UVB (150 mJ/cm^2) with various amounts of the extract (0.5-100 µg/mL) produced no signs of toxicity. The researchers concluded that phototoxic reactions of the skin would not be expected from the amounts of St. John's wort extract used in the treatment of depression since blood levels of hypericin would be insufficient (Bernd et al., 1999). Based on hypericin content, others have estimated that the amount of a commercial extract of St. John's wort required to increase the risk of photosensitization is approximately 2-4 g/day, or 5-10 mg/day of hypericin (Schulz, 2001).

Shiplochliev (1981) reported slight uterotonic effects of St. John's wort extract in animal cells in vitro.

Mutagenicity

Leuschner (1996) reported that no in vitro toxicity was found from St. John's wort extract (LI 160), and no in vivo mutagenic activity was found in feeding studies of the extract in rats and dogs administered 900 and 2,700 mg/kg p.o. for 26 weeks.

The constituent quercetin has been identified as a genotoxic component in cell-culture mutagenicity assays; however, mutagenicity assays using a 1:4 water extract containing 0.2% to 0.3% hypericin and 0.35% quercetin found no mutagenic potential in vivo or in vitro. Quercetin is practically ubiquitous in plants including food plants. Assessed by the International Agency for Research on Cancer, they concluded that no valid evidence exists for carcinogenicity of quercetin in humans. The amount of quercetin derived from the normal diet is many times higher than that ingested from the therapeutic use of herbs (Upton, 1997).

Toxicity in Animal Models

The no-effect single dose of LI 160 extract is greater than 5,000 mg/kg. In chronic dosage studies in rats and dogs receiving 900 and 2,700 mg/kg p.o., respectively, for 26 weeks, only nonspecific toxic effects were seen which were attributed to load damage: reduced body weight, slight changes in liver function (i.e., increased alanine aminotransferase and lactate dehydrogenase activity), kidney function, and the hemogram. A mild hypertrophy of the zona glomerulosa of the adrenal glands also occurred (Leuschner, 1996).

Garrett et al. (1982) fed rats finely ground, dried St. John's wort from fully blooming plants at 10% of their total diet for the first 12 days and at 5% of their diet for the next 107 days. The animals showed no tissue lesions, no decrease in life span, no direct adverse effects on levels of liver copper, and no major effects on liver levels of iron or zinc.

Toxicological concerns have centered on the potential photosensitizing effects of humans ingesting St. John's wort extract, since this is a well-known toxic effect in animals consuming large amounts of the fresh plant material (1% to 4% of body weight). Calves receiving up to 3 g/kg of St. John's wort herb have demonstrated no photosensitivity (Southwell and Campbell, 1991). In order of most to less susceptibility to toxicity from hypericin, horses are most sensitive, followed by cattle, sheep, then goats (Bourke, 1997).

Garrett et al. (1982) reported no adverse effects on fertility or reproduction in rats fed St. John's wort at 5% of total diet for 119 days. However, Gonzalez et al. (1998) tested an equivalent to the human dose of St. John's wort (uncharacterized preparation, 136 ± 3 mg/kg per day p.o.) and found "subtle toxic effects" in female mice administered the herb as part of their diet (0.75 mg/g), compared to controls not fed the herb. St. John's wort was administered 14 days prior to mating and for either another six weeks or through the gestation period. Litter size was significantly smaller in the St. John's wort group ($p = 0.02$), and neonates and fetuses were also smaller compared to the control group ($p = 0.03$). Yet using much higher dosages, Leuschner (1996) claimed no influence on post- and prenatal development, embryo development, or fertility was found from a St. John's wort extract (LI 160) administered to rats and dogs (900 and 2,700 mg/kg p.o., respectively) over a period of 26 weeks.

Rayburn et al. (2001) investigated the prenatal effect of St. John's wort on the physical maturation and long-term growth of CD-1 mouse offspring in a randomized placebo-controlled study. Adult female mice ($n = 40$) were administered food bars containing St. John's wort (Basic Organics Inc., Columbus, OH) at a dosage equivalent to the human dose of 900 mg/day (180 mg/kg per day) or placebo for a period of two weeks prior to mating and throughout the gestation period. The researchers reported that compared to placebo, St. John's wort had no effect on reproductive capability, growth and development of the offspring, perinatal outcomes, litter sizes, and gestational age at delivery, and that body length, body weight, and head circumference showed no difference in the two groups through their adulthood. Unfortunately, the nature of the herb employed in this study was not characterized by the researchers; however, given the dose it appears to have been an extract preparation. In another placebo-controlled feeding study, Rayburn et al. (2000) found no significant long-term differences in neurobehavior of antenatal CD-1 mice exposed to a standardized St. John's wort preparation at an amount equivalent to a human dose (0.75 mg/g of food).

REFERENCES

Alecu, M., Ursaciuc, C., Halalau, F., Coman, G., Merlevede, W., Waelkens, E., and de Witte, P. (1998). Photodynamic treatment of basal cell carcinoma and squamous cell carcinoma with hypericin. *Anticancer Research* 18: 4651-4654.

Ang-Lee, M.K., Moss, J., and Yuan, C.S. (2001). Herbal medicines and perioperative care. *Journal of the American Medicine Association* 286: 208-216.

Assalian, P. (2000). Sildenafil for St. John wort-induced sexual dysfunction. *Journal of Sex and Marital Therapy* 26(4): 357-358.

Baeuerle, P.A. and Henkel, T. (1994). Function and activation of NF-κB in the immune system. *Annual Review of Immunology* 12: 141-179.

Barone, G.W., Gurley, B.J., Ketel, B.L., and Abul-Ezz, S. (2001). Herbal supplements: A potential for drug interactions in transplant recipients. *Transplantation* 71: 239-241.

Barone, G.W., Gurley, B.J., Ketel, B.L., Lightfoot, M.L., and Abul-Ezz, S.R. (2000). Drug interaction between St. John's wort and cyclosporine. *Annals of Pharmacotherapy* 34(9): 1013-1016.

Bernd, A., Simon, S., Ramirez Bosca, A., Kippenberger, S., Diaz Alperi, J., Miquel, J., Villalba Garcia, J.F., Pamies Mira, D., and Kaufmann, R. (1999). Phototoxic effects of *Hypericum* extract in cultures of human keratinocytes compared with those of psoralen. *Photochemistry and Photobiology* 69: 218-221.

Bhatia, S.C. and Bhatia, S.K. (1997). Major depression: Selecting safe and effective treatment. *American Family Physician* 55: 1683-1694.

Bhattacharya, S.K., Chakrubarti, A., and Chatterjee, S.S. (1998). Active profiles of two hyperforin-containing *Hypericum* extracts in behavioral models. *Pharmacopsychiatry* 31(Suppl. 1): 22-29.

Biber, A., Fischer, H., Römer, A., and Chatterjee, S.S. (1998). Oral bioavailability of hyperforin from Hypericum extracts in rats and human volunteers. *Pharmacopsychiatry* 31(Suppl 1): 36-43.

Bilia, A.R., Bergonzi, M.C., Mazzi, G., and Vincieri, F.F. (2001). Analysis of plant complex matrices by use of nuclear magnetic resonance spectroscopy: St. John's wort extract. *Journal of Agricultural and Food Chemistry* 49: 2115-2124.

Biller, A. (1999). Letter to Kenneth Jones from Dr. Andreas Biller, Head of Clinical Research, Dr. Loges and Co., GmbH Ltd., Sept. 7, 1999.

Bingel, A.S., and Farnsworth, N.R. (1994). Higher plants as potential sources of galactogogues. In Wagner, H., Hikino, H., and Farnsworth, N.R. (Eds.), *Economic and Medicinal Plant Research,* Vol. 6 (pp. 1-54). New York: Academic Press.

Bladt, S. and Wagner, H. (1994). Inhibition of MAO by fractions and constituents of Hypericum extract. *Journal of Geriatric Psychiatry and Neurology* 7(Suppl. 1): S57-S59.

Bork, P.M., Bacher, S., Schmitz, M.L., Kaspers, U., and Heinrich, M. (1999). Hypericin as a non-antioxidant inhibitor of NF-κB. *Planta Medica* 65: 297-300.

Bourke, C.A. (1997). Effects of *Hypericum perforatum* (St. John's wort) on animal health and production. *Plant Protection Quarterly* 12: 91-92.

Bove, G.M. (1998). Acute neuropathy after exposure to sun in a patient treated with St. John's wort. *Lancet* 352 (Oct. 3): 1121-1122.

Breckenridge, A. (2000). Important interactions between St. John's wort *(Hypericum perforatum)* preparations and prescribed medicine, Medicine Controls Agency, Britain, February 29. Available online at: <http://www.open.gov.uk/mca/mcahome.htm>.

Breidenbach, Th., Hoffmann, M.W., Becker, Th., Schlitt, H., and Klempnauer, J. (2000). Drug interaction of St. John's wort with cyclosporin. *Lancet* 355 (May 27): 1912 (letter).

Breidenbach, Th., Kliem, V., Burg, M., Rafermacher, J., Hoffmann, M.W., and Klempnauer, J. (2000). Profound drop of cyclosporin A whole blood trough levels caused by St. John's wort *(Hypericum perforatum)*. *Transplantation* (Baltimore) 69: 2229-2230 (letter).

Brenner, R., Vadim, A., Madhusoodanan, S., and Pawlowska, M. (2000). Comparison of an extract of *Hypericum* (LI 160) and sertraline in the treatment of depression: A double-blind, randomized pilot study. *Clinical Therapeutics* 22: 411-419.

Brown, D. (1996). St. John's wort: Herbal alternative to prescription antidepressants. *Townsend Letter for Doctors and Patients* (April): 125.

Brown, D. (1998). Clinical efficacy of hyperforin-enriched St. John's wort extract. *Quarterly Review of Natural Medicine* (Fall): 203-204.

Budzinski, J.W., Foster, B.C., Vandenhoek, S., and Arnason, J.T. (2000). An in vitro evaluation of human cytochrome P450 3A4 inhibition by selected commercial herbal extracts and tinctures. *Phytomedicine* 7: 273-282.

Burstein, A.H., Horton, R.L., Dunn, T., Alfaro, R.M., Piscitelli, S.C., and Theodore, W. (2000). Lack of effect of St. John's wort on carbamazepine pharmacokinetics in healthy volunteers. *Clinical Pharmacology and Therapeutics* 68: 605-612.

Butterweck, V., Juergenliemk, G., Nahrstedt, A., and Winterhoff, H. (2000). Flavonoids from *Hypericum perforatum* show antidepressant activity in the forced swimming test. *Planta Medica* 66: 3-6.

Butterweck, V., Petereit, F., Winterhoff, H., and Nahrstedt, A. (1998). Solubilized hypericin and pseudohypericin from *Hypericum perforatum* exert antidepressant activity in the forced swimming test. *Planta Medica* 64: 291-294.

Calapai, G., Crupi, A., Firenzuoli, F., Inferrera, G., Gciliberto, G., Parisi, A., De Sarro, G., and Caputi, A.P. (2001). Interleukin-6 involvement in antidepressant action of *Hypericum perforatum*. *Pharmacopsychiatry* 34(Suppl. 1): S8-S10.

Chatterjee, S.S., Bhattacharya, S.K., Wonnemann, M., Singer, A., and Muller, W.E. (1998). Hyperforin as a possible antidepressant component of *Hypericum* extracts. *Life Sciences* 63: 499-510.

Chatterjee, S.S., Nölder, M., Koch, E., and Erdelmeier, C. (1998). Antidepressant activity of *Hypericum perforatum* and hyperforin: The neglected possibility. *Pharmacopsychiatry* 31(Suppl.): 7-15.

Chavez, M.L. and Chavez, P.I. (1997). Saint John's wort. *Hospital Pharmacy* 32: 1621-1632.

Coleta, M., Campos, M.G., Cotrim, M.D., and Proenca da Cunha, A. (2001). Comparative evaluation of *Melissa officinalis*, *Tilia europaea* L., *Passiflora edulis* Sims. and *Hypericum perforatum* L. in the elevated plus maze anxiety test. *Pharmacopsychiatry* 34(Suppl. 1): S20-S21.

Constantine, G.H. and Karchesy, J. (1999). Variations in hypericin concentrations in *Hypericum perforatum* L. and commercial products. *Pharmaceutical Biology* 36: 365-367.

Couldwell, W.T., Gopalkrishna, R., Hinton, D.R., He, S., Weiss, M.H., Law, R.E., Apuzzo, M.L., and Law, R.E. (1994). Hypericin: A potential antiglioma therapy. *Neurosurgery* 35: 705-710.

de Maat, M.M., Hoetelmans, R.M., Math, T.R.A., van Gorp, E.C., Meenhorst, P.L., Mulder, J.W., and Beijnen, J.H. (2001). Drug interaction between St. John's wort and nevirapine. *AIDS* 15: 420-421.

De Vry, J., Maurel, S., Schreiber, R., de Beun, R., and Jentzsch, K.R. (1999). Comparison of *Hypericum* extracts with imipramine and fluoxetine in animal models of depression and alcoholism. *European Neuropsychopharmacology* 9: 461-468.

Demisch, L., Nispel, J., Sielaff, T., Gebhart, C., Köhler, B., and Pflug, B. (1991). Influence of subchronic Hyperforat administration on melatonin production. *Pharmacopsychiatry* 24: 194 (abstract).

Denke, A., Schempp, H., Weiser, D., and Elstner, E.F. (2000). Biochemical activities of extracts of *Hypericum perforatum* L.: 5th communication: Dopamine-β-hydroxylase-product quantification by HPLC and inhibition by hyperpicins and flavonoids. *Arzneimittel-Forschung/Drug Research* 50: 415-419.

Department of Health, Great Britain (2000). New advice on St. John's wort, March 1. Available online at <http://www.doh.gov.uk/dhhome.htm>.

Di Matteo, V., Di Giovanni, G., Di Mascio, M., and Esposito, E. (2000). Effect of acute administration of *Hypericum perforatum*-CO_2 extract on dopamine and serotonin release in the rat central nervous system. *Pharmacopsychiatry* 33: 14-18.

Dimpfel, W., Schober, F., and Mannel, M. (1998). Effects of a methanolic extract and a hyperforin-enriched CO_2 extract of St. John's wort *(Hypericum perforatum)* on intracerebral field potentials in the freely moving rat (Tele-Stereo-EEG). *Pharmacopsychiatry* 31(Suppl.): 30-35.

Duke, J.A. (1985). *Handbook of Medicinal Herbs* (pp. 242-243). Boca Raton, FL: CRC Press.

Dürr, D., Stieger, B., Kullak-Ublick, G.A., Rentsch, K.M., Steinert, H.C., Meier, P.J., and Fattinger, K. (2000). St. John's wort induces intestinal P-glycoprotein/MDR1 and intestinal and hepatic CYP3A4. *Clinical Pharmacology and Therapeutics* 68(6): 598-604.

Eckert, G.P. and Müller, W.E. (2001). Effects of hyperforin on the fluidity of brain membranes. *Pharmacopsychiatry* 34(Suppl. 1): S22-S25.

Erdelmeier, C.A.J. (1998). Hyperforin, possibly the major non-nitrogenous secondary metabolite of *Hypericum perforatum* L. *Pharmacopsychiatry* 31(Suppl.): 2-6.

Ereshewsky, B., Gewertz, M., Larn, Y.W.F., Vega, L.M., and Ereshewsky, L. (1999). Determination of St. John's wort differential metabolism at CYP2D6 and CYP3A4, using dextromethorphan probe methodology. 39th Annual Meeting of the New Clinical Drug Evaluation Unit, Boca Raton, FL, June 1-4, poster 130.

Ernst, E. (1999). Second thoughts about safety of St. John's wort. *Lancet* 354 (December 11): 2014-2016.

Ernst, E., Rand, J.I., Barnes, J., and Stevinson, C. (1998). Adverse effects profile of the herbal antidepressant St. John's wort *(Hypericum perforatum* L.). *European Journal of Clinical Pharmacology* 54: 589-594.

Fornal, C.A., Metzler, C.W., Mirescu, C., Stein, S.K., and Jacobs, B.L. (2001). Effects of standardized extracts of St. John's wort on the single-unit activity of serotonergic dorsal raphe neurons in awake cats: Comparisons with fluoxetine and sertraline. *Neuropsychopharmacology* 25: 858-870.

Franklin, M. and Cowen, P.J. (2001). Researching the antidepressant actions of *Hypericum perforatum* (St. John's wort) in animals and man. *Pharmacopsychiatry* 34(Suppl. 1): S29-S37.

Gaind, K.N. and Ganjoo, T.N. (1959). Antibacterial principle of *Hypericum perforatum* L. *Indian Journal of Pharmacy* 21: 172-175.

Gambarana, C., Tolu, P.L., Masi, F., Rinaldi, M., Giachetti, D., Morazzoni, P., and De Montis, M.G. (2001). A study of the antidepressant activity of *Hypericum perforatum* on animals models. *Pharmacopsychiatry* 234(Suppl. 1): S42-S44.

Garrett, B.J., Cheeke, P.R., Miranda, C.L., Goeger, D.E., and Buhler, D.R. (1982). Consumption of poisonous plants *(Senecio jacobeae, Symphytum officinale, Pteridium aquilinum, Hypericum perforatum)* by rats: Chronic toxicity, mineral metabolism, and hepatic drug-metabolizing enzymes. *Toxicology Letters* 10: 183-188.

Gaster, B. and Holroyd, J. (2000). St. John's wort for depression. *Archives of Internal Medicine* 160: 152-156.

Gerloff, T., Störmer, E., Mrozikiewicz, A.P.M., and Roots, I. (2000). *Hypericum perforatum* (St. John's wort) has no effect on protein expression of intestinal P-glycoprotein (Mdr 1) in the rat. CPT 2000, Florence, Italy, abstract.

Gewertz, N., Ereshefsky, B., Lam, Y.W.F., Bonavides, R., and Ereshefsky, L. (1999). Determination of the differential effects of St. John's wort on the CYP1A2 and NAT2 metabolic pathways using caffeine probe methodology. 39th Annual Meeting of the New Clinical Drug Evaluation Unit, Boca Raton, FL, June 1-4, poster 131.

Gillis, M.C., Welbanks, L., Bergeron, D., Cormier-Boyd, M., Hachborn, F., Jovaisas, B., Pagotto, S., and Repchinsky, C. (Eds.) (1999). *Compendium of Pharmaceuticals and Specialties,* Thirty-Fourth Edition. Ottawa, Ontario, Canada: Canadian Pharmacists Association.

Glue, P. and Clement, R.P. (1999). Cytochrome P450 enzymes and drug metabolism—Basic concepts and methods of assessment. *Cellular and Molecular Neurobiology* 19: 309-323.

Gobbi, M., Moia, M., Pirona, L., Morazzoni, P., and Mennini, T. (2001). In vitro binding studies with two *Hypericum perforatum* extracts—hyperforin, hypericin and baipigenin—on 5-HT$_6$, 5-HT-$_7$, GABA$_A$/benzodiazepine, Sigma, NPY-Y$_1$/Y$_2$ receptors and dopamine transporters. *Pharmacopsychiatry* 34(Suppl. 1): S45-S48.

Gobbi, M., Valle, F.D., Ciapparelli, C., Diomede, L., Morazzoni, P., Verotta, L., Caccia, S., Cervo, L., and Mennini, T. (1999). *Hypericum perforatum* L. extract does not inhibit 5-HT transporter in rat brain cortex. *Naunyn-Schmiedeberg's Archives of Pharmacology* 360: 262-269.

Gonzalez, C.J., Stewart, J.D., Rayburn, W.F., and Christensen, H.D. (1998). Establishment of a relevant dose of antenatal *Hypericum* (St. John's wort) for neurobehavioral development study. *Neurotoxicology and Tetratology* 20: 369 (abstract NBTS 59).

Gordon, J. (1998). SSRIs and St. John's wort, possible toxicity? *American Family Physician* 62: 31.

Gray, D.E., Rottinghaus, G.E., Garrett, H.E.G., and Pallardy, S.G. (2000). Simultaneous determination of the predominant hypeforins and hypericins in St. John's wort (*Hypericum perforatum* L.) by liquid chromatography. *Journal of AOAC International* 83: 944-949.

Grush, L.R., Nierenberg, A., Keefe, B., and Cohen, L.S. (1998). St. John's wort during pregnancy. *Journal of the American Medical Association* 280: 1566 (letter).

Gulick, R.M., McAuliffe, V., Holden-Wiltse, J., Crumpacker, C., Liebes, L., Stein, D.S., Meehan, P., Hussey, S., Forcht, J., and Valentine, F.T. (1999). Phase I studies of hypericin, the active compound in St. John's wort, as an antiretroviral agent in HIV-infected adults. *Annals of Internal Medicine* 130: 510-514.

Haberlein, H., Tschiersch, K.P., Stock, S., and Hoelzl, J. (1992). [St. John's wort, *Hypericum perforatum* L. Part I. Identification of an additional napthodianthrone]. *Pharmazeutische Zeitung Wissenschaft* 137: 169-174.

Hale, T. (2000). *Medications and Mother's Milk* (pp. 407-408). Amarillo, TX: Pharmasoft Medical Publications.

Hansen, S.H., Jensen, A.G., Cornett, C., Bjornsdottir, I., Taylor, S., Wright, B., and Wilson, I.D. (1999). High-performance liquid chromatography on-line coupled to high-field NMR and mass spectrometry for structure elucidation of constituents of *Hypericum perforatum* L. *Analytical Chemistry* 71: 5235-5241.

Hänsgen, K.D., Vesper, J., and Ploch, M. (1994). Multicenter double-blind study examining the antidepressant effectiveness of the *Hypericum* extract LI 160. *Journal of Geriatric Psychiatry and Neurology* 7(Suppl. 1): S15-S18.

Harrer, G., Hübner, W.D., and Podzuweit, H. (1994). Effectiveness and tolerance of the *Hypericum* extract LI 160 compared to maprotiline: A multicenter double-blind study. *Journal of Geriatric Psychiatry and Neurology* 7(Suppl.):S24-S28.

Harrer, G., Schmidt, U., Kuhn, U., and Biller, A. (1999). Comparison of equivalence between St. John's wort extract LoHyp-57 and fluoxetine. *Arzneimittel-Forschung/Drug Research* 49: 289-296.

Harrer, G. and Schulz, V. (1994). Clinical investigation of the antidepressant effectiveness of *Hypericum*. *Journal of Geriatric Psychiatry and Neurology* 7(Suppl.): S6-S8.

Hobbs, C. (1989). St. John's wort. *HerbalGram* 18/19: 24-33.

Hübner, W.D., Lande, S., and Podzuwent, H. (1994). Hypericum treatment of mild depressions with somatic symptoms. *Journal of Geriatric Psychiatry and Neurology* 7(Suppl. 1): S12-S14.

Humphrey, S. (2001). Sheila Humphrey, RN, BSc, ICBLC, personal communication with INPR, September.

Jensen, A.G., Hansen, S.H., and Nielsen, E.Ø. (2001). Adhyperforin as a contributor to the effect of *Hypericum perforatum* L. in biochemical models of antidepressant activity. *Life Sciences* 68: 1593-1605.

Johne, A., Brockmöller, J., Bauer, S., Maurer, A., Langheinrich, M., and Roots, I. (1999). Interaction of St. John's wort with digoxin. *Clinical Pharmacology and Therapeutics* 66: 338-345.

Johnston, N. (1999). Sun trap. Keep a weather eye if you take herbal antidepressants. *New Scientist* (July 24): 24.

Kaehler, S.T., Sinner, C., Chatterjee, S.S., and Philippu, A. (1999). Hyperforin enhances the extracellular concentrations of catecholamines, serotonin and glutamate in the rat locus coeruleus. *Neuroscience Letters* 262: 199-202.

Karliova, M., Reichel, U., Malago, M., Frilling, A., Gerken, G., and Broelsch, C.E. (2000). Interaction of *Hypericum perforatum* (St. John's wort) with cyclosporin A metabolism in a patient after liver transplantation. *Journal of Hepatology* 33: 853-855.

Kasper, S. (1997). Treatment of seasonal affective disorder (SAD) with *Hypericum* extract. *Pharmacopsychiatry* 30(Suppl.): 89-93.

Kerb, R., Brockmoller, J., Staffeldt, B., Ploch, M., and Roots, I. (1996). Single-dose and steady-state pharmacokinetics of hypericin and pseudohypericin. *Antimicrobial Agents and Chemotherapy* 40: 2087-2093.

Khalifa, A.E. (2001). *Hypericum perforatum* as a nootropic drug: Enhancement of retrieval memory of a passive avoidance conditioning paradigm in mice. *Journal of Ethnopharmacology* 76: 49-57.

Kientsch, U., Bürgi, S., Ruedeberg, C., Probst, S., and Honegger, U.E. (2001). St. John's wort extract Ze 117 *(Hypericum perforatum)* inhibits norepinephrine and serotonin uptake into rat brain slices and reduces β-adrenoreceptor numbers on cultured rat brain cells. *Pharmacopsychiatry* 34(Suppl. 1): S56-S60.

Kim, H.L., Streltzer, J., and Goebert, D. (1999). St. John's wort for depression: A meta-analysis of well-defined clinical trials. *Journal of Nervous and Mental Disease* 187: 532-538.

Kleber, E., Obry, T., Hippeli, S., Schneider, W., and Elstner, E.F. (1999). Biochemical activities of extracts from *Hypericum perforatum* L. *Arzneimittel-Forschung/Drug Research* 49: 106-109.

Klusa, V., Germane, S., Noldner, M., and Chatterjee, S.S. (2001). *Hypericum* extract and hyperforin: Memory-enhancing properties in rodents. *Pharmacopsychiatry* 34(Suppl. 1): S61-S69.

Koytchev, R., Alken, R.G., and Dundarov, S. (1999). Hypericum-extract LI 160 for the therapy of *Herpes simplex genitalis* and *labialis:* Results of two placebo-controlled, randomized, double-blind clinical trials. *Zeitschrift für Phytotherapie* 20: 92 (abstract).

Krishtal, O., Lozovaya, N., Fisunov, A., Tsintsadze, T., Pankratov, Y., Kopanitsa, M., and Chatterjee, S.S. (2001). Modulation of ion channels in rat neurons by the constituents of *Hypericum perforatum. Pharmacopsychiatry* 34(Suppl. 1): S74-S82.

Kumar, V., Singh, P.N., Muruganandam, A.V., and Bhattacharya, S.K. (2000). Effect of Indian *Hypericum perforatum* Linn on animal models of cognitive dysfunction. *Journal of Ethnopharmacology* 72(1-2): 119-128.

Kunze, H. and Priebe, S. (1998). Assessing the quality of psychiatric hospital care: A German approach. *Psychiatric Service* 49: 794-796.

Kurth, H. and Spreemann, R. (1998). Phytochemical characterization of various St. John's wort extracts. *Advances in Therapy* 15: 117-128.

Laakmann, G., Schule, C., Baghai, T., and Kieser, M. (1998). St. John's wort in mild to moderate depression: The relevance of hyperforin for the clinical efficacy. *Pharmacopsychiatry* 31(Suppl.): 54-59.

Ladner, D.P., Klein, S.D., Steiner, R.A., and Walt, H. (2001). Synergistic toxicity of delta-aminolaevulinic acid-induced protoporphyrin IX used for photodiagnosis and *Hypericum* extract, a herbal antidepressant. *British Journal of Dermatology* 144: 916-918 (letter).

Lal, S. and Iskandar, H. (2000). St. John's wort and schizophrenia. *Canadian Medical Association Journal* 163: 262-263.

Lane-Brown, M.M. (2000). Photosensitivity associated with herbal preparations of St. John's wort *(Hypericum perforatum). Medical Journal of Australia* 172: 302.

Langosch, J.M., Zhou, X.Y., Heinen, M., Chatterjee, S.S., Nölder, M., and Walden, J. (2001). Effects of *Hypericum perforatum* L. on evoked potentials in guinea pig hippocampal slices. *Pharmacopsychiatry* 34(Suppl. 1): S83-S88.

Lantz, M.S., Buchalter, E., and Giambanco, V. (1999). St. John's wort and antidepressant drug interactions in the elderly. *Journal of Geriatric Psychiatry and Neurology* 12: 7-10.

Lavie, G., Mazur, Y., Lavie, D., Levin, B., Ittah, Y., and Meruelo, D. (1990). Hypericin as an antiretroviral agent. *Annals of the New York Academy of Sciences* 616: 556-562.

Lavie, G., Mazur, Y., Lavie, D., and Meruelo, D. (1995). The chemical and biological properties of hypericin—a compound with a broad spectrum of biological activities. *Medicinal Research Reviews* 15: 111-119.

Lavie, G., Mazur, Y., Lavie, D., Prince, A.M., Pascual, D., Liebes, L., Levin, B., and Meruelo, D. (1995). Hypericin as an inactivator of infectious viruses in blood components. *Transfusion* 35: 392-400.

Lenoir, S., Degenring, F.H., and Saller, R. (1999). A double-blind randomized trial to investigate three different concentrations of a standardized fresh plant extract obtained from the shoot tips of *Hypericum perforatum* L. *Phytomedicine* 6: 141-146.

Leuschner, J. (1996). Preclinical toxicological profile of Hypericum extract LI 160. *Phytomedicine* 3(Suppl. 1): 104.

Linde, K., Ramirez, G., Mulrow, C.D., Pauls, A., Weidenhammer, W., and Melchart, D. (1996). St. John's wort for depression—An overview and meta-analysis of randomized clinical trials. *British Medical Journal* 313: 253-258.

Lumpkin, M.M. and Alpert, S. (2000). Risk of drug interactions with St. John's wort and indinavir and other drugs. Center for Drug Evaluation and Research, FDA Public Health Advisory, February 10. Available online at <http://www.fda. gov/cder/drug/advisory/stjwort.htm>.

Mai, I., Kruger, H., Budde, K., Johne, A., Brockmoller, J., Neumayer, H.H., and Roots, I. (2000). Hazardous pharmacokinetic interaction of Saint John's wort *(Hypericum perforatum)* with the immunosuppressant cyclosporin. *International Journal of Clinical Pharmacology and Therapeutics* 38: 500-502.

Maisenbacher, P. and Kovar, K.A. (1992). Adhyperforin—a homologue of hyperforin from *Hypericum perforatum*. *Planta Medica* 58: 291-293.

Markowitz, J.S., DeVane, C.L., Boulton, D.W., Carson, S.W., Nahas, Z., and Risch, S.C. (2000). Effect of St. John's wort *(Hypericum perforatum)* on cytochrome P-450 2D6 and 3A4 activity in healthy volunteers. *Life Sciences* 66: PL133-PL139.

Martinez, B., Kasper, S., Ruhrmann, S., and Moller, H.J. (1994). Hypericum in the treatment of seasonal affective disorders. *Journal of Geriatric Psychiatry and Neurology* 7(Suppl.): S29-S33.

Mártonfi, P., Repcak, M., Ciccarelli, D., and Garbari, F. (2001). *Hypericum perforatum* L.—Chemotype without rutin from Italy. *Biochemical Sytematics and Ecology* 29: 659-661.

Maurer, A., Johne, A., Bauer, S., Brockmöller, J., Donath, F., Rppts, I., Langheinrich, M., and Hübner, W.D. (1999). Interaction of St. John's wort extract with phenprocoumon. *European Journal of Clinical Pharmacology* 55 (abstracts): A22.

Meier, B. (2001). Comparing phytopharmaceuticals: The example of St. John's wort. *Advances in Therapy* 18: 35-45.

Melzer, R., Fricke, U., and Hölzl, J. (1991). Vasoactive properties of procyanidins from *Hypericum perforatum* L. in isolated porcine coronary arteries. *Arzneimittel-Forschung/Drug Research* 41: 481-483.

Melzer, R., Fricke, U., Hölzl, J., Podehl, R., and Zylka, J. (1989). Procyanidins from *Hypericum perforatum* L. in isolated porcine coronary arteries. *Planta Medica* 55: 655-656.

Ming, D.S., Li, H.H., and Zhong, L.C. (2001). Three new hyperforin analogues from *Hyperforin perforatum*. *Journal of Natural Products* 64: 127-130.

Mirossay, A., Mojzis, J., Tothova, J., Hajikova, M., Lackova, A., and Mirossay, L. (2000). Hypocrellin and hypericin-induced phototoxicity of HL-60 cells: Apoptosis or necrosis? *Phytomedicine* 7: 471-476.

Misane, I. and Ögren, S.O. (2001). Effects of *Hypericum perforatum* (St. John's wort) on passive avoidance in the rat: Evaluation of potential neurochemical mechanisms underlying its antidepressant activity. *Pharmacopsychiatry* 34(Suppl. 1): S89-S97.

Moerman, D.E. (1998). *Native American Ethnobotany* (pp. 272-273). Portland, OR: Timber Press.

Moore, L.B., Goodwin, B., Jones, S.A., Wisely, G.B., Serabjit-Singh, C.J., Willson, T.M., Collins, J.L., and Kliewer, S.A. (2000). St. John's wort induces hepatic drug metabolism through activation of the pregnane X receptor. *Proceedings of the National Academy of Sciences USA* 97: 7500-7502.

Moses, E.L. and Mallinger, A.G. (2000). St. John's wort: Three cases of possible mania induction. *Journal of Clinical Psychopharmacology* 20: 115-117.

Moss, T.M. (1998). Herbal medicine in the emergency department: A primer for toxicities and treatment. *Journal of Emergency Nursing* 24: 509-513.

Müller, W.E., Rolli, M., Schäfer, C., and Hafner, U. (1997). Effects of *Hypericum* extract (LI 160) in biochemical models of antidepressant activity. *Pharmacopsychiatry* 30(Suppl.): 102-107.

Müller, W.E., Singer, A., and Wonnenmann, M. (2001). Hyperforin—antidepressant activity of a novel mechanism of action. *Pharmacopsychiatry* 34(Suppl. 1): S98-S102.

Müller, W.E., Singer, A., Wonnemann, M., Hafner, U., Rolli, M., and Schafer, C. (1998). Hyperforin represents the neurotransmitter reuptake inhibiting constituent of *Hypericum* extract. *Pharmacopsychiatry* 31(Suppl. 1): 16-21.

Murphy, J.M. (1999). Preoperative considerations with herbal medicines. *Association of Operating Room Nurses Journal* 69: 173-183.

Muruganandam, A.V., Ghosal, S., and Battacharya, S.K. (2000). The role of xanthones in the antidepressant activity of *Hypericum perforatum* involving dopaminergic and serotonergic systems. *Biogenic Amines* 15: 553-567.

Nahrstedt, A. and Butterweck, V. (1997). Biologically active and other chemical constituents of the herb of *Hypericum perforatum*. *Pharmacopsychiatry* 30(Suppl.): 129-134.

Nathan, P.J. (1999). The experimental and clinical pharmacology of St. John's wort (*Hypericum perforatum* L.). *Molecular Psychiatry* 4: 333-338.

Neary, J.T. and Bu, Y. (1999). Hypericum LI 160 inhibits uptake of serotonin and norepinephrine in astrocytes. *Brain Research* 816: 358-363.

Nebel, A., Schneider, B.J., Baker, R.K., and Kroll, D.J. (1999). Potential metabolic interaction between St. John's wort and theophylline. *The Annals of Pharmacotherapy* 33: 502 (letter).

Nielsen, A.C. III and Williams, T.A. (1980). Depression in ambulatory medical patients. *Archives of General Psychiatry* 37: 999-1004.

Nierenberg, A.A., Burt, T., Matthews, J., and Weiss, A.P. (1999). Mania associated with St. John's wort. *Biological Psychiatry* 46: 1707-1708.

Obach, R.S. (2000). Inhibition of human cytochrome P450 enzymes by constituents of St. John's wort, an herbal preparation used in the treatment of depression. *Journal of Pharmacology and Experimental Therapeutics* 294: 88-95.

O'Breasail, A.M. and Argouarch, S. (1998). Hypomania and St. John's wort. *Canadian Journal of Psychiatry* 43: 746-747 (letter).

Okpanyi, S.N. and Wiescher, M.L. (1987). Animal experiments on the psychotropic action of *Hypericum* extract. *Arzneimittel-Forschung/Drug Research* 37: 10-13.

Orth, H.C.J., Rentel, C., and Schmidt, P.C. (1999). Isolation, purity analysis and stability of hyperforin as a standard material from *Hypericum perforatum* L. *Journal of Pharmacy and Pharmacology* 51: 193-200.

Osterheider, M., Schmidtke, A., and Beckmann, H. (1992). Behandlung depressiver syndrome mit *Hypericum* (Johanniskraut)—eine placebokontrollierte doppelblindstudie [Treatment of depressive syndrome with *Hypericum* (St. John's wort)—a placebo-controlled double-blind study]. *Fortschritte der Neurologie, Psychiatrie* 60(Suppl. 2): 210-211 (abstract).

Öztürk, Y, Aydin, S., Baser, K.H.C., Kirimer, N., and Kurta-Öztürk, N. (1992). Hepatoprotective activity of *Hypericum perforatum* L. alcoholic extract in rodents. *Phytotherapy Research* 6: 44-46.

Panocka, I., Perfumi, M., and Massi, M. (2000). Effects of *Hypericum perforatum* extract on ethanol intake and on behavioral despair: A search for the neurochemical systems involved. *Pharmacology, Biochemistry and Behavior* 66: 105-111.

Panossian, A.G., Gabrielian, V., Manvelian, K., Jurcic, K., and Wagner, H. (1996). Immunosuppressive effects of hypericin on stimulated human leukocytes: Inhibition of the arachidonic acid release, leukotriene B4 and interleukin-1 (production, and activation of nitric oxide formation). *Phytomedicine* 3: 19-28.

Peebles, K.A., Baker, R.K., Kurz, E.U., Schneider, B.J., and Kroll, D.J. (2001). Catalytic inhibition of human DNA topoisomerase II alpha by hypericin, a naphthodianthrone from St. John's wort *(Hypericum perforatum)*. *Biochemical Pharmacology* 62: 1059-1070.

Pennachio, D.L. (2000). Drug-herb interactions: How vigilant should you be? *Patient Care* 19: 41-68.

Perloff, M.D., von Moltke, L.L., Störmer, E., Shader, R.I., and Grennblatt, D.J. (2001). Saint John's wort: An in vitro analysis of P-glycoprotein induction due to extended exposure. *British Journal of Pharmacology* 134: 1601-1608.

Perovic, S. and Müller, W.E.G. (1995). Pharmacological profile of *Hypericum* extract. Effect on serotonin uptake by postsynaptic receptors. *Arzneimittel-Forschung/Drug Research* 45: 1145-1148.

Petty, F., Kramer, G.L., Fulton, M., Moeller, F.G., and Rush, A.J. (1993). Low plasma GABA is a trait-like marker for bipolar illness. *Neuropsychopharmacology* 9: 125-132.

Petty, F., Kramer, G.L., Gullion, C.M., and Rush, A.J. (1992). Low plasma γ-aminobutyric acid levels in male patients with depression. *Biological Psychiatry* 32: 354-363.

Petty, F., Trivedi, M.H., Fulton, M., and Rush, A.J. (1995). Benzodiazepines as antidepressants: Does GABA play a role in depression? *Biological Psychiatry* 38: 578-591.

Philipp, M., Kohnen, R., and Hiller, K.O. (1999). Hypericum extract versus imipramine or placebo in patients with moderate depression: Randomized multicentre study of treatment for eight weeks. *British Medical Journal* 319: 1534-1538.

Philippu, A. (2001). In vivo neurotransmitter release in the locus coeruleus – effects of hyperforin, inescapable shock and fear. *Pharmacopsychiatry* 34(Suppl. 1): S111-S115.

Piscitelli, S.C., Burstein, A.H., Chaitt, D., Alfaro, R.M., and Fallon, J. (2000). Indinavir concentrations and St. John's wort. *Lancet* 355 (Feb. 12): 547-548.

Ploss, O., Petereit, F., and Nahrstedt, A. (2001). Procyanidins from the herb of *Hypericum perforatum*. *Pharmazie* 56: 509-511.

Prost, N., Tichadou, L., Rodor, F., Nguyen, N., David, J.M., and Jean-Pastor, M.J. (2000). [St. Johns wort-venlafaxine interaction]. *La Presse Medicale* (Paris) 29:1285-1286.

Raffa, R.B. (1998). Screen of receptor and uptake-site activity of hypericin component of St. John's wort reveals σ [Sigma] receptor binding. *Life Sciences* 62: 265-270 (pharmacology letter).

Rao, S.G., Laxminarayana, A.U., Saraswathi, I.U., Padma, G.M., Ganesh, R., and Kulkarni, D.R. (1991). *Calendula* and *Hypericum:* Two homeopathic drugs promoting wound healing in rats. *Fitoterapia* 6: 508-510.

Rayburn, W.F., Christensen, H.D., and Gonzalez, C.L. (2000). Effect of antenatal exposure to Saint John's wort *(Hypericum)* on neurobehaviour of developing mice. *American Journal of Obstetrics and Gynecology* 183: 1225-1231.

Rayburn, W.F., Gonzalez, C.L., Christensen, H.D., and Stewart, J.D. (2001). Effect of prenatally administered *Hypericum* (St John's wort) on growth and physical maturation of mouse offspring. *American Journal of Obstetrics and Gynecology* 184: 191-195.

Reuter, H.D. (1998). Chemistry and biology of *Hypericum perforatum* (St. John's wort). In Lawson, L.D. and Bauer, R. (Eds.), *Phytomedicines of Europe: Chemistry and Biological Activity, ACS Symposium Series 69* (pp. 287-298). Washington, DC: American Chemical Society.

Rey, J.M. and Walter, G. (1998). *Hypericum perforatum* (St. John's wort) in depression: Pest or blessing? *Medical Journal of Australia* 169: 583-586.

Roundtree, R. (1999). Herb-drug mix: Herbs and antidepressant drugs can cross paths, with careful use. *Herbs for Health* 4 (September/October): 32-34.

Rücker, G., Manns, D., Hartmann, R., and Bonsels, U. (1995). A C_{50}-hydroperoxide from *Hypericum perforatum*. *Archive der Pharmazie* 328: 725-730.

Ruschitzka, F., Meier, P.J., Turina, M., Luscher, T.F., and Noll, G. (2000). Acute heart transplant rejection due to St. John's wort. *Lancet* 355 (Feb. 12): 548-549 (research letter).

Schempp, C.M., Ludtke, R., and Simon, J.C. (2000). Effect of topical application of *Hypericum perforatum* extract (St. John's wort) on skin sensitivity to solar simulated radiation. *Photodermatology, Photoimmunology and Photomedicine* 16(3): 125-128.

Schempp, C.M., Pelz, K., Wittmer, A., Schopf, E., and Simon, J.C. (1999). Antibacterial activity of hyperforin from St. John's wort, against multiresistant *Staphylococcus aureus* and Gram-positive bacteria. *Lancet* 353 (June 19): 2129 (letter).

Schrader, D. (2000). Equivalence of St. John's wort extract (ZE 117) and fluoxetine: A randomized, controlled study in mild-moderate depression. *International Journal of Clinical Psychopharmacology* 15: 61-66.

Schrader, E., Meier, B., and Brattström, A. (1998). Hypericum treatment of mild-moderate depression in a placebo-controlled study. A prospective, double-blind, randomized, placebo-controlled, multicentre study. *Human Psychopharmacology* 13: 163-169.

Schulz, H. and Jobert, M. (1994). Effects of *Hypericum* extract on the sleep EEG in older volunteers. *Journal of Geriatric Psychiatry and Neurology* 7(Suppl.): S39-S43.

Schulz, V. (2001). Incidence and clinical relevance of interactions and side effects of *Hypericum* preparations. *Phytomedicine* 8: 152-160.

Serkedjieva, J., Manolova, N., Zgórniak-Nowosielska, I., Zawilinska, B., and Grzybek, J. (1990). Antiviral activity of the infusion (SHS-174) from flowers of *Sambucus nigra* L. aerial parts of *Hypericum perforatum* L., and roots of *Saponaria officinalis* L. against influenza and *Herpes simplex* viruses. *Phytotherapy Research* 4: 97-100.

Sharpley, A.L., McGavin, C.L., Whale, R., and Cowen, P.J. (1998). Antidepressant-like effect of *Hypericum perforatum* (St. John's wort) on the sleep polysomnogram. *Psychopharmacology* 139: 286-287.

Shelton, R.C., Keller, M.B., Gelenberg, A., Dunner, D.L., Hirschfeld, R., Thase, M.E., Russell, J., Lydiard, B., Crits-Crisoph, P., Gallop, R., et al. (2001). Effectiveness of St. John's wort in major depression. A randomized controlled trial. *Journal of the American Medical Association* 285: 1978-1986.

Shiplochliev, T. (1981). [Extracts from a group of plants enhancing uterine tonus]. *Veterinaro-Meditsiniski Nauki* 18: 94-96.

Silberman, H.C. (1996). Superstition and medical knowledge in an Italian herbal. *Pharmacy in History* 38: 87-94.

Simmen, U., Burkard, W., Berger, K., Schaffner, W., and Lundstrom, K. (1999). Extracts and constituents of *Hypericum perforatum* inhibit the binding of various ligands to recombinant receptors expressed with the Semliki forest virus system. *Journal of Receptor and Signal Transduction Research* 19: 59-74.

Singer, A., Wonnemann, M., and Müller, W.E. (1999). Hyperforin, a major antidepressant constituent of St. John's wort, inhibits serotonin uptake by elevating free intracellular Na^{+1}. *Journal of Pharmacology and Experimental Therapeutics* 290: 1363-1368.

Sloley, B.D., Urichuk, L.J., Ling, L., Gu, L.D., Coutts, R.T., Pang, P.K., and Shan, J.J. (2001). Chemical and pharmacological evaluation of *Hypericum perforatum* extracts. *Acta Pharmacologica Sinica* 21: 1145-1152.

Southwell, I.A. and Campbell, M.H. (1991). Hypericin content variation in *Hypericum perforatum* in Australia. *Phytochemistry* 30: 475-478.

Staffeldt, B., Kerb, R., Brockmoller, J., Ploch, M., and Roots, I. (1994). Pharmacokinetics of hypericin and pseudohypericin after oral intake of the *Hypericum perforatum* extract LI 160 in healthy volunteers. *Journal of Geriatric Psychiatry and Neurology* 7: S47-S53.

Stevenson, N.R. and Lenard, J. (1993). Antiretroviral activities of hypericin and rose Bengal: Photodynamic effects on Friend leukemia virus infection of mice. *Antiviral Research* 21: 119-127.

Stevinson, C., Dixon, M., and Ernst, E. (1998). *Hypericum* for fatigue—a pilot study. *Phytomedicine* 5: 443-447.

Takahashi, I., Nakanishi, S., Kobayashi, E., Nakano, H., Suzuki, K., and Tamaoki, T. (1989). Hypericin and pseudohypericin specifically inhibit protein kinase C: Possible relation to their antiretroviral activity. *Biochemical and Biophysical Research Communications* 165: 1207-1212.

Tekel'ová, D., Repcak, M., Zemkova, E., and Toth, J. (2000). Quantitative changes of dianthrones, hyperforin and flavonoids content in the flower ontogenesis of *Hypericum perforatum*. *Planta Medica* 66: 778-780.

Thiele, B., Brink, I., and Ploch, M. (1993). Modulation of cytokine expression by *Hypericum* extract. *Journal of Geriatric Psychiatry and Neurology* 7(Suppl. 1): 60-62.

Türi, M., Türi, E., Koljalg, S., and Mikelsaar, M. (1997). Influence of aqueous extracts of medicinal plants on surface hydrophobicity of *Escherichia coli* strains of different origin. *Acta Pathologica, Microbiologica et Immunologica Scandinavica* 105: 956-962.

Uehleke, B., Mueller, S.C., Uehleke, B., Woehling, H., Petzsch, M., Riethling, A.K., and Drewelow, B. (2000). Interaction of St. John's wort with digoxin in relation to dosage and formulation. *Phytomedicine* 7(Suppl. 2): 20 (abstract SL-33).

Upton, R. (Ed.) (1997). St. John's wort—*Hypericum perforatum*. American Herbal Pharmacopoeia and Therapeutic Compendium. *HerbalGram* (40) (Summer): 32 pp. insert.

Vandenbogaerde, A., Zanoli, P., Puia, G., Truzzi, C., Kamuhabwa, A., De Witte, P., Merlevede, W., and Baraldi, M. (2000). Evidence that total extract of *Hypericum perforatum* affects exploratory behavior and exerts anxiolytic effects in rats. *Pharmacology, Biochemistry and Behavior* 65: 627-633.

Verotta, L., Appendino, G., Belloro, E., Jakupovic, J., and Bombardelli, E. (1999). Furohyperforin, a prenylated phloroglucinol from St. John's wort *(Hypericum perforatum)*. *Journal of Natural Products* 62: 770-772.

Verotta, L., Appendino, G., Jakupovic, J., and Bombardelli, E. (2000). Hyperforin analogues from St. John's wort *(Hypericum perforatum)*. *Journal of Natural Products* 63: 412-415.

Vitiello, B. (1999). *Hypericum perforatum* extracts as potential antidepressants. *Journal of Pharmacy and Pharmacology* 51: 513-517.

Volz, H.P. (1997). Controlled clinical trials of hypericum extracts in depressed patients—an overview. *Pharmacopsychiatry* 30(Suppl.): 72-76.

Vorbach, E.U., Arnoldt, K.H., and Hubebner, W.D. (1997). Efficacy and tolerability of St. John's wort extract LI 160 versus imipramine in patients with severe depressive episodes according to ICD-10. *Pharmacopsychiatry* 30: 81-85.

Vorbach, E.U., Hübner, W.D., and Arnoldt, K.H. (1994). Effectiveness and tolerance of the *Hypericum* extract LI 160 in comparison with imipramine: Randomized double-blind study with 135 outpatients. *Journal of Geriatric Psychiatry and Neurology* 7(Suppl.): S19-S23.

Wang, Z., Gorski, C., Hamman, M.A., Huang, S.M., Lesko, L.J., and Hall, S.D. (2001). The effects of St. John's wort *(Hypericum perforatum)* on human cytochrome P450 activity. *Clinical Pharmacology and Therapeutics* 70: 317-326.

Weber, N.D., Murray, B.K., North, J.A., and Wood, S.G. (1994). The antiviral agent hypericin has in vitro activity against HSV-1 through non-specific association with viral and cellular membranes. *Antiviral Chemistry and Chemotherapy* 5: 83-90.

Wentworth, J.M., Agostini, M., Love, J., Schwabe, J.W., and Chatterjee, V.K.K. (2000). St John's wort, a herbal antidepressant, activates the steroid X receptor. *Journal of Endocrinology* 166(3): R11-R16.

Wheatley, D. (1997). LI 160, an extract of St. John's wort, versus amitriptyline in mildly to moderately depressed outpatients—A controlled 6-week clinical trial. *Pharmacopsychiatry* 30: 77-80.

Wilhelm, K.P., Biel, S., and Siegers, C.P. (2001). Role of flavonoids in controlling the phototoxicity of *Hypericum perforatum* extracts. *Phytomedicine* 8: 306-309.

Wirz, A., Simmen, U., Heilmann, J., Calis, I., and Sticher, O. (2000). Bisanthraquinone glycosides of *Hypericum perforatum* with binding inhibition to CRH-1 receptors. *Phytochemistry* 55: 941-947.

Woelk, H. (2000). Comparison of St. John's wort and imipramine for treating depression: Randomized controlled trial. *British Medical Journal* 321 (Sept. 2): 536-539.

Woelk, H., Burkhard, G., and Grünwald, J. (1994). Benefits and risks of the *Hypericum* extract LI 160: Drug monitoring study with 3,250 patients. *Journal of Geriatric Psychiatry and Neurology* 7(Suppl.): S34-S38.

Wonnemann, M., Singer, A., and Muller, W.E. (2000). Inhibition of synaptosomal uptake of 3H-L-glutamate and 3H-GABA by hyperforin, a major constituent of St. John's wort: The role of amiloride sensitive sodium conductive pathways. *Neuropsychopharmacology* 23(2): 188-197.

Wonnemann, M., Singer, A., Siebert, B., and Müller, W.E. (2001). Evaluation of synaptosomal uptake inhibition of most relevant constituents of St. John's wort. *Pharmacopsychiatry* 34(Suppl. 1): S148-S151.

Wood, S., Huffman, J., Weber, N., Andersen, D., North, J., Murray, B., Sidwell, R., and Hughes, B. (1990). Antiviral activity of naturally occurring anthraquinones and anthraquinone derivatives. *Planta Medica* 56: 651-652.

Wurglics, M., Westerhoff, K., Kaunzinger, A., Wilke, A., Baumeister, A., Dressman, J., and Schubert-Zsilavecz, M. (2001). Batch-to-batch reproducibility of St. John's wort preparations. *Pharmacopsychiatry* 34(Suppl. 1): S152-S156.

Yip, L., Hudson, J.B., Gruszecka-Kowlik, E., Zalkow, L.H., and Towers, G.H.N. (1996). Antiviral activity of a derivative of the photosensitive compound hypericin. *Phytomedicine* 3: 185-190.

Yu, D.K. (1999). The contribution of P-glycoprotein to pharmacokinetic drug-drug interactions. *Journal of Clinical Pharmacology* 39: 1203-1211.

Yu, P.H. (2000). Effect of *Hypericum perforatum* extract on serotonin turnover in the mouse brain. *Pharmacopsychiatry* 33: 60-65.

Yue, Q.Y., Berquist, C., and Gerden, B. (2000). Letter to the editor. *Lancet* 355 (Feb. 12): 576-577 (letter).

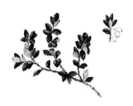

Uva Ursi

BOTANICAL DATA

Classification and Nomenclature

Scientific name: *Arctostaphylos uva-ursi* (L.) Sprengel; (synonym: *Arbutus uva-ursi* L.)

Family name: Ericaceae

Common names: uva ursi, bearberry, common bearberry, bear's grape, hog cranberry, mealberry, rockberry, sandberry, kinnikinnick, barentraube, raison d'ours (Bailey and Bailey, 1976; Brinker et al., 1995; De Smet et al., 1992; Willard, 1991)

Description

Arctostaphylos is a genus of woody plants containing an estimated 100 species and subspecies, of which probably 25-50 distinguishable taxa are known (Denford, 1981). Most are indigenous to the Western region of North America, although two species are native to circumpolar regions of Europe (Mabberley, 1993).

Chemotaxonomic studies indicate that taxa within the genus can be differentiated on the basis of chemical criteria, specifically flavonoids and flavonoid aglycones. These compounds can provide phytogeographic and taxonomic markers for biochemically "advanced" and "primitive" taxa within the genus (Denford, 1973, 1981). Variable distributions of myricetin, quercetin, and kaempferol derivatives (see Chemistry) were reported in 41 species, subspecies, and varieties. The data suggest that the distribution of certain glycosides corresponds to the formation of chemosystematic subdivisions within the genus (Denford, 1981).

Arctostaphylos uva-ursi is a small, prostate, creeping evergreen shrub found in the temperate regions of the Northern hemisphere (Anonymous,

1987; Leung and Foster, 1996) in Canada, Europe, and northern Asia (Bailey and Bailey, 1976). *Arctostaphylos uva-ursi* has the following characteristics: 15 cm in height (Leung, 1980) with small, dark green to brownish-green, fleshy, leathery leaves; obovate to spatulate, 2-3 cm long. The leaves have a coriaceous texture, are nearly glabrous, and the upper surface is shiny with sunken veinlets; the lower surface is lighter with one darker veinlet. The leaf blade gradually narrows to a very short petiole. The stems are creeping, short, woody, and decumbent. The flower is pale pink to white, waxy-looking, and bell-shaped; flowers appear in clusters in early summer and the plant blooms in May and June. The berry ripens in the fall (Leung and Foster, 1996; Grieve, 1931). The currant-size berries are juicy but generally are not used medicinally. They have an insipid taste that fades with cooking (Anonymous, 1987).

Named after its fruit, a small, red, glossy berry called the bearberry, *Arctostaphylos* literally means beargrape in Greek, while *uva-ursi* is the Latin term for the fruit (Brinker et al., 1995; Tyler, 1993). *Arctostaphylos uva-ursi* often spans vast areas of alpine coniferous forests up to 3,000 m in elevation (Thomson, 1983). An ecological study of the vast geographic distribution range of *A. uva-ursi* in Spain reveals that this species can adapt to diversified biogeographical and ecological habitats (Fromard, 1990). Several species of wildlife feed on the beargrape, including grouse, mountain sheep, black-tailed deer, and black bears (Brinker et al., 1995). Cattle, however, avoid the plant. *Arctostaphylos uva-ursi* grows abundantly on dry humus-rich sandy soils, rocks, and bare hills. Large colonies of the shrub as underbrush are common in open woods and on moors and heathlands throughout Europe, the northern United States, Canada, and Asia. The species provides a ground cover that can prevent soil erosion on slopes (Brinker et al., 1995; Leung and Foster, 1996; Johnson, 1884).

HISTORY AND TRADITIONAL USES

Arctostaphylos uva-ursi has a long history of medicinal use in many diverse cultures. Reportedly, in the thirteenth century, this species was part of the pharmacopoeia of the Welsh "Physicians of Myddfai." Clusius mentioned the therapeutic benefits of *A. uva-ursi* in 1601, as did Gerhard of Berlin in 1763. In the late 1600s New England herbalist John Josselyn wrote about the merits of bearberries against scurvy and the "fervor of hot diseases" (Vogel, 1970). Between 1790 and 1810 in the United States, several candidate medical doctors wrote their "inaugural dissertations" on indigenous botanical remedies of North America. Among these was the thesis of John S. Mitchell, MD, on the medicinal uses of *A. uva-ursi,* which he completed in 1803 (Brinker et al., 1995; Vogel, 1970). Dr. Barton, Dr. John Mitchell's mentor at the University of Pennsylvania, noted the plant as beneficial in the treatment of gonorrhea, nephritis, and kidney stones (Vogel, 1970). In the eighteenth century, Goethe received uva ursi following a diagnosis of urolithiasis; today in Germany the herb is recommended most often for prophylaxis of stone formation (Gross and Hummel, 1999).

Long recognized for its astringent and diuretic effects (Grieve, 1931), *Arctostaphylos uva-ursi* is also widely known for its use in the treatment of bladder and kidney diseases. Preparations made from the leaves are believed to have antiseptic properties and to help to strengthen the tone of the urinary passages (Tyler, 1993). Thus, the primary folk-medicinal uses of this species, both past and present, have been as remedies for inflammatory diseases of the urinary tract, including urethritis, chronic cystitis, nephritis, and urinary and renal calculi (kidney stones).

Over 12 American Indian tribes traditionally used *A. uva-ursi* (Willard, 1991), largely as an infusion for treating inflammation of the genitourinary tract and venereal disease (Brinker et al., 1995; Vogel, 1970). There were allegedly other uses as well. The leaves of this species, known by some tribes as sagackhomi, were added to herbal smoking mixtures, such as the ceremonial smoking compound of the Pueblo Indians. The Chippewa smoked sagackhomi as an intoxicant (Duke, 1985). Some Native American tribes used the fruits of *A. uva-ursi* for weight control (Willard, 1991). The Cheyenne applied the wet leaves topically to painful areas and prepared the aerial parts as a decoction ingested for stomach ailments and for bathing rheumatic conditions and sprained back; the latter was also treated by drinking an infusion of the leaves. In Virginia, the Rappahannock Indians treated swelling and sprains with a red clay poultice made from the leaves. In New Mexico, Hispanics employed an oral decoction of the plant primarily as a remedy for bladder infection, urethral inflammations, gout and swollen leg joints, a bath for rheumatism, and a sitz bath for vaginitis. In the northeastern United States, Anglo-American settlers relied on potions made from the leaves to treat many of these same ailments, as well as bronchitis. The astringent properties of the leaves were regarded as beneficial in treating profuse menses, bed-wetting, and diarrhea (Vogel, 1970). Similar uses were made of related species in the United States; *A. patula* in the western states by American Indians, and *A. pungens* in the southwest by Hispanics (Brinker et al., 1995).

In Canada, many of the coastal Indian tribes of British Columbia ate the berries in seal oil or some other grease and today eat them with butter (Turner, 1995). In southern British Columbia, the Thompson Indians used a decoction of the leaves and stems of "kinnickinnick" as an eyewash for sore eyes, and an infusion of the leaves as a diuretic and tonic for the bladder and kidneys, as well as a mouthwash to treat weak gums and canker sores. A decoction of the bark and root was taken internally in the treatment of bloody sputum. The berries were often cooked with salmon or trout and the dried leaves were smoked with wild tobacco (*Nicotiana attenuata* Torr.) (Turner et al., 1990). In northern Saskatchewan, the Dene drink a tea made from the roots to treat persistent cough. In northern Alberta, the Métis drink a decoction of the leaves for the treatment of bladder and kidney troubles and a decoction of the stems is drunk to induce menstruation, prevent miscarriage, and as an aid in recovering from childbirth (Marles et al., 2000).

In addition to its widespread use in folk medicine, *A. uva-ursi* has been an official part of the pharmacopoeias of several Western societies since the eighteenth century. In 1788 it was listed in the *London Pharmacopoeia* (Grieve, 1931), the *British Pharmaceutical Codex* (1934), the *British Herbal Pharmacopoeia* for 1983 and 1991, and in the official pharmacopoeias of Australia, Czechoslovakia, Egypt, France, Germany, Hungary, Japan, Russia, Switzerland, and Yugoslavia (Newall et al., 1996). *Arctostaphylos uva-ursi* (under its synonym *Arbutus uva-ursi*) was an official entry in the U.S. Pharmacopoeia between 1820 and 1936. The entry listed in the *United States National Formulary* (NF) was of a fluid extract made from the whole and powdered leaves (*National Formulary, 1935*). During the nineteenth century, homeopaths prescribed a remedy derived from the plant for painful urination and urination with burning. The homeopathic tincture was prepared from fresh leaves harvested during the fall (Brinker et al., 1995). *Arctostaphylos uva-ursi* is used homeopathically for cystitis, dysuria, hematuria, incontinence, pyelitis, urethritis, and urogenital disorders (Duke, 1985).

CHEMISTRY

The extract of *A. uva-ursi* is described as odorless with a bitter taste and astringent action (Evans, 1989). The leaves contain phenolic heterosides, flavonoid glycosides, and tannins. Secondary compounds are implicated in a wide range of therapeutic activities for this species. Certain compounds are found only in varietal species of *A. uva-ursi,* while others have only been isolated from plant material harvested from specific geographical regions.

Phenolic Compounds

Flavonoids

Flavonoids found in *A. uva-ursi* include ursolic acid (0.4% to 0.75%), quercitrin, quercetin (tetraoxyflavonol), isoquercetin (Willard, 1991), glycosides of quercetin (hyperoside, ca. 1.3%) and myricetin, phytosterols (Brinker et al., 1995; Moretti, 1977; Denford, 1973; Borkowski, 1960), and monotropein (Jahodar et al., 1978). Quercetin-3-galactoside is the most concentrated glycoside in *A. uva-ursi,* but its content varies by subspecies (Brinker et al., 1995). Similarly, the concentration of specific flavonoids is variable according to the geographical origin of the plant material. Veit et al.

(1992) reported that glycosides of both quercetin and myricetin are present in specimens of *A. uva-ursi* collected from North America (Colorado). By contrast, only quercetin glycosides were detected in samples of *A. uva-ursi* from the former USSR. An intermediate pattern of flavonoid distribution was seen in plants from Western Europe. Other flavonoids present in *A. uva-ursi* include the anthocyanidin derivatives delphinidin and cyanidin (Veit et al., 1992).

Tannins

The leaves of *A. uva-ursi* have been used in Sweden and Russia to tan leather (Uphof, 1968). The average concentration of tannins in *A. uva-ursi* is 10% to 20%, although the content can be as high as 40% for gallic acid-type tannins (Anonymous, 1987; Wahner et al., 1974). The primary compounds in this class are gallotannins, galloyl esters of glucose (Haslam et al., 1989; Britton and Haslam, 1965), ellagic acid, and catechin (Frohne, 1986). *Arctostaphylos uva-ursi* leaves contain about 0.25% phenolic acids in free form, primarily as gallic, *p*-coumaric, syringic (Dombrowicz et al., 1991), caffeic, and ellagic acids, and as catechol (Brinker et al., 1995). If the fluid extract is stored, the content of ellagic acid increases and forms a sediment of its crystalline precipitate (Brinker et al., 1995). Other tannins found in the leaves include tetragalloylglucose and trigalloylglucose (Kakiuchi et al., 1985).

The phenolic heterosides most concentrated in the leaves of *A. uva-ursi* are hydroquinone derivatives, particularly the hydroquinone β-D-glucopyranoside arbutin (4-hydroxyphenyl-β-D-glucopyranoside), and a phenolic glucoside (Brinker et al., 1995). Hydroquinone derivatives are calculated as anhydrous arbutin and expressed in terms of the dried plant material. Extensive phytochemical studies have been conducted on the variability of arbutin yields. The dried leaves contain a minimum of 5% to 6% anhydrous arbutin with maximum levels reaching between 17% (Shnyakina et al., 1981; Makarov, 1971), and 18.6% (Brinker et al., 1995). Others report a content in the dry plant of from 6% to 15%, although Kenndler et al. (1990), using capillary zone electrophoresis, detected from 6.4% to 7.6% arbutin in the dry leaves. Brinker et al. (1995) give the content of arbutin as 10.8% to 11.2% in the twigs and 14.4% to 14.6% in leaves, noting that the concentration of arbutin is lowest during flowering and highest when the fruit is ripe, particularly in well-lighted clearings. Arbutin was not detected in samples of the subspecies *A. uva-ursi stipitata* harvested in Canada, Alaska, and Colorado, and the concentration of arbutin found varied widely, depending on seasonality, geographical region, and varietal species (Brinker et al., 1995); however, Linnenbrink and Kraus (1986) found evidence from comparing outdoor planting and in vitro culture of *Arctostaphylos* spp. to suggest that arbutin concentration does not depend on geographical origin.

The leaves typically contain a small amount of methylarbutin (Frohne, 1986), calculated at 0.0% to 1.3% in one study, and 0.7% to 1.25% in another (Brinker et al., 1995). This compound was reportedly absent from the leaves of *A. uva-ursi* samples harvested from North America, Western Europe, and the former USSR (Anonymous, 1987; Wahner et al., 1974). However, no evidence suggests that the presence of methylarbutin can be used to differentiate a "chemotaxonomic race" (or varietal species) of *A. uva-ursi* by geographical origin or concentration of methylarbutin (Linnenbrink and Kraus, 1986). The aglycone of methylarbutin, *p*-methoxyphenol, occurs in trace amounts in fresh leaves and in relatively high amounts in the dried leaves (Jahodar and Leifertova, 1979).

Piceoside, a phenolic glucoside, was identified in a methanol extract of the dried leaves. The acetate, piceoside tetracetate, has been synthesized directly from 4-hydroxy-acetophenone and acetobromoglucose (Frohne, 1986; Karikas et al., 1987).

Terpenoid Compounds

Triterpenes

The dry leaf of *A. uva-ursi* contains 0.4% to 0.8% triterpenes, primarily ursolic acid, uvaol, lupeol, and amyrin derivatives (α-amyrin, β-amyrin, erythrodiol, and deamolic acid) (Leung and Foster, 1996; Proliac, 1980; Moretti, 1977).

Other Constituents

The leaves contain between a trace amount and 0.3% hydroquinone (Brinker et al., 1995). *Arctostaphylos uva-ursi* also contains small concentrations of ericinol (an ill-defined glucoside) (Grieve, 1931), ericolin, corilagin, pyroside (Tyler et al., 1981), a yellow-coloring principle resembling quercetin, allantoin, malic acid, galloyl acid, hyperin, corilagin pyroside, *O*-pyrocatechuic acid, trace volatile oil, resins, and waxes (Brinker et al., 1995; Leung and Foster, 1996; Britton and Haslam, 1965).

THERAPEUTIC APPLICATIONS

The leaves of *A. uva-ursi* are chiefly employed as an antiseptic in urinary tract infections. Remedies made from *A. uva-ursi* are traditionally administered as an infusion (Grieve, 1931), tea, or tincture (Leung and Foster, 1996). The vast majority of its uses in herbal medicine remain to be investigated scientifically: prostate problems, bronchitis, consumption, dysentery, dysmenorrhea, dysuria, hepatitis, menorrhagia, nephritis, pancreatitis, piles, polyuria, rheumatism, ulcers, diabetes, diarrhea, dysentery, profuse menstruation, fever, hemorrhoids, gonorrhea, spleen, and pancreatic conditions (Willard, 1991; Duke, 1985). Grieve (1931) recommended using only the green leaves collected during September and October and dried with gentle heat for therapeutic purposes; dried leaves should be tightly stored in wooden or tin boxes so that moisture from the open air will not be reabsorbed. Aqueous extracts must be boiled extensively to ensure that the principle active constituent, arbutin, can be thoroughly extracted from the tough leaves.

PRECLINICAL STUDIES

Digestive, Hepatic, and Gastrointestinal Functions

Hepatic Functions

Therapeutic and prophylactic activity from *A. uva-ursi* was shown against experimental hepatitis in albino rats by Azhunova et al. (1987, 1988). In male rats the leaf extract administered intraabdominally increased hepatic detoxification, increased the liver microsome content P-450 cytochrome, diminished the rate of detoxification enzyme inactivation, and shortened hexenal anesthesia (Azhunova et al., 1987). A patented preparation containing *A. uva-ursi* administered to white rats with carbon tetrachloride-induced hepato-renal syndrome normalized functional states of the liver and kidneys (Shantanov et al., 1997). In addition, ursolic acid derived from the fruits of *A. uva-ursi* prevented CCl_4-induced liver damage and improved recovery in mice (Brinker et al., 1995).

Endocrine and Hormonal Functions

Diabetes

In streptozotocin-induced diabetic mice, dried *A. uva-ursi* leaves as 6.25% by weight of a standard laboratory diet for nine days failed to improve hyperglycemia and insulinopenia (i.e., alter plasma glucose or insulin concentrations). However, the *A. uva-ursi*-supplemented feed significantly reduced streptozotocin-associated hyperphagia and polydipsia and significantly ($p < 0.05$) slowed the loss of body weight (Swanston-Flatt et al., 1989).

Genitourinary and Renal Functions

Renal Functions

Arbutin and its conjugate may be responsible for the diuretic activity shown in rabbits administered an extract of the leaves (Brinker et al., 1995).

Quercetin and ursolic acid (urson) exhibit a strong diuretic action at 1:100,000 dilution (Willard, 1991); isoquercetin may also be a contributing factor (Tyler, 1993).

In a study on the diuretic effect of *A. uva-ursi,* Beaux et al. (1999) administered a commercial aqueous extract of the leaves to male rats pretreated with hypotonic saline overload and compared the effect to that of hydrochlorozthiazide (HCT). A single dose of the leaf extract (50 mg/kg i.p.) produced significant diuresis which lasted from 2-24 h. and peaked at 8 h ($p < 0.001$). All of the hypotonic saline overload was excreted with 5.75 h versus a comparable 5.33 h after treatment with the reference diuretic, HCT. The excretion of potassium and sodium was not increased compared to controls and urinary pH was unchanged in all samples (pH 8.4-8.8).

Grases et al. (1994) examined seven herbal medicines reputed to be of use in treating kidney stones, including an infusion of *A. uva-ursi* leaves (3 g/L) prepared with ordinary tap water. Administered to groups of female rats on a standard rat diet as infusions in place of tap water, no differences were found after 12 days in diuresis and no effect was found on citraturia or calciuria. Urinary pH was not significantly changed relative to the control group (pH 7.8).

Immune Functions; Inflammation and Disease

Cancer

Cytotoxicity. That crude extracts of *A. uva-ursi* may be efficacious in the treatment of certain cancers is only suggested from activity of the constituents uvaol and ursolic acid in the PS-125 tumor system (Duke, 1985).

Infectious Diseases

Microbial infections. In the 1980s *A. uva-ursi* was found in most over-the-counter herbal urinary disinfectants (Anonymous, 1987). Multiple constituents may contribute to the antimicrobial activity of this botanical. Leaf preparations have shown antimicrobial activity against *Candida albicans, Staphylococcus aureus, Escherichia coli, Salmonella typhi,* and other pathogenic organisms (Jahodar et al., 1985). An extract of the aerial parts showed limited antimicrobial activity against *E. coli* and *Proteus vulgaris*—equal, at most, to 1/100 the activity of streptomycin (Holopainen et al., 1988). Against ten aggregative and ten nonaggregative different strains of *E. coli,* Türi et al. (1997) found that an undiluted decoction of leaves stopped the growth of every strain. From the diluted decoction (1:2), only one strain of *E. coli* showed any growth. In the salt aggregation test (SAT) used to examine the surface hydrophobicity of bacteria as a measurement of their ability to adhere to host-cell receptors, which can lead to bacterial aggregation, the leaf decoction caused a significant ($p < 0.01$) two- to tenfold increase in SAT titers in 15/15 strains of *E. coli*. In ten different aggregative and ten nonaggregative strains of *Acinetobacter haumannii*, the decoction increased salt aggregation titers in every strain and caused an increase in the aggregation of nonaggregative strains. The researchers concluded that the ability of the decoction to enhance both the aggregability and hydrophobicity of Gram-negative bacteria "suggests that in the case of urinary tract infections microbial particles might be more easily excreted" (Türi et al., 1997, p. 961).

Arbutin and its aglycone, hydroquinone, are held to be mainly responsible for the antimicrobial effects of the leaves. Arbutin is hydrolyzed to form hydroquinone, a urinary disinfectant, but arbutin is an effective antimicrobial agent only if the urine is alkaline (Frohne, 1970). Alkalized water (pH 7-8) extracts of the herb completely inhibited the growth of *Staphylococcus aureus* at a concentration of 2.0% to 3.0%. The increase in activity corresponded with an increase in the arbutin content of the extract (Karwowska et al., 1997).

Hydroquinone esters resulting from the hydrolyzation of arbutin by intestinal bacteria, particularly the sulfate esters (Kedzia, et al., 1975), are mildly astringent in alkaline urine and long speculated to be a source of antimicrobial activity (Schulz et al., 2001; Evans, 1989; Wallis, 1967; Wood and Osol, 1943). In whole-plant extracts of *A. uva-ursi*, ursolic acid also contributed to antibacterial activity (Brinker et al., 1995). Hydroquinone is most effective in alkaline urine with a low specific gravity. Maximum antibacterial action occurs about 3-4 h after *A. uva-ursi* has been ingested (Blumenthal et al., 1998). If the leaves are left to age for 6-12 months, arbutin and methylarbutin become decomposed, leading to an increased concentration of hydroquinone. Soaking the leaves in cold water for 12 h produces an effect similar to that of enhancing the yield of hydroquinone (Brinker et al., 1995). In vitro studies show that both arbutin and crude leaf extracts have mild antimicrobial activity. This suggests that arbutin may account for some of the antiseptic activity (Anonymous, 1987; Jahodar et al., 1985). Because pathogenesis caused by infection stimulates the enzymatic activity of β-glucosidase, Jahodar et al. (1985) theorized that arbutin could be hydrolyzed directly to the aglycone in the urinary tract by β-glucosidase activity. The minimum inhibitory concentration of an extract of *A. uva-ursi* leaves ranged from 0.4% to 0.8%, and correlated with β-glucosidase activity.

Parasitic infections. In low doses (50 ppm), an extract of *A. uva-ursi* showed molluscicidal activity against snail vectors *(Biomphalaria glabrata)* of tropical parasites (Willard, 1991).

Inflammatory Response

Several studies have shown anti-inflammatory activity from leaf extracts of *A. uva-ursi,* although more pronounced when the extracts were used in combination with pharmaceutical anti-inflammatory agents. A water extract of the leaves (1% or 2%) showed no inhibition of picryl chloride-induced contact dermatitis (PC-CD), nor carrageenan-induced paw edema; however, it enhanced the inhibitory action of dexamethasone ointment (0.005% or 0.025%) in allergic and inflammatory models (Matsuda et al., 1990).

Kubo et al. (1990) showed that when a single dose of a 50% methanolic extract of the leaves (100 mg/kg p.o. or more) was administered to mice 24 h after the application of PC-CD, the inhibitory effect of *A. uva-ursi* combined with prednisolone was significantly more potent than that of prednisolone administered alone, suggesting that arbutin may be responsible for the anti-inflammatory effect of *A. uva-ursi.* The mechanism of this synergistic effect was not elucidated.

Arbutin at certain doses may increase the inhibitory effect of prednisolone and dexamethasone on type-IV allergic reaction-induced immune inflammation. For example, against picryl chloride-induced contact dermatitis (PC-CD) and sheep blood red cell delayed-type hypersensitivity (SRBC-DTH)-induced inflammation, arbutin administered immediately before and 16 h after inflammation produced no inhibitory effect. However, administered 24 h after inflammation (10 and 50 mg/kg p.o.), it caused a rapid reduction of inflammatory symptoms associated with PC-CD and SRBC-DTH. In either model, the activity was stronger when arbutin was administered in combination with either prednisolone or dexamethasone, suggesting that it potentiates the anti-inflammatory effects of either agent. Administered alone, either agent diminished the weight of the spleen and thymus of mice, whereas these effects were not found with arbutin (Matsuda et al., 1990).

Metabolic and Nutritional Functions

Pharmacokinetics

After arbutin is hydrolyzed by intestinal flora within the gastric fluid to its aglycone, hydroquinone, the aglycone is metabolized to glucuronate and sulfate esters, which are excreted in the urine (Kedzia et al., 1975; Frohne, 1970). Arbutin is hydrolyzed in the kidneys because gallotannins block enzymatic activity that would normally metabolize arbutin in the gut (Brinker et al., 1995).

CLINICAL STUDIES

Genitourinary and Renal Disorders

Cystitis

Larsson et al. (1993) conducted a randomized, double-blind, placebo-controlled study on the prophylactic effect of UVA-E, a proprietary uva-ursi formulation (Medic Herb AB, Göteborg, Sweden), on recurrent cystitis. UVA-E tablets contain a hydroalcoholic extract of the leaves of uva-ursi (standardized to contain methylarbutin and arbutin) plus a hydroalcoholic extract of dandelion root *(Taraxacum officinale),* which serves as a mild diuretic (concentrations not stated). Fifty-seven otherwise healthy women (ages 32-63, para 0-4) were entered in the study, all of whom had experienced at least one episode of cystitis in the six months preceding the trial and at least three episodes over the past year. For one month, patients received either placebo or UVA-E (three tablets t.i.d.) and then underwent routine bacteriological and gynecological examinations after six and 12 months. At the end of the 12-month observation period, the results showed that 23% of those who received placebo had a recurrence of cystitis versus none in the UVA-E group. The difference was calculated to be significant in favor of the UVA-E group ($p < 0.05$), and no side effects were reported in either group. The researchers added that the voiding pattern showed no change.

Metabolic and Nutritional Disorders

Pharmacokinetics

When an aqueous extract of the tea of *A. uva-ursi* was consumed by six healthy volunteers, 53% of arbutin equivalents were eliminated in the urine during the first 3 h. During the following 3-6 h, an additional 14% was excreted. The study was designed to demonstrate that an herbal tea preparation is as effective as coated tablets of *A. uva-ursi* extract in promoting the release of hydroquinone derivatives to alkalinize the urine (Paper et al., 1993).

Neurological, Psychological, and Behavioral Functions

Receptor- and Neurotransmitter-Mediated Functions

Matsuda et al. (1996) reported that a 50% methanol extract of the leaves and arbutin effectively blocked the production of melanin in an in vitro tyrosinase assay. The extract blocked melanin synthesis through the inhibition of two pathways: tyrosinase-mediated production of melanin from dopa, and production of melanin by auto-oxidation of dopachrome. Although these findings suggested that extracts of the leaves may be effective as whitening agents (Matsuda et al., 1996; Matsuda et al., 1992), the arbutin metabolite hydroquinone or quinol has long been categorized as a depigmentor (Budavari et al., 1996) used topically in treating hyperpigmentation (Reynolds et al., 1996).

Respiratory and Pulmonary Functions

Bronchial Functions

Arbutin has shown antitussive activity in cats. At 50 mg/kg i.p. or p.o., arbutin caused a significant suppression of the cough reflex, cough frequency, cough attacks, and the number of efforts to cough. At 10 mg/kg i.p, arbutin was closest to codeine in antitussive effect; compared to the antitussive agent dropropizine, arbutin was more potent (Strapkova et al., 1991).

DOSAGE

In Europe, extracts of *A. uva-ursi* are prescribed as oral drugs in the form of an infusion, cold macerate, or solid formulation. Tyler (1993) recommends a dose of 1 g three to six times/day, assuming that the extract is made from dried leaves which contain at least 6.0% hydroquinone derivatives. In France, Fournier (1947-1948) gives the recommended dosage of the leaf infusion as 70 mg/kg. Robbers and Tyler (1999) advise that owing to the potential toxicity of hydroquinone, and the difficulty maintaining an alkaline urine, *A. uva-ursi* should be taken only for a few days at a time, at most. Paper et al. (1993) advise that the therapeutic regimen of the extract be followed for a maximum of seven days and not extend beyond this time without the advice of a knowledgeable physician. Paper and colleagues suggest that sodium hydrogen carbonate be administered with *A. uva-ursi* to ensure that a pH of 8 is maintained. Schulz et al. (2001) also advise that leaf preparation of *A. uva-ursi* not be taken for longer than seven days without the advice of a physician, and for not more than five one-week periods in a single year.

Commercial preparations consisting of crude and fluid extracts are typically expressed in weight-to-weight ratios and sometimes in arbutin contents (calculated as water-free arbutin and in relation to water-free plant material) (Leung and Foster, 1996; Blumenthal et al., 1998). A mean daily dosage of 10 g cut or powdered herb corresponds to 400-700 mg arbutin in 150 mL (0.75 cup) water consumed as a tea or cold maceration (Tyler, 1993; Robbers and Tyler, 1999).

The efficacy of *A. uva-ursi* depends on an alkaline urine; in the absence of this, the bioactivity of the preparation is compromised. Authorities therefore recommend monitoring the patient to ensure that the urine is alkalinized (at pH 8) (Blumenthal et al., 1998). It has been recommended that alkaline-promoting vegetables and fruits be added to the diet, while acidic fruits and foods be avoided (Paper et al., 1993).

SAFETY PROFILE

Most herbal remedies of *A. uva-ursi* deliver less than 1,000 mg of the crude herb per dose. Healthy individuals consuming up to 20 g showed no adverse pharmacological responses (Tyler et al., 1981).

Contraindications

According to the German Commission E monograph on *A. uva-ursi,* no contraindications for plant drugs derived from *A. uva-ursi* exist except for the use of *A. uva-ursi* in children under age 12 (Blumenthal et al., 1998); however, the *British Herbal Pharmacopoeia* indicates that the herb is contraindicated in kidney disorders (Bradley, 1992).

Drug Interactions

The 50% methanolic extract of the leaves may potentiate the activity of prednisolone (Kubo et al., 1990).

An acidic urine reduces the efficacy *A. uva-ursi.* If preparations of the leaves are taken with other herbal preparations, allopathic drugs, or foods that acidify the urine, the therapeutic effects of *A. uva-ursi* extracts may be abrogated. Acid-rich foods, including many fruits and their juices (e.g., cranberry), vitamin C, and sauerkraut should thus be avoided when taking preparations of this botanical; alkaline foods should be increased. By a simpler method, daily ingestion of sodium bicarbonate (6-8 g) will render the urine alkaline (Tyler, 1993).

Pregnancy and Lactation

One ethnobotanical record notes that in northern Alberta, the Métis drink a decoction of the stems to induce menstruation, prevent miscarriage, and as an aid in recovering from childbirth (Marles et al., 2000), inferring use during both pregnancy and early lactation. *Arctostaphylosuva-ursi* leaf extracts, especially in large doses, have oxytocic properties and can limit circulation to the uterus (Duke, 1985; Brinker et al., 1995; Brinker, 1998). The German Commission E monograph (Blumenthal et al., 1998) advises against use in pregnancy or lactation, noting that the presence of arbutin/hydroquinone in breast milk has not been researched. The amount of hydroquinone in milk is expected to be very small, as with other ingested substances. The *American*

Herbal Products Association's Botanical Safety Handbook (McGuffin et al., 1997) and Brinker (1998) caution against use during pregnancy but not lactation. No known documented cases of adverse reactions during lactation are known. Due to the potential toxicity of hydroquinone and empirical evidence of a greater sensitivity in children, guidance from a knowledgeable lactation expert should be sought before use during lactation. If used, a minimal dose and minimal length of therapy are strongly preferred for most mother/infant pairs. It is prudent to observe the infant for expected dose-related side effects such as vomiting or diarrhea (see Side Effects).

Side Effects

Excessive oral intake of extracts made from the leaves of *A. uva-ursi* can cause the urine to turn green, an effect which is harmless (Willard, 1991; Wood and Osol, 1943). Because the high tannin content of *A. uva-ursi* can produce gastric discomfort, precautionary measures should be taken to minimize the tannin content—for example, by soaking the leaves overnight in cold water (Tyler, 1993; Robbers and Tyler, 1999).

Extracts of *A. uva-ursi* consumed in excess can cause vomiting and diarrhea. If large doses are taken frequently (for more than one week at a time), the gastric mucosa can be irritated (Brinker et al., 1995). Nausea and vomiting sometimes occur in children and sensitive patients (Blumenthal et al., 1998), and children may be especially vulnerable to chronic liver damage from excessive dosing and long-term use (Brinker et al., 1995). Excessive ingestion of arbutin can produce tinnitus (ringing in the ears), delirium, convulsions, collapse, and even death (Leung and Foster, 1996). Arbutin taken orally in doses above 500 to 1,000 mg can result in skin eruptions (Brinker et al., 1995). Hydroquinone, the metabolite of arbutin, is responsible for toxicity resulting from excessive intake of arbutin.

Special Precautions

A medical practitioner should monitor the urine to ensure that it remains alkaline during the entire course of therapy.

It is speculated that if *A. uva-ursi* is used over a long period of time, especially in children, it may cause liver impairment (Brinker, 1998).

Toxicology

Mutagenicity

In the Ames method modified by using *Salmonella typhimurium* TA 98 and TA 100 in the absence or presence of rat liver S-9 mix, an extract of the leaf prepared using boiling water or methanol showed no mutagenic activity (Yamamoto et al., 1982; Morimoto et al., 1982). In the rec-assay with *Bacil-*

lus subtilis, a methanolic extract of the leaf showed no mutagenicity whereas a water extract did (Morimoto et al., 1982).

Toxicity in Animal Models

In large doses, the aglycone hydroquinone is toxic (oral LD_{50} in rats, 320 mg/kg) (Anonymous, 1987; Budavari et al., 1996).

REFERENCES

Anonymous (1987). Uva-ursi. *Lawrence Review of Natural Products,* September, pp. 1-3.

Azhunova, T.A., Sambueva, Z.G., Nikolaev, S.M., and Matkhanov, E.I. (1987). [The effect of an extract of *Arctostaphylos uva-ursi* (L.) Spreng. on the content of cytochrome P-450 and its inactivation rate]. *Rastitel' nye Resursy* 23: 259-261.

Azhunova, T.A., Sambueva, Z.G., Nikolaev, S.M., and Matkhanov, E.I. (1988). [Bile-expelling effect of *Arctostaphylos uva-ursi* (L.) extract]. *Farmatsiya* (Moscow) 37: 41-43.

Bailey, L.H. and Bailey, E.Z. (1976). *Hortus Third* (p. 101). New York: Macmillan General Reference.

Beaux, D., Fleurentin, J., and Mortier, F. (1999). Effect of extracts of *Orthosiphon stamineus* Benth, *Hieracium pilosella* L., *Sambucus nigra* L. and *Arctostaphylos uva-ursi* (L.) Spreng. in rats. *Phytotherapy Research* 13: 222-225.

Blumenthal, M.J., Busse, W.R., Goldberg, A., Gruenwald, J., Hall, T., Riggins, C.W., and Rister, R.S. (Eds.) (1998). *The Complete German Commission E Monographs* (pp. 224-225). Austin, TX: American Botanical Council.

Borkowski, B. (1960). Diuretische wirkung einiger flavondrogen [Diuretic activity of some flavone-containing drugs]. *Planta Medica* 8: 95-104.

Bradley, P. (Ed.) (1992). *British Herbal Compendium,* Vol. I (pp. 211-213). Bournemouth, Dorset, England: British Herbal Medicine Association.

Brinker, F. (1998). *Herb Contraindications and Drug Interactions,* Second Edition (pp. 34-35). Sandy, OR: Eclectic Medical Publications.

Brinker, F.J., Rosson, K.L., and Stoddart, N. (Eds.) (1995). *Eclectic Dispensatory of Botanical Therapeutics,* Vol. 2 (pp. 19-23). Sandy, OR: Eclectic Medical Publications.

British Pharmaceutical Codex (1934) (p. 1091). London, England: Pharmaceutical Press.

Britton, G. and Haslam, E. (1965). Gallotannins. Part XII. Phenolic constituents of *Arctostaphylos uva-ursi* L. Spreng. *Journal of the Chemical Society:* 7312-7319.

Budavari, S., O'Neil, M.J., Smith, A., Heckelman, P.E., and Kinneary, J.F. (Eds.) (1996). *The Merck Index,* Twelfth Edition (p. 825). Whitehouse Station, NJ: Merck Research Laboratories, Merck and Co., Inc.

De Smet, P.A.G.M., Keller, K., and Hänsel, R. (Eds). (1992). *Adverse Effects of Herbal Drugs*, Vol. 2. Berlin: Springer-Verlag.

Denford, K.E. (1973). Flavonoids of *Arctostaphylos uva-ursi*. *Experientia* 29: 939.

Denford, K.E. (1981). Chemical subdivisions within the genus *Arctostaphylos* based on flavonoid profiles. *Experientia* 37: 1287-1288.

Dombrowicz, E., Zadernowski, R., and Swiatek, L. (1991). Phenolic acids in leaves of *Arctostaphylos uva-ursi* L., *Vaccinium vitis idaea* L. and *Vaccinium myrtillus* L. *Pharmazie* 46: 680-681.

Duke, J.A. (1985). *Handbook of Medicinal Herbs* (pp. 55-56). Boca Raton, FL: CRC Press.

Evans, W.C. (1989). *Trease and Evans' Pharmacognosy,* Thirteenth Edition. London: Bailliere Tindall.

Fournier, P. (1947-1948). *Le Livre des Plantes Médicinales et Vénéneuses de France* [The book of medicinal and poisonous plants of France]. Paris, France: Lechevalier.

Frohne, D. (1970). Untersuchungen zur frage der harndesinfizierenden wirkungen von barentraubenblatt-extrakten [Research on the question of urine anti-infectionary effects of bearberry leaf extract]. *Planta Medica* 18: 1-25.

Frohne, D. (1986). *Arctostaphylos uva-ursi* (L.) Spreng.—die barentraube [*Arctostaphylos uva-ursi* (L.) Spreng.—the bearberry]. *Zeitschrift für Phytotherapie* 7: 45-47.

Fromard, F. (1990). *Arctostaphylos uva-ursi* (L.) Sprengel communities in the prePyrenees of Aragon (Spain): Ecology, phytosociology, and dynamics. *Documents Phytosociologiques* 12: 77-102.

Grases, F., Melero, G., Costa-Bauza, A., Prieto, R., and March, J.G. (1994). Urolithiasis and phytotherapy. *International Urology and Nephrology* 26: 507-511.

Grieve, M. (1931). *A Modern Herbal,* Vol. I (pp. 89-90). New York: Dover Publications.

Gross, A.J. and Hummel, G. (1999). Goethe almost died of urosepsis. *World Journal of Urology* 17: 421-424.

Haslam, E., Lilly, T.H., Cai, Y., Martin, R., and Magnolato, D. (1989). Traditional herbal medicines—The role of polyphenols. *Planta Medica* 55: 1-8.

Holopainen, M., Jahodar, L., Seppanen-Laakso, T., Laakso, I., and Kauppinen, V. (1988). Antimicrobial activity of some Finnish Ericaceous plants. *Acta Pharmaceutica Fennica* 97: 197-202.

Jahodar, L., Jilek, P., Patkova, M., and Dvorakova, V. (1985). [Antimicrobial action of arbutin and the extract from the leaves of *Arctostaphylos uva-ursi in vitro*]. *Ceskoslovenska Farmacie* 34: 174-178.

Jahodar, L. and Leifertova, I. (1979). The evaluation of *p*-methoxyphenol in the leaves of *Arctostaphylos uva-ursi*. *Die Pharmazie* 34: 188-189.

Jahodar, L., Leifertova, I., and Lisa, M. (1978). Investigation of iridoid substances in *Arctostaphylos uva-ursi*. *Die Pharmazie* 33: 536-537.

Johnson, L. (1884). *A Manual of the Medical Botany of North America.* New York: William Wood and Co.

Kakiuchi, N., Hattori, M., Namba, T., Nishiawa, M., Yamagishi, Y., and Okuda, T. (1985). Inhibitory effect of tannins on reverse transcriptase from RNA tumor virus. *Journal of Natural Products* 48: 614-621.

Karikas, G., Euerby, M., and Waigh, R. (1987). Isolation of piceoside from *Arctostaphylos uva-ursi*. *Planta Medica* 53: 307-308.

Karwowska, K., Stegman, J., Duszkiewicz-Reihnhard, W., and Dobrzeniecka, A. (1997). Studies on isolation and chemical composition of biologically active compounds of bearberry *(Arctostaphylos uva-ursi)* and bergenia *(Bergenia creassifolia).* Part IV. *Annals of Warsaw Agricultural University* (18): 115-121.

Kedzia, B., Wrocinski, T., Mrugasiewica, K., Gorechi, P., and Grzewinska, H. (1975). [Antibacterial action of urine containing arbutine metabolic products]. *Medycyna Doswiadczalna I Mikrobiologia* 27: 305-314.

Kenndler, E., Schwer, C., Fritsche, B., and Pohm, M. (1990). Determination of Arbutin in uvae-ursi folium (bearberry leaves) by capillary zone electrophoresis. *Journal of Chromatography* 514: 383-388.

Kubo, M., Ito, M., Nakata, H., and Matsuda, H. (1990). Pharmacological studies on leaf of *Arctostaphylos uva-ursi* (L.) Spreng: I. Combined effect of 50 percent methanolic extract from *Arctostaphylos uva-ursi* (L.) Spreng. (bearberry leaf) and prednisolone on immuno-inflammation. *Yakugaku Zasshi* 110: 59-67.

Larsson, B., Jonasson, A., and Fianu, S. (1993). Prophylactic effect of uva-e in women with recurrent cystitis: A preliminary report. *Current Therapeutic Research* 53: 441-443.

Leung, A.Y. (1980). *Encyclopedia of Common Natural Ingredients Used in Food, Drugs, and Cosmetics.* New York: John Wiley and Sons.

Leung, A.Y. and Foster, S. (1996). *Encyclopedia of Common Natural Ingredients Used in Foods, Drugs, and Cosmetics* (pp. 469-472). New York: John Wiley and Sons.

Linnenbrink, N. and Kraus, L. (1986). In vitro cultures of *Arctostaphylos* spp: III. Phytochemical comparison of in vitro cultures and outdoor plants. *Planta Medica* 6: 511.

Mabberley, D.J. (1993). *The Plant-Book: A Portable Dictionary of the Higher Plants.* Cambridge, England: Cambridge University Press.

Makarov, A.A. (1971). Chemical evaluation of *Arctostaphylos uva-ursi* (bearberries). *Uchenye Zapiski Yakutsk Gosudarstvennogo Universiteta* 18: 41-44.

Marles, R.J., Clavelle, C., Monteleone, L., Tays, N., and Burns, D. (2000). *Aboriginal Plant Use in Canada's Northwest Boreal Forest* (pp. 175-176). Vancouver, B.C., Canada: University of British Columbia Press.

Matsuda, H., Higashino, M., Nakai, Y., Iinuma, M., Kubo, M., and Lang, F.A. (1996). Studies of cuticle drugs from natural sources. IV. Inhibitory effects of some *Arctostaphylos* plants on melanin biosynthesis. *Biological and Pharmaceutical Bulletin* 19: 153-156.

Matsuda, H., Nakamura, S., and Shiomoto, H. (1992). Pharmacological studies on leaf of *Arctostaphylos uva-ursi* (L.) Spreng: IV. Effect of 50 percent methanolic extract from *Arctostaphylos uva-ursi* (L.) Spreng. (bearberry leaf) on melanin synthesis. *Yakugaku Zasshi* 112: 276-282.

Matsuda, H., Nakata, H., Tanaka, T., and Kubo, M. (1990). Pharmacological study on *Arctostaphylos uva-ursi* (L.) Spreng. II. Combined effects of arbutin and prednisolone or dexamethasone and immuno-inflammation. *Yakugaku Zasshi* 110: 68-76.

Moretti, V. (1977). [L'Uva ursina. Studio botanico, ricerca qualitativa e quantitativa dei principi attivi]. *Bollettino Societa Italiana Farm. Osp.* 23: 207-224, in *Chemical Abstracts* 88: 60105q.

Morimoto, I., Watanabe, F., Osawa, T., Okitsu, T., and Kada, T. (1982). Mutagenicity screening of crude drugs with *Bacillus subtilis* rec-assay and Salmonella/microsome reversion assay. *Mutation Research* 97: 81-102.

National Formulary, Sixth Edition (1935). Washington, DC: Committee on National Formulary, American Pharmaceutical Association.

Newall, C.A., Anderson, L.A., and Phillipson, J.D. (1996). *Herbal Medicines: A Guide for Health Care Professionals* (pp. 258-259). London: The Pharmaceutical Press.

Nikolayev, S.M., Shantanova, L.N., Mondodoyev, A.G., Rakshaina, M.T., Lonshakova, K.S., and Glyzin, V.I. (1996). [Pharmacological activity of the dry extract from the leaves of *Arctostaphylos uva-ursi* in experimental pyelonephritis]. *Rastitel'nye Ressursy* 32: 118-123.

Paper, D.H., Koehler, J., and Franz, G. (1993). Bioavailability of drug preparations containing a leaf extract of *Arctostaphylos uva-ursi (Uvae Ursi Folium)*. *Planta Medica* 59(Suppl.): A589.

Proliac, A. (1980). [Triterpenes *Arctostaphylos uva-ursi* Spreng]. *Plantes Medicinales et Phytotherapie* 14: 155-158.

Reynolds, J.E.F., Parfitt, K., Parsons, A.V., and Sweetman, S.C. (Eds.) (1996). *Martindale: The Extra Pharmacopoeia,* Twenty-First Edition (pp. 1086-1087). London: The Pharmaceutical Society of Great Britain.

Robbers, J.E. and Tyler, V.E.. (1999). *Tyler's Herbs of Choice: The Therapeutic Use of Phytomedicinals* (pp. 95-96). Binghamton, NY: The Haworth Herbal Press.

Schulz, V., Hänsel, R., and Tyler, V.E. (2001). *Rational Phytotherapy. A Physician's Guide to Herbal Medicine,* Fourth Edition (pp. 266-268). New York: Springer-Verlag.

Shantanov, L.N., Nikolaev, S.M., and Mondodoev, A.G. (1997). [The influence of a nephrophyte preparation on the functional state of liver and kidneys during intoxication by carbon tetrachloride]. *Rastitel'nye Resursy* 33: 76-81.

Shnyakina, G.P., Sedel'nikova, V., and Tsygankova, N.B. (1981). [Arbutin content in the leaves of some plants grown at Dal'nyi Vostok]. *Rastitel'nye Resursy* 17: 568-571.

Strapkova, A., Jahodar, L., and Nosalo'ova, G. (1991). Antitussive effect of arbutin. *Die Pharmazie* 46: 611-612.

Swanston-Flatt, S.K., Day, C., Baily, C.J., and Flatt, P.R.. (1989). Evaluation of traditional plant treatments for diabetes: Studies in streptozotocin diabetic mice. *Acta Diabetologica Latina* 26: 51-55.

Thomson, W.A. (1983). *Medicines from the Earth.* San Francisco, CA: Harper and Row.

Türi, M., Türi, E., Koljalg, S., and Mikelsaar, M. (1997). Influence of aqueous extracts of medicinal plants on surface hydrophobicity of *Escherichia coli* strains of different origin. *Acta Pathologica, Microbiologica et Imujnologica Scandinavica* 105: 956-962.

Turner, N.J. (1995). *Food Plants of Coastal First Peoples* (pp. 76-77). Victoria, B.C., Canada: Royal British Columbia Museum.

Turner, N.J., Thompson, L.C., Thompson, M.T., and York, A.Z. (1990). *Thompson Ethnobotany* (pp. 211-213, 287). Victoria, B.C., Canada: Royal British Columbia Museum.

Tyler, V.E. (1993). *Honest Herbal: A Sensible Guide to the Use of Herbs and Related Remedies,* Third Edition. Philadelphia, PA: George F. Stickley, Co.

Tyler, V.E., Brady, L.R., and Robbers, J.E. (1981). *Pharmacognosy,* Eighth Edition (pp. 77, 499). Philadelphia, PA: Lea and Febiger.

Uphof, J.C. (1968). *Dictionary of Economic Plants,* Second Edition (p. 46). New York: Verlag von J. Cramer.

Veit, M., van Rensen, I., Kirch, J., Geiger, H., and Czygan, F.C. (1992). HPLC analysis of phenolics and flavonoids in *Arctostaphylos uvae-ursi. Planta Medica* 58(Suppl. 1): A687-A688.

Vogel, V.J. (1970). *American Indian Medicine.* Norman, OK: University of Oklahoma Press.

Wahner, C., Schoenert, J., and Friedrich, H. (1974). Tannins of the leaves of the bearberry *(Arctostaphylos uva-ursi). Pharmazie* 29: 616.

Wallis, T.E. (1967). *Textbook of Pharmacognosy* (p. 128). London: J. and H. Churchill.

Willard, T.W. (1991). *The Wild Rose Scientific Herbal.* Calgary, Alberta, Canada: Wild Rose College of National Healing Ltd.

Wood, H.C. and Osol, A. (1943). *The Dispensatory of the United States of America,* Twenty-Third Edition (p. 1204). Montreal, Quebec: J.P. Lippincott.

Yamamoto, H., Mizutani, T., and Nomura, H. (1982). [Studies on the mutagenicity of crude drug extracts. I]. *Yakugaku Zasshi* 102: 596-601 (English abstract).

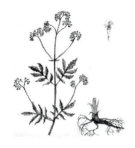

Valerian

BOTANICAL DATA

Classification and Nomenclature

Scientific name: *Valeriana officinalis* L., *Valeriana wallichii* DC.; synonym: *V. jatamansii* Jones

Family name: Valerianaceae

Common names: valerian, garden heliotrope, allheal, English valerian, German valerian, great wild valerian, vandalroot, fragrant valerian, dysentery root, tobacco root (Hobbs, 1994), and in Germany, baldrianwurzel. Whereas valerian is a generic term for the genus *Valeriana,* our use of the term in this review is specific to *Valeriana officinalis* unless otherwise indicated

Description

The name *Valeriana* comes from the medieval Latin valere, "to be healthy" or "courage," referring to its medicinal properties (Dweck, 1997). Valerian is native to Europe, but is naturalized in North America from Quebec west to Minnesota and south through New England to Ohio. Valerian is now widely cultivated for its root in Central and Northeastern Europe, as well as in the United States, Japan, and Australia. *Valeriana officinalis* thrives in damp places, such as streambanks and marshy meadows. Other species of valerian prefer limestone or mountain woods (Hobbs, 1994).

Valeriana officinalis has simple rhizomes, short and sometimes stoloniferous. The stems are 30-150 cm, rarely to 240 cm, usually solitary and robust. The leaves are usually pinnate with 3-25 leaflets, which are linear, lanceolate or elliptical, entire, or toothed. The inflorescence is compound; the flower is asexual and pink or white; the corolla tube is 2.5-5 mm long. The fruit is 2-5 mm long, hairy or glabrous (Morazzoni and Bombardelli, 1995).

Valeriana officinalis shows considerable morphological diversity, and diploid, tetraploid, and octaploid forms exist (Bernáth, 1997). *Valeriana officinalis* var. *latifolia* grows in Japan where the roots and rhizomes are traditionally used as the drug "Kesso" (Houghton, 1988). Today, this plant is known as *V. fauriei* Briq. (Houghton, 1997a). About 200 other species of valerian are found throughout the world, but only a few are known to have been used medicinally. *Valeriana wallichii* DC (syn. *V. jatamansii* Jones) from India and *V. edulis* Meyer from Mexico are currently used as commercial sources of active constituents of valerian (Morazzoni and Bombardelli, 1995).

HISTORY AND TRADITIONAL USES

In traditional herbal folklore, valerian is universally reputed to have sedative properties. It was known to the Greeks and Romans, to whom the plant may have been introduced from Northern Europe. They described it as bitter and aromatic, useful in the treatment of digestive disorders. Dioscorides and Galen in 2 A.D. extolled its virtues as an aromatic and diuretic, recommending it for the treatment of digestive problems, flatulence, nausea, "stagnant liver," and urinary tract disorders. Eleventh-century Saxons called it allheal. Fourteenth-century Arabs prescribed it to counter aggression. The plant is very attractive to cats and small animals, and it has often been said that valerian was used by the Pied Piper to lure rats from Hamelin. Medieval practitioners used it to treat epilepsy, and in the seventeenth to nineteenth centuries valerian was widely used to ease nervous disorders. The homeopathic materia medica lists valerian for treatments of hysteria, oversensitivity, spasms, cramps, rheumatic pains, spasmodic asthma, and insomnia (especially during pregnancy and menopause) (Hobbs, 1994; Duke, 1985). Valerian *(V. officinalis)* was listed in the *U.S. Pharmacopoeia* from 1820 to 1930 (Boyle, 1991). In World Wars I and II, tincture of valerian was used as a treatment for shell shock. Valerian is still listed in the British Pharmacopoeia and in the twelfth edition of the *Merck Index* as a sedative. Early in the twentieth century, pharmacologists proved that valerian exerted a sedative effect, so it was kept in use when many other vegetal drugs were discarded (Morazzoni and Bombardelli, 1995).

Generations have associated valerian with a penetrating smell, which many find extremely unpleasant. Yet in the sixteenth century the odor was considered pleasantly fragrant, and the root was placed in clothes as a deodorant (Leathwood et al., 1982). Later, it held a role in perfume manufacture (Dweck, 1997). The fresh root or freshly extracted drug does not have the characteristic smell which develops later due to an enzymatic hydrolysis giving rise to isovaleric acid (Morazzoni and Bombardelli, 1995). The odor of dried valerian has been described as similar to that of a tomcat (Dweck,

1997), which apparently resulted in the common name in France, "herbe aux chats." The characteristic of the dried root odor is ascribed to valerenic acid, a compound also found in the glandular secretion of some cat family members, which has been associated with their mating behavior; however, cats respond to the odor of the dried root much as they do to catnip *(Nepeta cataria),* and nepetalactone in the volatile oil of *Valeriana* spp. is believed to be the compound responsible, just as in catnip (Hölzl, 1997).

Valerian root has been traditionally used in the form of a tincture of the root (Morazzoni and Bombardelli, 1995). The rhizomes and roots, with and without stolons, are used for medicinal purposes and are best harvested in the autumn or spring. Immediately after harvest, the rhizomes and roots are rapidly washed with water to remove soil and dried at 40°C to prevent degradation of some active constituents (Morazzoni and Bombardelli, 1995).

CHEMISTRY

Chemical investigations of the Valerianaceae family have concentrated on the two major groups of constituents: the sesquiterpenes of the volatile oil and the iridoids. The drug also contains small amounts of flavonoids, triterpenes, and alkaloids, in addition to trivial compounds such as salts, sugars, organic acids, tannins, and resins (Morazzoni and Bombardelli, 1995; Houghton, 1997a).

The chief categories of active constituents have been summarized by Morazzoni and Bombardelli (1995). Readers interested in a complete tabulation of specific substituents represented by R_1, R_2, etc., in the structural diagrams shown below should consult Morazzoni and Bombardelli (1995) and Houghton (1997a).

In the 1900s, the therapeutic actions of valerian were attributed to its volatile oil content. With the isolation of the alkaloids morphine and quinine in 1891, it was supposed that valerian contained an alkaloid which acted on the central nervous system. The key constituent source of its action as a sedative has long been sought and has yet not been identified. The early assumption that the essential oil contributed to the sedative effect was later revised when it was discovered that the essential oil accounts for only one-third of the activity. Several groups of constituents have shown sedative activity, whereas others are spasmolytic and nervous system stimulants. At this point in research, it seems most likely that the therapeutic effects of the plant are the result of a synergistic action of constituents, rather than any one in particular (Valpiani, 1995).

Valerian root and rhizome preparations vary greatly in effectiveness, depending upon the type of preparation, age of the herb, age of the extract, species, variety, chemical race of the plant, growing conditions (Hobbs, 1994), and month of harvest (Bos, Woerdenbag, et al., 1998).

Lipid Compounds

Oils

The content of the volatile oil depends on many conditions, such as the soil and the harvesting period. Data reported in the literature on the content of the volatile oil vary considerably, from 0.1% to 2% or more in cultivated varieties (Morazzoni and Bombardelli, 1995). The main constituents of the essential oil are: valerenal, valerianol, borneol, bornyl acetate, kessane, valeranone, and cryptofauranol (Woerdenbag et al., 1997). The seed oil is rich in linoleic acid and other unsaturated fatty acids (Houghton, 1997a) and contains various sesquiterpenoids: γ-elemene, (+)-tamariscene (Paul et al., 2001), (–)-pacifigorgiol, germacrene D, alloaromadendrene, δ-cadinene α-ylangene, and others (Bos et al., 1986).

The volatile oil fraction contains six classes of compounds, as shown in Figure 1.

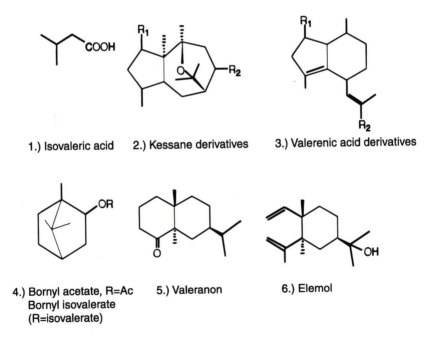

1.) Isovaleric acid   2.) Kessane derivatives   3.) Valerenic acid derivatives

4.) Bornyl acetate, R=Ac
Bornyl isovalerate
(R=isovalerate)

5.) Valeranon

6.) Elemol

FIGURE 1. Volatile Oil Constituents

Nitrogenous Compounds

Alkaloids

The alkaloids of valerian incorporate an iridoid ring structure, and valeranine and actinidine are quaternary alkaloids (see Figure 2).

Amino Acids

Valeriana officinalis contains the amino acids arginine, alanine, aspartate, asparagine, gamma-aminobutyric acid (GABA), glutamine, isoleucine, leucine, phenylalanine, serine, valine (Santos et al., 1994c), and tyrosine (Houghton, 1997a). Greater amounts of amino acids are found in aqueous extracts than in alcoholic extracts of the root (Houghton, 1999).

Phenolic Compounds

Flavonoids

Valeriana officinalis contains the flavonoid aglycones diosmetin, kaempferol, and luteolin; it also contains the phenolic acids caffeic, iso-ferulic, and cholorogenic acid (Houghton, 1997a).

Lignans

Valeriana officinalis root contains a group of four furanofuran lignans that are widely distributed in nature: (+)-1-hydroxypinoresinol, (+)-pin-oresinol-β-D-glucoside, (+)-pinoresinol, and (−)-pinoresinol. The lignan portion of the root extract can be determined by the presence of pinoresinol-β-D-glucoside (Bodesheim and Hölzl, 1997).

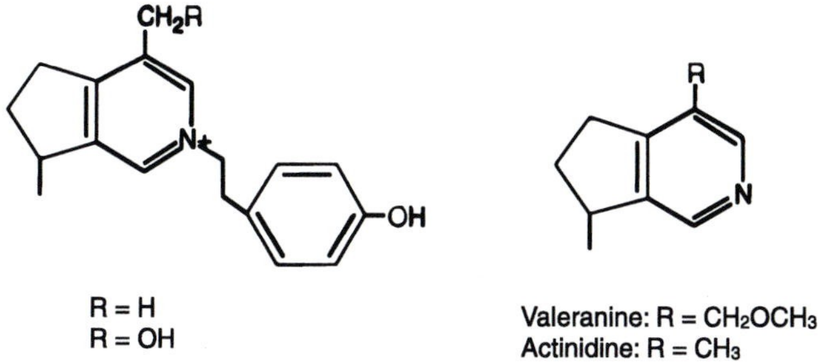

R = H
R = OH

Valeranine: R = CH₂OCH₃
Actinidine: R = CH₃

FIGURE 2. Valerian Alkaloid Structure

Terpenoid Compounds

Monoterpenes

Valepotriates identified in *V. officinalis* include acevaltrate, deacety-lisovaltrate, didrovaltrate, isovaltrate, IVHD-valtrate, kanokosides A, C, and D, valechlorine, valerisodatum, and valtrate (Houghton, 1997a). Greater quantities of the valpotriates are obtained in alcohol versus aqueous extract preparations (Houghton, 1999).

Failure to find a consistent correlation between essential oil components and sedative activity led to the investigation of nonvolatile components. Eventually, a series of iridoid derivatives, the valepotriates, were isolated that had the general structure shown in Figure 3.

Variations in the valepotriate structure include different acidic substituents esterifying the terpenoid moiety, the number of double bonds, presence or absence of the epoxy group, and presence or absence of sugar units. Over 37 different valepotriate derivatives have been identified, and the content in each species varies greatly (up to 14% in fresh roots of *V. thalictroides* and up to 1.2% in *V. officinalis*) (Morazzoni and Bombardelli, 1995). *Valeriana edulis* and *V. wallichii* mainly contain valepotriates (8% to 12% and 2.8% to 3.5%, respectively). The rhizomes and roots of *V. officinalis* contain mainly valepotriates (0.8% to 17%), valerenic acid, and derivatives thereof (0.1% to 0.5%) (Bos et al., 1996), which also show considerable variation in contents. Even in a single collection, the dried roots of 20 plants from a German cultivar of *V. officinalis* yielded 0.92-3.67 mg/g valpotriates and 3.01-12.34 mg/g of valerenic acid derivatives. Micropropagated plants of *V. officinalis* have shown considerably less variation in levels of these constituents than self-pollinated and open-pollinated plants (e.g., 2.21-3.63 mg/g valpotriates and 7.82-12.72 mg/g valerenic acids) (Gao and Björk, 2000).

The highest concentrations of valpotriates are found in the underground parts. The valepotriates are highly unstable and many of the compounds iso-

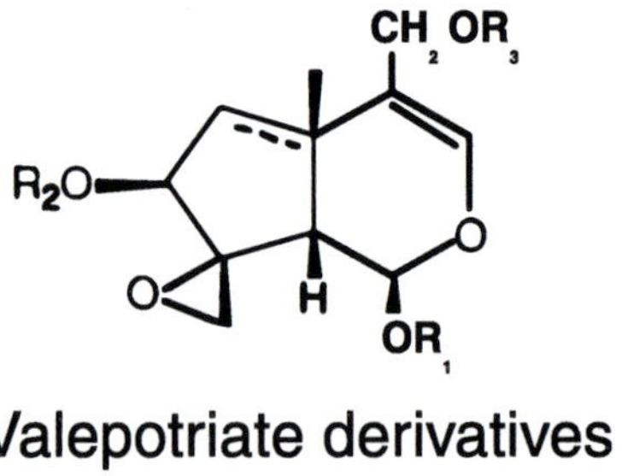

Valepotriate derivatives

FIGURE 3. Valepotriate Derivatives

lated may be artifacts. Some of the degradation products are formed on drying and processing and are major components of the processed roots (Morazzoni and Bombardelli, 1995). Despite an enormous amount of research on the valepotriates, it must be emphasized that it has not been unequivocally shown that they are responsible for the sedative activity of valerian (Bounthanh et al., 1981).

Sesquiterpenes

Valerian contains the sesquiterpenes α-curcumene, β-bisabolene, cryptofaurinol, faurinone, kessyl alcohol, (–)-pacifigorgiol, patchouli alcohol, valeranone, and various valerenic acid derivatives (Houghton, 1988; Bos, Woerdenbag, et al., 1998).

THERAPEUTIC APPLICATIONS

Double-blind experiments using pure valerian water extracts have demonstrated subjective and objective improvement in a variety of sleep parameters: decreased sleep latency (time it takes to fall asleep); improved sleep quality (subjective assessment), especially among elderly; and no effect on normal levels of nocturnal movement (Leathwood et al., 1982). These same studies concluded that valerian compares favorably with prescription sedatives (benzodiazapines and barbiturates) and can lessen or eliminate dependence upon them (Hobbs, 1994).

Preponderant evidence suggests that an alcoholic extract made from fresh roots of *V. officinalis* has a sedative effect. Research suggests that to a major extent this is due to the valepotriates and to the volatile oil constituents, notably the sesquiterpene valerenic acid found in most samples of European *V. officinalis* (Houghton, 1999, 1997a). *The European Pharmacopoeia* (1997) recognizes this constituent and, as one of its standards for valerian, requires the detection of both the valepotriates and the sesquiterpene valerenic acid in herbal extracts (Woerdenbag et al., 1997). While valerenic acids characterize *V. officinalis,* other species of *Valeriana* also contain valepotriates (Bos, Woerdenbag et al., 1998).

PRECLINICAL STUDIES

Immune Functions; Inflammation and Disease

Cancer

Cytotoxicity. Bounthanh et al. (1981) investigated the cytotoxic properties of valepotriate derivatives valtrat, baldrinal, and didrovaltrate in cultured rat hepatoma cells in vitro and in female mice with Krebs II ascitic tumors. The compounds were strongly cytotoxic to cultured hepatoma cells. Valtrate was the most potent: 100% cell mortality after 24-h exposure at a concentration of 33 µg/ml. In the mouse ascites tumors, the compounds were also highly active; a single peritoneal injection (i.p.) of didrovalerate (1.25 mg) led to an extension of the lifetimes of the treated animals versus the untreated of 15 days versus > 50 days, respectively, with apparently complete remission of the tumors in 3/5 treated mice.

Bos, Hendriks, et al. (1998) used the microculture tetrazolium or MTT assay to test three different species and constituents of *Valeriana* rhizomes and roots for in vitro cytotoxic activity against various cells lines of human cancers. In addition, they analyzed tinctures stored at room temperature for two months and freshly prepared tinctures (one part plant material:five parts ethanol, 70% w/v). Against human colorectal cancer cells (COLO 320) and human small-cell lung cancer cells (GLC_4), slightly higher cytostatic activity was found from either acevaltrate or valtrate (diene type valepotriates) than from cisplatin (IC_{50} 3 µM and 1 µM, respectively), a potent anticancer agent. Isovaltrate was only slightly less active. Valerenic acids and derivative compounds, which are peculiar to *V. officinalis,* were considerably less active than the baldrinals of valerian, among which the valpotriate isovaltral showed more potent activity against colorectal (IC_{50} 1.2 µM) and small-cell lung cancer cells (IC_{50} 0.4 µM) than any of the other valerian constituents tested (Bos, Hendriks, et al., 1998).

As for the three freshly prepared tinctures of valerian, the LD_{50} values for *V. officinalis* against GLC_4 and COLO 320 (1123 and 531 µM, respectively) showed this species to be approximately threefold and sevenfold more potent than *V. wallichii* and *V. edulis,* respectively. The stored tinctures showed even greater potency. Storage increased the cytotoxicity of *V. officinalis* 3.6-fold against GLC_4 and 3.7-fold against COLO 320. By comparison, the stored tincture of *V. wallichii* showed a 1.3-fold greater activity against either tumor cell line, and *V. edulis* a respective 4.6- and a 4.2-fold greater activity. *V. officinalis* was clearly the most potent. Bos, Hendriks, et al. (1998) concluded that most of the cytotoxic activity of these tinctures can be attributed to the valepotriates, which act as alkylating substances. A correspondingly greater increase in cytotoxicity against the tumor cells was found the more the valepotriates decomposed in the fresh tinctures during storage and, compared to the other stored tinctures, that of *V. officinalis* showed about 20% the level of valepotriates. Yet the stored tinctures of *V. edulis* and *V. wallichii* showed only low amounts of baldrinals (0.04-0.9 mg/100 mL), which form from the decomposition of the more potent diene valepotriates; *V. officinalis* showed no baldrinals, either in the crude plant material or the fresh or stored tincture.

Infectious Diseases

Fungal infections. Valtrate has shown activity against *Candida albicans* in solid culture. The minimum inhibitory concentration was 10 µg/mL. Growth inhibitory activity was also shown from valtrate against various plant pathogenic fungi (*Cladosporium cucumerium, Trichophyton menta-grophytes,* and *Aspergillus fumigatus*) and in vivo against the barley plant pathogen *Erysiphe graminis,* at which valtrate was comparable to Calixin in activity (Fuzzati et al., 1996).

Neurological, Psychological, and Behavioral Functions

Receptor- and Neurotransmitter-Mediated Functions

Varieties of valerian show significant pharmacological differences. Kessane derivatives with a particularly strong sedative effect (Hikino et al., 1980) are abundant in the Japanese valerian, *V. fauriei* Briq. (= *V. officinalis* var. *latifolia*) (Houghton, 1997a) and have shown antidepressant activity in mice (Oshima et al., 1995). The European variety of the same species is currently thought to be active due to the presence of the sesquiterpenes valerenic acid, valeranone, and valerenal (Houghton, 1988; Hobbs, 1994). Kesso compounds have been reported to occur in *V. officinalis,* although the essential oil was found to be devoid of them (Hazelhoff et al., 1979).

In studies with mice, Capasso et al. (1996) reported a significant reduction in motor coordination and locomotor activity from a valerian water extract (unstandardized, 25 mg/kg i.p.) prepared from the dried aerial parts. The extract also caused a significant reduction in stereotyped behavior and potentiation of pentobarbital-induced sleep. Similar results were obtained using a crude, unstandardized water extract of *V. adscendens* dried aerial parts, a plant originating in the northern Andes of Peru.

The sedative effect of valerian seems to be caused by a combination of depression of CNS center, and direct relaxation of smooth muscle (Houghton, 1988). Since their discovery, valepotriates have been generally acknowledged as the major active components of valerian. Yet valepotriates quickly break down in the presence of heat, moisture, or acid (such as hydrochloric acid in the stomach). Hobbs (1994) stressed that most commercial preparations of valerian contain very few of the originally active valepotriates. The derivatives baldrinal and homobaldrinal show activity, in some cases stronger than the parent valepotriates. Moreover, valepotriates are not water soluble, yet water extracts of valerian still show sedative effects in humans (Hobbs, 1994). This might perhaps be explained by the fact that the presence of water in ethanolic extracts allows valepotriates to decompose into baldrinals (Bos et al., 1996).

Hendriks et al. (1981) investigated the sedative activities of the essential oil and constituents in mice in a so-called syndrome test designed to detect largely central nervous system effects of the kind produced by either a depressant or muscle relaxant. At the lowest dose (50 mg/kg i.p.), valerenal decreased motor activity, abdominal muscle tone, and induced ataxia; valerenic acid induced ataxia. At the 100 mg/kg i.p. level, valerenal produced the same effects and decreased the respirational rate and rotarod performance; valerenic acid produced the same effects as from the lower dose and decreased the respirational rate and motor activity, decreased rotarod performance, and caused an absence of the righting reflex; valeranone decreased motor activity, the respirational rate, and rotarod performance, and caused an absence of pinnal (outer ear) reflex; the essential oil decreased motor activity and the respirational rate, and caused absence of the pinnal reflex. Isoeugenol-isovalerate was relatively inactive. In a further investigation, Hendriks et al. (1985) described the depressant activity of valerenic acid in a traction performance and rotarod test in mice. Valerenic acid only at relatively high doses (100 mg/kg i.p. or more) elicited responses indicative of a relatively nonspecific depressant activity, similar to that of pentobarbital. Valerenic acid (50 and 100 mg/kg i.p.) also prolonged pentobarbital-induced sleep in mice. Other sesquiterpenoid constituents of valerian that they tested (valeranone, valerenolic acid, acetylvalerenolic acid, patchouli-alcohol, and cryptofauronol) caused no impairment of performance in mice in the rotarod and truction test.

Veith et al. (1986) compared the efficacy of didrovaltratum and 4 degradation products (valtroxal, 8,9-didehydro-7-hydroxydolichodial, 11-ethoxyviburtanal, and baldrinal) on the inhibition of spontaneous motor activity following i.p. administration in light-dark synchronized mice. Valtroxal was the most potent with an ED_{50} of 59 μmol/kg. After oral administration, however, only slight activity was observed even after very high doses (120-760 μmol/kg).

Hiller and Zetler (1996) examined the neuropharmacological activity of fresh valerian root ethanolic extracts devoid of valepotriates in male mice. Compared to diazepam, valerian (100, 50, and 12.5 mg/kg i.p. as 1,000 mg equivalent to 4 g dry valerian root) exhibited no effect on body temperature, nociception, rearing, or locomotor activity (spontaneous running). Valerian extract (100 mg/kg i.p.), like diazepam (0.2 mg/kg i.p.), significantly prolonged anesthesia induced by the barbiturate thiopental. The extract antagonized the convulsive effects of picrotoxin derived from the seeds of *Anamirta cocculus,* protecting 7/8 mice at a dose of 50 mg/kg i.p. Diazepam protected all the mice from picrotoxin-induced convulsions at 0.5 mg/kg i.p. Further tests against picrotoxin showed that the ethanolic extract (1 g equivalent to 5 g valerian root) protected 80% of mice at 10 mg/kg i.p., whereas the aqueous fraction of the extract protected at most 60% from twice the dose. Based on its differences to diazepam against picrotoxin, Hiller and Zetler surmised that the ethanolic extract of valerian may exert its action through the chloride channel of the $GABA_A$-benzodiazepine receptor complex.

Others have examined the influence of valerian aqueous and hydroalcoholic extracts and constituents in blocking the breakdown of the inhibitory neurotransmitter γ-amino butyric acid (GABA). The aqueous extract of the root as well as the aqueous fraction of the hydroalcoholic extract showed affinity for $GABA_A$ receptors in vitro (Mennini et al., 1993). Valerenolic acid and acetyl-valerenolic acid inhibited the enzyme gabase (2-oxoglutarate-aminotransferase/semisuccinaldehyde oxidoreductase) by 20% and 38%, respectively, at 1 mmol concentration. Therefore, these components were relatively weak enzyme inhibitors; 1 mmol of L-glutamic acid produced an inhibition rate of 59% and chlorogenic acid of 69% (Riedel et al., 1982).

Using rat brain cortex synaptosomes, Santos et al. (1994a) showed that a standardized aqueous extract of valerian roots and rhizomes (Institute für Pharmacologische Biologie, University of Marburg, Germany, valerenic acid 55 mg/100 g dried extract) at 1 µg/mg could inhibit [^{3}H]-GABA reuptake by approximately 50%. Santos et al. (1994b) showed that the spontaneous release of [^{3}H]-GABA by rat brain (cerebral cortex) synaptosomes induced by the same standardized aqueous extract was shown to be largely Na^+ dependent, Ca^{2+} independent. Neither the uptake nor release of GABA was influenced by valerenic acid, but the amount of GABA found in the extract (5 mM) was sufficient to suggest that the majority of [^{3}H]-GABA released owed to the amino acid.

Because the blood-brain barrier is not easily penetrated by GABA, Santos et al. (1994c) suggested that valerian extract may exert its relaxant effects through peripheral tissues. They further suggested that the concentration of glutamine in the extract (approximately 14 mM) could explain the sedative activity of valerian in vivo since it can cross the blood-brain barrier and in GABAergic neurons becomes metabolized to GABA. However, Cavadas et al. (1995) determined that the effect of the amino acid was small in the [^{3}H]muscinol binding technique in crude synaptosomes from rat brain cortices and could not account for the "sedative" activity of the extract. From their own research, they concluded that the presence of GABA in the same aqueous extract as used by Santos et al. (1994c) was most likely responsible for the in vitro effects on $GABA_A$ receptors, although this activity could not explain the in vivo sedative effect of valerian extracts. While valerenic acid produced no displacement of [^{3}H]muscinol, both a hydroalcoholic and the aqueous extract displaced [^{3}H]muscinol at almost the same IC_{50} (4.7 and 4.6 × 10^{-3} mg/mL, respectively), even though glutamine, glutamate, asparagine, and serine were not present in the hydroalcoholic extract. Finally, in tests with amino acid mixtures at amounts found in the two kinds of extracts (aqueous and hydroalcoholic), Cavadas and co-workers showed that either mixture displaced [3H]muscinol in a manner similar to the total extracts, and the curves produced were similar to those obtained using GABA. (Houghton [1999] notes that higher concentrations of amino acids are found in aqueous extracts of the root, whereas valpotriates are found in greater concentration in alcoholic extracts.)

Nieves and Ortiz (1997) demonstrated that a crude ethanolic extract of the dried roots (commercially grown in Puerto Rico) completely inhibits the uptake of [3H]-GABA in vitro at the same time as potentiating [3H]-flunitrazepam binding. Both effects were dose dependent. A commercially available aqueous extract of valerian was less potent at inhibiting the uptake of [3H]-GABA, while constantly potentiating [3H]-flunitrazepam binding. The researchers concluded that valerian ethanolic extract is a "plausible GABAergic agent." Ortiz et al. (1999) subsequently confirmed that a crude ethanolic extract of valerian (1:40) exerts dose-dependent effects on $GABA_A$ receptors in vitro in mouse synaptosomes, significantly so at 0.3 mg/mL and higher concentrations. They also found that whereas low concentrations (EC_{50} 4.13×10^{-10} mg/mL) enhanced [3H]-flunitrazepam binding in rat cortical membranes, higher concentrations (IC_{50} 4.82×10^{-1}) inhibited binding. Despite its known occurrence in valerian root, the extract was devoid of endogenous GABA, which, in any case, does not cross the blood-brain barrier (Ortiz et al, 1999 citing Rosenstein, 1996). Likewise, they showed that the ethanol present in the extract had no effect on GABA uptake.

Bodesheim and Hölzl (1997), using radio-receptor assays, determined that among the four furanofuran lignins isolated from the root, in vitro affinity for the $GABA_A$ receptor and the benzodiazepine receptor were absent; nor was GABA-antagonist activity found. In tests for affinity to a serotonin receptor (5-hydroxytryptamine$_{1A}$ receptor), only weak affinities were found with the mixture of lignans. However, 1-hydroxypinoresinol showed an especially significant and concentration-dependent affinity to the 5-HT_{1A} receptor, showing an IC_{50} of 2.3 μM/L (= 0.88 μg/mL) (the mixture half-maximally at 25 μM/L). In contrast, the IC_{50} of serotonin is 6 nM/L. The lignan mixture also showed a concentration-dependent affinity to the μ-opioid receptor (half-maximally at 25 μM/L). The researchers noted that further experiments would be necessary to determine the bioavailability and metabolism of 1-hydroxypinoresinol and the lignans before the significance of these receptor affinities to the sedative activity of valerian root extracts can be known.

Balduini and Cattabeni (1989) reported that water-ethanolic extracts of valerian inhibited binding of the adenosine ligand [3H]-CHA (cyclohexyladenosine) to rat cortical membranes in a dose-dependent manner. The aqueous extracts, however, did not inhibit [3H]-CHA binding, nor did either type of extract inhibit binding of the benzodiazepine ligand [3H]-flunitrazepam, indicating a lack of interaction with benzodiazepam receptors.

These results are in conflict with those reported by Hölzl and Godau (1989), who found that a dichloromethane extract and a cyclohexane extract both significantly displaced the binding of [³H]-flunitrazepam in guinea pig cortical membranes. Two fractions separated from the total extract, one containing sesquiterpene alcohols and ketones and the other valepotriates, also significantly displaced binding of the radioligand and were approximately seven times more potent than the crude extracts.

CLINICAL STUDIES

Neurological, Psychological, and Behavioral Disorders

Psychological and Behavioral Disorders

Sleep disturbances. Stevinson and Ernst (2000) provided a systematic review of randomized, placebo-controlled double-blind trials of valerian on sleep, finding nine trials that met their inclusion criteria; however, of these only three were given maximum scores (see Leathwood and Chauffard, 1985; Leathwood et al., 1982; Vorbach et al., 1996). Owing to considerable differences in the quality of methodologies employed in the trials, contradictory results, and inconsistencies in patient selections and trial designs, Stevinson and Ernst concluded that the evidence for valerian as an effective treatment for insomnia has yet to be established. The first three of the following more recent trials (Donath et al., 2000; Quispe Bravo et al., 1997; Donath and Roots, 1996) were not included in their review. Double-blind, placebo-controlled randomized trials of valerian with less than 20 patients in each group are not included in our review unless a crossover design was employed.

Donath et al. (2000) conducted a randomized, double-blind, placebo-controlled crossover study of a valerian extract to assess both single-dose (short-term) and multiple-dose (long-term) effects on objective and subjective parameters of sleep. The trial was conducted in 16 patients between the ages of 22 and 55 (12 female and four male) with previously diagnosed psychophysiological insomnia according to ICSD code 1.A.1. In the first treatment period, they were instructed to take two 300-mg tablets 1 h before retiring to bed, which were either placebo or valerian extract (Sedonium tablets containing 300 mg of a dry extract of the roots; drug/extract ration 5:1). In the second treatment period, patients received the alternative tablets. After baseline polysomnographic (PSG) measurements during day one on placebo and short-term PSG on day two, subjects self-administered either the placebo or verum tablets from day two to day 15. On day 14 they underwent baseline PSG again, and once more on day 15 PSG to measure the long-term treatment effect. In addition, patients recorded their subjective perceptions of changes in sleep quality according to visual analogue scales before and after each PSG (evenings and mornings). However, the main target variable of the study was "objective sleep efficiency." The results showed that, compared to baseline placebo measurements for the two treatment periods, objective parameters showed no significant difference whereas the subjective parameter of sleep latency was significantly longer in the second treatment period ($p < 0.05$). From the single-dose treatment, the valerian extract failed to produce a significant difference on either subjective or objective parameters, and sleep efficiency increased throughout the trial, regardless of whether patients received placebo or valerian. In sleep microstructure, the arousal index also showed no significant difference in changes from valerian compared to placebo. However, slow-wave sleep (SWS) showed a significant decrease in latency ($p < 0.05$) in the valerian group compared to the placebo group after the long-term treatment and unlike placebo, the median SWS percentage was significantly higher compared to baseline. During treatment with valerian, most of the patients (10/16) showed a lower subjective sleep latency compared to treatment under placebo ($p < 0.001$ versus $p < 0.05$, respectively). Yet other subjective parameters showed no change in this study, including those of sleep quality, sleep time, daytime performance, and morning feeling. Twenty-one adverse events occurred which lasted one to three days—only three of them occurred during the valerian treatment and in only three patients (an accident during PSG, migraine attack in patient with previous migraine, and gastrointestinal complaints).

Quispe Bravo et al. (1997) summarized the results of their randomized, double-blind, placebo-controlled crossover study of a valerian extract (Sedonium, 600 mg/night for 14 nights) in the treatment of 16 insomniacs (mean age 44.9 ± 9.2). Polysomnographic tests were used to measure SWS latencies, REM latencies, sleep onset, total sleep time, and sleep stage distribution. Sleep length and latency were evaluated visually. The researchers reported that in objective measurements, valerian decreased SWS-latency (21.3 min versus 13.5 min) compared to placebo, and increased the duration of SWS compared to baseline. In the subjective results, the time to sleep onset was lessened under valerian compared to placebo (45 min versus 60 min, respectively).

Donath and Roots (1996) described the effects of a valerian extract (Sedonium) on EEG in single- (1,200 mg) and multiple-dose (600 mg/night for 14 nights) treatments of 16 healthy males in a double-blind, placebo-controlled, randomized crossover study. The single dose compared to placebo caused the power density of the theta band (temporo frontal leads) to significantly increase, which they associated with a decrease in the delta-band power density. Contrasting these results, their placebo group showed a significant increase in the power density of alpha1- and beta2-bands, which persisted throughout the time of measurement. From their multiple-dose results, the researchers reported that 3 h after the last dose of valerian extract on day 14, the alpha2-band power density significantly decreased and correlated with an increase in theta power (left frontal region). Donath and Roots concluded that the effects of the valerian extract on the power density of the resting EEG were time related and significant, whether from a single dose or from repeated doses, and that the changes in EEG approximated those produced by psychosedative anxiolytic compounds.

Kamm-Kohl et al. (1984) investigated the efficacy of valerian extract versus placebo in a randomized double-blind study of 80 hospitalized elderly patients with sleep disturbances of nervous origin and/or rapid fatigue. Patients received either placebo or a standardized valerian aqueous extract preparation over 14 days (Valdispert, three to nine tablets/day, each containing 45 mg of valerian aqueous extract). At the beginning of and following the treatment, patients were evaluated using Von Zarassen's Subjective Wellbeing Scale and the objective rating scale NOSIE (Nurse's Objective Rating Scale for Inpatient Evaluation). Statistically significant improvements in both the subjective well-being scale (mood) and behavioral disturbances (NOSIE scale, $p < 0.01$) were observed in the treated group in comparison to initial scores, but not in the placebo group. Patients treated with the extract reported improvements in their ability to fall asleep rapidly and to sleep through the night, as well as in their feelings of rapid fatigue, which the researchers assumed were related to the sleep disturbances.

In a multicenter, open-study in 11,168 patients treated by 982 general practitioners, the efficacy of a commercial valerian preparation (Baldrian-Dispert) in treating problems of falling asleep, problems sleeping through the night, and inner restlessness was evaluated. Subjects received tablets containing 45 mg of standardized extract and were evaluated over the course of ten days. Therapeutic outcomes were evaluated as good or very good in 72.1% of the falling-asleep disturbances, 75.5% of the sleeping-through disturbances, and 72.1% of the cases of inner restlessness. An additional 18% experienced some degree of improvement, while symptoms were unchanged in 6%. A remarkable feature of the results was the seeming rapidity of the response: most patients reported subjective improvements less than two days into the treatment (Schmidt-Voigt, 1986).

Combination products. In European phytotherapy, valerian is frequently used in combination with other calmative medicinal plants. A total of 16 different two-herb products containing hops (*Humulus lupulus* L.) and valerian were available in the German marketplace in 1998 (Schulz et al., 2001). The following samples of clinical trials on these combination products suggest equivalent or superior results may be obtained compared to valerian alone.

According to questionnaires, blood chemistry, hematology, and vital signs, Cerny and Schmid (1999) reported that a valerian/lemon balm (*Melissa officinalis* L.) preparation (Songha Night, Pharmaton, Bioggio/ Lugano, Switzerland, 120 mg valerian extract/80 mg lemon balm extract in coated tablet form) was well tolerated among 98 healthy volunteers of both sexes (ages 20-70) who participated in a double-blind, randomized, placebo-controlled, parallel group multicenter-design trial, taking a single 600-mg dose 30 min before bedtime daily for 30 days.

Schmitz and Jäckel (1998) compared the effects of a hops-valerian preparation (Hova, 245.7 mg/night; 45.5 mg hops extract 5.5:1, plus 200.2 mg valerian radix extract, 5:1) to those of benzodiazepine (Lexotanil, Roche, 3 mg bromazepam/tablet per night) in 46 middle-aged men (*n* = 9) and women (*n* = 37) diagnosed with nonpsychiatric and nonchronic sleep disorders according to the DSM-IV. The randomized, double-blind, controlled, parallel group design trial found that after two weeks of treatment, the health of the patients improved during treatment with either substance; however, the benefits seen diminished during cessation of therapy. The benzodiazepine group developed withdrawal symptoms while the hops-valerian group showed none. As for adverse drug reactions, individuals in both treatment groups reported only stomach complaints. The researchers concluded that the combination of hops and valerian represented "a sensible alternative to benzodiazepine" for treating patients with the types of sleep disorders they diagnosed (Schmitz and Jäckel, 1998, p. 292).

Bourin et al. (1997) tested a multicomponent preparation (Euphytose) containing a powder extract of valerian as the main constituent on adjustment disorder with anxious mood. The preparation, used in France as an anxiolytic since 1927, consists of powder extracts of the following herbs: 50 mg valerian *(V. officinalis)*, 40 mg passionflower (*Passiflora incarnata* L.), 15 mg kola nut (*Cola nitida* Schott. and Endl.), 15 mg guarana (*Paullinia cupana* Kunth.), 10 mg hawthorn (*Crataegus oxycantha* L.), and 10 mg black horehound (*Ballota foetida* Lam.; syn. *B. nigra* L.). The dosage of placebo or formula was two tablets t.i.d. for 28 days. The multicenter, double-blind, placebo-controlled general practice study included 182 outpatients randomized into two parallel groups who after a seven-day placebo treatment prior to active treatment continued to show a score of over 20 on the 14-item Hamilton anxiety scale (HAM-A). The Montgomery-Asberg depression rating scale was applied to exclude depressed patients. The results showed a significant decrease in the HAM-A scale on day 7 and on day 28 in scores of psychic anxiety (*p* = 0.025) and somatic anxiety (*p* = 0.011) compared to baseline, whereas no significant changes were found in the placebo group scores. Those scoring less than ten on the HAM-A scale at the end of the treatment period ("cured") numbered 23 (25.3%) in the placebo group versus 39 (42.9%) in the formula group. The physician scores using the Covi scale showed a significant difference on day 28 in favor of the formula versus the placebo ($p = 0.011$), as did the patient evaluation scores (Sheehan scale) compared to baseline and to placebo: 83% of the formula group reported an improved social life versus 65% of those in the placebo group. Adverse events occurred in four patients in the formula group and eight in the placebo group, none of which resulted in patient withdrawals from the trial. In the formula group, these consisted of one event each of dry mouth, headache, constipation, and drowsiness.

In a double-blind placebo-controlled study in 20 healthy volunteers, Dressling et al. (1992) studied the effects of a standardized preparation containing valerian and lemon balm on poor sleepers (Euvegal, Spitzner Arzneimittelfabrik GmbH, Ettlingen, Germany, 160 mg valerian extract/ 80 mg aqueous/ethanolic dry extract of lemon balm in coated tablet form). The results were compared with placebo and with the benzodiazepine triazolam (0.125 mg). During a prescreening procedure in which placebo was administered, subject groups were further subdivided into good and poor sleepers. Both triazolam and the valerian/lemon balm extract resulted in reduced sleep latency and a significant increase in sleep efficiency in sleep stages three and four (measured as a reduction in the percentage of time spent awake during the sleep period). They also produced an increase in sleep stages three and four in the group of poor sleepers. No rebound effects, daytime sedation, or impairments of concentration or performance were observed from either medication. Dressling and colleagues concluded that the valerian/lemon balm preparation was comparable to triazolam and that its use could be considered an effective alternative to conventional sleep pharmacotherapies.

In a multicenter drug monitoring study, Maisenbacher and Podzuweit (1992) examined the records of 2,395 patients taking a valerian and lemon balm product (Euvegal, Spitzner Arzneimittelfabrik GmbH, Ettlingen, Germany, 160 mg valerian extract and 80 mg lemon balm extract, two tablets in the morning and the evening preferentially by 58% of the patients) for acute or subacute psychophysical illness. They reported that over 66% were in complete remission, about 50% completely free from symptoms, and nearly all showed some improvement in individual somatic and psychological symptoms.

Lindahl and Lindwall (1989) evaluated the activity of a largely valepotriate-free valerian extract containing mainly sesquiterpenes, in a double-blind, placebo-controlled crossover study in 27 patients with sleep difficulties. The product under investigation (not stated) contained a full dose (400 mg) of a standardized extract containing only traces of valepotriates and a full complement of sesquiterpenes, in combination with 375 mg hops flowers (*Humulus lupulus* L.) and 160 mg lemon balm extract (*Melissa officinalis* L.). The placebo contained a full complement of lemon balm and hops but only

4 mg valerian extract so that any differences observed would be most likely to result from the valerian extract. Subjects were randomized to receive either the test preparation for two nights or the placebo for two nights; or placebo the first night and the herbal extract product on the subsequent night. Subjects were asked to evaluate their sleep quality for each of the nights on the second morning after the tests. Twenty-one of twenty-seven subjects rated the sleep preparation as better than the control, two rated them as equally effective, and four preferred the control. The differences were statistically significant ($p < 0.0001$), but no differences were found between those who took the test substance first and those who took the control first. Twenty-four of twenty-seven subjects reported improved sleep quality from the test preparation, while half as many (44%) reported "perfect sleep" after the test preparation. No side effects were observed and none of the subjects reported nightmares, which had occurred previously in some subjects after taking customary sedatives (Lindahl and Lindwall, 1989).

Kohnen and Oswald (1988) compared a valerian extract (100 mg) to propanolol (20 mg) and a combination of the valerian extract and propanolol (100 mg and 20 mg) in a double-blind placebo-controlled trial. Test substances were encapsulated, similar in taste, and equal in color and form. The low dosage of valerian was chosen based on a critical review of the literature from which the researchers postulated that in high doses valerian exhibits anti-convulsive-spasmolytic effects, while in low dosages it exhibits thymoleptic-sedative effects. Forty-eight healthy adults (ages 19-29) were subjected to stress-inducing settings (an arithmetical concentration test 150 min after dosing and a social call-up situation 90 min after dosing). No difference between placebo and the other treatments was found in the physiological activation induced by the mental arithmetic test in the call-up situation. The valerian extract was inactive at influencing physiological activation but significantly influenced subjective feelings of somatic arousal and without producing any sedative effects. The combination of propanolol and valerian and valerian alone reduced psychic strain both before and after the concentration and the call-up test situation; either treatment ameliorated the intensive "feelings of somatic arousal" while the stressful situations were occurring. Although valerian caused a slight improvement in the performance of the concentration test, under the combination or valerian alone a trend occurred toward impaired performance and the combination produced the lowest performance results. Although no drug interaction was found between propanolol and valerian, their combination favorably influenced both subjective and psychophysiological effects of stress, and psychic strain was reduced in both the concentration and social call-up test. The researchers concluded that the drugs acted independently and that their results support the hypothesized thymoleptic activity of valerian.

Leathwood et al. (1982) tested extracts of valerian on subjectively rated sleep parameters in 128 patients on a single-night basis. On three nights, each subject received nine encapsulated samples to test in a dosage of 400 mg: three containing placebo (brown sugar), three containing a nonproprietary aqueous extract of valerian root as freeze-dried powder, and three containing a proprietary OTC valerian preparation: an aqueous extract of valerian consisting of 60 mg valerian extract and 30 mg of hops flower extract (Hova). The coded samples were dispensed in random order and taken on nonconsecutive nights. Leathwood and colleagues reported that the nonproprietary valerian extract significantly decreased sleep latency scores and improved sleep quality compared to placebo, particularly in those who considered themselves poor sleepers or smokers and those who thought they had abnormally long sleep latencies. Night awakenings, dream recall, and somnolence the next morning were relatively unaffected by valerian. The proprietary preparation showed a significant effect only in the subjective reports of feeling more sleepy the next morning.

DOSAGE

In 1995, the German Commission E recommended a dosage for valerian root in the treatment of sleep disorders of 1-3 g/day (Kommission E, 1995, cited by Donath et al., 2000), which is lower than the 2-3 g/day recommended by the commission in 1990 (Blumenthal et al., 1998). It is interesting to note that in 1985 the Commission E gave uses for valerian in nervous excitation and spasmodic gastrointestinal pains resulting from nervous conditions in addition to its use for difficulty in falling asleep (Bradley, 1992).

Most clinical studies have used standardized extracts with the usual dose of approximately 400 mg taken 40-60 min before retiring. However, as the active constituents of valerian remain to be conclusively known, no accepted chemical marker exists by which to judge the quality of a standardized extract, and the presence and proportions of putative active ingredients may vary. Most commercial root extracts are standardized to 0.8% valerenic acid. The situation is somewhat more straightforward with tinctures. To be an effective sedative, valerian has to be prescribed in sufficient dosage. One authority gives this as a tincture, 1/2-1 tsp with up to 2 tsp at once if necessary (Hoffman, 1990).

The tincture of valerian root (1:5) is taken in a dosage of 1-3 mL as many as three times/day by adults. For children, the dosage is in accordance with their body weight and age or, for children ages three and older, 1/2 tsp of tincture in fruit juice or milk before bedtime (Schilcher, 1997). In European phytomedicine, valerian has also been taken in the form of a bath additive (Ammer and Melnizky, 1999; Weiss, 1996) using 100 g of root or an equivalent amount of an extract preparation to a full bath (Blumenthal et al., 1998).

SAFETY PROFILE

To assess the effects of a valerian root dry extract (600 mg/day, Lichtwer Pharma AG, LI 156) on impairments of concentration, reaction times, and alertness, Kuhlmann et al. (1999) conducted a randomized, placebo-controlled, group-comparison double-blind trial in healthy, nonsmoker volunteers made up of men and women ages 30 to 60 years. The reference control drug was flunitrazepam (FNZ, 1 mg/day) and all treatments were taken in the evening. As a secondary goal, they examined changes in sleep quality due to the use of valerian extract. Psychometric testing proceeded the morning after day 1 of the treatment period (section A) and, after a seven-day washout phase, the morning after the last dose of a 14-day treatment period (section B). These tests consisted of a validated standard, computer-aided instrument (Vienna Determination Test, VDT) used for testing aptitude and performance in sports, traffic, and pharmacopsychology. Changes in sleep quality were measured using questionnaires applied in the morning and before bedtime. In section A, the primary criterion of median reaction time showed a comparable decrease between the placebo ($n = 34$) and valerian ($n = 33$) groups and was significantly lower in the FNZ group ($n = 32$) compared to either of the other groups. Alertness levels were much the same in all three groups; however, the valerian group showed a significantly better performance speed compared to either of the other groups ($p < 0.01$). Hangover effect was noted in 59.4% of the FNZ group, 32.4% of the placebo group, and 30.3% of the valerian group. On day 1, adverse events were mild in all the groups, and only 1/11 events in the valerian group (dizziness) was judged as "probable" versus four in the FNZ group (dizziness, tiredness, "lack of concentration," and hypokinesis). The placebo group experienced 12 events. Global tolerance was rated as generally positive by both the subjects and the investigators in all the groups, although it was lower in the FNZ group compared to either of the other groups. After the 14-day treatment period (section B), the valerian group ($n = 47$) showed no significant difference compared to the placebo group ($n = 44$) in median reaction time. The researchers concluded that the valerian extract had no negative effect on alertness, concentration, or reaction time. Sleep quality in the valerian group was not significantly different compared to placebo, although a trend occurred toward improved quality versus placebo (+ 7.4% versus – 4.5%, respectively). In 80 subjects (39 placebo and 41 valerian), adverse events of a slight to moderate level were reported one or more times. Weakness and headache were reported with greatest frequency; however, in no case were the events probably caused by valerian. Finally, investigators evaluated the global tolerance of the valerian extract as moderate in 4.3%, good in 6.4%, and very good in 89.4% of the patients. Only minor differences in these evaluations were given by the patients.

Overdosage is unlikely, even with several doses of tincture (Hoffman, 1990). Overdose could be more of a problem in products manufactured from isolates rather than the whole root and rhizome (Valpiani, 1995). Very large doses may cause central paralysis and lessening of the heart rate and intestinal motility. A recommended first aid for this is gastric lavage, charcoal powder, and sodium sulfate. In case of accidental overdose (e.g., in the case of a child), an emetic can be given, as valerian is not corrosive (Hobbs, 1989). Symptoms of toxicity may include fatigue, tremor, and abdominal cramps. However, "only mild" symptoms were reported in the case of a nearly 25-g dose (Wells, 1995). In a systematic review of nine randomized, double-blind, placebo-controlled clinical trials of valerian in the treatment of sleep disturbances, Stevinson and Ernst (2000) found adverse events were scarce. Those reported were mild and considerably different compared to side effects in the placebo groups (Stevinson and Ernst, 2000). They mention the results of a postmarketing surveillance study in Europe of a valerian extract product that also contains hops arrived at much the same observation after monitoring 3,447 patients (Stevinson and Ernst, 2000 citing Lataster and Brattström, 1996). Whether the addition of hops altered the toxicity of valerian is unknown.

The long-term toxicity of valerian remains unknown.

Over the past 20 years, the use of purified and standardized extracts of valepotriates in western Europe has largely replaced the traditional tincture. The cytotoxicity of these compounds has given cause for concern and their absence from pharmaceuticals derived from crude valerian might be a future requirement. A survey for possible side effects in patients taking valerian over a period of time would be a useful indicator of the actual seriousness of the threat posed by the findings of cytotoxicity (Houghton, 1988).

Contraindications

None known (Bradley, 1992; Blumenthal et al., 1998).

Drug Interactions

Valerian may potentiate other CNS-depressant medications such as barbiturates and benzodiazepines (Brinker, 1998). Unlike other sedative drugs, valpotriates apparently do not act synergistically with alcohol (von Mayer and Springer, 1974).

Garges et al. (1998) reported the case of a 58-year-old man with a record of previous hypertension, cardiac failure, and congestive artery disease who, during an otherwise uneventful biopsy (lung nodule), required an increasing amount of oxygen after developing olguria and sinus tachycardia. After treatment with naloxone, he showed hypoxia, carbon dioxide retention, and tremulousness. Tests indicated he was experiencing delirium and high-output cardiac failure. His family revealed that in addition to his usual medications (vitamins, aspirin, benazepril, digoxin, furosemide, ibuprofen, isosorbide dinitrate, potassium, and a zinc supplement), which the attending physicians knew he was taking upon admission, he had for many years taken a valerian root extract (undefined; 530-2,000 mg times five/day) as a means to sleep and relax. Valerian was stopped, and three days later he was stable only after treatment with midazolam (11 mg over 17 h) followed by lorazepam (5 mg over 24 h), and clonazepam (0.5 mg b.i.d.). The patient remained stable at visits eight and 20 weeks after discharge. The researchers commented that, having ruled out other causes, the high-output cardiac failure may have been the result of abrupt withdrawal from valerian (24 h) after taking such a high dosage for many years; hypothetically, a "benzodiazepine-like withdrawal syndrome" since benzodiazepine administration reversed his symptoms. However, because the patient was taking a multitude of medications and underwent surgery, they could not make a causal link to valerian (Garges et al., 1998).

Drug interactions from the use of valerian product deliberately adulterated with sedative agents may be difficult to determine. Chan (1998) looked for "possible delayed adverse effects" from among 24 patients (ages 16-57) treated for overdose of valerian products in Hong Kong who had taken an OTC product containing hyoscine hydrobromide 0.25 mg, cyproheptadine hydrochloride 2 mg, and valerian dry extract 75 mg. For 23 patients, Chan estimated that the amount of valerian they had ingested was 150-4,500 mg. The symptoms treated were mainly anticholinergic poisoning and central nervous system depression. Unfortunately, for 13 of these cases still other substances were involved (i.e. alcohol, gasoline, hypnotics, and common cold medications). Seventeen patients underwent tests for liver function at admission or a day later and showed normal results; all 24 recovered completely and were not seen at any outpatient clinics. Chan concluded that severe adverse effects, such as delayed liver damage, were not likely because not one of the patients later presented with these problems. However, he could not rule out adverse effects of a milder nature or effects that received treatment outside the hospital region.

Because the GABAergic activity of valerian remains to be demonstrated with in vivo studies, additive or modulating effects with GABAergic drugs (e.g., gabapentin [Neurontin] remain unknown.

Pregnancy and Lactation

The German Commission E (Blumenthal et al., 1998) and the *American Herbal Products Association's Botanical Safety Handbook* (McGuffin et al., 1997) do not contraindicate use during pregnancy or lactation. McGuffin et al. further state, in editorial comment regarding valpotriates, that these constituents are poorly absorbed and easily degraded into less toxic metabolites and present little risk of acute adverse reaction. For lactation particularly, milk entry of constituents would thus be limited, and absorption of constituents by the infant further limited. The species *V. wallichii* is reputed to be an abortifacient and to interfere with menstrual cycles (Newall et al., 1996) (see Toxicity in Animal Models). No known incidents involving use during pregnancy or lactation have been documented.

Side Effects

Headache, excitability, uneasiness, insomnia, and disturbances of heart rhythm are suggested as possible concerns for constant use of valerian (Hobbs, 1989). No evidence suggests dependency/addiction in the literature on valerian; however, psychological dependency is possible since valerian has a subjective anxiety-reducing effect.

In an attempted suicide, an 18-year-old woman ingested 40-50 capsules of a 100% valerian root powder (Nature's Way, Springville, Utah, 470 mg valerian per capsule = 18.8-23.5 g). The manufacturer's recommended dosage was one to two capsules before bedtime. Thirty minutes later, she complained of fatigue, lightheadedness, tremors of the feet and hands, chest tightness, and abdominal pain and cramping. All tests, including liver function, blood pressure (BP), respiratory rate, and temperature, were normal. In the hospital, all symptoms resolved in 24 h (Mady et al., 1995).

Wells (1995) reported the case of a woman (age 25) who made a crude water extract of valerian root and, after self-injection of an unknown amount into her left antecubital vein, became lethargic with dilated pupils and stomach and chest pains. She was still responsive to voice and, while her blood pressure was unmeasurable, a femoral pulse remained. In the ER, she was still lethargic but could follow voice instructions. Other than her hair standing on end (piloerection), she showed no remarkable outward signs. Her pulse was 82 beats/min; her respiratory rate was 18 breaths/min; and her BP measured 60/40 mm Hg. Her mental status and BP returned to normal after 12 h. During hospitalization, tests showed hypokalemia, hypocalcemia, and hypophosphatemia. Wells concluded that the administration of valerian i.v. was unique and that the potential for resulting complications was great.

A diagnosis of acute hepatitis was reported in France in the case of a 63-year-old woman who presented with asthenia and jaundice and entered a hospital after noticing a change in the color of her urine. Extensive testing for diverse causes, including various retroviruses, turned up nothing. The only substance the investigators suspected as a possible cause was the valerian tea she had been taking regularly at bedtime in conjunction with homeopathic remedies, and only *V. officinalis* appeared to have been used in making the tea. Three months after stopping the tea she became asymptomatic and was discharged (Mennecier et al., 1999). Given the widespread use of valerian in Europe, in this case as in others (MacGregor et al., 1989;

Miskelly and Goodyer, 1992), toxicity caused by hepatotoxic adulterants (drugs, plants, etc.) and heavy metals must first be ruled out.

Special Precautions

McGuffin et al. (1997) note that registered valerian tinctures in Germany are required to carry a warning of reduced ability to drive or operate machinery. This warning appeared in the Commission E monograph on valerian of 1986 (Bradley, 1992); however, it does not appear in the Commission E monograph on valerian of 1990. Here the warning requirement is found for combination products of valerian containing hops *(Humulus lupulus)* plus passionflower *(Passiflora incarnata)*, and for valerian products containing hops plus lemon balm *(Melissa officinalis)*, but not for valerian plus hops (Blumenthal et al., 1998).

Toxicology

Mutagenicity

Valepotriates have inhibited protein and DNA synthesis in hepatoma cells in vitro, and dihydrovaltrate and isovaltrate have shown mutagenic activity in strains of *Escherichia coli* and in *Salmonella typhimurium* TA 100 with metabolic activation. Without metabolic activation, baldrinal and homobaldrinal caused mutation in strains of *Salmonella* (TA 98 and 100) and were directly cytotoxic in the SOS chromotest (von der Hude et al., 1986). If these potential toxicities are relevant in humans, the main sites of possible injury would be the liver and gastrointestinal tract (Bos et al., 1997).

Research has shown that the baldrinals and valepotriates undergo rapid metabolism in the body and the metabolites, baldrinal glucoronides, displayed no mutagenicity in the SOS chromotest, nor in the Ames test (Schilcher, 1997). Regardless, the best precautionary choice is for valerian products devoid of baldrinals and valepotriates (Bos et al., 1997) (e.g., tinctures stored for two months) (Bos, Hendriks, et al., 1998).

Toxicity in Animal Models

The acute oral LD_{50} of the valepotriates acevaltrate, didrovaltrate, and valtrate in mice is 4,600 mg/kg (Valpiani, 1995). The valepotriates are poorly absorbed in the gastrointestinal tract from oral administration (Bos et al., 1997); however, these compounds and the baldrinals forming from them as breakdown products have shown some alkylating, cytotoxic, and mutagenic activity (Hobbs, 1994; Bounthanh et al., 1981). The baldrinals, which are better absorbed and also sedating, have shown much less cytotoxic activity in vitro but more cytotoxicity in vivo (Hobbs, 1994).

Mice administered valerian extract, valeranone, valerenic acid, or the essential oil of valerian root showed an increased barbiturate-induced sleeping time (Bos et al., 1997).

A toxicity study in pregnant rats examined the effects of a mixture of valepotriates (5% acevaltrate, 15% valtrate, and 80% dihydrovaltrate) in doses of 6 mg/kg, 12 mg/kg, and 24 mg/kg p.o. daily for 30 consecutive days. Compared to controls, no changes were found in the average estrous cycle length or in the number of estrous phases; fertility showed no alteration; and body temperatures remained normal; however, intraperitoneal administration of the valepotriate mixture resulted in significant decreases in body temperature that lasted up to 4 h and ranged from 0.8°C to 1.9°C. Offspring showed no abnormalities externally, but internal examination revealed a significant number ($p < 0.001$) of abnormal fetuses in the 6 mg/kg group (2/22 rats), in the 12 mg/kg group (12/29), and in the 24 mg/kg dosage group (7/24) versus none in the control group. Between each of the dosage groups the differences were also significant (Tufik et al., 1994).

Although *V. officinalis* contains 800-1,700 mg/g valepotriates (mostly of valtrate and isovaltrate in a ratio of 1:1 to 1:4), no valepotriates are detected after valerian tinctures are left to sit for three weeks since they rapidly degrade. Teas made from the root using hot water were found to contain only little valepotriates (0.1%); as much as 60% remained in the root material (Bos et al., 1997).

REFERENCES

Ammer, K. and Melnizky, P. (1999). Medizinalbader zur therapie der generalisierten fibromyalgie [Medicinal baths for the treatment of generalized fibromyalgia]. *Forschende Komplementarmedizin* (Basel) 6: 80-85.

Balduini, W. and Cattabeni, F. (1989). Displacement of [³H]-cyclohexyladenosine [*sic*] binding to rat cortical membranes by an hydroalcoholic extract of *Valeriana officinalis. Medical Science Research* 17: 639-640.

Bernáth, J. (1997). Cultivation of valerian. In Houghton, P.J. (Ed.), *Valerian: The Genus Valeriana* (pp. 77-100). Amsterdam, the Netherlands: Harwood Academic.

Blumenthal, M., Busse, W.R., Goldberg, A., Gruenwald, J., Hall, T., Riggins, C.W., and Rister, R.S. (Eds.) (1998). *The Complete German Commission E Monographs* (pp. 226-227, 303-305). Austin, TX: American Botanical Council.

Bodesheim, U. and Hölzl, J. (1997). Isolierung, strukturaufklarung und radiorezeptorassays von alkaloiden und lignanen aus *Valeriana officinalis* L. [Isolation and receptor binding properties of alkaloids and lignans from *Valeriana officinalis* L.]. *Pharmazie* 52: 386-391.

Bos, R., Hendriks, H., Kloosterman, J., and Sipma, G. (1986). Isolation of the sesquiterpene alcohol (–)-pacifigorgiol from *Valeriana officinalis*. *Phytochemistry* 25: 1234-1235.

Bos, R., Hendriks, H., Scheffer, J.J.C., and Woerdenbag, H.J. (1998). Cytotoxic potential of valerian constituent and valerian tinctures. *Phytomedicine* 5: 219-225.

Bos, R., Woerdenbag, H.J., De Smet, P.A.G.M., and Scheffer, J.J.C. (1997). *Valeriana* species. In De Smet, P.A.G.M., Keller, K., Hänsel, R., and Chandler, R.F. (Eds.), *Adverse Effects of Herbal Drugs*, Vol. 3 (pp. 165-180). New York: Springer-Verlag.

Bos, R., Woerdenbag, H.J., Hendriks, H., Zwaving, J.H., De Smet, P.A.G.M., Tittel, G., Wikstrom, H.V., and Scheffer, J.J.C. (1996). Analytical aspects of phytotherapeutic valerian preparations. *Phytochemical Analysis* 7: 143-151.

Bos, R., Woerdenbag, H.J., van Putten, F.M.S., Hendriks, H., and Scheffer, J.J.C. (1998). Seasonal variation of the essential oil, valerenic acid and derivatives, and valepotriates in *Valeriana officinalis* roots and rhizomes, and the selection of plants suitable for phytomedicines. *Planta Medica* 64: 143-147.

Bounthanh, C., Bergmann, C., Beck, J.P., Haag-Berrurier, M., and Anton, R. (1981). Valepotriates, a new class of cytotoxic and antitumor agents. *Planta Medica* 41: 21-28.

Bourin, M., Bougerol, T., Guitton, B., and Broutin, E. (1997). A combination of plant extracts in the treatment of outpatients with adjustment disorder with anxious mood: Controlled study versus placebo. *Fundamental and Clinical Pharmacology* 11: 127-132.

Boyle, W. (1991). *Official Herbs. Botanical Substances in the United States Pharmacopoeias 1820-1990* (pp. 50-51). East Palestine, OH: Buckeye Naturopathic Press.

Bradley, P. (Ed.) (1992). *British Herbal Compendium,* Vol. I (pp. 214-217). Bournemouth, Dorset, England: British Herbal Medicine Association.

Brinker, F. (1998). *Herb Contraindications and Drug Interactions,* Second Edition (p. 163). Sandy, OR: Eclectic Medical Publications.

Capasso, A., De Feo, V., De Simone, F., and Sorrentino, L. (1996). Pharmacological effects of aqueous extract from *Valeriana adscendens*. *Phytotherapy Research* 10: 309-312.

Cavadas, C., Araujo, I., Cotrim, M.D., Amaral, T., Cunha, A.P., Macedo, T., and Ribeiro, C.F. (1995). In vitro study on the interaction of *Valeriana officinalis* L. extracts and their amino acids on $GABA_A$ receptor in rat brain. *Arzneimittel-Forschung/Drug Research* 45: 753-755.

Cerny, A. and Schmid, K. (1999). Tolerability and efficacy of valerian/lemon balm in healthy volunteers (a double-blind, placebo-controlled, multicentre study). *Fitoterapia* 70: 221-228.

Chan, T.Y.K. (1998). An assessment of the delayed effects associated with valerian overdose. *International Journal of Clinical Pharmacology and Therapeutics* 36: 569 (letter).

Donath, F., Quispe, S., Diefenbach, K., Maurer, A., Fietze, I., and Roots, I. (2000). Critical evaluation of the effect of valerian extract on sleep structure and sleep quality. *Pharmacopsychiatry* 33: 47-53.

Donath, F. and Roots, I. (1996). Effects of valerian extract (Sedonium®) on EEG power spectrum in male healthy volunteers after single and multiple application. *European Journal of Clinical Pharmacology* 50: 541 (abstract).

Dressling, H., Reimann, D., Löw, H., Schredl, M., Reh, C., Laux, P., and Müller, W.E. (1992). Baldrian-Melisse-kombinationen versus benzodiazepin: Bei schlafstörungen gleichwertig [Insomnia: Are valerian/melissa combinations of equal value to benzodiazepine]? *Therapiewoche* 42: 726-736.

Duke, J. (1985). *CRC Handbook of Medicinal Herbs* (pp. 503-504). Boca Raton, FL: CRC Press.

Dweck, A.C. (1997). An introduction to valerian *Valeriana officinalis* and related species. In Houghton, P.J. (Ed.), *Valerian: The Genus Valeriana* (pp. 1-19). Amsterdam, the Netherlands: Harwood Academic.

European Pharmacopoeia, Third Edition (1997). Strasbourg, France: Council of Europe.

Fuzzati, N., Wolfender, J.L., Hostettmann, K., Msonthi, J.D., Mavi, S., and Molleyres, L.P. (1996). Isolation of antifungal valepotriates from *Valeriana capense* and the search for valepotriates in crude Valerianaceae extracts. *Phytochemical Analysis* 7: 76-85.

Gao, X.Q. and Björk, L. (2000). Valerenic acid derivatives and valpotriates among individuals, varieties and species of *Valeriana*. *Fitoterapia* 71: 19-24.

Garges, H.P., Varia, I., and Doraiswamy, P.M. (1998). Cardiac complications and delirium associated with valerian root withdrawal. *Journal of the American Medical Association* 28: 1566-1567 (letter).

Hazelhoff, B., Smith, D., Malingre, T.M., and Hendriks, H. (1979). The essential oil of *Valeriana officinalis* L. s.l. *Pharmazeutisch Weekblad Scientific Edition* 114: 443-449.

Hendriks, H., Bos, R., Allersma, D.P., Malingre, T.M., and Koster, A.S. (1981). Pharmacological screening of valerenal and some other components of essential oil of *Valeriana officinalis*. *Planta Medica* 42: 62-66.

Hendriks, H., Bos, R., Woerdenbag, H.J., and Koster, A.S. (1985). Central nervous depressant activity of valerenic acid in the mouse. *Planta Medica* 46: 28-31.

Hikino, H., Hikino, Y., Kobinata, H., Aizawa, A., Konno, C., and Ohizumu, Y.(1980). Sedative principles of *Valeriana* roots. *Shoyakugaku Zasshi* 34: 19-24.

Hiller, K.O. and Zetler, G. (1996). Neuropharmacological studies on ethanol extracts of *Valeriana officinalis* L.: Behavioural and anticonvulsant properties. *Phytotherapy Research* 10: 145-151.

Hobbs, C. (1989). Valerian: A literature review. *HerbalGram* 21: 19-34.

Hobbs, C. (1994). *Valerian: The Relaxing and Sleep Herb*. Capitola, CA: Botanica Press.

Hoffman, D. (1990). *The Elements of Herbalism* (pp. 24-28). Longmead, Dorset, England: Element Books.

Hölzl, J. (1997). The pharmacology and therapeutics of *Valeriana*. In Houghton, P.J. (Ed.), *Valerian: The Genus Valeriana* (pp. 55-75). Amsterdam, the Netherlands: Harwood Academic.

Hölzl, J. and Godau, P. (1989). Receptor binding studies with *Valeriana officinalis* on the benzodiazepine receptor. *Planta Medica* 55: 642 (abstract).

Houghton, P.J. (1988). The biological activity of valerian and related plants. *Journal of Ethnopharmacology* 22: 121-142.

Houghton, P.J. (1997a). The chemistry of *Valeriana*. In Houghton, P.J. (Ed.), *Valerian: The Genus Valeriana* (pp. 21-54). Amsterdam, the Netherlands: Harwood Academic.

Houghton, P.J. (Ed.) (1997b). *Valerian: The Genus Valeriana*. Amsterdam, the Netherlands: Harwood Academic.

Houghton, P.J. (1999). The scientific basis for the reputed activity of valerian. *Journal of Pharmacy and Pharmacology* 51: 505-512.

Kamm-Kohl, A.V., Jansen, W., and Brockmann, P. (1984). Modern valerian therapy of nervous disorders in elderly patients. *MedWelt* 35: 1450-1454.

Kohnen, R. and Oswald, W.D. (1988). The effects of valerian, propanolol, and their combination on activation, performance, and mood of healthy volunteers under social stress conditions. *Pharmacopsychiatry* 21: 447-448.

Kommission E (1995). Valeriane radix/baldrianwurzel [Valerian root/baldrian root]. In *Kommission E (Phytopharmaka) of the Federal Institute for Drugs and Medical Devices* [Bundesinstitut für Arneimittel und Medizinprodukte] (p. 50). Berlin, Germany: Bundesanzeiger.

Kuhlmann, J., Berger, W., Podzuweit, H., and Schmidt, U. (1999). The influence of valerian treatment on "reaction time, alertness and concentration" in volunteers. *Pharmacopsychiatry* 32: 235-241.

Lataster, M.J. and Brattström, A. (1996). Die behandlung von patienten met schlafstörungen: Wirksamkeit und verträglichkeit von Baldrian-Hopfendragées [Therapy of patients with somnipathy: Effects and toleration of valerian-hops coated tablets]. *Notabene Medici* 4: 182-185.

Leathwood, P.D. and Chauffard, F. (1985). Aqueous extract of valerian reduced latency to fall asleep in man. *Planta Medica* 51: 144-148.

Leathwood, P.D., Chauffard, F., Heck, E., and Munoz-Box, R. (1982). Aqueous extract of valerian root (*Valeriana officinalis* L.) improves sleep quality in man. *Pharmacology, Biochemistry and Behavior* 17: 65-71.

Lindahl, O. and Lindwall, L. (1989). Double-blind study of a valerian preparation. *Pharmacology, Biochemistry, and Behavior* 32: 1065-1066.

Mady, S.P., Cobaugh, D.J., and Wax, P.M. (1995). Valerian overdose: A case report. *Veterinary and Human Toxicology* 37: 364-365.

Maisenbacher, J. and Podzuweit, H. (1992). Baldrian und melisse — milde psychopharmacka [Valerian and lemon balm—gentle psychoactive drugs]. *Therapiewoche* 42: 2140-2144.

McGregor, F.B., Abernethy, V.E., Dahabra, S., Cobden, I., and Hayes, P.C. (1989). Hepatotoxicity of herbal remedies. *British Medical Journal* 299: 1156-1157.

McGuffin, M., Hobbs, C., Upton, R., and Goldberg, A. (1997). *American Herbal Products Association's Botanical Safety Handbook.* Boca Raton, FL: CRC Press.

Mennecier, D., Saloum, T., Dourthe, P.M., Bronstein, J.A., Thiolet, C., and Farret, O. (1999). Hépatite aiguë et phytothérapie [Acute hepatitis and phytotherapy]. *La Presse Médicale* 28: 966 (letter), translation.

Mennini, T., Bernasconi, P., Bombardelli, E., and Morazzoni, P. (1993). In vitro study on the interaction of extracts and pure compounds from *Valeriana officinalis* roots with GABA, benzodiazepine and barbiturate receptors in rats brain. *Fitoterapia* 64: 291-300.

Miskelly, F.G. and Goodyer, L.I. (1992). Hepatic and pulmonary complications of herbal medicines. *Postgraduate Medical Journal* 68: 935 (letter).

Morazzoni, P. and Bombardelli, E. (1995). *Valeriana officinalis:* Traditional use and recent evaluation of activity. *Fitoterapia* 66: 99-112.

Newall, C.A., Anderson, L.A., and Phillipson, J.D. (1996). *Herbal Medicines: A Guide for Health Care Professionals.* London: The Pharmaceutical Press.

Nieves, J. and Ortiz, J.G. (1997). Effects of *Valeriana officinalis* extract on GABAergic transmission. *Journal of Neurochemistry* 69(Suppl.): S128 (abstract D).

Ortiz, J.G., Nieves-Natal, J., and Chavez, P. (1999). Effects of *Valeriana officinalis* extracts of [³H]flunitrazepam binding, synaptosomal [³H]GABA uptake, and hippocampal [³H]GABA release. *Neurochemical Research* 24: 1373-1378.

Oshima, Y., Matsuoka, S., and Ohisumi, Y. (1995). Antidepressant principles of *Valeriana fauriei* roots. *Chemical and Pharmaceutical Bulletin* 43: 169-170.

Paul, C., Konig, W.A., and Muhle, H. (2001). Pacifigorgianes and tamariscene as constituents of *Frullania tamarisci* and *Valeriana officinalis. Phytochemistry* 57: 307-313.

Quispe Bravo, S., Diefenbach, K., Donath, F., Fietze, I., and Roots, I. (1997). The influence of valerian on objective and subjective sleep in insomniacs. *European Journal of Clinical Pharmacology* 52(Suppl.): A170 (abstract 548).

Riedel, E., Hänsel, R., and Ehrke, G. (1982). [Inhibition of γ-amino butyric acid metabolism by valerenic acid derivatives]. *Planta Medica* 46: 219-220.

Rosenstein, J.M. (1996). Permeability of the blood-brain barrier to protein and [³H]GABA in intraparenchymal fetal CNS tissue grafts. *Experimental Neurology* 142: 66-79.

Santos, M.S., Ferreira, F., Cunha, A.P., Carvalho, A.P., and Macedo, T. (1994a). An aqueous extract of valerian influences the transport of GABA in synaptosomes. *Planta Medica* 60: 278-279.

Santos, M.S., Ferreira, F., Cunha, A.P., Carvalho, A.P., Ribeiro, C.F., and Macedo, T. (1994b). Synaptosomal GABA release as influenced by valerian root extract—Involvement of the GABA carrier. *Archives Internationales de Pharmacodynamie et de Therapie* 327: 220-231.

Santos, M.S., Ferreira, F., Faro, C., Pires, E., Carvalho, A.P., Cunha, A.P., and Macedo, T. (1994c). The amount of GABA present in aqueous extracts of valerian is sufficient to account for [^3H]GABA release in synaptosomes. *Planta Medica* 60: 475-476.

Schilcher, H. (1997). *Phytotherapy in Paediatrics. Handbook for Physicians and Pharmacists* (pp. 59, 167). Stuttgart, Germany: Medpharm Scientific.

Schmidt-Voigt, J. (1986). Treatment of nervous sleep disturbances and inner restlessness with a purely herbal sedative: Results of a study in general practice. *Therapiewoche* 36: 663-667.

Schmitz, M. and Jäckel, M. (1998). Vergleichsstudie zur untersuchung der lebensqualitat von patienten mit exogenen schladstorungen (vorubergehenden ein- und durchschlafstorungen) unter therapie mit einem hopfen-baldrian-praparat und einem benzodiazepin-praparat [Comparative study for assessing quality of life of patients with exogenous sleep disorders (temporary sleep onset and sleep interruption disorders) treated with a hops-valerian preparation and a benzodiazepine drug]. *Wein Medizinische Wochenschrift* 148: 291-298.

Schulz, V., Hänsel, R., and Tyler, V.E. (2001). *Rational Phytotherapy: A Physician's Guide to Herbal Medicine,* Fourth Edition (p. 103). New York: Springer-Verlag.

Stevinson, C. and Ernst, E. (2000). Valerian for insomnia: A systematic review of randomized clinical trials. *Sleep Medicine* 1: 91-99.

Tufik, S., Fujita, K., de Lourdes, M., Seabra, V., and Lobo, L.L. (1994). Effects of prolonged administration of valepotriates in rats on the mothers and their offspring. *Journal of Ethnopharmacology* 41: 39-44.

Valpiani, C. (1995). *ATOMS Journal: Publication of the Australian Traditional Medicine Society* 1: 57-62.

Veith, J., Schneider, G., Lemmer, B., and Willems, M. (1986). [The influence of some degradation products of valepotriates on the motor activity of light-dark synchronized mice]. *Planta Medica* 47: 179-183.

von der Hude, W., Scheutwinkel-Reish, M., and Braun, R. (1986). Bacterial mutagenicity of the tranquilizing constituents of Valerianaceae roots. *Mutation Research* 169: 23-27.

Von Mayer, B. and Springer, E. (1974). Psychoexperimentelle untersuchungen zur wirkung einer valpotriatkombination sowie zur kombinierten wirkung von valtratum und alcohol [Psychoexperimental study on the influence of a valpotriate combination and the combined effects of valtratum and alcohol]. *Arzneimittel-Forschung* 24: 2066-2070.

Vorbach, E.U., Gortelmeyer, R., and Bruning, J. (1996). Therapie von insomnien: Wirksamkeit und vertraglichkeit eines baldrianpraparats. *Psychopharmacotherapie* 3: 109-115.

Weiss, R.F. (1996). *Herbal Medicine* (p. 348). Beaconsfield, Bucks, England: Beaconsfield Publishers.

Wells, S.R. (1995). Intentional intravenous administration of a crude valerian root extract. *Journal of Toxicology, Clinical Toxicology* 33: 542 (abstract).

Woerdenbag, H.J., Bos, R., and Scheffer, J.J.C. (1997). Valerian: Quality assurance of the crude drug and its preparations. In Houghton, P.J. (Ed.), *Valerian: The Genus Valeriana* (pp. 101-128). Amsterdam, the Netherlands: Harwood Academic.

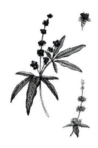

$\mathcal{V}itex$

BOTANICAL DATA

Classification and Nomenclature

Scientific name: *Vitex agnus-castus* L.

Family name: Verbenaceae

Common names: vitex, agnus castus, chasteberry, chaste tree, monk's pepper, monk's seed, pepper tree, agni casti fructus, wild pepper, hemp tree, Abraham's tree

Description

Vitex is a member of the Verbenaceae, a large family consisting of 1,900 species in 91 genera. The genus *Vitex* includes approximately 250 primarily tropical species and subspecies. *Vitex agnus-castus* is the only European species (Mabberley, 1990). Besides *V. agnus-castus,* other species used medicinally include *V. negundo* L. (China, India, Australia) (Stylian, 1996), *V. trifoliata* L. (India, Indonesia), *V. peduncularis* Wall. (India), *V. rotundifolia* L. (China, Japan) (Böhnert and Hahn, 1990), *V. trifolia* (Zhu, 1998), and *V. jeguado* L. var. *cannabifolia* (China) (Huang, 1999).

Vitex agnus-castus is a deciduous shrub 2-6 m in height, often of aromatic scent; leaves are opposite, divided into 5-7 linear lanceolate leaflets, 5-7 cm long, 1.2-4 cm wide, acute to acuminate; the entire base attenuates the young twigs and the underside of leaflets are covered with gray down. The leaves have a "sharp" taste (Böhnert and Hahn, 1990). The inflorescence is a thyrse, 1-2 cm long and terminal. The calyx is greyish-tomentose and the sepals are united to near apex. The corolla is sympetalous, blue to pink with stamens exherted; stigma is two-cleft (flowers with white variants), in dense racemes; blooming occurs in late summer. The fruits are drupes, 3-4 mm long (peppercorn size), globose, dark brown to reddish-black, with four seeds. The seeds smell and taste of black pepper. *Vitex* is native to the plains and low altitudes in the Mediterranean, Crimea, and Central Asia, and is found in dry soil along stream beds and river banks, often in association with oleander and tamarisk bushes. Propagation is by seed or soft wood cuttings (summer wood). In frost-free zones, *V. agnus-castus* is a garden ornamental and is naturalized in the United States from Maryland south to Florida and west to Texas (Snow, 1996), and in Nigeria, northern Brazil (Zoghbi et al., 1999), and undoubtedly other countries.

HISTORY AND TRADITIONAL USES

Vitex *(V. agnus-castus)* was widely used in antiquity. Reports mention its use in ancient Greek rituals, especially noting that the twigs were carried for protection against various dangers or to denote chastity. According to Greek mythology, the Greek goddess Hera, the protectress of marriage, was born under a Vitex bush. Its medicinal reputation is alluded to by Pausanias in the second century A.D., who described a statue of Asclepius, the Greek god of healing, carved of vitex wood. In the first century A.D., Pliny named the plant *vitex* from the ancient word *vei,* meaning "to bend or twine." Vitex twigs were often used in making wattle fences and baskets. The species name is usually described as being derived from a combination of the Greek name for the plant, *agnos* ("barren or unfruitful"), later corrupted to *agnus* (Latin for lamb), with *castus* derived from the Latin term for chastity *(castitas)* (Böhnert and Hahn, 1990). It is speculated that in southern Italian dialects the name *làgano* for the plant might be taken from the *lygos* told of by Homer (Russo and Galletti, 1996).

Hippocrates, in the fourth century B.C., suggested the use of the plant for inflammation, swelling of the spleen, and to help expel the placenta after birth (Snow, 1996). Dioscorides, in the first century A.D., described its use to "bring down the milk" and expel menstrual blood (plant part not specified). He also described the use of seed decoctions for "inflammation about the womb" (Duke, 1995). Pliny, also in the first century A.D., used vitex as an anaphrodisiac, to reduce fever and headache, to stimulate perspiration, and to increase lactation (Snow, 1996). He claimed that a beverage prepared from the seeds tasted like wine (Hobbs, 1991). Hippocrates suggested using vitex fruits to treat injuries and inflammations. Leaves steeped in wine were specified for hemorrhage and expelling the placenta after birth (Duke, 1995).

Renaissance herbalists drew heavily on the reputation of the plant to assist in treating inflammations of the uterus and as an emmenagogue (Hobbs, 1990). According to Arabian and Persian medical texts from 1200 A.D., vitex was used to cure insanity, madness, and epilepsy. Psychiatric uses persist in Egypt, where vitex fruits are currently given as an antidote for hysteria (Hobbs, 1991), and in southern Nigeria where the root bark and leaves are used as a treatment for depression and are recorded as having a sedative effect (Nwosu, 1999). Maintaining an older reputation as an aid to sustain chastity, during medieval times in Europe vitex was thought to suppress libido and was widely used as a ritual symbol of chastity and as a monasterial spice taken with the intention of suppressing libido (Böhnert and Hahn, 1990). Once famous, a syrup prepared from the seeds was distributed in convents to quel the passions; however, the French author Cazin, writing in the late 1800s, doubted its efficacy, believing it to be rather, "very stimulating" (Hobbs, 1991). In the sixteenth century, Lonicerus and Mattioli advised that the leaves and berries were effective as an emmenagogue (Russo and Galletti, 1996). Warnings were made against overdosing, even in times of antiquity, as Lonicerus wrote in the seventeenth century. Presently, vitex is used as a spice in southern Europe (Böhnert and Hahn, 1990).

Duke (1995) recounts various traditional uses of vitex. In Unani medicine, the plant is used as an abortifacient and emmenagogue, and the seeds are taken for dropsy, inflammation, to purify the brain and liver, and as a contraceptive. In Ayurvedic medicine, the seeds are classified as abortifacient, alexiteric, diuretic, heating and stomachic, and used for eye ailments and stomachache. Other Indian uses include the treatment of itch, thirst, and burning sensations (Duke, 1995). In Amazonian Brazil, where vitex was introduced by European settlers, the locals use the plant as an antiseptic, carminative, antispasmodic, emmenagogue, anaphrodisiac, and diuretic, and in the treatment of influenza, diarrhea, headache, stomach pains, and syphilis (Zoghbi et al., 1999).

CHEMISTRY

The chemical make up of vitex *(V. agnus-castus)* has yet to become well documented (Newall et al., 1996). Although standard extracts of the fruit have been extensively researched, the individual constituents are relatively unstudied. Information on the constituents of the leaf (LF), flower (FL), fruit (FR), and seed (SD) varies in completeness. Phytogeographic analyses indicate the existence of several chemotypes (Sorensen and Katsiotis, 1999).

Lipid Compounds

Oils

Essential oil composition and content shows considerable variation with regard to plant parts and growing area (Senatore et al., 1996; Males et al., 1998; Zoghbi et al., 1999). They varied from year to year in a Dalmation coastal population of vitex studied from 1981 to 1991 (Kustrak et al., 1992).

The researchers reported an overall essential oil content of 0.53% to 1.05% (LF), 0.4-0.8% (FL), and 1.13% to 1.64% (FR). Zwaving and Bos (1996) found that by hydrodistillation, a yield of only 0.71% essential oil was obtained from the fruits. From wild plants growing on the Island of Crete, Sorensen and Katsiotis (1999) obtained oil yields of 0.15% to 1.0% by hydrodistillation of the mature fruits. Chemotypically, the fruits were closer to profiles of vitex fruits of Mediterranean origin than those of other areas. From vitex plants growing in southern Italy, Senatore et al. (1996) reported that the yields of essential oils from hydrodistillation of the leaves, flowers, and fruits were in the range of 0.8% to 1.8% (dry weight basis).

Phenolic Compounds

Flavonoids

Orientin, iso-orientin, xyloside, vitexin, and isovitexin occur in the fruits and leaves, along with the main flavonoid, casticin (Gomaa et al., 1978), a quercitagenin derivative consisting of vitexin and vitexinine (Du Mee, 1993). Amounts of casticin in samples of commercial vitex extracts sold in Europe in 1995-1996 varied from 0.02% to 0.21% (Hoberg et al., 2000). Luteolin-7-glucoside and homo-orientin, the latter described by Koeppen (1964) as a C-glucopyranosyl derivative of luteolin, were identified in leaf extracts (Hänsel et al., 1965). Other flavonoids in *V. agnus-castus* include 6-hydroxykaempferol-3,6,7,4'-tetramethylether, 6-hydroxykaempferol 3,6,7-trimethylether, chrysosphenol-D, and penduletin (FR) (Gomaa et al., 1978; Wollenweber and Mann, 1983; Newall et al., 1996).

Four new cytotoxic flavonoids were recently isolated from the root bark: luteolin 6-C-(4"-methyl-6"-O-trans-caffeoylglucoside), luteolin 6-C-(6"-O-trans-caffeoylglucoside), luteolin 6-C-(2"-O-trans-caffeoylglucoside), and luteolin 7-O-(6"-p-benzoylglucoside) (Hirobe et al., 1997).

Tannins

In *V. agnus-castus* f. *rosea* growing wild in Dalmatia, the content of tannins (dry weight basis) was higher in the leaves (1.12% to 2.68%) than in the flowers (0.88% to 2.28%) or fruits (0.80% to 1.16%) (Males, 1998).

Polyphenolics

Total polyphenol contents of *V. agnus-castus* f. *rosea* growing wild in Dalmatia reached higher levels in the fruits and leaves (7.12% to 10.76%) than the flowers (4.88% to 8.72%), in which the content showed much less variation (8.08% to 8.48%) (Males, 1998).

Terpenoid Compounds

Iridoids

Iridoids reported in *V. agnus-castus* include aucubin (0.3%), agnuside (*p*-hydroxybenzoyl derivative of aucubin) (0.6%) (Du Mee, 1993; Gomaa et al., 1978) (LF, FR, FL), eurostoside (0.6%) (LF), unidentified glycosides (0.07%) (Newall et al., 1996), and iridoid glycosides (FL, LF) (Hänsel et al., 1965). Amounts of agnuside in commercial extracts sold in Europe in 1995-1996 showed high variability (0.007% to 0.207%) (Hoberg et al., 2000).

Monoterpenes

∝-pinene, 1,8-cineole, limonene (LF, FL, FR essential oil), α-terpineol, β-pinene, linalool, citronellol, *p*-cymene, camphene, and myrcene (LF essential oil) have been reported (Kustrak et al., 1992; Leung and Foster, 1996; Snow, 1996). In one study, out of 73 compounds identified in the essential oil of the fruit, 35% were monoterpenes largely made up of 4-terpinol, α-pinene, β-phellandrene, and sabinene (Zwaving and Bos, 1996). In wild, mature fruits on the island of Crete, sabinene and 1,8-cineole were the major monoterpenes detected (Sorensen and Katsiotis, 1999). In the leaves, flowers, and fruits of a population growing in southern Italy, the main monoterpenes in the essential oil were 1,8-cineole (20.6% in the fruit oil), α-terpinol (8.5% in the leaf oil), and terpinen-4ol (2.8% in the leaf oil) (Senatore et al., 1996). In a Dalmatian population in the area of Medici, the main components of the essential oil of the leaves, flowers, and fruits were monoterpenes, especially limonene, cineole (combined, 36.40% of the leaf oil), and sabinene (21.88% of the leaf oil) (Males et al., 1998).

Sesquiterpenes

Sesquiterpene compounds reported in vitex include β-caryophyllene, E-β-farnesene, caryophylline oxide (essential oil of LF, FR, FL) (Kustrak et al., 1992), cadinene, and ledol (LF essential oil) (Snow, 1996). Sesquiterpenes may constitute 52% of the essential oil of the fruits. In one population, they largely consisted of alloaromadendrene, β-caryophyllene, τ-cadinol, germacrene B, and spathulenol. The fruits of wild-grown plants in southern Italy were found to contain a larger amount of sesquiterpenes (39.8%) than the essential oil of the leaves (12.1%) (Galletti et al., 1996); in the mature fruits of wild vitex growing on Crete, the most abundant sesquiterpene detected was E-β-farnesene (Sorensen and Katsiotis, 1999). In another study of southern Italian vitex, the major sesquiterpenes in the oils of the leaves, flowers, and fruits were β-caryophyllene (9.7% in the flower oil), *cis*-β-farnesene (9.1% in the flower oil), and β-selinene (9.0% in the leaf oil) (Senatore et al., 1996).

Diterpenes

The fruits contain the labdan diterpenes, rotundifuran, vitexilactone, and a new diterpene (6β,7β-diacetoxy-13-hydroxy-labda-8,14-diene) (Hoberg et al., 1999). The content of these diterpenes in the fruits corresponded with contents of the main flavonoid, casticin. Quantitative analyses of commercial extract samples of vitex sold in Europe in 1995-1996 found total amounts of diterpenoids as high as 4.03%. Contents of individual diterpenes showed great variability. Rotundifuran was showed in amounts of between 0.04% and 2.22%, and in samples in the berries of between 1.04% and 2.23%. For vitexilactone, the contents were 0.01% to 1.00% in commercial extracts and 0.34% to 0.01% in berries. For the new diterpene, amounts varied in commercial extracts from 0.02% to 0.80% and in the berries from 0.02% to 0.10% (Hoberg et al., 2000). In a southern Italian population of vitex, Senatore et al. (1996) found the major diterpene in the oils of the leaves, flowers, and fruits was an alcohol, manool (2.1% in the flower oil).

Triterpenes

The triterpenic constituents reported are: 3-β-acetoxyolean-12-en-27-oic acid, 2-α,3-adihydroxyolean-5,12-dien-28-oic acid, 2-β,3-α-diacetoxyolean-5,12-dien-28-oic acid, and 2α-,3-β-diacetoxy-18-hydroxyolean-5,12-dien-28-oic acid (Leung and Foster, 1996).

Steroids

Progesterone, 17-αhydroxyprogesterone, testosterone, and epitestosterone were identified in the flowers, and androstenedione was found in the leaves. The report of ketosteroid in the leaf and flower must be treated cautiously (Saden-Krehula et al., 1990), and reports of progesterone-like activity of the seed (Belic et al., 1958) have been contested (Madaus Co., 1994).

Other Constituents

Castine, a bitter principle, has been isolated (Newall et al., 1996).

THERAPEUTIC APPLICATIONS

The first clinical studies of vitex sought to investigate the plant's ancient reputation as a galactogogue, and early animal experiments attempted to explain the plant's lactogenic reputation. However, at the time, precise concentrations of serum hormone levels could not be determined as sensitive detection methods had yet to be developed. Initial scientific investigations of vitex are attributed to Madaus Co. with the product Agnolyt in 1930, with which early work was limited to clinical investigations of galactogogue activity. By the late 1950s, research focused on utilizing vitex for menstrual difficulties. The German Commission E monograph (Blumenthal et al., 1998) lists the accepted applications of *Vitex agnus-castus* as: menstrual disturbances (with corpus luteum insufficiency), premenstrual syndrome, breast tenderness, menopausal complaints, and milk production stimulation.

A review of the available literature indicates some evidence of efficacy of vitex in the following conditions: hyperprolactinemia, corpus luteum insufficiency, infertility associated with corpus luteum insufficiency, mastodynia (breast discomfort), premenstrual syndrome (PMS), premenstrual tension syndrome (PMTS), premenopausal symptoms, uterine myomas, endometriosis adjunctive therapy, Parkinson's disease, and acne.

The Agnolyt package insert (Madaus Co., 1994) lists specific additional therapeutic applications in prophylaxis following curettage treatment of acyclic continuous bleeding and glandular-cystic hyperplasia of the endometrium; growth arrest of uterus myoma (uterine cysts) embedded in the muscle or subserous layer—"submucous myoma," however, must be treated surgically; and mild cases of endometriosis in the form of discomforts and symptoms that disappear with the onset of pregnancy and reappear at the end of the lactation period. The insert also states that "Agnolyt® is not effective for dysmenorrhea" (Madaus Co., 1994). Hobbs (1990) mentions the use of vitex after withdrawal of birth control pills, to "help stabilize the menstrual cycle and bring on ovulation more quickly."

Endocrine and Hormonal Functions

Hypothalamic and Pituitary Functions

Propping et al. (1988) recounted a study of women with normal prolactin levels who still suffered from menstrual difficulties. They referred to measured changes in the LH-RH (luteinizing hormone-releasing hormone) test after three months of vitex treatment and described vitex as effecting a "positive modification of LH-RH dynamics" (Propping et al., 1988). However, no mention of this effect is found in the reference they cite. Other evidence of an effect on gonadotropin-releasing hormone (Gn-RH) dynamics, independent of prolactin modulation by vitex, has not been found. Jarry et al. (1994) reported that gonadotropin secretion was not affected by the vitex extract at any concentration they tested, even under stimulated conditions of incubation with releasing hormone or with basal cells releasing follicle stimulating hormone (FSH) and luteinizing hormone-releasing hormone (LH-RH).

Notable also is the hypothesis that in lactating women, suckling may also stimulate β-endorphin release, which is associated with increased prolactin levels and perhaps with a second mechanism: a suppression of Gn-RH release (Lawrence, 1994). Information on the influence of vitex on β-endorphins is lacking, while interaction with opioid receptors has only recently come to light (Hoberg et al., 1999; Jarry et al., 2000; Meier et al., 2000). In this arena, it may be of interest to note that a recent study of women with PMS demonstrated an altered response to naloxone compared to women with no PMS (Rapkin et al., 1996). As yet incompletely understood, the role of stress in hypothalamic-pituitary function is currently an area of considerable research interest.

Reproductive Hormone Interactions

Eagon et al. (1997) examined the estrogenic activity of a vitex berry extract added to the diet of ovariectomized female rats on a standard liquid diet. The amount used was one-third the equivalent of a human dose (Eagon, 1999). After three weeks, the extract had caused uterine weight to increase and uterine *c-myc* mRNA expression (which is induced by estrogen) to increase and an increase in the hepatic estrogenic response, as evidenced by increased levels of hepatic ceruloplasmin mRNA levels. Eagon et al. (1998) have also reported that the berry extract, when tested in the same animals for a possible hypothalamic/pituitary response, was found to decrease LH levels significantly, by 31%.

Estrogenic activity of a methanolic extract of the berries was examined by Liu et al. (2001) using four types of in vitro assays. In estrogen receptor binding assays, the berry extract showed significant binding activity in both human recombinant α- and β-estrogen receptors. Although the berries were much less potent than methanolic extracts of red clover or hops, their affinities for the receptors showed no significant difference. The berry extract also stimulated progesterone receptor gene (PR) expression in estrogen-positive endometrial adenocarcinoma (Ishikawa) cells, yet alkaline phosphates activity as a measure of estrogenic activity was not affected by the extract. In an estradiol-sensitive line of breast cancer cells (S30 cells), the estrogen-inducible gene presenelin-2 (*pS2*) was up-regulated by the extract with a potency comparable to that of a methanolic extract of North American ginseng *(Panax quinquefolius)*.

Immune Functions; Inflammation and Disease

Cancer

Antiproliferative activity. The in vitro growth-inhibitory activity of vitex was examined in an estrogen- and progesterone-positive human breast cancer cell line, T-47D. Significant inhibitory activity from an extract of the berries was found from concentrations of 0.1% and 1%, producing 14% and 47% inhibitions of tumor growth, respectively (each $p < 0.001$) (Dixon-Shanies and Shaikh, 1999).

Infectious Diseases

Microbial infections. Vitex leaf has shown growth-inhibitory activity against *Pseudomonas aeruginosa, Escherichia coli, Bacillus subtilis,* and *Staphylococcus aureus.* Inhibitory activity was also found against aflatoxin production by *Aspergillus parasiticus,* and insecticidal activity was demonstrated as well (Snow, 1996). Ethanolic fluid extracts and an ether extract of the dried leaves were tested for antimicrobial activity using the broth dilution method. Growth inhibitory activity was found against *Candida krusei, E. coli, Penicillium viridactum, Staphylococcus aureus, Streptococcus faecalis* and, from lower concentrations of the dermatophytes, *Trichophyton mentagrophytes, Microsporum gypseum, M. canis,* and *Epidermophyton floccosum.* A 45% ethanol extract was less potent than a 90% ethanol extract, which was comparable in potency to an ether extract (Pepeljnjak et al., 1996). In the leaves and fruits, the iridoids agnoside and aucubin, and the flavonoids casticin, orientin, iso-orientin, vitexin, isovitexin, and xyloside have shown significant growth-inhibitory activity against *Bacillus megaterium, B. cereus,* and *S. aureus* (Gomaa et al., 1978). Volatile oils of the leaf are believed to be the antimicrobial and insecticidal principles (Snow, 1996). The efficacy of vitex in the treatment of acne vulgaris may be due in part to antibiotic activity, although hormonal influences may be primarily responsible (Werbach and Murray, 1994). Positive in vitro activity from the essential oil, iridoids, and ethanolic extracts of the flowers, fruits, and leaves of *V. agnus-castus* were found against the growth of *Bacillus subtilis, Candida albicans, E. coli,* and *Shigella sonei* (Kustrak et al., 1987).

Neurological, Psychological, and Behavioral Functions

Receptor- and Neurotransmitter-Mediated Functions

Vitex has long been used clinically for the relief of symptoms associated with the menstrual cycle, including PMS and PMTS, oligomenorrhea, polymenorrhea, infertility, and other associated conditions (e.g., acne). It has been hypothesized for several decades that the gynecological effects of vitex could not be explained by a direct hormone-like action, but could be explained through an indirect action on the hypothalmus-pituitary axis (Böhnert, 1997). Studies showed that vitex fruit extracts decreased the number of cystic and bloody follicles and increased the size of the corpus luteum in ovaries of experimentally altered guinea pigs. It was postulated that these effects were due to lowered levels of follicle-stimulating hormone (FSH) and increased levels of luteinizing hormone (LH). Researchers then also erroneously postulated that the increased corpus luteum in animals was evidence of increased prolactin levels (Böhnert, 1997).

It has now been demonstrated that vitex fruit extract has a dopamine-agonist action, in turn exerting an antiprolactin effect at the hypothalamus-pituitary level (Jarry et al., 1991; Sliutz et al., 1993; Jarry et al., 1994; Wuttke et al., 1995; Meier et al., 2000). The possibility of increased secretion of dopamine caused by vitex was ruled out (Wuttke et al., 1995).

Using Agnolyt (liquid extract of *V. agnus-castus*), Wuttke (1992) reported a concentration-dependent decrease in prolactin secretion in isolated rat pituitary cells in culture. Competition for dopamine receptors could be inferred from the interference of the dopamine agonist, as previously reported by Madaus Co. in 1994. Sliutz et al. (1993) demonstrated that an ethanol extract of vitex inhibited prolactin secretion in rat pituitary cells by directly binding to the dopamine receptor. Jarry et al. (1991), using an extract of vitex seeds, demonstrated dopamine D_2 receptor binding, accompanied by prolactin inhibition in rat pituitary cells. In vitro, LH and FSH release were unchanged. Using the rat striatum dopamine receptor assay, Jarry et al. (1994) demonstrated that at 0.5 and 1 mg/mL in vitro, a freeze-dried extract of the seeds (prepared using 60% ethanol) could significantly inhibit basal prolactin release by dopamine ($p < 0.05$). The D_2 tracer (radiolabeled D_2 receptor ligand sulpride, a D_2 antagonist) was significantly ($p < 0.05$) and dose-dependently displaced by the extract, which showed a competitive displacement otherwise found from approximately 10^{-5} M dopamine. Using the MTT test, they showed the effect was not due to cytotoxicity. In a separate in vitro experiment, they also showed that gonadotropin secretion was not affected by the vitex extract at any concentration they tested, even under stimulated conditions of incubation with releasing hormone or with basal cells releasing FSH and LH-RH (Jarry et al., 1994).

Wuttke et al. (1995) isolated three fractions from a water-soluble extract of vitex that contained 3.3 mg of water-soluble substances/mL. The fractions showed prolactin release-inhibitory activity in vitro, one with slight activity and two with comparably high potency in cultivated lactotropes (prolactin-producing cells in the pituitary which express the dopamine receptor D_2 subtype). Using specific radiolabeled D_2 receptor and D_1 receptor ligands, fraction R 5000 was able to displace both the D_2 and D_1 receptor subtype and was further fractionated to yield three active fractions, one of which again showed more potency than the others, an activity they confirmed in vitro and in vivo with rats. Like dopamine, these fractions proved highly thermolabile, showing loss of dopaminergic activity after storage at room temperature for 24 h. The researchers speculated that antioxidants, such as flavonoids in extracts of vitex, protect the dopaminergic principles.

Jarry et al. (2000) tested the prolactin-lowering activity of nine commercial samples of vitex sold in German pharmacies according to an in vitro dopaminergic activity assay. Although additives in two of the more potent extracts showed no significant activity, they found a tenfold difference in dopaminergic activity between the different formulations examined, thereby stressing the need for biological standardization and batch testing.

Recent research involving the berries has shown that their use in the treatment of diseases in which prolactin is oversecreted (e.g., PMS, corpus luteum insufficiency) may be attributed to dopaminergic activity specific to constituents that interact with the dopamine D_2 receptor (Meier et al., 2000). Since specific diterpene constituents in the berries were characterized that exhibit dopamine D_2 receptor activity and quantitatively corresponded with contents of the main flavonoid casticin (Hoberg et al., 1999), methods of standardization of vitex extracts will undoubtedly advance.

In a dopamine-D_2-receptor test for in vitro binding-inhibitory activity, Hoberg et al. (2000) identified the diterpenes rotundifuran and $6\beta,7\beta$-diacetoxy-13-hydroxy-labda-8,14-diene as active constituents, each exhibiting activity in bioactively possible ranges of concentration (IC_{50} 79 and 45 µg/mL, respectively), compared to butaclamol as the standard. Samples of commercial ethanolic extracts of the berries (Ze 440) showed comparable binding affinities (IC_{50} 40-70 µg/mL). When even greater potency was found from a hexane extract of the berries (IC_{50} 15 µg/mL), the researchers postulated that still other compounds in the extract may be acting synergistically with the diterpenes. These studies were elucidated by Meier et al. (2000) who reported that a concentrated powder extract of the berries (batch V23/95, prepared by extraction with ethanol, 60% v/v) exhibited in vitro binding-inhibition for the dopamine D_2 receptor with an IC_{50} of 40 ± 8 µg/ mL. Tests of subfractions prepared from a methanolic extract (80%) of the powder using hexane, butanol, chloroform, or water revealed that the hexane extract was the only active fraction and that it contained diterpenes and fatty acids. From this, inhibition of dopamine D_2 receptor binding was found from the two diterpenes and from linoleic acid (IC_{50} 40 ± 12 µg/mL), whereas constituents from the other solvent subfractions were inactive (i.e., aucubin, casticin, orientin, homoorientin, vitexin, isovitexin, and vitexilactone).

In further in vitro receptor-binding studies, Meier et al. (2000) found that the concentrated extract (V23/95) showed no significant inhibitory activity for the 5-HT transporter, nor for benzodiazepine, histamine H_1, or OFQ (orphanin-FQ) receptors; however, significant binding–inhibitory activity was found in kappa, mu, and delta opioid receptors (κ, μ, and δ) (IC_{50} 22, 36, and 194 µg/mL, respectively). Similar effects were observed from all the extracts on the kappa and mu receptors; however, little or no activity was exhibited for the delta receptor except by the water-soluble fraction (IC_{50} 58 mg/mL). Although no activity was found from the aqueous extract in an in vitro assay of norepinephrine release using functional α_2-adrenoreceptors, it showed a concentration-dependent inhibitory effect on acetylcholine release; an effect dose-dependently antagonized by a D_2 receptor antagonist (spiperone).

Reproductive Functions

Lactation Functions

The influence of vitex on lactation is currently unknown; human studies, performed in the 1940s and 1950s, claim lactogenic effects are disputable since the methodology used was inadequate by today's standards of lactation research. However, it must be kept in mind that full characterization of the activity of vitex at the D_2 receptor has yet to be elucidated; therefore, effects on lactation are still unknown. A summary of these earlier studies appears in the Clinical Studies section.

Studies of lactation performance in rats administered vitex were carried out by Winterhoff et al. (1991). Subcutaneous injection of vitex or saline solution for 14 days postpartum was associated with a rising cumulative mortality of the suckling rats. Vitex treatment was also associated with a reduced occurrence of "milk spots" in the suckling rats. These effects were attributed to lethal malnutrition due to prolactin inhibition (Madaus Co., 1994). Moreover, increased prolactin secretion resulting from ether-induced stress in male rats was markedly reduced by a water-soluble extract of vitex (60 mg i.v.) (Wuttke et al., 1995).

CLINICAL STUDIES

Endocrine and Hormonal Disorders

Hypothalamic and Pituitary Functions

The mammotropic neuropeptide prolactin is a pituitary hormone released by the pituitary under regulation by various factors, most notably by dopamine which inhibits pituitary prolactin release. Thyrotropin releasing hormone (TRH) and vasoactive intestinal peptide (VIP) stimulate prolactin release. In sleep, prolactin levels are at their highest during the last 60-120 min before awakening. During the deep phases of sleep and under stressful events, prolactin release is induced by a decrease in hypothalamic dopamine release and/or an increase in peptides released by the hypothalamus that stimulate prolactin release, thereby resulting in abnormally high levels of prolactin release. The result of high prolactin levels in women is increased lactation, and in mammary tissues, stimulation of lobuloaveolar growth; the latter resulting in painful breasts, premenstrual mastodynia, and premenstrual symptoms. In women who have "latent prolactinemia," stressful events and the deep phases of sleep result in higher serum prolactin levels, which persist for longer periods of time than found in normal controls (Biller, 1999). In women, hyperprolactinemia can also result in abnormal cyclic ovarian function, loss of libido, amenorrhea, occasional hirsutism, and an increased risk over the long-term of osteoporosis. In men, hyperprolactinemia can cause impotence, low sperm production, and loss of libido (Petty, 1999) and may be caused by antipsychotic medication (Dickson and Glazer, 1999). Experimental hyperprolactinemia in rats resulted in altered mitochondria of spermatozoa (Laszczynska et al., 1999) and hypogonadism (Huang et al., 1999).

Hyperprolactinemia may be caused by pregnancy, hypothyroidism (Biller, 1999), conventional antipsychotic medications (Lader, 1999), estrogens, opioids, thyroid-releasing factor, epilepsy, physical or psychic stress, herpes zoster infection, or surgery (Petty, 1999). Elevated levels of prolactin are associated with systemic lupus erythematosus (Ostensen, 1999; Chikanza, 1999), adult rheumatoid arthritis (Neidhart et al., 1999), stimulated immune function, autoimmune thyroiditis, cardiac allograft rejection (Chikanza, 1999), multiple sclerosis (Azar and Yamout, 1999), Sjogren's syndrome (Haga and Rygh, 1999), acne, infertility, headache, and pituitary tumors (prolactinomas). Prescription medications used to manage hyperprolactinemia are typically dopamine agonists such as pergolide, bromocriptine, and the more recent cabergoline, all of which commonly cause side effects of orthostatic dizziness or nausea (Biller, 1999).

Merz et al. (1996) surmised that based on the dopaminergic activity of vitex, new applications may come about for medical conditions for which an increased prolactin secretion might require higher dosages of the extract. For that reason they studied the dosage tolerance of a mostly water- and alcohol-free "thick" extract prepared from the ripe, dried fruits of *V. agnus-castus* (special extract BP1095E1) in 20 healthy male subjects, ages 20-32. Men were chosen because they show less variability in hormone status, even though their prolactin levels are lower compared to women. Because data was lacking on the tolerability and harmlessness of the high doses examined, blinding and randomization were obviated. The placebo-controlled clinical trial was run as an intraindividual and open comparison study of tolerance to three different daily doses of the extract (120 mg, 240 mg, and 480 mg), each taken daily in 40-mg soft gelatin capsules for 14 days at 8 a.m., 2 p.m., and 8 p.m. A washout phase of at least one week preceded each phase of the study. The study also sought to confirm the effect of the extract on prolactin secretion compared to placebo (soft gelatin capsules containing emulsifiers and vegetable oil). When individual variations measured as a sum from each phase were compared to that of the placebo phase sum using the *t*-test, the lowest dose of vitex appeared to decrease the 24-h serum prolactin level by more than 15%, then falling by a further 6% after the middle and highest dose to produce a final decrease in prolactin of 21% compared to placebo. However, because of individual differences in initial levels and the small number of participants, the researchers could not say for certain that the effect of the vitex extract on serum prolactin levels, which were minimal, was significant. The researchers found reason to suspect that the extract exerts both dopamine antagonistic and agonistic actions, with antagonistic action appearing more obvious at the lower dosage (Merz et al., 1996).

Overall, the three doses of extract were judged to be well tolerated. Temporary adverse effects were reported by a total of 13 subjects, including a sports injury in one subject taking placebo. The researchers found no evidence of dose dependency to any of the symptom complaints as a result of the increasing doses of vitex, and no one discontinued treatment. In most cases, the researchers could not ascertain a relation between the adverse event and the extract, although the number in which they could was not revealed. No changes in clinical chemistry were ascribable to the extract; nor were there any effects on serum concentrations of testosterone, FH, or FSH, and blood pressure and heart rate showed no change compared to placebo (Merz et al., 1996).

In women with normal menstrual cycles, gonadotrophin-releasing hormone (Gn-RH) is released in a pulsatile manner, leading to FSH release by the pituitary. FSH initiates follicle development. The developing follicle produces estradiol under the stimulus of LH, also released from the pituitary under Gn-RH control. The rise in estradiol triggers release of further LH and FSH surges at midcycle. The follicle then predominantly secretes progesterone until the oocyte is released (Lawrence, 1994). In lactating women, the pulsatile secretion of Gn-RH is altered or suppressed. The exact roles of suckling and associated higher prolactin levels in producing this effect are complex and not fully understood. It is observed, however, that follicle development is arrested at an early stage. Ultrasonic examination of the ovary of lactating, noncycling women shows no medium- or large-sized follicles during lactation. This suppression of follicle development is due to suppression of estradiol. Lawrence (1994) states, "it is clear that frequent suckling, which results in high prolactin levels, is closely associated with altered luteinizing hormone (LH) secretion and amenorrhea" (Lawrence, 1994, p. 450). It is known that nipple stimulation does result in an inhibition of dopamine secretion from the hypothalamus, with a resultant rise in prolactin levels, concurrent Gn-RH suppression, and resultant suppressed ovarian function, including lowered FSH, LH, and estrogen hormone levels. A separate proposed mechanism for lactational amenorrhea suggests that prolactin itself may also directly reduce ovarian response to gonadotrophins from the pituitary (Lawrence, 1994).

In contrast to the normal state of high prolactin and suppressed ovulatory function in breast-feeding women, women with hyperprolactinemia often present with symptoms associated with disordered follicular development and corpus luteum insufficiency. Over half of all women (62%) suffering from various menstrual problems have been found hyperprolactinemic (Böhnert, 1997). Conversely, hyperprolactinemic women almost always suffer various menstrual disorders (Neville and Neifert, 1983).

It has recently been postulated that vitex acts primarily to correct hyperprolactinemia, with a resultant reversal of the LH suppression, thus allowing full development of the corpus luteum during the luteal phase of the menstrual cycle (Böhnert, 1997). As the corpus luteum produces progesterone, levels of this hormone are also normalized. It has been verified in clinical studies that vitex does lower prolactin levels in hyperprolactinemic states, slightly lowers FSH levels, and increases LH and progesterone levels with concurrent alleviation of menstrual difficulties (Böhnert and Hahn, 1990; Böhnert, 1997). Women with hyperprolactinemia typically have abnormally low LH and progesterone levels that are now considered secondary to their abnormally high prolactin levels (Böhnert, 1997).

Vitex has often been described as "correcting" the estrogen/progesterone ratio in these women. It is apparent that vitex acts as a dopamine agonist, thus lowering prolactin levels to those of normal cycling women. This state is associated with increased gonadotrophin-releasing hormone (Gn-RH) function or release dynamics, with normal ovarian response to pituitary hormones. This would result in restoration of a normal pulsatile release of FSH and, subsequently, of LH and normal luteal development. The fully developed corpus luteum can then secrete normal amounts of estrogen and progesterone in the luteal phase of the menstrual cycle.

In a randomized, double-blind placebo-controlled study of 52 women with latent hyperprolactinemia, Milewicz et al. (1993) reported a lowered prolactin level after three months of treatment with a vitex extract (Strotan capsules, 20 mg/day). In these women, a shortened luteal phase and low progesterone levels had both normalized. At trial entry, they showed prolactin levels of 120 ng/mL at 30 min and 70 ng/mL at 15 min after thyrotropin-relleasing hormone (TRH) challenge at 200 μg, i.v. The luteal phase was found to have lengthened by five days. Midluteal progesterone levels, which were low before treatment, were found to be normal three months later ($p < 0.001$ versus placebo). All other hormonal parameters showed no change, with the exception of β-estradiol, which was significantly increased in the luteal phase of the women receiving vitex ($p < 0.001$ versus placebo). In addition, women in the vitex group who had PMS symptoms showed a significant reduction in symptoms. In this study, no side effects were noted and two out of 17 women in the vitex group became pregnant. No such changes were noted in the placebo group.

In a study using the vitex preparation Mastodynon N, 13 women with hyperprolactinemia and cyclic disorders were treated for three months. In all of the patients, prolactin levels were reduced, some to within normal range, and the menstrual cycle normalized (Roeder, 1994).

Integumentary, Muscular, and Skeletal Disorders

Skin Diseases

Acne. The Madaus Company Agnolyt information booklet (1994) describes several clinical studies of treating acne of various kinds with vitex, some of which were concurrent with PMS. In one study, 118 patients were treated with Agnolyt drops for 12-24 months. Their response was compared to a group of 43 patients with comparable acne who received "conventional acne treatment." The treatment group were reported to have healed more quickly with fewer recurrences. Madaus states that other German studies performed in the 1970s and 1980s confirmed these findings. Hobbs (1990) states that according to Madaus Company's information, both young men and women can be treated for acne with vitex, and Werbach and Murray (1994) include vitex as a treatment for acne.

Reproductive Disorders

The majority of clinical studies with vitex have been large, uncontrolled investigations to observe its effects as an initial intervention in menstrual disorders, including PMS, PMTS, hypermenorrhea, polymenorrhea, amenorrhea, oligomenorrhea, and infertility. Many of these conditions are described in the studies as related to corpus luteum insufficiency. Since this condition has recently become thought of as generally secondary to hyperprolactinemic states, the following review will focus first on studies of well-defined hyperprolactinemia treated with vitex before studies focusing on corpus luteum insufficiency (CLI), with and without concurrent hyperprolactinemia.

Other clinical studies of vitex, especially earlier ones, included women suffering from a wide spectrum of disorders related to the menstrual cycle: symptoms associated with hyperprolactinemia, CLI, PMS, PMTS, uterine fibroids, and premenopausal symptoms. However, the earliest clinical studies sought to explore the folk reputation of vitex as a galactogogue.

Infertility (Female)

Several studies have shown beneficial results with vitex in treating women with corpus luteum insufficiency (CLI). This condition is most easily defined by an abnormally low serum progesterone level three weeks after the onset of menstruation (less than 10-12 ng/mL). These levels are normal at puberty and at menopause, but pathological when arising between the ages of 20-40 years. Associated signs would be unduly curtailed or prolonged menstrual periods with or without menagorrhea. Anovulatory periods and resultant infertility often occur. Mastopathy and PMS may also occur. Although the vast majority of women with these symptoms may primarily suffer hyperprolactinemia, latent hypothyroidism or hyperandrogenemia (often related to obesity) may also be involved in cases showing signs of corpus luteum insufficiency (Propping and Katzorke, 1987; Propping et al., 1988).

Bubenzer (1983) recounted the results of a clinical trial by Dr. H. Kokemohr of Hamburg who conducted a placebo-controlled double-blind study of vitex extract in 52 women diagnosed with corpus luteum insufficiency and abnormal menstrual cycles. After the treatment (Strotan, 20 mg/day for three cycles), Kokemohr found the previous luteal phase, which averaged 5.5 days, had changed to 10.5 days; the previous 23.8-day extended-follicle phase had reduced to 18.5 days; and a highly significant reduction in the prolactin reserve had occurred, which reduced levels below those at baseline and compared to the placebo group. By comparison, the placebo group showed no such changes. A significant increase also occurred in progesterone and estrogen levels compared to placebo, and premenstrual complaints in the verum group became almost completely resolved. During the three-month treatment with the extract, three women who were previously unable to conceive became pregnant (Bubenzer, 1983).

An observatory study of vitex in the treatment of 120 patients with fairly heterogenic menstrual disorders was reported by Dr. J. Schnitker of Bielfeld, Germany. The results of treatment by 19 doctors using vitex preparations showed that, on average, 21% of the patients suffered from polymenorrheas for one year, 37% had premenstrual syndrome with various complaints and, while 42% were diagnosed with oligomenorrheas, 60% wished to become pregnant. Therapy consisted of a very low dosage of vitex (20 mg/day) for at most six cycles, or an average of four to five months. After treatment with vitex, cyclical phases normalized in 63% of the patients with pathologically extended follical phases and a similar number improved in terms of the luteal phase. After treatment, temperatures normalized in those who had disturbed temperature readings during their cycles (climbing type), yet only a mild improvement in hormonal changes was found. Collectively, progesterone levels rose from 6.5 ng/mL to 9.3 ng/mL, which was an advantage to those with very low levels at baseline. Patient evaluations of the vitex treatment showed that 50% felt the therapy was very good, while 75% felt it was acceptable. Side effects were reported by 5% to 10% of the patients who complained of feeling ill, headaches, or flatulence; however, 75% evaluated the treatment as being well tolerated (Bubenzer, 1983).

To evaluate the use of vitex in situations not apparently related to abnormal prolactin, thyroid, or androgen disorders, Propping and Katzorke (1987) carried out an open noncontrolled study of a select group of 18 infertile women of normal weight and childbearing age with normal prolactin values and normal thyroid function. All had abnormally low progesterone levels on day 20 of the menstrual cycle. After three months of treatment (Agnolyt, 40 drops/day), those parameters were remeasured. In seven patients, progesterone rose to normal levels and in four cases progesterone levels were increased more than two units above initial levels. Two women became pregnant. Basal body temperature, although not considered a reliable indicator of ovarian function, was observed to have a longer, more normal hyperthermic phase in all but four of the women. No side effects were noted (Propping and Katzorke, 1987). This study represents the first on vitex in which sensitive endocrinological assays were used in patient selection and monitoring.

Further clinical work on 48 more of this select population of women was described by Propping et al. (1988). Apparently, clients came to them for treatment of infertility of several years' duration. After eliminating other causes of sterility, and where ovulatory cycles were probably occurring as evidenced by progesterone levels greater than 7 ng/mL, vitex was used as the initial treatment. Propping and colleagues considered use of vitex as an initial treatment in this narrowly defined population to be desirable and described combining vitex therapy stepwise with synthetic hormones as needed, both to correct luteal insufficiency and to increase fertility; however, no published studies of such a combination therapy could be found.

Lactation Disorders

A number of small pilot galactogogue studies of vitex were done in Germany in the 1940s and early 1950s; though limited by very small sample sizes and judged at the time to be of inadequate design, they all yielded some evidence of galactogogue activity in women (Mohr, 1954). The most widely quoted study was that of Mohr (1954). This study was conducted with a total of 102 women treated with vitamin B_1 (at the time thought to assist milk production), 353 women treated with a vitex fruit extract ("Alyt"), and 362 women who received no treatment or placebo. A quantitative description of Alyt specifying degree of fruit extract concentration is not available. The researchers excluded those given vitamin B_1, as little response was seen. They also excluded women discharged home before 11 days, so the results were based only on those who remained hospitalized after birth due mainly to birth or lactation complications, including mastitis. Study results were based on 79 untreated women and 62 treated women who remained hospitalized over 11 days. The study was controlled but not blinded and suffers from lack of statistical testing; to modern eyes the lactation protocols were rudimentary at best. As a result, no scientific proof of efficacy or safety for the use of vitex during lactation can be derived from this study.

Despite these limitations, the study cannot be overlooked entirely as it is apparent that a definite trend in the data indicates galactogogue activity. Although it is difficult to have confidence in the authors' methodology for measuring milk production, the data comparing rates of duration of breast-feeding are probably reliable. The study period presumably ended on day 20 postpartum, as provided charts end on that day. Mohr (1954) found that among the 62 women who received vitex (45 drops of Alyt t.i.d.), all but one (1.6%) were breast-feeding upon discharge. This contrasts with 10 of the 79 untreated women (7.9%) who were no longer breast-feeding at discharge. Their conclusion: impairment of lactation due to puerperal complications was reversed by treatment with Alyt. Given the antibacterial activity documented for vitex, perhaps the herb helped in a more rapid resolution of mastitis; this possibility was not mentioned in the study. The authors report that urticarial rash and pruritis occurred in 15 patients, reversed with treatment withdrawal or medical intervention. Interestingly, they also noted that "some patients" had an early resumption of menses; unfortunately, no details are given on how long after birth this occurred. Normally, a non-lactating woman has no menses for six weeks, while the fully lactating woman may go many months or even years without resuming menstruation.

Mastalgia

Double-blind, placebo-controlled clinical trials of vitex (Mastodynon N) in the treatment of mastalgia conducted in small numbers of patients have reported good results (Kubista et al., 1983; Wuttke et al., 1995).

A randomized, placebo-controlled, double-blind multicenter trial of vitex extract (Mastodynon solution, 30 drops b.i.d.) in the treatment of cyclical mastalgia in 120 women (ages 23-40) was reported by Wuttke et al. (1997). The trial utilized a parallel group design and a double-dummy technique with tablet and liquid extract forms of the extract and corresponding placebos. All patients had experienced mastalgia for three or more cycles and suffered breast pain during a minimum of three days of the cycle. Patients reported changes in breast pain intensity using a linear analogue scale (VAS), and prolactin vales were obtained in cycles 0 and 3 after metoclopramide stimulation. The researchers found the following results compared to placebo: after cycle 1 the solution acted more quickly than the tablets; neither formulation showed any effect on FSH, LH, or progesterone; values for estradiol decreased only somewhat more from vitex; and basal levels of prolactin showed a significant decrease from the solution (4.35 ng/mL, $p = 0.039$) or the tablets (3.7 ng/mL, $p = 0.015$). Compared to placebo, premenopausal symptoms of headache, abdominal pains, psychological symptoms, and a tendency to edemas were more rarely indicated in both the tablet and solution groups; pain-free days increased in number by 15% for the vitex groups versus 8% for the placebo group; estradiol levels showed a stronger tendency to decrease in the vitex tablet and solution groups (25.7 and 28.5 pg/mL, respectively) compared to placebo (10.8 pg/mL); and prolactin levels between cycles 0 and 3 showed a significant decrease of 4.35 ng/mL (Mann-Whitney U test) compared to basal levels. Adverse events reported by the vitex groups were mostly of minor to medium severity, with 18 instances in 13 patients in the vitex solution group and nine patients reporting 20 events in the vitex tablet group. The placebo group results showed eight patients with 13 instances of adverse events (Wuttke et al., 1997).

Halaska et al. (1999) conducted a randomized, double-blind placebo-controlled trial of a vitex extract-containing solution in the treatment of 97 women diagnosed (ages 18-45) with cyclical mastalgia. The daily dose of the solution (30 drops b.i.d. for three menstrual cycles) provided the equivalent of 32.4 mg *Vitex agnus-castus* extract per day (10 g containing 20% mother tincture of vitex) and contained 53% alcohol. The only other ingredients in the solution were highly dilute homeopathic preparations consisting of 20% *Iris* (dilution D4) and 10% each of *Ignatia* (D6), *Cyclamen* (D4), *Caulophyllum thalictroides* (D4), and *Lilium tigrinum* (D3). With the same dosage used by Wuttke et al. (1997) and a similar study design, Halaska and colleagues set out to confirm both the efficacy and tolerability of the vitex extract-containing solution (VECS). Ninety-seven women (ages 18-45) who had suffered with cyclic mastalgia on a minimum of five days were allowed entry to the trial

1. if they had used hormonal contraceptives for six months preceding and would continue at the same dosage throughout the trial;
2. had cycles lasting a maximum of 35 days and a minimum of 25 days during the preceding three cycles;
3. were not pregnant or lactating;
4. were not receiving treatment with NSAIDS or analgesics;
5. had not received alcohol detoxification; and
6. had none of the following medical conditions: breast cancer, impending or recent breast surgery, intraductal papilloma, fibroadenoma, galactorrhea, severe endocrinopathy, or bloody or purulent nipple discharge.

Examinations were carried out on four successive cycles. Efficacy was assessed using the visual analog scale (VAS) in which patients made a record of the intensity of their mastalgia on premenstrual days and the intention to treat principle. Patients also recorded the intensity of their pain as absent, moderate, or severe. Eleven patients dropped out of the trial after randomization (five VECS and six placebo); one each from the placebo and VECS groups because of adverse events (continual tiredness in the VECS patient) and the rest because of noncompliance. Data from these patients were included in the final analysis if they had also received a trial medication. In the first cycle that patients received treatment, the VECS group showed a mean reduction in pain of 30% versus 11% in the placebo group. After the second cycle, the VECS group showed a mean reduction in pain intensity of 53% versus 25% in the placebo group ($p = 0.006$ vs. $p = 0.018$); half the VECS group was free from severe pain. After the third cycle, only a slight decrease in pain had occurred in the VECS group compared to placebo. At the end of the treatment, the VECS group showed a total reduction in pain intensity of 54% compared to 40% in the placebo group. According to VAS scale values, after two treatment cycles, 71.4% of the VECS group had an almost negligible level of pain whereas the placebo group still had pain; after the third cycle, 75% of the VECS group only had verve pain during < 10% of the days of their cycle. The difference during cycles 3 and 4 was significant compared to placebo ($p = 0.015$ versus $p = 0.021$) and corresponded with the increase in numbers of pain-free days. Adverse events, all only slight, were recorded by five in the VECS group and by four in the placebo group. Cyclic anomalies were reported by three patients in each group and coxarthritis and irregular bleeding were each reported by one patient in the placebo group. The only other adverse event reported was continual tiredness by an early dropout in the VECS group. The researchers concluded that the results of their trial justify the use of VECS for ≥ 3 months in women who have severe breast pain before considering the prescription of drugs with greater rates of side effects.

Menstrual Disorders

Many large "drug monitoring" clinical reports have been published on vitex, mostly using Agnolyt liquid extract and involving groups of women with a wide variety of menstrual difficulties, which will be briefly summarized. It is conceivable that in the drug monitoring studies from the 1990s many of the same women were included in more than one study.

Loch et al. (2000) described their findings of a multicentric open trial (noninterventional without control) on the efficacy and safety of a powder extract of vitex (Femicur capsules, Shaper & Brummer GmbH & Co. KG, Salzgitter, Germany) in 1,634 patients diagnosed with PMS. Patients had taken one capsule twice a day for the treatment of PMS; each capsule contained a concentrated, dried extract of the berries in an amount corresponding to 20 mg. The patients had suffered from the problem from less than 7 months to 6.3 years. Questionnaires designed to elicit information on efficacy and safety were given to 857 attending physicians to be completed from interviews with patients at the start of the therapy, and again after three menstrual cycles on the therapy. In addition, a qualitative and quantitative assessment of mastodynia was made on changes in its severity and frequency. After three months of treatment with the vitex extract, patients assessed their global improvement according to seven categories, ranging from very much worse to very much improved (Clinical Global Impression Scale 2). Patient compliance was 98%, and 90% of the attending physicians prescribed the recommended dosage. According to the self-assessments of the patients, 94% reported that their tolerance of the treatment was good to very good. Highly significant improvements were found in all categories of PMS and each symptom ($p < 0.001$), whether in complaints of a psychical nature (i.e. depression, symptoms of anxiety, sleep problems) or somatic complaints (i.e. headache/migraine, tiredness, vertigo, craving, bloating, joint/back pain, hyperhydration, pain/tension of the breasts, tachycardia, short-term weight gain at menstruation). Improvements in mastodynia were also reported highly significant ($p < 0.001$), whether in the number of patients still affected with the problem, which fell from 80.7% to 26.6% in three months, or in the particular symptoms of mastodynia (spontaneous pain of the breasts, tenderness, and tension). Symptoms of PMS decreased in 51% of the patients and 42% reported that they no longer suffered from the problem. Only 1% reported increased symptoms of PMS and for 6% there appeared to be no change at all. None of the patients were pregnant at entry to the trial; however, most of those who became pregnant (19/23 patients) were among the 8% of cases in the trial who were never able to become pregnant before (Loch et al., 2000).

Treatment was terminated by 7% of patients: 2.6% because of lack of improvement; 1.1% because of adverse events; 1.0% due to total recovery; 1.0% owing to substantial improvement; 0.8% because of pregnancy; 1.3% owing to other reasons; and for 0.3% no reason was given. None of the suspected symptoms or adverse events during the treatment were serious. The most commonly reported, made by 13 patients (0.8%), were epidermal or mucosal in nature, such as acne, allergic reaction, eczema, hair loss, itching, and urticaria. The next most common, reported by six patients (0.4%), were gastrointestinal symptoms, including diarrhea, stomach pain, nausea, vomiting, and abdominal distention. Incidences of patients reporting spotting, edema, vertigo, or nosebleeds were each less than 0.1% (Loch et al., 2000).

Christie and Walker (1997-1998) provided the results of a questionnaire on vitex use with responses from 153 members of the National Institute of Medical Herbalists practicing in England and Ireland in 1997. Among their findings, they reported that the vast majority (94.1%) prescribed vitex for the treatment of PMS, with 86.3% prescribing it for hot flashes and peri-menopausal complaints, and 98.6% believing the herb to be "very effective" or "effective" for treating hormonal imbalance syndromes in female patients. A majority of respondents (68.5%) claimed their patients showed responses to vitex in four to eight weeks. The majority also prescribed vitex for treating female infertility (89.5%) and female acne (79.7%). Prescribing vitex to patients taking conventional progestogenic or estrogenic drugs was avoided by 70.5%; yet 93.8% claimed they had found no drug interactions with vitex. The mean length of treatment with vitex in PMS was 4.8 months and for "menopausal symptoms," 7.1 months. Prescriptions of vitex to male patients was found in 17.1% of practitioners, with acne the most frequent (10.5%) symptom among male patients. The most common time of day for administration was morning (68.5%). Vitex "powdered herb preparations" were used by 9.2% (mean dosage 1,182 mg/day), fluid extracts by 28.1% (average dosage 13.9 drops/day, approximately equivalent to 700 mg/day dried vitex berries), and tinctures were used by 86.4% (mean dosage 2.2 mL/day equivalent to 440 mg of dried vitex berries). Scarcely any practitioners ($n = 5$) used standardized solid extracts of vitex (mean dosage 413 mg/day). As for side effects, 59.9% of respondents reported none; 15.6% reported minor side effects (e.g., headache and nausea); 13.6% reported single cases of minor side effects (headaches, nausea, heavier menstrual bleeding, length of cycle changed); and less (10.5%) reported the occurrence of minor side effects from dosages that were too high or that only appeared at the start of therapy.

A focused drug-monitoring study analysis of a mixed age population of 1,542 women diagnosed with PMS (as defined above) was carried out. In addition to PMS, some patients had diagnoses of CLI ($n = 1,016$), uterine fibroids ($n = 170$), menopausal symptoms ($n = 90$), or other diagnoses ($n = 493$). In addition, 603 women had previously been treated with other medications for these symptoms. Agnolyt drops (range 20-120 drops; average 42 drops/day) were taken over variable periods (7 days to 16 years). Efficacy was separately rated by patients and their doctors, although the dissatisfaction rate was about the same for both assessors: ~ 4.5%. Symptom improvement began after a mean of 25.3 ± 27 days (the scatter was very wide, ranging from one day to one year). Treatment was discontinued in only 58 cases (3.8%) because of inadequate effects. Thirty-two patients noted undesirable side effects (2.1%), but only 17 stopped treatment because of them. The most common occurring side effect noted within this population was nausea, which was reported in five patients. Other side effects, such as allergy, diarrhea, acne, pruritus, cardiac palpitation, heartburn, etc., occurred at a frequency of 1% to 3% of the participants, and "unknown side effects" occurred in seven (Dittmar et al., 1992).

Propping et al. (1991) reported the results of a multicenter (314 gynecologists) drug-monitoring study involving vitex tincture (Agnolyt) given to 1,592 women mainly for menstrual disorders and PMS, with CLI being the most prevalent diagnosis. Diagnoses of mastodynia (breast discomfort) and acne were included under PMS. The mean treatment was six months and the mean dose was 43 drops. The doctors reported a good or satisfactory response in 90% of the cases; only 6.5% of the women noted no response,

5.5% discontinued the study early for lack of response, and 4.4% (70 cases) became pregnant. Of the 145 patients who expressed the wish to have a child, 56 did become pregnant. Adverse effects were noted in 2.4% of the women, with nausea in seven cases, changes in menstrual rhythm in five cases, acne, skin rashes, and headache in three each, and dyspepsia and redness of the skin in two each. Fourteen out of the 39 patients with adverse effects discontinued treatment for these reasons.

Loch et al. (1991) reported on two drug-monitoring studies using Agnolyt drops on a total of 3,162 women, with 2,447 having menstrual disorders of some kind, in some cases for up to nine years. A total of 632 gynecologists took part. PMS was diagnosed in nearly half of the patients ($n = 1,016$) and CLI in 734 women with menstrual disturbances. Other diagnoses were uterine myomas ($n = 320$) and menopausal symptoms ($n = 167$). The mean duration of treatment was 153 days; the mean dose used was 42 drops/day. Efficacy was rated at 90%, variously rated by doctors and patients: good/very good response by doctors, 68%, with 31% of the women reporting complete disappearance of symptoms, with improvement starting after about one month (wide range); 2.9% of the women became pregnant; 1.0% of the women discontinued treatment due to side effects; and 2.3% ($n = 56$) reported side effects. Although details were not available on 13 of these cases, nausea was noted in eight cases, changes in period occurred in four, and diarrhea, weight increase, and headaches were reported in each of three cases. Other side effects were listed in one to two cases each (Loch et al., 1991).

Feldmann et al. (1990) investigated the use of vitex (Agnolyt tincture) for menstrual disturbances, which they related to CLI or ovarian dysfunction (hyperestrogenism/hyperfolliculinism). The sample was a total of 1,571 women. The average treatment lasted for 135 days and the mean dose was 40 drops of tincture/day taken on an empty stomach. No control group was used, in accordance with the concept of drug monitoring. The researchers report a response, as assessed by patient and doctor, to start at the end of 45.4 ± 28 days (range one to 365 days). They reported a response rate of "almost 90%." Failure to respond was the reason for premature withdrawal in 4.4% of the cases, and 10.9% were withdrawn by their physicians as they no longer had symptoms. Adverse effects were seen in 1.9% of the women: 12 cases of nausea, malaise, gastric symptoms, or diarrhea occurred. Single cases of allergy, weight gain, pyrosis, hypermenorrhea, and dizziness were also noted; 13 cases provided no details.

Attelman et al. (1972) reported on the use of vitex in over 2,000 cases of gynecological complaints, drawn from general and consulting practices of the researchers in Germany. The researchers described applications of vitex for PMS, polymenorrhea, hypermenorrhea due to uterine fibroids, headache associated with birth control pills, mastopathia, secondary amenorrhea, juvenile uterine bleeding, menopausal bleeding, sterility, and poor results with primary amenorrhea unless the patients were less than 15 years old. They report that in the treatment of menopausal symptoms, which they state occur with hyperfolliculinism and CLI secondarily, recurrent menopausal bleeding can seldom be avoided, even when continued after several months. They state that "only when Agnolyt begins to lose its effect is it necessary to change over to estrogens or other forms of treatment." The dose of Agnolyt tincture used was reported as 40 drops once daily, sometimes given t.i.d. after meals. One practitioner described 20 drops t.i.d. in refractory cases only. They noted that response to treatment begins not before three weeks, and sometimes only after six weeks. Most continued treatment for three to six months, and most felt at least three months of treatment was necessary to "consolidate the results." Side effects were noted as absent or rare in most practitioners' experience. One patient reported bilateral allergic varicophlebitis below the knee, which cleared up when Agnolyt was discontinued and did not recur.

Premenstrual Syndrome

PMS can be defined as a cyclic occurrence during the luteal phase of the menstrual cycle of a combination of symptoms—physical and/or psychological/behavioral—of such severity as to significantly interfere with normal activities and interpersonal relationships. Typically, such symptoms do not occur in the follicular phase and end abruptly with the onset of menstrual flow at the end of the luteal phase of menstruation. Over 100 different symptoms have been described in connection with PMS and a summary of the postulated causes of PMS is difficult. Dittmar et al. (1992) state that PMS is likely the outcome of a complex of poorly understood interactions between endocrine hormones, endogenous opiates, central and peripheral neurotransmitters, and prostaglandins. Psychological predisposition, lifestyle, stress, and stress response are also catalogued and undoubtedly play a role as well. Accordingly, this review reflects the fact that the treatment of PMS has been largely empirical.

Schellenberg (2001) reported excellent results from a vitex fruit extract (Ze 440, Zeller AG, Switzerland, a 60% ethanolic extract standardized to casticin content) in a randomized, double-blind, placebo-controlled parallel group design study performed over three menstrual cycles in 170 outpatients. Patients received the extract or an identical placebo in tablet form at a dosage of one 20-mg tablet/day. All patients entered into the trial were diagnosed with PMS according to the DSM-III-R and underwent a full examination, laboratory tests, and evaluation using CGI at the beginning of the first and at the end of the third cycle, when they also underwent self assessment, monitoring for adverse events, and checks for compliance. Although numerous exclusion criteria were implemented, use of oral contraceptives was permitted. Efficacy was primarily judged according to changes from baseline in combined scores of patient self-assessments of PMS symptoms (i.e., headache, irritability, mood swings, anger, bloating, breast fullness, and other menstrual symptoms). With the single exception of bloating and "other" menstrual symptoms that showed no change compared to placebo at the endpoint, major symptoms of PMS showed significant improvements, including mood swings, breast fullness, anger, irritability (each $p < 0.001$), and headache ($p < 0.002$). Also significant were improvement/deterioration scores, differences in self-assessment, and patients' overall assessment of benefit or risk (each $p < 0.001$). These assessments were corroborated by the attending physicians in evaluations of the CGI scale. Over half the patients experienced a 50% improvement in symptoms of PMS, and the few side effects noted were mild and, being prevalent in the population at large, may not have been related to treatment. Events were reported in only four patients (4.7%) in the vitex group (intermenstrual bleeding, acne, urticaria, multiple abscesses), and in three patients (4.8%) in the placebo group (gastric upset, acne, early menstrual period). One patient in the placebo group withdrew from the trial due to pregnancy whereas no withdrawals occurred in the vitex group. The researchers commented that the low incidence of adverse events may have been the result of knowledge by both patients and physicians that the treatments being administered were either placebo or "herbal."

Berger et al. (2000) conducted a prospective, multicenter trial on the efficacy of Ze 440 in the treatment of PMS. Fifty patients diagnosed with PMS according to the DSM-III received only one 20-mg tablet of Ze 440 daily for three menstrual cycles. Patients were assessed during two cycles at baseline and for three further cycles after the therapy phase, undergoing a minimum of three physical examinations and two laboratory evaluations, once at baseline and again at the end of the treatment phase. At baseline, plasma prolactin levels were normal. Of the 43 patients who completed the study, 13 were also taking oral contraceptives. Six left the study for reasons unrelated to the trial, and one left after four days of treatment because of headache and fatigue possibly related to the medication. The efficacy of the vitex preparation was mainly assessed using Moo's menstrual distress questionnaire (MMDQ), while secondary evaluations administered as patient self-assessments were made using a global impression scale and a visual analog scale. Similar to the trial by Schellenberg (2001), numerous exclusion criteria were applied, although use of oral contraceptives was allowed. At the end of the treatment period, significant benefits were found in MMDQ scores, which were 42.5% lower ($p < 0.001$) and remained about 20% lower than baseline at the end of the posttreatment period, a further three cycles after treatment was stopped ($p < 0.001$). Benefits were mainly found in reduced symptoms of fluid retention, pain, negative feelings, and behavioral changes. Twenty patients showed improvements of at least 50%. For these "responders," oral contraceptives had no effect on results, even in the posttreatment phase. The results were similar in the VAS score with a 47.2% reduction in symptoms persisting at 21.7% in the posttreatment phase (each $p < 0.001$), and oral contraceptives had no effect on the changes, nor on global efficacy, which was rated excellent by most of the patients (38/43) ($p < 0.001$) (Berger et al., 2000).

As for safety, adverse events were mild and of low incidence, including those in the patient who withdrew after reporting fatigue and headache. Berger et al. (2000) concluded that the treatment was "very well tolerated." Indeed, the most frequently reported adverse events were all those commonly reported by PMS patients regardless of the trial: acne ($n = 7$), headache ($n = 6$), spotting ($n = 5$), and gastrointestinal complaints ($n = 5$). In all, 37 events were reported by 20 patients over a total of 344 menstrual cycles in the study. Laboratory and medical examinations showed no influences of any kind relevant to the treatment. Serum prolactin levels showed no significant change compared to baseline when they were in all cases already at normal physiological levels (Berger et al., 2000)—a finding congruent with those of four other clinical trials in which vitex preparations decreased prolactin levels in patients with initially elevated levels. However, in three other trials of patients without elevated prolactin, basal levels were unaffected. Even so, symptoms of PMS improved after treatment with vitex (Blank et al., 2000).

Turner and Mills (1993) conducted a double-blind, placebo-controlled randomized trial of vitex in 600 women volunteers self-diagnosed with PMS, of whom only 217 completed the trial. Since the dropouts were evenly distributed among the placebo and verum groups, the researchers took this as an indication that the reasons for dropping out were unrelated to either treatment. No significant differences were found—between those withdrawing and those completing the trial—in age, employment, cycle lengths, or marital status. Evaluation was based on the Menstrual Distress Questionnaire. The results of the trial showed a statistically significant improvement in the vitex group in the symptom of "feel jittery or restless." No significant difference compared to placebo was found with respect to pain, fluid retention, or impaired concentration. The researchers concluded that for most of the symptoms associated with PMS, vitex was no more effective than placebo (soy based). However, they added that the albeit rigorous design of the trial showed some evidence of inadequately reflecting the total differences between the placebo and the vitex treatment (powdered *Vitex agnus castus* in 300-mg tablets, plant part not specified; 600 mg t.i.d. for three months and three cycles).

Premenstrual Tension Syndrome

A multicenter, randomized, double-blind controlled study of vitex focused on premenstrual tension syndrome (PMTS) (Lauritzen et al., 1997).

Of the 175 women who started, 105 fully completed the study. The control population received placebo twice daily during days 1 to 15 of the menstrual cycle and 100 mg pyridoxine (vitamin B_6) twice daily on days 16-35 of the cycle, a treatment of PMS symptoms that has some evidence of efficacy (Wyatt et al., 1999). The researchers decided that administering a placebo was unethical, given the degree of suffering in at least a third of the patient population. Therefore, the treated group took one capsule of vitex dried fruit extract (3.5-4.2 mg) and one capsule of placebo per day—placebo being included in the second daily capsule to preserve the double-blind nature of the study. The researchers claim that because the capsules looked identical and even the contents looked and tasted the same, the double-blind nature of the study was ensured. They sought to evaluate Agnolyt capsules, a new formulation from the Madaus Company. The treatment group received capsules standardized to agnuside, described as the most important 9-C-iridoid in the fruit extract, with HPLC analysis of Agnolyt liquid and capsule preparations having "corresponding peak patterns." The inclusion criteria for this study consisted of patients 18-45 years old with PMTS symptoms that consistently correlated with the luteal phase of the menstrual cycle and that were severe enough to interfere with quality of life. Patients also needed to be symptom free for at least a week during each cycle and not to have received during their three previous cycles a long inclusive list of medications, vitamins, phytopharmaceuticals, or minerals. However, no mention was made of diet (e.g., dietary sources of essential fatty acids, fish oils, etc.) (Lauritzen et al., 1997).

The Clinical Global Impression (CGI) scale showed that overall, efficacy was rated at 77.1% for vitex and 60.6% for pyridoxine. Investigators rated excellent efficacy at 24.6% for vitex and 12.1% for pyridoxine. In self-assessments, patients rated themselves free of symptoms in 36.1% of the vitex group and 21.1% of the pyridoxine group. The researchers concluded that while not statistically valid, these findings support the view that Agnolyt is "superior to pyridoxine with respect to these parameters." They also stated that to demonstrate any statistical significance, at least 100 subjects in each group were required, instead of the 105 in total that they used for analysis. It was the opinion of Lauritzen et al. (1997) that neither group suffered any "serious adverse events" and they concluded that the dried extract form of vitex (Agnolyt capsules) showed efficacy and safety in congruence with another study (Dittmar et al., 1992) performed with similarly defined PMTS patients treated with a Vitex liquid extract (Agnolyt drops).

The validity of the study by Lauritzen et al. (1997) is difficult to evaluate because no control group was used. Betz (1998) offers detailed criticisms of this study, commenting that trials of PMTS should be conducted using large numbers of patients with experimental and control cycles in which the subgroups are identified, including those with premenstrual dysphoric disorder (PMDD).

In a clinical study on the tolerance and effectiveness of a new dry extract form of vitex (Agnolyt capsules), Reuter et al. (1995) conducted a randomized, double-blind comparative trial using 175 mg/day against vitamin B_6 (pyridoxine, 200 mg/day). The two treatments were tested for three cycles in 175 women diagnosed with PMTS according to the PMTS scale; the scale was also used to evaluate the treatments according to six main symptoms of the syndrome along with the CGI scale and the evaluations of patients and physicians. The results showed that in the PMTS scale, points fell from an initial score of 15.2 before treatment to 5.1 after in the vitex groups, versus 11.9 points before treatment to 5.1 after in the vitamin B_6 group. With corresponding results in the CGI scale, the vitex group reported a greater diminishment of symptoms than the vitamin B_6 group in depressive moods, inner tension, headaches, edema, tension in the breasts, and constipation. Although for both treatment groups 80% of the physicians evaluated them as sufficient, only 12.1% evaluated vitamin B_6 as excellent versus 24.5% who gave vitex the same evaluation. Patient evaluations revealed that 21.3% in the vitamin B_6 group judged themselves free of symptoms, versus 36.1% in the vitex group. No serious side effects were reported by either group; however, five patients in the vitamin B_6 group and 12 in the vitex group noted short-term headaches, lower abdominal and gastrointestinal complaints, and skin phenomena. The researchers concluded that their study confirmed the harmlessness and effectiveness of the vitex extract (Reuter et al., 1995).

DOSAGE

Agnolyt liquid preparation: 58% alcohol, 100 g of solution containing 9 g tincture (1:5) of fruits, 40 drops/day (Madaus Co., 1994). This preparation is sometimes given in divided doses, 15 drops t.i.d. after meals, rarely 20 drops t.i.d. (Attelmann et al., 1972). Drops are taken for several months without interruption.

Agnolyt capsule: 175 mg dried vitex berries, 1:5 alcoholic extract capsule, taken once daily with liquid over several months without interruption (Madaus Co., 1994). Standardized preparations similar to this are currently being sold in the United States; for example, those containing 175 mg per capsule of a 20:1 fruit extract standardized to 0.5% agnusides. The recommended dose is one capsule per day. These dosage guidelines should be followed pending further clinical evaluations of the capsule formulation. Most clinical studies have used the Agnolyt liquid preparation, with doses averaging around 40 drops/day.

Strotan capsules (20 mg): alcoholic extract (50%-70% v/v), once daily (Milewicz et al., 1993) (Pharma Stroschein GmbH, Hamburg, Germany). No product literature is presently available.

Mastodyne N: detailed information is available in German only (Roeder, 1994). Mastodyne solution is described as an ethanol-water extract containing 55.4% ethanol by volume (Wuttke et al., 1997).

Ze 440 tablets (20 mg): 120-240 mg vitex berries, 6-12:1 ethanol (60% v/v), depending on individual tablet strength, one 20-mg tablet daily. Ze 440 is a new vitex preparation equivalent to V23/95, a dried ethanolic extract of vitex berries standardized to casticin content (Berger et al., 2000) as a marker of diterpene content (Hoberg et al., 1999). Similar to other extracts of vitex, it has shown activity in assays of dopamine D_2 receptor binding (Meier et al., 2000).

Femicur capsules (20 mg): 1.6-3.0 mg concentrated, dried extract of vitex berries, 6.7-12.5:1, one capsule b.i.d. Femicur is a new vitex preparation manufactured by Shaper & Brummer GmbH & Co. KG, Salzgitter, Germany (Loch et al., 2000).

SAFETY PROFILE

Although vitex preparations have been administered to large populations of human females for periods of months and even years, no definite significant or permanent adverse effects have been noted.

Contraindications

The German Commission E monograph (Blumenthal et al., 1998) reports no contraindications for vitex. Böhnert (1997) considers concomitant use of vitex with hormone therapy or oral contraceptives to be contraindicated, and states that vitex should be avoided during lactation due to its dopaminergic activity (see Pregnancy and Lactation). Brinker (1998, p. 55) speculates that vitex "may interfere with the efficacy of birth control pills."

Drug Interactions

The German Commission E monograph (Blumenthal et al., 1998) states that no drug interactions with *Vitex agnus-castus* are known.

Several clinical studies allude to treating menstrual disorders initially with vitex, then adding other treatments such as hormonal replacement as necessary. Studies of such combination therapies are lacking.

Recently documented reports of a dopamine agonist action, vitex may have the potential to interact with dopamine antagonists such as haloperidol and dopamine receptor-blocking agents, such as metoclopramide (Böhnert, 1997). As a speculative precaution based on dopaminergic activity, vitex may be contraindicated in patients taking MAOI, SSRI, or tricylic antidepressant agents.

Nocturnal seizures were reported by a 45-year-old woman taking evening primrose oil and black cohosh in addition to vitex (separate bottled products) to regulate her menstrual cycle. Yet her sister had taken the "same regimen" of herbs for one to two years apparently without incident. She experienced three nocturnal seizures in a span of three months and had been taking the herbal combination for about four months. She recalled that during the same period she had experienced facial flushing and fatigue. Although the seizures occurred only during sleep and she had no memory of them, they were noticed on two occasions by her boyfriend and once by her sister who together provided a description matching that of a "general tonic-clonic type of seizure." She awoke from the seizures in a confused state. After three days off the regimen, physicians found no positive signs; she was discharged with a prescription for carbamazepine to treat prophylaxis. The investigating pharmacist could find nothing in the literature to indicate central nervous system effects or seizures from any of the herbs, nor from the manufacturer of two of the products (Nature's Herbs, American Fork, Utah) (Shuster, 1996, p. 1554). The cause of the reported seizures was not resolved.

Pregnancy and Lactation

The American Herbal Products Association lists the berries of *Vitex agnus-castus* as an herb not to be used during pregnancy and for which the data available are not sufficient to make a classification of safety (McGuffin et al., 1997). Use of vitex during pregnancy was noted by Mohr (1954). He gave five women near term vitex drops with the intent of speeding up milk production after birth. He reported that the women soon started producing milk (premature lactogenesis), and that the milk leaking disappeared with discontinuation of the product.

Hobbs (1990) suggested that women may safely use vitex until after the first trimester, "which may help prevent miscarriage, according to research in Germany" (p. 13). No animal or human studies of vitex during pregnancy are available. Madaus Co. contraindicates vitex during pregnancy (Madaus Co., 1994). The German Commission E monograph (Blumenthal et al., 1998, p. 108) states there is "no application during pregnancy."

During unstimulated in vitro fertilization, following three hormonally normal cycles, a woman taking *Vitex agnus-castus* was reported to have developed disordered ovarian hormone and gonadotrophin measurements. Although pregnancy failed, she showed symptoms that would suggest a mild case of ovarian hyperstimulation syndrome in the luteal phase. Subsequently, her next two cycles were found endocrinologically normal (Cahill et al., 1994). One report attributed a negative outcome of in vitro fertilization in a patient concurrently using vitex (Fox et al., 1994).

It is not known if vitex constituents enter breast milk, though this is to be expected, similar to most other ingested substances. No reports of adverse effects on the infant are known from existing clinical trials (see Clinical Studies: Lactation Disorders) or elsewhere. The German Commission E monograph includes no contraindication for use during lactation; indeed, the authors indicate vitex as a galactogogue. However, this monograph was written before in vitro and in vivo dopaminergic, antiprolactin, and anti-lactogenic effects were documented. The effect of vitex on milk supply is very unclear at this time, with traditional and early experimental work supporting a galactogogue effect, while most in vitro, animal, and clinical studies of nonlactating women indicate an antigalactogogue effect. This seeming paradox can be solved only by further investigations of vitex with lactating animals given varying doses and for varying lengths of time. There is a distinct possibility that vitex may raise prolactin levels in low doses, or in the short term, while lowering prolactin levels at high doses, or with long-term use. Writing in the fourth century B.C., Hippocrates specified leaf preparations to "bring down the milk." This may indicate his awareness of the importance of dose, as the leaves contain less essential oils than the berries or seeds. The relationship of vitex with the hormone oxytocin or with the oxytocin receptor function is completely unexplored, as it is with most plants. Oxytocin is absolutely required for milk release in mammals, and is the main hormone orchestrating the expulsion of the fetus and placenta from the uterus during birth. It is pertinent to note that Hippocrates also describes use of vitex for what are clearly oxytocic effects: to "expel the placenta" as well as to "bring down the milk." Estrogenic influence of vitex on lactation is also not studied. Phytoestrogenic activity is common among reputed galactogogues and vitex is no exception (see Therapeutic Applications: Reproductive Hormone Interactions). The mechanisms by which phytoestrogens may increase milk production are not understood. Thus, it can be postulated that vitex may have a positive influence on lactation through estrogen and/or oxytocin and perhaps prolactin modulation. Despite research limitations, it is clear that Mohr (1954) was seeing rapid lactational responses only days after first administering vitex. This is in sharp contrast to vitex's influence on menstrual difficulties, where improvements occur only after three months or more, on average (see Reproductive Function: Lactation).

A study using rats indicated possible decreased milk supply as evidenced by lack of milk spots after maternal treatment with subcutaneous injection of vitex extract (Winterhoff et al., 1991), which the researchers attributed to lowered prolactin levels in the mother rats. In light of the recent in vitro characterization of vitex extract as a dopamine agonist with resultant suppression of prolactin (Jarry et al., 1991; Sliutz et al., 1993), vitex could have an unpredictable or negative effect on milk supply in nursing mothers, although not enough is known about dose response of prolactin to vitex to predict this effect with certainty (see Reproductive Function: Lactation). Use of vitex to slow milk production in cases of oversupply is unexplored and potentially valuable, though again, dose information is lacking.

Sustained use of vitex over several weeks during the early postpartum has been associated with premature return of the menses (Madaus Co., 1994; Mohr, 1954), representing a major loss of many benefits of lactational amenorrhea (LA) for the mother. These include the loss of the enjoyment of the normal LA state, loss of preventative benefits of low estrogen states associated with LA, including lowered risk of breast and ovarian cancer, and a premature need for birth control and increased risk of pregnancy. However, once a woman wishes to regain fertility, continued breast-feeding of the child is known to interfere with her ability to become pregnant. Use of vitex to help restore full ovulation and menstrual cycles may be preferable to either actively weaning the child or undergoing full medical infertility treatment. There is no evidence, other than empirical observations, to support the efficacy of this approach, however. Although vitex constituents are expected to enter milk, as most other ingested substances do, the amounts would be very small; adverse reactions in the nursing child would not be anticipated. It is anticipated that milk supply could be decreased, though late lactation is a time of normal prolactin levels, milk supply being primarily driven by autocrine control, not pituitary control. The alternative is weaning, so a lowered supply may be preferable. European physicians have been known to prescribe vitex for the purpose of reestablishing menses and ovulation after periods of lactation amenorrhea (personal communication Humphrey, 2001).

Side Effects

The German Commission E monograph (Blumenthal et al., 1998, p. 108) reports: "In rare cases, Vitex may cause an urticarial rash."

Madaus Co. (1994) lists "occasional occurrence of itching and urticarial exanthema" (pp. 1, 4). The summary of clinical information in this product insert indicates rare occurrences of nausea, allergic rash, diarrhea, weight gain, and headache. Serious side effects have not been observed.

Special Precautions

Liquid preparations of vitex are noted to contain over 50% alcohol. A typical dose range would deliver 0.8 g alcohol. According to Madaus Co. (1994, p. 1), "a health risk exists for patients with liver damage, alcoholics, epileptics and brain-damaged patients. The effectiveness of other medications can be affected." For others, the amount of alcohol does not present a health risk. Madaus Co. further recommends that the preparation not be used past the expiration date and that it should be kept out of the reach of children.

Medical diagnosis of breast pain, swelling, and discomfort should be made before vitex treatment.

Toxicology

In Vitro Toxicity

A recent report of cytotoxic flavonoids in the root bark of vitex is noted (Hirobe et al., 1997). The occurrence of these compounds in the leaves or fruit is unknown at this time. Jarry et al. (1991), in studies of cultured rat pituitary cells, found a negative MTT test, excluding the possibility of cytotoxic effects with vitex extracts in vitro.

Toxicity in Animal Models

Newall et al. (1996) noted the lack of toxicology studies on vitex. However, Madaus Co. (1994) reports LD_{50} studies with rat and mice, in which a single dose of over 7,000 mg/kg of Agnolyt had no toxic effects within 14 days following treatment. Doses ranging up to 3,500 mg/kg Agnolyt, representing approximately 1,400 times the therapeutic daily human dose, were given to eight male and eight female rats for over five weeks. No toxic effects were found.

Reports from antiquity warn against overdose (Böhnert and Hahn, 1990). Haller (1958) noted that very high doses of vitex given to guinea pigs caused complete inhibition of "prehypophyseal" gonadotropic function. Madaus Co. (1994) noted that Haller found this effect only after increasing the dose of vitex (Agnolyt) ten- to twenty-fold.

Winterhoff et al. (1991) reported signs of decreased milk intake and increased pup mortality in rats treated with vitex, which was attributed to a lack of prolactin.

REFERENCES

Attelmann, H., Bends, K., Hellenkemper, H., Reichert, J., and Warkalla, H.J. (1972). [Agnolyt® in the treatment of gynecological complaints]. *Zeitschrift für Praklinische Geriatrie* 2: 239-243 (translation).

Azar, S.T. and Yamout, B. (1999). Prolactin secretion is increased in patients with multiple sclerosis. *Endocrine Research* 25: 207-214.

Belic, J., Bergant-Dolar, D., Stucin, D., and Stucin, M. (1958). A biologically active substance from *Vitex agnus-castus* seeds. *Vestnik Slovenskega Kemliskega Drustva* 5: 63-67.

Berger, D., Schaffner, W., Schrader, E., Meier, B., and Brattstrom, A. (2000). Efficacy of *Vitex agnus castus* L. extract Ze 440 in patients with pre-menstrual syndrome (PMS). *Archives of Gynecology and Obstetrics* 264: 150-153.

Betz, W. (1998). Commentary—William Betz, Brussels. *Forschende Komplementarmedizin* (Basel) 5: 146-147 (in English).

Biller, B.M. (1999). Hyperprolactinemia. *International Journal of Fertility and Women's Medicine* 44: 74-77.

Blank, A., Maerz, R.W., and Gorkow, C. (2000). Evidence of efficacy of *Vitex agnus castus*. In 3rd International Congress on Phytomedicine, October 11-13, 2000, Munich, Germany, Abstracts. *Phytomedicine* 7(Suppl. 2): 9 (abstract SL-5).

Blumenthal, M., Busse, W.R., Goldberg, A., Gruenwald, J., Hall, T., Riggins, C.W., and Rister, R.S. (Eds.) (1998). *The Complete German Commission E Monographs* (p. 108). Austin, TX: American Botanical Council.

Böhnert, K.J. (1997). Clinical study on chaste tree for menstrual disorders. *Quarterly Review of Natural Medicine* (Spring): 19-21.

Böhnert, K.J. and Hahn, G. (1990). [Phytotherapy in gynecology and obstetrics. *Vitex agnus-castus* (chaste tree)]. *Erfahrungshielkunde* 9: 494-502 (translation).

Brinker, F. (1998). *Herb Contraindications and Drug Interactions,* Second Edition (p. 55). Sandy, OR: Eclectic Medical Publications.

Bubenzer, R.H. (1983). Therapie mit agnus castus: Dem monch von gestern, der frau von heute [Therapy with agnus castus: For the monk of yesterday, for the women of today]. *Therapiewoche* 43: 1705-1706 (translation).

Cahill, D.J., Fox, R., Wardle, P.G., and Harlow, C.R. (1994). Multiple follicular development associated with herbal medicine. *Human Reproduction* 9: 429-438.

Chikanza, I.C. (1999). Prolactin and neuroimmunomodulation: In vitro and in vivo observations. *Annals of the New York Academy of Sciences* 876: 119-130.

Christie, S. and Walker, A.F. (1997-1998). *Vitex agnus-castus* L.: (1) A review of its traditional and modern therapeutic use; (2) current use from a survey of practitioners. *The European Journal of Herbal Medicine* 3: 29-45.

Dickson, R.A. and Glazer, W.M. (1999). Hyperprolactinemia and male sexual dysfunction. *Journal of Clinical Psychiatry* 60: 125 (letter).

Dittmar, F.W., Bohnert, K.J., Peeters, M., Albrecht, M., Lamertz, M., and Schmidt, U. (1992). [Premenstrual syndrome treatment with a phytopharmaceutical]. *Therapiewoche Gynäkologie* 5: 60-68 (translation).

Dixon-Shanies, D. and Shaikh, N. (1999). Growth inhibition of human breast cancer cells by herbs and phytoestrogens. *Oncology Reports* 6: 1383-1387.

Du Mee, C. (1993). Vitex agnus-castus. *Australian Journal of Medical Herbalism* 5: 63-65.

Duke, J.A. (1995). Chasteberry. *The Business of Herbs* (November/December): 12-13.

Eagon, C.L., Elm, M.S., Teepe, A.G., and Eagon, P.K. (1997). Medicinal botanicals: Estrogenicity in rat uterus and liver. *Proceedings of the American Association for Cancer Research* 38: 293 (abstract 1967).

Eagon, P.K. (1999). University of Pittsburgh School of Medicine, personal communication with Kenneth Jones, August 23, 1999.

Eagon, P.K., Swafford, D.S., Elm, M.S., Ayer, H.A., Rich, C., Tress, N.B., and Eagon, C.L. (1998). Estrogenicity of medicinal botanicals. *Proceedings of the American Association for Cancer Research* 39: 386 (abstract 2624).

Feldmann, H.U., Albrecht, M., Lamertz, M., and Böhnert, K.J. (1990). [The treatment of corpus luteum insufficiency and premenstrual syndrome: Experience in a multicenter study under clinical practice conditions]. *Gyne* 12: 422-425 (translation).

Fox, R., Wardle, P.G., and Harlow, C.R. (1994). Multiple follicular development associated with herbal medicine. *Journal of Human Reproduction* 9: 1469-1470.

Galletti, G.C., Russo, M.T., and Bacchini, P. (1996). Essential oil composition of leaves and berries of *Vitex agnus-castus* L. from Calabria, Southern Italy. *Rapid Communications in Mass Spectrometry* 10: 1345-1350.

Gomaa, C.S., El-Moghazy, M.A., Halim, F.A., and El-Sayyad, A.E. (1978). Flavonoids and iridoids from *Vitex agnus-castus*. *Planta Medica* 33: 277.

Haga, H.J. and Rygh, T. (1999). The prevalence of hyperprolactinemia in patients with primary Sjogren's syndrome. *Journal of Rheumatology* 26: 1291-1295.

Halaska, M., Beles, P., Gorkow, C., and Sieder, C. (1999). Treatment of cyclical mastalgia with a solution containing a *Vitex agnus castus* extract: Results of a placebo-controlled double-blind study. *The Breast* 8: 175-181.

Haller, J. (1958). Tierexperimentelle untersuchungen am lipschutztier uber die einwirkung von sogennten "phytohormonen" auf die gonadotrope funktion des hypophysenvorderlappens, Kongress d. NWD-Gynakologen in Celle, pp. 1347-1353 (English summary).

Hänsel, R., Leuckert, C., Rimpler, H., and Schaaf, K.D. (1965). Chemotaxonomische untersuchungen in der gattung *Vitex* L. [Chemotaxonomic examinations in the genus *Vitex* L.]. *Phytochemistry* 4: 19-27.

Hirobe, C., Qiao, Z.S., Takeya, K., and Itokawa, H. (1997). Cytotoxic flavonoids from *Vitex agnus-castus*. *Phytochemistry* 46: 521-524.

Hobbs, C. (1990). *Vitex: The Women's Herb*. Capitola, CA: Botanica Press.

Hobbs, C. (1991). The chaste tree: *Vitex agnus castus*. *Pharmacy in History* 33: 19-24.

Hoberg, E., Meier, B., and Sticher, O. (2000). Quantitative high performance liquid chromatographic analysis of diterpenoids in agni-casti fructus. *Planta Medica* 66(4): 352-355.

Hoberg, E., Orjala, J., Meier, B., and Sticher, O. (1999). Diterpenoids from the fruits of *Vitex agnus-castus*. *Phytochemistry* 52: 1555-1558.

Huang, K.C. (1999). *The Pharmacology of Chinese Herbs,* Second Edition (p. 290). Boca Raton, FL: CRC Press.

Huang, W.J., Yeh, J.Y., Tsai, S.C., Lin, H., Chiao, Y.C., Chen, J.J., Lu, C.C., Hwang, S.W., Wang, S.W., Chang, L.S., et al. (1999). Regulation of testosterone by prolactin in male rats. *Journal of Cellular Biochemistry* 74: 111-118.

Humphrey, S. (2001). Sheila Humphrey, RN, BSc, ICBLC, personal communication with INPR, September.

Jarry, H., Leonhardt, S., Gorkow, C., and Wuttke, W. (1994). In vitro prolactin but not LH and FSH release is inhibited by compounds in extracts of *Agnus castus:* Direct evidence for a dopaminergic principle by the dopamine receptor assay. *Experimental and Clinical Endocrinology* 102: 448-454.

Jarry, H., Leonhardt, S., Wuttke, W., Behr, B., and Gorkow, C. (1991). [Agnus castus as a dopaminergic active principle in Mastodyn®N]. *Zeitschrift für Phytotherapie* 12: 77-82.

Jarry, H., Metten, M., and Wuttke, W. (2000). Comparison of the dopaminergic potency of various commercially available Agnus-castus preparations: The need for biological standardization. In 3rd International Congress on Phytomedicine, October 11-13, 2000, Munich, Germany, Abstracts. *Phytomedicine* 7(Suppl. 2): 10 (abstract SL-6b).

Koeppen, B.H. (1964). Structure of the glycosyl residues in orientin and homo-orientin. *South African Medical Journal* 38: 154.

Kubista, E., Müller, G., and Spona, J. (1983). Die konservative therapie der mastopathie [The conservative therapy of mastopathy]. *Zentralblatt für Gynäkologie* 105: 1153-1162.

Kustrak, D., Kuftinec, J., and Blazevic, N. (1992). The composition of the essential oil of *Vitex agnus-castus. Planta Medica* 58(Suppl. 1): A681.

Kustrak, D., Pepeljnjak, S., Antolic, A., and Blazevic, N. (1987). Antimicrobial activity of *Vitex agnus-castus. Pharmaceutisch Weekblad Scientific Edition* 9: 238 (abstract).

Lader, M. (1999). Some adverse effects of antipsychotics: Prevention and treatment. *Journal of Clinical Psychiatry* 60 (Suppl. 12): 18-21.

Laszczynska, M., Piasecka, M., and Kram, A. (1999). Alterations in the mitochondria of rat spermatozoa after experimental hyperprolactinemia. *Folia Histochemica et Cytobiologica* 37: 87-88.

Lauritzen, C.H., Reuter, H.D., Repges, R., Bohnert, K.J., and Schmidt, U. (1997). Treatment of premenstrual tension syndrome with *Vitex agnus-castus:* Controlled, double-blind study versus pyridoxine. *Phytomedicine* 4: 183-189.

Lawrence, R. (1994). *Breastfeeding: A Guide For The Medical Profession,* Fourth Edition. St. Louis, MO: Mosby Press.

Leung, A.Y. and Foster, S. (1996). *Encyclopedia of Common Natural Ingredients,* Second Edition (pp. 151-152). New York: Wiley-Interscience.

Liu, J., Burdette, J.E., Xu, H., Gu, C., van Breemen, R.B., Bhat, K.P., Booth, N., Constantinou, A.I., Pezzuto, J.M., Fong, H.H., et al. (2001). Evaluation of estrogenic activity of plant extracts for the potential treatment of menopausal symptoms. *Journal of Agricultural and Food Chemistry* 49: 2472-2479.

Loch, E.G., Bohnert, K.J., Peeters, M., Schmidt, U., and Lamertz, M. (1991). [The treatment of menstrual disorders with *Vitex agnus-castus tincture*]. *Der Fraunarzt* 32: 867-870 (translation).

Loch, E.G., Selle, H., and Boblitz, N. (2000). Treatment of premenstrual syndrome with a phytopharmaceutical formulation containing *Vitex agnus castus*. *Journal of Women's Health and Gender Medicine* 9: 315-320.

Mabberley, D.J. (1990). *The Plant Book*. Cambridge, MA: Cambridge University Press.

Madaus Co. (1994). Agnolyt®—The Natural Way for Hormone Imbalance. Package insert and research summary (translation).

Males, Z. (1998). Determination of the content of the polyphenols of *Vitex agnus-castus* L. f. *rosea*. *Acta Pharmaceutica* (Zagreb) 48: 215-218.

Males, Z., Blazevic, N., and Antolic, A. (1998). The essential oil composition of *Vitex agnus-castus* f. *rosea* leaves and flowers. *Planta Medica* 64: 286-287.

McGuffin, M., Hobbs, C., Upton, R., and Goldberg, A. (Eds.) (1997). *American Herbal Products Association's Botanical Safety Handbook* (pp. 123-124). Boca Raton, FL: CRC Press.

Meier, B., Berger, D., Hoberg, E., Sticher, O., and Schaffner, W. (2000). Pharmacological activities of *Vitex agnus-castus* extracts in vitro. *Phytomedicine* 7: 373-381.

Merz, P.G., Gorkow, C., Schrödter, A., Rietbrock, S., Sieder, C., Loew, D., Dericks-Tan, J.S., and Taubert, H.D. (1996). The effects of a special agnus castus extract (BP1095E1) on prolactin secretion in healthy male subjects. *Experimental and Clinical Endocrinology and Diabetes* 104: 447-453.

Milewicz, A., Gejdel, E., Sworen, H., Sienkiewicz, K., Jedrzejak, J., Teucher, T., and Schmitz, H. (1993). *Vitex agnus castus*-extrakt zur behandlung von regeltempoanomalien infolge latenter hyperprolaktinämie. Ergebnisse einer randomisierten plazebo-kontrollierten doppelblindstudie [*Vitex agnus-castus* extract for the treatment of menstrual irregularities due to latent hyperprolactinemia. A randomized, placebo-controlled, double-blind study]. *Arzneimittel-Forschung/Drug Research* 43: 752-756 (English summary).

Mohr, H. (1954). [Clinical investigations of means to increase lactation]. *Deutsche Medizinische Woehenschnift* 79: 1513-1516.

Neidhart, M., Gay, R.E., and Gay, S. (1999). Prolactin and prolactin-like polypeptides in rheumatoid arthritis. *Biomedical Pharmacotherapy* 53: 218-222.

Neville, M.C. and Neifert, M.R. (Eds.) (1983). *Lactation: Physiology, Nutrition and Breast Feeding*. New York: Plenum Press.

Newall, C.A., Anderson, L.A., and Phillipson, J.D. (1996). *Herbal Medicines: A Guide for Health Care Professionals* (pp. 19-20). London: The Pharmaceutical Press.

Nwosu, M.O. (1999). Herbs for mental disorders. *Fitoterapia* 70: 58-63.

Ostensen, M. (1999). Sex hormones and pregnancy in rheumatoid arthritis and systemic lupus erythematosus. *Annals of the New York Academy of Sciences* 876: 131-144.

Pepeljnjak, S., Antolic, A., and Kustrak, D. (1996). Antibacterial and antifungal activities of the *Vitex agnus-castus* L. extracts. *Acta Pharmaceutica* (Zagreb) 46: 201-206.

Petty, R.G. (1999). Prolactin and antipsychotic medications: Mechanism of action. *Schizophrenia Research* 35(Suppl.): S67-S73.

Propping, D., Bohnert, K.J., Peeters, M., Albrecht, M., and Lamertz, M. (1991). [*Vitex agnus-castus* treatment of gynecological syndromes]. *Therapeutikon* 5: 581-585 (translation).

Propping, D. and Katzorke, T. (1987). [Treatment of corpus luteum insufficiency]. *Zeitschrift für Allgemeinmedizin* 63: 932-933 (English translation).

Propping, D., Katzorke, T., and Belkien, L. (1988). [Diagnosis and therapy of corpus luteum deficiency in general practice]. *Therapiewoche* 38: 2992-3001 (translation).

Rapkin, A.J., Shoupe, D., Reading, A., Daneshgar, K.K., Goldman, L., Bohn, Y., Brann, D.W., and Mahesh, V.B. (1996). Decreased central opioid activity in premenstrual syndrome: Luteinizing hormone response to naloxone. *Journal of the Society for Gynecological Investigation* 3: 93-98.

Reuter, H.D., Bohnert, K.J., and Schmidt, U. (1995). Die therapie des prämenstruellen syndroms mit *Vitex agnus castus:* Kontrollierte doppelblindstudie gegen pyridoxin [The therapy of the premenstrual syndrome with *Vitex agnus castus:* Controlled double-blind study with pyridoxine]. *Zeitschrift für Phytotherapie* 7 (Abstracts volume): 7 (abstract, translation).

Roeder, D.A. (1994). [Therapy of cyclic disorders with *Vitex agnus-castus*]. *Zeitschrift für Phytotherapie* 15: 155-159 (English summary).

Russo, M. and Galletti, G.C. (1996). Medicinal properties and chemical composition of *Vitex agnus-castus* L.: A review. *Acta Horticulturae* 426: 105-112.

Saden-Krehula, M., Dustrak, D., and Blazevic, N. (1990). Delta 4-3-ketosteroids in flowers and leaves of *Vitex agnus-castus*. *Planta Medica* 56: 547.

Schellenberg, R. (2001). Treatment for the premenstrual syndrome with agnus castus fruit extract: Prospective, randomized, placebo controlled study. *British Medical Journal* 322: 134-137.

Senatore, F., Della Porta, G., and Reverchon, E. (1996). Constituents of *Vitex agnus-castus* L. essential oil. *Flavour and Fragrance Journal* 11: 179-182.

Shuster, J. (1996). ISMP adverse drug reactions. *Hospital Pharmacy* 31: 1553-1554.

Sliutz, G., Speiser, P., Schultz, A.M., Spona, J., and Zeillinger, R. (1993). Agnus castus extracts inhibit prolactin secretion of rat pituitary cells. *Hormone and Metabolic Research* 25: 253-255.

Snow, J.M. (1996). *Vitex agnus-castus* L. (Verbenaceae). *Protocol Journal of Botanical Medicine* (Spring): 20-23.

Sorensen, J.M. and Katsiotis, T.S. (1999). Variation in essential oil yield and composition of Cretan *Vitex agnus castus* L. fruits. *Journal of Essential Oil Research* 11: 599-605.

Stylian, G. (1996). Vitex negundo. *Australian Journal of Herbalism* 8: 34-39.

Turner, S. and Mills, S. (1993). A double-blind clinical trial on a herbal remedy for premenstrual syndrome: A case study. *Complementary Therapies in Medicine* 1: 73-77.

Werbach, M.R. and Murray, M.T. (1994). *Botanical Influences on Illness: A Sourcebook of Clinical Research.* Tarzana, CA: Third Line Press.

Winterhoff, H., Gorkow, C., and Behr, B. (1991). Die hemmung der laktation bei ratten als indirekter beweis fur die senkung von prolaktin durch agnus castus [Inhibition of lactation in rats as an indirect proof of prolactin lowering caused by agnus castus]. *Zietschrift für Phytotherapie* 12: 175-179.

Wollenweber, E. and Mann, K. (1983). Flavonols from fruits of *Vitex agnus-castus.* *Planta Medica* 48: 126-127 (English summary).

Wuttke, W. (1992). Zellbiologische untersuchungen mit Agnolyt®-praparationen (NH 246, NH 247) [Cellular biological examinations with Angolyt preparations]. *Personlich Keit Mittleilung* 8.7 (cited in Madaus Co., 1994).

Wuttke, W., Gorkow, C., and Jarry, H. (1995). Dopaminergic compounds in *Vitex agnus-castus.* In Loew, D. and Rietbrock, N. (Eds.), *Phytopharmaka un Forschung und Klinischer Anwendung* (pp. 81-91). Darmstatd, Germany: Steinkopff Verlag.

Wuttke, W., Splitt, G., Gorkow, C., and Sieder, C. (1997). Behandlung zyklusabhängiger brustschmerzen mit einem *Agnus castus*-haltigen arzneimittel [Treatment of cyclical mastalgia with *Agnus castus*: Results of a randomized, placebo-controlled, double-blind study]. *Geburtshilfe und Frauenheilkunde* 57: 569-574 (translation).

Wyatt, K.M., Dimmock, P.W., Jones, P.W., and Shaughn O'Brian, P.M. (1999). Efficacy of vitamin B-6 in the treatment of premenstrual syndrome: Systematic review. *British Medical Journal* 318: 1375-1381.

Zhu, Y.P. (1998). *Chinese Materia Medica. Chemistry, Pharmacology and Applications* (pp. 105-106). Amsterdam, the Netherlands: Harwood Academic.

Zoghbi, Marias das Gracas, B., Andrade, E.H.A., and Maia, J.G.S. (1999). The essential oil of *Vitex agnus-castus* L. growing in the Amazon region. *Flavour and Fragrance Journal* 14: 211-213.

Zwaving, J.H. and Bos, R. (1996). Composition of the essential fruit oil of *Vitex agnus-castus.* *Planta Medica* 62: 83-84 (letter).

Appendix I

A Note About Quality
in Botanical Supplements

Dennis J. McKenna

A significant portion of the natural dietary supplements currently on the market in the United States are derived from botanical sources. Botanicals, or botanical supplements, are widely available and are becoming increasingly popular for health maintenance, for the amelioration of a variety of conditions ranging from insomnia to menopause, and are even being used as natural alternatives to prescription medicines, such as antidepressants and tranquilizers.

With a large and growing segment of the consuming public coming to rely on botanical supplements as an integral part of health maintenance practices, two issues—safety and efficacy—become of paramount importance. Botanical extracts must be made as safe and efficaceous as possible, although neither of these criteria can ever be fulfilled with 100% assurance (as the rather spotty safety/efficacy track record of many prescription medicines illustrates). One of the major determinants of the efficacy of a botanical supplement is the manner in which it is formulated. Formulation also bears, though somewhat less directly, on safety, since an inefficacious supplement may ultimately lead to harm if it does not provide the expected therapeutic benefits.

Modern techniques utilized in the manufacture of phytopharmaceuticals are quite elaborate and every bit as sophisticated and technically challenging as similar practices in pharmaceutical manufacturing; in fact, they are often more challenging, since phytopharmaceutical formulations contain multiple active (as well as inactive) ingredients, as opposed to a single active ingredient, which is the norm in most pharmaceutical preparations. Phytopharmaceutical technologists sometimes refer to the "6 S" process— six key steps that are required to ensure the safety, purity, and efficacy of any phytomedicine:

- *Selection:* Product candidates are selected for development based on experience and knowledge.
- *Sourcing:* Commercial quantities of high-quality raw materials must be obtained from reputable and reliable producers.
- *Structural analysis:* Various analytical methods are applied to characterize the presence and nature of chemical components present in the phytomedicine.
- *Standardization:* Chemical analytical methods and sometimes pharmacological bioassays are applied to develop a formulation that consistently possesses a measurable, quantifiable, and replicable content of active constituents and/or biological activity.
- *Substantiation:* Claims for therapeutic efficacy should be substantiated through well-designed preclinical and clinical evaluation protocols. The results of such studies should be published in peer-reviewed scientific journals.
- *Safety:* Collection of data on the safety, as well as the efficacy, of a phytomedicine should be included as a part of well-designed preclinical or clinical evaluation studies.

**What Every Consumer Has a Right to Know
(or: Read the Label—It's Important!)**

Below are some guidelines for the kind of information that consumers should look for in comparing label information of botanical supplements:

- Statement of percentage standardization of the extract
- Statement describing which compounds are standardized
- Statement describing which parts of the plant are used in the formulation
- Extract ratio (the ratio of extract concentration to crude plant material, e.g., 1:4)
- Recommended daily dosage
- Weight and number of capsules or tablets per package
- Substantiated structure/function claims
- Product expiration date to confirm freshness
- A toll-free number and/or Web site address for company information and contact

---

The careful, consistent application of such procedures is the basis of the proper practice of phytopharmaceutical technology, the science and art of manufacturing botanical medicines (phytomedicines). Unfortunately, not all phytomedicines available on the market today have been evaluated according to the rigorous steps outlined above. This situation is changing, however; as consumers and health care professionals become more educated regarding botanicals, they are learning which questions to address to critically evaluate phytomedicinal products. Consumers have a right to expect that the phytomedicines they purchase are developed and manufactured with as much care as any conventional pharmaceutical products (see list). As phytomedicinal companies respond to the consumer-led demand for quality, overall quality standards for the industry are improving. Constraints of space prohibit the presentation here of a detailed technical discussion of phytopharmaceutical manufacturing technology, and readers interested in an in-depth look at this complex subject are urged to consult the appropriate technical literature (see e.g., List and Schmidt, 1989; Verall, 1996; Busse, 1999).

Plants, the ultimate source for botanical supplements, are complex organisms composed of thousands of organic compounds. Humans utilize plants as food, consuming them for their nutritional value, which can include vitamins, minerals, carbohydrates, protein, fats, etc.; in short, the whole gamut of plant constituents that provides nutritional support in our diet. When humans use plants as medicine, they are usually interested in the therapeutic benefits provided by one or more biologically active compounds present in the plant; consuming the plant as medicine may well provide additional nutritional support, but that is usually not the reason for consuming it. For as long as humans have utilized plants as medicine, they have made efforts to ensure efficacy, and their efforts have often involved the application of some kind of processing technology aimed at enhancing the potency of the botanical remedy. Usually, these efforts are intended to maximize the concentration of the (known or suspected) "active principles" in the plant, while reducing the volume of plant material that must be ingested. Some of these processing steps are quite simple and obvious and do not require any special expertise; making a tea, a hot-water infusion, is an example of one kind of processing step that almost anyone can carry out. Aqueous infusions frequently do represent a significant improvement over ingesting the whole herb, whether dried or fresh; teas often taste much better than the whole herb, and in many instances the active compounds are selectively extracted into the infusion, leaving inert ingredients, such as fiber, and sometimes bitter or unpleasant-tasting components, behind in the solid plant matrix. While the simple step of making tea does improve the therapeutic properties of many botanical remedies, as a rule, more elaborate extraction procedures are required.

The proper formulation of phytomedicines—the development of appropriate dosage forms—encompasses at least three of the six steps outlined previously: structural analysis must be applied to characterize the presence and nature of active ingredients; standardization techniques ensure that dosage forms are consistent from lot to lot and that active constituents are present in measurable, efficaceous quantities; and substantiation studies should (ideally) be conducted using the same dosage formulations as those used in commercial phytopharmaceutical products. The following sections provide a brief review of the various kinds of botanical formulations commonly used in commercial supplements and also discuss the relative merits of "standardized" botanical extracts versus "concentrated" extracts.

TYPES OF EXTRACTS

Medicinal plants can be processed by a variety of methods, which tend to be a reflection of empirical, practical techniques developed by apothecaries and herbalists over the centuries. Some methods are highly specialized and rarely used commercially—either because the resulting extracts are not suitable for large-scale commercial production technologies or because the methods are appropriate only for restricted applications—and often have been superseded by newer and more efficient methods.

Fresh Extracts

With a few exceptions, medicinal plant extracts are usually prepared from plant material that has been previously dried to a low moisture content (usually ≤ 10%), regardless of whether the form of the final extract preparation is a liquid or a solid. In some cases, however, the extract is prepared from the freshly harvested herb. Fresh herb extracts are rarely sold as dietary supplements in the United States, and are discussed only briefly here.

Fruit pulps are solid or pasty viscid preparations made by crushing the fruit and removing the hard parts. Fruit pulps are important in food processing but rarely used today in phytomedicines. An example is grapefruit juice concentrate.

Juices are liquid extracts obtained from plants by a variety of methods. They include the following subcategories:

- *Pressed juices* are obtained by expression of fresh fruits or other juice-rich parts of plants. Sometimes made with additional water and/or stimulated fermentation. An example is the pressed, flowering tops of echinacea, though this juice is commonly stabilized through the addition of some amount of alcohol.
- *Nonexpressed juices* are usually obtained as exudates or by "bleeding" from natural or artificial wounds. Examples are aloe juice and opium latex. Resinous plant exudates, such as gum arabic, myrhh, and Peru balsam, also fall into this category.

- *Artificial juices* are not obtained by expression or as an exudate. Artificial juices are usually concentrates of an aqueous extract. An example is licorice juice.

Syrups are liquid preparations with a high sugar content, which may contain juices or alcoholic plant extracts. Syrups are used primarily as flavorings but are used in some pharmaceutical formulations, such as cough syrups. Examples are currant syrup and raspberry syrup.

Alcoholates are prepared from fresh plant parts by maceration with 80-95% cold ethanol. Alcoholates are generally used in cases when the active ingredients would be lost or degraded by a drying process. "Stabilized alcoholates" are obtained by boiling fresh plant parts in alcohol under reflux. This denatures the plant enzymes, which may degrade some constituents.

Homeopathic preparations from fresh plants. The "mother tinctures" of most homeopathic preparations are obtained from fresh plants. Various methods are applied to their preparation, depending on juice content, moisture content, and the presence or nonpresence of essential oils or resins. Preparation procedures can be found in various homeopathic pharmacopoeias.

Liquid Extracts

Liquid extracts are prepared by extracting the plant, usually in a dried form, with water, ethanol, combinations of water and ethanol in various proportions, or other organic solvents, such as hexane or dichloromethane. When organic solvents other than ethanol are used, such extracts are almost always an intermediate step in the manufacture of dried, solvent-free extracts.

Aqueous Extracts

Aqueous extracts are plant extracts prepared using water as the solvent. Aqueous extracts of medicinal plants are usually intended to be used as soon as possible. The ratio of the volume of water to the volume of drug is usually 10:1, but exceptions do occur. Three main types of aqueous extracts are used.

- *Decoctions* are usually prepared from root bark and other woody parts. The shredded plant part is extracted in hot water (> 90° C) for 30 min to 1 h, stirring often. The mixture is then strained while still hot.
- *Chinese decoctions* are usually prepared with much larger quantities of herbs than are used in the West. Up to 150 g of dried herb are ex-

tracted in 1 liter of water, then reduced to 300-400 mL for three doses. The resulting mixture is very concentrated.

- *Infusions* are usually applied to leaves, flowers, and other soft or nonwoody plant parts. Infusions can be as simple as an herb tea; boiling water is poured over the dried herb (loose or in a tea ball or teabag) and allowed to steep for 5-15 min, then consumed after being allowed to cool. The West German Pharmacopoeia (DAB 8) describes a more formal way of making an infusion:

  One part drug in the prescribed comminution is kneaded several times in a mortar with 3-5 parts water and left to stand for 15 min. The rest of the boiling water is then poured onto the mixture, which is suspended in a container in a water bath and kept for 5 min with repeated stirring, at a temperature > 90 ° C. The mixture is covered and left to stand until cool. If the prescribed weight of infusion is not obtained after gentle expression of the drug residue, the required quantity of cold water is poured on the residue which is gently squeezed out again. This second extract is added to the main infusion to make it up to the prescribed weight. (List and Schmidt, 1989).

- *Macerates* are aqueous extracts made by pouring water at room temperature over the comminuted plant parts and allowing it to stand, with occasional stirring, for 30 min. The extract is then strained and made up to the required weight with the rinsings. Macerates are usually suitable for plant parts with a high mucous content, such as fruits and seeds.

Alcoholic Extracts

Alcohol, and combinations of alcohol and water, are the organic solvents chosen most frequently to prepare liquid plant extracts on the industrial scale. Many low molecular weight active constituents in plants are soluble to varying degrees in alcohol or alcohol-water mixtures. In addition to being an excellent solvent, alcohol is also an excellent preservative and antiseptic, and alcoholic extracts can be stable and free from microbial contaminants for prolonged periods. Because it is easily removed by evaporation or vacuum distillation, alcohol is also the solvent of choice for preparing liquid extracts, which are used as intermediates in the manufacture of solid, dried extracts. As with aqueous extracts, several types of alcoholic extracts are formally recognized:

- *Tinctures* are extracts made with ethanol/water combinations (25% to 80% ethanol, depending on the plant product) and are usually prepared in the ratio of 1:10 or 1:5, i.e., one weight unit of plant material to the specified amount of liquid. A 1:5 extract is 100 g in 500 ml of solvent, a 1:10 extract is 100 g of plant material in 1000 ml of solvent.

- *Fluid extracts* are liquid alcoholic extracts, only more concentrated. The usual ratio is 1:1, i.e., one part plant material to one part solvent. Tinctures can be prepared from fluid extracts by dilution.
- *Thin extracts,* now regarded as obsolete, are alcoholic extracts that have been concentrated to a honey-like consistency.
- *Viscous extracts* or *thick extracts,* another obsolete form, are produced by careful concentration of fluid extracts; they are solid at room temperature and become a thick, plastic mass on warming. They contain varying quantities of residual moisture and can be adjusted to a defined content of active substances by addition of inert materials, such as maltodextrin or lactose. Viscous extracts have been almost entirely replaced by dried extracts, because viscous extracts have low stability and are susceptible to microbial contamination.

Other Types of Liquid Extracts

Rarely used in commercial products and poorly suitable for industrial-scale manufacturing processes, other types of liquid extracts include *vinegars,* in which the plant material is extracted with dilute acetic acid, and *oil extracts,* in which medicinal substances are dissolved or suspended in edible oils, such as almond, peanut, or olive oil. They are obtained by maceration or digestion of the ground drug in the oil. An example, still encountered in some health food stores, is the reddish oil of St. John's wort.

Dry Extracts

Dry extracts are prepared by removal of the solvent from various types of liquid extracts. Usually hydroalcoholic liquid extracts are used as intermediates in the preparation of dry extracts, although extracts made with other organic solvents may also be used. In the latter instance, quality control measures are essential to ensure that the organic solvent is removed from the extract as completely as possible. Aqueous extracts are only rarely used in the manufacture of dry extracts. Often dry extracts are prepared by evaporating the extract over an inert carrier material, such as cellulose, maltodextrin, or even the pulverized, preextracted plant material itself. This helps to ensure uniformity and consistency in the extract and, in making standardized products, inert carrier substrates may also be added in calculated quantities to ensure that a specified level of active ingredients per unit weight of extract exists. As with liquid extracts, dry extracts are classified in the following different ways.

Native Extracts

The first step in the preparation of various kinds of solid extracts, native extracts are prepared by extracting the plant materials with an appropriate solvent and then removing the solvent by evaporation. The viscous, semisolid concentrate is called the native extract and can be used as an intermediate in the manufacture of solid, fluid, or powdered extracts. A native extract can be equivalent to an *oleoresin,* if the botanical contains resins or volatile oils, and a lipophilic solvent such as hexane is used in the extraction. Native extracts are also sometimes referred to as *soft extracts.*

Powdered Extracts

These are prepared from native extracts by dilution with an appropriate solid carrier substrate (e.g., maltodextrin) and/or an anticaking agent such as magnesium carbonate, followed by drying to yield a dry solid. The dried extract is then ground into a fine powder (of a specified mesh size) to yield a powdered extract. In other cases, it may be more coarsely granulated to yield a *granular extract.*

Solid Extracts

These are similar to powdered extracts, except that they are viscous liquids or semisolids, prepared by addition of viscous diluents such as liquid glucose or propylene glycol. Both solid extracts and powdered extracts can be manufactured to a specified strength by adjusting the amount of adjuvant carrier material that is added.

POTENCY OF BOTANICAL EXTRACTS

The potency of a botanical extract can be expressed in various ways.

Standardized Extracts

When the compound or compounds in the plant extract responsible for the therapeutic activity are known and can be quantified, then the extract can be standardized to a specified percentage of active ingredients by appropriate dilution with adjuvant carrier materials. In practice, most botanicals usually owe their activity to a group of structurally related active compounds rather than to a single compound, and the extract may be standardized according to its total content of active ingredients. For example, extracts of kava *(Piper methysticum)* are usually standardized to 30% or 55% total kavalactones, since kavalactones are known to be the constituents primarily responsible for the muscle-relaxing, anxiolytic properties of kava.

In some instances, when the compounds responsible for the activity are not completely known or are difficult to measure, the extract may be standardized based on its content of some other constituent that can be easily measured and quantified. The presumption is that when the extract is properly standardized to a key constituent, the other constituents in the extract which are responsible for the activity are also present in sufficient quantities. In these cases, the constituent in question is a marker compound; while not itself responsible for the activity, practical experience has shown that extracts containing the compound at a specified percentage have the desired activity (based on clinical studies or bioassay). An example is the herbal antidepressant, St. John's wort *(Hypericum perforatum);* most commercial St. John's wort extracts are standardized to contain 0.3% hypericin, even though most pharmacognosists now agree that hypericin is not the constituent primarily implicated in the antidepressant activity. Clinical trials have demonstrated that extracts standardized on hypericin are effective and that the compound is a good marker, because it is easy to detect and quantify. Both liquid and dried extracts may be standardized, although the practice is more commonly applied to dried extracts.

Concentrated Extracts (Drug Concentrates)

Not all dried extracts are standardized. In some cases, the strength of the extract is expressed as a ratio, e.g., 1:4 or 1:5. This means that the strength of the extract is based on its concentration relative to the crude, unextracted plant material. A 1:4 extract means that one part of the dried extract is equivalent to 4 parts of the crude drug. Occasionally, the numbers are reversed, owing to the fact that the notation has not been standardized: 4:1 has the same meaning as 1:4. In general, it is preferable to express strength as a standardized percentage of an active or marker compound, rather than as a concentration ratio. Owing to the variability in crude botanical materials (due to seasonal, geographic, varietal, agronomic, climatic, or other variables), it is actually possible to have, for example, a 1:4 concentrate that is completely lacking in active constituents! Standardization to a specified percentage at least ensures that the active compounds are present in the extract and also facilitates quality comparisons between extracts supplied by different manufacturers.

Although many types of botanical extracts are encountered today, most commercial dietary supplements sold into mainstream markets contain standardized extracts as the primary ingredient in capsule or tablet form. Occasionally, capsules or tablets are found that contain concentrates or even crude, unextracted plant materials. As larger manufacturers and companies accustomed to the application of pharmaceutical quality control procedures move into the dietary supplement market, standardized extracts are becoming the norm. This development is encouraging, since consumers and health

Appendix II

DSHEA: What Are the Key Provisions?

Dennis J. McKenna

INTRODUCTION

The explosive growth in the dietary supplement industry that has taken place recently has been fueled by three factors: (1) The large demographic segment of the population known as the baby boomers are increasingly turning toward alternative therapies and natural remedies, particularly botanicals, for health maintenance, disease prevention, and to slow or alleviate the debilitative effects of aging. This widespread change in attitude can be partially attributed to an increasing consumer disenchantment with managed health care and a common perception that conventional medicine is afflicted with an overreliance on synthetic pharmaceutical drugs with (real or imagined) adverse side effects. (2) Coverage of alternative therapies by the media has increased, including widespread information (as well as misinformation and disinformation) on the healing properties of botanical and other supplements. (3) The Dietary Supplement Health and Education Act (DSHEA) was passed in 1994, in response to an overwhelming grassroots lobbying effort directed at Congress. DSHEA has resulted in a fundamental restructuring of the regulatory environment with respect to the manner in which supplements and alternative remedies, including botanicals, can be manufactured, sold, and promoted.

The passage and implementation of DSHEA has provoked impassioned arguments on the merits of this legislation. Opponents have argued that DSHEA has effectively tied the hands of the FDA, making it more difficult, if not impossible, for the FDA to fulfill its mission of protecting the American people from unsafe foods, drugs, and dietary supplements. Proponents, on the other hand, argue just as vehemently that consumers should have a right to make their own decisions with regard to whether to use dietary supplements or alternative medicines, and that the FDA or any other regulatory agency should not be empowered to prevent any supplement from being marketed, provided no well-documented evidence can be found contraindicating its safety. Emotions on both sides of the issue run high, and the debate is likely to continue. Some of the issues raised by DSHEA will undoubtedly require further legislation to be resolved. Equally important, manufacturers and retailers of dietary supplement products, as well as consumers, must understand the key provisions of DSHEA and their implications. This overview offers a brief summary of DSHEA. Readers desiring a more in-depth analysis should consult the following references: AHPA, 1991; Appler, 1995; CDSL, 1997; McSweeney, 1995; and Merrill, 1995.

KEY PROVISIONS OF DSHEA

In his excellent review, Blumenthal (1994) discusses the key provisions of DSHEA with respect to dietary supplements. The summary presented here is derived from that article and some of the additional references provided.

Definition

DSHEA, Section 3, established the first legal definition of a dietary supplement as

> any product (other than tobacco) intended to supplement the diet that bears or contains one or more of the following ingredients: a vitamin; a mineral; an herb or other botanical; an amino acid; a dietary substance for use by man to supplement the total dietary intake; or a concentrate, metabolite, constituent, extract, or combination of any ingredient described [in the previous list].

In his review, Blumenthal notes that Section 3 also provides that a substance, initially sold as a dietary supplement that is subsequently sold as a drug, can continue to be sold as a dietary supplement as long as it is still deemed safe to do so. For example, standardized extracts of ginkgo are currently sold as dietary supplements by a number of companies; should one of those companies decide to apply to the FDA for permission to sell its ginkgo as an OTC product, this provision would ensure that other companies are not prohibited from continuing to sell their ginkgo products as dietary supplements after OTC status is granted for the petitioning company's product. Section 3 also prohibits the FDA from regulating botanicals and dietary supplements as food additives.

Safety

One of the most important provisions that DSHEA (Section 4) established involved situations in which a dietary supplement is suspected of being unsafe or adulterated: it is the responsibility of the FDA to provide evidence that the use of the product, in accordance with recommended use on the label, constitutes a significant or unreasonable risk of injury. If such a finding is made, the secretary of Health and Human Services (HHS) has the authority to order the supplement removed from the market; however, the government is required to convene hearings to review the evidence for taking such a measure.

Claim Substantiation

Another important new provision of DSHEA allows information derived from books or scientific papers to be used in connection with the sale of dietary supplements. The provision stipulates that the supporting information must

> not be false or misleading . . . does not promote a particular manufacturer or brand . . . present[s] a balanced view of the available scientific information . . . is physically separate from the dietary supplements . . . [and] does not have appended to it any information by sticker or any other method. (Section 5)

The provision also allows supplement retailers to sell books or publications as part of their normal business. As Blumenthal points out, the question of what is "balanced" and "not misleading" is an issue likely to be a source of considerable contention between opposing sides of the DSHEA debate.

Structure/Function Claims

Section 6 of DSHEA defines criteria for making "statements of nutritional support," sometimes referred to as "structure and function claims" by some industry lawyers. Under DSHEA, permitted structure/function claims for supplements can include the following:

1. Claims that a supplement can prevent a classical nutrient deficiency disease, e.g., "Vitamin C can help prevent scurvy."
2. Claims that a supplement or dietary ingredient can affect a structure or function in the body, e.g., "Calcium helps build strong bones."
3. Claims that describe or characterize the documented mechanism(s) by which a nutrient or ingredient acts to maintain structure or function, e.g., "Antioxidants can prevent damage to cells and tissues."
4. Claims that describe a general benefit resulting from consumption of a dietary supplement, e.g., "St. John's Wort can promote a positive mood."

Section 6 also mandates that the manufacturer have evidence that the claim is truthful and not misleading, and that the statement or label must prominently display the following disclaimer: *"This statement has not been evaluated by the Food and Drug Administration. This product is not intended to diagnose, treat, cure, or prevent any disease."* This subparagraph is intended to prevent therapeutic claims specifically related to diseases; manufactureres or retailers cannot claim that the product can be used to treat either the symptoms or the causes of any disease. The ambiguous distinction between therapeutic claims and structure/function claims is another issue that will probalby require litigation and/or further legislation to clarify. On making a structure/function claim, the manufacturer must notify the FDA within 30 days of making the claim.

Labeling Requirements

Section 7 of DSHEA stipulates that the term "dietary supplement" be displayed on the label, and each ingredient must be specified on the label by name and quantity. The label must specify all ingredients present in significant amounts or for which a recommended daily value has been established. Ingredients for which no daily values are established must be listed, and the fact that no daily value is defined must be noted. In the case of botanical ingredients, the part of the plant included must be stated.

New Dietary Supplements

DSHEA defines a "new dietary supplement" as a product or ingredient that has not been marketed before October 1, 1994. A new supplement may be marketed immediately if it is "an article used for food in a form in which the food has not been chemically altered." Under this definition, "chemically altered" does not include dehydration, lyophilization, milling, or creating a tincture, solution, or suspension (Anonymous, 1995). If the supplement does not qualify under this provision, the manufacturer must supply evidence of safety based on a "history of use" or other evidence that the product is safe when used under recommended conditions. This evidence must be furnished to the secretary of HHS at least 75 days before the product is introduced into interstate commerce. DSHEA does not provide the FDA with a basis for approving or rejecting a submission.

Good Manufacturing Practices

DSHEA mandates the creation of a set of good manufacturing practice (GMP) standards that specifically apply to dietary supplement products. Pharmaceutical and food GMP practices are not always easily applied or appropriate for supplements, particularly botanical supplements. Therefore, this provision of the DSHEA opens the door to the development of food GMP standards and methodologies that are appropriate for botanical supplements. This section of DSHEA also empowers the FDA to require expiration date labeling on dietary supplements "when necessary."

Conforming Amendments

Section 10 provides some protection for manufacturers by stipulating that a product that makes an appropriate structure and function claim in compliance with DSHEA will not result in its being treated as a drug solely because the label contains such a claim or other truthful and not misleading information. This provision also enables manufacturers to include recommended dosage information on the label as well as warnings of possible drug interactions or other contraindications without incurring the risk that inclusion of such information will constitute a therapeutic claim and thus identify the product as a drug.

Withdrawal of the Regulations and Advance Notice

In 1993, the FDA published an Advanced Notice of Proposed Rulemaking (ANPR) in the Federal Register in response to a report submitted to FDA Commissioner Kessler by the Task Force on Dietary Supplements in 1991 (the Dykstra Report). The ANPR outlined some of the FDA positions regarding the regulation of supplements and proposed regulating some supplements as drugs if the agency determined that they were being sold with an intent for therapeutic use. Section 11 of DSHEA specifically nullifies the ANPR issued on June 18, 1993.

Commission on Dietary Supplement Labels

DSHEA mandates the establishment of a presidential commission on dietary supplements, which will conduct a two-year study and issue a report on the regulation of label claims and statements for supplements. The provision specifies that appointees to the commission must have expertise in supplement manufacture, regulation, and usage and, very important for botanicals, one of three scientifically qualified members "shall have experience in pharmacognosy, medical botany, traditional herbal medicine, or other related sciences." Since the passage of DSHEA, the commission has completed its study, and its recommendations have been reviewed in *HerbalGram* (McCaleb and Blumenthal, 1997).

Office of Dietary Supplements

The final section of DSHEA mandates the secretary of HHS to establish an Office of Dietary Supplements within the National Institutes of Health (NIH) to "explore more fully the potential role of dietary supplements as a significant part of the efforts of the United States to improve human health," and "to promote scientific study of the benefits of dietary supplements in maintaining health and preventing chronic disease and other health related conditions." The director will also function in an advisory capacity to the Department of Health and Human Services, NIH, Centers for Disease Control and Prevention, and FDA on issues related to dietary supplements.

IMPLICATIONS OF DSHEA

DSHEA is not perfect, but then legislation crafted in the spirit of compromise and active debate that is characteristic of democratic societies is rarely, if ever, perfect, particularly if it is groundbreaking legislation not yet thoroughly tested in the real world of competing interests, points of view, and policy priorities. DSHEA is a step in the right direction. It represents a distinct improvement over the situation that formerly existed, in which manufacturers and retailers of dietary supplements could make virtually no claims or statements about their products. The regulatory limbo fostered in the pre–DSHEA era meant that consumers were afforded little guidance as to indications for usage, what doses were appropriate, and perhaps most important, what the risks, side effects, and contraindications might be for particular supplements. In its effort to prohibit the promulgation of false claims to an unsuspecting public, the FDA created an information vacuum; in doing so, it may have inadvertently increased the risks of inappropriate or unsafe use of dietary supplements.

Perhaps most important for the consumer, DSHEA benefits consumers by affording them readier access to truthful, balanced, and scientifically valid information about dietary supplements, including their risks as well as their benefits. It puts real information into the hands of consumers, enabling them, for the first time, to make informed decisions about whether to utilize dietary supplements and for what purposes. Such information, in the form of peer-reviewed scientific papers, review articles, books, and other media, was available in the pre–DSHEA era, but access was difficult; not everyone has the time or the inclination to go browsing through their local university medical library, and not everyone has access to a medical library. Now that DSHEA has made it permissible for supplement manufacturers and retailers to supply "true, balanced, and not misleading" third-party reference materials for the ingredients in their products, consumers have ready access to such information and, as a result, can make more intelligent and informed buying and usage decisions.

DSHEA has also proved beneficial for manufacturers and retailers of supplement products. For both of these industry segments, the allowance of structure/function claims has enabled them to make reasonable but not exaggerated claims for the benefits to be realized from using their products and has afforded a mechanism to convey information to consumers on the appropriate uses of supplement products. DSHEA has enabled responsible manufacturers of supplements (and most are responsible and as genuinely interested in the preservation of public health and safety as any regulatory agency) to put information on their labels as to who should *not* use their products as well as who should. This is good for the manufacturers as it protects them from liability; it is also good for consumers as it protects them from unsafe or inappropriate use. By mandating specific ingredient and labeling specifications, DSHEA has also been instrumental in raising the general quality of dietary supplements available on the market. Manufacturers must specify what ingredients and how much of each ingredient is in their products. This may be irritating for manufacturers who would rather not say, but DSHEA is specifically addressed to the majority of responsible manufacturers who are more than willing to describe their product specifications in detail. DSHEA also defines mechanisms that enable new dietary supplement products to be brought to the market, provided evidence exists to support their safety. This important provision allows for innovation within the industry and does not shut the door on innovation-stimulated growth of the industry.

DSHEA's stipulation to create a set of good manufacturing practices is also reasonable and of benefit to both consumers and manufacturers. Similar to the ingredient-labeling provisions, the mandating of GMP within the industry helps to ensure that higher-quality products are delivered to the market. At the same time, DSHEA recognizes that, often, neither pharmaceutical GMP protocols nor food GMP protocols are appropriate for dietary supplements. Here, again, DSHEA leaves open the door to innovation and provides the industry with incentives to develop new GMP standards that are specifically suited to dietary supplements.

By commissioning a presidential committee on dietary supplements, DSHEA provides a mechanism for discussion, revision, and resolution of some of the many unresolved issues resulting from the current DSHEA legislation. This wise provision recognizes that ongoing debate will occur; that DSHEA is a start, not the final solution; and that there needs to be a means for continuing the dialogue and enabling the legislation to mature into a carefully and thoughtfully crafted regulatory policy.

Finally, DSHEA establishes mandates and funding mechanisms enabling the government to sponsor research on dietary supplements and their potential "in maintaining health and preventing chronic disease and other health related conditions." This is not a statement by a government hostile to the notion that dietary supplements may have some value; on the contrary, this statement recognizes that a need exists for more and better research on dietary supplements and specifically establishes a mechanism for the government to facilitate such research. Few in the supplement industry would dispute the need for more and better research. The framers of the DSHEA legislation deserve credit for recognizing that this need exists and establishing an office within the NIH to coordinate it.

REFERENCES

American Herbal Products Association (AHPA) (1991). Botanical ingredient review proposal to the Food and Drug Administration. *HerbalGram* 25: 32-37.

Anonymous (1995). Dietary supplements: Recent chronology and legislation. *Nutrition Review* 53: 31-36.

Appler, W.D. (1995). New dietary supplement law provides marketing opportunities for retailers. *NFM's Nutrition Science News,* pp. 14ff.

Blumenthal, M. (1994). Congress passes dietary supplement health and education act of 1994. Herbs to be protected as supplements. *HerbalGram* 32:18-20.

Commission on Dietary Supplement Labels (CDSL) (1997). Report to the President, the Congress, and the Secretary of Health and Human Services. Available online at DHHS Web site: <http://web.health.gov/dietsupp>.

McCaleb, R. and Blumenthal, M. (1997). President's commission on dietary supplement labels issues final report. *HerbalGram* 41: 24-26, 57, 64.

McSweeney, D. (1995). Using information under DSHEA. *Vitamin Retailer* May, pp. 27-28.

Merrill, D. (1995). The Dietary Supplement Health and Education Act of 1994: What does it mean? *International Herb Association Newsletter* February, pp. 14-15.

Index

3,4-dihydroxyphenyl-acetic acid
(DOPAC)
  kava, 705, 706
St. John's wort, 705
5-hydroxyindolacetic acid (5HIAA),
  705, 706
5-lipoxygenase, and licorice, 744
6-mercaptopurine, 787
7-ethoxycoumarin *O*-deethylase, 894

abdominal distention
  milk thistle, 786
  schisandra, 907
  vitex, 1060
abdominal pain
  chamomile, 157
  ephedra, 298
  feverfew, 364
  green tea, 639-640
  horse chestnut, 684, 689
  milk thistle, 793
  schisandra, 907, 912
  valerian, 1027
  vitex, 1060
abortifacients
  ginger, 434
  kava, 697, 720
  valerian, 1029
Abraham's tree. *See* vitex
abscess, 1064
acetaminophen, 574-575, 772, 815
acetogenins, 926-927
acetylation, 742
acetylcholine, 1049-1050
acetyl-CoA carboxylase, 603
acetylenic compounds, 507
N-acetyltransferase, 552
Acinetobacter, 995
acne
  cat's claw, 131

acne *(continued)*
  saw palmetto, 863
  vitex, 1047, 1054, 1060, 1061, 1062,
    1064
actée a grappes. *See* black cohosh
active principle, 1081
adaptogens. *See* eleuthero; ginseng;
    schisandra
addiction
  ephedra, 303
  evening primrose oil, 333
  ginseng, 518
  to methamphetamine, 518
  to opioids, 518
  valerian, 1029
adenosine diphosphate, 358, 604
adenosine triphosphate, 423, 700
adhesion molecules, 580
adipose tissue, 327, 814
adrak. *See* ginger
adrenal glands
  capsicum, 72
  ephedra, 279-280, 284, 287-288
  ginseng, 511
  goldenseal, 551
  horse chestnut, 681
  saw palmetto, 862, 863
adrenergic receptors, 304-305
adrenocorticotropic hormone, 263, 511
aesculin. *See* horse chestnut
aflatoxins
  ginseng, 514
  horse chestnut, 689
  vitex, 1047
aggression, 956
aging
  cat's claw, 125-126
  eleuthero, 264
  ephedra, 285
  garlic, 389
  gingko biloba, 458-459, 471-473,
    478

THE HAWORTH HERBAL PRESS
Varro E. Tyler, PhD
Executive Editor

HERBAL MEDICINE: CHAOS IN THE MARKETPLACE by Rowena K. Richter (2002). "If you think dietary supplements are unregulated, this is the book for you . . . . Explains how we got into the current regulatory situation, describes the situation in detail, and provides suggestions as to how we might move forward." *Marilyn Barrett, PhD, Author,* The Handbook of Clinically Tested Herbal Remedies; *Founder, Pharmacognosy Consulting Services, San Carlos, CA*

BOTANICAL MEDICINES: THE DESK REFERENCE FOR MAJOR HERBAL SUPPLEMENTS, Second Edition by Dennis J. McKenna, Kenneth Jones, and Kerry Hughes (2002). "A detailed guide to the most common herbal supplements. An excellent resource for serious students, informed consumers, and health care professionals." *Andrew Weil, MD, Author,* Spontaneous Healing, Eight Weeks to Optimum Health, *and* Eating Well for Optimum Health

TYLER'S TIPS: THE SHOPPER'S GUIDE FOR HERBAL REMEDIES by George H. Constantine (2000). "George Constantine has given us a commonsense, easily read, well-organized shopper's guide to the most frequently utilized and best-documented herbal remedies." *Paul L. Schiff Jr., PhD, Professor of Pharmaceutical Sciences, School of Pharmacy, University of Pittsburgh, Pennsylvania*

HANDBOOK OF PSYCHOTROPIC HERBS: A SCIENTIFIC ANALYSIS OF HERBAL REMEDIES FOR PSYCHIATRIC CONDITIONS by Ethan B. Russo (2000). "Sound advice on the rational use of safe and effective herbs to help alleviate a wide range of neurological disorders. An authoritative guide in an area where solid, reliable information is often difficult to obtain." *Mark Blumenthal, Founder and Executive Director, American Botanical Council; Editor,* HerbalGram; *Senior Editor,* The Complete German Commission E Monographs

UNDERSTANDING ALTERNATIVE MEDICINE: NEW HEALTH PATHS IN AMERICA by Lawrence Tyler. "An eye-opening account of the emerging health paths in the United States and other parts of the Western world. . . . Contains thoughtful discussions on the perception of nonspecific factors in healing." *Mark Bender, Assistant Professor of Chinese, Department of East Asian Languages and Literatures, The Ohio State University, Columbus*

SEASONING SAVVY: HOW TO COOK WITH HERBS, SPICES, AND OTHER FLAVORINGS by Alice Arndt. "Well-written and wonderfully comprehensive exploration of the world of herbs, spices and aromatics—at once authorative and easy to use." *Nancy Harmon Jenkins, Author of* The Mediterranean Diet Cookbook

TYLER'S HONEST HERBAL: A SENSIBLE GUIDE TO THE USE OF HERBS AND RELATED REMEDIES, Fourth Edition by Steven Foster and Varro E. Tyler. "An up-to-date revision of the most reliable source for the layperson on herbal medicines. Excellent as a starting point for scientists who desire more information on herbal medicines." *Norman R. Farnsworth, PhD, Research Professor of Pharmacognosy, College of Pharmacy, University of Illinois at Chicago*

TYLER'S HERBS OF CHOICE: THE THERAPEUTIC USE OF PHYTOMEDICINALS, Second Edition by James E. Robbers and Varro E. Tyler. "The first edition of this book was a landmark publication. . . . This new edition will no doubt become one of the most often-used references by health practitioners of all types." *Mark Blumenthal, Founder and Executive Director, American Botanical Council; Editor,* HerbalGram

Order a copy of this book with this form or online at:
http://www.haworthpressinc.com/store/product.asp?sku=4527

BOTANICAL MEDICINES
The Desk Reference for Major Herbal Supplements, Second Edition

_____in hardbound at $169.95 (ISBN: 0-7890-1265-0)

_____in softbound at $79.95 (ISBN: 0-7890-1266-9)

COST OF BOOKS_____

OUTSIDE USA/CANADA/
MEXICO: ADD 20%____

POSTAGE & HANDLING_____
(US: $4.00 for first book & $1.50
for each additional book)
Outside US: $5.00 for first book
& $2.00 for each additional book)

SUBTOTAL_____

in Canada: add 7% GST____

STATE TAX____
(NY, OH & MIN residents, please
add appropriate local sales tax)

FINAL TOTAL____
(If paying in Canadian funds,
convert using the current
exchange rate, UNESCO
coupons welcome.)

☐ **BILL ME LATER:** ($5 service charge will be added)
(Bill-me option is good on US/Canada/Mexico orders only;
not good to jobbers, wholesalers, or subscription agencies.)

☐ Check here if billing address is different from
shipping address and attach purchase order and
billing address information.

Signature_____

☐ **PAYMENT ENCLOSED: $_____**

☐ **PLEASE CHARGE TO MY CREDIT CARD.**

☐ Visa ☐ MasterCard ☐ AmEx ☐ Discover
☐ Diner's Club ☐ Eurocard ☐ JCB

Account # _____

Exp. Date_____

Signature_____

Prices in US dollars and subject to change without notice.

NAME_____

INSTITUTION_____

ADDRESS_____

CITY_____

STATE/ZIP_____

COUNTRY_____ COUNTY (NY residents only)_____

TEL_____ FAX_____

E-MAIL_____

May we use your e-mail address for confirmations and other types of information?   Yes   No
We appreciate receiving your e-mail address and fax number. Haworth would like to e-mail ☐ fax s☐cial
discount offers to you, as a preferred customer. **We will never share, rent, or exchange your e-mail address
or fax number.** We regard such actions as an invasion of your privacy.

Order From Your Local Bookstore or Directly From
The Haworth Press, Inc.
10 Alice Street, Binghamton, New York 13904-1580 • USA
TELEPHONE: 1-800-HAWORTH (1-800-429-6784) / Outside US/Canada: (607) 722-5857
FAX: 1-800-895-0582 / Outside US/Canada: (607) 722-6362
E-mail: getinfo@haworthpressinc.com
PLEASE PHOTOCOPY THIS FORM FOR YOUR PERSONAL USE.
www.HaworthPress.com

BOF02